Hereditary Hearing Loss and Its Syndromes

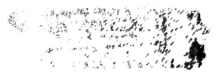

OXFORD MONOGRAPHS ON MEDICAL GENETICS

General Editors

ARNO G. MOTULSKY

MARTIN BOBROW

PETER S. HARPER

CHARLES SCRIVER

CHARLES J. EPSTEIN

JUDITH G. HALL

HEREDITARY HEARING LOSS AND ITS SYNDROMES

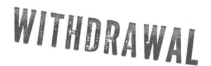

Second Edition

Edited by

HELGA V. TORIELLO, MS, PhD

Professor of Pediatrics/Human Development
Michigan State University
East Lansing, Michigan

WILLIAM REARDON, MD, MRCPI, DCH, FRCPCH, FRCP (LOND)

Consultant Clinical Geneticist
Our Lady's Hospital for Sick Children
Crumlin, Dublin, Ireland

ROBERT J. GORLIN, DDS, MS, DSc

Regent's Professor of Oral Pathology and Genetics
University of Minnesota
Minneapolis, Minnesota

OXFORD
UNIVERSITY PRESS
2004

OXFORD
UNIVERSITY PRESS

Oxford   New York
Auckland   Bangkok   Buenos Aires   Cape Town   Chennai
Dar es Salaam   Delhi   Hong Kong   Istanbul   Karachi   Kolkata
Kuala Lumpur   Madrid   Melbourne   Mexico City   Mumbai   Nairobi
São Paulo   Shanghai   Singapore   Taipei   Tokyo   Toronto

Published by Oxford University Press, Inc.
198 Madison Avenue, New York, New York, 10016
http://www.oup.com

Oxford is a registered trademark of Oxford University Press

Library of Congress Cataloging-in-Publication Data
Hereditary hearing loss and its syndromes /
edited by Helga V. Toriello, William Reardon, Robert J. Gorlin.—2nd ed.
p. ; cm. — (Oxford monographs on medical genetics ; no. 50)
Rev. ed. of: Hereditary hearing loss and its syndromes /
Robert J. Gorlin, Helga V. Toriello, M. Michael Cohen Jr. 1995.
Includes bibliographical references and index.
ISBN 978-0-19-513849-8
1. Deafness—Genetic aspects. I. Toriello, Helga V. II. Reardon, William, 1960-
III. Gorlin, Robert J., 1923- IV. Gorlin, Robert J., 1923- Hereditary hearing loss and its
syndromes. V. Series.
[DNLM: 1. Hearing Disorders—genetics. 2.
Abnormalities, Multiple—genetics. WV 270
H6788 2004]
RF292.H474 2004
617.8′042—dc21
2003049880

2 4 6 8 9 7 5 3

Printed in the United States of America
on acid-free paper

Foreword

Reports of genetic deafness began to appear in the middle of the nineteenth century. A good example is the 1858 report of Usher syndrome by Albrecht von Graefe (1828–1870), who was the first to describe retinitis pigmentosa in three deaf-blind brothers (9). He was able to do so only because a few years before the ophthalmoscope had become available for clinical application. An in-depth description of this syndrome was then published in 1861 by Richard Liebreich (1830–1917), a Berlin ophthalmologist (6). Liebreich performed a systematic examination of the deaf population in Berlin, which totaled 341 persons, and he was amazed by the relatively high incidence of retinitis pigmentosa among the deaf, particularly those with a Jewish background. Moreover, the consanguinity rate among the parents of the affected persons was strikingly high. The incidence of congenital deafness among Jews in Berlin at that time (1:368) was about four times higher than that among the remaining population (1:1477), the higher consanguinity rate among Jews thought to play a role in this. In 1880 Arthur Hartmann (1849–1931) reported that this disease had an "indirect way of transmission," which is now called an autosomal recessive mode of inheritance (4). Early in the twentieth century Mendel's laws (1865) were rediscovered and they explained the transmission pattern those early scientists had observed.

In 1922 Julia Bell (1879–1979) (1) split the Usher syndrome into two categories, recognizing a difference in an association with deaf-mutism (type I) and another with congenital hearing impairment (type II). In 1916 the British ophthalmologist Charles Usher described familial retinal pigment disorders and noted that 69 retinitis pigmentosa patients were also hearing impaired (7). In 1935 he described several of these families in the Bowman Lecture of the British Ophthalmologic Society, sharing his knowledge with a large, scientifically oriented audience (8). Later on his name became the eponym for this syndrome despite the previous important contributions by the Germans and by Julia Bell. With the development of gene linkage and gene identification techniques in the last years of the twentieth century, the Usher syndrome has been split into three main types (I–III) and at least 13 subtypes.

With regard to the splitting and lumping of several groups of syndromes and types of deafness in the first edition of *Genetic and Metabolic Deafness* (5), Bob Gorlin wrote to me in 1977, he thought he had "unfairly divided at times and then unfairly grouped in others. But that is the way it is the first time around and I am afraid the second, and third and fourth time around."

This first edition was edited and written by Bruce Koningsmark (1928–1973) and Bob Gorlin in 1976. The second edition appeared 19 years later, in 1995, under the title *Hereditary Hearing Loss and its Syndromes* with Bob Gorlin, Helga Toriello, and Michael Cohen (3) as editors and contributors. Now, 9 years later, the third edition, by Helga Toriello, Willie Reardon, and Bob Gorlin, is being published.

The application of gene linkage and gene identification techniques to several rare syndromes has contributed to our knowledge of genetic hearing loss, as has the study of nonsyndromic types of hearing impairment. In addition, we are beginning to understand some of the complex genetic mechanisms, such as role of modifier genes, involved in causing various forms of hearing loss. For example, mutations in myosin VIIA causes Usher syndrome 1B, autosomal recessive childhood-onset deafness (DFNB2), and the autosomal dominant hearing loss DFNA11. Mutations in wolframin cause the autosomal recessive Wolfram syndrome and the autosomal dominant nonsyndromic hearing loss, DFNA6/14. Mutations in *SLC26A4* can cause autosomal recessive nonsyndromic hearing loss (DFNB4), the enlarged vestibular aqueduct syndrome, and Pendred syndrome. Mutations in Noggin cause proximal symphalangism, multiple synostoses syndrome, and the Teunissen-Cremers (proximal symphalangism and deafness) syndrome (2).

Still, there remains much to learn about these genetic mechanisms. As in the nineteenth century, clinical studies of rare diseases will be essential in discerning previously unknown genetic mechanisms.

From careful clinical and molecular studies of various rare hearing loss syndromes, we are becoming better at the classification of these entities. But some element of uncertainty about lumping and splitting groups of syndromes remains in this edition, as predicted by Bob Gorlin many years ago.

Indirectly, this book is a gift to patients and their families as it will quickly guide their doctors to balanced up-to-date accounts of the rare conditions that affect them. The book contributes to a history of over 150 years of good clinical research. The field of the genetics of hearing impairment has expanded enormously in the last 10 years, making this new edition all the more welcome.

The production of a standard work like this in three editions represents a long-standing effort over decades. It is a labor of love done with a lot of compassion for those who are affected by hearing disorders. The enormous impact of that work may now become clear to those who could not foresee its value earlier. Biomedicine is profoundly indebted to Helga Toriello, Willie Reardon, and Bob Gorlin for editing this volume.

References

1. Bell J: Retinitis pigmentosa and allied diseases. In: *The Treasury of Human Inheritance*, Vol. 2, Pearson K (ed). Cambridge University Press, London, 1922, pp 1–29.
2. Cremers CWRJ: Hearing: cracking the code. *J Laryngol Otol* 114:6–16, 2000.
3. Gorlin RJ, Toriello HV, Cohen MM. *Hereditary Hearing Loss and Its Syndromes*. Oxford University Press, New York, 1995.
4. Hartmann A: *Taubstummheit und Taubstummenbildung nach den voorhanden Quellen sowie nach eigenen Beobachtungen und Erfahrungen*. Verlag Ferdinand Enke, Stuttgart, 1880.
5. Koningsmark BW, Gorlin RJ: *Genetic and Metabolic Deafness*. W.B. Saunders, Philadelphia, 1976.
6. Liebreich R: Abkunft aus Ehen unter Blutsverwandten als Grund von Retinitis pigmentosa. *Dtsch Arch Klin Med* 13:53–55, 1861.
7. Usher CH: On the inheritance of retinitis pigmentosa, with notes of cases. *R Lond Ophthalmol Hosp Rep* 19:130–236, 1916.
8. Usher CH: The Bowman lecture: on a few hereditary eye affections. *Trans Ophthalmol Soc UK* 55:164–170, 1935.
9. Von Graefe A: Vereinzelte Beobachtungen und Bemerkungen: exceptionelles Erhalten des Gesichtsfeldes bei Pigmentenartung der Netzhaut. *Von Graefe's Arch Ophthal* 4:250–253, 1858.

Cor W.R.J. Cremers, M.D., Ph.D.
Professor in Otology
University Medical Center St. Radboud, University of Nijmegen
Nijmegen, The Netherlands

Preface

There is an almost 20-year gap between the first and second versions of this book, but only an 8-year gap between the second and third. This is due, of course, in large part to the great strides that have been made in our understanding of the genetic causes of hearing loss. Ironically, almost as soon as the 1995 edition was published, a plethora of genetic discoveries were made that quickly outdated it. This led to our planning the current edition almost as soon as the ink was dry on edition two. Bob Gorlin asked me to lead the editorship of this edition. Because of other writing obligations, Mike Cohen had to decline participation. We were fortunate, however, that Willie Reardon was willing to join us in tackling this project.

Many colleagues contributed to this volume, and worked hard on their chapters. We are grateful to all of them. We would also like to acknowledge the contributors to the previous edition who laid the groundwork for several chapters: John Carey and Derin Westin for the renal chapter, William Dobyns for the chapter on nervous system disorders, Albert Schinzel for the chromosome chapter, and Michael Cohen for the chapters on syndrome delineation, genetic counseling, and musculoskeletal disorders. Many geneticists responded to my desperate pleas for photos: Wendy Smith, John Graham, John Carey, Judith Allanson, Robin Winter, Rhonda Scanlon, Margaret Rush, Jackie Robberson, Meg Hefner, and Lisa Shaffer. I also wish to thank Martha Nance and Cornelius Boerkoel who reviewed some of the entries for accuracy. To all a hearty thank you.

We have kept the overall format the same as in the previous edition, but have made some changes in the chapters. There is no longer a "miscellaneous" chapter; instead, we have included a new chapter on hearing loss conditions with associated heart defects. This chapter contains many of the previous miscellaneous entries. The other miscellaneous entries were placed in existing chapters. Some of these placements may appear arbitrary, but we tried to place them where they most logically belonged. We have also added cross-references at the end of each chapter. The greatest change is in the nonsyndromic chapter, which reflects an almost gene-a-week rate of discovery. Throughout the book we tried to sort entities on a clinical rather than molecular basis. That is why, for example, Waardenburg syndrome type 1 and the syndrome of nasal bone hypoplasia, hand contractures, and sensorineural hearing loss still have separate entries, even though both are caused by *PAX3* mutations. Similarly, we did not lump the KID (keratis-ichythosis-deafness) syndrome and nonsyndromic hearing loss, which are both caused by *Cx26* mutations. We also have separate entries for 22q deletion (velocardiofacial) syndrome and DiGeorge sequence, even though the vast majority of patients with DiGeorge sequence have 22q deletions.

Finally, we would like to acknowledge those individuals who operated behind the scenes. I wish to thank most of all Lois Huisman, our librarian, who must have blanched when she received my first batch of article requests numbering over 150. My genetic counselors also had to put up with my relative inaccessibility and occasional crabbiness, and I thank them for their patience. Of course, my family merits some thanks, although admittedly my daughters were clueless that I was even doing this. Willie Reardon wishes to thank his colleagues Robin Winter and Michael Baraitser, for their teaching and example, as well as his family, for their support. Bob Gorlin wishes to extend his deep thanks to individuals at his campus, particularly Dr. Guilan Norouzi, who has been responsible for Dr. Gorlin still having an office at the University of Minnesota. Last but not least, we want to thank Bob's longtime secretary, Carol Bauer Rose. She has been invaluable in putting the contributions from Minnesota in fine order, and for that I am eternally grateful.

H.V.T.
Grand Rapids, Michigan

Contents

7. Genetic Hearing Loss Associated with Eye Disorders, 126

William J. Kimberling

10. Genetic Hearing Loss Associated with Neurologic and Neuromuscular Disorders, 290

Helga V. Toriello

13. Genetic Hearing Loss Associated with Metabolic Disorders,   387

Michael L. Netzloff, Sarah H. Elsea, and Rachel A. Fisher

14. Genetic Hearing Loss Associated with Integumentary Disorders,   407

Helga V. Toriello

15. Genetic Hearing Loss Associated with Oral and Dental Disorders, 456

Robert J. Gorlin

16. Genetic Hearing Loss Associated with Chromosome Disorders, 462

Anne B. S. Giersch and Cynthia Morton

Cytogenic Disorders due to Aneuploidy, 462

Contents

Contributors

JUDITH ALLANSON, MB, CHB
Children's Hospital of Eastern Ontario
Ottawa, Ontario
Canada

HOLLY H. ARDINGER, MD
University of Kansas
Kansas City, Kansas

MARIA BITNER-GLINDZICZ, MRCP, PHD
Institute of Child Health
London, United Kingdom

ANGEL CAMPOS-BARROS, PHD
Hospital Universitario Niño Jesús
Madrid, Spain

DOUGLAS A. COTANCHE, PHD
Harvard Medical School
Boston, Massachusetts

CATHERINE A. DOWNS, MS
University of Michigan
Kellogg Eye Center
Ann Arbor, Michigan

SARAH H. ELSEA, PHD
Michigan State University
East Lansing, Michigan

RACHEL A. FISHER, PHD
Michigan State University
East Lansing, Michigan

ANNE B.S. GIERSCH, PHD
Brigham and Women's Hospital
Harvard Medical School
Boston, Massachusetts

ROBERT J. GORLIN, DDS, MS, DSc
University of Minnesota
Minneapolis, Minnesota

KAREN E. HEATH, PHD
Centro de Investigaciones Biologicas, CSIC
Madrid, Spain

WILLIAM J. KIMBERLING, PHD
Boys Town National Research Hospital
Omaha, Nebraska

ANGELA E. LIN, MD
Brigham and Women's Hospital
Boston, Massachusetts

CYNTHIA MORTON, PHD
Brigham and Women's Hospital
Harvard Medical School
Boston, Massachusetts

MICHAEL L. NETZLOFF, MD
Michigan State University
East Lansing, Michigan

WILLIAM REARDON, MD, MRCPI, DCH, FRCPCH,
 FRCP (LOND)
Our Lady's Hospital for Sick Children
Dublin, Ireland

SHELLEY D. SMITH, PHD
University of Nebraska
Omaha, Nebraska

KATHLEEN K. SULIK, PHD
University of North Carolina
Chapel Hill, North Carolina

R. THOMAS TAGGART, PHD
State University of New York, Buffalo
Buffalo, New York

HELGA V. TORIELLO, MS, PHD
Spectrum Health
Grand Rapids, Michigan

Hereditary Hearing Loss and Its Syndromes

Chapter 1
Genetic Hearing Loss—A Brief History

ROBERT J. GORLIN

References to hereditary hearing loss date from the sixteenth century. This chapter presents a very brief history of genetic hearing loss, but more comprehensive histories have been written by Stephens (26), Ruben (25), and Reardon (23). In the early seventeenth century Paulus Zacchias stated, "The deaf and dumb ought to abstain from marriage . . . for the good of the commonwealth, because there is evidence they beget children like themselves . . ." (7).

Autosomal dominant inheritance of hearing loss was described as early as the seventeenth century (32). In 1814 Adams (1) reported a kindred affected in four generations and recognized the hereditary nature of otosclerosis.

Autosomal recessive hearing loss was apparently first noted in the sixteenth century by Schenck, who described multiple affected sibs with profound congenital hearing loss who had normal parents (15). The importance of parental consanguinity in autosomal recessive hearing loss based on a prospective study was suggested by Wilde (33) in 1853, but denied by George Darwin (6) in 1875. An anonymous report (2) issued in 1877 pointed out that 60% of the population of Martha's Vineyard, all descended from one individual, were deaf. In 1880 Hartmann (17) presented evidence for both autosomal dominant inheritance and autosomal recessive inheritance of hearing loss, although obviously those terms were not used. Hartmann also emphasized the importance of parental consanguinity in recessive hearing loss.

In 1882 Politzer (22) stated that "the most frequent causes of congenital deafness are hereditary, including direct transmission, from parents as well as indirect transmission from forefathers, and marriage between blood relatives." The characteristic pattern of X-linked hearing loss was not recognized until 1930 by Dow and Poynter (10).

The first comprehensive study of genetic deafness was carried out in Norway in 1896 by Uchermann (28). He surveyed all children in Norway's schools for the deaf, specifically examining families for consanguinity through the census and church registers. Compared to parents of normal children, those with affected children had fourfold the rate of inbreeding. Further, Uchermann noted that those areas of Norway that had the highest frequency of hearing loss had the highest degree of consanguinity. In a retrospective study of 2262 congenitally deaf-mute individuals by Alexander Graham Bell (3) of later telephone fame, Bell noted that 55% had deaf relatives. After an address to the National Academy of Sciences (USA) in 1883 entitled "Memoir upon the Formation of a Deaf Variety of the Human Race," Bell became the darling of the eugenics movement, which embodied the philosophy of neo-Darwinism.

Bell sought to prevent intermarriage of the deaf. The reader may find it interesting that Bell's wife and mother were both deaf. He proposed that legislation be enacted to forbid marriage between persons who each had more than one profoundly congenitally deaf person in the family. He proposed the elimination of segregated schools for the deaf and less use of sign language through mainstreaming deaf students and giving them intensive oral education. Having won the Volta Prize for his invention of the telephone, Bell established the Volta Bureau in Washington, DC. In 1910 he advocated in the Bureau's journal (4) that American men be issued certificates of "fitness and unfitness." This was meant to allow women to better select husbands. Bell further wished to fund government employment only to the fit.

Ironically, a prospective study done by Fay (12) in 1898 entitled "Marriages of the Deaf in America" was funded by the Volta Bureau. In this study, involving 3078 marriages in which one or both partners were deaf, Fay sought to answer four questions: (a) Are marriages of deaf persons more likely to produce deaf children than marriages between hearing individuals? (b) Are children of two deaf partners more likely to be deaf than those from matings between a deaf and a hearing person? (c) Are certain classes of deaf individuals more likely to have deaf children? (d) Are marriages between two deaf individuals more stable than marriages between a deaf person and a hearing person? Fay found that deaf–deaf unions produced 9% deaf offspring while deaf–hearing marriages yielded 13.5% deaf children. Congenital deaf–congenital deaf unions yielded 25% deaf offspring versus 4% in the case of later-onset hearing loss from whatever cause. Lower rates of separation and divorce were found in the case of deaf–deaf marriages.

As pointed out by Ruben (25), the low point in eugenic attitudes occurred in Nazi Germany, where, after enactment in 1933 of a law for prevention of hereditary diseased offspring, 1600 deaf individuals were murdered and 17,000 were sterilized (5).

During the last decade of the twentieth century, through molecular genetic technology, the genes for type II Usher syndrome (18), Norrie syndrome (14), Waardenburg syndrome (11), X-linked mixed hearing loss with stapes fixation (31), and many others have been precisely located. It seems reasonable that by the year 2010 many dozen disorders of hearing loss will have been genomically mapped. When and how this information will be used, whether for heterozygote detection or for other reasons, cannot be predicted.

The earliest report of syndromal hearing loss is probably that of mandibulofacial dysostosis by Thomson (27) in 1846/7. Retinitis pigmentosa and hearing loss (Usher syndrome) were noted by Von Graefe (30) in 1858. Waardenburg syndrome may have been first noted by Rizzoli (24) in 1877 or Urbantschitsch (29) in 1910. Combined euthyroid goiter and congenital hearing loss was described by Pendred (21) in 1896 and its recessive pattern by Brain (6) in 1927. The combination of osteogenesis imperfecta, blue sclerae, and conductive hearing loss was noted by Dent (9) in 1900. A systematic approach to syndromal hearing loss was first attempted by Hammerschlag (16) in the years 1903 through 1905. This was followed by the extensive studies of Fraser (13) and Konigsmark and Gorlin (19), both published in 1976. In their text *Genetic and Metabolic Deafness*, Konigsmark and Gorlin described over 140 syndromes of hearing loss. Only one comparable text has subsequently been published (20). The recent vast expansion of knowledge in this area has made this edition necessary.

References

1. Adams J: *A Treatise on the Supposed Hereditary Properties of Diseases.* Callow, London, 1814.
2. Anonymous: Education of deaf-mutes. *Lancet* 1:221, 1877.
3. Bell AG: *Memoir Upon the Formation of a Deaf Variety of the Human Race.* National Academy of Sciences, Washington, DC, 1884.
4. Bell AG: A census of able-bodied. *Volta Rev* 12:403–406, 1910.
5. Biesold H, Friedlander H, Sayers W: *Crying Hands: Eugenics and Deaf People in Nazi Germany.* Gallaudet U. Press, Washington DC, 1999.
6. Brain WR: Heredity in simple goitre. *Q J Med* 20:303–319, 1927.
7. Cranefield PF, Federn W: Paulus Zacchias on mental deficiency and on deafness. *Bull NY Acad Med* 46:3–21, 1970.
8. Darwin GH: Marriages between first cousins in England and their effects. *J Stat Soc* 38:153–184, 1875.
9. Dent CT: Case of fragilitas ossium. *Trans Med Soc Lond* 20:339–340, 1900.
10. Dow GS, Poynter CI: The Dar family. *Eugen News* 15:128–130, 1930.

11. Fay C et al: Assignment of the locus for Waardenburg syndrome type I to human chromosome 2q37 and possible homology to the splotch mouse. *Am J Hum Genet* 46:1017–1023, 1990.

12. Fay EA: *Marriages of the Deaf in America*. Volta Bureau, Washington, DC, 1898.

13. Fraser GR: *The Causes of Profound Deafness in Childhood: A Study of 3,535 Individuals with Severe Hearing Loss Present at Birth or of Childhood Onset*. Johns Hopkins University Press, Baltimore, 1976.

14. Gal A et al: Norrie's disease: close linkage with markers from the proximal short arm of the X chromosome. *Clin Genet* 27:282–283, 1985.

15. Goldstein MA: *Problems of the Deaf*. Laryngoscope Press, St. Louis, 1933.

16. Hammerschlag V: Zur Kenntnis der hereditär-degenerativen Taubstummheit. *Z Ohrenheilkd* 45:329–344, 1903; 47:147–166, 1904; 50:87–96, 1905.

17. Hartmann A: *Taubstummheit und Taubstummenbildung, nach den vorhandenen Quellen, sowie nach eigenen Beobachtungen und Erfahrungen*. F. Enke, Stuttgart, 1880.

18. Kimberling WJ et al: Localization of Usher syndrome type II to chromosome 1q. *Genomics* 7:245–249, 1990.

19. Konigsmark BW, Gorlin RJ: *Genetic and Metabolic Deafness*. W.B. Saunders, Philadelphia, 1976.

20. Martini A et al: *Genetics and Hearing Impairment*. Whurr Publishers, London, 1996.

21. Pendred V: Deaf-mutism and goitre. *Lancet* 2:532, 1896.

22. Politzer A: *Lehrbuch der Ohrenheilkunde für praktische Ärtze und Studierende*, Vol. 2. F. Enke, Stuttgart, 1882.

23. Reardon W: Genetic deafness. *J Med Genet* 29:521–526, 1992.

24. Rizzoli F: Ciocca de capelli bianchi alla fronte congenita ed ereditaria. *Boll Soc Med Chir Bologna Ser* 5, 23:102, 1877.

25. Ruben RJ: The history of the genetics of hearing impairment. *Ann NY Acad Sci* 630:6–15, 1991.

26. Stephens SDG: Genetic hearing loss: a historical overview. *Adv Audiol* 3:3–17, 1985.

27. Thomson A: Notice of several cases of malformation of the external ear together with experiments on the study of hearing loss in such persons. *Monthly J Med Sci* 7:420–425, 727–738, 1846/7.

28. Uchermann VK: *De d vstumme i Norge*, Cammermeyer, Christiana, Norway, 1896.

29. Urbantschitsch E: Zur Ätiologie der Taubstummheit. *Verh Deutsche Otol Ges* 19:153–159, 1910.

30. Von Graefe A: Vereinzelte Beobachtungen und Bemerkungen. *Albrecht V Graefes Arch Klin Ophthalmol* 4:250–253, 1858.

31. Wallis C et al: X-linked mixed deafness with stapes fixation in a Mauritian kindred: linkage to Xq probe of pDP34. *Genomics* 3:299–301, 1988.

32. Werner H: *Geschichte des Taubstummenproblems bis ins 17. Jahrhundert*. G. Fischer, Jena, 1932.

33. Wilde W: *Practical Observations on Aural Surgery*. Blanchard and Lea, Philadelphia, 1853.

Chapter 2
Syndrome Diagnosis and Investigation in the Hearing-impaired Patient

WILLIAM REARDON

Among pediatricians, audiological physicians, otolaryngologists, and other non-dysmorphologists, the recognition of a specific syndrome is often assumed to be a reflex reaction on seeing the patient. In my bitter experience, few assumptions could be so factually ill-founded! Those occasional moments of euphoric dizziness when a gestalt (instant recognition) diagnosis is made in the waiting room are quickly submerged by the endless tide of patients whose abundance of distinctive clinical features should, one remorsefully feels, facilitate the identification of an underlying syndrome diagnosis that remains elusively unachievable. Gorlin has acknowledged the special qualities possessed by great diagnosticians and written of an ability "to intuit the answer to a clinical dilemma" (7). These individuals are the exceptions, possessed of a sixth sense. Most clinical geneticists and dysmorphologists approach the diagnosis of dysmorphic syndromes in a semistructured way that combines history taking, clinical examination, specialized investigation, training, intuition, inspiration, and exasperation in different measures according to the nature of the clinical problem represented by the patient in question and the experience and expertise of the clinician. Too often the unsatisfactory outcome of a consultation is the rueful acknowledgement that one does not recognize a syndrome in this case but would know this memorable malformation pattern if encountered in another patient in the future.

Understanding the basis of syndromes and related phenotypes

Despite the inevitable frustrations of diagnostic inadequacy in individual cases, remarkable steps have been made over the last few decades in classifying birth defects and their relationships, in syndrome delineation, in characterizing the underlying cause of individual malformation syndromes, and in the development of specific diagnostic investigations to confirm clinical diagnoses in malformation syndromes. These developments have combined seminal clinical observations with emerging biochemical, cytogenetic, and molecular technologies so that the diagnostic milieu for malformation syndromes is unrecognizable now compared to that of even a decade ago. A number of ironies have become apparent with these developments. Foremost among these is the observation that while a degree of rigidity in the clinical classification of syndromes has been central to the identification of an underlying genetic defect as the basis of specific malformation syndromes, a degree of clinical laxity may lead to the identification of clinically overlapping conditions also caused by genetic mutation at the same locus or a closely related locus. A good example of this phenomenon is represented by the autosomal dominant condition of Pfeiffer syndrome. In 1964, Pfeiffer described a syndrome of craniosynostosis, broad thumbs, broad halluces, and occasional soft tissue syndactyly of the hands segregating in an autosomal dominant manner (18). Similar pedigrees were later observed, one of which, reported by Baraitser and colleagues (3), was felt by some not to represent true Pfeiffer syndrome but a more variable craniosynostosis syndrome called Jackson-Weiss syndrome. The discussion was resolved in 1995 when a mutation of the *FGFR1* gene was discovered in families with Pfeiffer syndrome, including the Baraitser kindred (15). However, mutations at the related locus, *FGFR2*, were also identified in patients with Pfeiffer syndrome (22). Later, identifying families clinically thought to represent Pfeiffer syndrome in whom mutations at neither *FGFR1* nor *FGFR2* loci were identifiable, Bellus and colleagues (4) found mutations in families with a more variable form of craniosynostosis at the *FGFR3* locus on chromosome 4. The recognition of a more variable phenotype in this subgroup of patients with Pfeiffer syndrome led to the realization that patients with nonsyndromic or atypical forms of craniosynostosis could also harbor mutations at this locus (8,9,14,20) (Figs. 2–1 to 2–3).

Developing the theme of irony, Winter (25) noted that most malformation syndromes were the result of mutation in a new class of genes. The common characteristics of these genes were that clinical dysmorphologists had hardly ever heard of them and the developmental biologists working on these genes had neither heard of the syndromes nor predicted the phenotypic consequences of gene mutation at those loci. A steady flow of reports has continued to identify the mutational basis of genetic disorders, both syndromic and nonsyndromic. Frequently such reports simply presage subsequent observations of clinically overlapping disorders, as outlined above. More common in recent times has been the often perplexing observation of apparently clinically unrelated conditions caused by mutation at the same locus. A good example of this latter phenomenon is provided by the *COL11A2* gene, mutations in which cause both dominant and recessive osteochondrodysplasias (19,23). Patients with this disease spectrum, often referred to as nonocular Stickler syndrome, frequently demonstrate a high level of sensorineural hearing impairment, but also have depressed nasal bridge, midface hypoplasia, a high prevalence of cleft palate, and premature degenerative joint disease (2). However, mutation at this locus has also been established in nonsyndromic hearing loss of autosomal dominant type in two pedigrees without any evidence of joint disease, cleft palate, or facial malformation (12).

These remarks are as true of biochemical assays identifying particular syndromes as they are of molecular assays. Smith-Lemli-Opitz (S-L-O) syndrome is an autosomal recessive malformation syndrome in which a defect of cholesterol biosynthesis results in elevated levels of 7-dehydrocholesterol in affected individuals associated with a recognizable phenotype characterized by developmental delay, cleft palate, hypospadias, syndactyly and/or polydactyly and distinctive facial features (Figs. 2–4, 2–5). Central nervous system (CNS) abnormalities are part of the spectrum of malformations in this condition, specifically agenesis of the corpus callosum, cerebellar hypoplasia, anterior fusion of the cerebral hemispheres, and arhinencephaly. These CNS features are also described individually or collectively as elements of the holoprosencephaly (HPE) sequence. Additionally similar CNS malformations, sometimes resulting in frank HPE, are known to develop in the offspring of rats treated with agents known to inhibit cholesterol biosynthesis during pregnancy. From these observations, Kelley et al. (10) postulated that some patients presenting with HPE might have SLO syndrome as the basis of their clinical presentation. By screening patients with HPE for elevated 7-dehydrocholesterol levels, they identified patients with SLO in whom the presenting clinical picture was that of HPE rather than classical SLO, thus expanding the clinical phenotype of SLO and at the same time demonstrating the possible diagnostic value of this biochemical assay in a range of different clinical situations.

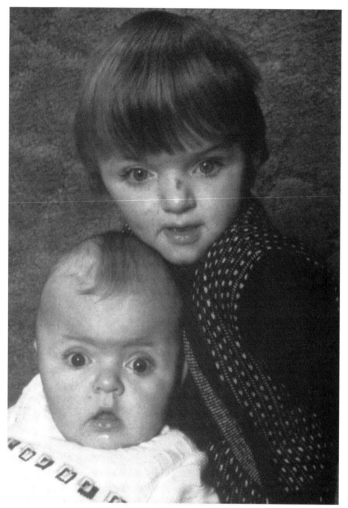

Figure 2–1. The brother and sister shown have craniosynostosis, as does their father. This combination of features led to a diagnosis of Pfeiffer syndrome, subsequently revised when *FGFR3* gene on chromosome 4 was shown to harbor the familial mutation (pro250 arg). [From Reardon et al. *J Med Genet* 34:632–636, 1997.]

The net effect of this remarkable growth in knowledge underpinning the practice of clinical dysmorphology is expansion of the investigative avenues available to the clinician in evaluating an individual patient. Increasingly, as new molecular and cytogenetic investigations specific to particular conditions become available, the challenge to the dysmorphologist is to identify the investigations appropriate to the patient, given the history and clinical profile. In this important respect, the practice of dysmorphology has changed significantly in recent years. Nonetheless, syndrome diagnosis, as emphasized by Aase, continues to rely heavily "upon the ability of the clinician to detect and correctly interpret physical and developmental findings and to recognise patterns in them" (1).

The initial delineation of syndromes

The improved investigative armamentary applies to patients whose syndromes are of known genesis. As outlined by Cohen (5), however, the process of syndrome delineation often involves an earlier period in which the genesis of the syndrome is unknown and may be unique to an individual patient or, if recognized in more than one individual, represents a recurrent pattern syndrome, the basis of which remains to be established. Elaborating diagnostic criteria for multiple congenital ab-

normality syndromes where the primary defect is unknown is difficult. Generally there is an identifiable process over time, beginning with the original report, which identifies a "new" syndrome as a pattern of phenotypic abnormalities. The next series of reports will usually be confined to cases exemplifying the central clinical features of the new condition. Thereafter the phenotype often becomes broader and features originally thought to be sentinel of the disorder are not noted in all cases. Sometimes syndromes described in different literatures by specialists representing different interests merge and a new entity which embraces previously disparate entities emerges.

Branchio-oto-renal (BOR) syndrome represents a case in point, with the earliest reports of familial occurrence of branchial anomalies dating to the 1830s, the relationship with hearing impairment being increasingly recognized in the 1930s, and the important report of Fourman and Fourman (6) documenting branchial fistulae, preauriculr pits, and sensorineural hearing loss in several affected individuals. Melnick (13) suggested the term *branchio-oto-renal syndrome* to emphasize the involvement of renal malformations. More recently the clinically overlapping condition of branchio-oto syndrome has been embraced within the phenotypic spectrum of BOR, as has oto-facio-cervical syndrome. This range of related phenotypes is now known to represent mutation at the *EYA1* locus on chromosome 8q.

Clinical anomalies are nonspecific

The identification of a clinical anomaly in a patient often triggers a series of diagnostic considerations and investigations to try to establish the underlying cause. It is worth recalling that individual clinical anomalies represent the final outcome of a range of different pathogenic possibilities during development. This is the phenomenon of heterogeneity, whereby a number of different and unrelated causes can result in the same clinical anomaly in different patients. Mondini malformation of the cochlea represents a case in point (Fig. 2–6). Table 2–1 lists several different clinical situations in which this radiological abnormality of the cochlea has been described over the last few years. In some of these reports the description of Mondini malformation is real and associated with syndromes of known genesis, both monogenic and chromosomal. In other situations, for instance, Kabuki syndrome, the observation of a Mondini malformation represents an emerging clinical feature of that syndrome, the syndrome itself being of unknown genesis at the time of writing. Other observations of Mondini malformation in association with the X-linked form of deafness, DFN3, are probably erroneous, representing radiological misinterpretation. Obviously the in-

Figure 2–2. Feet of father. Note broad halluces. [From Reardon et al. *J Med Genet* 34:632–636, 1997.]

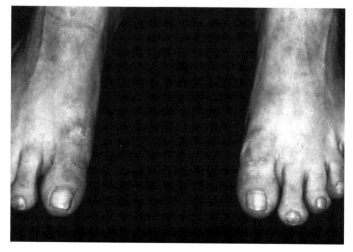

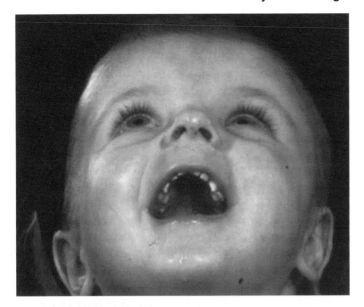

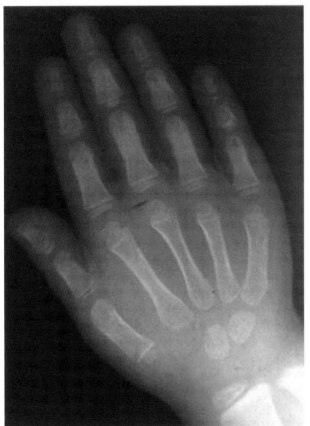

Figure 2–3. An alternative clinical presentation of the *FGFR3* pro250arg mutation is shown. The patient presented with a left-sided plagiocephaly due to left-sided coronal synostosis. This patient has no other clinical features but radiographs show cone-shaped epiphyses. [From Reardon et al. *J Med Genet* 34:632–636, 1997.]

vestigation of a patient with a Mondini malformation, and any genetic conclusion reached with respect to the underlying cause of that anomaly, will be determined by the presence of additional features consistent with the profile of one of the syndromes known to cause Mondini malformation or laboratory investigation designed to test a specific diagnostic hypothesis.

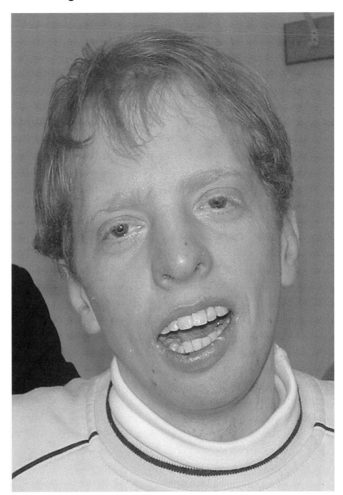

Figure 2–4. A 26-year-old male patient with Smith-Lemli-Opitz syndrome is illustrated. The facial features helpful in signaling the diagnosis are the bitemporal narrowing and ptosis. In addition, his feet show the typical 2/3 syndactyly seen in many patients with the condition. This patient also had severe hypospadias. Reproduced with the consent of the patient's family.

The patient with hearing loss

Hearing loss is often cited as a classic example in clinical genetics of the need to differentiate between syndromic and nonsyndromic forms of a presenting disorder. In clinical practice the answer to this question may not be enormously important in diagnostic or counseling terms and indeed too strict an approach may result in failure to recognize the diversity of phenotypes that can attend mutation at a locus for hearing

Figure 2–5. Gas chromatogram showing the elevated 7-dehydrocholesterol in the patient illustrated in Figure 2–4. In the normal population there is just a single large peak for cholesterol. Reproduced with kind permission of Professor Peter Clayton, Institute of Child Health, London.

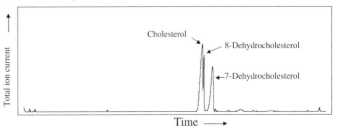

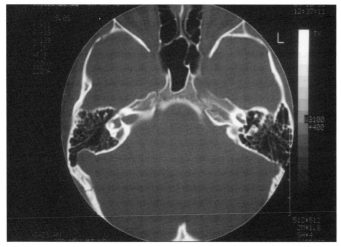

Figure 2–6. Axial CT scan of the petrous temporal bone in a patient with Pendred syndrome, showing a typical example of Mondini malformation. Only the basal coil is properly formed. Reproduced from Reardon and Phelps personal collection.

loss. Witness the example of Usher syndrome type I with typical autosomal recessive Usher phenotype characterized by profound congenital hearing loss, associated vestibular disturbance, and progressive retinal degenerative disease caused by mutation at the *MYOVIIA* locus on chromosome 11q. Yet, mutation at this same locus is established to cause both autosomal dominant and recessive forms of nonsyndromic hearing loss without associated retinal disease (11,24).

As with any clinical interaction, the patient's history will exert an enormous influence on the further examination and investigation of that patient. Aase (1) has established the basic elements of the history pertinent to the practice of dysmorphology as family history, parental history, pregnancy history, birth history, neonatal and subsequent history of the patient, as well as the corroboration of details where possible by examination of outside hospital records. The degree of hearing loss, whether there is evidence of progression on objective measurement, age at onset in the proband, evidence of others in the family similarly affected, and audiological confirmation of this. Clearly, in evaluating the history of hearing loss, the value of good audiological testing and the opportunity to discuss the findings with audiological colleagues can contribute significantly to the direction that the genetic assessment of an individual case may take.

The central importance of physical examination to any clinical dysmorphic consultation is the subject matter of specialized texts, not of this chapter. Hearing impairment is a nonspecific anomaly. It may be seen as an isolated finding (nonsyndromic) or, alternatively, may be an element of a condition with more widespread clinical effects (syndromic). The chapters in this book bear testimony to the range and degree of associated findings seen in patients with hearing impairment as an element of the clinical profile. Such is that spectrum of clinical abnormality that attempts at systematizing the investigative approach to individual patients with hearing loss are doomed to failure because each case needs to be addressed on its own merits and within the context of the history. There are, however, several basic investigations that are common to the patient without evidence of syndromic involvement.

Parker et al. (17) described the rather varied approach to investigation of hearing loss adopted by practicing consultant clinical geneticists in the United Kingdom, as ascertained by questionnaire. They also proposed an outline protocol that might be adopted for investigation of the hearing-impaired child (Table 2–2). In broad terms there is a logical sequence to the series of investigations they outlined, which warrants reflection. Four distinct elements may be divined:

1. Evaluation to characterise the nature and extent of the hearing loss
2. Basic screening of blood and urine
3. More focused investigations to be undertaken in conjunction with the clinical examination, the history, the knowledge that basic screening tests are normal, and the characteristics of the hearing loss as these emerge
4. Definitive investigations aimed at identifying a pathognomonic lesion on radiology, or a specific gene mutation.

Several modifications of Parker at al.'s. protocol might be deployed, depending on the individual circumstances presented by the patient, but most commentators would agree that these four elements represent a good and sensible approach to profiling genetically determined hearing loss. It may well become accepted that perchlorate discharge testing is not required for the diagnosis of Pendred syndrome, being less sensitive than petrous temporal bone radiology (21). Increasingly, specific diagnostic molecular investigations are becoming available, but their place in routine clinical practice, with the exception of connexin 26, remains unproven (16).

Table 2–1. Mondini malformation of the cochlea in association with "genetic" situations

General	Twinning
Known genesis	Pendred syndrome
	Meier-Gorlin syndrome
	Johanson-Blizzard syndrome
	DFN3
	Trisomy 13
	Trisomy 21
	Trisomy 22
Unknown genesis	Kabuki syndrome
	Goldenhar syndrome
	Fountain syndrome
	Wildervanck syndrome
	CHARGE association

Table 2–2. Suggested protocol for etiological investigation of congenital/early-onset sensorineural hearing loss

Audiology
Age appropriate, reliable audiological assessment, including tympanometry
Child/proband
Parents and siblings (if any clinical suspicion of hearing loss)

Urine analysis
CMV (first 2–3 weeks only)
Glucose
Microscopy
Organic and amino acids

Blood
Viral serology
  Rubella (first 6 months only)
  Toxoplasma
  Syphilis
DNA storage and investigation as appropriate
Cytogenetic analysis
T4 and TSH

EKG
Opthalmological assessment
ERG
CT/MRI petrous temporal bone
Vestibular function testing
Perchlorate discharge test
Renal ultrasound scan

CMV, cytomegalovirus; CT, computed tomography; EKG, electrocardiogram; ERG, electroretinogram; MRI, magnetic resonance imaging; TSH, thyroid-stimulating hormone.
Reproduced with permission from Parker et al. (17).

References

1. Aase J. *Diagnostic Dysmorphology.* Plenum Medical Book Company, New York, 1990.
2. Admiraal RJ et al: Hearing loss in the nonocular Stickler syndrome caused by a *COL11A2* mutation. *Laryngoscope* 110:457–461, 2000.
3. Baraitser M et al: Pitfalls of genetic counselling in Pfeiffer syndrome. *J Med Genet* 17:250–256, 1980.
4. Bellus GA et al: Identical mutations in three different fibroblast growth factor receptor genes in autosomal dominant craniosynostosis syndromes. *Nat Genet* 14:174–176, 1996.
5. Cohen MM Jr: *The Child with Multiple Birth Defects,* 2nd ed. Oxford Monographs on Medical Genetics, No. 31, Oxford University Press, New York, 1997.
6. Fourman P, Fourman J: Hereditary deafness in family with earpits (fistula auris congenita). *BMJ* 2:1354–1356, 1955.
7. Gorlin RJ: Foreword. In: *The Child with Multiple Birth Defects,* 2nd ed., Cohen MM (ed), Oxford Monographs on Medical Genetics, No. 31, Oxford University Press, New York, 1997.
8. Graham JM Jr: Syndrome of coronal craniosynostosis with brachydactyly and carpal/tarsal coalition due to Pro250Arg mutation in *FGFR3* gene. *Am J Med Genet* 77:322–329, 1998.
9. Gripp KW et al: Identification of the first genetic cause for isolated unilateral coronal synostosis: a unique mutation in *FGFR3. J Pediatr* 132:714–716, 1998.
10. Kelley RI et al: Holoprosencephaly in RSH/Smith-Lemli-Opitz syndrome: does abnormal cholesterol metabolism affect the function of *Sonic Hedgehog? Am J Med Genet* 66:478–484, 1996.
11. Liu X-Z et al: Autosomal dominant nonsyndromic deafness caused by a mutation in the MyosinVIIA. *Nat Genet* 17:268–269, 1997.
12. McGuirt WT et al: Mutations in *COL11A2* cause non-syndromic hearing loss (DFNA13). *Nat Genet* 23:413–419, 1999.
13. Melnick M et al: Autosomal dominant branchio-oto-renal dysplasia. A new addition to branchial arch syndromes. *Birth Defects* 11(5):121–128, 1975.
14. Moloney DM et al: Prevalence of Pro250Arg mutation of *FGFR3* in coronal craniosynostosis. *Lancet* 349:1059–1062, 1997.
15. Muenke M et al: A common mutation in the *FGFR1* gene in Pfeiffer syndrome. *Nat Genet* 8:269–274, 1994.
16. Navarro-Coy N et al: The relative ontribution of mutations in the DFNB loci to congenital/early childhood nonsyndromal sensorineural hearing impairment/deafness. *J Med Genet* 38(Suppl 1):abstract 1.31, 2001.
17. Parker MJ et al: Variations in genetic assessment and recurrence risks quoted for childhood deafness: a survey of clinical geneticists. *J Med Genet* 36:125–130, 1999.
18. Pfeiffer RA: Dominant erbliche Akrocephalosyndaktylie. *Z Kinderheilkd* 90:301–320, 1964.
19. Pihlajamaa T et al: Heterozygous glycine substitution in the *COL11A2* gene in the original patient with the Weissenbacher-Zweymüller syndrome demonstrates its identity with heterozygous OSMED (non-ocular Stickler syndrome). *Am J Med Genet* 80:115–120, 1998.
20. Reardon W et al: Craniosynostosis associated with *FGFR3* Pro250Arg mutation results in a range of clinical presentations including unisutural sporadic craniosynostosis. *J Med Genet* 34:632–636, 1997.
21. Reardon W et al: Enlarged vestibular aqueduct: a radiological marker of Pendred syndrome and mutation of the PDS gene. *Q J Med* 93:99–104, 2000.
22. Rutland P et al: Identical mutations in the *FGFR2* gene cause both Pfeiffer and Crouzon phenotypes. *Nat Genet* 9:173–176, 1995.
23. Vikkula M et al: Autosomal dominant and recessive osteochondrodysplasias associated with the COL11A2 locus. *Cell* 80:431–437, 1995.
24. Weil D et al: The autosomal recessive isolated deafness, DFNB2, and the Usher1B syndrome are allelic defects of the myosin VIIA gene. *Nat Genet* 16:191–193, 1997.
25. Winter RM: Recent molecular advances in dysmorphology. *Hum Mol Genet* 4:1699–1704, 1995.

Chapter 3
Epidemiology, Etiology, Genetic Patterns, and Genetic Counseling
WILLIAM REARDON, HELGA V. TORIELLO, AND CATHERINE A. DOWNS

Epidemiology

Wilson (58) estimated in 1985 that there were 70 million people in the world with a hearing loss of more than 55 dB. We have calculated that during the year 1985 between 2500 and 4500 profoundly deaf infants were born in the United States. It has been suggested that there are about 2 million deaf individuals and 12 million hearing-impaired individuals in the United States (15).

Many of the earlier epidemiologic studies carried out in both Europe and the United States indicate that at least one-third of all cases are hereditary. However, about 90% of people with congenital hearing loss have normal hearing parents. Since acquired forms of congenital and early-onset hearing loss comprise another one-third, it has been estimated that unknown factors are responsible for the remaining one-third. Estimates that one-third of cases are hereditary must be a minimal figure because a considerable proportion of isolated cases of unknown cause may, in reality, be hereditary. More recently the literature suggests that half of congenital hearing loss is genetic, and half is environmental (42). Among known hereditary examples, at least 15%–30% are syndromic, i.e., associated with other anomalies (10,11,13,14,19,36,37,40,42,47–50,55).

Etiology of hearing loss

Genetic hearing loss can be classified in many ways, including isolated, syndromic, congenital and early childhood (prelingual), later onset (postlingual), conductive, sensorineural, and mixed, among others. We will briefly examine the epidemiology of (*a*) congenital and early childhood hearing loss and (*b*) late-onset hearing loss.

Congenital and early childhood hearing loss. Konigsmark and Gorlin (26) pointed out that data regarding the causes of congenital and early-onset childhood hearing loss were disparate because of (*a*) varying completeness of examination of the different populations studied, (*b*) different years in which surveys were conducted, and (*c*) varying definitions regarding acceptance of one or another etiologic factor. For example, the frequencies of tuberculous meningitis, kernicterus, and rubella have markedly decreased in the last quarter-century (53,55). Therefore, in our present discussion we shall limit ourselves to surveys done during the last 30 years, with emphasis on those of the most recent decades. Readers who are interested in earlier studies are referred to Konigsmark and Gorlin (26) and to other comprehensive summaries (32,55,58). The only really large surveys of vestibular problems are those of Huygen and Verhagen (22) and Verhagen and Huygen (56).

Recent surveys have indicated that congenital hearing loss occurs with a prevalence of about 1/1000 births (12,14,30,34,36,47,52,55), a figure similar to that found in the 1960s (3,45,51,58). Hereditary factors account for about half of the cases and environmental factors for the other half (2,9,13,14,21,24,29,30,34,35,37–40,42,44,52,55,57). Within the group that is considered genetic, syndromic causes account for 30% and nonsyndromic, for 70% (42). Within the nonsyndromic group, approximately 77% are autosomal recessive in inheritance, 22% are autosomal dominant, and X-linked and mitochondrial inheritance account for the remaining 1% (33,43). Other investigators have obtained slightly different figures. For example, Majumder et al. (28) found that 85% were au-

tosomal recessive and 15% were autosomal dominant. Van Rijn (55), by contrast, noted that only 59% were autosomal recessive, 36% were autosomal dominant, and 5% were X-linked or other forms. Reardon (39) suggested that at least 4% of cases are X-linked. These data are similar to estimates made in the 1960–1975 period (3,4,16,33,43,45,52). In a 1993 survey, Marazita et al. (29) found that 75% of cases were autosomal recessive and 25% were autosomal dominant.

Late-onset hearing loss. Morton (32) pointed out that hearing impairment of more than 25 dB affects 15%–20% of the adult population, reaching a frequency of approximately 50% by age 80. Men are affected more often than women. At least 50% of men 65 years of age or older have a hearing loss of over 50 dB at 4000 Hz, sufficient to make understanding of speech difficult.

Late-onset hearing loss is considered multifactorial, with involvement of both genetic and environmental factors. One recent study using male twins suggested that heritability is approximately 50%, which means that half of the variance is caused by genetic differences (23). A second recent study examining sibling pairs and parent–child pairs found that heritability was 35%–55% (17). *DFNA5* has been an attractive candidate gene for late-onset hearing loss; however, Van Laer et al. (54) did not detect a significant association between *DFNA5* and late-onset hearing loss. Well-documented environmental factors involved in late-onset hearing loss include ototoxic drugs, infections, and environmental noise; the roles of cigarette smoking, exposure to solvents, and long-term use of certain drugs remain controversial (54). Because so little is known about the genetic factors involved, exploration of this topic is deferred to a future edition of this book.

Inheritance patterns

Because approximately half of congenital hearing loss is genetic, as noted above, and the contribution of genetic factors to late-onset hearing loss is significant, this section serves as a review of different modes of inheritance. These include (*a*) cytogenetics and chromosomal anomalies; (*b*) monogenetic inheritance patterns; (*c*) multifactorial inheritance; (*d*) sporadicity; and (*e*) nontraditional modes of inheritance (8).

Cytogenetics and chromosomal anomalies. Human chromosomes are grouped by size and centromere location; the latter may be metacentric, submetacentric, or acrocentric (Fig. 3–1). Characteristic banding patterns of the chromosomes permit identification of each individual chromosome (Fig. 3–2). Numerical abnormalities reflect the total number of chromosomes (Fig. 3–3). Sex chromosome aneuploidy is described both numerically and in the sex chromosome constitution.

Structural abnormalities of chromosomes include deletions (Fig. 3–4), duplications, inversions, and translocations. In these situations, the chromosome number may be normal, but detailed analysis reveals the abnormality.

Chromosome studies should be performed on all patients with a suspected chromosomal syndrome to confirm the diagnosis. Family studies may be indicated when structural rearrangements have been identified. For example, with translocation-type Down syndrome, it is important to know if the translocation arose *de novo* or if one parent is a translocation carrier. In the latter situation, the parent is at

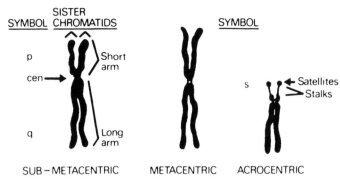

Figure 3–1. General morphology of human chromosomes. [From HA Lubs and PS Ing: Human cytogenetic nomenclature. In: *Principles and Practice of Medical Genetics*, Vol. 1, AEH Emery and DL Rimoin (eds), Churchill Livingstone, Edinburgh, 1983.]

increased risk for having another child with translocation-type Down syndrome.

Chromosome studies should also be carried out on any patient with multiple malformations when the overall diagnosis is unknown. The following generalizations should be kept in mind when using the criteria. First, chromosomal aberrations usually have adverse effects on many parts of the body. Consequently, an individual with only two anomalies, such as an atrial septal defect and clinodactyly, is unlikely to have a chromosome problem. Second, most people with unbalanced autosomes have growth deficiency of prenatal or postnatal onset and mental retardation. Thus, any individual with normal growth parameters and normal psychomotor development is not, as a rule, a candidate for chromosome study. Exceptions to both generalizations include some sex chromosome disorders that may have few, if any, recognizable anomalies. Other exceptions include very small deletions or duplications (46).

The field of human cytogenetics has passed through three phases. Chromosome analysis from 1956 to the late 1960s detected mostly abnormalities of chromosome number and a few structural aberrations. Discoveries during this period included conditions such as trisomies 13, 18, and 21; X-aneuploidy states such as Turner and Klinefelter syndromes; and deletions such as the cri du chat syndrome, Wolf-Hirschhorn syndrome, and deletion of the long arm of chromosome 18. In the 1970s, the introduction of banding techniques led to the discovery of a large number of interstitial and terminal deletions and duplications, double deletion, deletion-duplication, and double duplication. Examples include dup(5p) syndrome, del(11q) syndrome, mosaic tetrasomy 12p syndrome, del(16p) syndrome, and del(22q) syndrome, among many others. While this phase of discovery continues to the present time, a third stage was introduced during the 1980s—prometaphase staining and combining cytogenetic and molecular methods for identifying microdeletions and for gene mapping (6,46). Fluorescent in situ hybridization (FISH) techniques were introduced during the late 1980s and 1990s. It is these FISH techniques which are most useful for identifying microdeletions. Several common syndromes were fairly well delineated before their associated causative microdeletion was identified. Examples include velocardiofacial syndrome (22q−), Williams syndrome (7q−), and Miller-Dieker syndrome (17p−).

Monogenic inheritance patterns. Mendelian inheritance characterizes a number of disorders and syndromes with hearing loss. In medical genetics, autosomal dominant inheritance involves a rare gene, so that affected individuals are heterozygotes. An affected individual produces two kinds of gametes, one with a normal gene and one with an abnormal gene (Fig. 3–5). Thus, offspring of an affected individual have a 50% chance of being affected. An autosomal dominant pedigree is illustrated in Figure 3–6. Dominant disorders are transmitted from generation to generation without skips, and both sexes have an equal chance of being affected. Notice that there are two instances of male-to-male transmission, which rule out X-linked inheritance. The ability of an autosomal dominant gene to be transmitted from generation to generation

depends on the genetic fitness of the affected individual. For example, a pedigree similar to the one in Figure 3–6 might characterize a family with mandibulofacial dysostosis. In achondroplasia, the genetic fitness is reduced so that although some dominant pedigrees may be observed, most instances occur sporadically, resulting from new mutations. Fi-

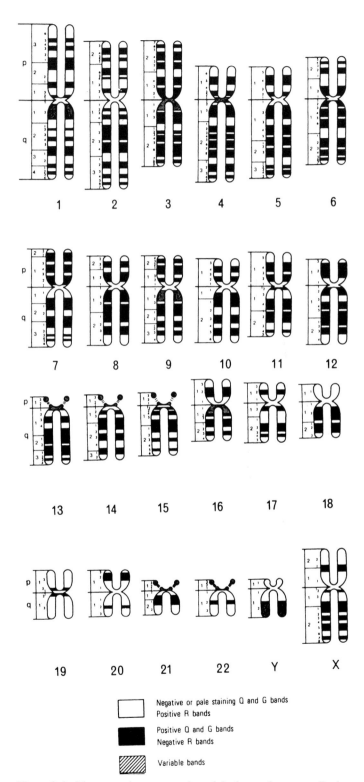

Figure 3–2. Diagrammatic representation of the human karyotype. Designations under the chromosomes indicate chromosome numbers and sex chromosomes. Numbers on the left-hand side of each chromosome refer to bands. Short arm of chromosome is indicated by p; long arm by q. [From Paris Conference on Chromosome Nomenclature, 1971.]

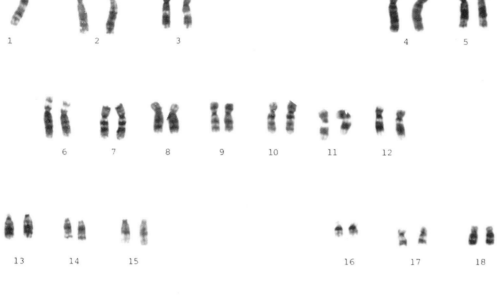

Figure 3–3. Human karyotype with banding showing Down syndrome (47,XY,+21). [From MM Cohen Jr, *The Child with Multiple Birth Defects*, 2nd ed, Oxford University Press, New York, 1997.]

nally, there are several forms of lethal skeletal dysplasia (e.g., thanatophoric dysplasia) in which an individual does not survive long enough to reproduce.

Other features frequently found with autosomal dominantly inherited genes are incomplete penetrance and variable expressivity. *Penetrance* refers to the gene's ability to be expressed at all; i.e., failure to exhibit any sign of the condition is referred to as "lack of penetrance." An isolated example of the disorder known to have autosomal dominant inheritance may represent a new mutation or, rarely, a misrepresentation of paternity. In Figure 3–7, an autosomal dominant pedigree is shown with two instances of incomplete penetrance. Although the incompletely penetrant individuals do not show the trait, they are so-called carriers for the disorder, with a 50% chance of transmitting the gene to their offspring. A genetic trait may be variably expressed, ranging from mild to severe. For example, a parent with mandibulofacial dysostosis might exhibit only mildly downslanting palpebral fissures and mild zygomatic hypoplasia. In contrast, an affected child might have severe downslanting of the palpebral fissures, absent zygomatic arches, severe microtia, and severe micrognathia. The child in this instance has inherited the same familial mutation as the affected parent, and the discrepancy in clinical severity is due to interindividual variation of gene expression. Finally, there are occasions when unaffected parents have more than one child with an autosomal dominant condition. In these situations one of the parents is likely a mosaic (that is, has some cells, including germ cells, that have the mutation and other cells that do not). Recur-

rence risk depends on the condition, but is generally between <1% and 7% (31).

With autosomal recessive inheritance, both parents are phenotypically normal but are heterozygous carriers for the abnormal gene. Parents produce two different kinds of gametes—one with a normal gene and one with the mutated form of the gene (Fig. 3–8). There is a 25% chance of two parents that are each carriers having an affected child. Of the phenotypically normal children, one would expect two-thirds to be heterozygous carriers for the disorder, like their parents.

Because offspring have a 25% chance of being affected, sibships of two or more affected children may be found (Fig. 3–9). Both sexes have an equal chance of being affected. More remote ancestors as well as the

Figure 3–5. In autosomal dominant inheritance, an affected individual has a 50% chance of having an affected offspring. (From MM Cohen Jr, *The Child with Multiple Birth Defects*, 2nd ed, Oxford University Press, New York, 1997.)

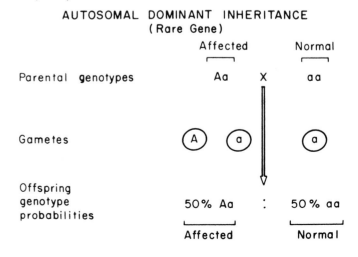

Figure 3–4. Deletion of long arm of chromosome 18 (right) del(18)(q22.1). [From MM Cohen Jr, *The Child with Multiple Birth Defects*, 2nd ed, Oxford University Press, New York, 1997.]

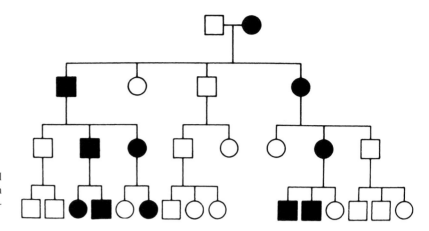

Figure 3–6. Autosomal dominant pedigree showing vertical transmission and male-to-male transmission. [From MM Cohen Jr, *The Child with Multiple Birth Defects*, 2nd ed, Oxford University Press, New York, 1997.]

parents are usually normal. An increased percentage of pedigrees may have consanguinity (i.e., parents are related to each other, and thus share some of their genes by virtue of common ancestry). The rarer the gene is in the population, the more likely that the clinical condition will be seen in consanguineous pedigrees for the most part. Figure 3–10 shows how consanguinity increases the probability of homozygosity for the abnormal gene. Examples of autosomal recessive disorders with hearing loss include Usher syndrome and Pendred syndrome.

Although two deaf parents who have profound autosomal recessive sensorineural hearing loss ought to have only deaf children, this is by no means the case. There are many clinically indistinguishable forms of autosomal recessive deafness. This range of possibilities derives from what is referred to as genetic heterogeneity. Empiric odds estimates take this into account (see Table 3–1).

In X-linked recessive inheritance, both parents are usually phenotypically normal. If the mother is a carrier for the abnormal gene, she is able to produce two kinds of gametes, one with a normal gene, the other with an abnormal gene. Offspring genotype probabilities are illustrated in Figure 3–11. Half of the males are affected and half of the females are phenotypically normal carriers for the gene. An X-linked recessive pedigree is shown in Figure 3–12A. The gene is transmitted from generation to generation in a diagonal pattern. Affected males do not produce affected offspring and are themselves the offspring of normal female carriers. However, all of their daughters are carriers. In the population as a whole, more males tend to be affected. When females are affected, they are the offspring of an affected father and a normal carrier mother. In such instances, the parents are often related.

Examples of X-linked recessive disorders with hearing loss are classic Alport syndrome, Norrie syndrome, and progressive mixed hearing loss with perilymphatic gusher. A typical X-linked pedigree is found in Figure 3–12A, showing affected males and female carriers. The same pedigree is slightly altered in Figure 3–12B to look more like an X-linked dominant pedigree. This pattern fits if the disorder is defined as expressing any degree of the syndrome. Since carrier mothers often do in fact have some expression of the disorder, they can be defined as being affected.

For X-linked dominant inheritance, parental genotypes, types of gametes, and offspring genotype probabilities are illustrated in Figures 3–13 and 3–14. A typical X-linked dominant pedigree is shown in Figure 3–15. Such a condition is transmitted from generation to generation without skips. All daughters of an affected male will be affected, but no sons of an affected male are affected. For affected females, offspring of either sex have a 50% chance of being affected. X-linked dominant conditions are usually more severely expressed in males than in females, and in the population as a whole, more females tend to be affected. An example of an X-linked dominant condition is vitamin D–resistant rickets.

Finally, the parental genotypes, types of gametes, and offspring genotype probabilities for X-linked dominant inheritance, lethal in the male, are illustrated in Figure 3–16. Only females are affected. The deficiency of affected males is expressed as an excess number of spontaneous abor-

Figure 3–8. In autosomal recessive inheritance, both parents are phenotypically normal carriers who have a 25% risk of having an affected offspring. [From MM Cohen Jr, *The Child with Multiple Birth Defects*, 2nd ed, Oxford University Press, New York, 1997.]

Figure 3–7. Autosomal dominant inheritance showing incomplete penetrance. Dots indicate genetic carriers for the abnormal gene who are phenotypically normal. [From MM Cohen Jr, *The Child with Multiple Birth Defects*, 2nd ed, Oxford University Press, New York, 1997.]

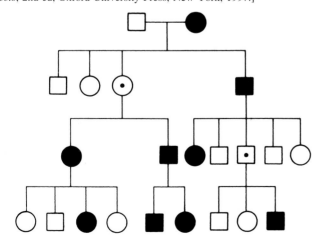

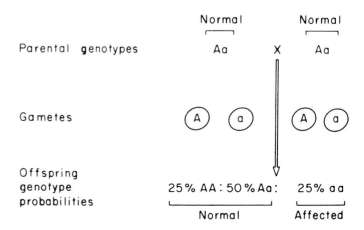

AUTOSOMAL RECESSIVE INHERITANCE

(Rare Gene)

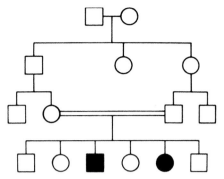

Figure 3–9. Autosomal recessive inheritance showing an affected brother and sister, normal parents, and normal grandparents. Note that the maternal grandfather and paternal grandmother are siblings, resulting in parental consanguinity indicated by the double horizontal line. [From MM Cohen Jr, *The Child with Multiple Birth Defects*, 2nd ed, Oxford University Press, New York, 1997.]

Table 3–1. Chance of recurrence of subsequent deaf offspring in various matings

Mating Types	No. of Deaf Offspring	No. of Tested Offspring (S)					
		0	1	2	3	4	5
Hearing × Hearing							
Positive family history	1	NA	0.20	0.19	0.17	0.16	0.14
Negative family history	1	NA	0.10	0.08	0.07	0.05	0.04
Deaf × Hearing							
All hearing children	0	0.07	0.04	0.03	0.02	0.01	0.01
At least 1 deaf child	>1	NA	0.41	0.41	0.41	0.41	0.41
Deaf × Deaf							
All hearing children	0	0.10	0.04	0.03	0.02	0.01	0.01
All deaf children	S	0.10	0.62	0.80	0.92	0.97	0.99
Deaf & hearing children	>0 < S	NA	NA	0.33	0.33	0.33	0.33

tions among the offspring of affected females. The condition is transmitted from mother to daughter. Examples of X-linked dominant conditions, lethal in the male, are the type I oral-facial-digital syndrome, Melnick-Needles syndrome, and incontinentia pigmenti.

Multifactorial inheritance. Multifactorial inheritance is thought to result from a combination of genetic and environmental factors. Distribution of the resultant phenotypes is primarily quantitative and continuous in nature. In the threshold model of multifactorial inheritance, the total liability of expression of the trait in question is reflected in the population as a normally distributed curve. Expression of the trait is restricted to those individuals who exceed a threshold of liability. Examples of multifactorial inheritance include cleft lip/palate and late-onset hearing loss.

Multifactorial traits have a number of characteristics. First, the recurrence in relatives is greater than the frequency of the disorder in the general population. Thus, first-degree relatives such as siblings and offspring are most likely to be affected, since, on average, they share 50% of their genes. Second-degree relatives such as aunts, uncles, nieces, and nephews are less likely to be affected, since they share only 25% of their genes. Third-degree relatives such as first cousins are even less likely to be affected, as they have only 12.5% of their genes in common.

Figure 3–10. Affected homozygote (aa), parental consanguinity indicated by the double horizontal line between two heterozygous parents, two heterozygous grandparents who are brother and sister, and the heterozygous great-grandmother. [From MM Cohen Jr, *The Child with Multiple Birth Defects*, 2nd ed, Oxford University Press, New York, 1997.]

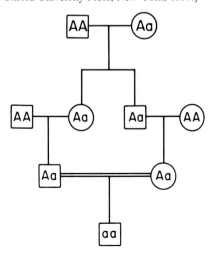

Second is that the chance of recurrence of the trait in question increases with each additional family member affected. The recurrence for a second affected child with a cleft lip/palate is approximately 4% if both parents are unaffected; the risk increases to approximately 10% if one parent is also affected. Third, the more severe the malformation, the greater the risk to the relatives. The odds for a second affected child are higher when the proband has bilateral cleft lip/palate than when the proband has unilateral cleft lip. Fourth, if sex differences exist in the frequency of the trait in question, the risk to relatives is greater when the trait occurs in the less frequently affected sex. For example, cleft palate occurs less frequently in males than in females. The odds of having cleft palate are greater in sibs of males with cleft palate than in sibs of females with cleft palate. Finally, an increase in parental consanguinity is to be expected in conditions with multifactorial causation (7,8).

Kurnit et al. (27) revolutionized our thinking about the role that chance may play in the occurrence of malformations. Their model may be applicable to malformations presently thought to have "low-risk multifactorial recurrence." Multifactorial explanations depend on the interaction between genetic and environmental factors. Thus, high discordance in monozygotic twins for major malformations such as ventricular septal defect has been ascribed to subtle environmental influences, for want of a better explanation. Kurnit et al. (27) suggested that this variability may be inherent in the role that chance itself plays in the process of development. Using computer simulations to describe endocardial cushion outgrowth and fusion, randomly walking cells were allowed to migrate, divide, and adhere with preset probabilities. On the basis of these simulations, a stochastic single gene model generated a continuous liability curve resembling the one obtained from a multifactorial threshold model. Outcomes were quite variable despite using identical genotypes and environments. Thus, segregation of a given malformation may be explained by a single defective gene that predisposes to, but does not necessarily result in, the malformation. Furthermore, the low penetrance and remarkably variable expressivity that characterize a number of presumed autosomal dominant malformation syndromes are possibly reflections of specific stochastic influences that are intrinsic to the embryonic process itself. Future studies may demonstrate that such syndromes arise predictably as a single gene disorder modified by the stochastic laws that govern growth (6).

Nontraditional modes of inheritance. Some types of genetic patterns are not explained by traditional Mendelian inheritance. Four con-

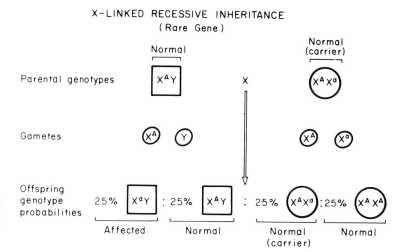

Figure 3–11. Parental genotypes, types of gametes, and offspring genotype probabilities in X-linked recessive inheritance. [From MM Cohen Jr, *The Child with Multiple Birth Defects*, 2nd ed, Oxford University Press, New York, 1997.]

cepts are discussed here: uniparental disomy, genomic imprinting, mitochondrial inheritance, and trinucleotide gene expansion.

Uniparental disomy. In uniparental disomy, two copies of a given chromosome come from one parent, and none come from the other parent. With DNA markers, it is possible to determine whether each member of a chromosome pair is inherited diparentally or uniparentally. In the latter case, it is likely that the chromosome in question was trisomic to begin with, followed by loss of a chromosome, leaving uniparental disomy (18). For example, cystic fibrosis, an autosomal recessive disorder resulting from the homozygous state of the gene on chromosome 7, has been shown in 0.02% of cases to have both copies of the gene maternally derived (4,18). However, 20%–30% of cases of Prader-Willi syndrome have their origin in this way.

Genome imprinting. In classic genetics, we are taught that the influence of a gene is independent of the source. But that is not strictly true. For example, in triploidy (where there are three complete sets of chromosomes), if the extra chromosome complement is from the father (diandry), a hydatiform mole is produced; if the extra set is maternal in origin, then there is a small undeveloped placenta without cystic changes and a growth-retarded embryo. In genomic imprinting, modifications in the genetic material occur depending on whether genetic information is maternally or paternally derived. Such modifications result in different phenotypes (18). For example, Prader-Willi syndrome and Angelman syndrome are caused by microdeletions in the same area of the long arm of chromosome 15. The deletions of the two syndromes are close to one another within the same band, but the phenotypes are very different. In Prader-Willi syndrome, the abnormal chromosome 15 is always paternally derived, and in Angelman syndrome, maternally derived.

Mitochondrial inheritance. Mitochondrial inheritance is characterized by transmission of the disorder from a mother to all of her sons and daughters. However, only females transmit the condition, since mi-

tochondria are contributed to the zygote only by the female. Male mitochondria, being located in the neck of the sperm, do not enter the zygote; only the head of the sperm does. Mitochondria replicate independently of their host cell and possess their own DNA, which differs from nuclear DNA.

However, we know that the expression of mitochondrially inherited disorders varies considerably and that not all of the children are affected. This has been explained by not all of the mitochondria having the mutation (heteroplasmy). If all of the mitochondria have the mutation, this is described as homoplasmy. Another factor may be modifying nuclear genes (5).

Disorders that have mitochondrial inheritance include certain encephalomyopathies, Leber's optic atrophy, rare forms of isolated sensorineural hearing loss, and aminoglycoside sensitivity.

Trinucleotide repeat disorders. Until recently, *anticipation* has been considered a genetic pseudophenomenon. The term is applied to the progressively earlier appearance and increasing severity of a disorder in successive generations (20). This phenomenon can be explained by the disorder being caused by repeated trinucleotide sequences within the gene. Below a certain number of repeats, the gene is considered stable. A small increase in the number of repeats leads to gene instability, but with little, if any, effect on the phenotype. This state is called premutation. Above a critical level (mutation), the condition becomes clinically evident. In some conditions, such as fragile X syndrome and myotonic dystrophy, the gene expansion occurs during female meiosis; in others, such as Huntington disease, it occurs during male meiosis.

Genetic counseling: definition and history

The term "genetic counseling" was first coined in 1949 (41). By the early 1950s hereditary disorders or hereditary counseling clinics were established across the United States in which geneticists saw patients

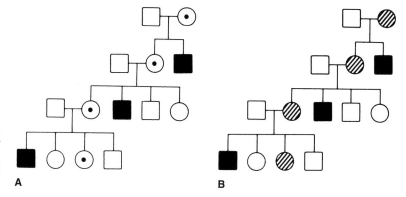

Figure 3–12. (A) X-linked recessive pedigree (dots indicate female carriers). (B) X-linked semidominant inheritance (disorder minimally defined so that female carriers are considered affected). [From MM Cohen Jr, *The Child with Multiple Birth Defects*, 2nd ed, Oxford University Press, New York, 1997.]

A

B

X-LINKED DOMINANT INHERITANCE
(Rare Gene)

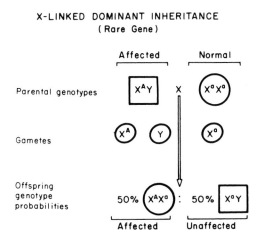

Figure 3–13. Parental genotypes, types of gametes, and offspring genotype probabilities in X-linked dominant inheritance (when the female is affected). [From MM Cohen Jr, *The Child with Multiple Birth Defects*, 2nd ed, Oxford University Press, New York, 1997.]

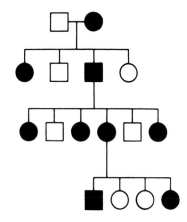

Figure 3–15. X-linked dominant pedigree. Note the vertical transmission and lack of male-to-male transmission. All daughters of an affected male are affected. [From MM Cohen Jr, *The Child with Multiple Birth Defects*, 2nd ed, Oxford University Press, New York, 1997.]

with positive family histories of genetic disorders. Although these pioneering genetic counseling sessions focused initially on the provision of recurrence risk figures, they have gradually embraced a wider role.

In 1975 the American Society of Human Genetics adopted the following definition of genetic counseling: "Genetic counseling is a communication process which deals with the human problems associated with the occurrence or risk of occurrence of a genetic disorder in a family. This process involves an attempt by one or more appropriately trained persons to help the individual or family to: (*1*) comprehend the medical facts including the diagnosis, probable course of the disorder, and the available management, (*2*) appreciate the way heredity contributes to the disorder and the risk of recurrence in specified relatives, (*3*) understand the alternatives for dealing with the risk of recurrence, (*4*) choose a course of action which seems to them appropriate in view of their risk, their family goals, and their ethical and religious standards and act in accordance with that decision, and (*5*) make the best possible adjustment to the disorder in an affected family member and/or to the risk of recurrence of that disorder." This definition is still in use today, almost 30 years after it was initially proposed (1).

From the time of its inception as a clinical subspecialty, a primary tenet underlying the practice of genetic counseling has been the concept of nondirectiveness. The most succinct definition of *nondirectiveness* in genetic counseling was proposed in 2001: "any procedure used

in genetic services that promotes the autonomy and self-directedness of the client." In contrast, *directiveness* encompasses "any procedure used in genetics services that uses one or more means to persuade a decision that might not otherwise have been made by the client" (25).

Goals of genetics evaluation and genetic counseling

Genetic counseling is an integral part of the genetic evaluation. The basic elements of the clinical genetics evaluation remain constant and include diagnosis, interpretation of genetic (molecular, cytogenetic, and biochemical) test results, etiology, recurrence risk, prognosis and treatment options, along with counseling directed toward the patient's clarification of concerns, assessment of family issues, processing of information, decision-making and coping strategies, and referrals for medical, psychological, and support group follow-up.

Working with deaf patients: unique considerations

It is sensible in counseling deaf patients to be aware of cultural identity factors that do not surround many other genetically determined conditions. Many deaf individuals see themselves as belonging to a Deaf community of entirely normal people whose method of communication differs from that of the general population. As a result, the agenda for

X-LINKED DOMINANT INHERITANCE
(Rare Gene)

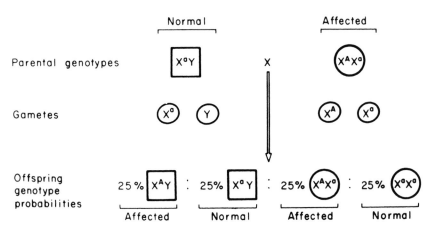

Figure 3–14. Parental genotypes, types of gametes, and offspring genotype probabilities in X-linked dominant inheritance (when the male is affected). [From MM Cohen Jr, *The Child with Multiple Birth Defects*, 2nd ed, Oxford University Press, New York, 1997.]

X-LINKED DOMINANT INHERITANCE
LETHAL IN THE MALE
(Rare gene)

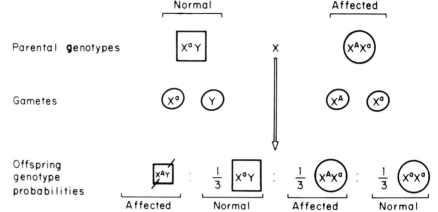

Figure 3–16. Parental genotypes, types of gametes, and offspring genotype probabilities in X-linked dominant inheritance (lethal in the male). Note that since the affected males are aborted, inheritance is from mother to daughter. An affected female has a one-third chance of having an affected daughter, a one-third chance of having a normal daughter, and a one-third chance of having a normal son. [From MM Cohen Jr, *The Child with Multiple Birth Defects*, 2nd ed, Oxford University Press, New York, 1997.]

such individuals attending a genetic counseling session may need to be clearly established, not just with respect to optimizing communication but also in terms of understanding the individual's questions and issues. Many other deaf individuals, however, see their condition as a medical condition and wish to have diagnosis, investigation, and counseling in line with a standard clinical genetic approach.

References

1. Baker DL et al: *A Guide to Genetic Counseling*. Wiley-Liss, New York, 1998.
2. Bliumina MG, Moskovkina AG: Genetic study of sensorineural hearing loss. *Genetika* 18:1012–1017, 1982.
3. Brown KS: Genetic and environmental factors in profound prelingual deafness. *Med Clin North Am* 53:741–772, 1969.
4. Chung CS, Brown KS: Family studies of early childhood deafness, ascertained through the Clarke School for the Deaf. *Am J Hum Genet* 22:630–644, 1970.
5. Clarke LA: Mitochondrial disorders in pediatrics. *Pediatr Clin North Am* 39:319–334, 1992.
6. Cohen MM Jr: Syndromology: an updated conceptual overview. *Int J Oral Maxillofac Surg* 18:333–338, 339–346, 1989; 19:26–32, 1990.
7. Cohen MM Jr: Dysmorphology, syndromology, and genetics. In: *Plastic Surgery*, Vol. 1, General Principles, McCarthy JG (ed), W.B. Saunders, Philadelphia, 1990, pp 69–112.
8. Cohen MM Jr: *The Child with Multiple Birth Defects*, 2nd ed, Oxford University Press, New York, 1997.
9. Cremers CWRJ: An approach to the causes of early childhood deafness. *Clin Otolaryngol* 3:21–26, 1978.
10. Das VK: Aetiology of bilateral sensorineural deafness in children. *J Laryngol Otol* 102:975–980, 1988.
11. Feinmesser M et al: Follow-up of 40,000 infants screened for hearing defect. *Audiology* 21:197–203, 1982.
12. Feinmesser M et al: Etiology of childhood deafness with reference to the group of unknown cause. *Audiology* 25:65–69, 1986.
13. Fraser GR: Profound childhood deafness. *J Med Genet* 1:118–161, 1964.
14. Fraser GR: *The Causes of Profound Deafness in Childhood*. Johns Hopkins University Press, Baltimore, 1976.
15. Fritsch MH, Sommer A: *Handbook of Congenital and Early Onset Hearing Loss*. Igaku-Shoin, New York, 1990.
16. Furusho T, Yasuda N: Genetic studies on inbreeding in some Japanese populations. XIII. A genetic study of congenital deafness. *Jpn J Hum Genet* 18:47–65, 1973.
17. Gates GA et al: Genetic associations in age-related hearing thresholds. *Arch Otolaryngol Head Neck Surg* 125:654–659, 1999.
18. Hall JG: Nontraditional inheritance. *Growth Genet Horm* 6:1–4, 1990.
19. Hall-Jones J: Congenital deafness—the aetiology and management of 100 cases. *J Laryngol Otol* 84:1003–1026, 1970.
20. Harper PS et al: Anticipation in myotonic dystrophy: new light on an old problem. *Am J Med Genet* 51:10–16, 1992.
21. Holton A, Parving A: Aetiology of hearing disorders at schools for the deaf. *Int J Pediatr Otorhinolaryngol* 10:229–236, 1985.
22. Huygen PL, Verhagen WI: Peripheral vestibular and vestibulo-cochlear dysfunction in hereditary disorders. A review of the literature and a report on some additional findings. *J Vestib Res* 4:81–104, 1994.
23. Karlsson KK et al: Description and primary results from an audiometric study of male twins. *Ear Hear* 18:114–120, 1997.
24. Kankkunen A: Pre-school children with impaired hearing in Göteborg 1964–1980. *Acta Otolaryngol Suppl* 391:1–124, 1982.
25. Kessler S: Psychological aspects of genetic counseling XIV. Nondirectiveness and counseling skills. *Genet Test* 5:187–191, 2001.
26. Konigsmark BM, Gorlin RJ: *Genetic and Metabolic Deafness*. W.B. Saunders, Philadelphia, 1976.
27. Kurnit D et al: Genetics, chance, and morphogenesis. *Am J Hum Genet* 41:979–995, 1987.
28. Majumder PP et al: On the genetics of prelingual deafness. *Am J Hum Genet* 44:86–99, 1989.
29. Marazita ML et al: Genetic epidemiological studies of early-onset deafness in the U.S. school-age population. *Am J Med Genet* 46:486–491, 1993.
30. Martin JAM et al: Childhood deafness in the European community. *Scand Audiol* 10:165–174, 1981.
31. Mettler G, Fraser FC: Recurrence risk for sibs of children with "sporadic" achondroplasia. *Am J Med Genet* 90:250–251, 2000.
32. Morton NE: Genetic epidemiology of hearing loss. *Ann NY Acad Sci* 630:16–31, 1991.
33. Nance WE: Genetic counseling of hereditary deafness: an unmet need. In: *Childhood Deafness: Causation, Assessment and Management*, Bass FH (ed), Grune & Stratton, New York, 1977, pp 211–216.
34. Newton VE: Aetiology of bilateral sensorineural hearing loss in young children. *J Laryngol Otol Suppl* 10:1–57, 1985.
35. Pabla HS et al: Retrospective study of the prevalence of bilateral sensorineural deafness in childhood. *Int J Pediatr Otorhinolaryngol* 22: 161–165, 1991.
36. Parving A: Epidemiology of hearing loss and aetiological diagnosis of hearing impairment in childhood. *Int J Pediatr Otorhinolaryngol* 5:151–165, 1983.
37. Parving A: Aetiologic diagnosis in hearing-impaired children—clinical value and application of a modern examination programme. *Int J Pediatr Otorhinolaryngol* 7:29–38, 1984.
38. Parving A: Hearing disorders in childhood: some procedures for detection, identification and diagnostic evaluation. *Int J Pediatr Otorhinolaryngol* 9:31–57, 1985.
39. Reardon W: Sex linked deafness: Wilde revisited. *J Med Genet* 27:376–379, 1990.
40. Reardon W, Pembrey M: The genetics of deafness. *Arch Dis Child* 65:1196–1197, 1990.
41. Reed SC: Counseling in Human Genetics, The Dight Institute of the University of Minnesota, bulletin no. 6, 1949, 1949, pp 7–21.
42. Resendes BL et al.: Review article: at the speed of sound: gene discovery in the auditory system. *Am J Hum Genet* 69:923–935, 2001.

43. Rose SP et al: Genetic analysis of childhood deafness. Causation, assessment and management. In: *Childhood Deafness*, Bass FH (ed), Grune & Stratton, New York, 1977, pp 19–35.

44. Ruben RJ, Rozycki DL: Clinical aspects of genetic deafness. *Ann Otol Rhinol Laryngol* 80:255–263, 1971.

45. Sank D: Genetic aspects of early total deafness. In: *Family and Mental Health Problems in a Deaf Population*, Rainer JD et al (eds), Columbia University, New York, 1963, pp 28–81.

46. Schinzel A: Microdeletion syndromes, balanced translocations, and gene mapping. *J Med Genet* 25:454–462, 1988.

47. Sehlin P et al: Incidence, prevalence and etiology of hearing impairment in children in the county of Västerbotten, Sweden. *Scand Audiol* 19:193–200, 1990.

48. Sellars S, Beighton P: Childhood deafness in southern Africa: an aetiological survey of 3,064 deaf children. *J Laryngol Otol* 97:885–889, 1983.

49. Sellars S et al: Aetiology of deafness in white children in the Cape. *S Afr Med J* 50:1193–1197, 1976.

50. Sellars S et al: Deafness in black children in Southern Africa. *S Afr Med J* 51:309–312, 1977.

51. Stevenson AC, Cheeseman EA: Hereditary deaf-mutism with particular reference to Northern Ireland. *Ann Hum Genet* 20:177–231, 1956.

52. Taylor IG et al: A study of the causes of hearing loss in a population of deaf children with special reference to genetic factors. *J Laryngol Otol* 89:899–914, 1975.

53. Upfold LF: Changes in the significance of maternal rubella as a factor in childhood deafness—1954 to 1982. *Med J Aust* 140:641–644, 1984.

54. Van Laer L et al: Is *DFNA5* a susceptibility gene for age-related hearing impairment? *Eur J Hum Genet* 10:883–886, 2002.

55. Van Rijn PM: Causes of Early Childhood Deafness. Ph.D. Thesis, Nijmegen, 1989.

56. Verhagen WIM, Huygen PLM: Central vestibulo-acoustic and oculomotor dysfunction in hereditary disorders. A review of the literature and a report on some additional findings. *J Vestib Res* 4:105–135, 1994.

57. Williamson I, Steel K: The aetiology of hearing impairment. *Hered Deafness Newsletter* 5:7–17, 1990.

58. Wilson J: Deafness in developing countries. Approaches to a global program of prevention. *Arch Otolaryngol* 111:2–9, 1985.

Chapter 4
Embryology of the Ear
KATHLEEN K. SULIK and DOUGLAS A. COTANCHE

Origin of the tissues that contribute to the ear

Embryonic development of the internal, middle, and external ear entails well-orchestrated temporal and spatial changes. Descriptions of these developmental changes, as presented here, are derived primarily from studies of mammalian development, although some data acquired from studies of other classes of vertebrates are included. As much descriptive and illustrative material from human embryos is presented as is possible, and most of the remainder is derived from studies of rodents. Although it must be done with caution, in many cases, extrapolation between species appears to be appropriate.

To aid our understanding of the developmental bases for malformations involving the ear, it is important to have a working knowledge of the origin of its tissues. This account of embryogenesis of the ear begins at the time in gestation when the embryo has implanted in the uterine wall and is beginning the process of gastrulation (during the third week post-fertilization in the human; see Table 4–1 for a temporal account of events in human ear development). At this stage of development, the embryo is establishing its definitive germ layers. The bilayered disk of cells that comprises the 2-week-old human conceptus is remodeled into a trilaminar configuration as a portion of the rapidly dividing "upper" or epiblast layer of cells migrates (gastrulates) through the caudal midline area known as the primitive streak to establish the mesoderm and to replace the primitive hypoblast with the definitive embryonic endoderm (Fig. 4–1). With the establishment of three cell (germ) layers, the term *ectoderm* replaces *epiblast* in reference to the "uppermost" cell layer. The gastrulating cells are laid down in a cranial-to-caudal sequence, with this process continuing at the caudal end of the embryo through the fourth week of human development. In the midsagittal region of the embryo, extending forward from the cranialmost aspect of the primitive streak, only two cell layers are present (Figs. 4–1, 4–2). The cells subjacent to the median ectoderm constitute the prechordal (prochordal) plate and the notochordal plate. The anterior rim of the prechordal plate indicates the region where the primitive oral cavity, the stomodeum, will form. Relative differences in growth rate result in a ventrocaudal displacement of the cardiogenic region, which is initially located anterior to the prechordal plate (Figs. 4–1 to 4–3).

The mesoderm located just lateral to the midline (paraxial mesoderm) in the developing cranial region is initially incompletely segmented into "somitomeres" (Fig. 4–4) (20). The somitomeres, which provide the first evidence of a segmental pattern for the head, are believed to be analogous to the more readily detectable mesodermal segments of the trunk, the somites. Seven somitomeres form in a cranial-to-caudal sequence from the region of the developing forebrain (prosencephalon) to the level of the otic placode, each one being associated with a specific portion of the cranial neural plate. Segmentation of the cephalic neural plate into the forebrain (prosencephalon), midbrain (mesencephalon), and hindbrain (rhombencephalon), with further subdivision of the midbrain into two neuromeres and the hindbrain into its initial upper four neuromeres (see Fig. 4–7), is, in fact, presaged by the somitomeres, each of which is located at the level of subsequent formation of the neuromeres. The forebrain develops in relationship to the first somitomere, etc. The somitomeric mesoderm gives rise to the muscle cells associated with the first and second visceral arches (including the tensor tympani and stapedius muscles), as well as to the skeletal tissue of a major portion of the calvaria (including major contributions to the otic capsule, occipital, parietal, petrous temporal, and basisphenoid cartilages and bones). Caudal to the otic placode, segmentation of the paraxial mesoderm results in formation of more readily distinguishable somites. The mesoderm positioned lateral to the paraxial mesoderm in the cranial region differs from its analogous component in the trunk, the lateral plate mesoderm, in that it does not separate into two distinct layers representing a splanchnopleure and somatopleure, but surrounds the aortic arch vessels.

The ectoderm is initially a columnar layer of cells. As this germ layer begins to differentiate, the ectoderm lateral to the neural plate, most of which forms the surface ectoderm, becomes a thinner (cuboidal to squamous) cell layer, while the neural ectoderm thickens. The ectoderm that will form the membranous labyrinth of the inner ear and its sensory neurons remains thick and is termed a *placode*. Using a number of experimental models, genes involved in placode formation and subsequent inner ear development have recently been identified (reviewed in Kiernan et al. [16]). The otic placodes are initially convergent medially with the hindbrain neural plate (Figs. 4–3, 4–4). By the time the anterior neural tube closes, thin ectoderm separates the otic placode from the neural epithelium, and the placodal epithelium thickens further (Fig. 4–5). Other "placodal" epithelia in the developing head are also involved in the development of sense organs and elements of the peripheral nervous system. These include the olfactory placodes for the sense of smell; the trigeminal placodes, which supply part of the trigeminal neurons; and epibranchial placodes, which supply sensory neurons for the seventh, ninth, and tenth cranial nerves (59) (Fig. 4–6).

As the neural folds elevate, but prior to their fusion at preotic levels in the mammal, neural crest cells located at the junction between the surface ectoderm and neural plate on each side begin to leave the ectodermal layer, becoming mesenchyme (i.e., forming loose connective tissue) (Fig. 4–4). The neural crest cells, for the most part, leave the neural folds in a cranial-to-caudal sequence, an exception being the slightly later emigration of the forebrain versus the midbrain-associated crest cells. The cells from the various levels of the neural folds populate specific regions (although there may be some overlap), with those from the forebrain and upper mesencephalic levels populating the region of the frontonasal prominence, and those from the lower mesencephalic and upper hindbrain regions populating the presumptive maxillary and mandibular regions, etc. (24,25,27,28,53,54). Most of the newly formed ectomesenchyme at cranial levels, as opposed to that in the trunk, is located immediately subjacent to the surface ectoderm. Neural crest cells do not move directly beneath the invaginating otic placode but migrate around its margins (Fig. 4–4e,f). Although the neural crest cells derived from all levels of the neural folds play a significant role throughout the body as they differentiate into pigment cells, nerve cells (both sensory and motor), and glial cells, they are of particular importance in the craniofacial region (6,15,21,29–31,47). In contrast to the trunk, where skeletal and connective tissues are mesodermally derived, in the head, much of the skeletal and connective tissue is neural crest derived. All of the skeletal and connective tissue components of the face (with the exception of the enamel of the teeth), including dentin, cartilage, bone, and the connective tissue surrounding blood vessels, glands, and muscle, and the dermis, smooth muscle, and adipose tissue of the skin are neural crest derived. As previously noted, neural crest cells contribute sen-

Table 4–1. Timetable of ear development

Mouse	Human	Description*
12–13 somites (9 days)	23 days	Otic placode evident
	24 days	Otic pit present
17 somites		Placode epithelium just starting to thicken; all ectoderm around placode thins
17–19 somites	26 days	Otic placode transforms into otic vesicle; geniculate ganglion is a cell mass located ventrorostral to otic anlage; ventral wall of otocyst contributes to SA ganglion
22–24 somites		Otocyst detached from surface
27 somites (10 days)	4 weeks	Otocyst is a closed sac; connecting stalk to surface is lost; medial wall is pseudostratified epithelium, 2–3 layers of nuclei; SA ganglion now identifiable caudal to geniculate ganglion but medial and somewhat rostral to the otocyst
12 days	5 weeks	Otocyst elongates and endolymphatic duct buds off the medial wall; pioneering nerve fibers begin to penetrate ventromedial wall of otocyst (otic capsule represented by condensed mesenchyme; auricular hillocks visible)
13 days	7 weeks	One-half coil of cochlear duct; fascicles of nerve fibers within walls of otocyst (otic capsule is cartilaginous and in direct contact with epithelial portions of the labyrinth; chondrification is beginning in Reichert's and Meckel's cartilages with malleus and incus identifiable); hair cells are differentiated in utricle and saccule
14 days	7 weeks	Cochlea at $1\frac{1}{4}$ turns; first definitive hair cells
15 days	7 weeks	Ductus reuniens starting to form; tectorial membrane has started (mouse)
16 days	8 weeks	Cochlea has $1\frac{1}{2}$ turns; perilymphatic spaces develop (external, middle, and internal ear assuming final form); many hair cells differentiate in utricle, saccule, and semicircular canals
18 days	9 weeks	$1\frac{3}{4}$ turns (full number in mouse); $2\frac{1}{2}$ turns (full number in human) but not full length in either; HC identifiable in mouse; development of cuticular plate occurs in mouse
	9–10 weeks	TM starting to form; vestibular HCs
	11–12 weeks	IHC visible throughout cochlea; OHC indistinguishable in apical 1 mm; stereocilia present on IHC and OHC; some cuticular plates are identifiable; synaptic specializations are present on HCs; efferent endings reach IHCs; perilymphatic spaces begin to develop in the human
6 DAB	4 months (16 weeks)	Tunnel of Corti appears in basal coil; membranous labyrinth has adult dimensions
10 DAB	4.5 months	Tunnel of Corti formation complete; efferent nerve endings appear
16 DAB	5 months (20–22 weeks)	Adult stereocilia configuration is on both IHC and OHC, but some kinicilia remain; tunnel of Corti appears in basal coil in human cochlea; periotic spaces are fully formed; ossicles have adult configuration
20 DAB	8 months	Cochlear structure is essentially similar to that of adult, including formation of Nuel spaces

*DAB, days after birth; HC, hair cell; IHC, inner hair cell; OHC, outer hair cell; SA, statoacoustic; TM, tectorial membrane.
Compiled from R O'Rahilly (32), LB Areay (2), and personal observations of the authors.

Figure 4–1. (a) Diagramatic representation of cross-sectional view of a human embryo at the beginning of third week post-fertilization. Cells of the inner cell mass have proliferated and become arranged as a bilayered disk. During the third week post-fertilization in the human, gastrulation begins, as cells from the epiblast migrate through the primitive streak as illustrated in (b). [Diagrams modified from H Tuchmann-Duplessis, *Illustrated Human Embryology*, 1975.]

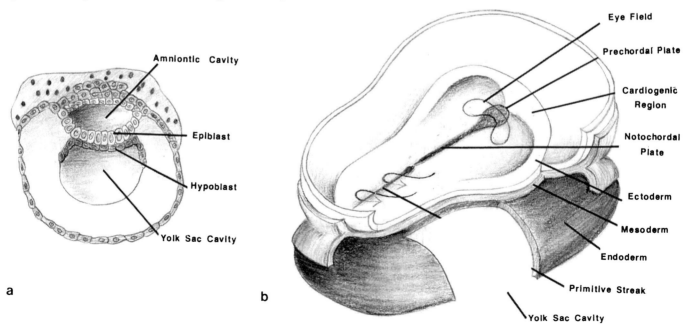

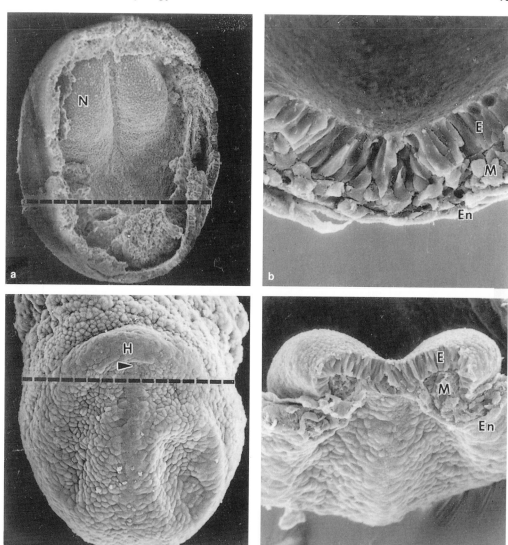

Figure 4–2. Scanning electron micrographs of gastrulation-stage mouse embryos. Dorsal view (a) illustrates the developing neural plate (N). A cut through the caudal end of the embryo at the position of the dotted line reveals morphology of the primitive streak as shown in (b). Ventral view of the embryo as shown in (c) illustrates the position of the cardiogenic area (H) anterior to the prechordal plate (arrowhead). A cut through the anterior end of the embryo as indicated by the dotted line reveals morphology as shown in (d). It is evident that a bilayer of cells occupies the midline. Ectoderm (E) is columnar, mesoderm (M) forms a relatively loose mesenchyme, and endoderm (En) is a squamous layer. [(a) from KK Sulik and MC Johnston, *Scanning Electron Microsc* 1:309, 1982; (b–d) from KK Sulik and GC Schoenwolf, *Scanning Electron Microsc* 4:1735, 1985.]

sory neurons to the craniofacial region. This includes some of the neurons of the trigeminal ganglia, as well as the neurons of the superior ganglia of the ninth and tenth cranial nerves. With specific reference to the ear, neural crest cells contribute glial and Schwann cells, cells that contribute to the formation of the otic capsule (30,58), tympanic ring, the tympanic membrane and external ear, and the middle ear ossicles (with the exception of the stapedial footplate and annulus, which are of mesodermal origin), and melanocytes associated with the inner ear.

Morphogenesis of visceral arches, middle ear, and external ear

The visceral (pharyngeal, branchial) arches form in a cranial-to-caudal sequence on the ventrolateral aspect of the developing face and neck (Figs. 4–5, 4–6). These bars of tissue (containing cells of both mesodermal and neural crest origin) are delineated from one another externally by grooves and internally by pouches (Fig. 4–7). The first visceral arch is readily apparent in embryo showing 13 somite pairs (approximately 4.5 weeks of human gestation). This arch (termed the *mandibular arch*) appears initially as a single prominence of tissue. By the time the embryo has 30 somite pairs (approximately the fifth week of human gestation), two distinct areas, the maxillary and mandibular prominences, are apparent. Dorsal to the groove that separates the second (hy-

oid) visceral arch from the third is the otic pit/otocyst. In the mammalian embryo, only four arches are visible externally, with an additional arch (the sixth) being present deep to the surface.

The sensory innervation of the structures associated with each of the visceral arches derives from neural crest cells and/or ectodermal placodes. Figure 4–6 illustrates the position of the ganglia and placodes associated with the arches, with the trigeminal (fifth cranial nerve) innervating the first arch, the facial (seventh cranial nerve) innervating the second arch, and the glossopharyngeal (ninth cranial nerve) and vagus (tenth cranial nerve) innervating the third and fourth arches, respectively. Recognizing this cranial-to-caudal sequence, and realizing that the otic placode (pit/otocyst) is in a craniocaudal position at the level between the second and third arches, it is logical that the eighth cranial nerve supplies the otic epithelium. The myoblasts of the muscles associated with each of the arches are mesodermally derived, while the connective tissue components of the muscles associated with the first and second arches (first arch—muscles of mastication, mylohyoid, and anterior belly of the digastric, tensor veli palatini, and tensor tympani; second arch—muscles of facial expression, posterior belly of the digastric, stylohyoid, and stapedius) are derived from neural crest cells. Connective tissue components of the laryngeal musculature are mesodermally derived. Motor supply to the visceral arch-associated musculature is by way of the corresponding cranial nerves.

The visceral arches initially serve as conduits for blood vessels, the aortic arch arteries (Fig. 4–7). The second arch vessel, the stapedial

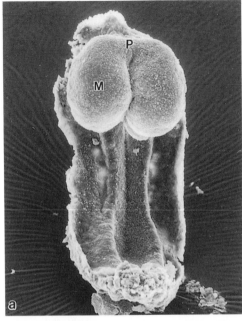

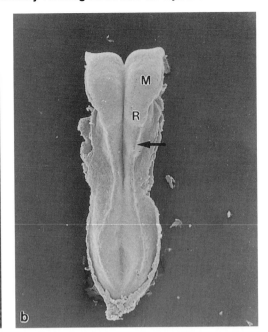

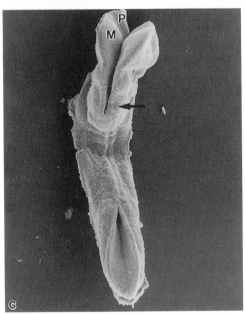

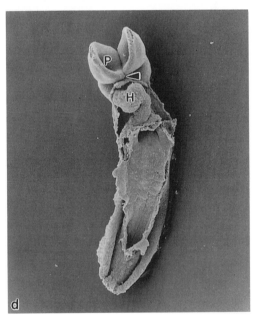

Figure 4–3. Scanning electron micrographs of neurulating mouse embryos. Three distinct regions of brain, forebrain (prosencephalon [P]), midbrain (mesencephalon [M]), and hindbrain (rhombencephalon [R]) become evident at a time corresponding to the fourth week postfertilization in the human. Dorsal views of sequentially older embryos (a–c) illustrate closure of neural folds and position of otic placode (arrow). A ventral view (d) of the embryo shown in (c) illustrates the developing heart (H), and primitive oral cavity (arrowhead), which is bounded laterally by first visceral arch, and cranially by developing frontonasal prominence and forebrain. [(a) from KK Sulik and MC Johnston, *SEM* 1:309, 1982; (b–d) from TW Sadler, *Langman's Medical Embryology*, 1990.]

artery, is of particular significance to the developing ear, as the stapes forms around it, the presence of this vessel resulting in the characteristic ring shape of this ossicle. The aortic arch vessels undergo a series of changes, with the first arch vessel contributing to the maxillary artery and the external carotid, the second arch vessel contributing to the proximal portion of the internal carotid and the distal part of the external carotid, and the third arch vessel eventually serving as the major conduit for arterial blood to the head—the common carotid and part of the internal carotid arteries. The fourth and sixth arch vessels contribute to the subclavian or aortic arch and the pulmonary arteries.

Each of the arches has a cartilaginous derivative. From the neural crest cells of the first arch comes Meckel's cartilage, around which the mandible forms, and from which is derived the head and neck of the malleus and the body and short crus of the incus, as well as the anterior ligament of the malleus and the sphenomandibular ligament. The anterior process of the malleus forms independently in membrane bone. Reichert's cartilage, the cartilage of the second arch, contributes the manubrium of the malleus and the long crus of the incus, as well as the head, neck, and crura of the stapes, the styloid process of the temporal

bone, the stylohyoid ligament, and the lesser horn and the cranial part of the body of the hyoid bone. Additionally, Reichert's cartilage provides a portion of the circumference of the labyrinthine and tympanic segments of the facial canal. The cartilages of the third, fourth, and sixth arches contribute to the hyoid and laryngeal apparatus. Scanning electron microscopic views of embryos that have been cut through the visceral arches in the coronal plane reveal the relationship between the visceral arches, pouches, and clefts (grooves) (Fig. 4–7). In addition, remnants of the buccopharyngeal membrane (tissue that is believed to be analogous to the anteriormost aspect of the prechordal plate), which has broken down to allow continuity between the primitive oral cavity (stomodeum) and the pharynx, can be observed. The epithelium on the stomodeal side of this membrane is ectodermally derived, whereas that on the pharyngeal side is endodermal in origin. The definitive position of this ectodermal–endodermal boundary is just in front of the palatine tonsils. The endoderm that lines the visceral pouches will definitively line the middle ear cavity and Eustachian or auditory tube (primarily the first pouch) and will contribute to glandular elements; the palatine tonsil (second pouch), the thymus and inferior parathyroids (third

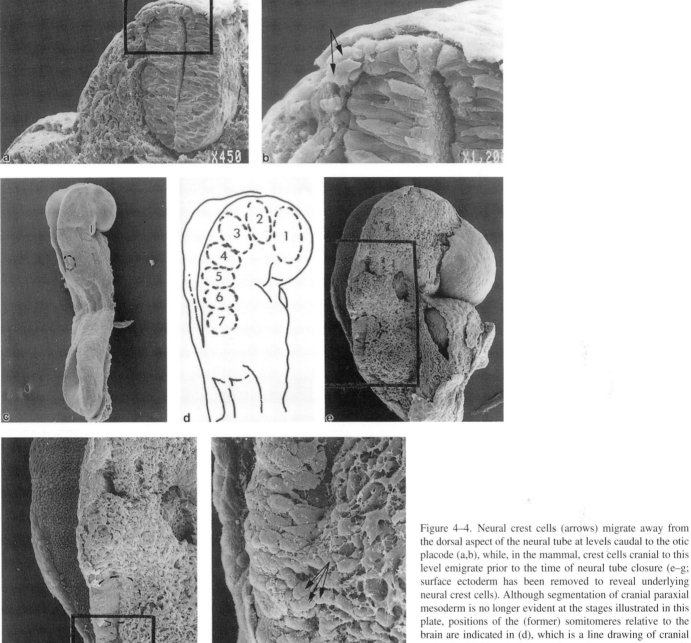

Figure 4–4. Neural crest cells (arrows) migrate away from the dorsal aspect of the neural tube at levels caudal to the otic placode (a,b), while, in the mammal, crest cells cranial to this level emigrate prior to the time of neural tube closure (e–g; surface ectoderm has been removed to reveal underlying neural crest cells). Although segmentation of cranial paraxial mesoderm is no longer evident at the stages illustrated in this plate, positions of the (former) somitomeres relative to the brain are indicated in (d), which is a line drawing of cranial region in (c). Boxed areas are those shown at higher magnification. The dotted line indicates the position of the otic placode. I, first visceral arch. [(a,b,e,g) from KK Sulik and MC Johnston, *Scanning Electron Microsc* 1:309, 1982; (c,d) from JR Siebert et al., *Holoprosencephaly: An Overview and Atlas of Cases*, 1990.]

pouch), the superior parathyroids (fourth pouch), and the ultimobranchial bodies (fifth pouch). The closing membranes between the arches are formed by apposition of the ectoderm and endoderm (Fig. 4–7c). It is these closing membranes that break down in fish, forming gill slits. The closing membranes in mammals do not undergo a major breakdown and are invaded by the neighboring mesenchyme. The tissue between the first and second arches forms the tympanic membrane as the tissue around the margins of the first groove grows, forming the external ear (described in further detail below). While the first and second arches undergo the changes resulting in the formation of the auricle, the more caudal visceral arches remain small and come to lie in a depression termed the *cervical sinus* (see Fig. 4–8). Under normal circumstances, this sinus is obliterated, but retention of some surface ectoderm, especially the ectoderm of the ninth and tenth cranial nerve placodes, i.e., the cervical vesicles (see Fig. 4–8a), may result in cervical cysts. Additionally, internal or external sinuses may result from persistence in whole or in part of the ectodermal clefts or endodermal pouches. Examination of Figure 4–8b allows one to readily see why the external sites for these abnormalities are inferior to the lobule of the ear and along the anterior border of the sternocleidomastoid muscle (Fig. 4–8d). Internally, the opening of a sinus is usually situated on the anterior aspect of the posterior pillar of the fauces, just behind the tonsil, and re-

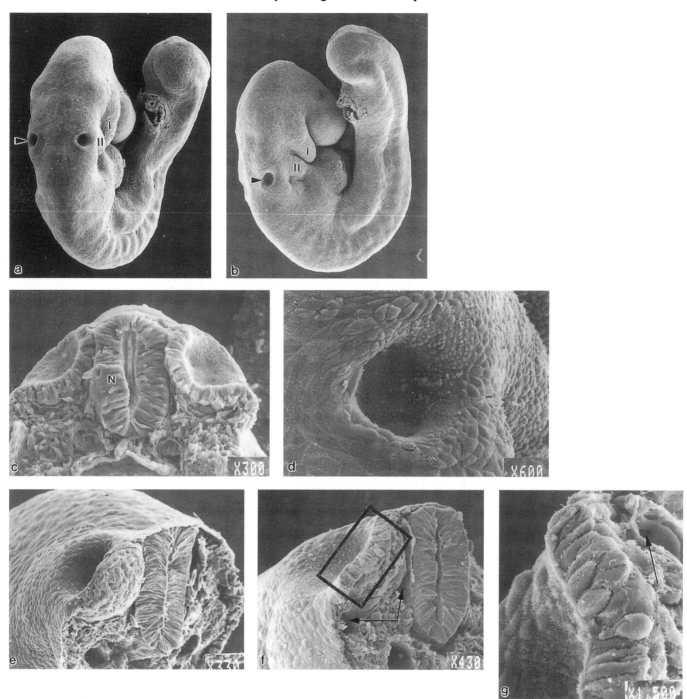

Figure 4–5. Dorsal (a) and lateral (b) views of embryo just following time of anterior neuropore closure illustrate position of otic pits (arrowheads) relative to midline and visceral arches (dorsal to the second cleft). Higher magnification views of otic pit and fractures made through the embryo at its level (c–g) show the close approximation of otic pits and neural tube (N) with intervening vascular network (arrows in f and g). Note the relative thicknesses of the surface, neural and otic epithelia. I, first visceral arch; II, second visceral arch. [(c) from JR Siebert et al., *Holoprosencephaly: An Overview and Atlas of Cases*, 1990.]

sults from persistence of the second pharyngeal pouch (Fig. 4–8e). A tract opening from the side of the neck, ascending and opening into the pharynx is termed a branchial fistula, a malformation that usually involves the second closing membrane.

The middle ear develops as the endoderm-lined dorsal aspect of the first pouch (and possibly part of the second and third dorsal pouches and the intervening pharyngeal wall) expands to become the tubotympanic recess, which surrounds the ossicles and their tendons and ligaments (Fig. 4–9). Later, backward expansion of the tympanic cavity gives rise to the tympanic antrum and, eventually, the mastoid air cells.

The tympanic cavity achieves its adult size by 37 weeks of gestation. During the later months of fetal life the endodermal mucosa of the tympanic cavity becomes thickened and edematous, almost obliterating the lumen. The cavity is again established shortly after birth.

Ossification of the middle ear bones begins in the fourth month of gestation. These bones achieve their adult size by the beginning of the sixth month and are the first bones in the body to attain their ultimate size. Around the footplate of the stapes, the cartilage of the otic capsule must break down to form the oval window. Developmental sequences involved in formation and ossification of the bones associated

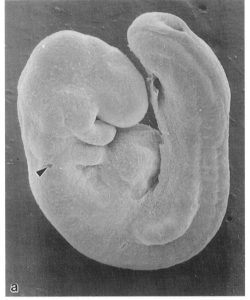

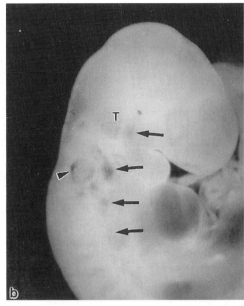

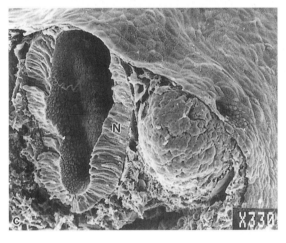

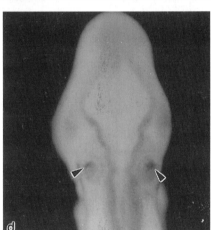

Figure 4–6. Separation of otic vesicle from surface ectoderm (arrowheads) is accompanied by physiological cell death. Staining with vital dye (Nile blue sulfate) allows localization of this, as well as other sites of cell death. These occur in normal embryos in the developing cranial ganglia (T, trigeminal ganglion) and their associated ectodermal placodes (arrows point, in a cranial-to-caudal order, to the trigeminal, facial, glossopharyngeal, and vagal placodes, respectively). In (c) and (d) note position of otic vesicle relative to neural tube (N), being located at the level of fifth hindbrain neuromere.

with both the middle ear and the inner ear have been extensively studied and reviewed (3,35).

As noted previously, the auricle of the external ear forms in the region around the first visceral groove. By the fifth week of gestation, the margins of the groove, which are initially smooth, become irregular as the auricular hillocks become recognizable. Although historically there have been differences of opinion regarding the relative contributions of each of the arches and their respective hillocks to the definitive auricle (45), scanning electron micrographs of human embryos of various gestational ages have helped to clarify the issue (Fig. 4–10). On the mandibular arch of 5-week embryos, the first hillock is distinct, while the second and third cannot be separately defined. On the hyoid (second) arch, the fourth and fifth hillocks are not separable as distinct entities, but the sixth hillock is. By the sixth week, each of the hillocks can be defined, as can the lobule that forms from the tissue of the second arch. In addition, it is clear that the second arch hillocks develop a furrow that will become the site of the scapha, with the hillocks contributing to the tissue on either side of this depression, i.e., helix and anthelix. The auricle in the eighth week of gestation has a conformation that can be readily related to the adult form. The contributions of each of the hillocks are as follows: hillock 1—tragus; hillock 2—crus helicus; hillock 3—ascending helix; hillock 4—horizontal helix, upper portion of scapha and anthelix; hillock 5—descending helix, middle portion of the scapha and anthelix; hillock 6—antitragus and inferior aspect of the helix. It is of interest that excessive numbers of epithelial cells mark the junction of hillocks 2 and 5 at the presumed former po-

sition of the first visceral cleft (Fig. 4–10g,h). It is also noteworthy that in the 5-week human embryo, the corner of the mouth is very close to the junction of the first and second auricular hillocks.

The external auditory meatus deepens by active proliferation of its ectoderm, forming a temporary epithelial plug that extends medially to the mesenchyme, in which the malleus will form and in which the chorda tympani is located (Fig. 4–9). This plug later breaks down in its central portion, canalizing the deeper portion of the meatus. The tympanic membrane, consisting of an outer ectoderm-derived epithelium, a central mesenchyme-derived fibrous layer, and the endoderm-derived inner epithelium, develops initially in a somewhat horizontal fashion, with its definitive upper margin tilting laterally. The neural crest–derived mesenchyme around the margin of the tympanic membrane begins to ossify in the third month, forming the (incomplete) tympanic "ring."

Morphogenesis of the internal ear

The epithelium of the inner ear, as well as its sensory neurons, is derived from the bilateral otic placodes. The placodes form early in the fourth week of development in the ectoderm lateral to the myelencephalon. As the ectoderm lateral to the rim of the neural tube begins to thin, the otic placodes thicken and then invaginate to form the otic pits (cups) and subsequently the vesicles (otocysts) (Figs. 4–5, 4–6). The dorsomedial margins of the otic pits are in close apposition to the hindbrain neuroepithelium, although mesenchymal cells and an exten-

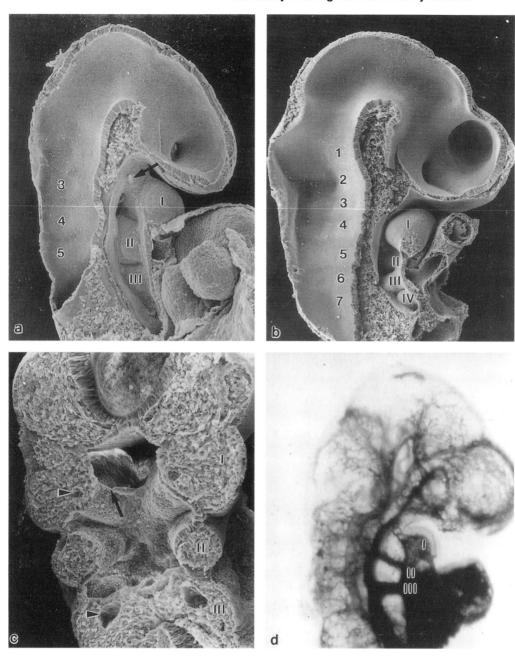

Figure 4–7. Midsagittal (a,b) and frontal (c) fractures through developing head and neck of mouse embryos illustrate relationships between the visceral arches (I, II, III, IV), pouches, and clefts. In (a) and (c) note remnants of buccopharyngeal membrane (arrows), which separate the ectoderm-covered stomodeum (primitive oral cavity) from the endoderm-lined pharynx. Numbers in (a) and (b) indicate hind-brain neuromeres. Following perfusion with India ink, aortic arch vessels, as well as the venous network, are apparent in mouse embryo having 29 somite pairs (d). Note corresponding first and third aortic arch vessels, which are evident in (c) (arrowheads).

sive vascular network are interposed between the two epithelial layers. It is noteworthy that the lateral rim of the otic pit is a site of extensive physiological cell death. The neurons of the statoacoustic ganglion are derived largely, if not exclusively, from the wall of the otic vessel. Migration of these cells from the ventral portion of the otic vesicle is evident in mammalian embryos having 21–29 somite pairs (fourth week of human gestation) (Fig. 4–11). Both vestibular and auditory neurons originate from a common area of otic epithelium that will later form the medial wall of the utricle (58). Thus, most of the neurons originate from a different site than the one they will eventually innervate. Apparently, attractant fields produced by areas of differentiating sensory cells act to guide the growing neurites to the appropriate regions. As previously noted, the statoacoustic ganglion has a dual origin, as neural crest cells contribute the satellite cells and Schwann cells.

Formation of the membranous labyrinth. Toward the end of the fourth week, the otic vesicle loses its attachment to the overlying ectoderm and becomes completely surrounded by mesenchyme (Fig. 4–12A). A shallow groove on the dorsolateral surface of the otocyst in-

dicates the site where it was formerly attached to the ectoderm. Just dorsal to this point there is a small evagination of the otocyst wall, which will eventually form the endolymphatic duct. Meanwhile, the rest of the otocyst enlarges, lengthening faster than it widens to form two pouches: a large, triangular vestibular pouch dorsally and a slender, flattened cochlear pouch ventrally (Fig. 4–12B). The area where the two pouches meet is the region that will eventually form utricle and saccule and has been termed the *atrium*. The triangular portion of the vestibular pouch dorsal to the atrium will give rise to the three semicircular canals. The ventral tip of the cochlear pouch concurrently begins to elongate and curve anteriorly. As the otocyst enlarges and separates into vestibular and cochlear pouches, the statoacoustic ganglion forms in the mesenchyme just medial and anterior to the otocyst.

The semicircular canals form during the fifth week from the three edges of the triangular dorsal surface of the vestibular pouch, with each edge of the triangle becoming a canal (Fig. 4–12C). The canals develop in sequence, with the superior forming first, followed by the posterior and lateral. Each edge of the triangle expands outwardly and forms a flattened pocket. The central area of each pocket collapses, the two lay-

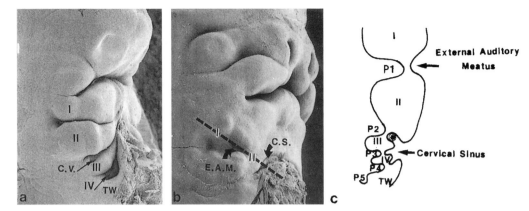

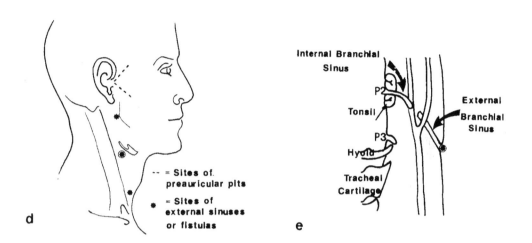

Figure 4–8. Normal human development from fifth (a) to sixth (b) weeks post fertilization results in disappearance of obvious branchial clefts. This occurs as growth of second arch overshadows that of more caudal arches. A cervical sinus (b,c) is formed, with the third and fourth arch tissue lying in a "depression" between the second arch and the developing thoracic body wall. Subsequent union of each of the adjacent arches with each other smoothes out this depression. Abnormal development in this region can result in formation of cysts, sinuses, or fistulas (d,e). Dotted line in (b) indicates plane of cut for (c).

ers fuse, and then they resorb so that an open lumen is left only at the periphery of the pocket. The ampullae of the semicircular canals form at the same time as the canals, with the superior and lateral ampullae growing at the anterior ends of their respective canals while the posterior ampulla arises at the posterior end of the posterior canal. During the fifth week, pioneering nerve fibers from the statoacoustic ganglion begin to penetrate the ventromedial wall of the otocyst.

The utricle and saccule develop during the sixth week by a division of the atrium into upper and lower parts (Fig. 4–12D). The division is formed by the ingrowth of a partition from the anterolateral wall of the atrium toward the opening of the endolymphatic duct on the posteromedial wall. This partition will eventually divide the entrance of the endolymphatic duct, leading to the formation of the utriculosaccular duct. As a result of the separation of the utricle and saccule, the semicircular canals remain associated with the upper part and open only into the lumen of the utricle. By the sixth week, the cochlear duct begins to separate from the posteroventral surface of the saccule. At this time the cochlea extends through about $\frac{1}{2}$ of a coil (Fig. 4–12D). By 8 weeks the cochlea has reached $1\frac{1}{2}$ turn, and by 9 weeks the full $2\frac{1}{2}$ turns of the coil have been achieved (Fig. 4–12E,F), although the length of the duct is only 20 mm (5). The full length of 33–37 mm is not reached until 16 weeks. The central axis, or modiolus, of the coiled cochlear duct is oriented in an anterior–posterior direction in the developing temporal bone, with the apex of the coil located anterior to the basal end.

The growth of the otocyst into the definitive membranous labyrinth is paralleled by the growth of the statoacoustic ganglion (Fig. 4–13). Initially, the ganglion forms a pars superior and a pars inferior at about the time when the otocyst is separated into a vestibular and cochlear pouch (44). Shortly thereafter, the pars inferior gives rise to a vestibular portion and a distinct cochlear spiral ganglion. As the membranous labyrinth and statoacoustic ganglion mature, the pars superior of the ganglion provides the peripheral neural connections to the superior and lateral ampullae and the utricle, while the pars inferioris innervates the

saccule and posterior ampulla. The spiral ganglion develops within the centrally located modiolus of the spiraling cochlear duct and sends fibers into the adjacent sensory epithelium.

Development of the sensory epithelium. During the development of the membranous labyrinth, the walls of the otocyst are composed of a pseudostratified epithelium that has two to three layers of cell nuclei. The cells in the epithelium are oriented so that their basal surfaces are directed out toward the exterior surface of the otocyst and their apical, or luminal, surfaces are directed in toward the lumen of the otocyst. The basal surfaces of the cells are separated from the surrounding mesenchymal tissues by a distinct basal lamina. At the earlier stages of development, the apical surfaces of all the cells in the otocyst are characterized by having numerous small microvilli and a single cilium, or kinocilium (18). As the membranous labyrinth attains its definitive structure, the various sensory regions begin to differentiate in the epithelium on the medial wall of the otocyst. Initially, the six regions of sensory epithelium are located close to one another, but as the labyrinth grows they spread out and become isolated into the three ampullae of the semicircular canals, the maculi of the utricle and saccule, and the organ of Corti in the cochlea. The differentiating sensory regions are first identified by an increase in the number of layers of cell nuclei. This is brought about by a period of intense cell division. Studies in the mouse have shown that most of the cell mitoses in the cochlea are completed by embryonic day 14 (39), a time equivalent to the seventh to eighth week of human development.

The sensory epithelium of the cochlear duct begins to develop in the medial wall of the duct during the seventh week, just as the duct is beginning to form its coils. Since the coiling of the cochlea occurs along an anterior–posterior axis with the apex of the duct lying anterior to the base, the medial wall of the cochlear outgrowth comes to lie on the posterior surface of the coiled duct. At this stage, the epithelium of the medial wall is composed of about six tightly packed layers of nuclei.

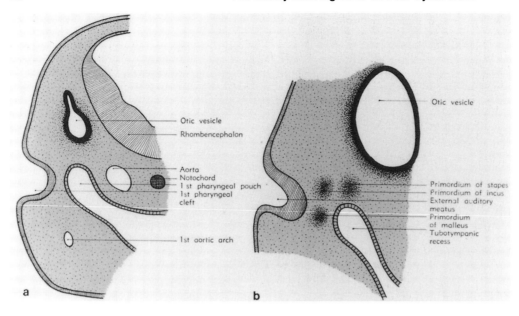

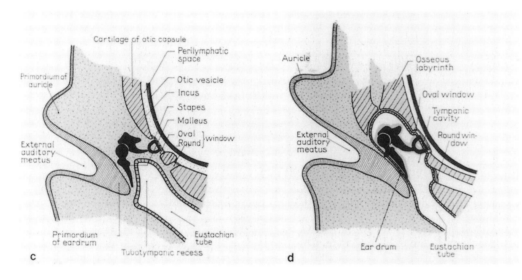

Figure 4–9. Schematic representation of the developing middle ear cavity. (From H Tuchmann-Duplessis, *Illustrated Human Embryology*, 1975.]

Growth of the cells in the sensory epithelium results in the formation of the embryonic precursor of the organ of Corti, the Kölliker's organ. This organ is composed of two ridges that spiral up the length of the cochlea. The two ridges have been identified as a greater epithelial ridge, located closest to the inner, or modiolar, edge of the duct, and a lesser epithelial ridge, located on the outer, or lateral, edge of the duct (6) (Fig. 4–14).

Kölliker's organ undergoes a rapid series of changes in the embryo so that only a portion of the cells in the two ridges end up as part of the mature organ of Corti (Fig. 4–14). The hair cells and supporting cells will eventually form from the cells located at the junction of the greater and lesser epithelial ridges. The inner hair cells will develop from the most lateral cells of the greater epithelial ridge, the pillar cells will arise at the junction of the greater and lesser ridges, and the outer hair cells and Deiters' cells will form from the most medial cells of the lesser epithelial ridge (59). The remainder of the cells in the greater ridge form a tall, dense pseudostratified layer that, from the eighth to the tenth weeks, secretes the material that will form the tectorial membrane. From the 10th through the 20th week, the epithelial cells in the lateral half of the greater epithelial ridge detach from the developing tectorial membrane and undergo an involution so that they end up as a flat layer of cuboidal cells, leaving a large space, the inner spiral sulcus. The cells in the medial half of the greater epithelial ridge, the interdental cells, remain attached to the tectorial membrane but become separated into longitudinally directed columns by the acellular "auditory teeth" of the spiral limbus. The cells in the lesser epithelial ridge that lie directly lateral to the outer hair cells will remain tall and columnar and become the Hensen's cells of the organ of Corti. The cells lateral to the Hensen's cells will involute to form the cells of Claudius, a low cuboidal layer that covers the floor of the outer spiral sulcus.

Although the Kölliker's organ begins to differentiate during the seventh week, presumptive hair cells are not seen in the epithelium until the 11th or 12th week of gestation (5,33). These initial hair cells can be identified because their nuclei lie closer to the lumen of the cochlear duct than do the nuclei of the supporting cells. Moreover, the microvilli on their luminal surfaces become organized into a round bundle that contains a single, eccentrically positioned kinocilium. At this time in development, the inner hair cells can be detected throughout all the turns of the cochlear duct, whereas the outer hair cells can only be definitively identified in the basal half of the duct. This observation defines a trend observed in many other aspects of cochlear development—i.e., that the basal region seems to develop ahead of the more apical regions (37). However, this gradient in development does not run in just one direction, for many researchers have found that the most basal portion of the cochlear duct appears to lag behind the mid-basal region. Moreover, a second gradient in development can be identified in the medial-to-lateral direction at each level of the cochlea, in which inner hair cell development precedes that of the outer hair cells.

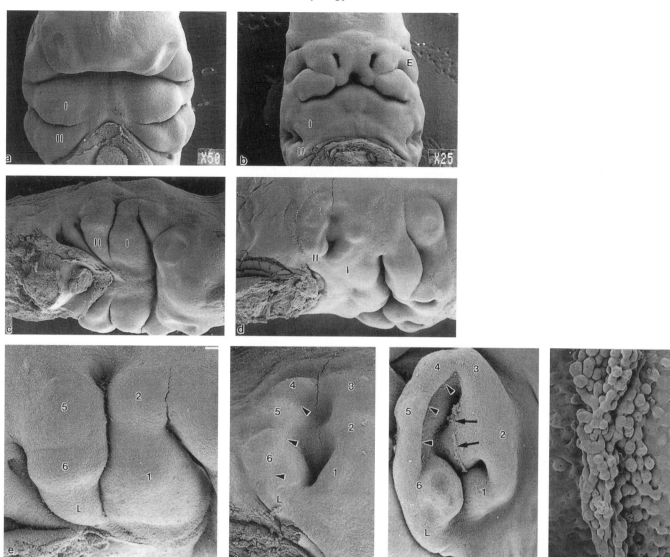

Figure 4–10. Human embryos of approximately 5 (a,c,e), 6 (b,d,f), and 8 weeks (g,h), examined with scanning electron microscopy, nicely illustrate the development of external ear. Note the relationship of external ears to lower jaw in (b). The auricular hillocks and their derivative portions of the external ear are numbered, with hillocks 1–3 originating from tissue of the first branchial arch (I) and hillocks 4–6 from the second arch (II). Note the groove that forms in hillocks 4–6, delineating the location of the scapha (arrowheads, f,g). Of interest is an "overgrowth" or piling up of surface ectoderm along the line that presumably represents the former position of the first closing membrane (arrows, g). E, eye; L, lobule.

Differentiated outer hair cells can be identified in the apical and basal tips of the cochlea by 16 weeks, and at this time there are normally only three rows of outer hair cells, with an occasional fourth row of cells, especially in the apical regions. By 17 weeks the total number of hair cells in the cochlea reaches the quantity found in the adult. The value is 3400 for inner hair cells and 13,400 for outer hair cells (5). Interestingly, the number of hair cells in the fourth row increases considerably in the apical half of the cochlea during the 19th to 24th weeks and remains constant throughout life. Thus, a fourth row of outer hair cells is quite common in the apical region of the cochlea in humans.

The supporting cells in the organ of Corti begin to develop in parallel with the hair cells. During the 11th week, the inner and outer pillar cells can be identified at the junction of the greater and lesser epithelial ridges. The tunnel of Corti, which is located between the two pillar cells, first appears in the mid-basal region at 20 weeks (5,10). The spaces of Nuel surround the outer hair cells and separate the bodies of the outer hair cells from the supporting cells. The Nuel spaces are formed by the overall growth in size of the organ of Corti and the constriction of the upper half of the cell bodies of the Deiters' cells to form the slender phalangeal processes. The first Nuel space, between the outer pillar cells and the first row of outer hair cells, is the earliest to form, and appears in the mid-basal turn somewhat earlier than the tunnel of Corti. The last Nuel space, often referred to as the *outer tunnel*, forms between the third row of outer hair cells and the Hensen's cells and is the last of the spaces to appear (Fig. 4–15B). As with the hair cells, the spaces first appear in the mid-basal region beginning at 20 weeks and spread apically and basally so that they finally extend throughout the length of the cochlea after 25 weeks.

Signal transduction in both inner and outer hair cells is brought about by a deflection of the stereociliary bundle on the apical surface of the cells. Stereocilia are modified microvilli and thus have a core of rigidly cross-linked actin filaments. In all hair cells the stereocilia are arranged in rows of increasing height, and the cells exhibit a directional sensitivity in their response that is oriented in the direction of the shortest to the tallest row of stereocilia. In the mammalian cochlea, the stereociliary bundles of the outer hair cells are arranged in a W-pattern, while those of the inner hair cells are in a straight line. For either cell type, however, there are usually only three rows of stereocilia, and the tallest

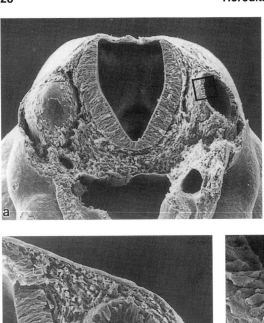

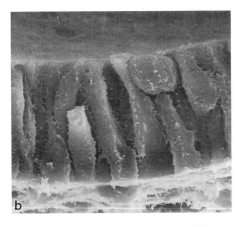

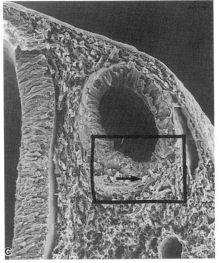

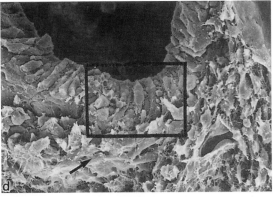

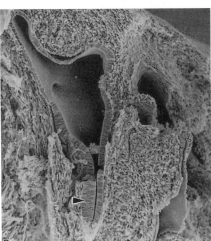

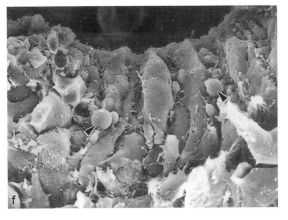

Figure 4–11. Scanning electron micrographs of developing mouse inner ear illustrate the epithelium that forms the walls of this hollow structure. Following separation of the otic vesicle from surface ectoderm, some of the cells at its ventral pole (arrows in c,d) migrate away from the vesicle to become sensory neurons of the eighth cranial nerve. Epithelium at this site contains numerous cellular fragments, which are probably the result of physiological cell death (arrowheads in f). As shown in (e), the change in form that occurs as the otocyst matures involves thinning of the epithelium dorsally, and thickening of the medial wall of the developing cochlear duct (arrowhead in e).

row of each bundle is located on the lateral side of the hair cell surface, i.e., farthest away from the modiolus. The development of the patterns in the stereociliary bundles is quite interesting, for it follows some very defined steps (19,20,55). When the hair cells first differentiate at 11 weeks, the entire cell surface is covered by short stereocilia, which are not much different in size from the microvilli on adjacent supporting cells. A single kinocilium is eccentrically located on the perimeter of each hair cell. Around the 13th week, the stereocilia closest to the kinocilium begin to increase in height so that they are taller than the remaining stereocilia (Fig. 4–16A). Then the rows farther away from the kinocilium begin to grow in progressive order so that a gradient in the heights of the rows is established. By about the 15th week the hair cells

still exhibit a round bundle of stereocilia, but the cells in the half of the bundle closest to the kinocilium are arranged in a staircase pattern of seven or eight rows, while those in the other half are still very short and similar in size to the supporting cell microvilli. This stage of development is followed by a period of restructuring in which the shortest stereocilia are resorbed, leaving a bundle on half of the cell surface (Fig. 14–16B). This bundle then reorganizes gradually into the W-pattern for the outer hair cells and the straight line for the inner hair cells (Fig. 14–16C). This reorganization includes an elimination of all but the three rows of stereocilia seen in the mature cell. Again, these developmental events exhibit the previously seen base-to-apex and the inner-to-outer hair cell gradient in maturation. In the mid-basal region, the inner hair

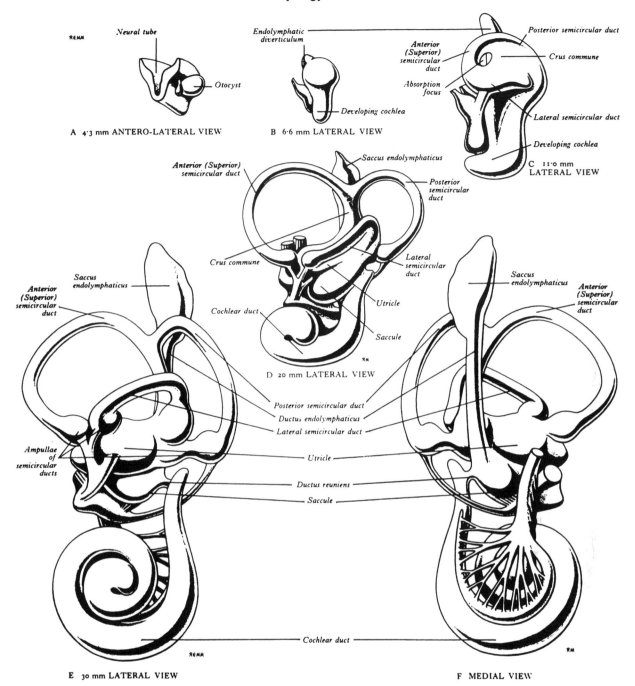

Figure 4–12. Development of the cochlear duct. A series of diagrams showing stages in development of the human membranous labyrinth. (A) Early fourth week. (B) Late fourth week. (C) Fifth week. (D) Sixth week. (E,F) Ninth week. [From Williams PL, Warwick R, Dyson M, and Bannister LH (eds), *Gray's Anatomy*, 37th ed. Churchill Livingstone, Edinburgh, 1989.]

cells appear fairly adult in structure by the 20th week, whereas the outer hair cells do not reach an adult configuration until the 22nd to 25th week.

As the stereociliary bundles on the hair cells are maturing, the other supporting cell surfaces also change their shape. Most significantly, the inner pillar cells expand in width so that the distance between the row of inner hair cells and the first row of outer hair cells increases. The tectorial membrane also undergoes a significant growth during this period (22,41). Initially, most of the tectorial membrane is secreted by the cells of the greater epithelial ridge. This process begins at about the ninth week. A second component of the tectorial membrane is secreted by the cells in the developing organ of Corti in the lesser epithelial ridge beginning by about the 10th or 11th week. As the major part of the

membrane grows, it expands outwardly over the lesser ridge and fuses with the component arising from the organ of Corti. Between the 10th and 20th weeks of development, the cells in the lateral part of the greater epithelial ridge involute and separate from the major part of the tectorial membrane, so that the membrane ends up being anchored to the interdental cells in the spiral limbus on the medial border of the cochlear duct (Fig. 4–17). Most of the tectorial membrane is thus suspended in the fluid of the scala media, and its very lateral edge is attached to the supporting cells in the reticular lamina and to the tallest row of stereocilia on the outer hair cells.

Innervation of the sensory epithelium. The coiling of the cochlear duct brings the sensory epithelium into close apposition with

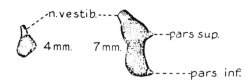

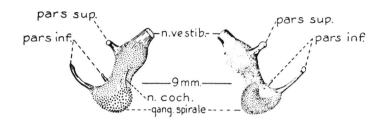

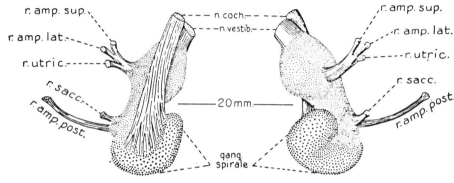

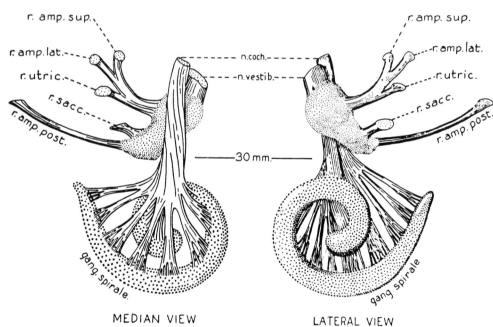

MEDIAN VIEW   LATERAL VIEW

Figure 4–13. Stages in differentiation of human acoustic nerve complex. Vestibular ganglion is shown by fine dots, and spiral ganglion by large dots. Embryonic ages range from fourth week (4 mm) to ninth week (30 mm). [From GL Streeter, *Contrib Embryol* 14:111, 1922.]

the cells of the spiral ganglion in the modiolus. The peripheral processes of the ganglion cells grow toward the region of the differentiating Kölliker's organ and begin to penetrate the basal surface of the epithelium during the seventh week. By the ninth week, the coiling of the duct is complete, and shortly thereafter nerve fibers can be seen entering the epithelium throughout the extent of the developing sensory epithelium. Most of the spiral ganglion nerve fibers pierce the middle region of the duct. By 20 weeks, both radial and spiral fibers are clearly identifiable in the spiral lamina (5).

In the epithelium of Kölliker's organ, several nerve endings can be seen at the bases and along the lateral membranes of the undifferenti-

ated cells during the ninth and tenth weeks (20,33). As soon as the hair cells begin to differentiate in the 11th week, synaptic endings of both afferent and efferent fibers can be identified on inner hair cells, while only afferent endings are seen in association with the outer hair cells (Fig. 4–18). At this time in development, both the afferent and efferent endings synapse directly on the body of the inner hair cell, and presynaptic bodies as well as postsynaptic cisterns can be found on the cytoplasmic side of the inner hair cell plasma membrane. This synaptic pattern changes as the hair cells and nerve endings mature, so that by 20 weeks only the afferent nerves synapse directly on the body of the inner hair cell. The efferent endings slowly retract from the inner hair

A 1DAB

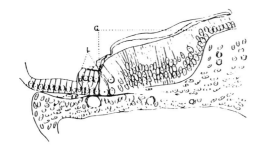

B 6DAB

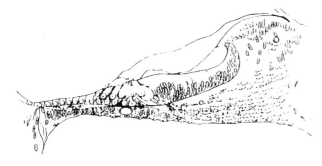

C 9DAB

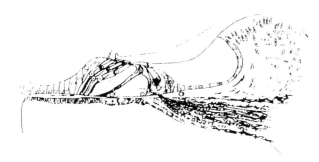

D 20DAB

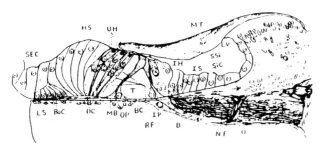

Figure 4–14. Development of Kölliker's organ in cochlea of albino rat. (A) One day after birth (DAB). (B) 6 DAB. (C) 9 DAB. (D) 20 DAB. [From T Wada, *Am Anat Mem* 10:3, 1923.]

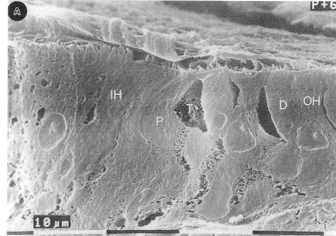

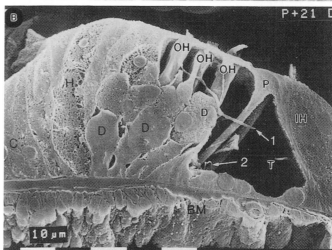

Figure 4–15. Development of tunnel of Corti and Nuel spaces in mouse cochlea. (A) Basal turn of 6-day-old mouse showing early stage of the formation of Corti's tunnel (T). (B) Apical turn of 21-day-old mouse showing well-developed Corti's tunnel and Nuel's spaces. 1, upper radial tunnel fibers; 2, basal radial tunnel fibers; IH, inner hair cell; D, Deiters' cells; OH, outer hair cells; P, pillar cells; T, Corti's tunnel. [From D Lim and M Anniko, *Acta Otolaryngol Suppl* 422:1, 1985.]

cell bodies and establish new synapses on the corresponding afferent dendrites of the hair cell. Concurrently, the postsynaptic cisterns in the inner hair cells disappear.

The synaptic pattern on the outer hair cells also undergoes a change during development. As mentioned earlier, only afferent terminals are found in association with the outer hair cells at the time when they first appear (Fig. 4–18). These afferent terminals form defined synapses on the hair cells, and presynaptic bodies can be seen in the hair cells across from the dendritic terminals. Shortly thereafter, the efferent endings begin to reach the outer hair cells, and they gradually displace the afferent endings and form efferent synapses on the base of the outer hair cells. Synaptic bodies in the hair cells become scarcer, and postsynaptic cisterns begin to form adjacent to the efferent terminals. At the time of the onset of hearing (20 weeks in the human), the outer hair cells have roughly an equal number of afferent and efferent endings, but as development proceeds, the efferent endings on the outer hair cells enlarge and push out all but a few small afferent endings. As with the developmental trends seen in other parts of the cochlea, the basal region of the cochlea undergoes these changes earlier than the apical end, and in each region the transition occurs progressively from the first to the third or fourth row of outer hair cells. It is interesting to note that the onset of auditory function occurs at about the time that the mature synap-

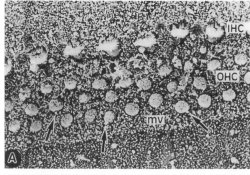

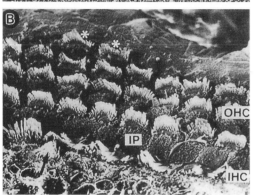

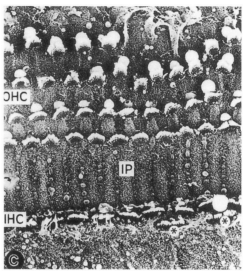

Figure 4–16. Development of stereociliary bundles on hair cells in human organ of Corti. (A) Stereocilia on inner (IHC) and outer (OHC) hair cells in apical turn of 13.5-week-old cochlea. Microvilli are on supporting cells (mv). (B) Basal turn of an 18-week-old human cochlea showing how someshorter stereocilia on IHC and OHC are resorbed, leading toward development of a W-shaped bundle. IP, inner pillar cells. (C) Hair cells in the basal turn of a 20-week-old human cochlea showing the organization of the stereociliary bundles and the separation of the OHC from the IHC by the IP cells. [From M Lavigne-Rebillard and R Pujol, *Anat Embryol* 174:369, 1986 and M Lavigne-Rebillard and R Pujol, *Acta Otolaryngol Suppl* 436:43, 1987.]

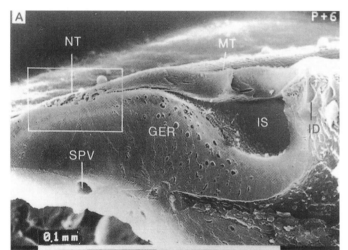

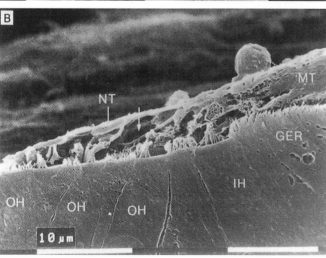

tic formation is achieved on inner hair cells, but long before the final patterns of innervation are reached on the outer hair cells (33).

Development of accessory structures on the cochlea. In addition to the organ of Corti, there are three major portions of the cochlear duct that are important for auditory function: the basilar membrane, the stria vascularis and Reissner's membrane. Two of these, the stria vascularis, and Reissner's membrane, develop from an interaction between the epithelium of the cochlear duct and the mesenchyme of the surrounding tissues. The basilar membrane develops directly below the organ of Corti and, except for the basal lamina of the cells in the cochlear epithelium, is produced by mesenchymal cells surrounding the duct. Unfortunately, there is almost no information on the development of these structures in human embryos. Therefore, the brief reviews outlined here are compiled primarily from studies of development in rodents.

The basilar membrane extends between the spiral limbus on the medial wall of the cochlear spiral and the spiral ligament on the lateral wall. In the adult, it is composed of a matrix of extracellular filaments and ground substance with a single layer of fibroblastic cells covering its lower (tympanic) surface. In the embryo, at about the time when the organ of Corti is differentiating in the cells of Kölliker's organ, the basilar membrane is thick and composed of many layers of cells. It can be divided into two components, an inner part under the greater epithelial ridge called the *zona arcuata* and an outer part under the lesser epithelial ridge called the *zona pectinata*. A large, longitudinally running blood

←

Figure 4–17. Development of tectorial membrane in the mouse organ of Corti. (A) In a 6-day-old mouse embryo, inner sulcus (IS) is created by receding greater epithelial ridge (GER). Tectorial membrane is immature and formed of thick major part (MT) and thin, poorly formed minor part (NT). ID, interdental cell; SPV, spiral vessel. (B) Enlargement of boxed area in (A) showing close-up view of minor tectorial membrane (NT) covering hair cells and anchoring to microvilli of supporting cells. IH, inner hair cell; OH, outer hair cell. [From D Lim and M Anniko, *Acta Otolaryngol Suppl* 422:1, 1985.]

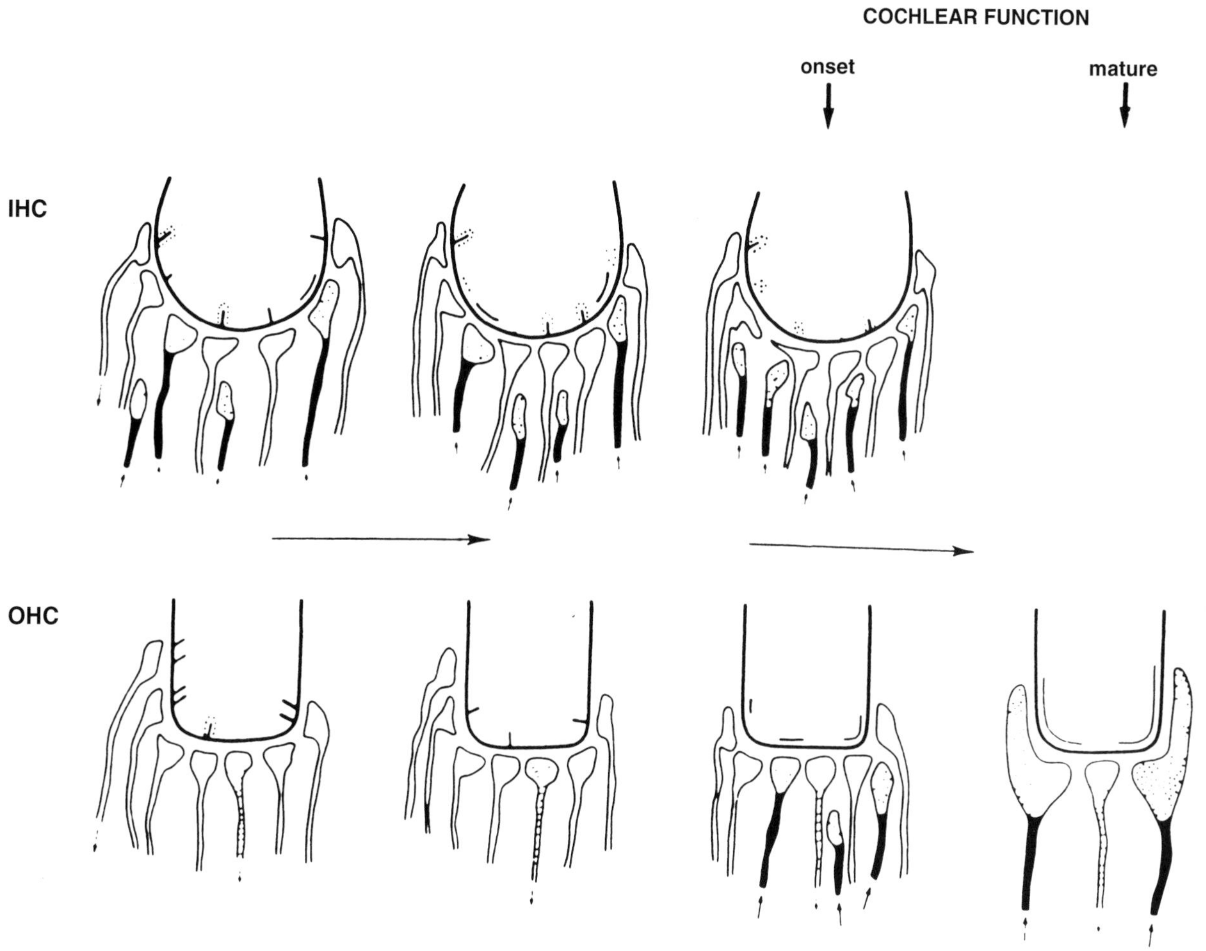

COCHLEAR FUNCTION

onset   mature

IHC

OHC

Figure 4-18. Synaptogenesis in mammalian cochlea. (Key to nerve endings: white or dashed = afferents; black and dotted = efferents.) Very few changes are seen at inner hair cell (IHC) level. In contrast, at the base of outer hair cells (OHC), abundant afferent endings are progressively replaced by efferents. [From R Pujol, *Acta Otolaryngol Suppl* 421:5, 1985.]

vessel, the spiral vessel, is found in the zona arcuata just below the developing pillar cells. As the cochlea develops toward maturity, the basilar membrane thins out and becomes acellular, with the exception of the layer of tympanic cells on its under surface. The spiral vessel decreases in size, but in some mammalian species it remains in the substance of the basilar membrane, especially in the basal regions. In most mammals, the adult basilar membrane is thin in the basal end of the duct but becomes progressively wider toward the apical end. In contrast, the thickness of the membrane is greatest in the basal end, but it gradually thins out toward the apex.

The stria vascularis on the lateral wall of the cochlear duct is thought to be responsible for the production of the unique ionic composition and the high positive endocochlear potential of the endolymphatic fluid. It is composed of three cell types plus an extensive capillary network. The three cell types, the marginal cells, intermediate cells, and basal cells, arise from at least two and possibly three different embryonic cell sources (13,17). The marginal cells are derived from the cells of the epithelium of the cochlear duct. At a time in development equivalent to 11 or 12 weeks in the human, the marginal cells are a single layer of cuboidal cells separated from the underlying mesenchyme by a basement membrane. Shortly thereafter, the basement membrane begins to break down and the marginal cells begin to extend basolateral processes through it to interdigitate with the cellular processes of the underlying intermediate cells. The intermediate cells appear to be a type of melanocyte, as they contain granules of melanin (13). This suggests that these cells are probably of neural crest origin. As the stria matures, the marginal cells express complex basolateral infoldings that interdigitate with processes of the intermediate cells, and the two cell types surround

and incorporate numerous capillaries that are developing in the mesoderm outside the lateral wall of the cochlear wall. A third cell type, the basal cell, is thought to be derived from either the surrounding mesenchyme or from nonpigmented neural crest cells. The basal cells form an underlying layer that separates the marginal cells, intermediate cells, and capillaries from the remaining tissues in the spiral ligament, although they do not have a basement membrane. Reissner's membrane is a thin, cellular layer that separates the scala media from the scala vestibuli. It is anchored medially to the spiral limbus just medial to the origin of the tectorial membrane and extends laterally and upwards to join the spiral ligament at the top of the stria vascularis. Reissner's membrane is composed of two flat cell layers separated by a basement membrane. The inner cell layer, facing the fluid of the scala media, is derived from the epithelium of the cochlear duct, while the outer cell layer, facing the scala vestibuli, arises from mesenchymal cells that condensed from the surrounding periotic mesenchyme (42).

Dysmorphogenesis of the ear

It is clear that malformations involving the ear are commonly associated with those involving other organ systems. To begin to comprehend the developmental bases for these associations, one must have a basic understanding of the overall developmental sequences occurring throughout the embryo concurrent with those of the developing ear. A full course in embryology is beyond the scope of this chapter, and the reader is referred to standard embryology texts for a review (2,12,26,40). Similarly, a detailed discussion of the various molecular mechanisms involved in the development of the ear would be exceptionally lengthy, and so the reader is referred to several review articles on the subject (1,7,36,38,46). Additionally, detailed knowledge of the sources of tissue and their cellular makeup, biochemical requirements, and the physiological activities that the various portions of the ear have in common with other organ systems will lead to a fuller understanding of genetic and environmentally induced multiorgan system malformations and/or dysfunction. That the development of the inner ear is considered to be relatively independent (based on location) of that of the external and middle ear explains the fact that malformations of all three portions of the ear are not always concurrent. However, the fact that there is temporal concurrence of significant developmental events, as well as many common sources of tissue for all portions of the ear, is of major significance.

A significant research resource relative to our understanding of congenital hearing loss and associated anomalies is the number of genetic mutant animals available. In a 1980 review, Deol (8) stated that about 50 mutant genes were known to affect the inner ear of the mouse. He divided these into two groups: those in which the morphogenesis of the ear is defective, and those that involve degeneration of previously formed structures. By 2002 that number had grown to 84 (1). Although tremendous strides have been made in our understanding of the developmental cascade that is involved in the development of the inner ear, work remains to be done to achieve full understanding of this process.

Technological advances in the fields of molecular genetics and cell biology will be invaluable in this regard. A prime example is identification of the genetic abnormality (deletion in the *Pax-3* gene) in mutant mice (Sp2H/Sp2H) that underlies dysgenesis of neural crest–

derived cell populations (9) and subsequent identification of the genetic abnormality in Waardenburg syndrome involving the human gene homologue (56). Inner ear abnormalities in Waardenburg syndrome patients are presumed to result from neural crest deficiencies.

Although genetic mutants with ear malformations have and will continue to supply valuable information, it is difficult to temporally pinpoint the initial dysmorphogenic events involved. This determination is, however, readily done in studies using acute teratogenic insult to the ear, allowing analysis of cell populations initially affected. For example, mouse models of malformations corresponding to some of those in the hemifacial microsomia spectrum (Fig. 4–19) as well as to mandibulofacial dysostosis (Treacher Collins syndrome) (Fig. 4–20) have shown that these malformations can be induced by acute teratogen exposure to retinoic acid at times corresponding respectively to approximately days 20–22 or 24–26 post-fertilization in the human (50–52,62). At the earlier treatment time, the embryos have approximately 3–5 somites—a stage when neural crest cells just begin to migrate into the first arch area, and have not yet begun to enter the second arch. Retinoid-induced deficiencies in these neural crest cell populations result in small mandibular prominences and very dysmorphic to virtually absent second arches (Fig. 4–19). This has the obvious result of affecting, to varying degrees, external and middle ear development (14). It is of interest that this treatment also results in the presence of tissue tags extending from the tragal area to the corner of the mouth, as is typical of some forms of hemifacial microsomia. The early proximity of the corner of the mouth to the tragal hillock and the early deficiency of the tissues in this area no doubt lead to the disorganized development inherent in the formation of these abnormal ap-

Figure 4–19. Retinoic acid–induced abnormalities of visceral arches/external ears in mouse embryos as illustrated in (b,d,e) resulting from acute exposure to this teratogen at the time that neural crest cells begin to leave neural folds to enter arches. Compare abnormal morphology of second arch in (b) to that of normal embryo of same developmental stage in (a), and morphology of external ear in (c) to mildly affected ear in (e) and more severely affected ear in (f). Also, in (e) and (f), note abnormal tags present in a line extending from corner of mouth to tragal region. E, eye.

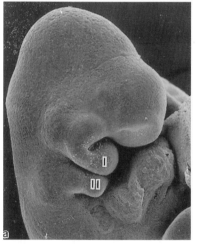
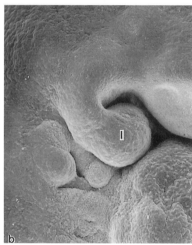
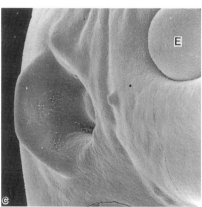
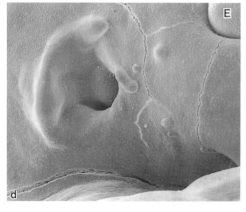
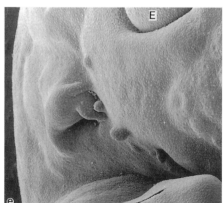

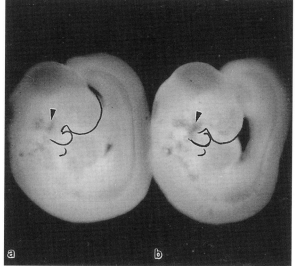
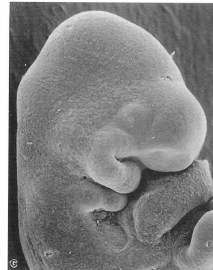
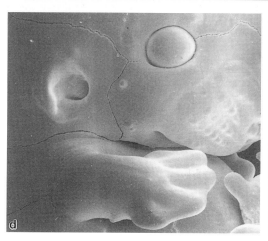
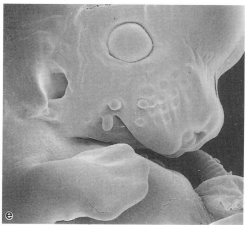

Figure 4–20. Retinoic acid–induced abnormalities of the visceral arches/external ear in mouse embryos as illustrated in (b,c,e) resulting from exposure to this teratogen when cells at dorsal aspect of the visceral arches (in region of ectodermal placodes and subjacent cells) are vulnerable to teratogen-induced excessive cell death. Compare dark (Nile blue sulfate) staining in first arch in (b) to that of a normal amount of physiological cell death in (a) (arrowheads). Comparison of (c) to a normal embryo of the same stage in Figure 4–19a illustrates deficiency at dorsal aspect of first arch and abnormal position of corner of mouth. At later stages of development, these deficiencies are apparent in the region of the mandibular ramus and zygoma as is typical of mandibulofacial dysostosis [compare normal fetus in (d) to abnormal one in (e)]. [(a,b) from KK Sulik et al., *Cleft Palate J* 26:209, 1989; (c,d) from KK Sulik et al., *Am J Med Genet* 27:359, 1987.]

pendages. This teratogen exposure time is also associated with inner ear malformation, including deficient coiling of the cochlea, as well as ocular and vertebral malformations.

In the mandibulofacial dysostosis model, teratogen exposure is at the time just after the neural crest cells have populated the upper visceral arches. The external ear malformations and deficiencies in the dorsal (proximal) aspect of the maxillary and mandibular regions appear to be related to cell loss (excessive teratogen-induced cell death) in the proximal aspect of the first and second arch (Fig. 4–20). It is noteworthy that, following this teratogen exposure time, the external ear malformations are not as severe as at the earlier time, detectable inner ear malformations are much less frequently induced, and tissue tags, though present, are located only at the corner of the mouth, not all along the oral–tragal line (14). It is also of interest that the induced maxillary deficiency places the corner of the mouth in an abnormal position relative to the developing auricular hillocks (compare Fig. 4–19a to Fig. 4–20c). Perhaps such abnormal relationships may account for the supratragal level of some auricular sinuses and fistulas.

It is obvious that teratogenesis studies involving acute exposures to single teratogens at a variety of known developmental stages can teach us a great deal about the genesis of malformations. Additionally, knowledge of the temporal sensitivity of a variety of organ systems to a number of teratogenic agents can provide some understanding of syndrome composition and clues to additional organ systems that should be examined in detail for suspected injury in animal models. For example, in mice, the limb and the urinary tract have been shown to be vulnerable to alcohol-induced teratogenesis when exposure occurs at virtually the same developmental stages as those at which retinoic acid induces

ear malformations (4,11,34,61). Obviously, some of the branchio-otorenal syndromes might arise from a genetic or environmental insult affecting this stage of development. Although it is more difficult to envision a genetically inherited malformation as arising from an acute time-related insult than it is for those of environmental origin, the possibility should not be discounted. No doubt, analyses of malformation spectra and gene expression patterns in animal models will, in addition to illustrating the basis for concurrence of specific malformations of various organ systems, allow one to appreciate the overlap that exists as one syndrome grades into another.

Acknowledgments

We are grateful to Danial Picard and Deborah Dehart for their generous assistance with the photography, and to Peter Bream for his help in preparation of the manuscript. This work was supported in part by NIH grant DC00412 (DAC).

References

1. Anagnostopoulos AV: A compendium of mouse knockouts with inner ear defects. *Trends Genet* 18:521–538, 2002.
2. Arey LB: *Developmental Anatomy: A Textbook and Laboratory Manual of Embryology*, 7th ed. W.B. Saunders, Philadelphia, 1974.
3. Austin DF: The ear: anatomy and embryology. In: *Diseases of the Nose, Throat, Ear, Head, and Neck*, Ballenger JJ (ed), Lea & Febiger, Philadelphia, 1985, pp 877–923.
4. Boggan WO et al: Effect of prenatal ethanol administration on the urogenital system in mice. *Alcohol Clin Exp Res* 13:206–208, 1989.
5. Bredberg G: Cellular pattern and nerve supply of the human organ of Corti. *Acta Otolaryngol Suppl* 236:127–135, 1989.
6. Bronner-Fraser M: Experimental analyses of the migration and cell linkage of avian neural crest cells. *Cleft Palate J* 27:110–120, 1990.

7. Bryant J et al: Sensory organ development in the inner ear: molecular and cellular mechanisms. *Br Med Bull* 63:39–57, 2002.

8. Deol SM: Genetic malformation of the inner ear in the mouse and man. *Birth Defects* 16(4):243–261, 1980.

9. Epstein DJ et al: Splotch (*SP2H*), a mutation affecting development of the mouse neural tube, shows a deletion within the paired homeodomain Pax-3. *Cell* 67:767–774, 1991.

10. Fujimoto S et al: Scanning and transmission electron microscope studies on the organ of Corti and stria vascularis in human fetal cochlear ducts. *Arch Histol Jpn* 44:223–235, 1981.

11. Gage WJ, Sulik KK: Pathogenesis of ethanol-induced hydronephrosis and hydroureter as demonstrated in a mouse model. *Teratology* 44:299–312, 1991.

12. Hamilton WJ et al: *Human Embryology*, Macmillan Press Ltd, London, 1976.

13. Hilding WJ, Ginzberg RD: Pigmentation of the stria vascularis. *Acta Otolaryngol* 84:24–37, 1977.

14. Jarvis BL et al: Congenital malformations of the external, middle and inner ear produced by isotretinoin exposure in fetal mice. *Otolaryngol Head Neck Surg* 102:391–401, 1990.

15. Johnston MC: A radioautographic study of the migration and fate of cranial neural crest cells in the chick embryo. *Anat Rec* 156:143–156, 1966.

16. Kiernan AE et al: Development of the mouse inner ear. In: *Mouse Development: Patterning, Morphogenesis, and Organogenesis*, Rossant J, Tam PPL (eds), Academic Press, San Diego, 2002, pp 539–566.

17. Kikuchi K, Hilding D: The development of the organ of Corti in the mouse. *Acta Otolaryngol* 60:207–222, 1965.

18. Kikuchi K, Hilding DA: The development of the stria vascularis in the mouse. *Acta Otolaryngol* 62:277–291, 1966.

19. Lavigne-Rebillard M, Pujol R: Development of the auditory hair cell surface in human fetuses: a scanning electron microscopy study. *Anat Embryol* 174:369–377, 1986.

20. Lavigne-Rebillard M, Pujol R: Surface aspects of the developing human organ of Corti. *Acta Otolaryngol Suppl* 436:43–50, 1987.

21. LeDouarin N: *The Neural Crest*, Cambridge University Press, Cambridge, 1982.

22. Lim D: Development of the tectorial membrane. *Hear Res* 28:9–21, 1987.

23. Lim D, Anniko M: Developmental morphology of the mouse inner ear: a scanning electron microscopic observation. *Acta Otolaryngol Suppl* 422:1–69, 1985.

24. Lumsden A et al: Segmental origin and migration of neural crest cells in the hindbrain region of the chick embryo. *Development* 113:1281–1292, 1991.

25. Meier S, Tam PPL: Metameric pattern development in the embryonic axis of the mouse. I. Differentiation of the cranial segments. *Differentiation* 21:95–108, 1982.

26. Moore KL, Persaud TVN: *The Developing Human*, 4th ed. W.B. Saunders, Philadelphia, 1993.

27. Nichols DH: Neural crest formation in the head of the mouse as observed using a new histological technique. *J Embryol Exp Morphol* 64:105–120, 1981.

28. Nichols DH: Formation and distribution of neural crest mesenchyme to the first pharyngeal arch region of the mouse embryo. *Am J Anat* 176:221–231, 1986.

29. Noden DM: The embryonic origins of avian cephalic and cervical muscles and associated connective tissues. *Am J Anat* 168:257–276, 1983.

30. Noden DM: Interactions and fates of avian craniofacial mesenchyme. *Development* (Suppl) 103:121–140, 1988.

31. Noden DM: Cell movements and control of patterned tissue assembly during craniofacial development. *J Craniofac Genet Dev Biol* 11:192–213, 1991.

32. O'Rahilly R: The timing and sequence of events in the development of the human eye and ear during the embryonic period proper. *Anat Embryol* 168:87–99, 1983.

33. Pujol R: Morphology, synaptology and electrophysiology of the developing cochlea. *Acta Otolaryngol Suppl* 421:5–9, 1985.

34. Randall CL, Anton RF: Aspirin reduces alcohol-induced prenatal mortality and malformations in mice. *Alcohol Clin Exp Res* 8:513–515, 1984.

35. Ricchany SF et al: The ear and the temporal bone: development and adult structure. In: *Otolaryngology*, Pearson BW (ed), Harper & Row, Philadelphia, 1987, pp 1–140.

36. Rinkwitz S et al: Development of the vertebrate inner ear. *Ann NY Acad Sci* 942:1–14, 2001.

37. Rubel EW: Ontogeny of structure and function in the vertebrate auditory system. In: *Handbook of Sensory Physiology*, Vol. 9, Jacobson M (ed), Springer-Verlag, Berlin, 1978, pp 135–137.

38. Rubel EW, Fritzsch B: Auditory system development: primary auditory neurons and their targets. *Annu Rev Neurosci* 25:51–101, 2002.

39. Ruben RJ: Development of the inner ear of the mouse: a radioautographic study of terminal mitoses. *Acta Otolaryngol Suppl* 220:4–44, 1967.

40. Sadler TW: *Langman's Medical Embryology*, 6th ed. Williams & Wilkins, Baltimore, 1990.

41. Sanchez-Fernandez JM et al: Early aspects of human cochlea development and tectorial membrane histogenesis. *Acta Otolaryngol* 95:460–469, 1983.

42. Sher AE: The embryonic and postnatal development of the inner ear of the mouse. *Acta Otolaryngol Suppl* 285:5–77, 1971.

43. Siebert JR et al: *Holoprosencephaly: An Overview and Atlas of Cases*, Wiley-Liss, New York, 1990.

44. Streeter GL: On the development of the membranous labyrinth and the acoustic and facial nerves in the human embryo. *Am J Anat* 6:139–165, 1906.

45. Streeter GL: Development of the auricle in the human embryo. *Contrib Embryol* 14:111–138, 1922.

46. Streit A: Extensive cell movements accompany formation of the otic placode. *Dev Biol* 249:237–254, 2002.

47. Sulik KK: Embryogenesis of the neural crest: a review. *Proc Greenwood Genet Ctr* 9:54–56, 1990.

48. Sulik KK, Johnston MC: Embryonic origin of holoprosencephaly: interrelationship of the developing brain and face. *Scanning Electron Microsc* 1:309–322, 1982.

49. Sulik KK, Schoenwolf GC: Highlights of craniofacial morphogenesis in mammalian embryos as revealed by scanning electron microscopy. *Scanning Electron Microsc* 4:1735–1752, 1985.

50. Sulik KK et al: Mandibulofacial dysostosis (Treacher Collins syndrome): a new proposal for its pathogenesis. *Am J Med Genet* 27:359–372, 1987.

51. Sulik KK et al: Teratogens and craniofacial malformations: relationships to cell death. *Development* (Suppl) 103:213–232, 1988.

52. Sulik KK et al: Pathogenesis of cleft palate in Treacher Collins, Nager, and Miller syndromes. *Cleft Palate J* 26:209–216, 1989.

53. Tan SS, Morriss-Kay GM: The development and distribution of cranial neural crest in the rat embryo. *Cell Tissue Res* 240:403–416, 1985.

54. Tan SS, Morriss-Kay GM: Analysis of cranial neural crest cell migration and early fates in postimplantation rat chimeras. *J Embryol Exp Morphol* 98:21–58, 1986.

55. Tanaka K et al: Organ of Corti in the human fetus: scanning and transmission electron microscope studies. *Ann Otol* 88:749–758, 1979.

56. Tassabehji M et al: Waardenburg's syndrome patients have mutations in the human homologue of the *Pax-3* paired box gene. Nature 355:635–636, 1992.

57. Tuchmann-Duplessis H: *Illustrated Human Embryology*, Springer-Verlag, New York, 1975.

58. Van De Water TR: Tissue interactions and cell differentiation: neurone–sensory cell interaction during otic development. *Development* (Suppl) 103:185–193, 1988.

59. Verwoerd CD, van Oostrom CD: Cephalic neural crest and placodes. *Adv Anat Embryol Cell Biol* 58:1–75, 1979.

60. Wada T: Anatomical and physiological studies on the growth of the inner ear of the albino rat. *Am Anat Mem* 10:3–174, 1923.

61. Webster WS et al: Someteratogenic properties of ethanol and acetaldehyde in C57B1/6J mice: implications for the study of the fetal alcohol syndrome. *Teratology* 27:231–243, 1983.

62. Webster WS et al: Isotretinoin embryopathy and the cranial neural crest: an in vivo and in vitro study. *J Craniofac Genet Dev Biol* 6:211–222, 1986.

Chapter 5
Genetic Hearing Loss with No Associated Abnormalities

SHELLEY D. SMITH and R. THOMAS TAGGART

On the basis of the number of known X-linked hearing loss genes, Morton (2) calculated that there would be about 120 different genes causing nonsyndromic hearing loss, 60 prelingual and 60 postlingual. More complicated estimates based on the analysis of mating types, inbreeding coefficients, and mutation rates have indicated that there may be about 36 recessive loci for hearing loss, most of them nonsyndromic. Although the assumptions behind these estimates were uncertain, the predictions appear to be quite accurate, as there are at least 67 Mendelian loci defined currently: 32 dominant (primarily postlingual), 31 recessive (primarily prelingual), and 4 X-linked. Additional loci are listed as "reserved," and information on those should be forthcoming. The Hereditary Hearing Loss Homepage, maintained by Guy Van Camp and Richard J.H. Smith (http://dnalab-www.uia.ac.be/dnalab/hhh/), provides an update on new loci as they are reported. A number of techniques have proven to be useful in localizing these genes, ranging from positional cloning in single large dominant pedigrees to consanguineous recessive pedigrees to the identification of mouse models and subsequent searches for human homologues. Candidate genes have also been identified through cDNA libraries from cochlear tissues in humans or other species, through homologies to other known genes, or through their involvement in syndromic forms of hearing loss. Identification of the genes involved in nonsyndromic hearing loss has helped dissect the molecular pathways for a variety of functions and structures in the inner ear: ion transfer, motility, membrane and extracellular matrix structure, mitochondrial energy generation, and gene regulation (Table 5–1).

In addition to genetic heterogeneity, there is also considerable variation in expression, with some nonsyndromic genes producing dominant, recessive, or syndromic phenotypes (Table 5–2). These variations have generally been attributed to the location and type of mutation within the gene. However, gene interactions have also been implicated in variations in expression—e.g., apparent digenic interaction of *DFNA2* and *TECTA* mutations, *GJB2* mutation and *GJB6* deletion, the interaction of the mitochondrial 1555A → G mutation and a recessive locus, and gene modification as exemplified by *DFNB26* and *DFNM1*.

Loci for nonsyndromic hearing loss are named according to mode of inheritance (DFN, X-linked; DFNA, dominant; DFNB, recessive), and then numbered within each type in the order of reporting.

Among cases of nonsyndromic hearing loss, approximately 22% are inherited in a dominant fashion, 77% are recessive, and 1% are X-linked or have other (primarily mitochondrial) modes of inheritance (2). These figures are based on studies of congenital severe-to-profound hearing impairment. If later-onset and milder forms of hearing loss are included, the proportion of dominant genes will be much greater. Accurate population genetic studies have not been completed, however. Within each mode of inheritance, the loci can be grouped into somewhat similar phenotypic subtypes, following the original clinical classification of Konigsmark and Gorlin in the first edition of this book. Because of the range of expression that is possible for several of the genes, however, the same locus may be associated with phenotypes in different sections. Table 5–3 summarizes all of the loci with a brief description of their phenotypes. In this table and in the text, the frequencies are divided into *low*, 250–500 Hz; *mid*, 500–2000 Hz; and *high*, above 2000 Hz. Severity of hearing loss is expressed as *mild* (thresholds between 25–40 dB SPL), *moderate* (41–69 dB), *severe* (70–94 dB), and *profound* (thresholds lower than 95 dB). The term *deafness* is generally used to refer to hearing loss in the severe to profound range, particularly in individuals who do not use speech for communication. Since this may be ambiguous in genetic studies, the term will not be used (1). Finally, the terms *prelingual* and *congenital* should be used carefully. In many cases, particularly when reliable testing has not been available for infants, it is not possible to determine if the hearing loss was present at birth, and the only indicator of early hearing loss is lack of speech development. In genetic conditions where there is clearly lack of progression of hearing loss, prelingual hearing loss is almost certainly congenital, but in cases where very early onset cannot be documented, the more conservative term *prelingual* is often used.

References

1. European Work Group on Genetics of Hearing Impairment: *Infoletter 2*, November 1996.
2. Morton NE: Genetic epidemiology of hearing impairment. *Ann NY Acad Sci* 630:16–31, 1991.

Autosomal Dominant Nonsyndromic Hearing Loss

Autosomal dominant progressive high-frequency hearing loss

This is a highly heterogeneous classification. All of the following show progressive cochlear hearing loss starting in the high frequencies, but differ in the age of onset, rate of progression, ultimate degree of hearing loss with age, and vestibular involvement. Diagnosis in all cases must first exclude other nongenetic causes of hearing loss as well as syndromic hearing loss. An autosomal dominant pattern is generally readily apparent.

DFNA2

- MIM: 600101 (DFNA2), 603537 (KCNQ4), 603324 (GJB3)
- Location, gene: 1p34; *KCNQ4* or *GJB3* (connexin 31) and at least one additional unidentified gene

At least nine families in the United States, Europe, and Japan have been reported with mutations in *KCNQ4* (4,7,10,11). Mutations in *KCNQ4* are one of the more common causes of dominant progressive

Table 5–1. Functions of genes causing nonsyndromic hearing loss

Function	Genes
Ion homeostasis	*GJB2, GJB3, GJB6, KCNQ4, CLDN14,* possibly *TCM1*
Cytoskeletal motility	*DIAPH1, MYO6, MYO7A, MYH9,* possibly *TMIE*
Cytoskeletal/extracellular matrix structure	*TECTA, COL11A2, CDH23, USHIC,* possibly *COCH, DSPP*
Protease	*TMPRSS3*
Gene regulation	*EYA4, POU4F3, TFCP2L3*
Mitochondrial function	12S rRNA, tRNA$^{Ser(UCN)}$, tRNA$^{Leu(UUR)}$

Table 5–2. Hearing loss genes with variable expression

Gene	Dominant Locus	Recessive Locus	Syndrome
CDH23		DFNB12	Usher syndrome ID
COCH			Ménière's disease
COL11A2	DFNA13		Nonocular Stickler syndrome, OSMED syndrome
DSPP	DFNA39		Dentinogenesis imperfecta
GJB2	DFNA3	DFNB2	Palmoplantar keratodermia, Vohwinkel syndrome
GJB3	DFNA2		Erythrokeratodermia variabilis
GJB6	DFNA3	DFNB2	Hidrotic ectodermal dysplasia
MYH9	DFNA17		May-Hegglin anomaly, Fechtner, Epstein, and Alport-like syndromes
MYO7A	DFNA11	DFNB2	Usher syndrome IB
PCDH15		DFNB23	Usher syndrome IF
SLC26A4		DFNB4	Pendred syndrome, enlarged vestibular aqueduct syndrome
TCM1	DFNA36	DFNB7/11	
TECTA	DFNA8/12	DFNB21	
USH1C		DFNB18	Usher syndrome IC
WFS	DFNA6/14/38		Wolfram syndrome

OSMED, otospondylomegaepiphyseal dysplasia.

hearing loss in families of European descent (11). Two Chinese families have been reported with mutations in *GJB3* (connexin 31) (14), and two familes, one Indonesian and one American, have been reported, which link to the DFNA2 region but do not have mutations in either gene (4,5,10).

Auditory findings. For individuals with *KCNQ4* mutations, sensorineural hearing loss was usually detected in the high frequencies before age 10 and gradually progressed to severe to profound loss in all frequencies in the fifth to sixth decade. However, there was some variation in onset and rate of progression within and between families. Tinnitus was infrequent. Speech discrimination was somewhat better than that in individuals with mutations in the *COCH* gene who had similar degrees of hearing loss; this may be due to the relative lack of expression of *KCNQ4* in the basal cochlea (2).

The families with *GJB3* mutations showed much later age of onset, with subjects generally noting high-frequency sensorineural hearing loss around age 40, preceded by tinnitus. Thresholds sloped to the moderate range (60 dB).

The Indonesian kindred described in the first report of linkage to the DFNA2 region showed hearing loss intermediate between the two other genes, with onset after 10 years of age and accompanied by tinnitus. It progressed from the high frequencies to include all frequencies, with moderately severe to profound loss by age 40 (3). Both linkage mapping and mutation analysis have excluded the *KCNQ4* and *GJB3* genes in that kindred. Similarly, an American kindred with high-frequency hearing loss beginning in the first and second decade and progressing to a severe to profound sloping loss showed linkage to the DFNA2 region, but no mutations in *KCNQ4* or *GJB3* were found (5,10).

Vestibular findings. Generally, vestibular dysfunction has not been associated with any of the DNFA2 genes. However, some members of one family (later found to have a *KCNQ4* mutation) showed an increased vestibulo-ocular reflex, indicative of vestibular hyper-reactivity (8).

Radiology/pathology. The CT scan of the temporal bones was normal.

Molecular studies. Animal studies have shown that *KCNQ4*, a voltage-gated potassium channel gene, is expressed in inner and outer hair cells and the spiral ganglia of the cochlea, as well as in type 1 vestibular cells and some brain stem nuclei (6). There appears to be a gradient of activity along the cochlea, ranging from more expression in inner hair cells in the basal region to more expression in the outer hair cells apically (1). *KCNQ4* was localized to 1p36 by Kubisch et al. (7) and mutations were found in two small French families. Subsequently, at least nine families in the United States, Europe, and Japan have been

reported with mutations in *KCNQ4* (4,7,11,12). Most mutations have been in the pore region of the molecule (13).

GJB3 produces the gap junction protein connexin 31, which combines with other connexin molecules into hexameric complexes, or *connexons*, which connect adjacent cells and allow passage of ions and small molecules (see DFNB1, below, for more complete discussion of connexins and hearing loss). *GJB3* is expressed in the supporting cells of the organ of Corti and in the fibroblasts of the spiral ganglion of the rat. Two Chinese families with dominant inheritance of hearing loss due to mutations in *GJB3* have been reported; one had a missense mutation, 547G → A, resulting in an E183L change, and the other had a 538C → T, producing a stop codon at amino acid position 180 (R180X). Both of these nucleotides were found to be highly conserved, and a somewhat similar E186K mutation of *GJB1* causes X-linked Charcot-Marie-Tooth disease. Reduced penetrance was noted in one female with the mutation from each family, although one apparently unaffected mutation carrier was in her early 40's, around the age that hearing loss was first detected by most family members (14). These mutations affected the second extracellular domain of the protein. In contrast, missense mutations that were located more 5′, in the amino terminal and the transmembrane domains, were also found in some families with erythrokeratodermia variabilis (9).

Heredity. In families with *KCNQ4* mutations and in the two families with unknown mutations, inheritance was autosomal dominant with complete penetrance. Penetrance may be incomplete in *GJB3* families.

Prognosis. In individuals with *KCNQ4* mutations, high-frequency hearing loss starts in the first decade and progresses to moderate loss in the low and mid frequencies and profound loss in the high frequencies in the fifth decade. In individuals with *GJB3* mutations, high-frequency hearing loss is noticeable in the fifth decade, progressing to moderate to severe sloping hearing loss.

In families showing linkage of hearing loss to DFNA2 but no mutations in *KCNQ4* or *GJB3*, hearing loss began in the second decade and progressed to moderate to severe hearing loss in the fifth decade.

Summary. There are at least three genes in the DFNA2 region that cause high-frequency progressive sensorineural nonsyndromic hearing loss, with mutations of *KCNQ4* being the most common. The phenotypes produced by these genes differ in age of onset and severity, and vestibular function has been normal.

References

1. Beisel KW et al: Longitudinal gradients of *KCNQ4* expression in spiral ganglion and cochlear hair cells correlate with progressive hearing loss in DFNA2. *Brain Res Mol Brain Res* 82:137–149, 2000.

Table 5–3. Summary of nonsyndromic loci

Locus	Location	Gene	Onset	Frequencies	Final Severity	Progression	Vestibular Involvement	Inner Ear Abnormalities
DFNA1	5q31	DIAPH1	5–30 years	Low, then all	Profound	Yes	1 child with unilateral dysfunction	No
DFNA2	1p34	KCNQ4, GJB3, plus 1 unknown	KCNQ4: 1st–2nd decade; GJB3: 40 years; Unknown: 2nd decade	High, then all	KCNQ4: profound; GJB3: moderate	Yes	KCNQ4: some with asymmptomatic hyperreflexia; GJB3 ?	No
DFNA3	13q12	GJB2, GJB6	Congenital in nonprogressive types; 10–20 years in progressive types	All frequencies in nonprogressive forms; high, then mid and low	Moderate to profound	Yes, in some	?	?
DFNA4	19q13.3–q13.4	Unknown	<10–20 years	All	Moderate to profound	Yes, fluctuating	?	?
DFNA5	7p15	DFNA5	5–15 years	High, then all	Severe	Yes	No	?
DFNA6/14/38	4p16.3	WFS1	Congenital or early childhood	Low, then high	Moderate to severe	Yes	Asymptomatic hyperreflexia	No
DFNA7	1q21–23	Unknown	>5 years	High	Moderate	Yes, with initial asymmetry	No	?
DFNA8/12	11q22–24	TECTA	Prelingual in some families; 9 or 19 years in later-onset families	Primarily mid frequencies in prelingual, nonprogressive families; high to all in progressive families	Moderate to severe in prelingual, nonprogressive families; mild to profound in progressive families	Yes in some	Symptoms in some progressive families	No
DFNA9	14q12–13	COCH	20 or 36–62 years	High, then all	Profound	Yes; fluctuation and asymmetry in some	Yes, with possible Ménière symptoms	Degeneration of cochlear structures with acidophilic deposits
DFNA10	6q22–q23	EYA4	<10–40 years	Mid, then all	Moderate to severe	Yes	Yes in 2 of 42 individuals	?
DFNA11	11q13.5	MYO7A	<10–20 years	High, then all	Moderate	Yes	No symptoms; 2 with decreased responses on calorics	Disorganization of stereocilia in mouse model shaker-1
DFNA13	6p21.3	COL11A2 plus unknown	Prelingual or 10–30 years	Mid, then all	COL11A2, moderate to severe	Yes in some	Yes, asymptomatic areflexia in some	Histological abnormalities of tectorial membrane in mouse knockout
DFNA15	5q31.q33	POU4F3	20–40 years	High or all	Unknown: profound; Severe	Yes	No symptoms	?
DFNA16	2q23–q24.3	Unknown	1st decade	High	Profound	Yes; sudden onset, frequent fluctuation	Some with vertigo	No
DFNA17	22q12.2–q13.3	MYH9	10 years	High to all	Severe to profound	Yes	No symptoms	Cochleosaccular dysplasia
DFNA18	3q22	Unknown	<10 years	High to all	Severe	Yes	No	?
DFNA19	10 pericentric	Unknown	Congenital	All	Mild to moderate	No	?	?
DFNA20	17q25	Unknown	10–30 years	High to all	Severe to profound	Yes	No	?
DFNA21	6p21.3	Unknown	Prelingual to 45 years	Mid to all	Moderate to severe	Yes	No	?
DFNA22	6q13	MYO6A	6–8 years	High to all	Profound	Yes	No	Fusion of stereocilia in snell's waltzer mouse
DFNA23	14q21–q22	Unknown	Prelingual	All; sloping	Moderate to profound	No	?	?
DFNA24	4q	Unknown	Prelingual	All; sloping	Severe to profound	No	?	?
DFNA25	12q21–24	Unknown	20–50 years	High	?	Yes	?	?

Table 5–3. Summary of nonsyndromic loci (*continued*)

Locus	Location	Gene	Onset	Frequencies	Final Severity	Progression	Vestibular Involvement	Inner Ear Abnormalities
DFNA26	17q25 (overlaps with DFNA20)	Unknown	?	?	?	Yes	?	?
DFNA27	4q12	Unknown	10–30 years	?	Profound	Yes	?	?
DFNA28	8q22	TFCP2L3	7 years	High or mid	Moderate to severe	Yes	?	?
DFNA29	Reserved							
DFNA30	15q25–26	Unknown	10–40 years	High to mid and high	?	Yes	?	?
DFNA31	Withdrawn							
DFNA32	11p15	Unknown	?	?	?	Yes	?	?
DFNA33	Reserved							
DFNA34	1q44	Unknown	20–40 years	?	?	Yes	?	?
DFNA35	Reserved							
DFNA36	9q13–21	TMC1	5–10 years	High to all	Profound	Yes	No	Normal morphology in *Beethoven* mouse model, with progressive loss of hair cells.
DFNA37	1p21	Unknown	5 years	Low and high	Moderate	Yes	No	No
DFNA38	See DFNA6/14/38							
DFNA39	4q2	DSPP	20–30 years	High	Severe to profound	Yes	Symptoms in 1	?
DFNA40	Reserved							
DFNA41	12q24–qter	Unknown	20–30 years	All	Severe to profound	Yes	No	?
DFNB1	13q12	GJB2	Congenital	All	Moderate to profound	Yes in some	No symptoms	No
DFNB2	11q13.5	MYO7A	Congenital to 16 years	All	Severe to profound	Yes in some	Yes	No
DFNB3	17p11.2	MYO15	Congenital	All	Severe to profound	No	No symptoms	Shortened stereocilia, disorganized actin cores in *shaker-2* mouse
DFNB4	7q31	SLC26A4 (PDS)	Congenital	Variable	Variable	Very likely	Yes in some	EVA or Mondini malformations
DFNB5	14q12	Unknown	Congenital	All	Severe to profound	No	?	?
DFNB6	3p14–p21	TMIE	Congenital	All	Severe to profound	No	Delayed walking reported in 1 family	Abnormal maturation of stereocilia in *spinner* mouse
DFNB7/11	9q13–q21	TMC1	Congenital	All	Profound	No	?	Postnatal degeneration of inner and outer hair cells in *deafness* mouse
DFNB8/10	21q22	TMPRSS3	Congenital or 10–12 years	All	Severe or profound, depending on type of mutation	Yes, with some mutations	No symptoms	?
DFNB9	2p22–p23	OTOF	Congenital	All	Severe to profound	No	No symptoms	?
DFNB12	10q21.q22	CDH23	Congenital	Variable	Moderate to profound	May be progressive in some families	No symptoms	Delayed maturation and disorganization of stereocilia in *waltzer* mouse
DFNB13	7q34–q36	Unknown	Childhood	?	Profound	Yes	?	?
DFNB14	7q31	Unknown	Prelingual	All	Profound	No	?	?
DFNB15	3q21–q25 or 19p13	Unknown	Prelingual	All	Profound	No	?	?

DFNB16	15q15–q22	STRC plus unknown	Childhood	Sloping	Severe to profound	No	?	?
DFNB17	7q31	Unknown	Prelingual	All	Profound	No	?	?
DFNB18	11p15.1	USH1C	Prelingual	All	Severe to profound	No	Probably no	?
DFNB19	18p11	Unknown	Congenital	All	Profound	No	?	?
DFNB20	11q25–qter	Unknown	Prelingual	All	Moderate or profound	No	?	?
DFNB21	11q22–q24	TECTA	Prelingual	All	Severe to profound	No	?	?
DFNB22	16p12.2	OTOA	?	?	Moderate to severe	No	?	?
DFNB23	10p11.2–q21	Unknown	?	?		?	?	?
DFNB24	11q23	Unknown	?	?		?	?	?
DFNB25	4p15.3–q12	Unknown				?	?	?
DFNB26	4q31	Unknown	Congenital	All	Severe to profound	No	?	?
DFNB27	2q23–q31	Unknown	Prelingual	?	Severe to profound	No	?	?
DFNB28	22q13	Unknown	Prelingual	All	Severe to profound	No	?	?
DFNB29	21q22	CLDN14	Congenital	All	Profound	No	No symptoms	?
DFNB30	10p11.1	MYO3A	10–20 years	All, sloping	Moderate low; severe mid and high	Yes	No symptoms	?
DFNB31	9q32–q34	Unknown	Prelingual	All	Profound	No	?	?
DFNB32	1p13.3–p22.1	Unknown	?	?	?	?	?	?
DFNB33	9q34.3	Unknown		All	Severe	No	?	?
DFN1	Xq22	TIMM8A; syndromic	Early childhood					
DFN2	Xq22	Unknown	Congenital	Males: all; Females: high	Males: profound; Females: mild to moderate	No	?	No
DFN3	Xq21.1	POU3F4	Congenital in males	Males: all; Females: high	Males: moderate to profound; Females: mild to moderate	Yes	Enlarged internal auditory meatus, thinning of temporal bones, Mondini dysplasia	
DFN4	Xp21.2	Unknown	Congenital in males	Males: all; Females: high	Males: profound; Females: mild to moderate	Yes in females	No	No
DFN5	Withdrawn							
DFN6	Xp22	Unknown	Males: 5–7 years; Females, 30–40 years	Males: high to all; Females: high	Males: profound; Females: moderate	Yes	No	?
DFN7	Withdrawn							
DFN8	Reserved							

2. Bom SJH et al: Speech recognition scores related to age and degree of hearing impairment in DFNA2/KCNQ4 and DFNA9/COCH. *Arch Otolaryngol Head Neck Surg* 127:1045–1048, 2001.
3. Coucke P et al: Linkage of autosomal dominant hearing loss to the short arm of chromosome 1 in two families. *N Engl J Med*, 331:425–431, 1994.
4. Coucke PJ et al: Mutations in the *KCNQ4* gene are responsible for autosomal dominant deafness in four DFNA2 families. *Hum Mol Genet* 8:1321–1328, 1999.
5. Goldstein JA, Lalwani AK: Further evidence for a third deafness gene within the DFNA2 locus. *Am J Med Genet* 108:304–309, 2002.
6. Kharkovets T et al: *KCNQ4*, a K⁺ channel mutated in a form of dominant deafness, is expressed in the inner ear and the central auditory pathway. *Proc Natl Acad Sci USA* 97:4333–4338, 2000.
7. Kubisch C et al: *KCNQ4*, a novel potassium channel expressed in sensory outer hair cells, is mutated in dominant deafness. *Cell* 96:437–446, 1999.
8. Marres H et al: Inherited nonsyndromic hearing loss. An audiovestibular study in a large family with autosomal dominant progressive hearing loss related to DFNA2. *Arch Otolaryngol Head Neck Surg* 123:573–577, 1997.
9. Richard G et al: The spectrum of mutations in erythrokeratodermias—novel and de novo mutations in *GJB3*. *Hum Genet* 106:321–329, 2000.
10. Stern RE, Lalwan AK: Audiologic evidence for further genetic heterogeneity at DFNA2. *Acta Otolaryngol* 122:730–735, 2002.
11. Talebizadeh Z et al: A novel mutation in the *KCNQ4* gene in a large kindred with dominant progressive hearing loss. *Hum Mutat* 14:493–501, 1999.
12. Van Camp G et al: A mutational hot spot in the *KCNQ4* gene responsible for autosomal dominant hearing impairment. *Hum Mutat* 20:15–19, 2002.
13. Van Hauwe P et al: Mutations in the *KCNQ4* K⁺ channel gene, responsible for autosomal dominant hearing loss, cluster in the channel pore region. *Am J Med Genet* 93:184–187, 2000.
14. Xia JH et al: Mutations in the gene encoding gap junction protein beta-3 associated with autosomal dominant hearing impairment. *Nat Genet* 20:370–373, 1998.

DFNA3

- MIM: 601544 (DFNA3), 121011 (GJB2), 604418 (GJB6)
- Location, gene: 13q12; *GJB2* (connexin 26) or *GJB6* (connexin 30)

Mutation of *GJB2* (connexin 26) is the most common cause of recessive nonsyndromic hearing impairment (DFNB1), and will be covered in the section on recessive hearing loss below. One family has been described with a dominant mutation of *GJB2* causing dominant progressive nonsyndromic hearing loss (5). Other mutations of *GJB2* have been reported to cause dominant congenital nonprogressive hearing loss, which will be reviewed in that section. Finally, dominant progressive hearing loss and keratoderma (a form of Vohwinkel syndrome) (4) can also be caused by *GJB2* mutations. Mutation of the closely linked GBJ6 gene has been reported as the cause of dominant and sometimes progressive hearing loss in one small Italian family (2). Deletions of *GJB6* can also cause recessive hearing loss in individuals who are homozygous for the deletion or who are compound heterozygotes for the deletion and a mutation in *GJB2* (1) (see DFNB1, below).

Auditory findings. The large dominant family with progressive hearing impairment and a *GJB2* mutation had onset of high-frequency loss in late childhood, between the ages of 10 and 20, with progression to include the mid frequencies by age 50 (5). There was considerable variation among family members in the rate of progression of the hearing loss, however, and severity ranged from moderate to profound.

In the Italian family with the *GJB6* mutation, the three affected individuals (parent and two offspring) also showed a wide phenotypic range. Two family members (parent and one child) had mid- and high-frequency hearing loss with evidence of progression in one of them, and the other had a severe to profound hearing loss.

Vestibular findings. No vestibular testing was reported.

Radiology/histology. No studies have been reported.

Molecular studies. Connexin molecules form hexameric transmembrane structures, *connexons*, that combine with corresponding con-

nexons in adjacent cells to form gap junctions for the passage of ions (see DFNB1, below, for more complete discussion of connexin structure and function). In the family with a *GJB2* mutation, all affected members were heterozygous for a 605G → T mutation, resulting in a C202F substitution. This affects the fourth transmembrane domain of the protein and may interfere with the formation of the connexons. In the Italian family with the *GJB6* mutation, a T5M mutation removed a hydrophilic residue and increased the probability of the formation of a helix in that region. A resulting dominant-negative interference with function was suggested by functional studies in *Xenopus* oocytes (5).

Dominant progressive hearing loss due to a mutation in *GJB2*, 176G → C (Q59A), has also been observed in association with palmoplantar keratoderma (3).

Heredity. Inheritance was autosomal dominant with complete penetrance in both families.

Prognosis. For the *GJB2* 605G → T mutation, hearing loss onset was in late childhood and was progressive, but there was considerable variability within the family. Similarly, given the wide variability of hearing loss in the three reported individuals with the *GJB6* mutation, it is not possible to reliably predict the degree of hearing loss in a mutation carrier.

Summary. In the DFNA3 region, mutations in both *GJB6* and *GJB2* can cause dominant nonsyndromic hearing loss. Mutations in both genes can also cause dominant hearing loss with keratoderma and/or ichthyosis.

References
1. del Castillo I et al: A deletion involving the connexin 30 gene in nonsyndromic hearing impairment. *N Engl J Med* 346:243–249, 2002.
2. Grifa A et al: Mutations in *GJB6* cause nonsyndromic autosomal dominant deafness at DFNA3 locus. *Nat Genet* 23:16–18, 1999.
3. Heathcote K et al: A connexin 26 mutation causes a syndrome of sensorineural hearing loss and palmoplantar hyperkeratosis (MIM 148350). *J Med Genet* 37:50–51, 2000.
4. Maestrini E et al: A missense mutation in connexin26, *D66H*, causes mutilating keratoderma with sensorineural deafness (Vohwinkel's syndrome) in three unrelated families. *Hum Mol Genet* 8:1237–1243, 1999.
5. Morle L et al: A novel C202F mutation in the connexin26 gene (*GJB2*) associated with autosomal dominant isolated hearing loss. *J Med Genet* 37:368–370, 2000.

DFNA4

- MIM: 600652
- Location, gene: 19q13.3–q13.4; gene unknown

At least three European and American families have shown linkage to the 19q region (1,3,4). At this time, the causal gene has not been identified.

Auditory findings. Onset of hearing loss has been reported to be in the first to second decade with fluctuation and progression to the moderate to profound range across all frequencies by age 40. The audiograms are only gently sloping, since all frequencies are involved to some extent.

Vestibular findings. No evaluations have been reported.

Radiology/histology. No studies have been reported.

Molecular studies. A maximum LOD score of 4.05 was found at marker D19S246 with $\theta = 0.00$. The critical region spanned 14 cM, flanked by D19S412 and D19S571. Mutation analysis has excluded the mitochondrial seryl-tRNA synthetase (*SARSM*), mitoribosomal protein S12 (*RPMS12*), and *BAX* genes (3,4). The myotonic dystrophy protein kinase gene (*DMPK*) has also been suggested as a candidate (2).

Heredity. Inheritance is autosomal dominant with complete penetrance.

Prognosis. Onset of hearing loss is in the first to second decade, progressing to moderate to profound hearing loss in the fourth to fifth decade.

Summary. This form of hearing loss involves all frequencies, with somewhat greater loss in the high frequencies. Unlike most other forms of dominant progressive hearing loss, fluctuation has been observed. The gene or genes in this region have not been identified.

References

1. Chen AH et al: Linkage of a gene for dominant non-syndromic deafness to chromosome 19. *Hum Mol Genet* 4:1073–1076, 1995.
2. McGuirt WT et al: Characterization of autosomal dominant non-syndromic hearing loss loci. *Adv Otorhinolaryngol* 56:84–96, 2000.
3. Mirghomizadeh F et al: Second family with hearing impairment linked to 19q13 and refined DFNA4 localisation. *Eur J Hum Genet* 10:95–99, 2002.
4. Shah ZH et al: Novel coding-region polymorphisms in mitochondrial seryl-tRNA synthetase (*SARSM*) and mitoribosomal protein S12 (RPMS12) genes in DFNA4 autosomal dominant deafness families. *Hum Mutat* 17:433–434, 2001.

DFNA5

- MIM: 600994 (DFNA5)
- Location, gene: 7p15; DFNA5 (aka *ICERE-1*). Since the protein function is unknown, it is also called DFNA5.

This localization was found in one large Dutch family, which is one of the first dominant progressive hearing loss families reported (1 [MIM 124800], 3). A deletion was found in a gene of unknown function, designated DFNA5 (4).

Auditory findings. Onset of high-frequency hearing loss was between ages 5 and 15. This progressed to a severe hearing loss involving the remaining frequencies by 40–50 years of age (Fig. 5–1).

Vestibular findings. Vestibular function was normal, and there were no reports of tinnitus.

Radiology/histology. No studies were reported.

Molecular studies. A maximum LOD score of 10.07 was found for marker D7S516 at $\theta = 0.00$, although there were four other markers in that region that also had LOD scores over 3 with no recombination (3). Addition of more family members narrowed the critical region to 600–850 kb between D7S3076 and D7S1821. In searching this region for candidate genes, van Laer et al. (4) identified a novel gene that was expressed in the cochlea. An intronic insertion/deletion was found in affected members that produced skipping of the eighth exon and premature termination. Sequence homology studies identified this gene as the same as the previously reported "inversely correlated with estrogen receptor expression" (*ICERE-1*) gene, which had been found by differential display analysis comparing expression of estrogen receptor positive vs. negative breast carcinoma cells. However, since the relationship of this gene with breast cancer had not been established, it was thought that the relationship with the estrogen receptor could be a secondary effect, and the gene was renamed DFNA5. Subsequent transfection studies by Lage et al. (2) showed that decreased *DFNA5* expression was associated with increased resistance to the antineoplastic drug etoposide in melanoma cells, and they hypothesized that the gene was directly or indirectly involved in apoptosis pathways. The relationship between these possible functions and hearing loss is not known.

Heredity. Inheritance is autosomal dominant with complete penetrance.

Prognosis. Progressive high-frequency hearing loss starts before age 15 and leads to a severe loss involving all frequencies by the fifth to sixth decades.

Summary. DFNA5 has been identified in one very large Dutch pedigree showing dominant progressive sensorineural hearing loss beginning in the high frequencies. The DFNA5 gene has been identified and is the same as *ICERE-1*, but the function in the cochlea is unknown.

References

1. Huizing EH et al: Studies on progressive hereditary perceptive deafness in a family of 335 members. I. Genetical and general audiological results. *Acta Otolaryngol* 61:35–41, 1966.
2. Lage H et al: DFNA5 (*ICERE-1*) contributes to acquired etoposide resistance in melanoma cells. *FEBS Lett* 494:54–59, 2001.
3. Van Camp G et al: Localization of a gene for non-syndromic hearing loss (DFNA5) to chromosome 7p15. *Hum Mol Genet* 4:2159–2163, 1995.
4. Van Laer L et al: Nonsyndromic hearing impairment is associated with a mutation in DFNA5. *Nat Genet* 20:194–197, 1998.

DFNA7

- MIM: 601412
- Location, gene: 1q21–23; gene unknown
  This locus was discovered in one Norwegian family (1,3).

Auditory findings. Individuals in the Norwegian DFNA7 family showed variable onset of hearing loss, but none showed onset before age 4–5. Periods of rapid progression were noted in childhood, and the hearing loss was sometimes greater in one ear during those times, with later progression of the other ear so that ultimately the hearing loss was symmetrical and in the moderate range. The audiograms showed sloping high-frequency hearing loss, with preservation of the low and mid frequencies, and speech was unaffected in most individuals. Tinnitus was not present.

Vestibular findings. Caloric testing was normal in five affected family members.

Radiology/histology. No studies were reported.

Molecular studies. Linkage analysis defined a 22 cM region between D1S104 and D1S466, with a maximum LOD score of 7.65 for marker D1S196 at $\theta = 0.00$. Preliminary mutation analysis of the myelin protein zero gene (P_o) by SSCP did not show any mutations. *GJA8* (connexin 50) is also located at 1q21.1, but was apparently excluded by linkage analysis. The gene *DFNM1*, which modifies the expression of the recessive DFNB26, was also within the critical region, and the gene *PMX1* (paired mesoderm homeobox 1) has been suggested as a candidate for that gene and possibly DFNA7 as well (2).

Heredity. Inheritance is autosomal dominant with complete penetrance.

Prognosis. Hearing loss is completely penetrant, but the age of onset, rate of progression, and degree of hearing loss cannot be predicted reliably, and close audiological monitoring is necessary. The hearing loss remains confined to the high frequencies until old age, however, and generally does not interfere with oral communication.

Summary. This form of high-frequency progressive hearing loss is distinguished by periods of rapid progression of the hearing loss and by the sparing of low and mid frequencies. It may be allelic to *DFNM1*, which has been shown to modify hearing loss caused by the DFNB26 locus.

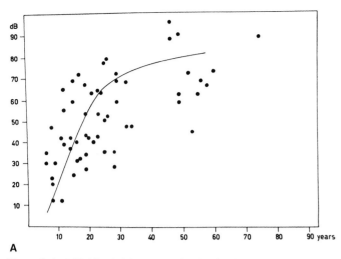

A

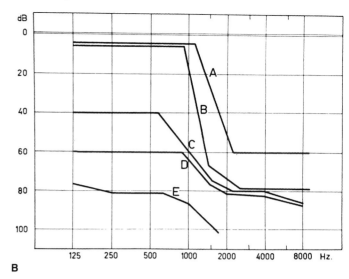

B

Figure 5–1. *DFNA5*. (A) Mean perceptive hearing loss as a function of age. Note rapid increase of impairment in first three decades. (B) Characteristic audiometric stages of progression of impairment from childhood (curve A) to greater than 45 years (curve E). [From EH Huizing et al., *Acta Otolaryngol* 61:35, 1966.]

References

1. Fagerheim T et al: Identification of a new locus for autosomal dominant non-syndromic hearing impairment (DFNA7) in a large Norwegian family. *Hum Mol Genet* 5:1187–1191, 1996.
2. Riazuddin S et al: Dominant modifier *DFNM1* suppresses recessive deafness DFNB26. *Nat Genet* 26:431–434, 2000.
3. Tranebjaerg L et al: DFNA7. *Adv Otorhinolaryngol* 56:97–100, 2000.

DFNA8/12

- MIM: 601543 (DFNA8), 601842 (DFNA12), 602574 (TECTA)
- Location, gene: 11q22–24; *TECTA* (α-tectorin)

Several families have been reported with dominant hearing loss due to *TECTA* mutations, and the degree of hearing loss has differed. Two families had congenital, nonprogressive hearing loss (3 [initially described as DFNA8],6) and will be described in that section below, while two other families have been found to have progressive hearing loss (1,2). An autosomal recessive phenotype has also been reported, DFNB21 (5).

Auditory findings. Alloisio et al. (1) described a French family in which bilateral sensorineural hearing loss had a prelingual onset and was slowly progressive, resulting in a mild to moderate high-frequency loss. A Swedish family reported by Balciuniene et al. (2) showed two phenotypes: either a hearing loss with onset around age 9, progressing to a profound high-frequency loss, or an onset around 19 years, resulting in a mild high-frequency loss.

Vestibular findings. Vestibular dysfunction was indicated in several affected individuals in the French family who did not walk until age 2, but further testing was not reported (1).

Radiology/histology. No studies have been reported.

Molecular studies. Alpha-tectorin is a major component of the non-collagenous matrix of the tectorial membrane, which is an extracellular matrix that overlies the stereocilia of the outer hair cells in the organ of Corti. The hair cells themselves are part of the basilar membrane, and movement of the basilar membrane in response to sound creates a shearing effect on the stereocilia, resulting in mechanosensory transduction of the sound through the hair cells to the auditory nerve. The *TECTA* gene has three domains with similarities to different proteins: an entactin G1 basement membrane–type domain, a zonadhesin domain with von Willebrand factor type D repeats, and a zona pellucida domain (4). These form polypeptides that crosslink to each other via disulfide bonds and combine with β-tectorin (7).

The mouse *tecta* gene was mapped to a region homologous to the critical region on chromosome 11 for DFNA8/12, and mutation analysis was performed in the original Belgian and Austrian families that defined the locus (7). Both of those families had prelingual hearing loss, and will be reviewed in the section on dominant nonprogressive hearing loss. In the French family with progressive hearing loss, a 4857G $\rightarrow$ C mutation was found, creating a missense C1619S change in the protein (1). In the Swedish family, a 3170C $\rightarrow$ T mutation was found in all family members with more severe, earlier-onset hearing loss, but also in several (but not all) individuals with the milder type of hearing loss. This created a missense C1057S alteration. Both of these mutations occurred in the zonadhesin domain of the protein; in contrast, mutations associated with dominant congenital hearing loss (reviewed below) occurred in the zona pellucida domain.

The phenotypic variation in the Swedish family was attributed to either variable expression of the mutation, with hearing loss caused by other factors in the affected individuals who did not carry the mutation, or to the digenic effect of a gene in the DFNA2 region. All individuals with the severe phenotype also carried the same haplotypes for the DFNA2 region, while those with the milder phenotype carried either the *TECTA* mutation or the DFNA2-shared haplotypes. No mutations were found in either *KCNQ4* or *GJB3*, so identification of a third gene in the DFNA2 region will be needed to determine if this is truly an example of digenic segregation in the family (2).

DFNB21 is also caused by mutation in *TECTA*, in this case a splice site mutation, causing truncation of the protein (4). Since this would produce haploinsufficiency for the product, the authors hypothesized that dominant hearing loss resulted from dominant-negative mechanisms, implying that a-tectorin must form homo- or heteromeric structures.

Heredity. Inheritance was autosomal dominant with variation in severity in one of the two families.

Prognosis. The prognosis is for progressive high-frequency hearing loss, although severity cannot be predicted.

Summary. It appears that mutations in different parts of the *TECTA* gene are associated with different hearing loss phenotypes, with mutations in the zonadhesin domain uniquely associated with progressive hearing loss. There may also be interaction with the unidentified DFNA2 gene, causing a more severe, earlier-onset hearing loss.

References

1. Alloisio N et al: Mutation in the zonadhesin-like domain of alpha-tectorin associated with autosomal dominant non-syndromic hearing loss. *Eur J Hum Genet* 7:255–258, 1999.
2. Balciuniene J et al: Alpha-tectorin involvement in hearing disabilities: one gene—two phenotypes. *Hum Genet* 105:211–216, 1999.
3. Kirschhofer K et al: Autosomal-dominant, prelingual, nonprogressive sensorineural hearing loss: localization of the gene (DFNA8) to chromosome 11q by linkage in an Austrian family. *Cytogenet Cell Genet* 82:126–130, 1998.
4. Legan PK et al: The mouse tectorins. Modular matrix proteins of the inner ear homologous to components of the sperm–egg adhesion system. *J Biol Chem* 272:8791–9801, 1997.
5. Mustapha M et al: An alpha-tectorin gene defect causes a newly identified autosomal recessive form of sensorineural pre-lingual non-syndromic deafness, DFNB21. *Hum Mol Genet* 8:409–412, 1999.
6. Verhoeven K et al: A gene for autosomal dominant nonsyndromic hearing loss (DFNA12) maps to chromosome 11q22–24. *Am J Hum Genet* 60:1168–1173, 1997.
7. Verhoeven K et al: Mutations in the human α-tectorin gene cause autosomal dominant non-syndromic hearing impairment. *Nat Genet* 19:60–62, 1998.

DFNA9

- MIM: 601369 (DFNA9), 603196 (COCH)
- Location, gene: 14q12–q13; *COCH* (cochlin)

Hearing loss due to mutation of the *COCH* (coagulation factor C homology) gene has been reported in multiple families in the United States, Europe, and Australia.

Auditory findings. The age of onset and rate of progression differ according to the *COCH* mutation in a family. In the American and Australian families, high-frequency hearing loss was noted around 20 years of age, with progression to anacousis in all frequencies in the 40's (4,7,9). Families from Belgium and Holland had a later age of onset, around age 36–62, with rapid progression to profound hearing loss. Fluctuation and asymmetry of the hearing loss were both noted in some affected individuals in these families, several of whom shared the same mutation (2,11). Word recognition abilities also declined with age, more than would be expected for the degree of hearing loss (1), but it was not clear if this represented an additional central component. Cochlear

implantation has been successful in individuals with profound hearing loss (7).

Vestibular findings. Vestibular symptoms have been noted at the same time as the onset of hearing loss. Instability and movement-dependent oscillopsia were noted along with the onset of hearing loss in all individuals in a family with the P51S mutation (2); and serious progressive vestibular deficits, including complete areflexia, were also seen in some affected individuals in that family and in families with other mutations as well. Symptoms included positional vertigo, instability in the dark, feelings of light-headedness or a "drunken" feeling, and characteristics of Ménière disease (hearing loss, aural fullness, tinnitus, and vertigo), although hearing loss did not worsen noticeably during attacks, and was in the high frequencies rather than in the low-frequencies usually associated with Ménière disease (3,12). In one large Belgian family with the common P51S mutation, 9 of 60 affected individuals could be diagnosed as having Ménière disease. Age of onset was after 35 in all of them (12).

Radiology/histology. Histologic studies were quite distinctive, and had been observed in early studies of temporal bone pathology (Fig. 5–2). Acidophilic mucopolysaccharide deposits were identified in various regions and supporting structures of the cochlear and vestibular systems, accompanied by loss of cellularity and degeneration. This included deposits in the proximal basilar membrane of the cochlea with variable loss of inner and outer hair cells, as well as patchy areas of atrophy in the stria vascularis, loss of cell bodies and peripheral processes of spiral ganglion cells and of Scarpa's ganglion, deposits and degeneration of cells in the spiral ligament and spiral limbus, loss of hair cells of the vestibular system with degeneration of the stroma of the maculae and cristae and of the otolithic membrane, and loss of dendritic processes of the cochlear and vestibular nerves. (5,7–9). Endolymphatic hydrops has also been observed in some cases, characteristic of Ménière disease (5,8).

Molecular studies. The *COCH* gene was initially identified by Robertson et al. (9) in a fetal cochlear library and mapped to 14q11.2–q13, which made it a candidate for the DFNA9 locus that had already been identified by Manolis et al. (7). Mutations were confirmed in several families and tended to cluster around a group of cysteines in the amino terminus, including V66G, G88E, W117R, and I109N (4,9). A P51S mutation was found to be common to several Dutch and Belgian families, and haplotype analysis indicated a founder effect (2). The

Figure 5–2. *DFNA9.* (A) Midmodiolar section shows acidophilic deposit in spiral ligament, spiral limbus, and spiral lamina of all three turns of the cochlea. Degeneration of dendrites is severe. (B) Membranous and osseous spiral lamina, spiral limbus, and spiral ligament are saturated with homogeneous acidophilic deposit. Loss of spiral limbus and spiral limbus cellularity is severe. [From U Khetarpal et al., *Arch Otolaryngol Head Neck Surg* 117:1032, 1991.]

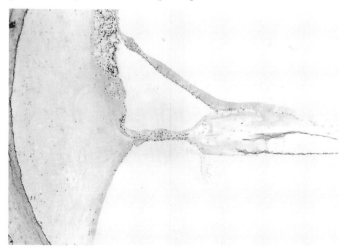

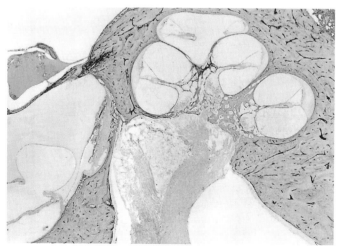

A

B

sequence of the *COCH* gene contains an LCCL domain, with homology the lipopolysaccharide-binding coagulation factor of Limulus polymorphus, or Limulus factor C, and all of the known mutations have been found in this region. Factor C proteins are generally involved in clotting and are activated by lipopolysaccharide binding. There are also two von Willebrand factor type A domains, which are often found in secreted proteins and can bind fibrillar collagens, as well as being involved in complement system (9). The function of the protein product, cochlin, is unknown, but it is structurally similar to the VIT1 protein in the vitreous of the eye, and may serve to bind and stabilize collagen fibrils in extracellular matrix. Mutations of the gene are likely to interfere with folding or binding of the protein, which might affect collagen stability and also result in accumulation of bound polysaccharides. A role in immune function might also make individuals more susceptible to recurrent inner ear infections (6,9,10).

Heredity. Inheritance is fully penetrant autosomal dominant transmission of hearing loss, with variable penetrance of vestibular dysfunction. One homozygote for the P51S mutation has been identified, with earlier onset (age 24) and more severe hearing loss than that of heterozygous family members (11).

Prognosis. Hearing loss is progressive and may result in anacousis for all frequencies. Cochlear implantation may be considered. There is also risk of progressive vestibular dysfunction, including Ménière disease.

Summary. This type of hearing loss is distinctive in two major respects: it is one of the few nonsyndromic hearing loss disorders to include vestibular dysfunction, including Ménière disease, and acidophilic deposits are seen histologically.

References

1. Bom SJH et al: Speech recognition scores related to age and degree of hearing impairment in DFNA2/*KCNQ4* and DFNA9/*COCH*. *Arch Otolaryngol Head Neck Surg* 127:1045–1048, 2001.
2. de Kok YJ et al: A Pro51Ser mutation in the *COCH* gene is associated with late onset autosomal dominant progressive sensorineural hearing loss with vestibular defects. *Hum Mol Genet* 8:361–366, 1999.
3. Fransen E et al: High prevalence of symptoms of Ménière's disease in three families with a mutation in the *COCH* gene. *Hum Mol Genet* 8:1425–1429, 1999.
4. Kamarinos M et al: Identification of a novel *COCH* mutation, I109N, highlights the similar clinical features observed in DFNA9 families. *Hum Mutat* 17:351, 2001.
5. Khetarpal U: Autosomal dominant sensorineural hearing loss. Further temporal bone findings. *Arch Otolaryngol Head Neck Surg* 119:106–108, 1993.
6. Liepinsh E et al: NMR structure of the LCCL domain and implications for DFNA9 deafness disorder. *EMBO J* 20:5347–5353, 2001.
7. Manolis EN et al: A gene for non-syndromic autosomal dominant progressive postlingual sensorineural hearing loss maps to chromosome 14q12–13. *Hum Mol Genet* 5:1047–1050, 1996.
8. Merchant SN et al: Histopathology of the inner ear in DFNA9. *Adv Otorhinolaryngol* 56:212–217, 2000.
9. Robertson NG et al: Mutations in a novel cochlear gene cause DFNA9, a human nonsyndromic deafness with vestibular dysfunction. *Nat Genet* 20:299–303, 1998.
10. Robertson NG et al: Inner ear localization of mRNA and protein products of *COCH* mutated in the sensorineural deafness and vestibular disorder, DFNA9. *Hum Mol Genet* 10:2493–2500, 2001.
11. Verhagen WI et al: Familial progressive vestibulocochlear dysfunction caused by a *COCH* mutation (DFNA9). *Arch Neurol* 57:1045–1047, 2000.
12. Verstreken M et al: Hereditary otovestibular dysfunction and Ménière's disease in a large Belgian family is caused by a missense mutation in the *COCH* gene. *Otol Neurotol* 22:874–881, 2001.

DFNA11

- MIM: 601317 (DFNA11), 276903 (MYO7A)
- Location, gene: 11q13.5; *MYO7A* (myosin VIIA)

Mutation of *MYO7A* as a cause of dominant nonsyndromic hearing impairment has been described in one Japanese family (2,4). Other mutations in this gene also cause the nonsyndromic recessive hearing loss DFNB2 (see below), and Usher syndrome type IB, as well as the recessive *shaker-1* mutation in the mouse.

Auditory findings. In the one reported family, the hearing loss was sensorineural with onset of hearing loss in the first to second decade, with gradual progression to gently sloping or flat audiograms in the moderate range of hearing loss. Acoustic reflex thresholds and short increment sensitivity tests were consistent with cochlear involvement, and otoacoustic emissions were absent.

Vestibular findings. No vestibular symptoms were reported, but caloric testing on three of five tested individuals indicated vestibular dysfunction (6).

Radiology/histology. The CT scans showed normal middle and inner ear structures (5).

Molecular studies. Myosin VIIA is one of the class of unconventional (non-muscle) myosins. It has a head, neck, and tail region, with the head region of the molecule being highly conserved and moving along actin filaments through hydrolysis of ATP. The tail region contains a membrane-binding motif. In studies of the homologuous mouse gene, myosin VIIA localized to the crosslinks between hair cell stereocilia, and disorganization of the stereocilia bundles was seen in the mouse mutant *shaker-1*. Defective endocytosis was also seen in cochlear cells, as well as defective transport of organelles and melanosomes in the retinal epithelium, indicating a role in intracellular transport (1,3). Individuals with Usher syndrome IB have profound hearing impairment, vestibular areflexia, and retinitis pigmentosa, indicating the necessity of *MYO7A* in the hearing, balance, and visual systems.

Family members with progressive hearing loss were all found to be heterozygous for a 9 base-pair deletion in exon 22 that was in-frame, deleting an alanine and two lysines between positions 886 and 888. It was not found in 60 control samples (2). This is within the coiled-coil domain of the protein, and is the first report of a mutation in this region. Myosin VIIA, which is an unconventional myosin, forms head-to-tail dimers, and it is thought that the deletion would act in a dominant-negative manner to disrupt both homodimers and heterodimers containing the mutant protein. This would still leave some functional homodimers from the normal allele, and presumably this is what preserves vision and lessens the hearing and vestibular deficits in this family (5).

Heredity. Inheritance is autosomal dominant with complete penetrance.

Prognosis. Hearing loss is gradually progressive, affecting all frequencies, ultimately resulting in moderate hearing loss. There are no reports of visual symptoms. Electroretinograms of affected family members are normal, so vision should be unaffected. Although vestibular function may be abnormal, this is also asymptomatic.

Summary. One family has been reported with this mutation, and is the only reported example of a mutation of *MYO7A* causing dominant nonsyndromic hearing loss.

References

1. Liu X et al: Mutant myosin VIIa causes defective melanosome distribution in the RPE of *shaker-1* mice [letter]. *Nat Genet* 19:117–118, 1998.
2. Liu, X-Z et al: Autosomal dominant non-syndromic deafness caused by a mutation in the myosin VIIA gene. *Nat Genet* 17:268–269, 1997.
3. Self T et al: Shaker-1 mutations reveal roles for myosin VIIA in both development and function of cochlear hair cells. *Development* 125:557–566, 1998.
4. Tamagawa Y et al: A gene for a dominant form of non-syndromic sensorineural deafness (DFNA11) maps within the region containing the DFNB2 recessive deafness gene. *Hum Mol Genet* 5:849–852, 1996.
5. Tamagawa Y et al: Phenotype of DFNA11: a nonsyndromic hearing loss caused by a myosin VIIA mutation. *Laryngoscope* 112:292–297, 2002.
6. Tamagawa Y et al: Sensorineural hearing impairment, non-syndromic, dominant DFNA11. *Adv Otorhinolaryngol* 56:103–106, 2000.

DFNA15

- MIM: 602459 (DFNA15), 602460 (POU4F3)
- Location, gene: 5q31–q33; *POU4F3*, *BRN3C* (POU domain class 4, transcription factor 3)

Mutation in the transcription factor *POU4F3* has been identified in one large Israeli-Jewish family, Family H, which traced its origins back to Italy, but migrated through Libya, Tunisia, and Egypt, and now has branches in Belgium and the United States (3).

Auditory findings. Hearing loss in the family was variable. Onset of progressive sensorineural hearing loss was between age 20 and 40 with sloping, high-frequency audiological configuration or a flat loss, generally in the severe range. Otoacoustic emissions were abnormal and ABR findings indicated normal central pathways, indicating a cochlear hearing loss. Of 12 affected individuals, 1 reported tinnitus, and 2 individuals had additional conductive hearing loss. (1,2).

Vestibular findings. No vestibular symptoms were reported by the affected individuals.

Radiology/histology. No studies have been reported.

Molecular studies. *POU4F3* is a member of the POU domain family of transcription factors, which are involved in early development. *POU4F3* is specifically involved in cochlear development, as determined by detection in fetal cochlea cDNA. In contrast, no expression was found in other human tissues. Since the hearing loss is progressive, *POU4F3* may also be necessary for maintenance of hair cells (3). Another gene in the same family, *POU4F3* on the X chromosome, also produces hearing loss along with stapes dysfunction and perilymphatic gusher. Homologs of *POU4F3* are known in *C. elegans* and in the mouse, and targeted deletion of this gene in the mouse produces profound deafness and vestibular dysfunction. In Family H, an 8-nucleotide deletion (884del8) was found in the second exon of the gene, producing a frameshift that resulted in a stop codon and truncation of the protein at amino acid position 299 (3). This presumably acts in a dominant-negative fashion to interfere with DNA binding and gene regulation (1).

Heredity. Inheritance is autosomal dominant with complete penetrance by age 40.

Prognosis. Prediction of age of onset and degree of hearing loss is complicated by intrafamilial variation, but some degree of hearing loss is identifiable by age 40.

Summary. Hearing loss in this family had a relatively late onset and had either a flat or high-frequency configuration, with worst loss in the severe range. Frydman et al. (2) noted that the variability in the hearing loss and clinical similarity to other genetic types of nonsyndromic hearing loss made it impossible to diagnose DFNA15 on clinical grounds alone.

References

1. Avraham KB: DFNA15. *Adv Otorhinolaryngol* 56:107–115, 2000.
2. Frydman M et al: Clinical characterization of genetic hearing loss caused by a mutation in the *POU4F3* transcription factor. *Arch Otolaryngol Head Neck Surg* 126:633–637, 2000.
3. Vahava O et al: Mutation in transcription factor *POU4F3* associated with inherited progressive hearing loss in humans. *Science* 279(5358):1950–1954, 1998.

DFNA16

- MIM: 603964
- Location, gene: 2q23-q24.3; gene unknown

This localization was made in one four-generation Japanese family (1).

Auditory findings. This form of hearing loss appears to be unique in that it is characterized by sudden onset and fluctuations, with or without tinnitus. Onset of fluctuations appeared to be around age 10, although high-frequency hearing loss was occasionally present before then. In episodes of hearing loss, the high-frequency hearing loss became more pronounced, reaching as far as the profound range. Exacerbation appeared to be related to physical stress, illness, or pregnancy. Hearing loss improved with steroid treatment, which could indicate an autoimmune component, but testing for the 68 kDa antibody which has been described in cases of fluctuating hearing loss with Ménière-like symptoms was negative during episodes of hearing loss in individuals from this family. There was no other evidence of autoimmune disease in the family, so the apparent response to steroid treatment may have been coincidental (1).

Vestibular findings. Two family members reported episodes of vertigo, but not associated with drops in hearing.

Radiology/histology. The CT scans of the temporal bone in two individuals with documented fluctuations in hearing were normal with no evidence of dilated vestibular aqueduct, which is sometimes associated with fluctuating hearing loss.

Molecular studies. Linkage analysis produced a critical region spanning 3.5 cM between D2S354 and D2S124, with a multipoint LOD score of 4.08 at D2S345 at a θ of 0.00. Two voltage-gated sodium channel genes in the region, *SCN2A* and *SCN3A*, were screened in the family, but no mutations were found (2). The region overlaps with the critical region of DFNB27, which is a prelingual recessive hearing loss.

Heredity. Inheritance is autosomal dominant.

Prognosis. All affected family members reported fluctuating hearing loss after about age 10.

Summary. This is a unique form of high-frequency hearing loss characterized by sudden onset and dramatic fluctuations in hearing, without inner ear malformation, and no convincing evidence of autoimmune disease. The gene for DFNB27 is in the same region.

References

1. Fukushima K et al: A gene for fluctuating, progressive autosomal dominant nonsyndromic hearing loss, DFNA16, maps to chromosome 2q23–24.3. *Am J Hum Genet* 65:141–150, 1999.
2. Kasai N et al: Genomic structures of *SCN2A* and *SCN3A*—candidate genes for deafness at the DFNA16 locus. *Gene* 264:113–122, 2001.

DFNA17

- MIM: 603622 (DFNA17), 160775 (MYH9)
- Location, gene: 22q12.2-q13.3; *MYH9* (nonmuscle myosin heavy chain IIA)

Mutation in the *MYH9* gene has been described in one five-generation American family (2). Mutations of this gene also cause a collection of conditions that are now known to be part of a spectrum: May-Hegglin anomaly, Sebastian syndrome, Fechtner syndrome, Epstein syndrome, and Alport-like syndrome with macrothrombocytopenia. These conditions are characterized by giant platelets, thrombocytopenia, and leukocyte inclusions. Fechtner syndrome, Epstein syndrome, and Alport-like syndrome also include nephritis, cataracts, and sensorineural hearing loss (1).

Auditory findings. High-frequency hearing loss was first noted around age 10, with progression to moderate to severe hearing loss by the 20's. The proband, who was 61 when he died, had profound hearing loss (2).

Vestibular findings. No vestibular symptoms were described.

Radiology/histology. Histology of the temporal bones in the proband showed Scheibe-type cochleosaccular dysplasia, which includes degeneration of the organ of Corti, the saccular epithelium, and the stria vascularis. Gliosis was also noted in the inferior olivary nucleus. Immunohistology of rat cochlear preparations showed that *MHY9* was expressed in the outer hair cells, the subcentral region of the spiral ligament, and Reissner's membrane, but not in the stria vascularis nor in vestibular tissues. The lack of expression in the stria vascularis was especially notable, since dysfunction of the stria has been postulated to be a cause of cochleosaccular degeneration (2).

Molecular studies. Affected members from the family ascertained by Lalwani and colleagues (2) were found be heterozygous for a 2114G → A mutation in *MYH9*, resulting in an R705H missense alteration. This is within a highly conserved linker region between two helical domains in the myosin head, SH1 and SH2, which are critical to the conformational changes that must occur during force generation in the myosin motor domain. Although the function of *MYH9* in the cochlea is unknown, hypotheses include involvement in the cytoarchitecture of Reissner's membrane, leading to its degeneration and resulting disruption of cochlear ion homeostasis, and/or maintenance of tension in the basilar membrane. Interestingly, an adjacent R702H mutation, as well as an R702C mutation, have been described in the Fechtner, Epstein, and Alport-like conditions, and all cases of these mutations included hearing loss (1).

Heredity. Inheritance is autosomal dominant with complete penetrance.

Prognosis. High-frequency sensorineural hearing loss progresses to a flat hearing loss.

Summary. This form of progressive hearing loss is characterized by Sheibe cochleosaccular degeneration. Alternate mutations of the gene are involved with macrothrombocytopenia/deafness/nephritis syndromes.

References

1. Heath KE et al: Nonmuscle myosin heavy chain IIA mutations define a spectrum of autosomal dominant macrothrombocytopenias: May-Hegglin anomaly and Fechtner, Sebastian, Epstein, and Alport-like syndromes. *Am J Hum Genet* 69:1033–1045, 2001.
2. Lalwani AK et al: Human nonsyndromic hereditary deafness DFNA17 is due to a mutation in nonmuscle myosin *MYH9*. *Am J Hum Genet* 67:1121–1128, 2000.

DFNA18

- MIM: 606012
- Location, gene: 3q22; gene unknown

This localization was found in one large German family with dominant progressive hearing loss (1).

Auditory findings. Onset of hearing loss was noted in the first decade, with gradual inclusion of the mid and low frequencies, ultimately resulting in a flat hearing loss in the 80 dB range. No tinnitus was reported, and otoacoustic emissions were absent.

Vestibular findings. No vestibular symptoms were reported.

Radiology/histology. No studies were reported.

Molecular studies. A maximum LOD score of 3.77 was found with marker D3S1292, with a 10 cM critical region between D3S1589 and D3S1309. This region excluded DFNB15 and Usher syndrome type III, but it did include the myotonic dystrophy and proximal myotonic myopathy loci (*DM2/PROMM*) (1). DM2 has been since been found to be due to mutation in a zinc finger protein, *ZNF9*, but hearing loss has not been described in these families. Members of the DFNA18 family did not show any evidence of muscle disease on neurological examination.

Heredity. Inheritance is autosomal dominant with complete penetrance.

Prognosis. Sensorineural hearing loss progresses to the severe-to-profound range across all frequencies.

Summary. This is a fairly severe form of progressive hearing loss, ultimately including all frequencies. *ZNF9* may be a candidate gene.

References

1. Bonsch D et al: A novel locus for autosomal dominant, non-syndromic hearing impairment (DFNA18) maps to chromosome 3q22 immediately adjacent to the DM2 locus. *Eur J Hum Genet* 9:165–170, 2001.

DFNA20

- MIM: 604717
- Location, gene: 17q25; gene unknown

This gene was identified through a genome screen in a large three-generation U.S. family from Michigan (2,3). DeWan et al (1) described a second family.

Auditory findings. Onset of the hearing loss in the high frequencies was as early as early teens in some family members, and was present in all affected family members by their 20's. The hearing loss progressed in all frequencies but maintained a sloping configuration. Hearing loss eventually was severe to profound.

Vestibular findings. Findings were normal on neurological exam at age 65.

Radiology/histology. No studies were reported.

Molecular studies. Linkage analysis produced a maximum LOD score of 6.62 at $\theta = 0.0$ for the marker D17S784. A 12 cM critical region was defined by D17S1806 and D17S668. This overlaps with the region defined by DFNA26. Several candidate genes expressed in the inner ear were identified in the candidate region including *ACTG1* (actin, gamma 1), *ARHGDIA* (rho GDP dissociation inhibitor α) and *P4HB* (prolyl 4-hydroxylase). Mutation analysis of *P4HB* did not detect any mutations that segregated with the hearing loss in this family. Mustapha et al. (4) have placed the Usher type IG gene in this region as well. Dewan et al (1) narrowed the critical region to 6.05 cm, within the DFNA20 and DFNA26 interval.

Heredity. Inheritance is autosomal dominant.

Prognosis. Sensorineural hearing loss ultimately progresses to the severe to profound range.

Summary. In younger individuals, the hearing loss had a configuration similar to that of noise-induced loss, and at an older age it resembled presbycusis. The authors pointed out that identification of this gene could give clues to the etiology of either of these conditions. The critical region overlaps with DFNA26 and with USHIG, and DFNA20 may be allelic with either or both of these.

References

1. DeWan AT et al. A second kindred linked to DFNA20 (17q25.3) reduces the genetic interval. *Clin Genet* 63:39–45, 2003.
2. Elfelbein JL et al: Audiologic aspects of the search for DFNA20: a gene causing late-onset, progressive sensorineural hearing loss. *Ear Hear* 22:279–288, 2001.
3. Morell RJ et al: A new locus for late-onset, progressive, hereditary hearing loss DFNA20 maps to 17q25. *Genomics* 63:1–6, 2000.
4. Mustapha M et al: A novel locus for Usher syndrome type I, USH1G, maps to chromosome 17q24–25. *Hum Genet* 110:348–350, 2002.

DFNA22

- MIM: 606346 (DFNA22), 600970 (MYO6)
- Location, gene: 6q13; *MYO6* (myosin VI)

This localization was made by a full genome search in an Italian family. *MYO6* was a candidate because of the involvement of mouse *Myo6* in the *Snell's waltzer (sv)* mutation, which includes deafness and vestibular dysfunction (1).

Auditory findings. Onset of hearing loss could be detected between 6 and 8 years of age, and progressed to profound hearing impairment by the 50's. Configuration of the hearing loss was sloping, although all frequencies were ultimately involved.

Vestibular findings. Vestibular function was reported to be normal.

Radiology/histology. No studies were reported. Studies of the *Snell's waltzer* mouse showed normal stereocilia at birth, but subsequently progressive fusion was seen by day 1, starting at the base and resulting in giant stereocilia and degeneration of the hair cells by day 20 postnatally (2).

Molecular studies. Myosin VI is an unconventional myosin, with a motor domain that binds actin and hydrolyses ATP to facilitate movement. As in mice, *MYO6* is expressed at the base of the stereocilia of inner and outer hair cells in humans, and is probably involved in the changes in shape that occur in the hair cells during signal transduction. It is distinguishable from other myosins in that it appears to move in the opposite direction along actin filaments (3).

All affected family members were heterozygous for a missense 1325G $\rightarrow$ A mutation in exon 12 of *MYO6*, creating a C442Y substitution. This cysteine is in the motor domain and is conserved in many species, as well as in other myosins, and it was hypothesized that its replacement by the larger tyrosine would destablize the molecule.

Heredity. Inheritance is autosomal dominant.

Prognosis. Progressive sensorineural hearing loss leads to severe to profound hearing loss.

Summary. Although its involvement with the *Snell's waltzer* mouse model made *MYO6* a candidate for human hearing loss, this is the only family that has been reported to date with a mutation.

References

1. Melchionda S et al: *MYO6*, the human homologue of the gene responsible for deafness in *Snell's Waltzer* mice, is mutated in autosomal dominant nonsyndromic hearing loss. *Am J Hum Genet* 69:635–640, 2001.
2. Self T et al: Role of myosin VI in the differentiation of cochlear hair cells. *Dev Biol* 214:331–341, 1999.
3. Wells AL et al: Myosin VI is an actin-based motor that moves backwards. *Nature* 401:505–508, 1999.

DFNA25

- MIM: 605583
- Location, gene: 12q21–24; gene unknown

This locus was identified through a genome scan in a large U.S. family of Czech descent (1).

Auditory findings. Onset of sensorineural hearing loss was variable, ranging from before 20 years to between 20 and 50 years of age. Hearing loss was primarily in the high frequencies and was progressive. Two individuals in their 60's who carried the affected haplotypes had hearing loss that was not greater than would be expected from presbycusis or their history of noise exposure, so they may have been nonpenetrant. Examination of the pedigree suggested that modifier genes in some branches of the family might affect the penetrance or age of onset of the hearing loss. One individual was apparently a phenocopy, having a hearing loss but not the affected haplotypes. He also had a history of noise exposure.

Vestibular findings. No vestibular evaluations were reported.

Radiology/histology. No studies were reported.

Molecular studies. A maximum single point LOD score of 6.82 with $\theta = 0.041$ was found for marker D12S1030. The critical region spanned from D12S327 to D12S84, about 20 cM. Candidate genes included *ATP2A2* and *ATPB1*, both Ca^{2+} transporting ATPases. Mutations in *ATP2A2* cause Darier-White disease, which involves skin disease with much the same mechanism of some of the connexin genes. In the mouse, *Atp2b2* causes the mutation *deafwaddler (dfw)*. Other candidates include *UBE3B* (E3 ubiquitin ligase) and *VR-OAC* (vanilloid receptor–related osmotically activated channel).

Heredity. Inheritance is autosomal dominant with reduced penetrance.

Prognosis. Progressive high-frequency hearing loss occurs with a wide range in severity and age of onset.

Summary. In some older individuals, it was very difficult to distinguish this form of hearing loss from presbycusis or noise-induced hearing loss. This could indicate that mutations in this gene could have a role in these common conditions (1).

References

1. Greene CC et al: DFNA25, a novel locus for dominant nonsyndromic hereditary hearing impairment, maps to 12q21–24. *Am J Hum Genet* 68:254–260, 2001.

DFNA26

- MIM: Not assigned
- Location, gene: 17q25; gene unknown

This localization was made in two families from the United States (2).

Auditory findings. Hearing loss was progressive. Since this was reported in abstract form, no further information was available.

Vestibular findings. No evaluations have been reported.

Radiology/histology. No studies have been reported.

Molecular studies. Maximum LOD scores of 3.20 and 5.06 were obtained for the two families. According to the Hereditary Hearing Loss Homepage (http://dnalab-www.uia.ac.be/dnalab/hhh/), markers D17S784, D17S914, and D17S970 can be used to screen for this region. The critical region overlaps with DFNA20, and Mustapha et al. (1) have localized Usher syndrome type IG to this region. They note that the mouse mutant *jackson shaker (js)* also maps to the same area.

Heredity. Inheritance is autosomal dominant.

Prognosis. Progressive hearing loss occurs.

Summary. This family appears to be phenotypically similar to DFNA20, and the critical regions overlap. It is possible that these conditions are allelic, and either or both may also be allelic with USH1G.

References

1. Mustapha M et al: A novel locus for Usher syndrome type I, USH1G, maps to chromosome 17q24–25. *Hum Genet* 110:348–350, 2002.

2. Yang T, Smith R: A novel locus DFNA26 maps to chromosome 17q25 in two unrelated families with progressive autosomal dominant hearing loss [abstract]. *Am J Hum Genet* 67:300, 2000.

DFNA27

- MIM: not assigned
- Location, gene: 4q12; gene unknown

Auditory findings. Onset of hearing loss was noted from between the preteen years to the late 20's. It progresses from moderate to profound hearing loss before age 40 to profound in older individuals (1).

Vestibular findings. No evaluations have been reported.

Radiology/histology. No studies have been reported.

Molecular studies. A maximum LOD score of 4.76 at $\theta = 0.0$ was found for the marker D4S3248. The critical region is about 15 cM, between D4S428 and D4S392 (1).

Heredity. Inheritance is autosomal dominant.

Prognosis. Sensorineural hearing loss with variable age of onset progresses to the profound range after age 40.

Summary. Although some details are unpublished, this form of hearing loss appears to be similar in phenotype to DFNA4 and DFNA20, and possibly DFNA26.

References
1. Fridell RA et al: DFNA27, a new locus for autosomal dominant hearing impairment on chromosome 4 [abstract]. *Am J Hum Genet* 66:A249, 1999.

DFNA28

- MIM: not assigned
- Location, gene: 8q22; *TFCP2L3* (transcription factor cellular promotor 2-like 3)
  This gene was localized and identified in a large U.S. family (1,2).

Auditory findings. Onset of hearing loss was noted as early as age 7, and gradually progressed to the moderate to severe range by the 40's. The configuration of the hearing loss was variable, with either high frequencies or mid frequencies involved to the greatest extent. Normal speech discrimination scores implied a cochlear defect (1).

Vestibular findings. No studies were reported.

Radiology/histology. No studies were reported.

Molecular studies. *TFCP2L3* is a transcription factor in the TFCP2 family, which includes the *Drosophila* mutation *grainyhead*. It is widely expressed in epithelial tissues, but its target genes in the inner ear are not known. The mouse homologue, *Tfcp2l3*, is expressed in epithelial tissues lining the scala media during embryonic stages. Involvement in later-onset progressive hearing loss would imply that it is also important for maintenance of function.

Peters et al. (2) identified a heterozygous insertion of a C (1609–1610insC) in affected family members, which occurs just prior to the donor splice site in the 13th exon. If translated, this would produce a stop codon in the 14th exon of the 16 exon gene, which would eliminate part of the dimerization domain of the molecule.

Heredity. Inheritance is autosomal dominant.

Prognosis. Progressive sensorineural hearing loss occurs with the predominant effect being in either the mid- or high-frequencies.

Summary. Although some autosomal dominant forms of nonsyndromic hearing loss show variability in age of onset or rate of progression, most are consistent in the frequencies that are primarily involved. This form of hearing loss differs from others in the inclusion of both mid- and high-frequency audiological configurations. The role of the transcription factor *TFCP2L3* is currently unknown.

References
1. Anderson DW et al: A new locus for autosomal dominant hearing loss DFNA28 mapped to chromosome 8q22 [abstract]. *Am J Hum Genet* 66:A241, 1999.
2. Peters LM et al: Mutation of a transcription factor, *TFCP2L3*, causes progressive autosomal dominant hearing loss, DFNA28. *Hum Mol Genet* 11:2877–2885, 2002.

DFNA30

- MIM: 606451
- Location, gene: 15q25–26; gene unknown
This localization was made in a four-generation Italian family (1).

Auditory findings. There was a very wide range in the age of onset of hearing loss in this family, from 10 to 40 years. High frequencies were involved first, with progression to the mid frequencies.

Vestibular findings. No evaluations were reported.

Radiology/histology. No studies were reported.

Molecular studies. A maximum LOD score of 4.12 was found for the marker D15S1004 at $\theta = 0.0$. Haplotype analysis placed the critical region between D15S151 and D15S130, and multipoint analysis produced a maximum LOD of 4.34 between these markers. This defined a critical region of 18 cM, which was telomeric to the DFNB16 gene, *STRC* (2). One individual with the affected haplotypes did not have hearing loss, indicating decreased penetrance. Candidate genes in this region included *AGC1* (aggrecan) and *PTD014*, both expressed in the cochlea. Direct sequence analysis of these genes did not find any causal mutations. The critical region also included the otosclerosis (*OTS*) gene.

Heredity. Inheritance is autosomal dominant with a wide range in age of onset and decreased penetrance.

Prognosis. Progressive, sloping hearing loss occurs with initial involvement of high frequencies and gradual inclusion of the mid frequencies as well.

Summary. The wide range in age of onset as well as the occurrence of nonpenetrance may indicate the presence of modifier genes that affect the expression of the DNFA30 gene. The authors also suggested that it may be allelic to the otosclerosis gene.

References
1. Mangino M et al: Mapping of a new autosomal dominant nonsyndromic hearing loss locus (DFNA30) to chromosome 15q25–26. *Eur J Hum Genet* 9:667–671, 2001.
2. Verpy E et al: Mutations in a new gene encoding a protein of the hair bundle cause non-syndromic deafness at the DFNB16 locus. *Nat Genet* 29:345–349, 2001.

DFNA32

- MIM: not assigned
- Location, gene: 11p15; gene unknown
  This localization was made in a U.S. family (1).

Auditory findings. Hearing loss was progressive.

Vestibular findings. No vestibular studies were reported.

Radiology/histology. No studies were reported.

Molecular studies. A maximum LOD score of 4.1 was found with the marker D11S1984. The region is distal to DFNB18 and USH1C (Usher syndrome type IC).

Heredity. Inheritance is autosomal dominant.

Prognosis. Hearing loss is progressive.

Summary. Phenotypic details of this form of hearing loss await publication.

References

1. Li X et al: A new gene for autosomal dominant nonsyndromic sensorineural hearing loss (DFNA32) maps to 11p15 [abstract]. *Am J Hum Genet* 67:312, 2000.

DFNA34

- MIM: not assigned
- Location, gene: 1q44; gene unknown

This locus has been identified through genome screening in a single family studied in the United States (3).

Auditory findings. Hearing loss in this family was detected in their 20's and 30's, with gradual progression.

Vestibular findings. No evaluations were reported.

Radiology/histology. No studies were reported.

Molecular studies. A maximum LOD score of 3.33 was obtained with marker D1S2836 at $\theta = 0.00$. The gene *MWS*, which causes Muckle-Wells syndrome (urticaria-deafness-amyloidosis syndrome), is within the critical region. Hearing loss in that syndrome is sensorineural and progressive. Muckle-Wells syndrome, as well as familial cold urticaria and CINCA syndrome, have since been found to be due to mutations in the *CIAS1* gene (2). Dode et al. (1) found that the same mutation of *CIAS1* can cause different diseases, suggesting that modifiers exist that affect the expression of the gene. Thus, the *CIAS1* gene would be a candidate for DFNA34.

Heredity. Inheritance is autosomal dominant.

Prognosis. Hearing loss has onset in the third or fourth decade with gradual progression.

Summary. This phenotype has a relatively late onset, similar to DFNA4 and DFNA15 (*POU4F3*). The *CIAS1* gene is a candidate.

References

1. Dode C et al: New mutations of *CIAS1* that are responsible for Muckle-Wells syndrome and familial cold urticaria: a novel mutation underlies both syndromes. *Am J Hum Genet* 70:1498–1506, 2002.
2. Hoffman HM et al: Mutation of a new gene encoding a putative pyrin-like protein causes familial cold autoinflammatory syndrome and Muckle-Wells syndrome. *Nat Genet* 29:301–305, 2001.
3. Kurima K et al: Genetic map localization of DFNA34 and DFNA36, two autosomal dominant nonsyndromic deafness loci [abstract]. *Am J Hum Genet* 67:300, 2000.

DFNA36

- MIM: 606705 (DFNA36), 606706 (TMC1)
- Location, gene: 9q13–q21; *TMC1* (transmembrane cochlear-expressed gene 1)

DFNA36 was localized in a large five-generation U.S. family (3). The causal mutation in *TMC1* was found in this family and in families with DFNB7 and DFNB11 by Kumira et al. (2). Mutation of mouse *Tmc1* causes the dominant phenotype Beethoven (Bth) and the recessive deafness (dn).

Auditory findings. Onset of hearing loss in the high frequencies was observed between 5 and 10 years of age, with rapid progression to profound hearing loss over all frequencies in the next 10–15 years.

Vestibular findings. No vestibular deficits were noted by history or examination.

Radiology/histology. No studies were available from family members, but histological studies with an antisense probe of *Tmc1* in the mouse showed specific hybridization to cochlear inner and outer hair cells and to neurosensory epithelia of the vestibular system. In the *Beethoven* dominant mouse mutation, progressive loss of hair cells was noted after postnatal day 30, with almost complete degeneration of inner hair cells in the middle turn of the cochlea by day 35 (5).

Molecular studies. Linkage analysis had positioned DFNA36 in the same region as the recessive DFNB7/11 locus. Analysis of the DFNB7/11 families identified a 3 Mb critical region within the critical region defined by DFNA36, so the smaller region was searched for candidate genes. Known genes were excluded by mutation analysis, so the region was put to BLAST analysis to identify homologous genes. This process detected sequence similarity to a predicted gene (later termed *TCM2*) on chromosome 20. The shared sequences were used to probe a fetal brain cDNA library to identify a transcript. This led to the sequence of the cDNA, and the sequence of both human and mouse genomic DNA was developed. The function of the *TCM1* gene is unknown, and sequence analysis produced no significant homologies to known genes. There appear to be six transmembrane domains, and both the amino and carboxyl terminal regions would be cytoplasmic.

In the mouse, histologic studies with an antisense probe to *Tcm1* localized expression to cochlear hair cells and to the vestibular neuroepithelium. mRNA expression levels as determined by quantitative polymerase chain reaction (PCR) showed activity after the second week of embryogenesis, with increased levels through 3 weeks postnatally (3).

Tcm1 mutations were found to cause the dominant *Beethoven* mouse, which also has progressive hearing loss. Recessive mutations produce the deafness (dn) phenotype of profound congenital deafness. Early microscopic studies of the cochlea in *dn* mice showed normal hair cell embryonic development but later degeneration, indicating that the mutation may have a physiologic rather than structural effect (1,4). This, plus the presence of transmembrane domains, suggested to Kurima et al. (3) that the *TCM1* gene could function for ion transport.

Affected members of the DFNA36 family were found to be heterozygous for a missense mutation, 1714G $\rightarrow$ A, resulting in a substitution of asparagine for a conserved aspartic acid (D572N) in a cytoplasmic loop of one of the transmembrane domains. Similarly, the dominant Beethoven phenotype was found to be due to an M412K mutation in an extracellular loop (5). In contrast, recessive *deafness* mutations were found to be either truncations or missense mutations in the transmembrane domain (2).

Heredity. Inheritance is autosomal dominant with complete penetrance.

Prognosis. Sensorineural hearing loss occurs with onset between 5 and 10 years and rapid progression to profound hearing loss.

Summary. This form of hearing loss is notable for its early onset and rapid progression. *TCM1* mutations cause both recessive and dominant hearing loss in humans and in mice. The function of *TCM1* is unknown, but it is likely to be involved in ion transport (2).

References

1. Bock GR, Steel KP: Inner ear pathology in the deafness mutant mouse. *Acta Otolaryngol* 96:39–47, 1983.
2. Kurima K et al: Dominant and recessive deafness caused by mutations of a novel gene, *TMC1*, required for cochlear hair-cell function. *Nat Genet* 30:277–284, 2002.
3. Kurima K et al: Genetic map localization of DFNA34 and DFNA36, two autosomal dominant nonsyndromic deafness loci [abstract]. *Am J Hum Genet* 67:300, 2000.
4. Pujol R et al: Early degeneration of sensory and gangion cells in the inner ear of mice with uncomplicated genetic deafness (*dn*): preliminary observations. *Hear Res* 12:57–63, 1983.
5. Vreugde S et al: Beethoven, a mouse model for dominant, progressive hearing loss DFNA36. *Nat Genet* 30:257–258, 2002.

DFNA39

- MIM: 605594 (DNFA39), 125485 (DSPP)
- Location, gene: 4q21; *DSPP* (dentin sialophosphoprotein)

High-frequency progressive hearing loss showed cosegregation with dentinogenesis imperfecta in two out of three Chinese families (2). They did not have other features of osteogenesis imperfecta, such as blue sclerae, fractures, or short stature.

Auditory findings. Hearing loss was in the high frequencies. Examination of sample audiograms suggested preservation of hearing in the low and mid frequencies, while hearing loss could reach the severe to profound range in the high frequencies.

Vestibular findings. No vestibular evaluations were reported.

Radiology/histology. No studies were reported.

Molecular studies. *DSPP* encodes two proteins, dentin sialoprotein, which is expressed in odontoblasts and ameloblasts and may be important for dentinogenesis, and dentin phosphoprotein, which may be involved in mineralization of the dentin matrix. Although previous immunohistochemistry studies had not found evidence of *DSPP* in mouse tissue samples (1), transcripts of *DSPP* were found in total RNA from mouse inner ear, demonstrating that it is active there. The co-occurrence of hearing loss and dentinogenesis imperfecta in some forms of osteogenesis imperfecta suggested that either or both proteins may interact with the type I collagens. The two families with hearing loss and dentinogenesis imperfecta, as well as a third family which had only dentinogenesis imperfecta, had mutations in the dentin sialoprotein portion of the gene. One family with hearing loss had a 49C → A mutation producing a P17T missense, and the other had a 52G → T mutation, resulting in a V18F substitution. These adjacent amino acids are both highly conserved and are in the transmembrane domain. In the family with dentinogenesis imperfecta alone, a G → A mutation was found at the donor splice site of intron 3, which was hypothesized to result in skipping of exon 3 in dentin sialoprotein.

Heredity. Inheritance is autosomal dominant with complete penetrance.

Prognosis. Dentinogenesis imperfecta produces discoloration of primary and permanent dentitions. The hearing loss is in the high frequencies and is progressive.

Summary. Since a nonauditory system is involved, this could be considered a syndromic form of hearing loss. Both phenotypes are fairly mild, so the cosegregation of the hearing loss and dentinogenesis imperfecta may have been missed in some pedigree studies concentrating on either hearing or dental anomalies (1).

References

1. Patel PI: Soundbites. *Nat Genet* 27:129–130, 2001.

2. Xiao S et al: Dentinogenesis imperfecta 1 with or without progressive hearing loss is associated with distinct mutations in *DSPP*. *Nat Genet* 27:201–204, 2001.

DFNA41

- MIM: not assigned
- Location, gene: 12q24–qter; gene unknown

This localization was made in a large Chinese kindred (1).

Auditory findings. Onset of hearing loss was in the third decade, with gradual progression to severe to profound levels. All frequencies were involved.

Vestibular findings. No symptoms were evident in affected family members.

Radiology/histology. No studies were reported.

Molecular studies. An LOD score of 6.56 was obtained at $\theta = 0.0$ for the marker D12S343, with the critical region spanning 15 cM between D12S1609 and the telomere of the long arm of chromosome 12. This places the locus distal to DFNA25. Candidate genes included *FZD10*, homologous to the *Drosophila frizzled* family of transmembrane receptors.

Heredity. Inheritance is autosomal dominant, with sex difference in age of onset.

Prognosis. Adult-onset hearing loss progresses to the severe to profound range over all frequencies.

Summary. This form of dominant progressive hearing loss is somewhat similar to DFNA15 in age of onset and ultimate severity. The critical region does not overlap DFNA25.

References

1. Blanton SH et al: A novel locus for autosomal dominant non-syndromic deafness (DFNA41) maps to chromosome 12q24–qter. *J Med Genet* 39:567–570, 2002.

Autosomal dominant mid-frequency hearing loss

The European Work Group on Genetics of Hearing Impairment (1996) has defined mid-frequency hearing loss (sometimes termed a "cookie bite" configuration) as encompassing the frequencies of 500 Hz to 2000 Hz with at least a 15 dB difference between the poorest mid-frequency threshold and the best thresholds in the low and high frequencies. Temporal bone studies have shown atrophy of the stria vascularis, organ of Corti, and ganglion cells, but these have not been attributed to a specific locus (Fig. 5–3).

DFNA10

- MIM: 601316 (DFNA10); 603550 (EYA4)
- Location, gene: 6q22–q24; *EYA4*

Mutations in the *EYA4* gene have been found to be responsible for progressive mid-frequency hearing loss in two families, one from the United States and one from Belgium (5). A third Norwegian family may also link to this region (3).

Auditory findings. In the U.S. and Belgian families, onset of hearing loss was noted within the first and fourth decades. In the Belgian family, the youngest affected individual was 6 years old, and the oldest unaffected (who carried the affected haplotypes) was 36 years old. Hearing loss involved all frequencies and was flat or sloping, although individuals from the Belgian and Norwegian families in particular

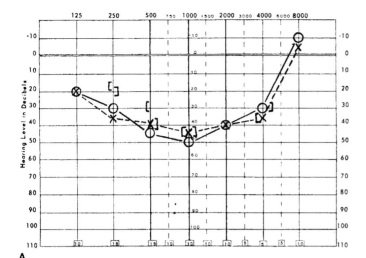

A

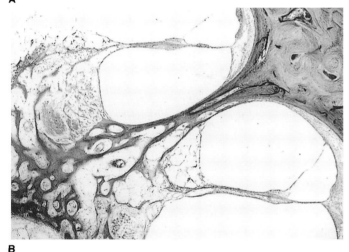

B

Figure 5–3. *Autosomal dominant mid-frequency hearing loss.* (A) Mother and son had almost identical audiograms. (B) Temporal bone shows marked loss of ganglion cells, atrophy of stria vascularis, and degeneration of organ of Corti. [(A) from F Williams, LA Roblee, *Arch Otolaryngol* 75:69, 1962; (B) from MM Paparella et al., *Arch Otolaryngol* 90:44, 1969.]

showed initial loss in the mid frequencies. Continued loss was noted in the high frequencies, but analysis of the progression indicated that the hearing loss due to the DFNA10 locus was in the severe range and stable after age 30, primarily affecting the mid frequencies with further loss in the high frequencies felt to be due to superimposed presbycusis (1,3,4). Tinnitus was reported in 35% of affected individuals from the Belgian family (4).

Vestibular findings. Of 42 affected individuals in the U.S. and Belgian families, two reported episodic vertigo (1,4).

Radiology/histology. No studies have been reported.

Molecular studies. *EYA4* is a member of the "eyes absent" family of transcription factors, first defined in *Drosophila*, that are active in embryonic development. Expression of *EYA4* was demonstrated by reverse-transcription polymerase chain reaction (RT-PCR) in a human fetal cochlear DNA library, and in situ hybridization in rat cochlear sections showed expression in the neuroepithelia during embryonic development, starting with precursors of Reissner's membrane and the stria vascularis, and later involving the developing spiral limbus, organ of Corti, and spiral prominence. For the first 2 weeks after birth, expression of *Eya4* was seen in the cochlear capsule, during the ossification

process. Its function in maintenance of cochlear function in later life is unknown.

EYA4 was found to be within the critical region defined by linkage analysis of the three known families and was considered to be a likely candidate because a related gene, *EYA1*, is known to cause a syndromic form of hearing loss, branchio-oto-renal (BOR) syndrome. Mutation analysis of the gene in the U.S. family revealed a heterozygous insertion of two alanines at nucleotide position 1468, producing a frameshift and termination in exon 14. Affected individuals in the Belgian family were heterozygous for a 2200C → T mutation, creating a stop codon in exon 20. These are both in the C-terminal eya-homologous region, eyaHR, which is highly conserved and is important in its protein-binding functions (5). This section of *EYA1* is also mutated in BOR syndrome, but no other syndromic features are seen in these families. It is interesting, however, that *EYA4* is expressed in heart tissues and families with a condition involving dalated cardiomyopathy and progressive hearing loss also map to this region. In that condition, hearing loss onset is during school age, with most individuals showing a moderate to severe hearing loss, although a few had profound hearing loss. A sample audiogram with moderate to severe thresholds suggests slightly more loss in the mid frequencies (2).

Heredity. Inheritance is autosomal dominant with apparently complete penetrance.

Prognosis. Mid-frequency hearing loss progresses to the severe range, although age of onset is widely variable within families.

Summary. Although hearing loss affects the mid frequencies more than others, all frequencies are affected, and the differences between them are not great. In older individuals, a sloping audiogram may be seen, presumably secondary to presbycusis. The syndrome of dilated cardiomyopathy and hearing loss may be allelic.

References

1. De Leenheer EMR et al: The DFNA10 phenotype. *Ann Otol Rhinol Laryngol* 110:861–866, 2001.
2. Schonberger J et al: Dilated cardiomyopathy and sensorineural hearing loss: a heritable syndrome that maps to 6q23–24. *Circulation* 101:1812–1818, 2000.
3. Verhoeven K et al: Refined localization and two additional linked families for the DFNA10 locus for nonsyndromic hearing impairment. *Hum Genet* 107:7–11, 2000.
4. Verstreken M et al: Audiometric analysis of a Belgian family linked to the DFNA10 locus. *Am J Otol* 21:675–681, 2000.
5. Wayne S et al: Mutations in the transcriptional activator *EYA4* cause late-onset deafness at the DFNA10 locus. *Hum Mol Genet* 10:195–200, 2001.

DFNA13

- MIM: 601868 (DFNA13); 120290 (*COL11A2*)
- Location, gene: 6p21.3; *COL11A2* (α-2 (IX) collagen), plus one unknown gene

Four families have shown linkage to this region, two U.S. and two Dutch. Mutations in *COL11A2* have been documented in one of the Dutch and one of the U.S. families (5). One Dutch family had not been screened at the time of publication (3), and mutation in *COL11A2* was excluded in the other U.S. family (6).

Auditory findings. Hearing loss was primarily in the moderate to severe range in the mid frequencies in the U.S. family with a *COL11A2* mutation and in the two Dutch families. Onset was thought to be prelingual and possibly congenital in the U.S. family, with no significant progression aside from later high-frequency loss attributable to presbycusis (2). In contrast, only 4 of 21 affected individuals from the Dutch family with a *COL11A2* mutation had a clear childhood onset, with most reporting that they noticed symptoms in the second to third decades. One of these had documented hearing loss at 4 years of age with rapid progression. However, young children were not tested audiometrically and serial audiograms were only available on two individuals, so age of onset and progression could not be directly assessed in other family members. High-frequency hearing loss did appear with age, but was indistinguishable from presbycusis (4). In the other Dutch family, serial audiograms were also unavailable for all but one individual, but reports from family members and statistical analysis across age groups suggested that the hearing loss was not prelingual and was noted around age 30, initially involving the mid frequencies, and was progressive in all frequencies, although superimposed presbycusis created additional high-frequency hearing loss.

Tinnitus was present in about a third of affected family members from the two Dutch families (3,4). The U.S. family without a detectable *COL11A2* mutation appears phenotypically different, in that it is probably congenital (detected as young as 6 months), initially presenting as a relatively flat moderate to severe hearing loss, with gradual progression to the severe to profound range in the high frequencies by the third decade (6).

Vestibular findings. Asymptomatic vestibular abnormalities were found with caloric testing in some individuals from the two Dutch families and the U.S. family with the *COL11A2* mutation. No vestibular abnormalities were found in the other linked Dutch family, nor in the U.S. family without a *COL11A2* mutation.

Radiology/histology. No studies of the inner ear are reported. Cephalometric analysis of X-rays from two individuals showed normal craniofacial features (5).

Molecular studies. Linkage analysis in the four families localized to the 6p21.3 region, and the *COL11A2* gene was within the critical region for all four. Type XI collagen is a fibrillar collagen, composed of heterotrimers of type XI α-1, type XI α-2, and type XI α-3, which is actually transcribed from the *COL2A1* gene. These molecules combine to form a rope-like triple helical structure and interact with type II collagen. Mutations in type XI and type II collagen can both cause syndromes that are part of a spectrum of disorders that include osteochondrodysplasia with auditory, craniofacial, and sometimes ocular symptoms (Stickler syndrome, Kniest syndrome, spondyloepiphyseal dysplasia (SED), Marshall syndrome, and otospondylomegaepiphyseal dysplasia (OSMED). All of these syndromes are dominantly inherited except for some recessive OSMED phenotypes, and include progressive hearing loss to some degree. In situ hybridization of an antisense probe to *Col11a2* in mouse cochlear sections showed expression in the otic capsule in the embryo and in the spiral limbus and lateral wall of the cochlea in 5-day-old mice. Mice with a homozygous knockout of *Col11a2* showed a slightly abnormal structure of the tectorial membrane with disorganization of its collagen fibrils and had hearing loss, while heterozygous mice had normal hearing (5). This could be expected if haploinsufficiency is not pathogenic.

The American family originally described by Brown et al. (1) and later by DeLeenheer et al. (2) was found to have a heterozygous C → T mutation resulting in a missense R549C. Cysteines are notably absent in the helical region of the collagen protein, so the substitution of a cysteine could be expected to disrupt the molecule, and in fact other cysteine substitutions in other fibrillar collagens are pathogenic. In the Dutch family, affected individuals were heterozygous for a G → A transition that produces a G323E substitution. Glycines are critical in the propagation of the triple helix, and their replacement is also often pathogenic. The authors pointed out that mutations located more toward the 5′ end of the gene cause less severe phenotypes than those that are 3′, since post-translational modification proceeds 3′ to 5′; consistent with this, a G955E mutation causes a severe dominant condition similar to the OSMED phenotype (5). Both of these mutations would act in a dominant-negative fashion.

Heredity. Inheritance is autosomal dominant.

Prognosis. For those with a *COL11A2* mutation, hearing loss is primarily mid frequency and may be stable in adulthood in some families, aside from an overlay of presbycusis.

Summary. Mutations of type XI and the associated type II collagen molecules have usually been associated with dominant syndromes, although there is a wide range of expression—so wide that separate syndromes have been defined, and the mildest, Stickler syndrome, may be difficult to diagnose in some cases. The families in these reports demonstrate that the phenotype can be so mild that only auditory symptoms are seen. Age of onset and rate of progression are unclear, however. There may be variability based on different mutations, but early ascertainment and longitudinal follow-up of affected individuals will be required to be certain.

References

1. Brown MR et al: A novel locus for autosomal dominant nonsyndromic hearing loss, DFNA13, maps to chromosome 6p. *Am J Hum Genet* 61:924–927, 1997.
2. De Leenheer EMR et al: Autosomal dominant inherited hearing impairment caused by a missense mutation in *COL11A2* (DFNA13). *Arch Otolaryngol Head Neck Surg* 127:13–17, 2001.
3. Ensink RJH et al: A Dutch family with progressive autosomal dominant nonsyndromic sensorineural hearing impairment linked to DFNA13. *Clin Otolaryngol* 26:310–316, 2001.
4. Kunst H et al: The phenotype of DFNA13/*COL11A2*: nonsyndromic autosomal dominant mid-frequency and high-frequency sensorineural hearing impairment. *Am J Otol* 21:181–187, 2000.
5. McGuirt WT et al: Mutations in *COL11A2* cause non-syndromic hearing loss (DFNA13). *Nat Genet* 23:413–419, 1999.
6. Talebizadeh Z et al: Mutation analysis of alpha 1 chain in type XI collagen (*COL11A1*) in a kindred with dominant progressive hearing loss linked to chromosome 1p21. Presented to the 23rd Annual Midwinter Meeting of the Association for Research in Otolaryngology, St. Petersburg, FL, February 20, 2000.

Autosomal dominant low-frequency hearing loss

DFNA1

- MIM: 124900 (DFNA1); 602121 (DIAPH1)
- Location, gene: 5q31; *DIAPH1* (also called *HDIA1*) (human homologue to *Drosophila*) diaphanous

Mutation in the *DIAPH1* gene has been found as a cause of hearing loss in a large Costa Rican kindred. This has been referred to as "Kindred M," or Monge deafness, after an ancestor born in Costa Rica in 1713 (3,4,7).

Auditory findings. Onset of hearing loss can be as early as 5 years or as late as 20 years, with variability seen within sibships (5). It starts with a mild loss in the low frequencies, and may be accompanied by tinnitus. The loss progresses to the mid and high frequencies, resulting in a flat severe to profound hearing loss. Exact age of onset and rate of progression are variable, however, even among siblings, but all affected individuals have at least a 50 dB low-frequency loss by age 30. In one child who had low-frequency hearing loss, otoacoustic emissions were present in the high frequencies with preserved hearing but absent in conjunction with hearing loss, and auditory brain stem responses had normal configurations. Electrocochleography was consistent with endolymphatic hydrops, which can be associated with low-frequency hearing loss (2).

Vestibular findings. Evaluations, including clinical assessment, electonystagmography, and calorics, were normal in two adults. An 8-year-old child showed unilateral vestibular weakness on caloric stimulation (2).

Radiology/histology. The CT scan of the temporal bones was normal in an affected adult.

Molecular studies. Diaphanous is part of the formin-homology family of genes and is involved in cytokinesis and cell division. It functions to establish polarity of the cell in limb development in the mouse. Studies of mutation of the gene in *Drosophila* confirmed that these actions are mediated through the actin cytoskeleton and that the protein may be involved in signaling pathways to organize and anchor actin (1). *DIAPH* is expressed in multiple human tissues as assessed by Northern hybridization, and RT-PCR of cochlear mRNA confirmed cochlear expression (7).

Seventy-eight affected members of the M kindred were found to be heterozygous for a G → T substitution in the splice donor site of the penultimate exon of *DIAPH*. This results in use of a cryptic splice site and a frameshift insertion, leading to 21 missense codons and a stop codon with premature truncation of the last 32 amino acids of the protein. The mutation segregated completely with the hearing loss in the family and was not found in controls of the same ethnic background. It was hypothesized that the mutation would interfere with actin polymerization in hair cells, affecting either the amplification of sound by the outer hair cells or the structure of the stereocilia. Defective diaphanous protein might affect the ability of the hair cells to protect themselves from noise exposure (7). Alternatively, the finding of electrophysiological signs of endolymphatic hydrops suggests that the protein may be involved with intracellular protein trafficking and maintenance of endolymphatic homeostasis (2). If defects in repair mechanisms indeed contribute to the progression of hearing loss, protection from noise exposure may help affected individuals preserve some hearing longer (6).

A homologue of *DIAPH1*, *DIAPH2*, was localized to the X-chromosome and was proposed as a candidate for DFN2 (7).

Heredity. Inheritance is autosomal dominant with complete penetrance by age 30.

Prognosis. Although there was considerable variability in age of onset and range of progression, all affected individuals ultimately had a severe to profound hearing loss with a flat audiological configuration.

Summary. This form of low-frequency hearing loss is distinguished from the more common type caused by mutation of *WFS1* by its more rapid progression and greater severity of the hearing loss.

References

1. Afshar K et al: Functional analysis of the *Drosophila* Diaphanous FH protein in early embryonic development. *Development* 127:1887–1897, 2000.
2. Lalwani AK et al: Further characterization of the DFNA1 audiovestibular phenotype. *Arch Otolaryngol Head Neck Surg* 124:699–702, 1998.
3. León PE et al: Low frequency hereditary deafness in man with childhood onset. *Am J Hum Genet* 33:209–214, 1981.
4. León PE et al: The gene for an inherited form of deafness maps to chromosome 5q31. *Proc Natl Acad Sci USA* 89:5181–5184, 1992.
5. León PE, Lalwani AK: Auditory phenotype of DFNA1. *Adv Otorhinolaryngol* 61:34–40, 2002.
6. Lynch ED, León PE: Non-syndromic dominant DFNA1. *Adv Otorhinolaryngol* 56:60–67, 2000.
7. Lynch ED et al: Nonsyndromic deafness DFNA1 associated with mutation of the human homolog of the *Drosophila* gene diaphanous. Science 278:1315–1318, 1997.

DFNA6/14/38

- MIM: 600965 (DFNA6/14/38), 606201 (WFS1)
- Location, gene: 4p16.3; *WFS1* (wolframin)

In 1968, the Vanderbilt University Hereditary Deafness Study Group published a detailed description of autosomal dominant low-frequency hearing loss in two kindreds that were probably related to each other. This was one of the first clinical descriptions of dominant nonsyndromic low-frequency hearing loss. Because of a second report by Konigsmark et al. (6), this is sometimes referred to as Konigsmark type.

Auditory findings. In the families reported by the Vanderbilt Study Group (12), moderate hearing loss was present in the low frequencies as early as age 4, with mild to normal hearing thresholds above 1000 Hz (Fig. 5–4). No mention was made of progression, except for loss in the high frequencies in older adults, which could have been the overlay of presbycusis. Subsequently, Konigsmark et al. (6) described three more families. Affected individuals from these families showed very

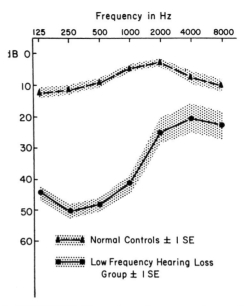

Figure 5–4. *DFNA6/14/38*. Comparison of mean pure-tone audiograms in patients with hereditary low-frequency hearing loss and their normal relatives. [From Vanderbilt Group, *Arch Otolaryngol* 88:242, 1965.]

similar low-frequency losses with a wide age range at which the hearing loss was diagnosed. However, progression of the loss was noted in some, and it was hypothesized that the hearing loss was generally present in childhood with gradual progression until it was clinically noticeable. Many affected individuals also experienced progressive high-frequency hearing loss with age, and finally loss of mid-frequency hearing as well. A large Dutch family that was subsequently found to have the same molecular basis as the Vanderbilt kindred also showed suggestive evidence of either congenital hearing loss or gradual progression of the low-frequency hearing loss in childhood, followed by a period of stability, with subsequent high-frequency loss being due to presbycusis. Almost half of affected individuals noted tinnitus (7,11). Bille et al. (3) described a Norwegian family with "Konigsmark deafness" and concluded that the hearing loss may be congenital. Serial audiograms were available for some individuals between the ages of 13 and 21 years, and a 13–17 dB progression of loss in the low frequencies was documented. Hearing loss could be detected in preschool-aged children from a family with low-frequency hearing loss in Newfoundland, Canada, and was observed to be slowly progressive in the low frequencies. However, this family also showed involvement of the mid frequencies in the second decade, whereas the mid frequencies were often preserved in other families, even after the onset of presbycusis (13).

Vestibular findings. Vestibular function studies in 17 affected individuals from the Dutch kindred suggested that about a third had evidence of vestibular hyperreactivity. However, none of the family members had symptoms of vestibular dysfunction (7).

Radiology/histology. Temporal bone tomography (3,12) and magnetic resonance imaging (MRI) studies (7) showed normal middle and inner ear structures.

Molecular studies. Linkage studies of the Vanderbilt kindred showed localization of the gene to 4p16.3 (8), and this was given the designation DFNA6. Initially, analysis of that family and the Dutch family suggested that there were two separate loci, and the second locus was named DFNA14. However, careful phenotype comparisons showed strong similarities between the two families, and it was recognized that they might be due to the same gene, despite the genetic evidence to the contrary (11). This was confirmed when expansion of the DFNA6 family produced evidence of a recombination event that excluded the previously defined region. This suggested that an individual who had contributed the critical recombination event that excluded the DFNA14 region was actually a phenocopy. With this change, the regions for DFNA6 and DFNA14 were overlapping, and the gene for Wolfram syndrome type 1 became a candidate for both (2). Simultaneously, the hearing loss in a separate family from Newfoundland was found to localize to 4p16 and a mutation in *WFS* was found. This locus was initially given the name DFNA38 (13).

Wolfram syndrome (also called DIDMOAD) is an autosomal recessive condition of diabetes insipidus, diabetes mellitus, optic atrophy, and deafness. It is genetically heterogeneous, with a second recessive locus, *WFS2*, located at 4q22–q24 (5), and some families with *WFS1* have also had mitochondrial abnormalities (1). This genetic variation likely contributes to the phenotypic variation, which can include mental retardation, renal dysfunction, ataxia, peripheral neuropathy, and brain stem atrophy. In addition, there appears to be a high risk of psychiatric disorder, including depression and psychosis. Interestingly, hearing loss in individuals with Wolfram syndrome is generally in the high frequencies, but obligate heterozygotes for Wolfram syndrome had been noted to have a risk of hearing loss and diabetes (9). Risk for psychiatric problems has also been suggested, but none of the family members in the Vanderbilt family showed evidence of psychiatric symptoms (2). The function of the *WFS1* protein, wolframin, is unknown, but it has nine transmembrane domains and is located in the endoplasmic reticulum, so it may be involved with membrane trafficking, protein processing, or calcium homeostasis. Expression is ubiquitous, but some localization to limbic system neurons was noted, which may account for some of the psychiatric characteristics (10).

Sequence analysis of the *WFS1* gene in affected members of the original Vanderbilt family showed heterozygosity for a 2656T → C mutation, resulting in an L829P substitution. A Dutch family had a 2266C → T (T699M) mutation, while another Dutch family and an Irish family both had a 2316G → A (A716T) mutation. These were on different haplotypes backgrounds, so presumably were independent events. Two additional small families with low-frequency hearing loss had a 2662G → A mutation, producing a G831D amino acid substitution, and a 2506G → A mutation, producing a V778M substitution. All of these mutations were in exon 8, which encodes the cytoplasmic C-terminal domain of the protein (2). The Newfoundland family was reported to have a 2146G → A mutation (A716T). Further analysis of a total of 10 *WFS1* mutations causing low-frequency hearing loss concluded that none of the mutations caused protein terminations or inactivations, while 64% of Wolfram syndrome mutations cause inactivation of the protein (4). Interestingly, however, a child homozygous for the A716T mutation presented with insulin-dependent diabetes mellitus at age 3 (13).

Heredity. Inheritance is autosomal dominant with complete penetrance.

Prognosis. Low-frequency hearing loss is present in early childhood (possibly congenitally) and may progress slowly. High-frequency loss may occur in later adulthood, possibly secondary to presbycusis. In some but not all families, hearing in the mid frequencies is preserved.

Summary. Mutation of the *WFS1* gene is the most common cause of low-frequency dominant nonsyndromic hearing loss. Affected individuals do not appear to have any of the features of Wolfram syndrome aside from hearing loss.

References

1. Barrientos A et al: A nuclear defect in the 4p16 region predisposes to multiple mitochondrial DNA deletions in families with Wolfram syndrome. *J Clin Invest* 97:1570–1576, 1996.
2. Bespalova IN et al: Mutations in the Wolfram syndrome 1 gene (*WFS1*) are a common cause of low frequency sensorineural hearing loss. *Hum Mol Genet* 10:2501–2508, 2001.
3. Bille M et al: Two families with phenotypically different hereditary low frequency hearing impairment: longitudinal data and linkage analysis. *Scand Audiol* 30:246–254, 2001.
4. Cryns K et al: Mutations in the *WFS1* gene that cause low-frequency sensorineural hearing loss are small non-inactivating mutations. *Hum Genet* 110:389–394, 2002.
5. El-Shanti H et al: Homozygosity mapping identifies an additional locus for Wolfram syndrome on chromosome 4q. *Am J Hum Genet* 66:1229–1236, 2000.
6. Konigsmark BW et al: Familial low frequency hearing loss. *Laryngoscope* 81:759–771, 1971.
7. Kunst H et al: Autosomal dominant non-syndromal low-frequency sensorineural hearing impairment linked to chromosome 4p16 (DFNA14): statistical analysis of hearing threshold in relation to age and evaluation of vestibulo-ocular functions. *Audiology* 38:165–173, 1999.
8. Lesperance MM et al: A gene for autosomal dominant nonsyndromic hereditary hearing impairment maps to 4p16.3. *Hum Mol Genet* 4:1967–1972, 1995.
9. Ohata T et al: Evidence of an increased risk of hearing loss in heterozygous carriers in a Wolfram syndrome family. *Hum Genet* 103:470–474, 1998.
10. Takeda K et al: WFS1 (Wolfram syndrome 1) gene product: predominant subcellular localization to endoplasmic reticulum in cultured cells and neuronal expression in rat brain. *Hum Mol Genet* 10:477–484, 2001.
11. Van Camp G et al: A gene for autosomal dominant hearing impairment (DFNA14) maps to a region on chromosome 4p16.3 that does not overlap the DFNA6 locus. *J Med Genet* 36:532–536, 1999.
12. Vanderbilt University Hereditary Deafness Study Group: Dominantly inherited low-frequency hearing loss. *Arch Otolaryngol* 88:242–250, 1968.
13. Young T-L et al: Non-syndromic progressive hearing loss DFNA38 is caused by heterozygous missense mutation in the Wolfram syndrome gene *WFS1*. *Hum Mol Genet* 10:2509–2514, 2001.

DFNA37

- MIM: not assigned
- Location, gene: 1p21; gene unknown
  This gene was localized in a four-generation U.S. family (1).

Auditory findings. Onset of hearing loss was noted in the low or mid frequencies as early as age 5 years, with gradual progression to include the high frequencies. In some cases, there was a "reverse cookie bite" configuration with low- and high-frequency loss greater than the mid-frequency loss. Hearing loss generally was in the moderate range.

Vestibular findings. Vestibular studies were normal for individuals in one branch of the kindred.

Radiology/histology. The CT scan of the temporal bones was normal.

Molecular studies. A maximum LOD score of 8.29 was obtained at $\theta = 0.0$ for marker D1S495, with a 13 cM critical region bounded by D1S2793 and D1S2651. Two individuals who did not share the hearing loss phenotype characteristic of the rest of the family and had been coded as phenotype unknown were found to carry the affected haplotype. The genes *COLllA1* and *KCNC4* were eliminated as candidates by mutation analysis. The region containing the gene for DFNB32 appears to overlap with DFNA37.

Heredity. Inheritance is autosomal dominant with reduced penetrance.

Prognosis. Sensorineural hearing loss is progressive.

Summary. In several individuals in this family, DFNA37 is very similar in phenotype to DFNA6/14, and may represent a third locus for low-frequency hearing loss. DFNA37 may be allelic to DFNB32.

References

1. Talebizadeh Z et al: A new locus for dominant progressive hearing loss, DFNA37, mapped to chromosome 1p21 [abstract]. *Am J Hum Genet* 67:314, 2000.

Autosomal dominant nonprogressive hearing loss

DFNA3

- MIM: 601544 (DFNA3); 121011 (GJB2)
- Location, gene: 13q12; *GJB2* (connexin 26)

Mutation of *GJB2* is a rare cause of dominant hearing loss; in contrast, mutations of this gene are the most common cause of recessive hearing loss (see DFNB1, below). Although the causative role of some mutations in this gene is in dispute, there is convincing evidence in at least two French families (2). Mutation of a second gene in the DFNA3 region, *GJB6*, causes dominant progressive hearing loss.

Auditory findings. Hearing loss was present before the age of 3 years, sloping across all frequencies from the moderate to profound range. Otoacoustic emissions were absent in frequencies of hearing loss.

Vestibular findings. No studies were reported.

Radiology/histology. No studies were reported.

Molecular studies. In both French families, affected individuals were heterozygous for a G → C transversion, resulting in a W44C substitution. This tryptophan is in the first extracellular loop of connexin 26 and is highly conserved, and the extra cysteine could also be expected to complicate disulfide bonding within the molecule. When incorporated with normal proteins in a connexon, this would be expected to have a dominant-negative effect (3). Subsequently, a third family has been described with the same W44C mutation (6).

Heterozygosity for a D66H mutation was found to produce dominant congenital hearing loss, but accompanied by mutilating palmoplantar keratoderma (Vohwinkel syndrome) (4). The KID syndrome (keratitis-icthyosis-deafness) also includes congenital hearing impairment and can be due to heterozygous *GJB2* mutations (5).

Another *GJB2* mutation, M34T, had been reported to be associated with dominant hearing loss, but subsequently it has been shown to be present in individuals with normal hearing; moreover, homozygosity for the M34T allele does not appear to contribute to recessive hearing loss (1).

Heredity. Inheritance is autosomal dominant with complete penetrance.

Prognosis. Hearing loss is present very early in life and is either very slightly progressive or nonprogressive.

Summary. In contrast to its contribution to recessive nonsyndromic hearing loss, mutation of *GJB2* appears to be a rare cause of dominant non-sydromic hearing loss.

References
1. Cucci RA et al: The M34T allele variant of connexin 26. *Genet Test* 4:335–344, 2000.
2. Denoyelle F et al: Connexin 26 gene linked to a dominant deafness. *Nature* 393:319–320, 1998.
3. Denoyelle F et al: DFNA3. *Adv Otorhinolaryngol* 56:78–83, 2000.
4. Maestrini E et al: A missense mutation in connexin26, D66H, causes mutilating keratoderma with sensorineural deafness (Vohwinkel's syndrome) in three unrelated families. *Hum Mol Genet* 8:1237–1243, 1999.
5. Richard G et al: Missense mutations in *GJB2* encoding connexin-26 cause the ectodermal dysplasia keratitis-ichthyosis-deafness syndrome. *Am J Hum Genet* 70:1341–1348, 2002.
6. Tekin M et al: W44C mutation in the connexin 26 gene associated with dominant non-syndromic deafness. *Clin Genet* 59:269–273, 2001.

DFNA8/12

- MIM: 601543 (DFNA8), 601842 (DFNA12), 602574 (TECTA)
- Location, gene: 11q22-24; *TECTA* (α-tectorin)

While several families have been reported with dominant progressive hearing loss due to mutations in the *TECTA* gene (see above), the two original families that defined the locus both had prelingual, nonprogressive hearing loss (1,2). Mutation in this gene also causes DFNB21.

Auditory findings. In both families, the hearing loss was presumed to be prelingual and probably congenital and no progression was observed from cross-sectional studies and serial audiograms. For example, average brain stem response (ABR) testing of one child at 3 months of age showed evidence of hearing loss that was unchanged at 5 years (1). The loss was moderate to severe, with slightly more involvement of the mid frequencies in both families (1,2).

Vestibular findings. The Austrian family had vestibular testing which was apparently normal (1).

Radiology/histology. The CT scans of the temporal bones in the Austrian family were apparently normal (1).

Molecular studies. As reviewed above under dominant progressive hearing losses, α-tectorin is a major constituent of the noncollagenous extracellular matrix of the tectorial membrane of the cochlea. The Austrian family had a 5876A → T missense mutation in the *TECTA* gene producing a Y1870C change. The Belgian family showed two cosegregating mutations, 5725C → T (L1820F) and 5738G → A (G1824D), either or both of which could have been pathogenic. All three mutations in these families were in highly conserved amino acids in the zona pellucida domain of the protein, which may account for the more severe presentation in these families. These mutations are presumed to interfere with the interaction of the polypeptides in the extracellular matrix, resulting in a dominant-negative effect (3).

Heredity. Inheritance is autosomal dominant with complete penetrance.

Prognosis. Nonprogressive moderate to severe hearing loss occurs.

Summary. Mutations of the *TECTA* gene cause a variety of phenotypes that vary in the mode of inheritance (dominant or recessive), age of onset (prelingual, first decade, or second decade), and presence or absence of progression. The phenotypes appear to depend upon the location of the mutation, the mechanism of action (dominant negative vs. haploinsufficiency), and possibly also the effects of modifying loci. The nonprogressive form is unique in that the mid frequencies are somewhat more severely involved than the high and low frequencies.

References
1. Kirschhofer K et al: Autosomal-dominant, prelingual, nonprogressive sensorineural hearing loss: localization of the gene (DFNA8) to chromosome 11q by linkage in an Austrian family. *Cytogenet Cell Genet* 82:126–130, 1998.
2. Verhoeven K et al: A gene for autosomal dominant nonsyndromic hearing loss (DFNA12) maps to chromosome 11q22–24. *Am J Hum Genet* 60:1168–1173, 1997.
3. Verhoeven K et al: Mutations in the human α-tectorin gene cause autosomal dominant non-syndromic hearing impairment. *Nat Genet* 19:60–62, 1998.

DFNA19

- MIM: not assigned
- Location, gene: 10 centromere; gene unknown

This locus was identified by a full genome screen in a five-generation European family (1). It was given the tentative designation of DFNA18, but the official name was later determined to be DFNA19.

Auditory findings. Mild to moderate congenital sensorineural hearing loss occurs, averaging 40 dB in the speech frequencies.

Vestibular findings. No vestibular evaluations were reported.

Radiology/histology. No studies have been reported.

Molecular studies. Details have not been published.

Heredity. The linkage to chromosome 10 was found using a model of autosomal dominant inheritance with reduced penetrance.

Prognosis. Stable mild to moderate hearing loss occurs.

Summary. This form of nonprogressive dominant hearing loss appears to be less severe than the other reported forms.

References

1. Green G et al: Identification of a new locus—DFNA18—for dominant hearing impairment. Presented at the Molecular Biology of Hearing and Deafness, Bethesda, MD, October 8, 1998, Abstract 107.

DFNA23

- MIM: 605192
- Location, gene: 14q21–q22; gene unknown

This localization was made in a three-generation Swiss-German family (2).

Auditory findings. The hearing loss in this family appeared to be prelingual and probably congenital. The configuration of the loss was sloping, but with a range of severity, from normal to mild loss in the low frequencies to moderate to profound loss in the high frequencies. Little progression was noted over as much as 32 years of audiograms. Five out of 10 affected individuals also had a conductive component in the low frequencies, but tympanometry was not reported, so it is not clear if this could have been due to middle ear disease.

Vestibular findings. No vestibular evaluations have been reported.

Radiology/histology. No studies have been reported.

Molecular studies. A maximum multipoint LOD score of 5.1 was found with marker D14S290. Several candidate genes expressed in fetal cochlea were noted to be within the 9.4 cM critical region, which was flanked by D14S980 and D14S1046. The best candidates were proposed to be *ACTN1* (α-actinin α 1), *NID2* (nidogen 2), and *KTN1* (kinectin). *ACTN1* is known to be expressed in rat cochlea and, as an actin-associated protein, is similar in function to *DIAPH1*, which causes DFNA1. *NID2* binds collagen IV, and mutations of members of the collagen IV family cause Alport syndrome. *KTN1* is similar in structure to the myosin II family, and myosin mutations cause several different forms of syndromic and nonsyndromic hearing loss. Other candidates were *PRKCH* (protein kinase C-η), *RTN1* (reticulon), *HSPE1* (heatshock 10-KD protein), *HIF1A* (hypoxia-inducible factor 1), *BMP4* (bone morphogenic protein 4), and *OTX2* (homologue of *Drosophila* orthodenticle).

Heredity. Inheritance is autosomal dominant with complete penetrance.

Prognosis. Early-onset hearing loss with sloping configuration occurs, with little to no progression.

Summary. This form of hearing loss is phenotypically similar to DFNA24, described by the same authors in the same ethnic population (1), except that a conductive hearing loss is not noted in DFNA24.

References

1. Häfner FM et al: A novel locus (DFNA24) for prelingual nonprogressive autosomal dominant nonsyndromic hearing loss maps to 4q35–qter in a large Swiss German kindred. *Am J Hum Genet* 66:1437–1442, 2000.

2. Salam AA et al: A novel locus (DFNA23) for prelingual autosomal dominant nonsyndromic hearing loss maps to 14q21–q22 in a Swiss German kindred. *Am J Hum Genet* 66:1984–1988, 2000.

DFNA24

- MIM: 606282
- Location, gene: 4q35–qter; gene unknown

This gene was localized by full genome screen in a large Swiss-German kindred (1).

Auditory findings. Bilaterally symmetrical sensorineural hearing loss had prelingual onset and was possibly congenital. The audiograms had a sloping configuration with a range of severity, from mild to moderate in the low frequencies to severe to profound loss in the high frequencies. When serial audiograms were available, there was no evidence of progression.

Vestibular findings. No vestibular evaluations were reported.

Radiology/histology. No studies were reported.

Molecular studies. A maximum multipoint LOD score of 11.6 was found with marker D4S1652. The critical region spanned about 7.8 cM, flanked by markers D4S408 and D4S1523. The gene for fascioscapulohumeral muscular dystrophy (which includes early-onset high-frequency progressive hearing loss) is in the *DFNA24* region. Although the family had no clinical signs of muscle weakness, this remains a good candidate gene. Another candidates is *ArgBP2*, which the authors cite as being associated with the actin cytoskeleton. Caspase-3 is also in this region, and mutation of this gene has been found to cause progressive hearing loss in mice, making it an additional candidate (2).

Heredity. Inheritance is autosomal dominant with complete penetrance.

Prognosis. Early-onset sloping hearing loss occurs with no progression.

Summary. This phenotype is very similar to DFNA23.

References

1. Häfner FM et al: A novel locus (DFNA24) for prelingual nonprogressive autosomal dominant nonsyndromic hearing loss maps to 4q35–qter in a large Swiss German kindred. *Am J Hum Genet* 66:1437–1442, 2000.

2. Morishita H et al: Deafness due to degeneration of cochlear neurons in caspase-3–deficient mice. *Biochem Biophys Res Commun* 284:142–149, 2001.

Autosomal Recessive Nonsyndromic Hearing Loss

Nearly all recessive loci are associated with severe to profound hearing impairment that is prelingual (probably congenital) in origin. However, most studies of recessive hearing loss have been targeted toward populations with profound hearing impairment, and in many cases only one kinded is described, so the range of phenotypic expression may be unknown. Also, many of the loci have been described in kindreds from areas in which full diagnostic evaluations are not possible, so details of audiologic progression, vestibular function, and other clinical parameters may not be available. In particular, age of onset may be confounded by the age at which the hearing loss was clinically detectable. It is possible that diagnosis was delayed in some individuals with some residual hearing, and this may explain some cases in which age of onset appears to be after birth, but no progression is noted. For these reasons, the only phenotypic separation of these loci has been by clear presence or absence of progression. Histologic studies of mouse models for several known recessive hearing loss genes have shown cochlear abnormalities including loss of hair cells; and although these abnormalities have also been observed in temporal bones from humans with recessive hearing loss, they have not been definitively associated with specific gene mutations (Fig. 5–5).

Autosomal recessive congenital/prelingual profound hearing impairment loss

DFNB1

- MIM: 220290 (DFNB1), 121011 (GJB2), 604418 (GJB6)
- Location, gene: 13q12; *GJB2* (connexin 26), *GJB6* (connexin 30)

DFNB1 was initially localized in a Tunisian kindred (45). The responsible gene was found to be *GJB2* (connexin 26), and mutation of this gene has since been found to be the most common cause of recessive hearing loss.

Auditory findings. Although the first kindreds studied had severe to profound hearing impairment, mutation screening of unselected families with recessive nonsyndromic hearing loss has demonstrated the wide range of hearing loss that is possible, from mild to profound and including flat or sloping configurations. In addition, about one-third of cases have gradually progressive hearing loss. Variation is not mutation-specific and is observed within sibships (15,16,25,83).

Vestibular findings. Vestibular function is normal.

Radiology/histology. The CT scans of the temporal bones have been normal.

Molecular studies. The genomic knockout of connexin 26 is lethal in the mouse, so to study gene expression in vivo, a targeted, tissue-specific knockout of connexin 26 had to be created that eliminated the expression in the epithelial cells of the inner ear (14). Testing and histological examination showed that there were no vestibular abnormalities, but hearing loss was detectable by ABR in 3-week-old mice. Inner ear development appeared normal until 2 weeks postnatally. After that point, the organ of Corti began to collapse, and there was loss of the outer hair cells, the supporting cells around the hair cells, and the interdental cells of the spiral limbus. The inner hair cells appeared nor-

mal, but abnormalities of their synapses suggested immaturity. Not surprisingly, the endocochlear potential was also normal until postnatal day 14, when apparently connexin 26 gap junctions become essential. Subsequently, the endocochlear potential was decreased, along with decrease in K^+ concentrations in the endolymph. Since the damage in the cochlea was observable immediately upon onset of hearing at day 14, it was hypothesized that the normal response of the inner hair cells to sound generated an increase in K^+ in the perilymph, but the absence of connexin 26 gap junctions prevented the circulation of the potassium ions. This in turn would affect glutamate transport, which would lead to inhibition of glutathione. Glutathione acts as an antioxidant, and it is thought that accumulation of free radicals is a cause of noise damage to the inner ear. Thus, lack of connexin 26 could make the cochlea extremely sensitive to noise-induced hearing loss and lead to the types of cell damage and death that were observed.

Connexin gap junctions facilitate the cell-to-cell transfer of a variety of small molecules (<1 kDa) between adjacent cells (60,68,90). Gap junctions can form aggregates of hundreds to even thousands of intercellular contacts between cells. The primary determinant of differences in their specificity involves regulatory domains, which, in combination with highly conserved transmembrane domains, are responsible for maintenance of the dynamic intercellular flow of ions, cellular metabolites, and second messengers within adjacent cells (10,65,66,109,131,132). Understanding the pathogenic role of specific connexin gene mutations within the neural–auditory network is complicated by several factors: the multimeric structure of the assembled channels, the potential for heteromorphic interaction of different connexin subunits, the coordinate control of the expression of functionally related connexins, and, most importantly, the wide diversity of connexin mutations found among individual connexins (61). Indeed, due to the extensive molecular genetic heterogeneity of connexin gap junctions segregating in most populations, they are consistently found to be a major component of human hereditary deafness (19,54,64,99).

There are 20 different types of connexins, which are classified by molecular weight and similarity in subunit structure into one of four homology groups—α, β, γ, or unclassified (6,31,32,46,70,71,126). Variants associated with hearing loss involve the α- and β-connexin genes. There are at least seven human α-connexins—*GJA1, GJBA3–GJA5, GJA7, GJA8,* and *GJA10* (Cx43, Cx46, Cx37, Cx40, Cx45, Cx50, and Cx59)—and six human β-connexins—*GJB1–GJB6* (Cx32, Cx26, Cx32, Cx30.3, Cx31.1, Cx30). Each connexin exhibits different specificities, although many closely related connexins have similar tissue distribution and function. The basic structure of the α- and β-connexin genes is evolutionarily conserved. All involve a single exon encoding the protein subunit in combination with one or two 5′ upstream noncoding exons. During intracellular assembly, six connexin subunits combine to form a transmembrane channel protein called a connexon, which can be composed of the same or different types of connexins expressed in a specific cell type. Thus individual connexons can be homomeric (all the same connexin) or heteromeric (different connexin subunits). Upon docking of the hexameric connexon with its counterpart on an adjacent cell, the two connexons that join can be identical (homotypic channel) or nonidentical (heterotypic channel). Studies have demonstrated that both types of gap junction channels can be formed, which suggests the possibility for an additional level of complexity for unraveling the pathologic role of individual connexin mutations (70,71,99,112).

Connexins have four transmembrane domains that form the intercellular channel. The opening of gap junction channels is regulated by several factors including phosphorylation, voltage, and acidification. Interactions between different domains of transmembrane regions are critical for the permeability of the respective gap junctions. Several factors modulate gap junction permeability to produce three different types of gap junction channels (fast, intermediate, and long term). The amino and carboxyl termini of connexins and the region between the second and third transmembrane domains lies in the cytoplasm. Mutations that affect regulation of the connexins are most common within the cytoplasmic domains, which are critical in the regulation of the channel activity. The tissue distribution and temporal expression of each type of connexin are varied, although many appear to exhibit somewhat over-

Figure 5–5. *Autosomal recessive nonsyndromic hearing loss.* In a temporal bone section taken from a patient with autosomal recessive congenital severe hearing loss, a section from the basal turn of the cochlea shows atrophy of stria vascularis and degeneration of hair cells of organ of Corti. [From E Guli, U Bonetti, *Folia Hered Pathol (Milano)* 5:102, 1956.]

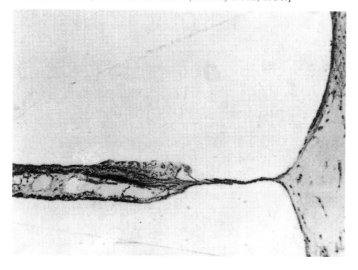

lapping specificities, tissue distribution, and shared functions within the auditory–neural axis and other tissues (34,97,99,120).

Willecke et al. (126) first assigned the genes for connexins 26, 32, 37, 40, 43, and 46 to human chromosomes, 13, X, 1, 6, and 13, respectively, by mapping on human–mouse somatic cell hybrids with rat cDNA probes. Subchromosomal assignments were deduced for Cx32 gene to Xq13–p11, for Cx37 and Cx40 genes to 1pter–q12, and for Cx43 to 6q14–qter. Additional studies confirmed and extended these assignments to include Cx43 (*GJA1*) on chromosome 6 and Cx32 (*GJB1*) on chromosome Xp11–q22 (32,110). Mignon and coworkers (85) assigned Cx26 (*GJB2*) and Cx46 (*GJA3*) genes to human chromosome 13q11–q12 and the homologous mouse chromosome 14D1-E1 by in situ hybridization. Kelley and coworkers (56) demonstrated that Cx26 and Cx30 were located with ~30 kb on chromosome 13q12. Cx26 and Cx30 were found to lie on the same large fragment PAC (P1 derived artificial chromosome) genomic clone that hybridized to chromosome 13q12. Human connexin 26 and connexin 30 are expressed in the same cells of the cochlea. Cx26 and Cx30 share 77% identity in amino acid sequence but Cx30 has an additional 37 amino acids at its C terminus. Cx50, also known as MP70, is expressed in the lens and was mapped to 1q21.1 by fluorescence in situ hybridization (FISH) to human chromosomes (38). Sequencing of the human genome and mapping of expressed sequences from a variety of tissues have facilitated the mapping and identification of human connexin genes, specifically as related to nonsyndromic hearing loss and syndromic hearing. These are presented in Table 5–4. This information is updated continuously and is available from online Web sites linked to the National Center for Biotechnology Information (NCBI) (http://www.ncbi.nlm.nih.gov/ Entrez/). Additional information on connexins related to deafness is available on several Web sites (http://www.crg.es/deafness/, http:// www.geneclinics.org/, http://www.uia.ac.be/dnalab/hhh, and http:// www.cdc.gov/genomics/hugenet/reviews/GJB2.htm).

The chromosomal assignment of deafness loci and connexin genes synergistically lead to the identification of mutations in Cx32 (*GJB1*) in X-linked Charcot-Marie-Tooth disease (12,13,18,50,91) as well as connexin 26 associated with nonsyndromic deafness (11,24,58,134). Mutations in connexin 26 (Cx26) are the predominant cause of both sporadic and hereditary childhood-onset nonsyndromic deafness (11,21,24,36,37,39,40,55,57,58,62,95,98,111,115). Over 70 different mutations within the Cx26 gene (*GJB2*; chromosome 13q12) are known (64,99,134). In most populations studied, there is usually a relatively high carrier frequency (>1%) for a single predominant recessive mutation. This includes the 35delG (2%–3%) in some Caucasian populations, 167delT in Ashkenazi Jews (4%), and 235delC in Asian populations (1%) (1,30,67,69,72,75,78,86,96,99,116,118,121). In general, the mutations involving loss of function (deletions, frame shift, splicing or unstable transcripts) are almost exclusively associated with severe to profound nonsyndromic deafness, although, depending on the site and nature of amino acid substitutions, there may or may not be associated pathological changes (syndromic) beyond hearing loss. There has not been a clear genotype–phenotype correlation for autosomal recessive *GJB2* mutations (15,16,25,29,75,87,88). In practical terms, the extensive heterogeneity of mutations creates a challenge to define the phenotype of a rare or private mutation (35,98). Moreover, there is a relatively wide variability of hearing impairment even among individuals with the same mutation and in the same family (52,98).

While Cx26 mutations are predominantly associated with nonsyndromic deafness, others lead to deafness associated with skin disorders or neurological disorders (17,27,28,48,57,60,64,73,82,101,106,119, 122). These relatively rare or private Cx26 missense mutations are detected in families with autosomal dominant inheritance (25,51,105,117). Many of these mutations are located within the extracellular domain or are located near boundaries of transmembrane domains. The generality with regard to Cx26-associated deafness is that most cases of prelingual deafness are caused by the lack of Cx26, and adult-onset hearing loss and skin disorders are mainly caused by missense Cx26 mutations in regions that are crucial for assembly or gating polarity of connexons. The dominant negative effect of the missense mutation on the normal connexin channels is thought to occur by disruption of docking or assembly of the gap junction. Finally, in a fashion common to most recessive conditions, there is a wide array of relatively rare or private recessive missense mutations dispersed among the remainder of the molecule, which in combination with the predominant loss of function mutations (i.e., 35delG, 167delT) result in nonsyndromic deafness (2–5). One incompletely resolved situation is the M34T Cx26 variant that was originally suggested to represent a causative mutation (20,39,40,42). This variation occurs relatively frequently in as many as 2%–2.5% of subjects with normal hearing, yet it does not occur among deaf individuals at increased frequency, as observed for the 35delG mutation (49). If the M34T substitution were a recessive mutation one would expect that it would occur as frequently as the 35delG mutation among deaf individuals, as either homozygotes or compound heterozygotes with the 35delG mutation. In fact, the M34T is not observed at increased frequency in deaf individuals beyond that observed in the normal hearing population (125). In vitro studies of M34T alleles in transfected cell lines suggest the channel has altered properties, although the actual formulation of heterotypic or homotypic gap junctions within the inner ear remains unclear (22,84,93). At present there is no compelling evidence that the M34T variant is a major contributor to hereditary deafness (43,44,64,125).

A major complication for clinical application of diagnostic tests for nonsyndromic congenital deafness is the finding that as many as 40%–50% of patients identified with a *GJB2* mutation are apparent heterozygotes for otherwise recessive mutations (39,40,63,64,83,92, 100,114,127). The single Cx26 mutation in a child with congenital deafness presents a difficult dilemma for diagnostic evaluation (8,81,83,108,113). The single Cx26 mutation associated with the hearing loss could be due to chance, since from 1% to 3% of normal hearing individuals are carriers of Cx26 mutations. Alternatively, it could indicate the presence of another yet undetected mutation in *GJB2* or possible interactions with mutations in other loci. This diagnostic problem is complicated by the observation that three different connexins (Cx26, Cx30, and Cx31) exhibit similar distributions and temporal patterns of expression within the inner ear, specifically within the regions of the spiral limbus, spiral ligament, and stria vacularis that are responsible for the recycling of K^+ ions in the endolymph. Each of these connexins could be a cause of hearing loss associated with an otherwise single Cx26 mutation. (56,77,79,80,123,124,129,130).

In some populations the apparent excess of Cx26 heterozygotes has been associated with a novel large 342 kb deletion that includes the closely linked Cx30 gene (*GJB6*) on the other non-Cx26 mutation chromosome (23,76,94). The 342 kb deletion does not extend into *GJB2*.

Table 5–4. Connexin genes, locations, and association with nonsyndromic and syndromic deafness loci

Connexin	Locus	Location	NSD	Syndrome	Reference No.
Cx43	GJA1	6q21–q23	DFNBG		77
Cx32	GJB1	Xq13.1		CMTX	7,9,47,50,133
Cx26	GJB2	13q11–q12	DFNB1	PPK, VS	30,37,48,58,64,74,100,101,106,134
			DFNA3		
Cx31	GJB3	1p34	DFNA2	EKV	77,128
Cx30	GJB6	13q11–q12	DFNB1	HED	26,41,56,76,94
			DFNA3		

Abbreviations: CMTX, X-linked Charcot-Marie-Tooth disease; EKV, erthrokeratodermia variabilis; HED, hidrotic ectodermal dysplasia; NSD, nonsyndromic deafness; PPK, palmoplantar keartodermia; VS, Vohwinkel syndrome.

Cx26 and Cx30 are very similar in amino acid sequence with nearly identical temporal and tissue distribution within the structures of the inner ear (53), and mutations in *GJB6* are also associated with hearing loss (41). Three independent reports have identified what appears to be the same deletion mutation (delGJB6:D13S1830) among Spanish, French, and Ashkenazi Jewish populations (23,76,94). The del-GJB6:D13S1830 mutation does not directly involve the nearby GJB2 transcript; however, it is postulated the deletion of the Cx30 transcript may cause nonsyndromic deafness in association with a single *GJB2* mutation through depletion of heterotypic channels (digenic interaction) or alternatively by disruption of the tissue-specific coordinate expression of the *GJB2* gene. This deletion mutation appears to account for one-half to two-thirds of previously undetected mutations in Cx26 heterozygotes of Spanish origin (23); it appears to be the second mutation in only about 10% of Cx26 heterozygotes in Caucasians in the United States and Northern Europe. Other mutations and deletions may be segregating in these populations. The complexity of genetic heterogeneity involving connexins is multifaceted and most likely involves heterotypic interaction of functionally related subunits, novel yet undetected mutations in the *GJB2–GJB6* region, and possibly other epigenic factors involved in the regulation and modulation of the respective gap junctions in the auditory–neural network (89,102). The discovery and identification of novel genes expressed in the cochlea will assist in future studies attempting to unravel these genotypic interactions (103). In addition, novel approaches will be required to understand the functional significance of sequence variations in genes expressed in the ear that affect hearing and are also expressed in alternative tissues more accessible for study, such as in the case of connexin expressed both within the ear and the skin (101,104,107).

Heredity. Inheritance is autosomal recessive.

Prognosis. Because of the wide variation in phenotype, it is difficult to predict the extent of hearing loss or the stability.

Summary. Mutation of *GJB2* accounts for as much as half of recessive nonsyndromic hearing loss. Since there are still a significant number of affected individuals with one *GJB2* mutation, additional mutations of *GJB2* or other genes await discovery.

References

1. Abe S et al: Prevalent connexin 26 gene (*GJB2*) mutations in Japanese. *J Med Genet* 37:41–43, 2000.
2. Angeli S et al: *GJB2* gene mutations in childhood deafness. *Acta Otolaryngol* 120:133–136, 2000.
3. Antoniadi T et al: Mutation analysis of the *GJB2* (connexin 26) gene by DGGE in Greek patients with sensorineural deafness. *Hum Mutat* 16:7–12, 2000.
4. Baris I et al: Frequency of the 35delG mutation in the connexin 26 gene in Turkish hearing-impaired patients. *Clin Genet* 60:452–455, 2001.
5. Bason L et al: Homozygosity for the V37I connexin 26 mutation in three unrelated children with sensorineural hearing loss. *Clin Genet* 61:459–464, 2002.
6. Bennett MV et al: The connexins and their family tree. *Soc Gen Physiol Ser* 49:223–233, 1994.
7. Bissar-Tadmouri N et al: Mutational analysis and genotype/phenotype correlation in Turkish Charcot-Marie-Tooth type 1 and HNPP patients. *Clin Genet* 58:396–402, 2000.
8. Bitner-Glindzicz M: Hereditary deafness and phenotyping in humans. *Br Med Bull* 63:73–94, 2002.
9. Bondurand N et al: Human connexin 32, a gap junction protein altered in the X-linked form of Charcot-Marie-Tooth disease, is directly regulated by the transcription factor SOX10. *Hum Mol Genet* 10:2783–2795, 2001.
10. Bruzzone R et al: Connections with connexins: the molecular basis of direct intercellular signaling. *Eur J Biochem* 238:1–27, 1996.
11. Carrasquillo MM et al: Two different connexin 26 mutations in an inbred kindred segregating non-syndromic recessive deafness: implications for genetic studies in isolated populations. *Hum Mol Genet* 6:2163–2172, 1997.
12. Chance PF, Lupski JR: Inherited neuropathies: Charcot-Marie-Tooth disease and related disorders. *Baillieres Clin Neurol* 3:373–385, 1994.
13. Cochrane S et al: X linked Charcot-Marie-Tooth disease (CMTX1): a study of 15 families with 12 highly informative polymorphisms. *J Med Genet* 31:193–196, 1994.
14. Cohen-Salmon M et al: Targeted ablation of connexin26 in the inner ear epithelial gap junction network causes hearing impairment and cell death. *Curr Biol* 12:1006–1111, 2002.
15. Cohn ES, Kelley PM: Clinical phenotype and mutations in connexin 26 (DFNB1/GJB2), the most common cause of childhood hearing loss. *Am J Med Genet* 89:130–136, 1999.
16. Cohn ES et al: Clinical studies of families with hearing loss attributable to mutations in the connexin 26 gene (*GJB2*/DFNB1). *Pediatrics* 103:546–550, 1999.
17. Common JE et al: Functional studies of human skin disease- and deafness-associated connexin 30 mutations. *Biochem Biophys Res Commun* 298:651–656, 2002.
18. Corcos IA et al: Refined localization of human connexin32 gene locus, *GJB1*, to Xq13.1. *Genomics* 13:479–480, 1992.
19. Cremers FP: Genetic causes of hearing loss. *Curr Opin Neurol* 11:11–16, 1998.
20. Cucci RA et al: The M34T allele variant of connexin 26. *Genet Test* 4:335–344, 2000.
21. Dahl HH et al: Prevalence and nature of connexin 26 mutations in children with non-syndromic deafness. *Med J Aust* 175:191–194, 2001.
22. D'Andrea P et al: Hearing loss: frequency and functional studies of the most common connexin26 alleles. *Biochem Biophys Res Commun* 296:685–691, 2002.
23. del Castillo I et al: A deletion involving the connexin 30 gene in nonsyndromic hearing impairment. *N Engl J Med* 346:243–249, 2002.
24. Denoyelle F et al: Prelingual deafness: high prevalence of a 30delG mutation in the connexin 26 gene. *Hum Mol Genet* 6:2173–2177, 1997.
25. Denoyelle F et al: Connexin 26 gene linked to a dominant deafness. *Nature* 393:319–320, 1998.
26. Denoyelle F et al: Clinical features of the prevalent form of childhood deafness, DFNB1, due to a connexin-26 gene defect: implications for genetic counselling. *Lancet* 353:1298–1303, 1999.
27. Di WL et al: Connexin 26 expression and mutation analysis in epidermal disease. *Cell Adhes Commun* 8:415–418, 2001.
28. Di WL et al: Defective trafficking and cell death is characteristic of skin disease–associated connexin 31 mutations. *Hum Mol Genet* 11:2005–2014, 2002.
29. Engel-Yeger B et al: The effects of a connexin 26 mutation—35delG—on oto-acoustic emissions and brainstem evoked potentials: homozygotes and carriers. *Hear Res* 163:93–100, 2002.
30. Estivill X et al: Connexin-26 mutations in sporadic and inherited sensorineural deafness. *Lancet* 351:394–398, 1998.
31. Evans WH, Martin PE: Gap junctions: structure and function (review). *Mol Membr Biol* 19:121–136, 2002.
32. Fishman GI et al: The human connexin gene family of gap junction proteins: distinct chromosomal locations but similar structures. *Genomics* 10:250–256, 1991.
33. Forge A et al: Gap junctions and connexin expression in the inner ear. *Novartis Found Symp* 219:134–150, 1999.
34. Forge A et al: Connexins and gap junctions in the inner ear. *Audiol Neurootol* 7:141–145, 2002.
35. Fuse Y et al: Three novel connexin26 gene mutations in autosomal recessive non-syndromic deafness. *Neuroreport* 10:1853–1857, 1999.
36. Gabriel H et al: Mutations in the connexin26/*GJB2* gene are the most common event in non-syndromic hearing loss among the German population. *Hum Mutat* 17:521–522, 2001.
37. Gasparini P et al: High carrier frequency of the 35delG deafness mutation in European populations. Genetic Analysis Consortium of GJB2 35delG. *Eur J Hum Genet* 8:19–23, 2000.
38. Geyer DD et al: Regional mapping of the human *MP70* (Cx50; connexin 50) gene by fluorescence in situ hybridization to 1q21.1. *Mol Vis* 3:13, 1997.
39. Green GE et al: Carrier rates in the midwestern United States for *GJB2* mutations causing inherited deafness. *JAMA* 281:2211–2216, 1999.
40. Green GE et al: Genetic testing to identify deaf newborns. *JAMA* 284:1245, 2000.
41. Grifa A et al: Mutations in *GJB6* cause nonsyndromic autosomal dominant deafness at DFNA3 locus. *Nat Genet* 23:16–18, 1999.
42. Griffith AJ: Genetic analysis of the connexin-26 M34T variant. *J Med Genet* 38:E24, 2001.
43. Griffith AJ, Friedman TB: Auditory function and the M34T allele of connexin 26. *Arch Otolaryngol Head Neck Surg* 128:94, 2002.
44. Griffith AJ et al: Autosomal recessive nonsyndromic neurosensory deafness at DFNB1 not associated with the compound-heterozygous *GJB2*

(connexin 26) genotype M34T/167delT. *Am J Hum Genet* 67:745–749, 2000.

45. Guilford P et al: A nonsyndromic form of neurosensory, recessive deafness maps to the pericentromeric region of chromosome 13q. *Nat Genet* 6:24–28, 1994.

46. Haefliger JA et al: Four novel members of the connexin family of gap junction proteins. Molecular cloning, expression, and chromosome mapping. *J Biol Chem* 267:2057–2064, 1992.

47. Hahn AF et al: Genotype/phenotype correlations in X-linked dominant Charcot-Marie-Tooth disease. *Ann NY Acad Sci* 883:366–382, 1999.

48. Heathcote K et al: A connexin 26 mutation causes a syndrome of sensorineural hearing loss and palmoplantar hyperkeratosis (MIM 148350). *J Med Genet* 37:50–51, 2000.

49. Houseman MJ et al: Genetic analysis of the connexin-26 M34T variant: identification of genotype M34T/M34T segregating with mild-moderate non-syndromic sensorineural hearing loss. *J Med Genet* 38:20–25, 2001.

50. Ionasescu V et al: Point mutations of the connexin32 (GJB1) gene in X-linked dominant Charcot-Marie-Tooth neuropathy. *Hum Mol Genet* 3:355–358, 1994.

51. Janecke AR et al: De novo mutation of the connexin 26 gene associated with dominant non-syndromic sensorineural hearing loss. *Hum Genet* 108:269–270, 2001.

52. Janecke AR et al: Progressive hearing loss, and recurrent sudden sensorineural hearing loss associated with *GJB2* mutations—phenotypic spectrum and frequencies of *GJB2* mutations in Austria. *Hum Genet* 111:145–153, 2002.

53. Kammen-Jolly K et al: Connexin 26 in human fetal development of the inner ear. *Hear Res* 160:15–21, 2001.

54. Keats BJ, Berlin CI: Genomics and hearing impairment. *Genome Res* 9:7–16, 1999.

55. Kelley PM et al: Novel mutations in the connexin 26 gene (*GJB2*) that cause autosomal recessive (DFNB1) hearing loss. *Am J Hum Genet* 62:792–799, 1998.

56. Kelley PM et al: Human connexin 30 (*GJB6*), a candidate gene for non-syndromic hearing loss: molecular cloning, tissue-specific expression, and assignment to chromosome 13q12. *Genomics* 62:172–176, 1999.

57. Kelley PM et al: Connexin 26: required for normal auditory function. *Brain Res Brain Res Rev* 32:184–188, 2000.

58. Kelsell DP et al: Connexin 26 mutations in hereditary non-syndromic sensorineural deafness. *Nature* 387:80–83, 1997.

59. Kelsell DP et al: Connexin mutations associated with palmoplantar keratoderma and profound deafness in a single family. *Eur J Hum Genet* 8:141–144, 2000.

60. Kelsell DP et al: Connexin mutations in skin disease and hearing loss. *Am J Hum Genet* 68:559–568, 2001.

61. Kelsell DP et al: Human diseases: clues to cracking the connexin code? *Trends Cell Biol* 11:2–6, 2001.

62. Kemperman MH et al: Hearing loss and connexin 26. *J R Soc Med* 95:171–177, 2002.

63. Kenna MA et al: Connexin 26 studies in patients with sensorineural hearing loss. *Arch Otolaryngol Head Neck Surg* 127:1037–1042, 2001.

64. Kenneson A et al: *GJB2* (connexin 26) variants and nonsyndromic sensorineural hearing loss: a HuGE review. *Genet Med* 4:258–274, 2002.

65. Kikuchi T et al: Potassium ion recycling pathway via gap junction systems in the mammalian cochlea and its interruption in hereditary nonsyndromic deafness. *Med Electron Microsc* 33:51–56, 2000.

66. Kikuchi T et al: Gap junction systems in the mammalian cochlea. *Brain Res Brain Res Rev* 32:163–166, 2000.

67. Kitamura K et al: Deafness genes. *J Med Dent Sci* 47:1–11, 2000.

68. Krutovskikh V, Yamasaki H: Connexin gene mutations in human genetic diseases. *Mutat Res* 462:197–207, 2000.

69. Kudo T et al: Novel mutations in the connexin 26 gene (*GJB2*) responsible for childhood deafness in the Japanese population. *Am J Med Genet* 90:141–145, 2000.

70. Kumar NM: Molecular biology of the interactions between connexins. *Novartis Found Symp* 219:6–16, 1999.

71. Kumar NM, Gilula NB: Molecular biology and genetics of gap junction channels. *Semin Cell Biol* 3:3–16, 1992.

72. Kupka S et al: Frequencies of *GJB2* mutations in German control individuals and patients showing sporadic non-syndromic hearing impairment. *Hum Mutat* 20:77–78, 2002.

73. Lamartine J et al: Mutations in *GJB6* cause hidrotic ectodermal dysplasia. *Nat Genet* 26:142–144, 2000.

74. Lench N et al: Connexin-26 mutations in sporadic non-syndromal sensorineural deafness. *Lancet* 351:415, 1998.

75. Lerer I et al: Contribution of connexin 26 mutations to nonsyndromic deafness in Ashkenazi patients and the variable phenotypic effect of the mutation 167delT. *Am J Med Genet* 95:53–56, 2000.

76. Lerer I et al: A deletion mutation in *GJB6* cooperating with a *GJB2* mutation in *trans* in non-syndromic deafness: a novel founder mutation in Ashkenazi Jews. *Hum Mutat* 18:460, 2001.

77. Liu XZ et al: Mutations in connexin31 underlie recessive as well as dominant non-syndromic hearing loss. *Hum Mol Genet* 9:63–67, 2000.

78. Liu XZ et al: The prevalence of connexin 26 (*GJB2*) mutations in the Chinese population. *Hum Genet* 111:394–397, 2002.

79. Lopez-Bigas N et al: Connexin 31 (GJB3) is expressed in the peripheral and auditory nerves and causes neuropathy and hearing impairment. *Hum Mol Genet* 10:947–952, 2001.

80. Lopez-Bigas N et al: R32W variant in connexin 31: mutation or polymorphism for deafness and skin disease? *Eur J Hum Genet* 9:70, 2001.

81. Lucotte G, Mercier G: Meta-analysis of *GJB2* mutation 35delG frequencies in Europe. *Genet Test* 5:149–152, 2001.

82. Maestrini E et al: A missense mutation in connexin26, D66H, causes mutilating keratoderma with sensorineural deafness (Vohwinkel's syndrome) in three unrelated families. *Hum Mol Genet* 8:1237–1243, 1999.

83. Marlin S et al: Connexin 26 gene mutations in congenitally deaf children: pitfalls for genetic counseling. *Arch Otolaryngol Head Neck Surg* 127:927–933, 2001.

84. Martin PE et al: Properties of connexin26 gap junctional proteins derived from mutations associated with non-syndromal hereditary deafness. *Hum Mol Genet* 8:2369–2376, 1999.

85. Mignon C et al: Assignment of connexin 26 (*GJB2*) and 46 (*GJA3*) genes to human chromosome 13q11 → q12 and mouse chromosome 14D1-E1 by in situ hybridization. *Cytogenet Cell Genet* 72:185–186, 1996.

86. Morell RJ et al: Mutations in the connexin 26 gene (*GJB2*) among Ashkenazi Jews with nonsyndromic recessive deafness. *N Engl J Med* 339:1500–1505, 1998.

87. Mueller RF et al: Congenital non-syndromal sensorineural hearing impairment due to connexin 26 gene mutations—molecular and audiological findings. *Int J Pediatr Otorhinolaryngol* 50:3–13, 1999.

88. Murgia A et al: Cx26 deafness: mutation analysis and clinical variability. *J Med Genet* 36:829–832, 1999.

89. Nance WE et al: Relation between choice of partner and high frequency of connexin-26 deafness. *Lancet* 356:500–501, 2000.

90. Nicholson SM, Bruzzone R: Gap junctions: getting the message through. *Curr Biol* 7:R340–R344, 1997.

91. Orth U et al: X-linked dominant Charcot-Marie-Tooth neuropathy: valine-38-methionine substitution of connexin32. *Hum Mol Genet* 3:1699–1700, 1994.

92. Orzan E et al: Connexin 26 preverbal hearing impairment: mutation prevalence and heterozygosity in a selected population. *Int J Audiol* 41:120–124, 2002.

93. Oshima A et al: Roles of M34, C64, and R75 in the assembly of human connexin 26: implication for key amino acid residues for channel formation and function. *J Biol Chem* 15:15, 2002.

94. Pallares-Ruiz N et al: A large deletion including most of GJB6 in recessive non-syndromic deafness: a digenic effect? *Eur J Hum Genet* 10:72–76, 2002.

95. Pampanos A et al: Prevalence of *GJB2* mutations in prelingual deafness in the Greek population. *Int J Pediatr Otorhinolaryngol* 65:101–108, 2002.

96. Park HJ et al: Connexin26 mutations associated with nonsyndromic hearing loss. *Laryngoscope* 110:1535–1538, 2000.

97. Plum A et al: Unique and shared functions of different connexins in mice. *Curr Biol* 10:1083–1091, 2000.

98. Prasad S et al: Genetic testing for hereditary hearing loss: connexin 26 (*GJB2*) allele variants and two novel deafness-causing mutations (R32C and 645-648delTAGA). *Hum Mutat* 16:502–508, 2000.

99. Rabionet R et al: Molecular genetics of hearing impairment due to mutations in gap junction genes encoding beta connexins. *Hum Mutat* 16:190–202, 2000.

100. Rabionet R et al: Molecular basis of childhood deafness resulting from mutations in the *GJB2* (connexin 26) gene. *Hum Genet* 106:40–44, 2000.

101. Rabionet R et al: Connexin mutations in hearing loss, dermatological and neurological disorders. *Trends Mol Med* 8:205–212, 2002.

102. Read AP: Hereditary deafness: lessons for developmental studies and genetic diagnosis. *Eur J Pediatr* 159 Suppl 3:S232–S235, 2000.

103. Resendes BL et al: Gene discovery in the auditory system: characterization of additional cochlear-expressed sequences. *J Assoc Res Otolaryngol* 3:45–53, 2002.

104. Richard G: Connexins: a connection with the skin. *Exp Dermatol* 9:77–96, 2000.

105. Richard G et al: Functional defects of Cx26 resulting from a heterozygous missense mutation in a family with dominant deaf-mutism and palmoplantar keratoderma. *Hum Genet* 103:393–399, 1998.

106. Richard G et al: Missense mutations in *GJB2* encoding connexin-26 cause the ectodermal dysplasia keratitis-ichthyosis-deafness syndrome. *Am J Hum Genet* 70:1341–1348, 2002.

107. Risek B et al: Multiple gap junction genes are utilized during rat skin and hair development. *Development* 116:639–651, 1992.

108. Robin NH et al: Pediatric otolaryngologists' knowledge and understanding of genetic testing for deafness. *Arch Otolaryngol Head Neck Surg* 127:937–940, 2001.

109. Ruch RJ: The role of gap junctional intercellular communication in neoplasia. *Ann Clin Lab Sci* 24:216–231, 1994.

110. Schwarz HJ et al: Chromosomal assignments of mouse genes for connexin 50 and connexin 33 by somatic cell hybridization. *Somat Cell Mol Genet* 20:243–247, 1994.

111. Scott DA et al: Identification of mutations in the connexin 26 gene that cause autosomal recessive nonsyndromic hearing loss. *Hum Mutat* 11:387–394, 1998.

112. Shibata Y et al: Diversity and molecular anatomy of gap junctions. *Med Electron Microsc* 34:153–159, 2001.

113. Skvorak Giersch AB, Morton CC: Genetic causes of nonsyndromic hearing loss. *Curr Opin Pediatr* 11:551–557, 1999.

114. Smith RJH: Mutation screening for deafness: more than simply another diagnostic test. *Arch Otolaryngol Head Neck Surg* 127:941–942, 2001.

115. Smith RJH, Van Camp G: Non-syndromic hearing impairment: gene linkage and cloning. *Int J Pediatr Otorhinolaryngol* 49 Suppl 1:S159–S163, 1999.

116. Sobe T et al: High frequency of the deafness-associated 167delT mutation in the connexin 26 (*GJB2*) gene in Israeli Ashkenazim. *Am J Med Genet* 86:499–500, 1999.

117. Tekin M et al: W44C mutation in the connexin 26 gene associated with dominant non-syndromic deafness. *Clin Genet* 59:269–273, 2001.

118. Usami S et al: Molecular diagnosis of deafness: impact of gene identification. *Audiol Neurootol* 7:185–90, 2002.

119. Uyguner O et al: The novel R75Q mutation in the *GJB2* gene causes autosomal dominant hearing loss and palmoplantar keratoderma in a Turkish family. *Clin Genet* 62:306–309, 2002.

120. Van Hauwe P et al: The DFNA2 locus for hearing impairment: two genes regulating K$^+$ ion recycling in the inner ear. *Br J Audiol* 33:285–289, 1999.

121. Van Laer L et al: A common founder for the 35delG *GJB2* gene mutation in connexin 26 hearing impairment. *J Med Genet* 38:515–518, 2001.

122. van Steensel MA et al: A novel connexin 26 mutation in a patient diagnosed with keratitis-ichthyosis-deafness syndrome. *J Invest Dermatol* 118:724–727, 2002.

123. Wangemann P: K(+) cycling and the endocochlear potential. *Hear Res* 165:1–9, 2002.

124. Wenzel K et al: Human gap junction protein connexin31: molecular cloning and expression analysis. *Biochem Biophys Res Commun* 248:910–915, 1998.

125. Wilcox SA et al: High frequency hearing loss correlated with mutations in the *GJB2* gene. *Hum Genet* 106:399–405, 2000.

126. Willecke K et al: Six genes of the human connexin gene family coding for gap junctional proteins are assigned to four different human chromosomes. *Eur J Cell Biol* 53:275–280, 1990.

127. Wu BL et al: Effectiveness of sequencing connexin 26 (*GJB2*) in cases of familial or sporadic childhood deafness referred for molecular diagnostic testing. *Genet Med* 4:279–288, 2002.

128. Xia JH et al: Mutations in the gene encoding gap junction protein beta-3 associated with autosomal dominant hearing impairment. *Nat Genet* 20:370–373, 1998.

129. Xia AP et al: Expression of connexin 31 in the developing mouse cochlea. *Neuroreport* 11:2449–2453, 2000.

130. Xia A et al: Expression of connexin 30 in the developing mouse cochlea. *Brain Res* 898:364–367, 2001.

131. Yamasaki H et al: Connexin genes and cell growth control. *Arch Toxicol Suppl* 18:105–114, 1996.

132. Yamasaki H et al: Role of connexin (gap junction) genes in cell growth control and carcinogenesis. *C R Acad Sci III* 322:151–159, 1999.

133. Yoshimura T et al: Mutations of connexin32 in Charcot-Marie-Tooth disease type X interfere with cell-to-cell communication but not cell proliferation and myelin-specific gene expression. *J Neurosci Res* 51:154–161, 1998.

134. Zelante L et al: Connexin26 mutations associated with the most common form of non-syndromic neurosensory autosomal recessive deafness (DFNB1) in Mediterraneans. *Hum Mol Genet* 6:1605–1609, 1997.

DFNB2

- MIM: 600060 (DFNB2), 276903 (MYO7A)
- Location, gene: 11q13.5; *MYO7A* (myosin VIIA)

Nonsyndromic recessive hearing impairment due to mutation in *MYO7A* has been described in 3 families, one Tunisian (2) and two Chinese (3). Mutations of *MYO7A* also cause DFNA11 and Usher syndrome type 1B.

Auditory findings. By report, onset of hearing loss was variable within the large, inbred Tunisian kindred, ranging from birth to 16 years of age, although all individuals had severe to profound hearing loss across all frequencies when tested.

Vestibular findings. Zina et al. (6) re-examined the Tunisian kindred and found absent vestibular function in some affected individuals.

Radiology/histology. No studies were reported.

Molecular studies. DFNB2 was localized to 11q13 by linkage studies with the Tunisian and Chinese families, and it was noted that the region overlapped that of Usher syndrome 1B. The homologous region in the mouse contains the locus for *shaker-1*, a mutant phenotype with vestibular abnormalities and deafness, but without obvious retinopathy. When mutation of myosin VIIA was found to be the cause of *shaker-1*, it was immediately tested in individuals with Usher 1B (4). Subsequently, the Tunisian kindred was studied and a homozygous 1797G → A mutation was found at the last nucleotide of exon 15, producing an M599I substitution. This mutation is in the motor domain of the molecule, so the effect could be either on motility or splicing efficiency (5). In the two Chinese families studied, one was found to be homozygous for a 731G → C mutation, producing a R244P change, also in the motor domain. The other family showed compound heterozygosity; one mutation was an insertion of a T at nucleotide position 3596 in the tail region, producing an aberrant amino acid and a frameshift, leading to truncation 28 amino acids downstream, and the other mutation was an acceptor splice site mutation in intron 3 (3). Astuto et al. (1) have noted that there is no discernable difference between mutations that can cause Usher syndrome and those that are nonsyndromic, and have questioned whether the cases of DFNB2 are truly nonsyndromic. In partial support of this, follow-up of the Tunisian kindred indicated that some individuals had mild retinal degeneration and retinal pigmentation (6). However, members of the Chinese families had normal electroretinogram studies, which suggest that if there is retinal involvement in the DFNB2 families, it may be considerably delayed.

Heredity. Inheritance is autosomal recessive with complete penetrance.

Prognosis. Profound sensorineural hearing loss and vestibular dysfunction occur. The hearing loss may be progressive in childhood, but this has not been clearly documented. If retinopathy exists, it appears to be either asymptomatic or late onset.

Summary. Myosins are extremely important in the function of the inner ear, as evidenced by three hearing loss phenotypes produced by mutations of *MYO7A* (DFNA11, DFNB2, USH1A), as well as hearing loss caused by *MYO3* (DFNB30), *MYO6* (DFNA22), and *MYO15* (DFNB3).

References

1. Astuto LM et al: Searching for evidence of DFNB2. *Am J Med Genet* 109:291–297, 2002.

2. Guilford P et al: A human gene responsible for neurosensory, nonsyndromic recessive deafness is a candidate homologue of the mouse *sh-1* gene. *Hum Mol Genet* 3:989–993, 1994.

3. Liu XZ et al: Mutations in the myosin VIIA gene cause nonsyndromic recessive deafness. *Nat Genet* 16:188–190, 1997.

4. Weil D et al: Defective myosin VIIA gene responsible for Usher syndrome type 1B. *Nature* 374:60–61, 1995.

5. Weil D et al: The autosomal recessive isolated deafness, DFNB2, and the Usher 1B syndrome are allelic defects of the myosin-VIIA gene. *Nat Genet* 16:191–193, 1997.
6. Zina ZB et al: From DFNB2 to Usher syndrome: variable expressivity of the same disease. *Am J Med Genet* 101:181–183, 2001.

DFNB3

- MIM: 600316 (DFNB3), 602666 (MYO15A)
- Location, gene: 17p11.2

DFNB3 was described in individuals from Bengkala, Bali, in Indonesia. In this population, 2% of the people were hearing impaired, presumably from this autosomal recessive condition (1). Two additional families from India and three from Pakistan have also been reported (2,4).

Auditory findings. Deafness was congenital and in the severe-to-profound level in all individuals tested.

Vestibular findings. There were no symptoms of vestibular dysfunction.

Radiology/histology. No studies were reported.

Molecular studies. Like myosin VIIA, myosin XV is also an unconventional (non-muscle) myosin. Mutation in the homologous gene in the mouse, *Myo15*, causes the shaker-2 (sh2) phenotype with vestibular deficits and deafness in the homozygote. In this mutant, cochlear hair cells had shortened stereocilia and their actin cores appeared disorganized. A C → A point mutation, creating a cysteine-to-tyrosine substitution, was found in the motor domain of Myo15 (5). Also in the mouse, Myo15 expression was detected in the cochlear and vestibular sensory epithelium and was seen by immunofluorescence in the cuticular plate at the base of the stereocilia, as well as in the stereocilia themselves. Thus, the function of Myo15 appears to be in the actin structure and anchoring of the stereocilia. As there is also expression in pituitary tissues, the authors cautioned that there could be associated symptoms of pituitary dysfunction with DFNB3, although these have not been observed clinically (3).

In all of the families studied, mutations were homozygous in affected individuals. In the Bengkala kindred, a 2674A → T transversion created an I892F substitution in the MyTH4 domain in the tail region of the protein. Both Indian families also had mutations in the tail region—one had a 3898A → T mutation that produced a stop codon (K1300X), while the other had a 2668A → T mutation (N890Y) in the MyTH4 region (6). One of the Pakistani families had an 8486G → T transversion producing a Q2716H substitution in another domain of the tail, the FERM domain. Although the exact functions of these regions in *MYO15* are unknown, the tail is presumed to be involved in binding to membranes or to other macromolecular structures for transport. Mutations in the other two Pakistani families were different—a 4023C → T mutation producing a stop codon in exon 3 of the motor domain, and a mutation of a splice site donor in intron 4, also in the motor domain (4). Interestingly, Liburd et al. (4) also noted that the *MYO15* gene was included in the chromosomal deletion in a child with Smith-Magenis syndrome who had a moderate to severe high-frequency loss, and suggested that haploinsufficiency for myosin XV gene may be the cause of hearing loss observed in some children with the syndrome.

Heredity. Inheritance is autosomal recessive with complete penetrance.

Prognosis. Severe to profound congenital hearing impairment occurs. Although pituitary dysfunction has not been observed, expression of *MYO15* in pituitary tissues suggests that this possibility should be considered.

Summary. Myosin XV is one of the group of unconventional myosins required for hair cell and stereocilia structure and function.

Through a contiguous deletion, this gene may also account for hearing loss in individuals with Smith-Magenis syndrome.

References

1. Friedman TB et al: A gene for congenital, recessive deafness DFNB3 maps to the pericentromeric region of chromosome 17. *Nat Genet* 9:86–91, 1995.
2. Liang Y et al: Genetic mapping refines DFNB3 to 17p11.2, suggests multiple alleles of DFNB3, and supports homology to the mouse model *shaker-2*. *Am J Hum Genet* 62:904–915, 1998.
3. Liang Y et al: Characterization of the human and mouse unconventional myosin XV genes responsible for hereditary deafness DFNB3 and Shaker 2. *Genomics* 61:243–258, 1999.
4. Liburd N et al: Novel mutations of *MYO15A* associated with profound deafness in consanguineous families and moderately severe hearing loss in a patient with Smith-Magenis syndrome. *Hum Genet* 109:535–541, 2001.
5. Probst FJ et al: Correction of deafness in *shaker 2* mice by an unconventional myosin in a BAC transgene. *Science* 280:1444–1447, 1998.
6. Wang A et al: Association of unconventional myosin *MYO15* mutations with human nonsyndromic deafness DFNB3. *Science* 280:1447–1451, 1998.

DFNB5

- MIM: 600792
- Location, gene: 14q12; gene unknown

Linkage of hearing impairment to 14q12 was found in a consanguineous family from India using homozygosity mapping (1). In the publication, this locus was referred to as DFNB4, but it later officially became DFNB5.

Auditory findings. The three affected children in this family all had severe to profound congenital hearing impairment.

Vestibular findings. No evaluations were reported.

Radiology/histology. No studies were reported.

Molecular studies. Linkage analysis and haplotype mapping placed the region containing the DFNB5 gene between D14S70 and D14S288, which was estimated to cover 2–6 cM (by current maps, the estimate is 7–8 cM; see http://www.ncbi.nlm.nih.gov/cgi-bin/Entrez/map_search).

Heredity. Inheritance is autosomal recessive with complete penetrance.

Prognosis. Congenital severe to profound hearing impairment occurs.

Summary. This is one of many recessive genes causing nonsyndromic hearing impairment that are phenotypically indistinguishable. The technique used to map this gene exploits the value of consanguineous families in identifying these genes.

References

1. Fukushima K et al: Consanguineous nuclear families used to identify a new locus for recessive non-syndromic hearing loss on 14q. *Hum Mol Genet* 4:1643–1648, 1995.

DFNB6

- MIM: 600971 (DFNB6); 607237 (TMIE)
- Location, gene: 3p21; *TMIE* (transmembrane inner ear–expressed gene)

DFNB6 was first localized by homozygosity mapping in a consanguineous Indian family (1). Four additional consanguineous families were identified that showed linkage to the same region (3).

Auditory findings. All individuals had congenital severe to profound hearing loss.

Vestibular findings. Affected individuals in one family were delayed in learning to walk, which could reflect vestibular abnormality. Further clinical studies could not be done.

Radiology/histology. No studies were reported.

Molecular studies. Because of chromosomal homology with the linked region, the mouse mutant *spinner* is a candidate for DFNB6. The *spinner* mouse has deafness and vestibular dysfunction, and histologic studies show abnormal maturation of the stereocilia of the cochlear hair cells. The causal gene for *spinner* was found to be *Tmie*, a novel gene that has no sequence similarities to known genes. Two possible transmembrane domains, one of which overlaps a predicted signal peptide, have been identified. This, along with the histologic studies, suggests a function similar to the unconventional myosins in development and maintenance of stereocilia (2).

Mutation analysis of *TMIE* in the five identified families showed homozygosity for a different mutation. These included three missense mutations involving arginine in exon 3—R84W, R81C, and R92W. These are expected to be in the cytoplasmic domain of the molecule. The other two mutations may inactivate the protein. One was a 4 bp insertion in exon 2 which produced a frameshift with 72 aberrant amino acids before reaching a stop codon; and the other was deletion/insertion in the intron between exons 1 and 2, altering the acceptor splice site (3).

Heredity. Inheritance is autosomal dominant.

Prognosis. Profound congenital hearing impairment occurs.

Summary. The genetic mutation underlying this form of recessive congenital hearing loss may have functional homology to other disorders that affect the structure and function of the stereocilia.

References

1. Fukushima K et al: An autosomal recessive nonsyndromic form of sensorineural hearing loss maps to 3p-DFNB6. *Genome Res* 5:305–308, 1995.
2. Mitchem KL et al: Mutation of the novel gene *Tmie* results in sensory cell defects in the inner ear of *spinner*, a mouse model of human hearing loss DFNB6. *Hum Mol Genet* 11:1887–1898, 2002.
3. Naz S et al: Mutations in a novel gene, *TMIE*, are associated with hearing loss linked to the DFNB6 locus. *Am J Hum Genet* 71:632–636, 2002.

DFNB7/11

- MIM: 600974 (DFNB7 and 11), 606707 (TMC1)
- Location, gene: 9q13–q21; *TMC1* (transmembrane cochlear-expressed gene 1)

DFNA7 was localized in two consanguineous Indian families (1), and DFNA11 was found in two inbred Israeli Bedouin kindreds (3). The critical regions were adjacent, and with identification of the *TMC1* gene, it was shown that the two loci were the same. Mutation in this gene also causes the autosomal dominant DFNA36 phenotype.

Auditory findings. All affected individuals had congenital profound hearing impairment.

Vestibular findings. No studies have been reported.

Radiology/histology. No studies have been reported.

Molecular studies. (See DFNA36, above, for a description of *TCM1* structure and expression.) *TCM1* is homologous to *Tcm1* in the mouse, and mutations in that gene produce the dominant Beethoven (Bth) and recessive deafness (dn) phenotypes, as well as the human dominant DFNA36. The function of the gene is unknown, but six transmembrane loops are recognizable. *TCM1* was analyzed for mutations in 11 consanguineous multiplex DFNB7/11 families from India and Pakistan. Five Pakistani families had a 100C → T mutation that substituted a stop codon for an arginine, and haplotype analysis indicated that this

most likely came from a common founder. Two additional families had point mutations that would be predicted to result in terminations: a 1534C → T (R512X), and a deletion of an alanine at nucleotide 295. An eighth family had a 26.7 kb deletion that would include exons 4 and 5, and another had an intronic mutation that would be expected to affect a splice donor site. Thus all of these mutations could be null alleles. A tenth family had a 1960A → G missense mutation that would produce a M654V substitution. This methionine was conserved in *TCM2* and *Tcm1* and would be in a transmembrane domain. If it disrupted the structure of the protein, it could also be a functional null. The last family had an intronic mutation that affected a splice acceptor, but the effects of the mutation could not be determined. Overall, the mutations found in the recessive families fit with the prediction that null alleles would produce normal phenotypes in the heterozygotes but have severe effects in the homozygote, while mutations with less effect on structure could have a dominant-negative effect (2).

Heredity. Inheritance is autosomal recessive.

Prognosis. Congenital profound hearing impairment occurs.

Summary. The variety of mutations in both humans and mice indicate that *TCM1* has an important function in the cochlea. Further studies are needed to determine the function of the gene and genotype–phenotype correspondences.

References

1. Jain PK et al: A human recessive neurosensory nonsyndromic hearing impairment locus is a potential homologue of the murine deafness (dn) locus. *Hum Mol Genet* 4:2391–2394, 1995.
2. Kurima K et al: Dominant and recessive deafness caused by mutations of a novel gene, *TMC1*, required for cochlear hair-cell function. *Nat Genet* 30:277–284, 2002.
3. Scott DA et al: An autosomal recessive nonsyndromic-hearing-loss locus identified by DNA pooling using two inbred Bedouin kindreds. *Am J Hum Genet* 59:385–391, 1996.

DFNB8/10

- MIM: 601072 (DFNB8), 605316 (DFNB10), 605511 (TMPRSS3)
- Location, gene: 21q22; *TMPRSS3* (also called ECHOS1) (transmembrane protease, serine 3)

DFNB8 was localized in a large consanguineous kindred from Pakistan (4), and DFNA10 was localized in a Palestinian kindred (1). Initially, it was not clear whether the critical regions overlapped, particularly since there were phenotypic differences between the two kindreds, but identification of the *TMPRSS3* gene showed that they are allelic.

Auditory findings. In the Pakistani (DFNB8) kindred, hearing loss was noted between ages 10 and 12, and it rapidly progressed to profound hearing impairment within 4–5 years. In the Palestinian (DFNB10) kindred, hearing loss was congenital (with detection confirmed at 1 week of age) and in the severe range, with no progression.

Vestibular findings. There were no vestibular symptoms in the DFNB10 family. No results are reported for the DFNB8 family.

Radiology/histology. No studies have been reported.

Molecular studies. TMPRSS3 was identified through the search for the causal gene for DFNA8/10. It was found to be expressed in fetal cochlea, and sequence analysis indicated a transmembrane low-density lipoprotein receptor domain, a scavenger-receptor cysteine-rich domain (both of which could bind cell surface or extracellular molecules), and an extracellular serine protease domain. Its function in the inner ear is unknown, but it could be associated with the turnover of glycosylated acidic proteins in the endolymph (3).

Mutation analysis of the DFNB8 kindred with childhood-onset hearing impairment indicated a pathogenic intronic mutation, IVS4-6A → G, which would create an alternate splice acceptor site. In vitro studies of the effects of such a mutation indicated that a 4 bp insertion would result, which would be expected to result in a null allele. However, some splice acceptor mutations allow a degree of normal splicing, and it is possible that this accounts for the later onset of hearing loss in this kindred. In contrast, the DFNB10 kindred revealed an 8 bp deletion and insertion of eighteen 68 bp β-satellite repeats. Fluorescent in situ hybridization studies indicated that the β-satellite repeat sequences were homologous to those in the short arms of acrocentric chromosomes. This is the first description of such an insertion in an active gene (3). Unlike the DFNB8 mutation, this would be expected to completely disrupt gene function. Homozygosity for two different missense mutations, W251C and P404L, have been identified in two Tunisian families with congenital profound hearing loss. Both of these were predicted to alter the active site of the serine protease domain (2).

To determine the contribution of *TMPRSS3* mutations to hearing loss in Caucasian populations, mutation analysis was done in 448 individuals with severe to profound prelingual hearing impairment who did not have the *GJB2* 35delG mutation. One Spanish individual was found to be homozygous for a single base pair deletion (207delC) with a resulting frameshift and termination close to an exon border. Depending on the use of an alternative splice site, this could result in protein truncation. A Greek individual also showed the 207delC mutation as well as a missense mutation (D103G), which was predicted to alter a Ca^{2+} binding site. These were the only possibly pathogenic mutations found in the sample, leading to the conclusion that mutation of *TMPRSS3* is a rare cause of profound congenital hearing loss in Caucasians (5).

Heredity. Inheritance is autosomal recessive.

Prognosis. Sensorineural hearing loss occurs, with the onset and degree of hearing loss being dependent on the mutation.

Summary. While complete loss of *TMPRSS3* function causes congenital profound hearing loss characteristic of many recessively inherited mutations, partial expression produces a unique presentation with later onset but rapid progression to profound hearing loss.

References

1. Bonné-Tamir B et al: Linkage of congenital recessive deafness (gene DFNB10) to chromosome 21q22.3. *Am J Hum Genet* 58:1254–1259, 1996.
2. Masmoudi S et al: Novel missense mutations of *TMPRSS3* in two consanguineous Tunisian families with non-syndromic autosomal recessive deafness. *Hum Mutat* 18:101–108, 2001.
3. Scott HS et al: Insertion of beta-satellite repeats identifies a transmembrane protease causing both congenital and childhood onset autosomal recessive deafness. *Nat Genet* 27:59–63, 2001.
4. Veske A et al: Autosomal recessive non-syndromic deafness locus (DFNB8) maps on chromosome 21q22 in a large consanguineous kindred from Pakistan. *Hum Mol Genet* 5:165–168, 1996.
5. Wattenhofer M et al: Mutations in the *TMPRSS3* gene are a rare cause of childhood nonsyndromic deafness in Caucasian patients. *J Mol Med* 80:124–131, 2002.

DFNB9

- MIM: 601071 (DFNB9), 603681 (OTOF)
- Location, gene: 2p22–p23; *OTOF* (otoferlin)

The initial localization of DFNB9 was made in a consanguineous family from Lebanon (1). Although termed DFNB6 in the publication, it was given the official designation of DFNB9.

Auditory findings. Affected individuals have congenital severe to profound hearing loss (1–3). There is also a preliminary report of families with less severe hearing losses who have auditory neuropathy (5).

Vestibular findings. There was no evidence of vestibular symptoms (1).

Radiology/histology. No studies were reported.

Molecular studies. In the search for a candidate gene within the DFNB9 region, extension and sequencing of expressed sequence tags (ESTs) and comparison with transcripts from mouse cochlear libraries identified a candidate gene. Sequence analysis of the putative protein product revealed homology with the *C. elegans FER-1* gene, a spermatogenesis factor, and with the human dysferlin protein. Accordingly, it was named otoferlin. It was predicted to have a cytoplasmic amino terminus, a transmembrane domain, and a hydrophobic C terminus, with most homology with FER-1 and dysferlin being in the C terminus. Either three or six C2 domains can be found in this region, forming short or long isoforms, respectively (7). C2 regions form β sheets and can interact with phospholipids and proteins in membrane trafficking and fusion. The last four C2 regions in *OTOF* are capable of binding Ca^{2+}, indicating a possible role in neurotransmitter release. In situ hybridization in the mouse from E19.5 to P20 indicated *Otof* expression primarily in inner hair cells and neuroepithelium of the vestibular utricle, saccule, and semicircular canals. This led to the hypothesis that otoferlin may be involved in synaptic vesicle trafficking and fusion (6).

Mutation analysis in four Lebanese kindreds (the original kindreds described by Chaib et al. [1], plus three new families) detected homozygosity for a 2416T $\rightarrow$ A mutation that produces a stop codon (Y730X) in the second C2 domain (6). This mutation would affect Ca^{2+} binding in both short and long isoforms. An Indian family was found to have an intronic mutation that would affect an acceptor splice site, causing skipping of exon 9 and a premature termination, which would affect the long isoform but not the short one (7). Similarly, a large Turkish kindred (originally described in Leal et al. [2]), was found to have two missense mutations that only affected the long isoform. These mutations, P490Q and I515T, were both predicted to disrupt the C2 structure by inserting two α helices, removing one of the β sheets and creating a new myrisylation site.

Recently, it has been reported that several families with hearing loss and recessively inherited auditory neuropathy have been found to have *OTOF* mutations (5). Auditory neuropathy is generally defined as hearing loss with abnormal auditory brain stem responses but normal outer hair cell function (as determined by otoacoustic emissions or cochlear microphonics), indicating that the hearing loss is peripheral but not cochlear. In individuals with residual hearing, this can create the paradox of poorer speech discrimination than would be expected for the degree of hearing loss, and such individuals may not obtain benefit from conventional hearing aids. Some have responded well to cochlear implantation, however. Some individuals lose their normal otoacoustic emissions over time, so this may not be detectable in adulthood (4). This would be consistent with a defect in the synaptic vesicles rather than in hair cell function itself, and may indicate that the level of hearing loss is much broader than originally determined by selection of families with profound congenital hearing loss.

Heredity. Inheritance is autosomal recessive.

Prognosis. Hearing loss is not progressive. If auditory neuropathy is indeed a component, cochlear implantation may be particularly helpful in individuals with residual hearing who do not benefit from conventional hearing aids.

Summary. The localization of the molecular defect to the synaptic vesicles may indicate that this is a unique form of hearing loss. Although some mutations produce severe to profound congenital hearing loss, there may be individuals with lesser degrees of hearing loss who have characteristics of auditory neuropathy.

References

1. Chaib H et al: A gene responsible for a sensorineural nonsyndromic recessive deafness maps to chromosome 2p22–23. *Hum Molec Genet* 5:155–158, 1996.

2. Leal SM et al: A second Middle Eastern kindred with autosomal recessive non-syndromic hearing loss segregates DFNB9. *Eur J Hum Genet* 6:341–344, 1998.
3. Mirghomizadeh F et al: Substitutions in the conserved C2C domain of otoferlin cause DFNB9, a form of nonsyndromic autosomal recessive deafness. *Neurobiol Dis* 10:157–164, 2002.
4. Starr A et al: The varieties of auditory neuropathy. *J Basic Clin Physiol Pharmacol* 11:215–230, 2000.
5. Varga R et al: Non-syndromic recessive auditory neuropathy is the result of mutations in the otoferlin (*OTOF*) gene. *J Med Genet* 40:45–50, 2003.
6. Yasunaga S et al: A mutation in *OTOF*, encoding otoferlin, a FER-1-like protein, causes DFNB9, a nonsyndromic form of deafness. *Nat Genet* 21:363–369, 1999.
7. Yasunaga S et al: *OTOF* encodes multiple long and short isoforms: genetic evidence that the long ones underlie recessive deafness DFNB9. *Am J Hum Genet* 67:591–600, 2000.

DFNB12

- MIM: 601386 (DFNB12), 605516 (CDH23)
- Location, gene: 10q21–q22; *CDH23* (cadherin 23)

DFNB12 was localized in a consanguineous kindred from Syria (4). Five additional families were ascertained and mutations were found in *CDH23*, which also causes Usher syndrome type 1D (3), and the mouse homologue *Cdh23* causes the waltzer phenotype. Astuto et al. (1) have described eight additional families with nonsyndromic hearing loss with homozygous or heterozygous *CDH23* mutations.

Auditory findings. Hearing loss was congenital and profound in the families reported by Chaib et al. (4) and Bork et al. (3). Families ascertained by Astuto et al. (1) were unselected by phenotype and had a wider range, including moderate to severe hearing loss in some families and progression noted in some families.

Vestibular findings. No clinical symptoms were evident.

Radiology/histology. No studies were reported.

Molecular studies. The cadherins are cell adhesion proteins that facilitate cell–cell connections and interactions with extracellular matrices. *CDH23* has a signal peptide and 27 extracellular cadherin repeats that bind Ca^{2+}, followed by a helical transmembrane domain, with the carboxyl terminus being intracellular (2). In situ hybridization of the homologous RNA in mouse cochleae indicated expression confined to inner and outer hair cells at postnatal day 4. Examination of the hair cells in *waltzer* mice, who have deafness and vestibular dysfunction due to a mutation in the *Cdh23* gene, showed delayed maturation and disorganization of the stereocilia. This implies that *Cdh23* is involved in the organization of the stereocilia, perhaps as a component of the cross-links (5). This has been supportive of findings of Siemens et al. (6) showing complexes between *CHD23* and harmonin, the protein mutated in Usher syndrome type 1C and DFNB18. Involvement with cross-links has also been proposed for *MYO7A*, which causes Usher syndrome type 1B. Usher syndrome 1D was found to be caused by two mutations in *CDH23* in one family: one was a missense mutation associated with milder retinitis pigmentosa (RP), and the other was a truncation mutation with more severe RP (2). Four other families with Usher type 1D also had mutations that could have major effects on the protein, with two nonsense mutations and two intronic splice site mutations, although individuals with one of the splice site mutations had a milder phenotype with later-onset RP.

Five families with recessive congenital profound hearing impairment, linkage to DFNB12, and no evidence of RP were screened for mutations in *CDH23*. Missense mutations were found in all five; four were homozygous for mutations D188N, D1243N, D1400N, and P2257T, and one showed compound heterozygosity for an I2148N and an R2154C mutation. All but the P2257T mutation occurred in extracellular cadherin domains (3). These results were similar to those found by Astuto et al. (1), in which all of the mutations associated with non-

syndromic hearing loss were missense mutations. This study noted that there was a wide range in auditory and visual phenotypes, with mild phenotypes seen in some individuals with Usher syndrome ID, and some nonsyndromic individuals showing very equivocal findings on fundoscopic examinations or electroretinograms.

In contrast to mutations in *MYO7A*, then, it appears that missense mutations are more likely to cause nonsyndromic hearing loss, while more severely disruptive mutations cause retinitis pigmentosa and vestibular dysfunction characteristic of Usher syndrome. The phenotypic range may be broad, however.

Heredity. Inheritance is autosomal recessive.

Prognosis. Congenital moderate to profound hearing loss occurs. Since some mutations produce symptoms of Usher syndrome, vestibular and retinal studies should be done.

Summary. Further studies with more varied phenotypes will determine the spectrum of effect of mutations in *CDH23*, from nonsyndromic hearing loss to varying degrees of severity of Usher syndrome.

References

1. Astuto LM et al: *CDH23* mutation and phenotype heterogeneity: a profile of 107 diverse families with Usher syndrome and nonsyndromic deafness. *Am J Hum Genet* 71:262–275, 2002.
2. Bolz H et al: Mutation of *CDH23*, encoding a new member of the cadherin gene family, causes Usher syndrome type 1D. *Nat Genet* 27:108–112, 2001.
3. Bork JM et al: Usher syndrome 1D and nonsyndromic autosomal recessive deafness DFNB12 are caused by allelic mutations of the novel cadherin-like gene *CDH23*. *Am J Hum Genet* 68:26–37, 2001.
4. Chaib H et al: Mapping of *DFNB12*, a gene for a non-syndromal autosomal recessive deafness, to chromosome 10q21–22. *Hum Mol Genet* 5:1061–1064, 1996.
5. Di Palma F et al: Mutations in *Cdh23*, encoding a new type of cadherin, cause stereocilia disorganization in *waltzer*, the mouse model for Usher syndrome type 1D. *Nat Genet* 27:103–107, 2001.
6. Siemens J et al: The Usher syndrome proteins cadherin 23 and harmonin form a complex by means of PDZ-domain interactions. *Proc Natl Acad Sci USA* 99:14946–14951, 2002.

DFNB14

- MIM: 603678
- Location, gene: 7q31; gene unknown

This localization was made in a Lebanese kindred (1).

Auditory findings. All individuals had profound prelingual hearing loss, detectable by ABR as early as 1 year and likely congenital.

Vestibular findings. No evaluations were reported.

Radiology/histology. No studies were reported.

Molecular studies. Linkage was initially done with candidate loci already known to be involved in hereditary hearing loss, and positive results were obtained for the DFNB4/PDS region. Fine mapping indicated a critical region of 15 cM between D7S527 and D7S3074. Because of the proximity to the DFNB4/PDS locus, thyroid studies, including perchlorate discharge, were performed on three affected individuals and mutation screening of the PDS gene (now called *SLC26A4*) was done. These studies were normal, indicating a separate locus.

Heredity. Inheritance is autosomal recessive.

Prognosis. Profound prelingual hearing loss, probably congenital, occurs.

Summary. It has been observed that DFNB14 may overlap DFNB17; however, with the distances between DFNB4, DFNB14, and

DFNB17 being close, and map locations being refined, these may need to be re-evaluated. Phenotypically, DFNB14 and DFNB17 are alike.

References

1. Mustapha M et al: Identification of a locus on chromosome 7q31, DFNB14, responsible for prelingual sensorineural non-syndromic deafness. *Eur J Hum Genet* 6:548–551, 1998.

DFNB15

- MIM: 601869
- Location, gene: 3q21–q25 or 19p13; gene unknown

Linkage analysis with a consanguineous family from India gave maximum LOD scores of 2.78 for both 3q and 19p, so the responsible locus could be in either region, or in both (1).

Auditory findings. All affected individuals had profound prelingual hearing impairment.

Vestibular findings. No symptoms were observed on examination.

Radiology/histology. No studies were reported.

Molecular studies. A genome-wide screen resulted in two localizations. On 3q, the critical region spanned 39 cM between D3S1290 and D3S1282, and on 19p, the critical region covered 32 cM between D19S209 and D19S411. On chromosome 3, the gene for Usher syndrome type III is within the region, and three mouse mutations are in the homologous region on mouse chromosome 3: *flaky tail (ft)*, *deafwaddler (dfw)*, and *spinner (sr)*. The region on chromosome 19 includes *MYO1F*, which is an unconventional myosin whose family members *MYO7A, MYO15,* and *MYO3A* cause hearing loss, and *NOTCH*, whose homologues in birds have been associated with inner ear development. The human homologue to the mouse mutant *mocha (mh)* may also be in the region. The *mocha* mouse shows postnatal cochlear degeneration. Mutation analysis of *MYO1F* showed no pathogenic mutations (2).

While either locus could be responsible for hearing loss in this family, the authors also brought up the possibility that both loci could be involved through digenic inheritance.

Heredity. Inheritance is autosomal recessive, although digenic inheritance is a possibility.

Prognosis. Profound prelingual hearing impairment occurs.

Summary. Further studies will be needed to resolve the locus and mode of inheritance responsible for this form of hearing loss. Given the very large critical regions, this will require either additional families with similar linkage results or mutation analysis of candidate genes.

References

1. Chen A et al: New gene for autosomal recessive non-syndromic hearing loss maps to either chromosome 3q or 19p. *Am J Med Genet* 71:467–471, 1997.
2. Chen AH et al: *MYO1F* as a candidate gene for nonsyndromic deafness, DFNB15. *Arch Otolaryngol Head Neck Surg* 127:921–925, 2001.

DFNB16

- MIM: 603720 (DFNB16), 606440 (STRC)
- Location, gene: 15q15; *STRC* (stereocilin) plus one unknown gene

This form of hearing loss was localized in three consanguineous kindreds from Pakistan, Palestine, and Syria (1). A fourth family from France was reported by Villamar et al. (3).

Auditory findings. Hearing loss was recognized in early childhood (3–5 years) in the Pakistani family and in the French family. The audiometric configuration was sloping, with severe to profound loss in the mid and high frequencies, and was not progressive (2,3). Although full details were not given, the other two kindreds were presumably similar, with severe to profound hearing loss.

Vestibular findings. No evaluations were reported.

Radiology/histology. No studies were reported.

Molecular studies. Initial linkage studies were somewhat ambiguous as to the critical region for DFNB16. The first report cited a 12–14 cM region between D15S132 and D15S155, as defined by the third of the three families studied (1). In the French family, a somewhat different region was defined between D15S994 and D15S132, which includes the region of the first two families reported by Campbell et al. (1), but not the smaller region defined in the third (3). In a search for candidate hearing loss genes expressed in subtracted mouse inner ear cDNA libraries, Verpy et al. (2) identified a novel gene that maps to 15q15. The gene, *STRC*, was characterized and mutation analysis was done for all four families. Mutations were found in two of the four families, the first Pakistani family and the French family. The other two families did not have mutations in *STRC* and appeared to map distally to it. This suggests a second DFNB16 locus at 15q21.1 between D15S161 and D15S126.

STRC (stereocilin) did not show homology to any known proteins. Sequence analysis predicted a signal peptide followed by several hydrophobic regions, but it was unclear whether it was membrane-bound or secreted. Immunofluorescence with mouse inner ear indicated expression in the hair cells, particularly the stereocilia, of both the coclear and vestibular systems. Developmentally, expression was seen in cochlear inner hair cells before outer hair cells between postnatal days 6 and 20. The *STRC* gene was found to be duplicated, with the two copies about 100 kb apart. The two copies were virtually identical except for some intronic variations or silent substitutions, and one contained a stop codon that might indicate that it was a pseudogene. Hearing-impaired individuals from the Pakistani family had a homozygous insertion of a cytosine (3157insC), creating 19 aberrant amino acids and a termination signal in exon 13; and a homozygous deletion of 4 base pairs (2171–2174delTTTG) was found in the French family, resulting in five aberrant amino acids and a stop codon in exon 5. These were found in the presumably functional copy of *STRC* and would produce an inactive product (2).

Heredity. Inheritance is autosomal recessive.

Prognosis. Severe to profound sloping hearing loss occurs, with no progression. Diagnosis is in early childhood, which could indicate prelingual or congenital onset.

Summary. This form of hearing loss appears to have somewhat more residual hearing in the low frequencies than in other recessive nonprogressive forms. There appears to be a second locus in this region, and the characteristics of the hearing loss in the families defining the second locus are unclear.

References

1. Campbell DA et al: A new locus for non-syndromal, autosomal recessive, sensorineural hearing loss (DFNB16) maps to human chromosome 15q21-q22. *J Med Genet* 34:1015–1017, 1997.
2. Verpy E et al: Mutations in a new gene encoding a protein of the hair bundle cause non-syndromic deafness at the DFNB16 locus. *Nat Genet* 29:345–349, 2001.
3. Villamar M et al: Deafness locus DFNB16 is located on chromosome 15q13–q21 within a 5-cM interval flanked by markers D15S994 and D15S132 (Letter). *Am J Hum Genet* 64:1238–1241, 1999.

DFNB17

- MIM: 603010
- Location, gene: 7q31; gene unknown

This localization was made in a family from India (1).

Auditory findings. All affected individuals had profound prelingual hearing impairment.

Vestibular findings. No symptoms were observed on examination.

Radiology/histology. No studies were reported.

Molecular studies. Linkage analysis mapped DFNB17 to a 3 cM region between D7S486 and D7S2529, which would place it telomeric to DFNB4/PDS. A second Indian family was also described in which the candidate gene was localized to DFNB4 but there was no detectable mutation in *SLC26A4* (1).

Heredity. Inheritance is autosomal recessive.

Prognosis. Prelingual profound hearing impairment occurs.

Summary. As noted in the discussion of DFNB14, the exact locations of DFNB4, DFNB14, and DFNB17 are uncertain. DFNB14 and DFNB17 are phenotypically the same, but may not overlap, and it appears that there may be a nonsyndromic locus that overlaps DFNB4 but is not due to mutation in *SLC26A4*.

References

1. Greinwald JH et al: Localization of a novel gene for nonsyndromic hearing loss (DFNB17) to chromosome region 7q31. *Am J Med Genet* 78:107–113, 1998.

DFNB18

- MIM: 602092 (DFNB18), 605242 (USH1C)
- Location, gene: 11p15.1; *USH1C* (harmonin)

DFNB18 was localized in a consanguineous family from India (2), and subsequently a Chinese family with a homozygous mutation in harmonin was described (4).

Auditory findings. Hearing impairment was prelingual and profound in all affected family members.

Vestibular findings. There were no vestibular symptoms on clinical evaluation, including calorics, in hearing-impaired members of the Indian family (2). Vestibular testing could not be performed with the Chinese family, although one subject complained of vertigo (4).

Radiology/histology. No studies were reported.

Molecular studies. Initial linkage studies placed DFNB18 within the region for Usher syndrome 1C, so electroretinograms were performed on two hearing-impaired family members of ages 18 and 19. The results were normal and vestibular evaluation was negative, thus a diagnosis of Usher syndrome was ruled out in the Indian kindred (2). Discovery of the gene causing Usher syndrome type 1C, harmonin (6), led to its testing in nonsyndromic families.

The *USH1c* gene produces at least eight isoforms in the mouse inner ear, with all but two of the longer isoforms also expressed in eye. This has led to the conjecture that mutations that selectively affect those isoforms would cause nonsyndromic hearing loss without retinal abnormalities. The isoforms all have piperazinedione two (PZD) domains followed by a coiled-coil domain. Longer isoforms have an additional PZD domain, and in the longest form, expressed only in ear, there is an additional coiled-coil domain followed by a proline-serine-threonine rich (PST) domain, followed by another PZD domain. PZD domains are found in "scaffolding proteins" involved in organization of macromolecular complexes, so that protein signaling and interactions are coordinated. Typically, they bind to specific cytoskeletal proteins. It has been hypothesized that harmonin may allow a complex of myosins to slide along the actin cytoskeleton of the stereocilia, releasing tension of the tip-links between stereocilia after their deflection by sound (3). It has

also been shown that harmonin complexes with CDH23. Since defects in CDH23 lead to splayed stereocilia, involvement with structures that connect the stereocilia is also suggested (5).

Mutation analysis of harmonin in the Indian family with DFNB18 revealed homozygosity for an intronic mutation that causes skipping of exon 12 with a resulting frameshift producing a stop codon in exon 13. This should disrupt isoforms in the retina as well as the ear. However, expression studies have shown that normally spliced protein is also produced, indicating that this is a "leaky" mutation. It is possible that enough product is formed to sustain activity in the eye but not the ear (1). In contrast, the mutation found in the Chinese family supports the hypothesis that mutations in isoforms expressed only in the ear will cause nonsyndromic hearing loss. Homozygosity was found for a missense mutation producing an R608P change in exon "D," which is only found in the long isoforms. Interestingly, mutation screening in individuals with nonsyndromic hearing loss from a variety of ethnic backgrounds revealed heterozygous mutations in three American probands. Two of these were in exon D and one was in another alternatively spliced exon, exon B. It is not clear whether these have clinical significance or if a second mutation could be in a regulatory region or in another gene (4).

Heredity. Inheritance is autosomal recessive.

Prognosis. Prelingual severe to profound hearing loss occurs. Since there may be a spectrum of expression from nonsyndromic to Usher syndrome, visual and vestibular function should be evaluated.

Summary. Study of harmonin has revealed an important mechanism underlying the presentation of a mutation as syndromic or nonsyndromic, namely the presence of the mutation in alternatively expressed isoforms.

References

1. Ahmed ZM et al: Nonsyndromic recessive deafness DFNB18 and Usher syndrome type 1C are allelic mutations of *USH1C*. *Hum Genet* 110:527–531, 2002.
2. Jain PK et al: A gene for recessive nonsyndromic sensorineural deafness (DFNB18) maps to the chromosomal region 11p14–p15.1 containing the Usher syndrome type 1C gene. *Genomics* 50:290–292, 1998.
3. Montell C: A PDZ protein ushers in new links. *Nat Genet* 26:6–7, 2000.
4. Ouyang XM et al: Mutations in the alternatively spliced exons of *USH1C* cause non-syndromic recessive deafness. *Hum Genet* 111:26–30, 2002.
5. Siemens J et al: The Usher syndrome proteins cadherin 23 and harmonin form a complex by means of PDZ-domain interactions. *Proc Natl Acad Sci USA* 99:14946–14951, 2002.
6. Verpy E et al: A defect in harmonin, a PDZ domain–containing protein expressed in the inner ear sensory hair cells, underlies Usher syndrome type 1C. *Nat Genet* 26:51–55, 2000.

DFNB19

- MIM: not assigned
- Location, gene: 18p11; gene unknown

This locus was identified in a consanguineous family with four children with hearing loss (1).

Auditory findings. All of the affected children had profound congenital hearing loss.

Vestibular findings. No evaluations were described.

Radiology/histology. No studies were reported.

Molecular studies. Linkage analysis resulted in an LOD score of 3.0 for marker D18S842, with a critical region between D18S62 and D18S1163.

Heredity. Inheritance is autosomal recessive.

Prognosis. Profound congenital hearing loss occurs.

Summary. At this time, this form of hearing loss would be indistinguishable from most others in this category.

References

1. Green GE et al: Identification of a novel locus (DFNB19) for non-syndromic autosomal recessive hearing loss in a consanguineous family. Presented at the Molecular Biology of Hearing and Deafness Meeting, Bethesda, MD, October 8, 1998, Abstract 108.

DFNB20

- MIM: 604060
- Location, gene: 11q25–qter; gene unknown

This locus was identified in a consanguineous Pakistani family. This region of chromosome 11 was specifically examined in a population of families with recessive hearing loss because of the localization of a syndromic form of hearing loss, histiocytosis with joint contractures, and deafness (MIM 602782) (1).

Auditory findings. Hearing loss was detected between 3 months and 1 year of age, but there was variability in the severity of the hearing loss. Out of the four affected children, two had a moderate hearing loss and two had a profound loss. The study of this family did not state if the degree of hearing loss is related to age, but the order of the children in the pedigree would suggest that it is not, and there was no reference to progression of the loss.

Vestibular findings. No evaluations were reported.

Radiology/histology. No studies were reported.

Molecular studies. Linkage analysis showed a multipoint LOD score of 3.3 for the region from D11S969 to the telomere of the long arm of chromosome 11. This included the region containing the gene for histiocytosis, joint contractures, and deafness, suggesting that these might be allelic. Hearing impairment in that condition begins in childhood and progresses to profound loss. Mapping excluded the region containing the TECTA gene.

Heredity. Inheritance is autosomal recessive.

Prognosis. Congenital/prelingual hearing loss occurs, ranging from moderate to profound in severity.

Summary. The variation in the degree of hearing loss associated with this locus is distinctive. It may be allelic to the histiocytosis/joint contractures/deafness gene localized to the same region.

References

1. Moynihan L et al: DFNB20: a novel locus for autosomal recessive, non-syndromal sensorineural hearing loss maps to chromosome 11q25–qter. *Eur J Hum Genet* 7:243–246, 1999.

DFNB21

- MIM: 603629 (DFNB21), 602574 (TECTA)
- Location, gene: 11q23–q25; TECTA (tectorin)

Linkage analysis with a Lebanese kindred resulted in linkage to the region containing the TECTA gene, and mutation of that gene was confirmed (1).

Auditory findings. All affected family members had prelingual severe to profound hearing impairment.

Vestibular findings. No evaluations were reported.

Radiology/histology. No studies were reported.

Molecular studies. A brief description of the a-tectorin protein and its function is given under autosomal dominant progressive hearing loss, DFNA8/12. In this family, affected family members were found to be homozygous for a G → A transition in the donor splice site of intron 9. This would be expected to result in the skipping of exon 9 and a frameshift resulting in a stop codon at amino acid 972, in one of the von Willebrand repeat regions of the zonadhesin domain. This would presumably result in a nonfunctional product. In contrast, dominant hearing loss due to mutations in α-tectorin are not inactivating mutations and appear to act in a dominant negative fashion, interfering with normal proteins in heteromeric or homomeric combinations (1).

Heredity. Inheritance is autosomal recessive.

Prognosis. Prelingual severe to profound hearing loss occurs.

Summary. The critical role of α-tectorin in the hearing process is clear from the variety of phenotypes produced by mutations in the TECTA gene: autosomal recessive prelingual severe to profound, dominant prelingual moderate to severe, and dominant progressive.

References

1. Mustapha M et al: An alpha-tectorin gene defect causes a newly identified autosomal recessive form of sensorineural pre-lingual non-syndromic deafness, DFNB21. *Hum Mol Genet* 8:409–412, 1999.

DFNB22

- MIM: 607039 (DFNB22), 607038 (OTOA)
- Location, gene: 16p12.2; OTOA (otoancorin)

The OTOA gene was identified through analysis of transcripts from a subtracted inner ear library. The gene was localized to 16p12.2, and linkage analysis in a population of families with hearing loss was used to identify a Palestinian family whose hearing loss was localized to that region. Mutation analysis of that gene confirmed that disruption of OTOA led to hearing loss (1).

Auditory findings. Affected family members had moderate to severe prelingual hearing loss.

Vestibular findings. No evaluations were reported.

Radiology/histology. No studies were reported.

Molecular studies. OTOA was found to be expressed only in the inner ear, making it a candidate gene for hearing loss. Judging by the protein sequence, otoancorin has a signal peptide at the amino terminus, followed by 11 putative N-glycosylation sites and a hydrophobic carboxyl terminus, suggesting that it is bound to a membrane. Immunofluorescent studies indicated that it is expressed in precursors of the inner and outer hair cells of the cochlea, and later is found along the surface of cells adjacent and medial to the inner hair cells as well as the vestibular hair cells. Expression in a Tecta mutant mouse cochlea determined that otoancorin was not part of the tectorial membrane. Thus it was deduced that otoancorin forms a connection between the sensory epithelial cells (but not the stereocilia) and the tectorial membrane or similar acellular structures in the vestibular system.

OTOA was localized to chromosome 16p12.2 between markers D16S3046 and D16S412 by homology to a BAC clone sequence from that region. Analysis for linkage to that region was performed in 200 families with recessive hearing loss, identifying a Palestinian family. Mutation analysis of the OTOA gene revealed a T → C transition which affects the donor splice site at the exon 12 intron junction. This would be predicted to lead to skipping of exon 12 or use of an alternate cryptic splice site.

Heredity. Inheritance is autosomal recessive.

Prognosis. Moderate to severe prelingual hearing loss occurs. Given the expression in the vestibular system, vestibular evaluation should be done.

Summary. The hearing loss in this family is somewhat less severe than in most other recessive prelingual hearing losses, although this could be due to a bias of selection in other studies.

References

1. Zwaenepoel I et al: Otoancorin, an inner ear protein restricted to the interface between the apical surface of sensory epithelia and their overlying acellular gels, is defective in autosomal recessive deafness DFNB22. *Proc Natl Acad Sci USA* 99:6240–6245, 2002.

DFNB23

- MIM: not assigned
- Location, gene: 10p11.2–q21; gene unknown

Details of this localization by R.J.H. Smith are unpublished, but the critical region overlaps that of Usher syndrome 1F, which is caused by mutation of the protocadherin 15 gene (PCDH15: MIM 605514) (1).

References

1. Van Camp G, Smith RJH: Hereditary Hearing Loss Homepage, http://dnalab-www.uia.ac.be/dnalab/hhh/, 2002.

DFNB24

- MIM: not assigned
- Location, gene: 11q23; gene unknown

Details of this locus, identified by R.J.H. Smith, are unpublished; the *TECTA* and *MYO7A* regions have been excluded (1).

References

1. Van Camp G, Smith RJH: Hereditary Hearing Loss Homepage, http://dnalab-www.uia.ac.be/dnalab/hhh/, 2002.

DFNB25

- MIM: not assigned
- Location, gene: 4p15.3–q12; gene unknown

Details of this localization by R.J.H. Smith are unpublished (1).

References

1. Van Camp G, Smith RJH: Hereditary Hearing Loss Homepage, http://dnalab-www.uia.ac.be/dnalab/hhh/, 2002.

DFNB26

- MIM: 605428
- Location, gene: 4q31; gene unknown
- Modifier: DFNM1
- MIM: 605429
- Location, gene: 1q24; gene unknown

This localization was made in a large consanguineous Pakistani kindred, but was significant only when affected individuals were included in the linkage analysis. The presence of unaffected individuals with the same homozygous haplotype led to the discovery of a second modifier locus, *DFNM1*, which suppresses the expression of hearing loss.

Auditory findings. Affected members of this family had severe to profound congenital hearing loss. Individuals with the affected haplotype but with the modifier gene had hearing levels that were indistinguishable from those of unaffected family members, including normal otoacoustic emissions (1).

Vestibular findings. No evaluations were reported.

Radiology/histology. No studies were reported.

Molecular studies. Linkage analysis localized the hearing loss gene in this family to chromosome 4q, but haplotype analysis revealed that eight affected individuals and seven unaffected individuals shared the same homozygous haplotype. When only the affected members were used, a LOD score of 8.10 was obtained for marker D4S1610 at $\theta = 0.0$, with a critical region of 1.5 cM. The nonpenetrance trait in the seven unaffected haplotype carriers linked to 1q24 with an autosomal dominant model of inheritance (LOD 4.31, $\theta = 0$ for D1S2850) for a 5.6 cM critical region bounded by D1S2658 and D1S2790. This includes the region of DFNA7. Involvement of common mitochondrial loci was ruled out by sequence analysis (1).

Heredity. Inheritance is autosomal recessive with reduced penetrance in the presence of an autosomal dominant modifier.

Prognosis. Severe to profound congenital hearing loss occurs, except in the presence of the modifier gene.

Summary. This is the first description of a recessively inherited hearing loss that is made completely nonpenetrant by a separate modifier gene. The very large size of this kindred made linkage detection possible, and it could be missed in smaller pedigrees.

References

1. Riazuddin S et al: Dominant modifier DFNM1 suppresses recessive deafness DFNB26. *Nat Genet* 26:431–434, 2000.

DFNB27

- MIM: 605818
- Location, gene: 2q23–q31; gene unknown

This localization was made in a large consanguineous kindred in the United Arab Emirates (1).

Auditory findings. All affected family members had prelingual hearing impairment, presumably severe to profound, although this is not stated.

Vestibular findings. No evaluations were reported.

Radiology/histology. No studies were reported.

Molecular studies. Linkage analysis resulted in an LOD score of 5.18 at $\theta = 0$ for the marker D2S2257, and haplotype analysis defined a critical region of 17 cM between D2S2157 and D2S326. This overlaps with the region for the DFNA16 locus. However, one individual who married into the family and was thought to be unrelated carried part of the affected haplotype; if this haplotype is actually identical by descent to the haplotype in the affected individuals, a recombinant event excludes DFNA16.

Heredity. Inheritance is autosomal recessive.

Prognosis. Prelingual hearing loss occurs.

Summary. Although the degree of hearing loss is not specified, use of the term "prelingual deafness" implies that it was severe to profound, as with most recessive loci described. This may be allelic with DFNA16, although some information from the family excludes that locus.

References

1. Pulleyn LJ et al: A new locus for autosomal recessive non-syndromal sensorineural hearing impairment (DFNB27) on chromosome 2q23–q31. *Eur J Hum Genet* 8:991–993, 2000.

DFNB28

- MIM: not assigned
- Location, gene: 22q13; gene unknown
  This localization was made in a consanguineous Palestinian kindred (1).

Auditory findings. The hearing loss was prelingual, severe to profound.

Vestibular findings. No evaluations were reported.

Radiology/histology. No studies were reported.

Molecular studies. Linkage analysis produced a multipoint LOD score of 5.23 for the 6.5 Mb region between D22S1045 and D22S282. This is within the DFNA17 region, but analysis of MYH9 is not included in the abstract. DFNB28 is not in the region of 22q typically deleted in the velocardiofacial syndrome.

Heredity. Inheritance is autosomal recessive.

Prognosis. Severe to profound prelingual hearing loss occurs.

Summary. This locus would be indistinguishable phenotypically from other recessive loci producing severe to profound prelingual hearing loss. *MYH9* (DFNA17) would be a candidate.

References
1. Walsh TD et al: DFNB28, a novel locus for prelingual nonsyndromic autosomal recessive hearing loss, maps to 22q13 in a large consanguineous Palestinian kindred [abstract]. *Am J Hum Genet* 67 (Suppl 2):368, 2000.

DFNB29

- MIM: 605608 (CLDN14)
- Location, gene: 21q22; *CLDN14* (claudin 14)
  Mutations in the *CLDN14* gene were found to cause hearing loss in two large consanguineous Pakistani kindreds (1).

Auditory findings. Hearing loss in affected family members was congenital and profound.

Vestibular findings. Affected family members had no symptoms of vestibular dysfunction.

Radiology/histology. No studies were reported.

Molecular studies. Claudins interact with other proteins to form tight junctions, or seals, around cells to regulate their permeability. This is required to separate extracellular compartments that differ in ion concentrations, such as the chambers of the cochlea, to maintain cell polarity. They have four transmembrane domains, and the carboxyl terminus is capable of binding to PZD domains of "scaffolding proteins." In situ hybridization and immunofluorescence in mouse cochlea showed that claudin-14 is expressed postnatally, concentrating in the supporting cells of the organ of Corti and in the vestibular sensory neuroepithelium, with the timing of expression corresponding to the development of the endocochlear potential. Thus it appears that claudin-14 functions to maintain an electrochemical gradient between the endolymph and the tissues of the organ of Corti (1).

Two different mutations in *CLDN14* were found in the two families in which linkage to 21q22 was known. In one family, a deletion of a thymine (398delT) resulted in a frameshift producing 23 aberrant amino acids before ending in a stop codon in the third transmembrane domain. In the other family, a missense mutation was found (T254A) that produced a V85D substitution. Valine is hydrophobic and neutral while aspartic acid is hydrophobic and negatively charged, which would be predicted to disrupt the structure of the transmembrane domain. Since this is in the critical region for the Down syndrome phenotype, it may also contribute to the early-onset presbycusis seen in individuals with Down syndrome.

Heredity. Inheritance is autosomal recessive.

Prognosis. Congenital profound hearing loss occurs. Although *CLDN14* is also expressed in vestibular, renal, and hepatic tissues, there appear to be no signs of dysfunction in these tissues with the mutations that were identified. (1)

Summary. The requirement for claudin-14 in hearing is another example of the critical importance of ionic gradients in the function of the cochlea. Overexpression of *CLDN14* may be related to the high incidence of early presbycusis in Down syndrome.

References
1. Wilcox ER et al: Mutations in the gene encoding tight junction claudin-14 cause recessive deafness DFNB29. *Cell* 104:165–172, 2001.

DFNB31

- MIM: 607084
- Location, gene: 9q32–q34; gene unknown
  The DFNB31 locus was identified in a consanguineous Palestinian family living in Jordan (1).

Auditory findings. All affected individuals had profound prelingual hearing impairment.

Vestibular findings. No evaluations were reported.

Radiology/histology. No studies were reported.

Molecular studies. A genome screen for linkage resulted in positive results for marker D9S1776. Additional markers were typed, and a multipoint LOD score of 6.14 was obtained for the region D9S1824 to D9S1682. Flanking markers were D9S289 and D9S1881, defining a region of 15 cM. This region is orthologous to the mouse region containing the *whirler* (wi) phenotype, which includes deafness and vestibular dysfunction.

Heredity. Inheritance is autosomal recessive.

Prognosis. Profound prelingual hearing loss occurs.

Summary. The mouse mutation *whirler* may be a model for DFNB31. It is otherwise indistinguishable phenotypically from other profound prelingual recessive hearing loss loci.

References
1. Mustapha M et al: DFNB31, a recessive form of sensorineural hearing loss, maps to chromosome 9q32–34. *Eur J Hum Genet* 10:210–212, 2002.

DFNB32

- MIM: not assigned
- Location, gene: 1p13.3–p22.1; gene unknown
  This localization by Hamadi Ayadi is unpublished (1).

References
1. Van Camp G, Smith RJH: Hereditary Hearing Loss Homepage, http://dnalab-www.uia.ac.be/dnalab/hhh/, 2002.

DFNB33

- MIM: 607239
- Location, gene: 9q34.3; gene unknown
  This localization was made in a consanguineous family from Jordan (1).

Auditory findings. Affected members had severe hearing loss with onset in early childhood.

Vestibular findings. No evaluations were reported.

Radiology/histology. No studies were reported.

Molecular studies. A genome search for linkage gave an LOD score of 3.38 at $\theta = 0.0$ for the marker D9S905. Flanking markers as determined by homozygosity were D9S1826 and D9S1838, spanning a region of 6.3 cM. The *CLIC3* (chloride intracellular channel 3) gene was in this region, but mutation of this gene was excluded by direct genomic sequencing.

Heredity. Inheritance is autosomal recessive.

Prognosis. Severe hearing loss occurs with onset in childhood.

Summary. This form of hearing loss appears to be slightly less severe than other forms of recessive hearing impairment. This may contribute to its apparent later age of onset, since detection may not be as easy in a very young child.

References

1. Medlej-Hashim M et al: Non-syndromic recessive deafness in Jordan: mapping of a new locus to chromosome 9q34.3 and prevalence of DFNB1 mutations. *Eur J Hum Genet* 10:391–394, 2002.

Autosomal recessive progressive hearing loss

DFNB4

- MIM: 600791 (DFNB4), 603545 (enlarged vestibular aqueduct syndrome), 605646 (SLC26A4)
- Location, gene: 7q31; *SLC26A4* or *PDS* (pendrin)

DFNB4 was first described in a large Druze kindred from the Middle East (1). It was later determined that it was allelic to Pendred syndrome (hearing loss and thyroid dysfunction) and to the enlarged vestibular aqueduct syndrome, and follow-up of the Druze kindred revealed that some individuals had goiter (4). Mutations of the *SLC26A4* gene may be the most common cause of inner ear malformations, either nonsyndromic or with thyroid enlargement (Pendred syndrome). Pendred syndrome was initially thought to be one of the most common causes of hearing loss, and even then it became clear that the criteria that had been used (goiter or perchlorate discharge testing) were resulting in underdiagnosis (5). With the current understanding of the phenotypic range of *SLC26A4* mutations, the contribution of this gene to syndromic and nonsyndromic hearing loss is considerable.

Auditory findings. In the original Druze kindred, all affected family members had congenital severe to profound hearing impairment involving all frequencies (1). As the phenotype has expanded to include families with mutation in *SLC26A4* and enlarged vestibular aqueduct (EVA) or Mondini malformation, the corresponding hearing loss shows great variability. Generally, hearing loss is congenital and in the high frequencies initially, but there is often fluctuation and progression of hearing loss (9).

Vestibular findings. Vestibular dysfunction, particularly episodes of vertigo, are reported with EVA or Mondini malformations and can be associated with drops in hearing.

Radiology/histology. Mondini malformation of the cochlea (hypoplasia of the apical turns of the cochlea) and/or enlarged vestibular aqueduct are common. The EVA may be the most accurate marker for mutation in *SLC26A4* (6); however, not all individuals with EVA have detectable *SLC26A4* mutations (8).

Molecular studies. *SLC26A4* is a member of a solute carrier family that transports chloride and iodide (7). It was identified as the cause

of Pendred syndrome (thus the original gene name of *PDS*) (2) and noted to have 11 transmembrane domains. Studies in the mouse *Pds* homolog indicated that it is expressed in areas that appear to be involved with endolymphatic fluid homeostasis, including the external sulcus of the cochlea, the endolymphatic duct and sac, and in utricle and saccule of the vestibular system (3). To study the effects of complete loss of pendrin, a knockout mouse was developed, which revealed the mechanism of action of the anion transport defect on structural development. Inner ear development was normal for the first 2 weeks of gestation, but at embryonic day 15, there were signs of dilation of the endolymphatic duct and sac, followed by dilation of the cochlea and sometimes the semicircular canals. Thus it would appear that alterations of the anion balance cause pressure changes that damage the developing inner ear structures. These same imbalances, compounded by the abnormal inner ear structures, are presumably responsible for the fluctuations and progression of hearing seen in humans. Accordingly, continuing degeneration of cochlear and vestibular structures was seen in postnatal knockout mice as far as day 45. As with humans within the same sibship, the knockout mice showed variability in the extent of inner ear damage. Since the effects of the *Pds* knockout were similar to endolymphatic hydrops, the authors questioned whether this condition, as well as Ménière disease, might be related to defects in the *PDS* gene.

Many different mutations have been described in *SLC26A4*, and attempts have been made to correlate genotypes with the variable phenotypes of thyroid defect, Mondini malformation, or EVA. Although the phenotypic variation within and between pedigrees indicates that other genes and environmental factors contribute to the phenotype, functional studies have indicated that the most common mutations causing Pendred syndrome cause loss of the ability to transport iodide and chloride, while mutations that caused EVA without thyroid defect retained some transport ability. This suggests that mutations that totally disrupt anion transport result in thyroid dysfunction and Pendred syndrome, but that mutations that maintain a level of transport sufficient for thyroid function show nonsyndromic hearing loss with inner ear malformation (6). It is notable that in many studies of mutation of the *SLC26A4* gene, individuals are found who have only one detectable mutation. Presumably the second mutation is in a regulatory region, particularly in families with clear recessive inheritance that are consistent with linkage to 7q31. In other families, digenic inheritance would also be a possibility.

Heredity. Inheritance is autosomal recessive with variable expression.

Prognosis. The variability in expression makes prediction of the degree of hearing loss difficult; however, progression is very likely. This same variability also affects distinction between syndromic and nonsyndromic forms, so thyroid function should be assessed through testing and monitoring for enlargement, according to guidelines for Pendred syndrome.

Summary. Mutations of the *SLC26A4* gene affect inner ear structure and, in some cases, thyroid function. When thyroid function is clinically detectable through goiter or perchlorate discharge testing, the term *Pendred syndrome* is applied. Screening for this gene at the population level is complicated by the variety of mutations, but it appears to be one of the more common causes of syndromic and nonsyndromic hearing loss. It is readily distinguishable by the findings of inner ear malformations on CT or MRI scans.

References

1. Baldwin CT et al: Linkage of congenital, recessive deafness (DFNB4) to chromosome 7q31 and evidence for genetic heterogeneity in the Middle Eastern Druze population. *Hum Mol Genet* 4:1637–1642, 1995.
2. Everett LA et al: Pendred syndrome is caused by mutations in a putative sulphate transporter gene (*PDS*). *Nat Genet* 17:411–422, 1997.
3. Everett LA et al: Expression pattern of the mouse ortholog of the Pendred syndrome gene (*Pds*) suggests a key role for pendrin in the inner ear. *Proc Natl Acad Sci USA* 96:9727–9732, 1999.
4. Li XC et al: A mutation in *PDS* causes non-syndromic recessive deafness (letter). *Nat Genet* 18:215–217, 1998.

5. Reardon W et al: Pendred syndrome—100 years of underascertainment? *Q J Med* 90:443–447, 1997.
6. Reardon W et al: Enlarged vestibular aqueduct: a radiological marker of Pendred syndrome, and mutation of the *PDS* gene. *Q J Med* 93:99–104, 2000.
7. Scott DA et al: The Pendred syndrome gene encodes a chloride-iodide transport protein. *Nat Genet* 21:440–443, 1999.
8. Scott DA et al: Functional differences of the *PDS* gene product are associated with phenotypic variation in patients with Pendred syndrome and non-syndromic hearing loss (DFNB4). *Hum Mol Genet* 9:1709–1715, 2000.
9. Usami S-I et al: Non-syndromic hearing loss associated with enlarged vestibular aqueduct is caused by *PDS* mutations. *Hum Genet* 104:188–192, 1999.

DFNB8/10

- MIM: 601072 (DFNB8), 605316 (DFNB10), 605511 (TMPRSS3)
- Location, gene: 21q22; *TMPRSS3* (also called *ECHOS1*) (transmembrane protease, serine 3)

As noted above in the section on recessive congenital profound hearing loss, some mutations of *TMPRSS3* result in rapidly progressive hearing loss.

Auditory findings. In a Pakistani kindred with progressive hearing loss, the loss was noted between ages 10 and 12, and rapidly progressed to profound hearing impairment within 4–5 years (1).

Vestibular findings. No evaluations were reported.

Radiology/histology. No studies reported.

Molecular studies. (See discussion of DFNB8/10 under recessive congenital profound hearing loss.) The mutation of *TMPRSS3* that caused progressive hearing loss affected an intronic splice acceptor (2). It is possible that use of a cryptic splice site would make this a "leaky" mutation, resulting in a less severe phenotype.

Heredity. Inheritance is autosomal recessive.

Prognosis. Sensorineural hearing loss occurs, with the onset and degree of hearing loss being dependent on the mutation.

Summary. Although the onset of hearing loss is in late childhood, the progression is rapid.

References

1. Bonné-Tamir B et al: Linkage of congenital recessive deafness (gene DFNB10) to chromosome 21q22.3. *Am J Hum Genet* 58:1254–1259, 1996.
2. Scott HS et al: Insertion of beta-satellite repeats identifies a transmembrane protease causing both congenital and childhood onset autosomal recessive deafness. *Nat Genet* 27:59–63, 2001.

DFNB13

- MIM: 603098
- Location, gene: 7q34–q36; gene unknown

This localization was made in a large consanguineous kindred in Lebanon (1).

Auditory findings. Audiologic testing was done with five siblings who ranged in age from 8 to 26. The younger children had severe hearing loss, while the older sibs had profound hearing loss; this suggests that the loss is progressive. Since this was the first time any of the subjects had been formally tested, age of onset and rate of progression were not available.

Vestibular findings. No evaluations were reported.

Radiology/histology. No studies were reported.

Molecular studies. Linkage analysis with a genome search resulted in an LOD score of 4.5 for markers on chromosome 7, and fine mapping narrowed the region to between D7S2505/D7S2468 and D7S2439, a distance of about 17 cM.

Heredity. Inheritance is autosomal recessive.

Prognosis. Severe hearing loss occurs in childhood, progressing to profound by the third decade.

Summary. This is one of the rare forms of recessive hearing loss that is progressive. It appears to be more severe than the progressive hearing loss caused by mutation of *MYO3A* (DFNB30).

References

1. Mustapha M et al: A sensorineural progressive autosomal recessive form of isolated deafness, DFNB13, maps to chromosome 7q34–q36. *Eur J Hum Genet* 6:245–250, 1998.

DFNB30

- MIM: 607101 (DFNB30), 606808 (MYO3A)
- Location, gene: 10p11.1; *MYO3A* (myosin IIIA)

Mutations in this gene as a cause of progressive hearing loss were found in an extended Jewish kindred that had emigrated to Israel from an ancient Iraqi community (1).

Auditory findings. Onset of hearing loss was generally in the second decade, although there was variation in the age of onset even within sibships. Progression led to a sloping hearing loss that was moderate in the low frequencies and severe in the mid and high frequencies by age 50.

Vestibular findings. Clinical vestibular evaluation was normal in affected individuals.

Radiology/histology. No studies were reported.

Molecular studies. Myosin IIIA is homologous to the *NINAC* gene in *Drosophila*, where it interacts with actin filaments and *INAD*, a PDZ-containing scaffolding protein to form a phototransduction signaling complex in the eye. Type III myosins have an N-terminal kinase domain followed by the usual head/neck/tail configuration of myosins. The tail domain is specific to class III myosins and the function is not clear, although it is quite conceivable that it also binds to PDZ domains and forms an analogous signaling complex in the mammalian ear. In situ hybridization of Myo3a antisense probes in mouse cochlea showed expression only in inner and outer hair cells. Interestingly, *InaD*, the mouse homologue to *INAD*, was also expressed in cochlea.

Three different myosin IIIA mutations segregated in this family, with affected individuals being homozygotes or compound heterozygotes. All heterozygous individuals had normal hearing, a finding supporting an autosomal recessive mode of inheritance. One of the mutations was a nonsense mutation, and the other two were intronic mutations affecting splice acceptor sites. The nonsense mutation created a stop codon at amino acid 1043, truncating the protein after the head domain. One intronic mutation in the splice acceptor site of exon 17 led to loss of exon 18 followed by a frameshift and truncation at codon 668 in the head domain. The other mutation, in the eighth intron, apparently led to an unstable product, since no expression was detectable with RT-PCR from transformed lymphocytes.

Genotype–phenotype correlation could be demonstrated in the age of onset and initial progression of the hearing loss, in that individuals who were homozygous for the nonsense mutation had more severe hearing loss between the ages of 25 and 50 than did individuals with other genotypes. Ultimate severity did not differ between genotypes, however.

Heredity. The best-fitting model for the mode of inheritance for this family was autosomal recessive with age-related penetrance, although a dominant model could not be excluded. The molecular findings support the autosomal recessive hypothesis.

Prognosis. Progressive hearing loss begins between ages 10 and 20, with severe mid- and high-frequency hearing loss occurring by age 50. Although *MYO3A* is expressed in retina, there appears to be no retinal pathology, and since there have been no localizations of Usher syndrome to this region, there is no indication at this time that mutations of this gene are a cause of Usher syndrome.

Summary. This form of progressive recessive hearing loss is distinguishable from DFNB13 by its later age of onset and less severe outcome. All of the recessive mutations were inactivating, and it will be interesting to see if other types of *MYO3A* mutations act in a dominant fashion.

References

1. Walsh T et al: From flies' eyes to our ears: mutations in a human class III myosin cause progressive nonsyndromic hearing loss DFNB30. *Proc Nat Acad Sci USA* 99:7518–7523, 2002.

X-linked Nonsyndromic Hearing Loss

DFN1

- MIM: 304700 (Mohr-Tranebjaerg syndrome, Dystonia-Deafness-Optic Atrophy), 300356 (TMM8A, dystonia deafness peptide)
- Location, gene: Xq22; *TMM8A* (translocase of inner mitochondrial membrane 8)

This locus was originally described in a Norwegian kindred as nonsyndromic (1). Hearing loss onset was in early childhood and was rapidly progressive. The family was re-ascertained and affected members were found to have developed neuromotor and vision problems with mental deterioration (2). Thus it is not actually nonsyndromic and will not be covered here. However, this does emphasize the importance of continued surveillance to be sure that hearing loss is not just the initial presentation of a more complex disorder.

References

1. Mohr J, Mageroy K: Sex-linked deafness of a possibly new type. *Acta Genet Statist Med* 10:54–62, 1960.
2. Tranebjaerg L et al: A new X linked recessive deafness syndrome with blindness, dystonia, fractures, and mental deficiency is linked to Xq22. *J Med Genet* 32:257–263, 1995.

DFN2

- MIM: 304500
- Location, gene: Xq22; gene unknown

The designation of DFN2 was initially made for any family with X-linked nonsyndromic congenital profound hearing impairment. It is now recognized that this is a heterogenous classification, and now the DFN2 appellation has been given to the locus on Xq22 that was localized in a large British-American kindred. A second phenotypically similar family did not exclude the DFN2 region but was too small to provide statistical significance for or against linkage (1).

Auditory findings. Hearing impairment was congenital and profound in affected males. Obligate female carriers had a mild to moderate high-frequency hearing loss; however, at least two females who were at risk had normal hearing but decreased otoacoustic emissions. Affected women were generally unaware of their hearing loss.

Vestibular findings. No evaluations were reported.

Radiology/histology. The CT scans of the temporal bones in affected males were normal.

Molecular studies. Linkage to DFN3 and DFN4 was excluded. An LOD score of 2.91 was obtained for marker DXS1106 and for a marker within *COL4A5*. Flanking markers were DXS990 and DXS1001. There were no features of Alport syndrome in the family, but *COL4A5* itself would still be a candidate gene. The *TIMM8A* gene is also in this region, and it is possible that this could represent a nonsyndromic allele of the Mohr-Tranebjaerg syndrome. Other candidates included the Pelizaeus-Merzbacher gene (now known to be *PLP-1*, proteolipid protein-1) and *COL4A6*.

In a second phenotypically similar family the entire DFN2 region was not excluded, but the family was too small to provide statistical significance for or against linkage. The *COL4A5* gene itself was excluded, however.

Heredity. Inheritance is X-linked dominant with milder expression in females.

Prognosis. Profound congenital hearing loss occurs in males, mild to moderate hearing loss in females.

Summary. This locus is phenotypically similar to DFN4.

References

1. Tyson J et al: Mapping of DFN2 to Xq22. *Hum Mol Genet* 5:2055–2060, 1996.

DFN3

- MIM: 304400 (DFN4), 300039 (POU3F4)
- Location, gene: Xq21.1; *POU3F4* (POU domain class 3, transcription factor 4)

This condition was originally characterized as conductive or mixed (sensorineural and conductive) hearing loss with stapes fixation and perilymphatic gusher (9). The importance of recognizing this condition prior to attempts to surgically release the apparently fixed footplate was emphasized, because of the high risk of a sudden leakage ("gusher") of perilymph or cerebral spinal fluid from the inner ear (5). It has since been recognized that the sensorineural component can be significant and even mask the conductive component, or that the hearing loss may be sensorineural alone (3). This gene is also involved in the contiguous deletion syndrome of choroideremia, deafness, and mental retardation (10).

Auditory findings. Hearing loss in males is moderate to profound and sensorineural or mixed, with progression of the sensorineural component. Milder sensorineural or mixed loss may also be seen in carrier females and may also be progressive (5) (Fig. 5–6).

Vestibular findings. Vestibular function is impaired in affected males (11) but not in carrier females (4).

Radiology/histology. Radiologic studies have confirmed a thinning of the bone between the basal turn of the cochlea and the internal auditory canal (IAC), with dilation of the lateral end of the IAC and communication between the IAC and labyrinth occurring through an enlarged vestibule (Fig. 5–7). This abnormal communication leads to fluctuations in pressure in the perilymph, with extreme intracochlear pressure resulting in damage to the neuroepithelium.

Carrier females may have milder dilation of the IAC (Fig. 5–7C) (11). Cremers (4) has pointed out that the stapes may not be fixed in actuality; the malformation may produce increased pressure in the cochlea leading to turgor at the round window, resulting in decreased movement of the footplate. Although initially it was thought that other inner ear malformations were indicative of a separate X-linked gene, Mondini-type dysplasias have also been found to be due to mutations in *POU3F4* (1,13).

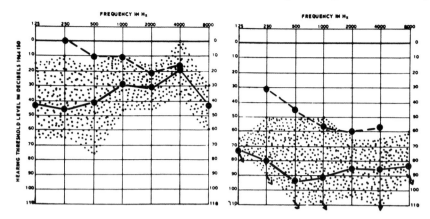

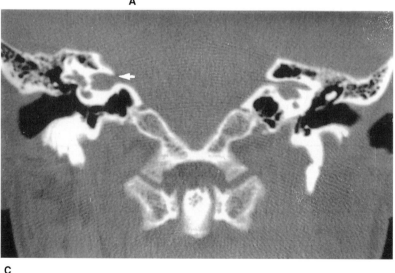

Figure 5–6. *DFN3*. Audiograms showing comparison of average air and bone conduction thresholds in four carrier females (left) and six affected males (right). Stippled area indicates range of air conduction thresholds. [From WE Nance et al., *Birth Defects* 7(4):64, 1971.]

Molecular studies. Mutations of *POU3F4* were found to cause X-linked hearing loss with stapes fixation and perilymphatic gusher (6). *POU3F4* is a transcription factor of the POU family, related to *POU4F3*, which is the causal gene for DFNA15. Members of the family have two domains, a POU homeodomain of 60 amino acids and a POU-specific domain of about 75 amino acids that confers specificity of binding. Targeted deletion of the mouse homologue, *Pou3f4* (also known as *Brn4*), has allowed visualization of the regions of expression and developmental changes of the mutant gene. Expression was seen in the devel-

oping inner ear starting around embryonic day 10 and was found throughout the otic capsule by day 12.5. In the adult male mouse, the inner ear malformations were reminiscent of those seen in humans, with hypoplasia of the cochlea, especially in the basal turn, as well as a decreased number of turns. The hair cells themselves appeared normal, but the spiral limbus and the fibrocytes of the spiral ligament were smaller than normal, and there appeared to be evidence of cochlear hydrops. The footplate of the stapes was flattened and thinner than usual, but mobility was unimpaired. In the vestibular system, there was con-

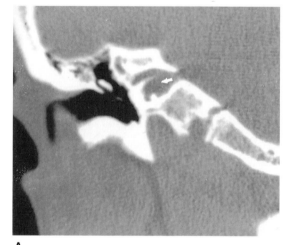

A

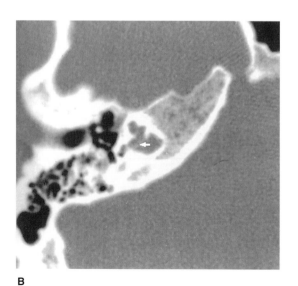

B   C

Figure 5–7. *DFN3*. (A,B) Affected male. Coronal and axial CT shows bulbous internal auditory meatus and poor or incomplete bony separation from coils of cochlea (arrows). [From PD Phelps, *Neuroradiology* 33:326, 1991.]

striction of the superior semicircular canal. The temporal bones showed dilation of the internal auditory meatus and thinning of bones surrounding the cochlea and vestibular structures. The nature of the malformations suggested an effect on mesenchymal cells. Female carrier mice had normal inner ears (12). The fibrocytes of the spiral ligament are thought to be involved in the circulation of K$^+$ ions through the stria vascularis to the endolymph, and accordingly the endocochlear potential was found to be decreased in mutant mice (8). This could also explain the hydrops that was observed, and it is possible that the hearing loss is due to a combination of ionic imbalances and hydrolic pressure variations. Testing of female carrier mice at 1 year documented progressive hearing loss in about one-third, which was also attributed to alterations in ion transport (14).

Identification of the genes within the contiguous gene deletion syndrome of choroideremia, deafness, and mental retardation led to the localization of DFN3 (2,10). *POU3F4* was identified as the gene that was deleted, and mutations within *POU3F4* were identified in males with nonsyndromic mixed deafness. The mutations were in either the homeodomain or the POU-specific domain (which comprise 35% of the *POU3F4* coding region) and resulted in truncations of the gene product (6). Subsequently, it has been found that about half of the cases of DFN3 are associated with deletions of the region proximal to *POU3F4*, but not including the gene itself. Some of these have been located as far as 800 kb from the gene (7). These indicate either deletion of regulatory regions for *POU3F4* or presence of a second gene with indistinguishable phenotypic effects.

Heredity. Inheritance is X-linked dominant with milder expression in some females consistent with Lyonization.

Prognosis. Progressive sensorineural or mixed hearing loss results in profound loss in males, and progressive sensorineural hearing loss occurs in some carrier females.

Summary. Mutations in *POU3F4* account for about 50% of X-linked deafness. The radiological findings allow clinical diagnosis, which is particularly important when there is a conductive component and surgical intervention is contemplated.

References

1. Arellano B et al: Sensorineural hearing loss and Mondini dysplasia caused by a deletion at locus DFN3. *Arch Otolaryngol Head Neck Surg* 126:1065–1069, 2000.
2. Bach I et al: Microdeletions in patients with gusher-associated, X-linked mixed deafness (DFN3). *Am J Hum Genet* 50:38–44, 1992.
3. Bitner-Glindzicz M et al: Further mutations in brain 4 (*POU3F4*) clarify the phenotype in the X-linked deafness, DFN3. *Hum Mol Genet* 4:1467–1469, 1995.
4. Cremers CWRJ.: The X-linked recessive progressive mixed hearing loss syndrome with perilymphatic gusher during stapes surgery (DFN3). In: *Genetics and Hearing Impairment,* Martini A, Read A, Stephens D (eds), Singular Publishing, San Diego, 1996, pp 236–243.
5. Cremers CWRJ et al: Clinical features of female heterozygotes in the X-linked mixed deafness syndrome (with perilymphatic gusher during stapes surgery). *Int J Pediatr Otorhinolaryngol* 6:179–185, 1983.
6. de Kok YJM et al: Association between X-linked mixed deafness and mutations in the POU domain gene *POU3F4. Science* 267:685–688, 1995.
7. de Kok YJM et al: Identification of a hot spot for microdeletions in patients with X-linked deafness type 3 (DFN3) 900 kb proximal to the DFN3 gene *POU3F4. Hum Mol Genet* 5:1229–1235, 1996.
8. Minowa O et al: Altered cochlear fibrocytes in a mouse model of DFN3 nonsyndromic deafness. *Science* 285:1408–1411, 1999.
9. Nance WE et al: X-linked mixed deafness with congenital fixation of the stapedial footplate and perilymphatic gusher. *Birth Defects* VII(4):64–69, 1971.
10. Nussbaum RL et al: Isolation of anonymous DNA sequences from within a submicroscopic X chromosomal deletion in a patient with choroideremia, deafness, and mental retardation. *Proc Natl Acad Sci USA* 84:6521–6525, 1987.
11. Phelps PD et al: X-linked deafness, stapes gushers, and a distinctive defect of the inner ear. *Neuroradiology* 33:326–330, 1991.
12. Phippard D et al: Targeted mutagenesis of the POU-domain gene *Brn4/Pou3f4* causes developmental defects in the inner ear. *J Neurosci* 19:5980–5989, 1999.
13. Piussan C et al: X-linked progressive mixed deafness; a new microdeletion that involves a more proximal region in Xq21. *Am J Hum Genet* 56:224–230, 1995.
14. Xia A-P et al: Late-onset hearing loss in a mouse model of DFN3 non-syndromic deafness: morphologic and immunohistochemical analyses. *Hear Res* 166:150–158, 2001.

DFN4

- MIM: 30030
- Location, gene: Xp21.2; gene unknown

Lalwani et al. (2) used linkage analysis in a four-generation kindred to distinguish X-linked deafness without inner ear malformation, DFN4, from DFN3. A second family from Turkey narrowed the critical region containing the gene (4).

Auditory findings. Affected males in the family had congenital profound hearing loss. Some carrier females in the original family described by Lalwani et al. (2) developed later-onset, high-frequency mild to moderate progressive hearing loss. Affected females in the Turkish family had a stable moderate high-frequency hearing loss (4).

Vestibular findings. Vestibular function testing was normal in affected males in the Turkish family (4).

Radiology/histology. The CT scans indicated normal temporal bones.

Molecular studies. Significant linkage with DXS997 localized DFN4 to the region of the Duchenne muscular dystrophy (*DMD*) gene. Fine mapping with additional markers excluded the DFN3 region, and analysis of recombination localized the gene between DXS992 and DXS1068. This includes part of the region 5′ to *DMD*, extending to intron 50 (2). Information from the Turkish family indicated that the region was between DXS992 and intron 44, within the *DMD* locus. None of the family members had any clinical features of muscular dystrophy, and creatinine phosphokinase (CPK) blood level was normal in the one male that was tested. Screening of the *DMD* gene for pathologic deletions and duplications was also normal (4).

Dystrophin isoforms are expressed in the cuticular plate, cytoskeleton, and synaptic regions of the inner and outer hair cells of the cochlea (3). The *mdx* mouse, which has a mutation in the homologue of the *DMD* gene, is particularly susceptible to noise exposure (1), and an electroretinographic abnormality similar to that seen in patients with Duchenne muscular dystrophy has been observed in affected individuals from the Turkish family (5). Thus, while it is possible that DFN4 is due to a separate gene imbedded within the DMD locus, it is also possible that a cochlear-specific isoform or intronic regulator of *DMD* is mutated in DFN4.

Heredity. Inheritance is X-linked dominant with decreased penetrance and milder expression in females.

Prognosis. Congenital profound hearing loss occurs in males, progressive mild to moderate hearing loss occurs in some females.

Summary. Hearing loss in DFN4 is very similar to that in DFN2 in both males and females. Mutation involving the structure or regulation of the Duchenne muscular dystrophy gene is likely.

References

1. Chen TJ et al: Increased vulnerability of auditory system to noise exposure in mdx mice. *Laryngoscope* 112:520–525, 2002.
2. Lalwani AK et al: A new nonsyndromic X-linked sensorineural hearing impairment linked to Xp21.2. *Am J Hum Genet* 55:685–694, 1994.
3. Michalak M, Opas M: Functions of dystrophin and dystrophin associated proteins. *Curr Opin Neurol* 10:436–442, 1997.
4. Pfister MHF et al: A second family with nonsyndromic sensorineural hearing loss linked to Xp21.2: refinement of the DFN4 locus within *DMD. Genomics* 53:377–382, 1998.

5. Pfister MH et al: Clinical evidence for dystrophin dysfunction as a cause of hearing loss in locus DFN4. *Laryngoscope* 109:730–755, 1999.

DFN6

- MIM: 300066
- Location, gene: Xp22; gene unknown
This locus was defined in a five-generation Spanish kindred (1).

Auditory findings. Onset in affected males was around 5–7 years, starting in the high frequencies and progressing to profound loss in adulthood. In females, a moderate high-frequency loss was observed with onset between 30 and 40 years.

Vestibular findings. Vestibular functions were normal.

Radiology/histology. No studies were reported.

Molecular studies. Linkage was detected to marker DXS8036 with an LOD score of 5.30 at $\theta = 0.0$. Haplotype analysis placed the critical region between DXS7108 and DXS7105, covering about 15 cM.

Heredity. Inheritance is X-linked dominant with decreased penetrance and milder expression in females.

Prognosis. High-frequency childhood hearing loss progresses to profound loss in males and adult-onset, moderate high-frequency hearing loss in females.

Summary. This locus is unique among X-linked forms in its later onset and progression.

References

1. del Castillo I et al: A novel locus for non-syndromic sensorineural deafness (DFN6) maps to chromosome Xp22. *Hum Mol Genet* 5:1383–1387, 1996.

Mitochondrial Nonsyndromic Hearing Loss

Table 5–5 summarizes mitochondrial mutations that have been associated with nonsyndromic hearing loss.

The hearing loss caused by these mutations shows some consistencies; it is generally high frequency and progressive, and there is considerable variation in penetrance. The mutations that cause hearing loss are in rRNA and highly conserved regions of mitochondrial tRNA genes as opposed to the proteins coding genes, with the exception of large deletions that include all types of genes (1,2). Within the multisystem syndromes, the only manifestation of the phenotype may be hearing loss (1); conversely, individuals with a nonsyndromic mitochondrial mutation may have normal hearing. This is not solely due to variations in

Table 5–5. Mitochondrial mutations with hearing loss

Mutation	Gene	Phenotype
961T → C	12S rRNA	Ototoxicity
1095T → C	12S rRNA	Nonsyndromic HL or ototoxicity
1445G → A	12S rRNA	Ototoxicity
1555A → G	12S rRNA	Nonsyndromic HL and ototoxicity
3243A → G	tRNALeu(UUR)	Diabetes/HL or MELAS
7445A → G	tRNASer(UCN)/CO1 junction	Palmoplantar keratoderma/HL
7472insC	tRNASer(UCN)	Nonsyndromic HL or late-onset neuromuscular disease/HL
7510T → C	tRNASer(UCN)	Nonsyndromic HL
7511T → C	tRNASer(UCN)	Nonsyndromic HL

HL, hearing loss; MELAS, *m*itochondrial *e*ncephalopathy, *l*actic *a*cidosis, and *s*troke-like episodes.

the proportions of mutant mitochondria, since the nonsyndromic mutations are often homoplasmic (3).

Fischel-Ghodsian (3) suggested that part of the variation is due to interaction with environmental factors. This is most evident with the 1555A → G mutation, which confers an increased susceptibility to aminoglycoside ototoxicity, as do several other mutations in this gene.

References

1. Ensink RJH et al: Early-onset sensorineural hearing loss and late-onset neurological complaints caused by a mitochondrial mutation at position 7472. *Arch Otolaryngol Head Neck Surg* 124:886–891, 1998.
2. Fischel-Ghodsian N: Mitochondrial RNA processing and translation: link between mitochondrial mutations and hearing loss? *Mol Genet Metab* 65:97–104, 1998.
3. Fischel-Ghodsian N.: Mitochondrial deafness mutations reviewed. *Hum Mutat* 13:261–270, 1999.

12SrRNA

- MIM: 561000 (MTRNR1), 580000 (streptomycin ototoxicity)
- Gene: Mitochondrial 12S ribosomal RNA
Certain individuals have an extreme sensitivity to the ototoxic effects of streptomycin or other aminoglycosides (kanamycin, gentamycin, tobramycin, neomycin), resulting in profound deafness. This was observed to run in families, but not in a Mendelian fashion. Clear demonstration of maternal transmission was made by Higashi (7).

Early-onset nonsyndromic hearing loss can also occur without aminoglycoside exposure. One large Arab-Israeli family has been described in which hearing loss resulted from the presence of the 1555A → G mutation and an autosomal modifying gene, *MDMI* (2). In addition, a child with early onset severe to profound hearing loss was found to have a 1095T → C mutation.

Audiology. Susceptible individuals develop hearing loss as much as 3 months after the administration of an aminoglygoside antibiotic. Degree of hearing loss varies but may involve primarily the high frequencies, or it may be profound. Tinnitus may be constant (13). Family members with the 1555A → G mutation who are not exposed to an aminoglycoside or the modifying gene are still at risk for developing an adult-onset nonsyndromic progressive hearing loss (3).

In the Arab-Israeli family with the 1555A → G mutation and the autosomal recessive *MDMI*, individuals inheriting both factors had an early-onset progressive hearing impairment resulting in a severe to profound loss (Fig. 5–8) (9).

The 1095T → C mutation was associated with severe to profound hearing loss in the proband, with less severe hearing losses in maternal relatives unless there had been exposure to aminoglycosides.

Vestibular findings. Vestibular function remains normal in susceptible individuals who receive normal doses of aminoglycosides. This is in contrast to individuals who receive large doses of amnioglycosides, which then are vestibulotoxic as well as ototoxic (1).

Molecular studies. Three mutations have been identified that confer susceptibility to aminoglycoside ototoxicity. By far the most common is the 1555A → G mutation; screening of individuals from the United States with aminoglycoside-induced hearing loss revealed that it was present in 17% (5,6), and it appears to be even more common in Japan, with fully 3% of individuals with hearing loss attending an otolarynogology clinic having the mutation (13). The mutation is homoplasmic. The location of this mutation in the rRNA molecule is homologous to the aminoglycoside binding position in bacterial rRNA, and the mutation serves to make the human rRNA equally available for binding (8). Other mutations in the 12SrRNA that produce susceptibility to aminoglycosides are deletion of a thymine and insertion of multiple cytosines (961T → Cn) (4) and 1445G → A (10).

In the Arab-Israeli family with a five-generation history of early-onset hearing loss, segregation analysis was consistent with a digenic model including an autosomal recessive locus and a mitochondrial lo-

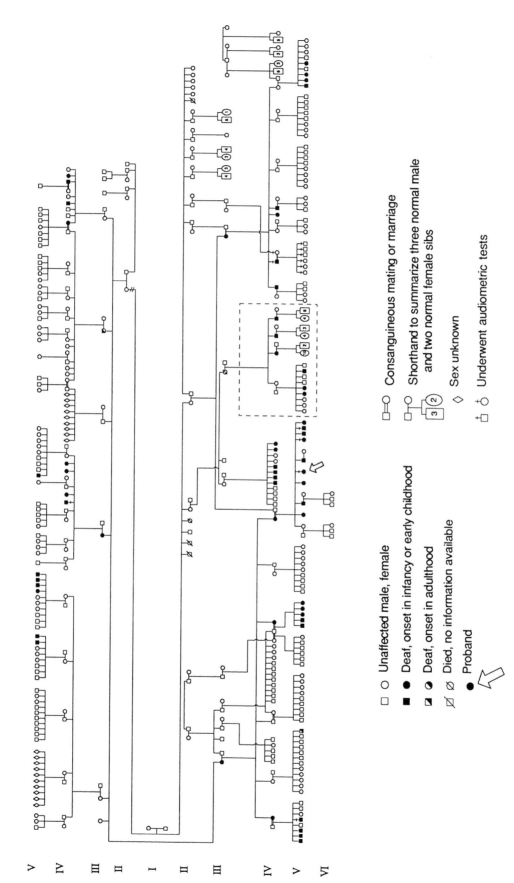

V

IV

III

II

I

II

III

IV

V

VI

○—○ Unaffected male, female

● Deaf, onset in infancy or early childhood

◐ Deaf, onset in adulthood

⌀ Ø Died, no information available

● Proband

○—○ Consanguineous mating or marriage

○—□ Shorthand to summarize three normal male and two normal female sibs

◇ Sex unknown

□ ○ Underwent audiometric tests

Figure 5–8. Kindred showing mitochondrial inheritance. [From L Jaber et al., *J Med Genet* 29:86, 1992.]

cus, and it was found that affected individuals were homoplasmic for the 1555A → G mutation (11). Additional families from Spain, Italy, and Norway were ascertained, and linkage analysis localized the autosomal recessive locus to chromosome 8. An LOD score of 4.0 was obtained for markers D8S277, D8S561, and D8S1819 at 8p23 (2).

In a screen of children with hearing loss compatible with mitochondrial inheritance, Tessa et al. (12) identified a child with a 1095T → C mutation. This was found to be homoplasmic in the child, but more mildly affected maternal relatives were found to be heteroplasmic, although some had more severe hearing loss after aminoglycoside exposure.

Heredity. Homoplasmy for the mutations in the mitochondrial 12SrRNA creates a pattern of maternal inheritance for the susceptibility to ototoxic aminoglycosides or adult-onset progressive hearing loss. Early-onset progressive hearing loss requires the combination of homozygosity for mutation in *MDMI* and the 1555A → G mitochondrial mutation.

Prognosis. Exposure to an aminoglycoside antibiotic in a susceptible individual can produce a progressive hearing loss that may be profound. In the absence of aminoglycoside exposure, hearing loss has a later adult onset with slow progression. When inherited with *MDMI*, hearing loss has an onset in childhood and is progressive. No other systems are affected.

Summary. The nonsyndromic hearing loss resulting from mitochondrial mutations can be quite variable, even within families. The source of this variation can be genetic or environmental, as illustrated by the interactions of these mutations, particularly the 1555A → G mutation, with both aminoglycoside administration or a nuclear gene. Assay for this mutation should be made in a child with hearing loss and a history of aminoglycoside exposure, especially in the presence of normal vestibular function, so that other susceptible family members can be identified.

References

1. Braverman I et al: Audiovestibular findings in patients with deafness caused by a mitochondrial mutation and precipitated by an inherited nuclear mutation or aminoglycosides. *Arch Otolaryngol Head Neck Surg* 122:1001–1004, 1996.
2. Bykhovskaya Y et al: Modifier locus for mitochondrial DNA disease: linkage and linkage disequilibrium mapping of a nuclear modifier gene for maternally inherited deafness. *Genet Med* 3:177–180, 2001.
3. Estivil X et al: Familial progressive sensorineural deafness is mainly due to the mtDNA A1555G mutation and is enhanced by treatment with aminoglycosides. *Am J Hum Genet* 62:27–35, 1998.
4. Fischel-Ghodsian N.: Genetic factors in aminoglycoside toxicity. *Ann NY Acad Sci* 884:99–109, 1999.
5. Fischel-Ghodsian N et al: Mitochondrial ribosomal RNA gene mutation associated with aminoglycoside ototoxicity. *Am J Otolaryngol* 14:399–403, 1993.
6. Fischel-Ghodsian N et al: Mitochondrial gene mutations: a common predisposing factor in aminoglycoside ototoxicity. *Am J Otolaryngol* 18:173–178, 1997.
7. Higashi K: Unique inheritance of streptomycin-induced deafness. *Clin Genet* 35:433–436, 1989.
8. Hutchin T et al: A molecular basis for human hypersensitivity to aminoglycoside antibiotics. *Nucleic Acids Res* 21:4174–4179, 1993.
9. Jaber L et al: Sensorineural deafness inherited as a tissue specific mitochondrial disorder. *J Med Genet* 29:86–90, 1992.
10. Maguire DJ et al: A possible new mtrRNA mutation site for aminoglycoside-induced deafness syndrome. In: *Oxygen Transport to Tissue XXI*, Eke A, Delpy DT (eds), Kluwer Academic/Plenum, New York, 1999, pp 411–417.
11. Prezant TR et al: Mitochondrial ribosomal RNA mutation associated with both antibiotic-induced and non-syndromic deafness. *Nat Genet* 4:289–294, 1993.
12. Tessa A et al: Maternally inherited deafness associated with a T1095C mutation in the mDNA. *Eur J Hum Genet* 9:147–149, 2001.
13. Usami S-I et al: Sensorineural hearing loss associated with the mitochondrial mutations. *Adv Otorhinolaryngol* 56:203–211, 2000.

tRNALeu(UUR)

- MIM: 590050 (MTTL1)
- Gene: Mitochondrial transfer RNA, leucine, 1

The 3243A → G mutation has been associated with the maternally inherited syndrome of late-onset diabetes and deafness, as well as MELAS (*m*itochondrial *m*yopathy, *e*ncephalopathy, *l*actic *a*cidosis, and *s*troke-like episodes). There is considerable phenotypic variability within families with these conditions, and there are also a few reports of apparently nonsyndromic hearing loss (4). However, careful follow-up is important to monitor for the development of additional symptoms.

Audiology. Hearing loss generally starts in adulthood, initially in the high frequencies, and is progressive. Ultimate severity is variable, although it may reach the profound range. Tinnitus is often present (3).

Vestibular function. With a few exceptions with diminished caloric responses, vestibular function is usually normal (2).

Molecular studies. In contrast to the 12SrRNA mutations, individuals with the 3243A → G mutation are heteroplasmic. The percent of mutant mitochondria in cochlear tissues is likely to contribute to the variability in hearing loss, but this is difficult to estimate since it is not necessarily reflected by the percent of mutant mitochondria in blood or other tissues.

In a screen of 100 Japanese individuals with hearing loss, 3 were found to be heteroplasmic for the 3243A → G mutation. The characteristics of the hearing loss were quite different, with one subject showing onset of high-frequency loss and tinnitus at 61 years, another having a history of fluctuating loss starting at age 33, and the third presenting with moderate to severe hearing loss at 6 years of age, and it was questioned whether the loss was actually prelingual (1).

Heredity. Inheritance is maternal with variation in expression, including syndromic features.

Prognosis. Progressive hearing loss occurs, with risk of developing syndromic complications.

Summary. Purely nonsyndromic hearing loss resulting from the 3243A → G mutation may be rare, with neurological or endocrinological complications arising later in life.

References

1. Oshima T et al: Hearing loss with a mitochondrial gene mutation is highly prevalent in Japan. *Laryngoscope* 109:334–338, 1999.
2. Tamagawa Y et al: Audiologic findings in patients with point mutation at nucleotide 3,243 of mitochondrial DNA. *Ann Otol Rhino Laryngol* 106:338–342, 1997.
3. Usami S-I et al: Sensorineural hearing loss associated with the mitochondrial mutations. *Adv Otorhinolaryngol* 56:203–211, 2000.
4. van den Ouweland JMW et al: Mutation in mitochondrial tRNALeu (UUR) gene in a large pedigree with maternally transmitted type II diabetes mellitus and deafness. *Nat Genet* 1:368–371, 1992.

tRNASer(UCN)

- MIM: 590080 (MTTS1)
- Gene: Mitochondrial transfer RNA, serine 1

Several mutations in tRNASer(UCN) have been associated with nonsyndromic hearing loss, including 7445A → G (5), 7472insC (1), 7510T → C (4), and 7511T → C (7).

Audiology. Age of onset is variable, is gradually progressive, and may ultimately reach the severe range.

Vestibular function. No symptoms were reported.

Molecular studies. The 7445A → G mutation is actually at the 3′ end of the tRNASer(UCN) gene and affects the rate of transcription rather than the structure of the product (3). This mutation was identified in a Scottish kindred (5), a New Zealand kindred (2), and a Japanese kindred (6). The hearing loss was more highly penetrant in the New Zealand kindred, and this was attributed at least in part to additional mitochondrial mutations. In the study by Sevior et al. (6), it was noted that the hearing loss was accompanied by palmoplantar keratoderma, and reevaluation of both the New Zealand and Scottish kindreds confirmed these findings in those families as well (8). Thus the 7445 mutation may actually be syndromic, but the dermatologic manifestations may not always be appreciated.

Other mutations of the tRNASer(UCN) gene are presumed to affect the highly conserved acceptor arm of the molecule. The phenotypic effects of the 7472Cins mutation vary from nonsyndromic hearing loss to a syndrome of associated neurological disorders such as ataxia, myoclonic epilepsy, or cognitive impairment, with variation seen within families. Some relationship is seen with the degree of heteroplasmy, with individuals who appear to be homoplasmic showing neurological symptoms in addition to hearing loss, but there may also be nuclear modifiers (1,9).

Family members with the 7511T → C mutation were heteroplasmic or homoplasmic in blood. While there was no clinical evidence of myopathy, muscle biopsy did show partial cytochrome C oxidase deficiency, but no ragged red fibers (7). As with the other mitochondrial mutations, hearing loss was progressive and age of onset was variable.

An adjacent mutation, 7510C → T, has also been described. The phenotype was similar and affected individuals were homoplasmic (4).

Heredity. Inheritance is maternal, with variation in expression and penetrance presumably affected by degree of cochlear heteroplasmy and/or mitochondrial or nuclear modifier genes.

Prognosis. Hearing loss is progressive and age of onset is variable. Palmoplantar keratoderma may be present. Neurologic signs may develop with age.

Summary. While hearing loss due to mutations in and around the tRNASer(UCN) gene can be nonsyndromic, other syndromic manifestations may develop.

References

1. Ensink RJH et al: Early-onset sensorineural hearing loss and late-onset neurological complaints caused by a mitochondrial mutation at position 7472. *Arch Otolaryngol Head Neck Surg* 124:886–891, 1998.
2. Fischel-Ghodsian N et al: Mitochondrial mutation associated with nonsyndromic deafness. *Am J Otolaryngol* 16:403–408, 1995.
3. Guan MX et al: The deafness-associated mitochondrial DNA mutation at position 7445, which affects tRNASer(UCN) precursor processing, has long-range effects on NADH dehydrogenase subunit ND6 gene expression. *Mol Cell Biol* 18:5868–5879, 1998.
4. Hutchin TP et al: A novel mutation in the mitochondrial tRNASer(UCN) gene in a family with non-syndromic sensorineural hearing impairment. *J Med Genet* 37:692–694, 2000.
5. Reid FM et al: A novel mitochondrial point mutation in a maternal pedigree with sensorineural deafness. *Hum Mutat* 3:243–247, 1994.
6. Sevior KB et al: Mitochondrial A7445G mutation in two pedigrees with palmoplantar keratoderma and deafness. *Am J Med Genet* 75:179–185, 1998.
7. Sue CM et al: Maternally inherited hearing loss in a large kindred with a novel T7511C mutation in the mitochondrial DNA tRNA[Ser(UCN)] gene. *Neurology* 52:1905–1908, 1999.
8. Van Camp G, Smith RJH: Maternally inherited hearing impairment. *Clin Genet* 57:409–414, 2000.
9. Verhoeven K et al: Hearing impairment and neurological dysfunction associated with a mutation in the mitochondrial tRNASer(UCN) gene. *Eur J Hum Genet* 7:45–51, 1999.

Glomus tympanicum (non-chromaffin paragangliomas, chemodectomas, familial glomus tumors) and hearing loss

Non-chromaffin paragangliomas (NCP) may be isolated or familial. In the head and neck region, familial NCP most often involve the tympanic and jugular glomera (glomus jugulotympanicum) (23%), glomus vagale (6%), and carotid glomus (84%). Multiple sites may be involved, especially in familial (50%) but not nonfamilial (5%) cases (14). Guild (5), in 1941, and Rosenwasser (15), in 1945, first described the glomus jugulotympanicum, and Linn and Proctor (10) first described familial jugular and vagal body tumors. In 1982, Van Baars et al (19), reviewed 32 reports of familial NCP encompassing 160 patients Several other series of isolated and familial cases have been described (4,8,9,11–13,16–18).

Auditory findings. Pulsative tinnitus occurs in over 50%–75%, with hearing loss in about 30%–50%. Less common are otalgia (7%–18%), aural fullness (4%–18%), and otorrhea (3%–8%) (8,12,16). Mean duration of symptoms prior to diagnosis is 30 months. Hearing loss can be conductive, mixed, or sensorineural, most often being conductive (8,12). Hearing loss has ranged from minor to total (4). Presentation usually occurs in midlife (range 20–88 years). Symptoms suggestive of a secretory tumor have not been present. The form of presentation and symptomology do not differ between isolated and familial cases.

Pathology. The retrotympanic glomus tympanicum tumors occur along the tympanic branch of the glossopharyngeal nerve (Jacobson's nerve) or, less often, the auricular branch of the vagus nerve (Arnold's nerve), sparing the jugular bulb (7). The tumors are reddish-blue in color. The cells are arranged in clusters, or "cell-balls" (Fig. 5–9).

Diagnosis. The tumors are usually retrotympanic, although rarely they may protrude through the eardrum into the external ear canal. Spontaneous pulsation of the tumor, auricle, or region of the neck below the ear is found in about 35% (4).

High-resolution CT is currently the radiographic study of choice to determine whether the jugular bulb is involved (12,14). A thorough imaging work-up is mandated before surgical intervention because of the not uncommon location of the internal carotid artery in such cases and the possibility of its injury during the biopsy procedure.

Figure 5–9. *Glomus tympanicum (non-chromaffin paragangliomas, chemodectomas, familial glomus tumors) and hearing loss.* Carotid body tumor. Note classic "cell-ball" pattern. [From MR Abell et al., *Hum Pathol* 1:503, 1970.]

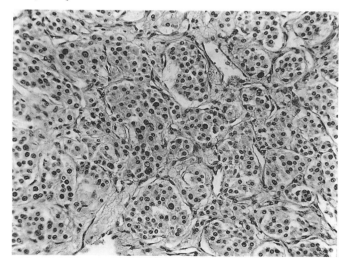

Heredity. Among isolated cases, there appears to be a marked female predilection (8). However, in familial cases, there is no sex predilection. Penetrance for this autosomal dominant gene is 100% over the age of 45 years (19).

Heutink et al. (6) mapped the gene for hereditary paragangliomas of the head and neck to 11q23–qter. They found evidence suggestive of genomic imprinting in that affected individuals inherited the disease gene from their fathers but expression of the phenotype was not observed in the offspring of affected females until subsequent transmission through a male carrier (6,20). Mutations have been reported in the *SDHD* gene on chromosome 11, which encodes a subunit of cytochrome B in succinate-ubiquinone oxidoreductase (3). Surprisingly, no evidence for imprinting has been shown. Badenhop et al. (2) reported mutations in four families with carotid body paragangliomas and sensorineural deafness and/or tinnitus. Mutations in the related gene *SDHB* are reported in cases of cervical and extra-adrenal pheochromocytoma, but no association with deafness was seen in these families (1).

Summary. Characteristics include (*1*) autosomal dominant inheritance, (*2*) non-chromaffin paragangliomas, and (*3*) hearing loss that is sensorineural, conductive, or mixed.

References

1. Astuti D et al: Gene mutations in the succinate dehydrogenase subunit *SDHB* cause susceptibility to familial pheochromocytoma and to familial paraganglioma. *Am J Hum Genet* 69:49–54, 2001.
2. Badenhop RF et al: Novel mutations in the *SDHD* gene in pedigrees with familial carotid body paraganglioma and sensorineural hearing loss. *Genes Chromosome Cancer* 31:255–263, 2001.
3. Baysal BE et al: Mutations in *SDHD*, a mitochondrial complex II gene, in hereditary paraganglioma. *Science* 287:848–851, 2000.
4. Brown LA: Glomus jugulare tumor of the middle ear: clinical aspects. *Laryngoscope* 63:281–292, 1953.
5. Guild SR: A hitherto unrecognized structure, the glomus jugularis, in man [abstract]. *Anat Rec* 79:28, 1941.
6. Heutink P et al: A gene subject to genomic imprinting and responsible for hereditary paragangliomas maps to chromosome 11q23–qter. *Hum Mol Genet* 1:7–10, 1992.
7. House WF, Glasscock ME III: Glomus tympanicum tumors. *Arch Otolaryngol* 87:550–554, 1968.
8. Jackson CG et al: Glomus tympanicum tumors: contemporary concepts in conservation surgery. *Laryngoscope* 99:875–884, 1989.
9. Lawrence RC et al: Familial chemodectomas. *Int J Radiol Oncol Biol Phys* 7:949–952, 1981.
10. Linn HJ, Proctor B: Tumor of the ganglion nodosum of the vagus nerve. *Laryngoscope* 66:1577–1581, 1956.
11. Macre F, Casatta MD: Tumori glomici multipli con recorrenza famigliare. *Otorinolaringologia* 39:541–545, 1989.
12. O'Leary MJ et al: Glomus tympanicum tumors: a clinical perspective. *Laryngoscope* 101:1038–1043, 1991.
13. Ophir D: Familial multicentric paragangliomas in a child. *J Laryngol Otol* 105:376–380, 1991.
14. Phelps PD, Stansbie JM: Glomus jugulare or tympanicum? The role of CT and MR imaging with gadolinium DTPA. *J Laryngol Otol* 102:766–776, 1988.
15. Rosenwasser H: Carotid body tumor of the middle ear and mastoid. *Arch Otolaryngol* 41:64–67, 1945.
16. Spector GJ et al: Glomus tumors in the middle ear: An analysis of 46 patients. *Laryngoscope* 83:1652–1672, 1973.
17. Tali ET et al: Magnetic resonance imaging of bilateral familial paragangliomas. *Ann Otol Rhinol Laryngol* 102:473–477, 1993.
18. Van Baars F et al: Familial non-chromaffin paragangliomas: clinical aspects. *Laryngoscope* 91:988–996, 1981.
19. Van Baars F et al: Genetic aspects of nonchromaffin paraganglioma. *Hum Genet* 60:305–309, 1982.
20. Van der Mey AGL et al: Genomic imprinting in hereditary glomus tumors: evidence for new genetic theory. *Lancet* 2:1291–1294, 1989.

Chapter 6
Genetic Hearing Loss Associated with External Ear Abnormalities
JUDITH ALLANSON

In the first edition of this book, 10 hereditary deafness syndromes with external ear abnormalities were described. Two of those syndromes—ear malformations, cervical fistulas or nodules, and mixed hearing loss; and preauricular pits, branchial fistulas, and sensorineural hearing loss—have been unified into the branchio-oto-renal syndrome. In the second edition, 30 distinctive hereditary syndromes of hearing loss with external ear changes were described. The external ear abnormalities ranged from anotia to large, cupped, simple auricles.

Several syndromes with hearing loss and external ear anomalies are not covered in this chapter because other aspects of the syndromes warrant their inclusion elsewhere, including two conditions that were part of this chapter in the second edition. In this third edition, a handful of new conditions are described. Measurements, proportions, architecture, and placement of the pinna are now well established (2–4), and isolated anomalies of the auricle have been well reviewed (1,5,6).

References

1. Davis J: Surgical embryology. In: *Aesthetic and Reconstructive Otoplasty,* Davis J (ed), Springer-Verlag, Berlin, 1987, pp 93–125.
2. Farkas LG: *Anthropometry of the Head and Face in Medicine.* Elsevier, New York, 1981.
3. Farkas LG: Otoplastic architecture. In: *Aesthetic and Reconstructive Otoplasty,* Davis J (ed), Springer-Verlag, Berlin, 1987, pp 13–52.
4. Hall JG et al: *Handbook of Physical Measurements.* Oxford University Press, New York, 1989.
5. Jaffe BF: Pinna anomalies associated with congenital conductive hearing loss. *Pediatrics* 57:332–341, 1976.
6. Lange G: Familienuntersuchungen über die Erblichkeit metrischer und morphologischer Merkmale des äusseren Ohres. *Z Morphol Anthropol* 57:111–167, 1961.

Mandibulofacial dysostosis (Treacher Collins syndrome)

Although mandibulofacial dysostosis was probably first described by Thomson (52) and Toynbee (53) in 1846–1847, credit for its discovery is usually given to Berry (4) or, especially, to Treacher Collins (55) (the name is often erroneously hyphenated), who described the essential components of the syndrome. Franceschetti and coworkers (11,12) extensively reviewed the disorder and coined the term *mandibulofacial dysostosis.* Perhaps 400 or more cases have been published and the condition is said to occur with an incidence of 1 in 50,000 livebirths (46).

Craniofacial findings. Facial abnormalities are bilateral and usually symmetric, but not always (58). The nose appears large but this appearance is really secondary to hypoplastic supraorbital rims and hypoplastic zygomas (22). The face is narrow. Downward-sloping palpebral fissures, depressed cheekbones, malformed pinnae, receding chin, and large downturned mouth are characteristic (Fig. 6–1A–F). About 25% of patients manifest a tongue-shaped process of hair that extends toward the cheek (44) (Fig. 6–1G).

The palpebral fissures are short and slope laterally downward, and often (75%) there is a coloboma in the outer third of the lower lid (Fig. 6–1H). About half of the patients have deficiency of cilia medial to the coloboma. Iris colobomas may also occur. The lower lacrimal points may be absent as well as the Meibomian glands and intermarginal strip (13,30).

The nasofrontal angle is usually obliterated, and the bridge of the nose raised. The nose appears large (22) because of the lack of malar development and hypoplastic supraorbital ridges. The nares are often narrow, and the alar cartilages are hypoplastic. Choanal atresia has been reported (28,34,47). Obstructive sleep apnea is not rare (20).

The pinnae are often malformed, crumpled forward, or misplaced toward the angle of the mandible. In the survey of Stovin et al. (50), 51 of 63 patients had anomalous pinnae. Kolar et al. (22) found microtia in 60%. Extra ear tags and blind fistulae may occur anywhere between the tragus and the angle of the mouth. In one case, blind fistulae were found behind the ear lobes (15).

The palate is cleft in about 35% (11,35,38,50). Congenital palatopharyngeal incompetence (agenesis of soft palate, foreshortened soft palate, submucous palatal cleft, immobile soft palate) has been found in an additional 30%–40% (38). Rarely, cleft lip–palate has been noted. Macrostomia, observed in about 15%, may be unilateral or bilateral. The elevator muscles of the upper lip are deficient (17). The parotid glands may be absent or hypoplastic (17,31,33). Pharyngeal hypoplasia, a constant finding, may explain cases of neonatal death (48).

Radiographic findings. The calvaria is essentially normal, but radiographic studies reveal that the supraorbital ridges are poorly developed (32,35,50). The body of the malar bones may be totally absent but more often is grossly and symmetrically underdeveloped, with nonfusion of the zygomatic arches. The zygomatic process of the frontal bone is hypoplastic, as are the lateral pterygoid plates and muscles (Fig. 6–1I,J). The mastoids are not pneumatized and are frequently sclerotic. The paranasal sinuses are often small and may be completely absent. The orbits are hyperteloric (22). The lower margin of the orbit may be defective and the infraorbital foramen is usually absent. The cranial base is progressively kyphotic (37). The reader is referred to several articles for detailed craniofacial measurements (1,10,23).

The mandibular condyle is severely hypoplastic. The neck is short and the condyle malformed. The undersurface of the body is often quite concave. The angle is more obtuse than normal and the ramus is often deficient. The coronoid and condyloid processes are flat or even aplastic. There is no articular eminence and the articular area is atypically medial (14,15,34,44) (Fig. 6–1K).

Central nervous system. Intelligence is usually normal. However, Stovin et al. (50) reviewed 63 patients and found 4 who were mentally deficient. Other investigators have also noted mild mental retardation in their patients (15).

Auditory system. The auditory ossicles and cochlear and vestibular apparatus have been observed to be absent or severely malformed (18,25,29,30,33,39,42). Radiographic and surgical studies have shown agenesis or hypoplasia of the mastoid and mastoid antrum, absence of the external auditory canal, narrowing or agenesis of the middle ear cleft, agenesis or malformation of the malleus and/or incus, monopodal stapes, absence of stapes and oval window, ankylosis of stapes in oval window, deformed suprastructure of stapes, and complete absence of middle ear and epitympanic space (Fig. 6–1L–N). The space may be filled with connective tissue (18,25,30,33). The inner ear is usually normal (29). Bilateral hearing loss has been found in at least 55% (40). In a computed tomography (CT) study, Pron et al. (42) found that normal,

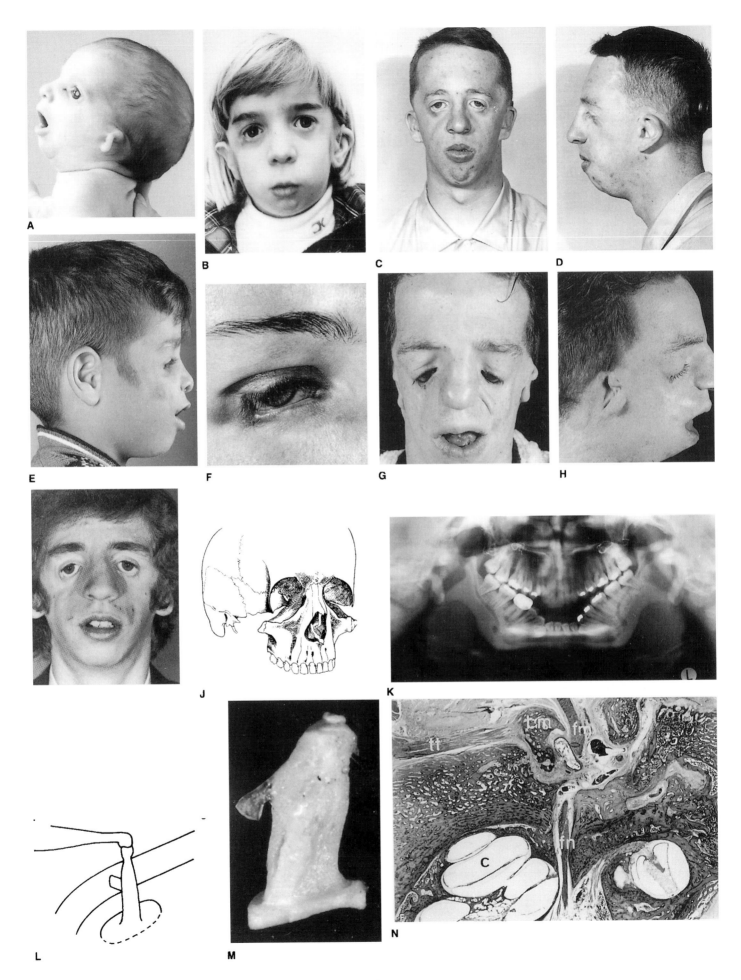

stenotic, and atretic external canals were associated with 44, 54, and 62 dB loss, respectively. Those without ossicles had flat conductive loss, whereas those having ankylosed or hypoplastic ossicles had flat (60%) or sloping (40%) audiograms.

Pathogenesis. There have been several excellent anatomic and embryologic studies (2,3,6,17,26,33,41). Histological studies in animal phenocopies indicate abnormalities of neural crest when teratogenic doses of vitamin A and isotretinoin are given during pregnancy (25,51,57).

Heredity. The syndrome has autosomal dominant inheritance with variable expressivity (30,46,50,56). Among the roughly 60% that represent new mutations, fathers tend to be older (21). The locus was mapped to the 5q31.3–q33.3 region (8,9,19). In 1996, a Collaborative Group led by Dixon (54) isolated the gene (*TCOF1*) and called the protein Treacle. Subsequent family studies have detected loss-of-function mutations throughout the gene (49). Almost all mutations result in a truncated protein; the majority are deletions; however, insertion, splice-site, and nonsense mutations are reported (49). No genotype–phenotype correlation has emerged (49). One study reported a mutation detection rate of 93%; genetic heterogeneity for the phenotype was suggested as an explanation for the lack of mutation detection in two families (49). Treacle is known to be a nucleolar phosphoprotein, the correct dosage of which seems to be essential for survival of cephalic neural crest cells (7), lending credence to the teratologic studies of phenocopies.

Diagnosis. Oculo-auriculo-vertebral spectrum is easily excluded. Nager acrofacial dysostosis closely resembles mandibulofacial dysostosis. The thumbs are hypoplastic or absent, the radius and ulna may be fused, or there may be absence or hypoplasia of the radius and/or one or more metacarpals. Dominantly inherited and X-linked maxillofacial dysostosis consists of bilateral hypoplasia of malar bones, downward-slanting palpebral fissures, without colobomas, maxillary hypoplasia, open bite, and relative mandibular prognathism. A similar facial phenotype has been seen in an autosomal recessive disorder found in Hutterites (27), in an autosomal dominant osteosclerotic disorder (24), and in a father and son with ectrodactyly. Richieri-Costa et al. (43) reported an autosomal recessive mandibulofacial dysostosis, as did Stovin et al. (50). Hedera et al. (16) described a family with an autosomal dominant mandibulofacial dysostosis with ptosis in which linkage to *TCOF1* was excluded.

Prenatal diagnosis. Mid-trimester ultrasonographic (2,3,5) and fetoscopic diagnoses (36) have been accomplished.

←————————

Figure 6–1. *Mandibulofacial dysostosis (Treacher Collins syndrome).* (A–F) Note variable phenotype in individuals of different age. Especially note downslanting palpebral fissures, micrognathia, and varying degrees of microtia. (G) Note hair tongue extending to cheek. (H) Observe coloboma in lower lid with absence of cilia medial to coloboma. (I,J) Note agenesis of zygomata. (K) Panoramic radiographic showing prominent antegonial notching and open bite. (L) Schematic diagram of dwarfing of stapes deformity. The stapes, columnar in form, has its footplate ankylosed in oval window. (M) Stapes showing crurae fused into monopodal structure onto neck of which stapedius tendon was inserted. (N) The tensor tympani muscle (tt) of right ear is attached to bony ossicular mass (bm) in mesotympanum. These structures are covered laterally only by soft tissue and not by bone. The facial nerve (fn) exits almost directly laterally from its position in internal auditory meatus. It curves in the middle ear around bony ossicular mass (bm) before leaving the temporal bone. The bone between cochlea (c) and tensor sympani (tt) is markedly thickened. [(E,F) courtesy of VA McKusick, Baltimore, Maryland; (G) from BO Rogers, *Br J Plast Surg* 17:109, 1964; (I,J) courtesy of P Tessier, Paris, France; (L) from G Keerl, *Ophthalmology* 143:5, 1962; (M) from WG Edwards, *J Laryngol Otol* 78:152, 1964; (N) from I Sands et al., *Trans Am Acad Ophthalmol Otolaryngol* 72:913, 1968.]

Prognosis. There is no progression of hearing loss.

Summary. Characteristics of this syndrome include (*1*) autosomal dominant transmission with variable expressivity; (*2*) hypoplastic zygomas with resultant downslanting palpebral fissures, coloboma of the lower eyelids, and lack of cilia medial to the colobomas; (*3*) mandibular hypoplasia; (*4*) malformed pinnae, external canals, and middle ear structures; and (*5*) conductive hearing loss.

References

1. Arvystas M, Shprintzen RJ: Craniofacial morphology in Treacher Collins syndrome. *Cleft Palate Craniofac J* 28:226–231, 1991.
2. Behrents RG et al: Prenatal mandibulofacial dysostosis (Treacher Collins in man). *Arch Oral Biol* 20:265–282, 1975.
3. Behrents RG et al: Prenatal mandibulofacial dysostosis (Treacher Collins syndrome). *Cleft Palate J* 14:13–34, 1977.
4. Berry GA: Note on a congenital defect (coloboma?) of the lower lid. *R Lond Ophthalmol Hosp Rep* 12:255–257, 1889.
5. Crane JP, Beaver HA: Midtrimester sonographic diagnosis of mandibular dysostosis. *Am J Med Genet* 25:251–255, 1986.
6. Dahl E et al: A morphologic description of a dry skull with mandibulofacial dysostosis. *Scand J Dent Res* 83:257–266, 1975.
7. Dixon J et al: Increased levels of apoptosis in the prefusion neural folds underlie the craniofacial disorder, Treacher Collins syndrome. *Hum Mol Genet* 9:1473–1480, 2000.
8. Dixon MJ et al: The gene for Treacher Collins syndrome maps to the long arm of chromosome 5. *Am J Hum Genet* 48:274–280, 1991.
9. Dixon MJ et al: Genetic and physical mapping of the Treacher Collins syndrome locus: refinement of the localization to chromosome 5q32–33.2. *Hum Mol Genet* 1:249–253, 1992.
10. Figueroa AA et al: Neurocranial morphology in mandibulofacial dysostosis (Treacher Collins syndrome). *Cleft Palate Craniofac J* 30:369–375, 1993.
11. Franceschetti A, Klein D: Mandibulo-facial dysostosis: new hereditary syndrome. *Acta Ophthalmol (Kbh)* 27:143–224, 1949.
12. Franceschetti A et al: Dysostose mandibulo-facial unilatérale avec déformations multiples du squelette (Processus paramastöide, synostose des vertebres, sacralisation, etc.) et torticollis clonique. *Ophthalmologica* 118:796–814, 1949.
13. Franceschetti A et al: La dysostose mandibulo-faciale dans le cadre des syndrome du premier arc branchial. *Schweiz Med Wochenschr* 89:478–483, 1959.
14. Garner LD: Cephalometric analysis of Berry-Treacher Collins syndrome. *Oral Surg* 23:320–327, 1967.
15. Grönvall H, Olsson Y: Dysostosis mandibulofacialis. *Acta Ophthalmol (Kbh)* 31:245–252, 1953.
16. Hedera P et al: Novel autosomal dominant mandibulofacial dysostosis with ptosis: clinical description and exclusion of TCOF1. *J Med Genet* 39:484–488, 2002.
17. Herring SE et al: Anatomical abnormalities in mandibulofacial dysostosis. *Am J Med Genet* 3:225–259, 1979.
18. Hutchinson JC Jr et al: The otologic manifestations of mandibulofacial dysostosis. *Trans Am Acad Ophthalmol* 84:520–528, 1977.
19. Jabs EW et al: Mapping the Treacher Collins syndrome locus to 5q31.3–5q33.3. *Genomics* 11:193–198, 1991.
20. Johnston C et al: Obstructive sleep apnea in Treacher Collins syndrome. *Cleft Palate J* 18:39–44, 1981.
21. Jones KL et al: Older paternal age and fresh gene mutation: data on additional disorders. *J Pediatr* 86:84–88, 1976.
22. Kolar JC et al: Surface morphology in Treacher Collins syndrome: an anthropometric study. *Cleft Palate J* 22:266–274, 1985.
23. Kreiborg S, Dahl E: Cranial base and face in mandibulofacial dysostosis. *Am J Med Genet* 47:753–760, 1993.
24. Lehman RAW: Familial osteosclerosis with abnormalities of the nervous system and meninges. *J Pediatr* 90:49–54, 1977.
25. Lloyd GAS, Phelps PD: Radiology of the ear in mandibulofacial dysostosis–Treacher Collins syndrome. *Acta Radiol Diagn* 20:233–240, 1979.
26. Lockhart RD: Variants coincident with congenital absence of zygoma (zygomatic process of temporal bone). *J Anat* 63:233–236, 1928–1929.
27. Lowry RB et al: Mandibulofacial dysostosis in Hutterite sibs: a possible recessive trait. *Am J Med Genet* 22:501–512, 1985.
28. Lübke F von: Über die Beobachtung einer Dysostosis mandibulofacialis. *Z Geburtsch Gynäkol* 156:235–246, 1961.
29. Mafee MF et al: Radiographic features of the ear-related developmental anomalies in patients with mandibulofacial dysostosis. *Int J Pediatr Otolaryngol* 7:229–238, 1984.

30. Mann I, Kilner TP: Deficiency of the malar bones with defect of the lower lids. *Br J Ophthalmol* 27:13–20, 1943.

31. Markitzin A et al: Major salivary glands in branchial arch syndromes. *Oral Surg* 58:672–677, 1984.

32. Marsh JL et al: The skeletal anatomy of mandibulofacial dysostosis (Treacher Collins syndrome). *Plast Reconstr Surg* 78:460–468, 1986.

33. McKenzie J, Craig J: Mandibulo-facial dysostosis (Treacher Collins syndrome). *Arch Dis Child* 30:391–395, 1955.

34. McNeill KA, Wynter-Wedderburn L: Choanal atresia: a manifestation of the Treacher Collins syndrome. *J Laryngol Otol* 67:365–369, 1953.

35. Nager FR, deReynier JP: Das Gehörorgan bei den angeborenen Kopfmissbildungen. *Pract Otorhinolaryngol (Basel) Suppl* 2, 10:1–128, 1948.

36. Nicolaides KH et al: Prenatal diagnosis of mandibulofacial dysostosis. *Prenat Diagn* 4:201–205, 1984.

37. Peterson-Falzone S, Figueroa AA: Longitudinal changes in cranial base angulation in mandibulofacial dysostosis. *Cleft Palate J* 26:31–35, 1989.

38. Peterson-Falzone S, Pruzansky S: Cleft palate and congenital palato-pharyngeal incompetency in mandibulofacial dysostosis: frequency and problems in treatment. *Cleft Palate J* 13:354–360, 1976.

39. Phelps PD et al: The ear deformities in mandibulofacial dysostosis. *Clin Otolaryngol* 6:15–28, 1981.

40. Pinsky L: Penetrance and variability of major malformation syndromes associated with deafness. *Birth Defects* 15(5B):207–226, 1979.

41. Poswillo D: The pathogenesis of the Treacher Collins syndrome (mandibulofacial dysostosis). *Br J Oral Surg* 13:1–26, 1975.

42. Pron G et al: Ear malformations and hearing loss in patients with Treacher Collins syndrome. *Cleft Palate Craniofac J* 30:97–103, 1993.

43. Richieri-Costa A et al: Mandibulofacial dysostosis: report on two Brazilian families suggesting autosomal recessive inheritance. *Am J Med Genet* 46:659–664, 1993.

44. Roberts FG et al: An X-radiocephalometric study of mandibulofacial dysostosis in man. *Arch Oral Biol* 20:265–282, 1975.

45. Rogers BO: Berry-Treacher Collins syndrome: a review of 200 cases. *Br J Plast Surg* 17:109–137, 1964.

46. Rovin S et al: Mandibulofacial dysostosis: a familial study of five generations. *J Pediatr* 65:215–221, 1964.

47. Sahawi E: Beitrag zur Dysostosis mandibulofacialis. *Z Kinderheilkd* 94:1195–1201, 1965.

48. Shprintzen RJ et al: Pharyngeal hypoplasia in Treacher Collins syndrome. *Arch Otolaryngol* 105:127–131, 1979.

49. Splendore A et al: High mutation rate in *TCOF1* among Treacher Collins syndrome patients reveals clustering of mutations and 16 novel pathogenic changes. *Hum Mutat* 16:315–322, 2000.

50. Stovin JJ et al: Mandibulofacial dysostosis. *Radiology* 74:225–231, 1960.

51. Sulik K et al: Mandibulofacial dysostosis (Treacher Collins syndrome): a new proposal for its pathogenesis. *Am J Med Genet* 37:359–372, 1987.

52. Thomson A: Notice of several cases of malformation of the external ear, together with experiments on the state of hearing in such persons. *Monthly J Med Sci* 7:420, 1846–1847.

53. Toynbee J: Description of a congenital malformation in the ears of a child. *Monthly J Med Sci* 1:738–739, 1847.

54. Treacher Collins Collaborative Group: Positional cloning of a gene involved in the pathogenesis of Treacher Collins syndrome. *Nat Genet* 12:130–136, 1996.

55. Treacher Collins E: Cases with symmetrical congenital notches in the outer part of each lid and defective development of the malar bones. *Trans Ophthalmol Soc UK* 20:190–192, 1900.

56. Wildervanck LS: Dysostosis mandibulo-facialis (Franceschetti-Zwahlin) in four generations. *Acta Genet Med Gemellol (Roma)* 9:447–451, 1960.

57. Wiley MJ et al: Effects of retinoic acid on the development of the facial skeleton in hamsters: early changes involving cranial neural crest cells. *Acta Anat* 116:180–192, 1983.

58. Wilkinson WB, Poswillo DE: Asymmetry in mandibulofacial dysostosis. *J Craniofac Genet Dev Biol* 11:41–47, 1991.

Nager acrofacial dysostosis syndrome (preaxial acrofacial dysostosis)

Nager acrofacial dysostosis is a mandibulofacial dysostosis associated with radial defects. Since the original description of the syndrome by Nager and DeReynier (36) in 1948, over 70 cases have been reported (1–10,12–23,26–30,32,34–38,42,43,48,49,53,57). A comprehensive review is provided by McDonald and Gorski (33).

Physical findings. Occasional growth retardation is noted (5,6,14,57).

Craniofacial findings. Abnormalities of the cranium have been described in 25% of patients (12,14,19). Hypoplasia of zygomata, maxilla, and mandible are almost constant features. The palpebral fissures are downslanting. About 30% of patients have absence of the medial third of the lower eyelashes (4,10,18,23,24,26,30,34,37,56,57), with coloboma of the lower lid being noted in almost 20% (14,18,24,56,57). A high nasal bridge with upturned nasal tip is relatively common. A tongue-like extension of hair onto the cheek is seen occasionally (18,23,24). Limited jaw movement secondary to functional ankylosis of the temporomandibular joints is present in about 25% of patients (4,14,23,27,34,37,49). Over 20% have macrostomia (15,23,24,27,43,49), occasionally in association with lateral facial clefts (15,24). Abnormalities of the palate are frequent, and include cleft palate in over 30%, agenesis or partial agenesis of soft palate (9,22), short palate (4,7,30), highly arched palate (10,24), submucous cleft palate (18), and bifid uvula (18,56) (Fig. 6–2A–E). Bilateral lateral palatine fistulae (30), broad palatine ridges (1), and hypoplasia of the epiglottis (7,28) have also been reported. Dental anomalies include enamel hypoplasia and oligodontia (30). Facial asymmetry is rare (34). Groeper et al. (17) discuss the anesthetic implications of Nager syndrome, as related to craniofacial manifestations.

Musculoskeletal system. Radial ray abnormalities are a common feature of Nager syndrome (12,19). Varying degrees of thumb hypoplasia or aplasia are seen in 75% of cases (Fig. 6–2F–I). Other thumb anomalies include stiff metacarpophalangeal joint (18), triphalangeal thumb (6), symphalangism (42), double thumb (13), and syndactyly between thumb and index finger with associated thumb hypoplasia (4,20). Radial hypoplasia or aplasia has been described in 40%, with radioulnar synostosis in 25%. These malformations frequently lead to reduced extension at the elbow. Marked reduction in size of the forearm is rare (53), but when present is usually associated with hypoplasia of humerus and ulna (5,20,43). Total absence of the forearm has rarely been reported (15,19,24). Other upper limb anomalies include synostosis of carpal bones (4,5,18), hypoplasia of thenar eminence (4,18,43), camptodactyly (24,28,34,52), and clinodactyly (7,24,34,42). Mild abnormalities of the lower limb include talipes (14,18,19,26), duplication of proximal hallucal phalanx (44), hypoplastic hallux (19), absent toe (18), and absence of the distal interphalangeal creases of the toes (34). A few patients have been described with more significant lower limb anomalies, including absence of the tibia and fibula (15) and frank phocomelia with hypoplasia of the pelvis (24). Scoliosis (18,56), tightness of trapezius muscles leading to pseudopterygium colli and Sprengel deformity (18), hip dislocation (14,28,34), pes cavus (18), pectoral muscle hypoplasia (19), and pectus excavatum (14) are rare features.

Genitourinary system. Vesico-ureteric reflux (18), unilateral renal agenesis (43), duplication of a ureter (24), and bicornuate uterus (24) have each been noted in one patient.

Cardiovascular system. Tetralogy of Fallot (15,52), ventriculoseptal defect (24), and patent foramen ovale (49) rarely occur.

Central nervous system. Intelligence is usually normal, but intellectual handicap has been reported (6,41). However, many affected individuals were either stillborn or died in the newborn period.

External ear. The auricles are dysplastic in 80% of cases. Hypoplasia of the anthelix (18), tragus (4,18), antitragus (18), and helix (12,30) have been described. The ears are occasionally simple and small (14,19) with a preauricular tag (19,24,30,57), and are frequently low-set and posteriorly angulated (6,20,28,34). In almost 50%, there is narrowing or atresia of the external auditory canal.

Auditory system. Conductive hearing loss, frequently congenital (19) and usually moderate (18), is noted in 50% of patients. Unilateral mixed hearing loss was described by Burton and Nadler (5).

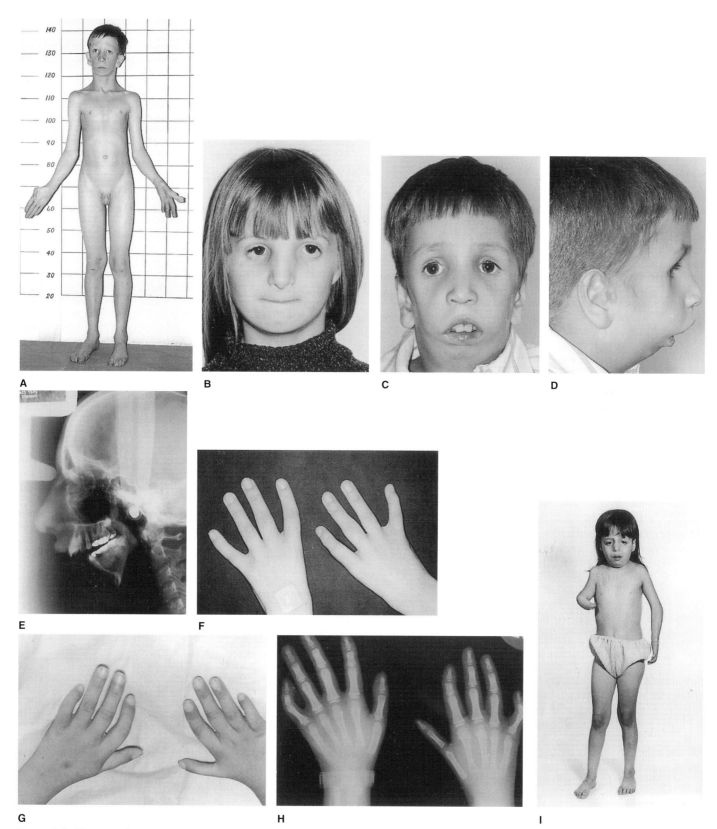

Figure 6–2. *Nager syndrome.* (A) Note downslanting palpebral fissures, somewhat unusual pinnae, cubitus valgus, and hypoplastic thumbs with preaxial duplication in patient's left hand. (B) Malar hypoplasia, deficiency of eyelashes, downslanting palpebral fissures. (C,D) Severe micrognathia. (E) Radiograph showing severe micrognathia. (F) Absence of thumbs. (G,H) Hypoplasia of thumbs and associated metacarpals as well as hypoplasia of multiple phalanges of fifth fingers. (I) Hypoplasia of entire radius. [(A) from P Bowen and F Harley, *Birth Defects* 10(5):109, 1974; (B,F) from FA Walker, *Birth Defects* 10(8):135, 1974.]

Pathology. Ossicular defects have been confirmed at autopsy. These have included deformation of ossicles (4), absent incus with fused ossicular mass (30), stapedial footplate fixed to oval window (28), and absence of ossicles with rudimentary semicircular canals (15). Autopsy has also revealed hypoplasia of the larynx and epiglottis (28) and abnormal septation of lungs (24,28). Although the gene has not been identified, presumably it has a role in programmed cell death (51).

Heredity. Most cases of Nager acrofacial dysostosis have been sporadic. Mildly to moderately affected sibs with apparently normal parents have been described (7,20,37,56), a finding suggesting autosomal recessive inheritance. Single cases with consanguineous parents have lent some support to this concept (5,24,43). Transmission from parent to child has also been reported (2,19,26,57). One family with six affected individuals covering four generations was briefly presented (57). Advanced paternal age in sporadic cases has supported autosomal dominant inheritance (4,30,32). Manifestations within a family may be markedly consistent, as in the mildly to moderately affected father and son reported by Aylsworth et al (2). In contrast, Hall (19) described extreme intrafamilial variability: a mildly to moderately affected mother, whose son died minutes after birth with severe phocomelic Nager acrofacial dysostosis. Bonthron et al. (3) reported minor changes in parents.

Genetic heterogeneity clearly challenges both diagnosis and counseling. Apparent recessive inheritance could represent nonpenetrance or germinal mosaicism. Alternatively, both autosomal dominant and recessive forms of the disorder may exist. However, one cannot assume that mild to moderate cases are more likely to be recessive while severe cases are dominant. After the birth of one affected child, a couple should be offered high-resolution ultrasonography in a subsequent pregnancy. Chromosome analysis should always be performed; a 1q12q21.3 deletion and chromosome translocation (X;9)(p22.1;q32) have been reported (54,59).

Diagnosis. Several entities must be considered in the differential diagnosis of Nager acrofacial dysostosis. In Miller syndrome, acrofacial dysostosis is associated with postaxial limb defects, and both upper and lower limbs are usually involved (35,39). Distinctive features include cup-shaped ears, cleft lip and/or palate, and accessory nipples. Although postaxial limb defects are most common, preaxial defects may be seen to a lesser degree, and abnormal thumbs, and shortness of radius and ulna with or without radioulnar synostosis have all been described. Reynolds et al. (45) reported an autosomal dominant acrofacial dysostosis syndrome with both pre- and postaxial involvement. There was mild congenital mixed hearing loss. Patients with Fontaine syndrome (11) have abnormal ears, retromicrognathia, cleft palate, and split foot with normal upper limbs. They do not show downward-slanting palpebral fissures, coloboma of the eyelids, or hearing loss.

Distal 2q duplication syndrome shares some of the features of Nager acrofacial dysostosis, such as downslanting palpebral fissures, dysplastic external ears, and micrognathia (55,58). However, malar hypoplasia and defects of the external ear canal are absent, and hypertelorism and nystagmus, which are not seen in Nager acrofacial dysostosis syndrome, are frequent. Acral anomalies in the distal 2q duplication syndrome are usually limited to clinodactyly and camptodactyly of the fifth digit. No thumb defects have been described.

Oculo-auriculo-vertebral spectrum may occasionally include radial defects but can usually be differentiated by the unilateral involvement of the ear, eye, face, and mandible, and the presence of epibulbar dermoids and vertebral anomalies. Sugiura (50) described a 6-year-old boy with hemifacial microsomia, absence of left radius and thumb, ventricular septal defect, and crossed renal ectopia. Gorlin et al. (16) described a female infant with oculo-auriculo-vertebral spectrum phenotype and absence of the first left metacarpal with hypoplasia of the corresponding thumb. In 1971, Mandelcorn et al. (31) reported a boy with hemifacial microsomia and acral anomalies, consisting of short ulna, four metacarpals, and four fingers on the left, with hypoplastic humerus, short ulna, three metacarpals, and two fingers on the right side.

The facial features of Nager acrofacial dysostosis are similar to those in isolated mandibulofacial dysostosis (Treacher Collins syndrome). The presence of preaxial limb defects distinguishes the two. External ear defects and cleft palate are more common in Nager syndrome, while lower lid colobomata are more frequent in mandibulofacial dysostosis.

In 1977, Kelly et al. (25) described three males, two of them brothers, with preaxial limb anomalies and mild mandibulofacial hypoplasia. In addition, they showed intrauterine growth retardation with subsequent short stature, mental retardation, and genitourinary anomalies. All had sensorineural hearing loss. Autosomal recessive or X-linked recessive inheritance seems likely. The acrofacial dysostosis triphalangeal thumb syndrome described by Richieri-Costa et al. (46) can be distinguished from Nager acrofacial dysostosis by the rarity of cleft lip and the presence of triphalangeal thumb in the latter syndrome. In 1983, Poissonnier et al. (44) described a single male whose facial features were consistent with mandibulofacial dysostosis. In addition, there was hypoplastic scapulae and right humerus, hypoplastic or absent ulnae and fibulae, and absent fifth digitometacarpal rays, in association with aplasia of the left hemidiaphragm and atrial and ventricular septal defects.

In 1990, Rodriguez et al. (47) described an apparently new autosomal recessive syndrome in three sibs with acrofacial dysostosis, predominantly preaxial limb deficiencies, rare postaxial limb anomalies, and cardiac and central nervous system (CNS) malformations. The third sib showed marked similarity to Nager syndrome (47). Opitz et al. (40) and Arens et al. (1) described still other forms of acrofacial dysostosis. The reader is referred to the comprehensive review of this subject by Opitz et al. (40).

Prognosis. When provided with early and appropriate hearing aids, patients with Nager acrofacial dysostosis seem to function within the normal range (4,12,27,30,34,56). Developmental delay, mostly apparent in the first 2 years of life, is due to feeding difficulties, hearing loss, and surgical procedures to correct the ear and palate anomalies. Premature delivery and perinatal mortality are relatively high in this syndrome, especially in sporadic cases. Death within the neonatal period (6,7,19,20,23,24,28,49,52) and stillbirth (32) are well documented.

Summary. Characteristics of this syndrome include (*1*) usually sporadic, with occasional autosomal dominant and perhaps autosomal recessive inheritance; (*2*) malformations of the external ear; (*3*) abnormalities of the radial ray, particularly thumb aplasia or hypoplasia and radial aplasia or hypoplasia; (*4*) characteristic facial appearance with downslanting palpebral fissures, malar and zygomatic hypoplasia, cleft palate, and retromicrognathia; and (*5*) conductive hearing loss.

References

1. Arens R et al: A new form of postaxial acrofacial dysostosis? *Am J Med Genet* 41:438–443, 1991.
2. Aylsworth AS et al: Nager acrofacial dysostosis: Male-to-male transmission in two families. *Am J Med Genet* 41:83–88, 1991.
3. Bonthron DT et al: Nager acrofacial dysostosis—minor manifestations support dominant inheritance. *Clin Genet* 43:127–131, 1993.
4. Bowen P, Harley F: Mandibulofacial dysostosis with limb malformations (Nager's acrofacial dysostosis). *Birth Defects* 10(5):109–115, 1974.
5. Burton BK, Nadler HL: Nager acrofacial dysostosis. *J Pediatr* 91:84–86, 1977.
6. Byrd LK et al: Nager acrofacial dysostosis in four patients including monozygous twins. *Proc Greenwood Genet Ctr* 7:30–35, 1988.
7. Chemke J et al: Autosomal recessive inheritance of Nager acrofacial dysostosis. *J Med Genet* 25:230–232, 1988.
8. Chou YC: Mandibulofacial dysostosis. *Chin Med J* 80:373–375, 1960.
9. El Faki HMA: Unilateral hypoplasia of the soft palate. *Eur J Plast Surg* 13:176–177, 1990.
10. Fernandez AD, Ronis ML: The Treacher Collins syndrome. *Arch Otolaryngol* 80:505–520, 1964.
11. Fontaine G et al: Une observation familiale du syndrome ectodactylie et dysostose mandibulofaciale. *J Genet Hum* 22:289–307, 1974.
12. Gellis SS et al: Nager's syndrome (Nager's acrofacial dysostosis). *Am J Dis Child* 132:519–520, 1978.
13. Gingliani R, Pereira CH: Nager's acrofacial dysostosis with thumb duplication. *Clin Genet* 26:228–230, 1984.

14. Golabi et al: Nager syndrome: report of seven new cases and a follow up report of two previously reported cases. *Proc Greenwood Genet Ctr* 4:127–128, 1985.

15. Goldstein DJ, Mirkin LD: Nager acrofacial dysostosis: evidence for apparent heterogeneity. *Am J Med Genet* 30:741–746, 1988.

16. Gorlin RJ et al: Oculoauriculovertebral dysplasia. *J Pediatr* 63:991–999, 1963.

17. Groeper K et al: Anaesthetic implications of Nager syndrome. *Paediatr Anaesth* 12:365–368, 2002.

18. Halal F et al: Differential diagnosis of Nager acrofacial dysostosis syndrome: report of 4 patients with Nager syndrome and discussion of other related syndromes. *Am J Med Genet* 14:209–224, 1983.

19. Hall BD: Nager acrofacial dysostosis: autosomal dominant inheritance in mild to moderately affected mother and lethally affected phocomelic son. *Am J Med Genet* 33:394–397, 1989.

20. Hecht JT et al: The Nager syndrome. *Am J Med Genet* 27:965–969, 1987.

21. Herrmann J et al: Acrofacial dysostosis type Nager. *Birth Defects* 11(5):341, 1975.

22. Jackson IT et al: A significant feature of Nager's syndrome: palatal agenesis. *Plast Reconstr Surg* 84:219–226, 1989.

23. Jones RG: Mandibulofacial dysostosis. *Cent Afr J Med* 14:193–200, 1968.

24. Kawira EL et al: Acrofacial dysostosis with severe facial clefting and limb reduction. *Am J Med Genet* 17:641–647, 1984.

25. Kelly TE et al: Acrofacial dysostosis with growth and mental retardation in three males, one with simultaneous Hermansky-Pudlak syndrome. *Birth Defects* 13(3B):45–52, 1977.

26. Kim HJ et al: Nager syndrome with autosomal dominant inheritance [abstract]. Presented at March of Dimes Clinical Genetics Conference, 1987.

27. Klein D et al: Sur une forme extensive de dysostose mandibulofaciale (Franceschetti) accompagnée de malformations des extremites et d'autres anomalies congénitales chez une fille dont le frere né presente qu'une forme fruste du syndrome (fistula auris congenita retrotragica). *Rev Otoneuroophtalmol* 42:432–440, 1970.

28. Krauss CM et al: Anomalies in an infant with Nager acrofacial dysostosis. *Am J Med Genet* 21:761–764, 1985.

29. Le Merrer M et al: Acrofacial dysostosis. *Am J Med Genet* 33:318–322, 1989.

30. Lowry RB: Nager syndrome (acrofacial dysostosis): evidence for autosomal dominant inheritance. *Birth Defects* 13(3C):195–220, 1977.

31. Mandelcorn MS et al: Goldenhar's syndrome and phocomelia. *Am J Ophthalmol* 72:618–621, 1971.

32. Marden PM et al: Congenital anomalies in the newborn infant, including minor variations. *J Pediatr* 64:357–371, 1964.

33. McDonald MT, Gorski JL: Syndrome of the month: Nager acrofacial dysostosis. *J Med Genet* 30:779–782, 1993.

34. Meyerson MD et al: Nager acrofacial dysostosis: early intervention and long-term planning. *Cleft Palate J* 14:35–40, 1977.

35. Miller M et al: Postaxial acrofacial dysostosis syndrome. *J Pediatr* 95:970, 1979.

36. Nager FR, DeReynier JP: Das Gehörorgan bei den angeborenen Kopfmissbildungen. *Pract Oto-Rhino-Laryng (Basel)* (Suppl 2)10:1–128, 1948.

37. Neidhart E: Die Dysostosis mandibulofacialis (Franceschetti-Zwahlen-Klein-Syndrom) in Kombination mit Missbildungen der oberen Extremitäten. Inaug. Dissertation, Zürich, 1968.

38. O'Connor CB, Conway ME: Treacher Collins syndrome (dysostosis mandibulofacialis). *Plast Reconstr Surg* 5:419–425, 1950 (case 1).

39. Opitz JM: Nager "syndrome" versus "anomaly" and its nosology with the postaxial acrofacial dysostosis syndrome of Genée and Wiedemann. *Am J Med Genet* 27:959–963, 1987.

40. Opitz JM et al: Acrofacial dysostoses: review and report of a previously undescribed condition: the autosomal or X-linked dominant Catania form of acrofacial dysostosis. *Am J Med Genet* 47:660–678, 1993.

41. Palomeque A et al: Nager anomaly with severe facial involvement, microcephaly and mental retardation. *Am J Med Genet* 36:356–357, 1990.

42. Pavone L et al: Acrofacial dysostosis of Nager and ocular abnormalities. *Ophthalmol Paediatr Genet* 3:115–119, 1986.

43. Pfeiffer RA, Stoess H: Acrofacial dysostosis (Nager syndrome): synopsis and report of a new case. *Am J Med Genet* 15:255–260, 1983.

44. Poissonnier M et al: Dysostose mandibulofaciale et ulno-fibulaire lethale. *Ann Pediatr* 30:713–717, 1983.

45. Reynolds JF et al: A new autosomal dominant acrofacial dysostosis syndrome. *Am J Med Genet* (Suppl) 2:143–150, 1986.

46. Richieri-Costa A, Silveira Pereira SC: Short stature, Robin sequence, cleft mandible, pre/postaxial hand anomalies and clubfoot: a new autosomal recessive syndrome. *Am J Med Genet* 42:681–687, 1992.

47. Rodriguez JI et al: New acrofacial dysostosis syndrome in 3 sibs. *Am J Med Genet* 35:484–489, 1990.

48. Ruedi L: The surgical treatment of the atresia auris congenita: a clinical and histological report. *Laryngoscope* 64:666–684, 1954.

49. Schönenberg H: Die differential Diagnose der radialen Defektbildungen. *Paediatr Prax* 7:455–467, 1968.

50. Sugiura Y: Congenital absence of the radius with hemifacial microsomia, ventricular septal defect and crossed renal ectopia. *Birth Defects* 7(7):109–116, 1971.

51. Sulik KK et al: Pathogenesis of cleft palate in Treacher Collins, Nager and Miller syndromes. *Cleft Palate J* 26:209–216, 1989.

52. Thompson E et al: The Nager acrofacial syndrome and the tetralogy of Fallot. *J Med Genet* 22:408–410, 1985.

53. van Goethem H et al: Nager's acrofacial dysostosis. *Acta Paediatr Belg* 34:253–256, 1981.

54. Waggoner DJ et al: Deletion of 1q in a patient with acrofacial dysostosis. *Am J Med Genet* 82:301–304, 1999.

55. Wagner SF, Cole J: Nager syndrome with partial duplication of the long arm of chromosome 2. *Am J Hum Genet* 31:116A, 1979.

56. Walker FA: Apparent autosomal recessive inheritance of the Treacher Collins syndrome. *Birth Defects* 10(8):135–139, 1974.

57. Weinbaum M et al: Autosomal dominant transmission of Nager acro-facial dysostosis. *Am J Hum Genet* 33:93A, 1981.

58. Zankl M et al: Distal 2q duplication: report of two familial cases and an attempt to define a syndrome. *Am J Med Genet* 4:5–16, 1979.

59. Zori RT et al: Preaxial acrofacial dysostosis (Nager syndrome) associated with an inherited and apparently balanced X;9 translocation. *Am J Med Genet* 46:379–383, 1993.

Postaxial acrofacial dysostosis, cupped ears, and conductive hearing loss (Miller syndrome, Genée-Wiedemann syndrome)

In 1969, Genée (10) reported an infant with postaxial limb deficiency, cup-shaped ears, and malar hypoplasia. Wiedemann (27), in 1973, and Wildervanck (28), in 1975, noted similar patients. In 1979, Miller et al. (14) presented details of three similar unrelated patients, one of which was previously reported by Smith et al. (25) in 1975. An affected sib of a patient described by Miller et al. (14) was briefly reported by Fineman (8). At least 25 patients have been described (2–6,8–23,25,28).

Physical findings. Malar hypoplasia and lower lid ectropion are extremely common. Ectropion tends to become more obvious with age. Eyelid colobomata and eyelash anomalies are occasionally noted. Micrognathia is a constant finding (Fig. 6–3A,B). Cleft lip and/or palate is found in several cases (23). Other patients appear to have a long philtrum. Supernumerary nipples are seen in almost 50% of cases (6,13,17).

Musculoskeletal system. Almost all patients have bilateral absence of the fifth finger including the fifth metacarpal. Varying degrees of hypoplasia of the thumbs and syndactyly are occasionally noted. Forearm anomalies are extremely common, with ulnar hypoplasia being the most characteristic (Fig. 6–3C). Radioulnar synostosis has also been reported (16). It is possible that some patients have no digital anomalies (20). Absence of the toes on the lateral border of the feet has been observed with rare exception (4,20) (Fig. 6–3D). The fifth toe was always involved, with occasional hypoplasia or absence of the third and fourth toes. Severe limb anomalies, rarely described, have included absent fibula, phocomelia, and hypoplasia of the pectoral girdle. Supernumerary vertebrae, vertebral and sternal segmentation anomalies, cervical ribs, and pectus excavatum have also been noted. Sulik et al. (26) postulated involvement of the apical ectodermal ridge of limb buds.

Other systems. Ogilvy-Stuart and Parsons (16) described midgut malrotation, gastric volvulus, and renal tract anomalies (reflux, hydronephrosis).

External ear. The ears, remarkably similar in reported cases, are small, simple, and cupped. Stenosis of the external auditory canal was noted in two cases.

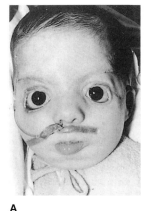
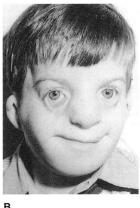
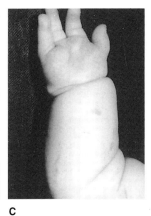
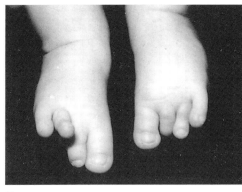

A   B   C   D

Figure 6–3. *Genée-Wiedemann syndrome.* (A,B) Compare facies. Note extensive lower lid ectropion and mild malar hypoplasia. (C,D) Postaxial hypogenesis in both the hands and feet. [(A,C,D) from E. Genée, *J Genet Hum* 17:42, 1969; (B) courtesy of MM Cohen Jr, Halifax, Nova Scotia, Canada.]

Auditory system. Hearing loss has been found in several patients (8,16,23). Middle ear hypoplasia has been mentioned.

Laboratory findings. Radiographs confirmed the presence of the skeletal anomalies described above.

Heredity. Sibling pairs with normal parents have been reported (8,11,14–17). The parents of a sporadic case were fifth cousins (21); thus it appears that the syndrome is transmitted in an autosomal recessive manner.

Diagnosis. Several disorders must be distinguished from this acrofacial malformation syndrome. The facial appearance is similar to that described in Treacher Collins syndrome, but distal limb anomalies are not part of that autosomal dominant condition. Nager acrofacial dysostosis includes preaxial hand deficiencies, normal feet, and a Treacher Collins–like face (3,24). The distal limb anomalies in Nager syndrome are most frequently hypoplasia or absence of the thumb and/or radius, as opposed to the predominantly postaxial limb anomalies in this condition. De Lange syndrome, Weyers syndrome, femur-fibula-ulna syndrome, and Schinzel syndrome have ulnar ray defects, but differ in facial appearance and other clinical features. Allanson and McGillivray (1) and Falace and Hall (7) reported autosomal dominant inheritance of a syndrome of ectropion, facial clefting, and dental anomalies. The patient with four digits reported by Ruedi (24) appears to have mandibulofacial dysostosis. The child reported by Danziger et al. (5) has features of both Miller and Nager syndrome.

Opitz et al. (18) have thoroughly reviewed the many different acrofacial dysostoses.

Summary. The major characteristics of this syndrome include (*1*) probable autosomal recessive inheritance; (*2*) craniofacial dysostosis, including malar hypoplasia with ectropion, long philtrum, micrognathia, and cleft palate; (*3*) postaxial limb anomalies affecting all four limbs; (*4*) cupped simple ears; and (*5*) occasional conductive hearing loss.

References

1. Allanson JE, McGillivray BC: Familial clefting syndrome with ectropion and dental anomaly with limb anomalies. *Clin Genet* 27:426–429, 1985.
2. Barbuti D et al: Postaxial acrofacial dysostosis or Miller syndrome. *Eur J Pediatr* 148:445–446, 1989.
3. Bowen P, Harley F: Mandibular dysostosis with limb malformations (Nager's acrofacial dysostosis). *Birth Defects* 10(5):109, 1974.
4. Chrzanowska KH et al: Phenotype variability in the Miller acrofacial dysostosis syndrome: report of two further patients. *Clin Genet* 35:157–160, 1989.
5. Danziger I et al: Nager's acrofacial dysostosis. Case report and review of the literature. *Int J Pediatr Otorhinolaryngol* 20:225–240, 1990.
6. Donnai D et al: Postaxial acrofacial dysostosis (Miller) syndrome. *J Med Genet* 24:422–425, 1987.
7. Falace PB, Hall BD: Congenital euryblepharon with ectropion and dental anomaly: an autosomal dominant clefting disorder with marked variability of expression. *Proc Greenwood Genet Ctr* 8:208, 1989.
8. Fineman RM: Recurrence of the postaxial acrofacial dysostosis syndrome in a sibship: implications for genetic counseling. *J Pediatr* 98:87–88, 1981.
9. Fryns JP, Van den Berghe H: Brief clinical report. Acrofacial dysostosis with postaxial limb deficiency. *Am J Med Genet* 29:2005–2008, 1988.
10. Genée E: Une forme extensive de dysostose mandibulofaciale. *J Genet Hum* 17:42–52, 1969.
11. Grannotti A et al: Familial postaxial acrofacial dysostosis syndrome. *J Med Genet* 29:752, 1992.
12. Lenz W: Genetische Syndrome mit Aplasie ulnare und/oder fibularer Randstrahlen. Klinische Genetik in der Pädiatrie. 2nd Symposium, Mainz, 1979.
13. Meinecke P, Wiedemann H-R: Letter to the editor. Robin sequence and oligodactyly in mother and son. Probably a further example of the postaxial acrofacial dysostosis syndrome. *Am J Med Genet* 27:953–956, 1987.
14. Miller M et al: Postaxial acrofacial dysostosis syndrome. *J Pediatr* 95:970–975, 1979.
15. Neumann et al: A new observation of two cases of acrofacial dysostosis type Genee-Wiedemann in a family—remarks on mode of inheritance: report on two sibs. *Am J Med Genet* 64:556–562, 1996.
16. Ogilvy-Stuart AL, Parsons AC: Miller syndrome (postaxial acrofacial dysostosis): further evidence for autosomal recessive inheritance and expansion of the phenotype. *J Med Genet* 28:695–700, 1991.
17. Opitz JM, Stickler GB: The Genée-Wiedemann syndrome, an acrofacial dysostosis—further observation. *Am J Med Genet* 27:971–975, 1987.
18. Opitz JM et al: Acrofacial dysostoses: review and report of a previously undescribed condition: the autosomal or X-linked dominant Catania form of acrofacial dysostosis. *Am J Med Genet* 47:660–678, 1993.
19. Pashayan H, Finegold M: Case report 28. *Synd Ident* 3:7–8, 1975.
20. Piper HG: Augenärztliche Befunde bei frühkindlicher Entwicklungsstörungen. *Monatschr Kinderheilkd* 105:170–176, 1957.
21. Richards M: Miller's syndrome: anaesthetic management of postaxial acrofacial dysostosis. *Anaesthesia* 42:871–874, 1987.
22. Richieri-Costa A, Guion-Almeida ML: Postaxial acrofacial dysostosis: report of a Brazilian patient. *Am J Med Genet* 33:447–449, 1989.
23. Robinow M, Chen H: Genée-Wiedemann syndrome in a family. *Am J Med Genet* 37:393, 1990.
24. Ruedi L: The surgical treatment of the atresia auris congenita. *Laryngoscope* 64:666–670, 1954.
25. Smith DW et al: Case report 28. *Synd Ident* 3:7–13, 1975.
26. Sulik KK et al: Pathogenesis of cleft palate in Treacher Collins, Nager and Miller syndrome. *Cleft Palate J* 26:209–216, 1989.
27. Wiedemann H-R: Milsbildungs-Retardierungs-Syndrom mit Fehlen des 5. Strahls an Händen und Füssen, Gaumenspalte, dysplastischen Ohren und Augenlidern und radioulnarer Synostose. *Klin Padiatr* 185:181–186, 1973.
28. Wildervanck LS: Case report 28. *Synd Ident* 3:11–13, 1975.

Oculo-auriculo-vertebral spectrum (hemifacial microsomia, Goldenhar syndrome)

This complex is a predominantly unilateral malformation of craniofacial structures that develop from the first and second branchial arches. The many terms used for this complex indicate the wide spectrum of anomalies described and emphasized by various authors. This entity has been known as hemifacial microsomia, oculo-auriculo-vertebral dysplasia (OAV), Goldenhar syndrome, Goldenhar-Gorlin syndrome, first arch syndrome, first and second branchial arch syndrome, and lateral facial dysplasia. The term *oculo-auriculo-vertebral spectrum* is the most inclusive term. The first recorded cases may were those of Canton (15) in 1861 and von Arlt (3) in 1881. There are numerous more recent important reviews (2,6,8,14,17,18,21,24–26,28,31,38,45,47,53,63,64,66, 68,73,76,81).

Craniofacial findings. Marked facial asymmetry is present in 20% of patients, with some degree of asymmetry evident in 65% (74). The asymmetry may be more apparent with increasing age. The maxillary, temporal, and malar bones on the more severely involved side are somewhat reduced in size and flattened (Fig. 6–4A,C). About 10%–30% of patients have bilateral involvement (14,31,66). Even so, the disorder is almost always more severe on one side, more often the right side.

Aplasia or hypoplasia of the mandibular ramus and condyle may be found in association with macrostomia or pseudomacrostomia, usually of mild degree (30). It is more common (3:2) for the right side to be involved. Unilateral or bilateral cleft lip and/or cleft palate occurs in 7%–15% (6,66). Occasionally, there may be parotid salivary gland agenesis. Malocclusion is frequent (Fig. 6–4D).

Ocular system. Eye anomalies are common. Epibulbar dermoids are found in 35% of cases (6,28,31) (Fig. 6–4B). Blepharoptosis or narrowing of the palpebral fissure occurs on the affected side in about 10%. Clinical anophthalmia or microphthalmia has been described in several patients and may be correlated with the presence of mental retardation (1,6,16,48,73,84). Unilateral colobomas of the upper lid are noted in about 20%, and are bilateral in possibly 3% (6).

Central nervous system. A wide range of neurological defects may be associated. Lower facial nerve weakness occurs in 10%–20% of patients, probably related to bony involvement in the region of the facial canal (5,31). Nearly all cranial nerves have occasionally been involved (2). The range of skull defects includes cranium bifidum, microcephaly, dolichocephaly, and plagiocephaly (1,13,30). In the so-called expanded OAV spectrum, brain malformations occur. Intracranial anomalies may include encephalocele, hydrocephaly, lipoma, dermoid

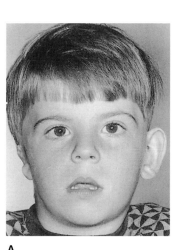
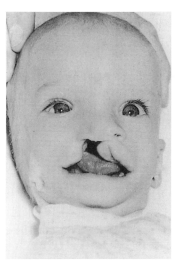
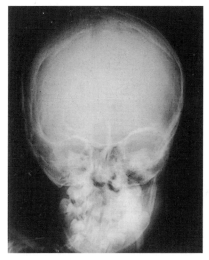

A   **B**   **C**

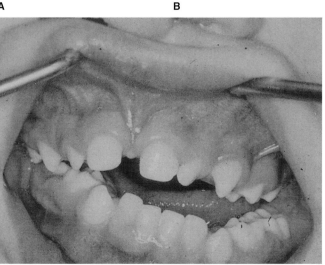
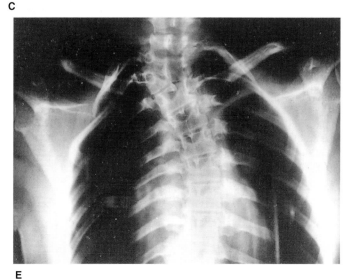

D   **E**

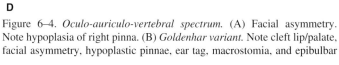

Figure 6–4. *Oculo-auriculo-vertebral spectrum.* (A) Facial asymmetry. Note hypoplasia of right pinna. (B) *Goldenhar variant.* Note cleft lip/palate, facial asymmetry, hypoplastic pinnae, ear tag, macrostomia, and epibulbar dermoid. (C) Unilateral hypoplasia of mandible. (D) Malocclusion. (E) Hemivertebra with compensating scoliosis.

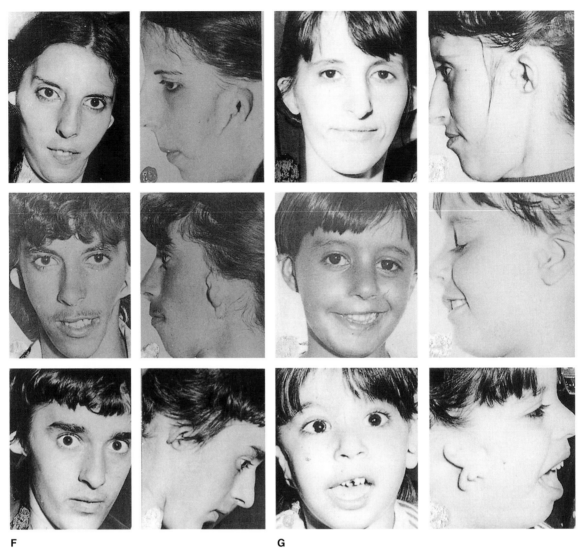

F   G

Figure 6–4. *Continued.* (F,G) Numerous members of kindred exhibiting rare autosomal dominant form of oculo-auriculo-vertebral spectrum. Note variable degrees of facial hypoplasia, dysplastic pinnae, macrostomia, and epibulbar dermoid. [(B) courtesy of *BGA ter Haar,* Nijmegen. The Netherlands; (F,G) from *L Regenbogen et al., Clin Genet* 21:161, 1982.]

cyst, teratoma, Arnold-Chiari malformation, lissencephaly, arachnoid cyst, holoprosencephaly, unilateral arhinencephaly, and hypoplasia of the corpus callosum (2). Estimates of the frequency of mental deficiency range from 5% to 15% (38,73). Those infants and toddlers at particularly increased risk appear to be those with abnormal muscle tone, bilateral involvement, and cervical vertebral anomalies (19).

Cardiovascular system. Various forms of heart anomalies have been recorded (27,30,32,59,66,73,81,84) and are found in 5%–58% of patients. Ventricular septal defect (VSD) and tetralogy of Fallot account for half these anomalies although no single cardiac lesion is characteristic.

Musculoskeletal system. Cervical spine and cranial base anomalies occur with increased frequency. Skull defects have also been noted (17,34,49,54) and may be associated with a poorer prognosis (84). Cervical vertebral fusions occur in 20%–35% of cases, while platybasia and occipitalization of the atlas are found in about 30%. Spina bifida, hemivertebrae, butterfly vertebrae, fused and hypoplastic vertebrae, Klippel-Feil anomaly, scoliosis, and anomalous ribs occur in at least 30% (4,36) (Fig. 6–4E). Talipes equinovarus has been reported in about 20% (30). Radial limb anomalies have been noted in about 10% (68). These may take the form of hypoplasia or aplasia of radius and/or thumb and bifid or digitalized thumb.

Pulmonary system. Pulmonary anomalies range from incomplete lobulation to hypoplasia to agenesis. They may be unilateral or bilateral, with absent lung usually being ipsilateral to the facial anomalies (11,30,46,55,60). Tracheoesophageal fistula has also been documented (11).

Renal system. Renal anomalies have included renal agenesis, double ureter, crossed renal ectopia, renovascular abnormalities, hydronephrosis, and hydroureter (12,65,73).

Gastrointestinal system. Imperforate anus with or without rectovaginal fistula has been described (12).

External ear. Abnormality of the external ear may vary from anotia to an ill-defined mass of tissue that is displaced anteriorly and inferiorly to a mildly dysmorphic ear. The anomaly is occasionally bilateral. Preauricular tags of skin and cartilage are extremely common and may be unilateral or bilateral. Supernumerary ear tags may appear anywhere from the tragus to the angle of the mouth. They are more commonly seen in patients with macrostomia and/or aplasia of the parotid gland and epibulbar dermoids. Preauricular sinuses may be observed. Narrow external auditory canals are found in milder cases. Atretic canals are seen in more severe examples. At times, small auricles with normal architecture are seen. Isolated microtia is considered by some to be a microform of OAV spectrum (7).

Auditory system. Both conductive hearing loss and, less frequently, sensorineural hearing loss have been reported in over 50% of cases (6,13,21,51,83,85). The etiology of hearing loss is diverse and includes anomalies of the middle and external ears, hypoplasia or agenesis of ossicles, aberrant facial nerves, patulous eustachian tube, and abnormalities of the skull base (70).

Heredity. The OAV spectrum occurs with a frequency of approximately 1/5600 births (31). The male/female ratio is at least 3:2 (30,66,75,84). The vast majority of cases are sporadic, but familial instances may also be observed. Expression varies within families. For example, there are reports of ear and mandibular involvement in two first-degree relatives, and reports of isolated microtia or preauricular tags in one first-degree relative of a patient with ear and mandibular involvement (64). These reports support the suggestion that isolated microtia or preauricular tags may represent the mildest expression of the gene in some families (30,31,48,64,66,81). Affected individuals in successive generations have been observed (17,31,37,52,57,61,62,64, 72,78,79,82). Affected sibs with normal parents have also been reported (31,41,42,71). This suggests that etiologic heterogeneity is likely. Overall, recurrence is 2%–3%. However, in some families, which represent 1%–2% of cases, autosomal dominant inheritance is likely (37,61,78) (Fig. 6–4F,G). Therefore, evaluation of first-degree relatives is important to look for mild facial manifestations of this spectrum and various extracranial anomalies. Recurrence risk counseling should be provided on an individual-family basis.

Discordance in monozygotic twins has been reported frequently (9,10,14,20,22,23,29,31,56,58,64,72,77). Rarely, concordance with variable expression has been documented in monozygotic twins (64,69,80). The rarity of reports of concordance of the defect in twins supports the suggestion that the condition is sporadic in most families. The interested reader is referred to the excellent segregation analyses of Burck (14) and Kaye et al. (40).

Diagnosis. First and second branchial arch anomalies, often combined with facial palsy, have been observed in infants born to pregnant women exposed to thalidomide (44,50,67), primidone (35), and retinoic acid (43). The OAV phenotype has also been noted in infants born to diabetic mothers (33,39). Several chromosomal anomalies have been associated, including del(5p), del(6q), trisomy 7 mosaicism, del(8q), trisomy 9 mosaicism, trisomy 18, recombinant chromosome 18, del(18q), ring 21 chromosome, del(22q), 49,XXXXY, and 47,XXY. Although the overwhelming majority of cases are nonsyndromal, it is essential to exclude several syndromes with overlapping features such as Townes-Brocks syndrome, branchio-oto-renal syndrome (65), mandibulofacial dysostosis, maxillofacial dysostosis, Nager acrofacial dysostosis, and Miller postaxial acrofacial dysostosis. Characteristics of VATER association, CHARGE association, and MURCS association overlap with the OAV spectrum.

Prognosis. Prognosis obviously depends on the severity of the phenotype and the presence or absence of associated mental retardation.

Summary. This syndrome is characterized by (*1*) usually sporadic but rare autosomal dominant inheritance (1%–2% of cases); (*2*) anomalies of aural, oral, and mandibular development, generally unilateral but occasionally bilateral, and of varying severity; (*3*) congenital heart defects; (*4*) anomalies of cervical spine; (*5*) mental retardation in 5%–15% of cases; and (*6*) conductive or occasionally sensorineural hearing loss.

References

1. Aleksic S et al: Unilateral arrhinencephaly in Goldenhar-Gorlin syndrome. *Dev Med Child Neurol* 17:498–504, 1975.
2. Aleksic S et al: Intracranial lipomas, hydrocephalus and other CNS anomalies in oculo-auriculo-vertebral dysplasia (Goldenhar-Gorlin syndrome). *Childs Brain* 11:285–297, 1984.
3. Arlt F von: *Klinische Darstellung der Krankheiten des Auges.* W. Braunmüller, Vienna, 1881.
4. Avon SW, Shively JL: Orthopedic manifestations of Goldenhar syndrome. *J Pediatr Orthop* 8:683–686, 1988.
5. Bassila MK, Goldberg R: The association of facial palsy and/or sensorineural hearing loss in patients with hemifacial microsomia. *Am J Med Genet* 26:289–291, 1989.
6. Baum JL, Feingold M: Ocular aspects of Goldenhar's syndrome. *Am J Ophthalmol* 75:250–257, 1973.
7. Bennum RD et al: Microtia: a microform of hemifacial microsomia. *Plast Reconstr Surg* 76:859–863, 1985.
8. Berkman MD, Feingold M: Oculoauriculovertebral dysplasia (Goldenhar's syndrome). *Oral Surg* 25:408–417, 1968.
9. Bock RH: Ein Fall von epibulbarem Dermolipome mit Missbildungen einer Gesichtshälfte. Diskordantes Vorkommen bei einem eineiigen Zwillingspaar. *Ophthalmologica* 155:86–90, 1961.
10. Boles DJ et al: Goldenhar complex in discordant twins: a case report and review of the literature. *Am J Med Genet* 28:103–109, 1987.
11. Bowen AD, Parry WH: Bronchopulmonary foregut malformation in the Goldenhar anomalad. *AJR Am J Roentgenol* 134:186–188, 1980.
12. Bowen DI et al: Clinical aspects of oculo-auriculo-vertebral dysplasia. *Br J Ophthalmol* 55:145–154, 1971.
13. Budden SS, Robinson GC: Oculoauricular vertebral dysplasia. *Am J Dis Child* 125:431–433, 1973.
14. Burck U: Genetic aspects of hemifacial microsomia. *Hum Genet* 64:291–296, 1983.
15. Canton E: Arrest of development of the left perpendicular ramus of the lower jaw, combined with malformation of the external ear. *Trans Pathol Soc Lond* 12:237–238, 1861.
16. Coccaro PJ et al: Clinical and radiographic variations in hemifacial microsomia. *Birth Defects* 11(2):314–324, 1975.
17. Cohen MM Jr: Variability versus "incidental findings" in the first and second branchial arch syndrome: unilateral variants with anophthalmia. *Birth Defects* 7(7):103–108, 1971.
18. Cohen MM Jr et al: Oculoauriculovertebral spectrum: an updated critique. *Cleft Palate J* 26:276–286, 1989.
19. Cohen MS et al: Neurodevelopmental profile of infants and toddlers with oculo-auriculo-vertebral spectrum and the correlation of prognosis with physical findings. *Am J Med Genet* 60:535–540, 1995.
20. Connor JM, Fernandez C: Genetic aspects of hemifacial microsomia. *Hum Genet* 68:349, 1984.
21. Converse JM et al: On hemifacial microsomia. The first and second branchial arch syndrome. *Plast Reconstr Surg* 51:268–279, 1973.
22. Cordier J et al: Syndrome de Franceschetti-Goldenhar discordant chez deux jumelles monozygotes. *Arch Ophtalmol (Paris)* 30:321–328, 1970.
23. Ebbesen F, Petersen W: Goldenhar's syndrome: discordance in monozygotic twins and unusual anomalies. *Acta Paediatr Scand* 71:685–687, 1982.
24. Figueroa AA, Pruzansky S: The external ear, mandible and other components of hemifacial microsomia. *J Maxillofac Surg* 10:200–211, 1982.
25. Feingold M, Baum J: Goldenhar's syndrome. *Am J Dis Child* 132:136–138, 1978.
26. François M, Baum J: Goldenhar's syndrome. *Ann Ocul* 187:340–368, 1954.
27. Friedman S, Saraclar M: The high frequency of congenital heart disease in oculo-auriculo-vertebral dysplasia (Goldenhar's syndrome). *J Pediatr* 85:873–874, 1974.
28. Goldenhar M: Associations malformatives de l'oeil et de l'oreille, en particulier le syndrome dermoide epibulbaire-appendices auriculaires-fistula auris congenita et ses relations avec la dysostose mandibulo-faciale. *J Genet Hum* 1:243–282, 1952.
29. Gomez Garcia A et al: Sindrome de Goldenhar. Discordancia en gemelos monocigotos. *An Esp Pediatr* 20:400–402, 1984.
30. Gorlin RJ et al: Oculoauriculovertebral spectrum. In: *Syndromes of the Head and Neck*, 4th ed. Oxford University Press, New York, 2001, pp 790–798.
31. Grabb WC: The first and second branchial arch syndrome. *Plast Reconstr Surg* 36:485–508, 1965.
32. Greenwood RD et al: Cardiovascular malformations in oculoauriculovertebral dysplasia. *J Pediatr* 85:816–818, 1974.
33. Grix A Jr: Malformations in infants of diabetic mothers. *Am J Med Genet* 13:131–137, 1982.
34. Gupta JS et al: Oculo-auriculo-cranial dysplasia. *Br J Ophthalmol* 52:346–347, 1968.
35. Gustavson EE, Chen H: Goldenhar syndrome, anterior encephalocele and aqueductal stenosis following fetal primidone exposure. *Teratology* 32:13–17, 1985.
36. Helmi C, Pruzansky S: Craniofacial and extracranial malformations in the Klippel-Feil syndrome. *Cleft Palate J* 17:65–88, 1980.

37. Herrmann J, Opitz JM: A dominantly inherited first arch syndrome. *Birth Defects* 5(2):110–112, 1969.
38. Hollwich F, Verbeck B: Zur Dysplasia oculoauricularis (Franceschetti-Goldenhar). *Klin Monatsbl Augenheilkd* 154:430–443, 1969.
39. Ide CH et al: Familial facial dysplasia. *Arch Ophthalmol* 84:427–433, 1970.
40. Kaye CI et al: Oculoauriculovertebral anomaly: segregation analysis. *Am J Med Genet* 43:913–917, 1992.
41. Kirke DK: Goldenhar's syndrome: two cases of oculo-auriculo-vertebral dysplasia occurring in full-blood Australian aboriginal sisters. *Aust Paediatr J* 6:213–214, 1970.
42. Krause VH: The syndrome of Goldenhar affecting two siblings. *Acta Ophthalmol (Kbh)* 48:494–499, 1970.
43. Lammer ES et al: Retinoic acid embryopathy. *N Engl J Med* 313:837–841, 1985.
44. Livingston G: Congenital ear abnormalities due to thalidomide. *Proc R Soc Med* 58:493–497, 1965.
45. Mansour AM et al: Ocular findings in the facio-auriculo-vertebral sequence (Goldenhar-Gorlin syndrome). *Am J Ophthalmol* 100:555–559, 1985.
46. Margolis S et al: Retinal and optic nerve findings in Goldenhar-Gorlin syndrome. *Ophthalmology* 91:1327–1333, 1984.
47. Melnick M: The etiology of external ear malformations and its relation to abnormalities of the middle ear, inner ear and other organ systems. *Birth Defects* 16(4):303–331, 1980.
48. Melnick M, Myrianthopoulos NC: External ear malformations: epidemiology, genetics and natural history. *Birth Defects* 15(9):27–29, 1979.
49. Michaud C, Sheridan S: Goldenhar's syndrome associated with cranial and neurological malformations. *Can J Ophthalmol* 9:347–350, 1974.
50. Miehlke A, Partsch CJ: Ohrmissbildung, Facialis- und Abducenslähmung als Syndrom der Thalidomidschädigung. *Arch Ohrenheilkd* 181:154–174, 1963.
51. Miyamoto RT et al: Goldenhar syndrome associated with submandibular gland hyperplasia and hemihypoplasia of the mobile tongue. *Arch Otolaryngol* 102:313–314, 1976.
52. Moeschler J, Clarren SK: Familial occurrence of hemifacial microsomia with radial limb defects. *Am J Med Genet* 12:371–375, 1982.
53. Mounoud RL et al: A propos d'un cas de syndrome de Goldenhar. *J Genet Hum* 23:135–154, 1975.
54. Murphy MJ et al: Intracranial dermoid cyst in Goldenhar's syndrome. *J Neurosurg* 53:408–411, 1980.
55. Opitz JM, Faith GC: Visceral anomalies in an infant with the Goldenhar syndrome. *Clin Genet* 5:104–105, 1969.
56. Papp Z et al: Probably monozygotic twins with discordance for Goldenhar syndrome. *Clin Genet* 5:86–90, 1974.
57. Par MM et al: A propos d'une observation familiale de syndrome de Franceschetti-Goldenhar. *Bull Soc Ophtalmol Fr* 63:705–707, 1963.
58. Perez Alvarez F et al: Sindrome otocraneofacial asimetrico (microsomia hemifacial) en gemelos monocigoticos discordantes. Aspectos otologicos. *An Esp Pediatr* 21:769–773, 1984.
59. Pieroni D: Goldenhar's syndrome associated with bilateral Duane's retraction syndrome. *J Pediatr Ophthalmol* 6:16–18, 1969.
60. Pierpont MEM et al: Congenital cardiac, pulmonary and vascular malformations in oculoauriculovertebral dysplasia. *Pediatr Cardiol* 2:297–302, 1982.
61. Regenbogen L et al: Further evidence for an autosomal dominant form of oculoauriculovertebral dysplasia. *Clin Genet* 21:161–167, 1982.
62. Robinow M et al: Hemifacial microsomia, ipsilateral facial palsy, and malformed auricle in two families: an autosomal dominant malformation. *Am J Med Genet* (Suppl) 2:129–133, 1986.
63. Rollnick BR: Oculoauriculovertebral anomaly: variability and causal heterogeneity. *Am J Med Genet* (Suppl) 4:41–53, 1988.
64. Rollnick BR, Kaye CI: Hemifacial microsomia and variants: pedigree data. *Am J Med Genet* 15:233–253, 1983.
65. Rollnick BR, Kaye CI: Hemifacial microsomia and the branchio-oto-renal syndrome. *J Craniofac Genet Dev Biol* (Suppl) 1:287–295, 1985.
66. Rollnick BR et al: Oculoauriculovertebral dysplasia and variants: phenotypic characteristics of 294 patients. *Am J Med Genet* 26:361–375, 1987.
67. Rosenal TH: Aplasia-hypoplasia of the otic labyrinth after thalidomide. *Acta Radiol* 3:225–236, 1965.
68. Ross RB: Lateral facial dysplasia (first and second branchial arch syndrome, hemifacial microsomia). *Birth Defects* 11:51–59, 1975.
69. Ryan CA et al: Discordance of signs in monozygotic twins concordant for the Goldenhar anomaly. *Am J Med Genet* 29:755–761, 1988.
70. Sando I, Ikeda M: Temporal bone histopathology findings in oculo-auriculovertebral dysplasia. Goldenhar's syndrome. *Ann Otol Rhinol Laryngol* 95:396–400, 1986.
71. Saraux MH, Besnainou L: Les syndrome maxillooculaires. *Ann Ocul* 198:953–964, 1965.
72. Setzer ES et al: Etiologic heterogeneity in the oculoauriculovertebral syndrome. *J Pediatr* 98:88–91, 1981.
73. Shokeir MHK: The Goldenhar syndrome: a natural history. *Birth Defects* 13(3C):67–83, 1977.
74. Smakel Z: Craniofacial changes in hemifacial microsomia. *J Craniofac Genet Dev Biol* 6:151–170, 1986.
75. Smith DW: Facio-auriculo-vertebral spectrum. In: *Recognizable Patterns of Human Malformation*, 3rd ed. W.B. Saunders, Philadelphia, 1982, pp 497–500.
76. Stark RB, Saunders DE: The first branchial syndrome: the oral-mandibular-auricular syndrome. *Plast Reconstr Surg* 29:229–239, 1967.
77. Stoll C: Discordance for skeletal and cardiac defect in monozygotic twins. *Acta Genet Med Gemellol* 33:501–504, 1984.
78. Summitt R: Familial Goldenhar syndrome. *Birth Defects* 5(2):106–109, 1969.
79. Taysi K et al: Familial hemifacial microsomia. *Cleft Palate J* 2:47–53, 1983.
80. Ter Haar B: Oculo-auriculo-vertebral dysplasia (Goldenhar's syndrome). Concordant in identical twins. *Acta Med Genet Gemellol (Roma)* 21:116–124, 1972.
81. Tenconi R, Hall BD: Hemifacial microsomia: phenotypic classification, clinical implications and genetic aspects. In *Treatment of Hemifacial Microsomia*, Harvold EP (ed), Alan R. Liss, New York, 1983, pp 39–49.
82. Thomas P: Goldenhar syndrome and hemifacial microsomia: observations in three patients. *Eur J Pediatr* 133:287–292, 1980.
83. Wells MD et al: Oculo-auriculo-vertebral dysplasia. *J Laryngol Otol* 97:689–696, 1983.
84. Wilson GN: Cranial defects in Goldenhar's syndrome. *Am J Med Genet* 14:435–443, 1983.
85. Zeitzer LD, Lindeman RC: Multiple branchial arch anomalies. *Arch Otolaryngol* 93:562–567, 1971.

Townes-Brocks syndrome (lop ears, imperforate anus, triphalangeal thumbs, and sensorineural hearing loss)

In 1972, Townes and Brocks (30) described a family in which a father and five of his seven children displayed a syndrome of "satyr" ears, imperforate anus, triphalangeal thumbs, and sensorineural hearing loss. Similarly affected families or individuals have subsequently been described (2,3,5–8,9,14–16,24,26,32) and the spectrum of anomalies has been expanded to include renal and cardiac defects. At least 60 cases have been published. Powell and Michaelis provide an excellent review (22).

Gastrointestinal system. Anorectal anomalies constitute the most characteristic hallmark of this condition. Imperforate anus (usually high) has been found in 21 of 44 patients. It was associated with rectoperitoneal or rectovaginal fistula in 65% of these cases (21). A midline perineal raphe extended from the site of the anal orifice to the scrotum (5,24). Anal anomalies may also include anterior placement (seven females), anal stenosis (15%) (21), or excess perianal skin without functional disturbance (six males) (21).

Musculoskeletal system. The skeletal anomalies are variable, but radial ray anomalies are present in over 50% of cases, with triphalangeal thumbs, bifid thumbs, broad thumbs, hypoplastic thumbs, supernumerary thumbs, and distal ulnar deviation of thumbs all described (Fig. 6–5E–G). Variable syndactyly of the second to fourth fingers has been seen (5,6). Absence of third toes, syndactyly of third and fourth toes, overlapping of second to fourth toes, clinodactyly of fifth toes, and pes planus have been noted in about 25%.

Genitourinary system. Although renal anomalies were not part of the original description, seven patients have been reported with a variety of findings including renal hypoplasia, unilateral renal agenesis, posterior urethral valves, ureterovesical reflux, meatal stenosis, and glandular hypospadias (5,9,17) (Fig. 6–5D).

Cardiovascular system. On rare occasions patients have congenital heart defects including tetralogy of Fallot, atrial septal defect, truncus arteriosus, and ventricular septal defect (2,6,9,19).

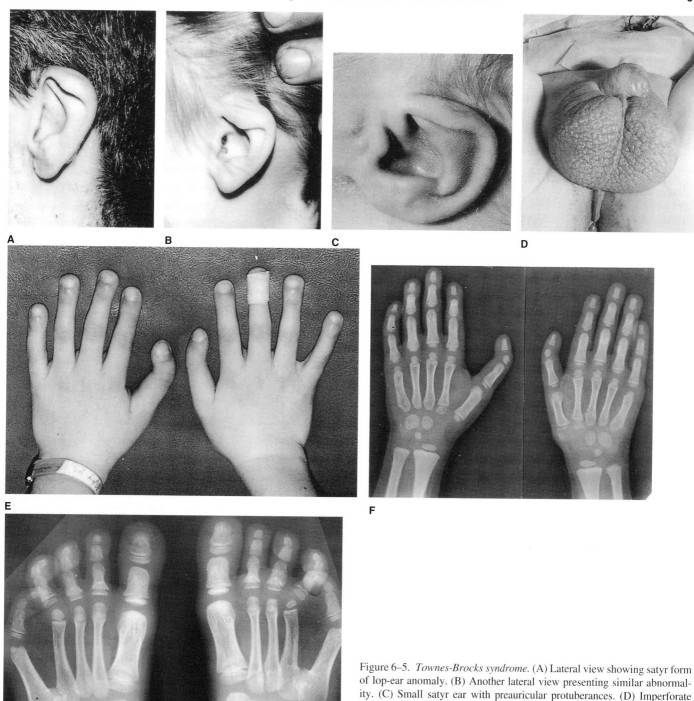

Figure 6–5. *Townes-Brocks syndrome.* (A) Lateral view showing satyr form of lop-ear anomaly. (B) Another lateral view presenting similar abnormality. (C) Small satyr ear with preauricular protuberances. (D) Imperforate anus, prominent perineal raphé, scrotum bifidum, and glandular hypospadias. (E) Deviation of distal phalanges of thumb. (F) Note triphalangeal thumbs. Supernumerary thumbs had been surgically excised. Note accessory carpal bone and absence of triquetral bones. (G) Radiograph of feet. Note lateral displacement and fusion of proximal ends of fourth and fifth metatarsals. Also observe cone-shaped epiphyses at proximal end of first metatarsals and at proximal phalanges of second and third toes. [(A,B,E–G) from PL Townes and ER Brocks, *J Pediatr* 81:321, 1972; (C,D) from MACS de Vries-Van der Weerd et al., *Clin Genet* 34:195, 1988.]

External ears. The satyr form of lop-ear anomaly with folding of the superior helix has been found in 35% (20) (Fig. 6–5A–C). Additional ear anomalies include preauricular skin tags (30%), preauricular pits (5%), and microtia (2,17,21).

Central nervous system. Mental retardation has been noted in a few patients (3,31).

Auditory system. Among those with dysmorphic pinnae, 13 of 44 (30%) patients had unilateral or bilateral sensorineural hearing loss of 40–60 dB (21). Occasionally, hearing loss is severe to profound. Ossicular anomalies can be found (6).

Radiographic findings. Hand radiographs have demonstrated pseudoepiphysis of the second metacarpal, absent triquetral and/or navicular bones, fused triquetrum and hamate, and short or fused metatarsals (5,6,9,30,32).

Heredity. The syndrome clearly demonstrates autosomal dominant inheritance with variable expressivity. Cytogenetic findings suggest that the causative gene is mapped to chromosome 16q. Mutations in *SALL1* have been identified in a family with vertical transmission of Townes-Brocks syndrome and in a sporadic case (13). The *SALL1* gene codes for a protein homologous to a *Drosophila* developmental regulator and is thought to be a zinc-finger transcription factor. The mutations identified result in a prematurely truncated protein lacking all putative DNA-binding domains (13).

Diagnosis. The incidence of anal/rectal malformations varies from 1/1500 to 1/5000 live births (29). Most isolated malformations are sporadic although, in rare instances, autosomal dominant, autosomal recessive, and X-linked recessive inheritance have been reported (4,12,27,31,34). In approximately 50% of affected individuals, associated congenital anomalies can be found (6). Imperforate anus may be part of a complex association of vertebral defects, cardiac defects, tracheoesophageal fistula with esophageal atresia, and radial and renal defects known as VATER or VACTERL association (18,20). Auricular defects were present in 3 of the first 19 patients described. This association of anal malformations (55%), renal dysplasia or agenesis (45%), congenital heart anomalies (75%), ear anomalies (40%), and thumb anomalies (30%) shows considerable overlap with Townes-Brocks syndrome (33). Quan and Smith (23) proposed that defective differentiation of mesoderm, prior to 35 days gestation, might be the pathogenetic mechanism in VATER or VACTERL association. Such a mechanism may be the basis for the clinical manifestations of Townes-Brocks syndrome as well.

Triphalangeal and/or bifid thumb may be inherited as an isolated dominant trait (28) or in association with cardiovascular anomalies in the Holt-Oram syndrome (10) and Blackfan-Diamond syndrome (18). Aase and Smith (1) described a combination of congenital anemia and triphalangeal thumbs as an autosomal recessive syndrome. Triphalangeal thumbs have also been reported in association with hearing loss. What appears to be autosomal dominant oculo-auriculo-vertebral spectrum with anal stenosis has been labeled Townes-Brocks syndrome (11). The association of anorectal malformation with end-stage renal disease and sensorineural hearing loss in several members of a three-generation family was reported by Lowe et al. (17) but the association may have been one of chance. Finally, many of the features of Townes-Brocks syndrome, including preauricular tags, anal atresia, cardiac and renal malformations, are also seen in partial duplication 22 (cat eye syndrome), so careful chromosome studies are indicated, particularly if ocular anomalies are present (25).

Prognosis. The hearing loss appears very early in life and in most cases is probably congenital. At least one report documents onset of hearing loss at age 6 years. There is no evidence to suggest that the hearing loss is progressive.

Summary. This syndrome is characterized by (*1*) autosomal dominant inheritance with variable expressivity; (*2*) satyr ears, often accompanied by preauricular tags and occasional pits; (*3*) imperforate anus with rectovaginal or rectoperineal fistula, or occasionally anterior or stenosed anus; (*4*) triphalangeal thumbs and various other bony anomalies; (*5*) renal anomalies; (*6*) congenital heart defects; and (*7*) sensorineural hearing loss.

References

1. Aase J, Smith DW: Congenital anemia and triphalangeal thumbs. *J Pediatr* 74:471–474, 1961.
2. Barakat AY et al: Townes-Brocks syndrome: report of three additional patients with previously undescribed renal and cardiac abnormalities. *Dysmorph Clin Genet* 2:104–108, 1988.
3. Cameron TH et al: Townes-Brocks syndrome in two mentally retarded youngsters. *Am J Med Genet* 41:1–4, 1991.
4. Cozzi F, Wilkinson AW: Familial incidence of congenital anorectal anomalies. *Surgery* 64:669–671, 1968.
5. De Vries-Van der Weerd MACS et al: A new family with Townes-Brocks syndrome. *Clin Genet* 34:195–200, 1988.
6. Ferraz FG et al: Townes-Brocks syndrome. Report of a case and review of the literature. *Ann Genet* 32:120–123, 1989.
7. Friedman PA et al: Six patients with the Townes-Brocks syndrome including five familial cases and an association with a pericentric inversion of chromosome 16. *Am J Hum Genet* 41(Suppl):A60, 1987.
8. Hasse W: Associated malformations with anal and rectal atresiae. *Prog Pediatr Surg* 9:99–103, 1976.
9. Hersh JH et al: Townes syndrome: a distinct multiple malformation syndrome resembling VACTERL association. *Clin Pediatr* 25:100–102, 1986.
10. Holmes LB: Congenital heart disease and upper-extremity deformities. *N Engl J Med* 272:437–444, 1965.
11. Johnson JP, Sherman S: Townes-Brocks syndrome: three generations with variable expression. *Proc Greenwood Genet Ctr* 8:200, 1989.
12. Kaijser K, Malmstrom-Groth A: Ano-rectal abnormalities as a congenital familial incidence. *Acta Paediatr Scand* 46:199–200, 1957.
13. Kohlhase J et al: Mutations in the *SALL1* putative transcription factor gene cause Townes-Brocks syndrome. *Nat Genet* 18:81–83, 1998.
14. König R et al: Townes-Brocks syndrome. *Eur J Pediatr* 150:100–103, 1990.
15. Kotzot D et al: Townes-Brocks-Syndrom. *Monatschr Kinderheilkd* 140:343–345, 1992.
16. Kurnit DM et al: Autosomal dominant transmission of a syndrome of anal, ear, renal and radial congenital malformations. *J Pediatr* 93:270–273, 1978.
17. Lowe J et al: Dominant ano-rectal malformation, nephritis and nerve deafness: a possible new entity? *Clin Genet* 24:191–193, 1983.
18. Minagi H, Steinbach HL: Roentgen appearance of anomalies associated with hypoplastic anemias of childhood: Fanconi's anemia and congenital hypoplastic anemia. *AJR Am J Roentgenol* 97:100–109, 1966.
19. Monteiro de Pina-Neto J: Phenotypic variability in Townes-Brocks syndrome. *Am J Med Genet* 18:147–152, 1984.
20. Nora AH, Nora JJ: A syndrome of multiple congenital anomalies associated with teratogenic exposure. *Arch Environ Health* 30:17–21, 1975.
21. O'Callaghan M, Young ID: The Townes-Brocks syndrome. *J Med Genet* 27:457–461, 1990.
22. Powell CM, Michaelis RC: Townes-Brocks syndrome. *J Med Genet* 36:89–93, 1999.
23. Quan L, Smith DW: The VATER association. *J Pediatr* 82:104–107, 1973.
24. Reid IS, Turner G: Familial anal abnormality. *J Pediatr* 88:992–994, 1976.
25. Schinzel A et al: The "cat eye" syndrome. *Hum Genet* 57:148–158, 1981.
26. Silver W et al: The Holt-Oram syndrome with previously undescribed associated anomalies. *Am J Dis Child* 124:911–914, 1972.
27. Suckling PV: Familial incidence of congenital abnormalities of the anus and rectum. *Arch Dis Child* 24:75–76, 1949.
28. Swanson AB, Brown KS: Hereditary triphalangeal thumb. *J Hered* 53:259–265, 1962.
29. Teixiera OHP et al: Cardiovascular anomalies with imperforate anus. *Arch Dis Child* 58:747–749, 1983.
30. Townes PL, Brocks ER: Hereditary syndrome of imperforate anus with hand, foot and ear anomalies. *J Pediatr* 81:321–326, 1972.
31. Van Gelder DW, Kloepfer HW: Familial anorectal anomalies. *Pediatrics* 27:334–336, 1961.
32. Walpole IR, Hockey AH: Syndrome of imperforate anus, abnormality of hands and feet, satyr ears, and sensorineural deafness. *J Pediatr* 100:250–252, 1982.
33. Weaver DD et al: The VATER association. Analysis of 46 patients. *Am J Dis Child* 140:225–229, 1986.
34. Weinstein ED: Sex-linked imperforate anus. *Pediatrics* 35:715–718, 1965.

Branchio-oto-renal (BOR) syndrome (branchio-oto syndrome, ear-pit hearing loss syndrome)

The term *branchio-oto-renal syndrome* (BOR) was first used in 1975 by Melnick et al. (55) to refer to patients with branchial cleft, fistulas, or cysts; otologic anomalies, including malformed pinnae, preauricular pits or sinuses, and hearing loss; and renal anomalies of various types. Many other clinical features have subsequently been noted. Its prevalence is about 1/40,000 and it is thought to occur in about 2% of profoundly affected children (23). Excellent reviews by Fraser et al. (22) and Cremers and Fikkers-van Noord (14) are available. The first summary descriptions were published in the nineteenth century (3,34,65,66).

Initially the branchio-oto (BO) syndrome was considered to be distinct from the BOR syndrome because of the absence of reported renal anomalies and type of hearing loss (54,57). The earpit hearing loss syndrome was also considered a distinct entity (50). This distinction was based largely on early reports of patients in whom complete renal and/or branchial evaluations were not undertaken (19,21,51,53,73,88). Once families were reported in which individual members had either BO or BOR involvement, and had either conduction, sensorineural, or mixed hearing loss, the BO and BOR syndromes began to be considered a single condition with variable expression (14,22,33,81). We suspect that the syndrome of renal pelviocalyceal dysmorphism and sensorineural hearing loss is the same as BOR syndrome (59).

Craniofacial findings. Facial shape is frequently long and narrow with a "constricted" palate and deep overbite (12,22,55,56). Facial nerve paralysis has been described in less than 10% of cases (14,33,71). Aplasia or stenosis of the lacrimal duct has been reported in approximately 10% (14,22,57). Rarely, clinical features suggestive of lacrimal duct stenosis are actually due to misdirected seventh cranial nerve enervation leading to gustatory lacrimation (67). Occasionally, facial or mandibular asymmetry is found (33,60,71). Facial nerve anomalies are documented in less than 5% of affected individuals (9,28). Rollnick and Kaye (71,72) reported a family and two additional probands with manifestations of both BOR syndrome and oculo-auriculo-vertebral spectrum. They hypothesized that the hemifacial microsomia (HFM) phenotype may constitute a severe form of BOR in some families. Heimler and Lieber (33) reported one individual in a large BOR pedigree affected with both BOR and HFM, a finding lending support to this hypothesis.

Branchial cysts/fistulas. Branchial cysts or fistulas are reported in approximately 60% of patients (9,14,22). Branchial cleft cysts, fistulas, or sinuses, usually bilateral, may be present on the external lower third of the neck, usually at the median border of the sternomastoid muscle. The fistulas may rarely open internally into the tonsillar fossa; they may drain fluid or become infected. Nipple-like cartilage rests can also be found (Fig. 6–6B–D,G,H).

Genitourinary system. Between 12% and 20% of affected individuals reported in the early literature had diagnosed structural anomalies of the renal system (22; Allanson, unpublished data, 1989). One systematic study of 19 patients by intravenous pyelography showed that 75% had a structural anomaly and 33% had functional anomalies of the renal system (14). Another study of 16 patients found 100% to have structural or functional renal manifestations (87). A recent review reported renal anomalies in around 80% of affected persons (9).

Some renal anomalies can remain asymptomatic (14); most are minor. If renal agenesis or severe hypoplasia is not present in infancy, the anomalies are not progressive (87). Only 6% are reported to have symptomatic severe renal involvement (23,69).

Severe renal anomalies include bilateral renal agenesis (8,19, 20,29,57), polycystic kidneys (14,56), and enlarged blunted kidneys (87). Structural anomalies can range from mild to severe and include hypoplastic kidneys (10,19,54,87), vesicoureteric reflux (12,33), crossed renal ectopia (8), bilateral bifid renal pelvis (33), ureteropelvic junction obstruction (33), extrarenal pelvis (33), fetal lobulation (33), abnormal rotation of the kidney (87), and calyceal diverticuli or distorted calyceal system (22,56,87).

Mild structural anomalies include slight blunting of the calyces, blunted calyceal fornices without pyelonephritis or papillary necrosis, segmented hypoplasia of the superior pole, reduced renal parenchymal volume (14), and outpouching of the renal pelvis on the medial border of the kidney (14,56) (Fig. 6–6E,F).

With regard to renal function, a small number of patients have disturbed concentration capacity and proteinuria, or reduced clearance of creatinine and diminished glomerular filtration rates (14,87). Histological studies may reveal prominent glomerular lesions (16,87) and irregularly shaped tubuli with swollen tubular epithelial cells (87). Segmental and focal hyalinization with dense immunoglobulin deposits of

IgG, IgM, IgA, and C3 along the basement membrane and in the mesangium has been observed (16).

Neither the presence or absence nor the severity of the renal defect may run true within families (8,19,20,29). Fraser et al. (24) described a family with duplication of the collecting system, which he termed the branchio-oto-ureteral (BOU) syndrome. This almost certainly represents variable expression of the BOR syndrome, based on the pedigree of Heimler and Lieber (33) in which several affected individuals in a family with BOR syndrome had double collecting system, while other affected family members had other renal anomalies. Konig et al. (41) described a family in which individuals had symptoms of BOR, BOU, or BO.

External ears. Anomalies of the external ear occur in 30%–60% of patients (22, Allanson, unpublished data, 1989). These range from severe microtia to minor anomalies of the pinnae, variously described as cup shaped, flaplike, lopped, flattened, or hypoplastic (Fig. 6–6A). The external canal may be narrow, "malformed," or slanted upward. Helical or preauricular pits are present in 70%–80% (22, Allanson, unpublished data, 1989). The pits are shallow, pinhead sized, with blind depressions in the helix of the ear near its upper attachment, or in the skin anterior to this site (14,33,56). Rarely, they communicate with the tympanic cavity (13).

Auditory system. Hearing loss has been reported in about 75% of cases (14,22, Allanson, unpublished data, 1989). Conductive hearing loss is found in 30%, sensorineural loss in 20%, and mixed hearing loss in 50% (14,15,26). Cremers et al. (15) noted absence of stapedius muscle reflexes and reduced tympanic membrane mobility. Age of onset varies from early childhood to young adulthood. Hearing loss may be progressive or nonprogressive (9,25). All three types of hearing loss have been observed in different members of the same family who are affected with variable manifestations of the BOR syndrome and include individuals with only branchial or otologic features. In several individuals the type of hearing loss differs between the two ears (20,87). These observations have led to the conclusion that there is no distinction between the BO and BOR syndromes based on type of hearing loss (14,22,33).

Vestibular system. The vestibular apparatus has rarely been examined. However, Cremers and Fikkers-van Noord (14) evaluated 11 members of a family with no vestibular complaints. Reduced or abolished caloric response was established with certainty in 7 of 11. One patient showed congenital nystagmus (jerk type).

Laboratory findings. Tomography of the temporal bones will usually identify anomalies (9,14). The most common outer ear abnormalities are stenosis and atresia of the external auditory canal. Middle ear anomalies include malformation, malposition, dislocation or fixation of the ossicles, and reduction in size or malformation of the middle ear cavity (9). In the inner ear, cochlear hypoplasia was most common, with one and a half or two coils of the cochlea being more likely than the normal two and a half turns (9,64). Dysplasia of the horizontal semicircular canal, dilation of the vestibular aqueduct, bulbous internal auditory canals, deep posterior fossae, and acutely angled promontories are all commonly desribed (9,64).

Pathology. Many anomalies of the middle ear have been described. Malformations of the ossicles, including unconnected or fused stapes and incus (14,15,33), temporal bone anomalies (19), and a small mastoid process with a reduced number of aerated air cells (22), have been reported. A mother and daughter with congenital cholesteatoma have been noted (44). Two additional cases validate the link between congenital cholesteatoma and this syndrome (28,91). Inner ear malformations include unilateral or bilateral malformed cochlea (14,20,22,56,62,78). The cochlea is often hypoplastic, with an acutely angled basal turn and a reduced number of coils (39,62,78,90). This is similar to but not characteristic of Mondini defect. Mondini dysplasia of the inner ear has also been reported in this condition (20,26,56). A

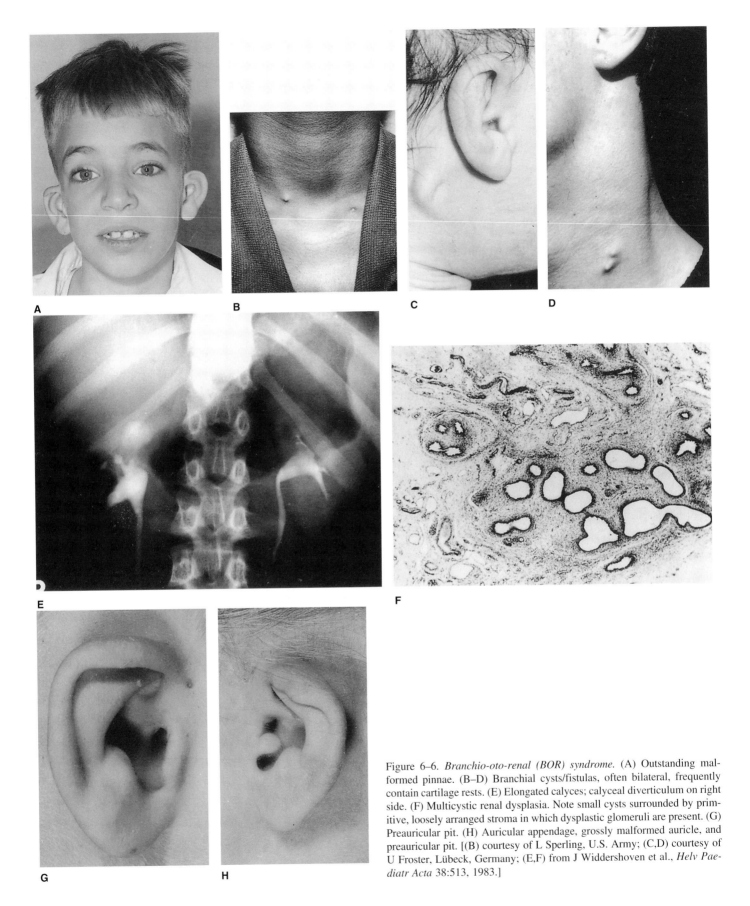

Figure 6–6. *Branchio-oto-renal (BOR) syndrome.* (A) Outstanding mal-formed pinnae. (B–D) Branchial cysts/fistulas, often bilateral, frequently contain cartilage rests. (E) Elongated calyces; calyceal diverticulum on right side. (F) Multicystic renal dysplasia. Note small cysts surrounded by prim-itive, loosely arranged stroma in which dysplastic glomeruli are present. (G) Preauricular pit. (H) Auricular appendage, grossly malformed auricle, and preauricular pit. [(B) courtesy of L Sperling, U.S. Army; (C,D) courtesy of U Froster, Lübeck, Germany; (E,F) from J Widdershoven et al., *Helv Pae-diatr Acta* 38:513, 1983.]

detailed description of the pathology of the cochlea is reported by Fitch et al. (20).

Heredity. The syndrome has autosomal dominant inheritance with variable expressivity (22,37,39,56,60). Penetrance is very high (14, 22,23,61) but probably not complete (33). Linkage to chromosome 8q was established in 1992 (42,80). One of the original hints was a report of a three-generation family in which a complex rearrangement of chromosome 8q segregated with both tricho-rhino-phalangeal syndrome and BOR syndrome (31). Among eight affected family members, seven had preauricular pits, five had branchial remnants, seven had hearing loss, and none had evidence of renal disease. Another child with deleted 8q had unilateral preauricular pit and branchial sinus (5). In 1997, Abdelhak et al. identified a gene with homology to the *Drosophila absent eyes (EYA1)* gene by positional cloning (1). Deletions and mutations likely leading to haploinsufficiency have been demonstrated in families with BOR and BO syndromes (1,84,92).

Pathogenesis. Malformations of the external and middle ear arise from growth and differentiation anomalies of the first and second branchial arches. Such anomalies may lead to microtia or preauricular fistulas, which seem to result from incomplete fusion of the mesodermal buttons originating from the branchial arches (47). Aplasia, dysplasia, or fusion of the ossicular chain components may also be due to defects in differentiation of the first branchial arch. It is generally accepted that dysplasia and fixation of the footplate of the stapes are the result of altered differentiation of the otic capsule, or failure of the stapedial lamina to separate from it (47). The presence of lateral cervical sinuses, fistulas, and cysts is thought to reflect abnormal differentiation of the first and second branchial arches and the first and second branchial clefts (54). The concomitant occurrence of paralysis of the facial nerve can be explained by the fact that the facial nerve is the nerve of the second branchial arch. The sensorineural hearing loss, however, cannot be explained simply as a branchial arch malformation, because the inner ear is derived from the otocyst and not the branchial arch system proper (25). However, experiments in avian and rat embryos have shown that the branchial arch tissues and the root ganglia of several cranial nerves are of neural crest origin. Johnston and Listgarten (38) have emphasized the important role played by neural crest elements. In BOR syndrome, the genetic defect may interfere with normal development of the neural crest with secondary involvement of not only the branchial system but also interruption of migration of melanocytes to the stria vascularis of the inner ear. This could account for the sensorineural hearing loss (35).

The association of ear and renal malformations has long been recognized (36,68). The renal anomalies in the BOR syndrome can be explained as aberrant inductive interaction between the ureteric bud and the metanephrogenic mesenchymal mass (27). This may arise because of a constitutional cell deficiency and/or late arrival of these cells. It is becoming increasingly apparent that cell interactions play a critical role in the choosing of new developmental pathways by embryonic cells and that genetically programmed cell surface components are instrumental in governing such cellular interactions (57). The embryologic events underlying the BOR syndrome most likely represent failure of directed cell movement and/or cellular spatial organization. This could be associated with an alteration in the character of cell recognition surface proteins. The resultant abnormal cell numbers and/or arrangement in the mesenchymal components of the branchial arches and metanephrogenic masses could alter the temporal sequence of interactions between differentiated regions in their attempt to initiate secondary pattern formation. This relationship appears to be particularly strong between the stria vascularis of the inner ear and the renal glomeruli (2) (see Alport syndrome). Saito et al. (74) observed renal agenesis and absence of the stria vascularis in the basal turn of the cochlea in a neonate with Potter syndrome. Fitch and Srolovitz (19) observed atrophy and dysplasia of the stria vascularis in histopathological examination of the temporal bones of a child with BOR syndrome. Johnston and Listgarten (38) provided much evidence of dynamic ectomesenchymal migration from the neural crest over and around the head. The derivatives of the neural crest form

most of the major components of the face. Ectomesenchymal deficiency in the area of the first and second branchial arches can lead to external ear and ossicular deformities, whereas deficiency of this tissue in the neck can result in branchial cleft fistula. Ectomesenchymal deficiency may produce an unreinforced bilaminar branchial membrane that splits apart, or a disruption of coordinated inductive interactions. These consequences may be associated with constitutional deficiency of ectomesenchyme or late, rather than normally programmed arrival of that tissue. Aberrant interactions may be similar to that postulated in the renal anomalies.

Tissue expression patterns of *EYA1* suggest a direct role for this gene in the development of all components of this syndrome (1). The type of DNA modifications reported suggests that BOR syndrome results from a reduced gene dosage, implying that the amount of protein encoded by *EYA1* is critical for the normal development of branchial arches, ear, and kidney. *EYA1* may be one of several developmental genes with a normal activity close to a threshold level required for the appearance of clinical defects. Such threshold dosage effects may explain the variable expression and incomplete penetrance within the same family (1).

Diagnosis. Minor ear malformations occur relatively frequently in the general population. For example, preauricular tags occur in 0.2% of live births and preauricular pits or sinuses in 0.8%. Nonsyndromic preauricular pits or sinuses are far more common in blacks than in whites (54). Approximately 1/200 children with a preauricular pit has profound hearing loss (21,46). Autosomal dominant inheritance of isolated preauricular pits is well described (11,40,49,86). Penetrance in familial cases has been estimated to be 85% (30). Preauricular pits and renal disease have been reported in a family in which there was no evidence of branchial anomalies or other features of the BOR syndrome (43). Some individuals had only preauricular pits, others had only renal disease, while a third group had a combination of the two.

Branchial cleft sinuses are relatively common congenital anomalies that generally occur as isolated defects but may have autosomal dominant transmission (6,17,30,32,44,45,63,76,79,83,85). Several families have been reported in which the combination of preauricular pits and branchial fistulas is dominantly inherited without mention of hearing loss (7,48,58,60,75), although this was not ruled out audiometrically. Autosomal dominant preauricular pits and sensorineural hearing loss (21); autosomal dominant malformed auricles, preauricular tags or preauricular pits, and moderate conduction hearing loss (77,88); and branchial fistulas, malformed auricles, and hearing loss (51) have been reported. These may represent variable expression of the BOR syndrome rather than distinct entities.

The BOU syndrome (24) likely represents variable expression of the BOR syndrome, particularly as Heimler and Lieber (33) have described a family in which some affected individuals have duplication of the collecting system and others have renal anomalies more characteristically associated with BOR syndrome. Although Fraser et al. (24) proposed this as a separate genetic defect, it is almost certainly the same entity. The branchio-oto-costal syndrome will be distinguished from BOR only by molecular analysis.

There is marked overlap between BOR syndrome and otofaciocervical syndrome (18), which is discussed later in this chapter. The latter lacks preauricular tags and lacrimal duct stenosis and has, in addition to features of BOR syndrome, unusual sloping shoulders, short stature, and characteristic facies. It now seems likely that otofaciocervical syndrome is a contiguous gene deletion syndrome involving *EYA1* (70).

Stratakis et al. (82) described a family with features very similar to BOR syndrome, but in which the ear malformation was separate and distinctive. Facial asymmetry was relatively common. Linkage to *EYA1* was not found. Several syndromes have been described with ear and renal anomalies including autosomal dominant dysmorphic pinnae-polycystic kidney syndrome (36), autosomal dominant dysmorphic pinnae-hypospadias-renal dysplasia syndrome (36), and autosomal recessive oto-renal-genital syndrome (89). The syndrome described in 1994 by Marres et al. (46) has considerable overlap with the BOR syndrome, but is separated from it by the presence of commissural lip pits, absence of linkage to 8q13, and linkage to 1q (see Marres syndrome, at conclusion of this chapter).

Prenatal diagnosis. At-risk pregnancies examined by direct real-time ultrasonography may identify more severe renal involvement (29). Diagnostic errors in non–real-time ultrasonography have been noted (8). Measurement of maternal serum alpha-fetoprotein as an indicator of fetal renal agenesis has been reported (4) but may not be a reliable prenatal diagnostic technique in all cases (8). In familial cases where the mutation is known, molecular analysis will provide the ideal method for prenatal diagnosis.

Prognosis. Hearing loss may be progressive (9,23). Only about 6% of individuals are reported to have severe renal involvement (23) and/or renal failure (8,19,20,57).

Summary. Characteristics of this syndrome include (*1*) autosomal dominant transmission with variable expressivity; (*2*) unilateral or bilateral preauricular pits; (*3*) unilateral or bilateral branchial fistulas; (*4*) hearing loss that may be sensorineural, conductive, or mixed; (*5*) anomalies of the external ear; and (*6*) renal abnormalities of varying severity.

References

1. Abdelhak S et al: A human homologue of the *Drosophila eyes absent* gene underlies branchio-oto-renal (BOR) syndrome and identifies a novel gene family. *Nat Genet* 15:157–164, 1997.
2. Arnold W: Inner ear and renal disease. *Ann Otol Rhinol Laryngol* 93:119–123, 1984.
3. Ascherson FM: *De fistulis colli congenitis* adjecta fissuraeum branchialium in mammalibus avibusque historia succincta. CH Jonas, Berolini, 1832, pp 1–21.
4. Balfour RP, Laurence KM: Raised serum AFP levels and fetal renal agenesis. *Lancet* 1:317, 1980.
5. Beighle C et al: Small structural changes of chromosome 8. Two cases with evidence for deletion. *Hum Genet* 38:113–121, 1977.
6. Bhalla V et al: Familial transmission of preauricular fistula in a seven generation Indian pedigree. *Hum Genet* 48:339–341, 1979.
7. Binns PM, Lord OC: Five cases of bilateral branchial fistulae in three generations of a family. *J Laryngol Otol* 79:455–456, 1965.
8. Carmi R et al: The branchio-oto-renal (BOR syndrome): report of bilateral renal agenesis in three sibs. *Am J Med Genet* 14:625–627, 1983.
9. Chen A et al: Phenotypic manifestations of branchiootorenal syndrome. *Am J Med Genet* 58:365–370, 1995.
10. Chitayat D et al: Branchio-oto-renal syndrome: further delineation of an underdiagnosed syndrome. *Am J Med Genet* 43:970–975, 1992.
11. Connon FE: Inheritance of ear pits in six generations of a family. *J Hered* 32:413–414, 1941.
12. Coté A, O'Regan S: The branchio-oto-renal syndrome. *Am J Nephrol* 2:144–146, 1982.
13. Cremers CWRJ: Congenital pre-auricular fistula communicating with the tympanic cavity. *J Laryngol Otol* 97:749–753, 1983.
14. Cremers CWRJ, Fikkers-van Noord M: The earpits-deafness syndrome. Clinical and genetic aspects. *Int J Pediatr Otorhinolaryngol* 2:309–322, 1980.
15. Cremers CWRJ et al: Otological aspects of the earpit-deafness syndrome. *ORL J Otolaryngol Relat Spec* 43:223–239, 1981.
16. Dumas R et al: Glomerular lesions in the branchio-oto-renal (BOR) syndrome. *Int J Pediatr Nephrol* 3:67–70, 1982.
17. Ewing MR: Congenital sinuses of the external ear. *J Laryngol Otol* 61:18–23, 1946.
18. Fara M et al: Dismorphia otofaciocervicalis familiaris. *Acta Chir Plast (Praha)* 9:255–268, 1967.
19. Fitch N, Srolovitz H: Severe renal dysgenesis produced by a dominant gene. *Am J Dis Child* 130:1356–1357, 1976.
20. Fitch N et al: The temporal bone in the preauricular pit, cervical fistula, hearing loss syndrome. *Ann Otol Rhinol Laryngol* 85:268–275, 1976.
21. Fourman P, Fourman J: Hereditary deafness in family with earpits (fistula auris congenita). *BMJ* 2:1354–1356, 1955.
22. Fraser FC et al: Genetic aspects of the BOR syndrome-branchial fistulas, ear pits, hearing loss and renal anomalies. *Am J Med Genet* 2:241–252, 1978.
23. Fraser FC et al: Frequency of the branchio-oto-renal (BOR) syndrome in children with profound hearing loss. *Am J Med Genet* 7:341–349, 1980.
24. Fraser FC et al: Autosomal dominant duplication of the renal collecting system, hearing loss, and external ear anomalies: a new syndrome? *Am J Med Genet* 14:473–478, 1983.
25. Gimsing S: The BOR syndrome as a possible neurocristopathy. *Ear Nose Throat J* 66:154–158, 1987.
26. Gimsing S, Dyrmose J: Branchio-oto-renal dysplasia in 3 families. *Ann Otol Rhinol Laryngol* 95:421–426, 1986.
27. Gluecksohn-Waelsch S: Genetic control of mammalian differentiation. In: *Genetics Today, Vol 2, Proceedings of the XIth International Congress of Genetics, 1963,* Pergamon Press, The Hague, pp 209–219.
28. Graham GE, Allanson JE: Congenital cholesteatoma and malformations of the facial nerve: rare manifestations of the BOR syndrome. *Am J Med Genet* 86:20–26, 1999.
29. Greenberg CR et al: The BOR syndrome and renal agenesis—prenatal diagnosis and further clinical delineation. *Prenat Diagn* 8:103–108, 1988.
30. Gualandri V: Ricerche genetiche sulla fistula auris congenita. *Acta Genet Med Gemell* 18:51–68, 1969.
31. Haan EA et al: Tricho-rhino-phalangeal and branchio-oto-renal syndromes in a family with an inherited rearrangement of chromosome 8q. *Am J Med Genet* 32:490–494, 1989.
32. Hall JG, Zimmer J: Congenital preauricular communicating fistulas: diagnosis, complications and treatment. *Acta Otolaryngol* 49:213–220, 1958.
33. Heimler A, Lieber E: The branchio-oto-renal-syndrome: reduced penetrance and variable expressivity in four generations of a large kindred. *Am J Med Genet* 25:15–27, 1986.
34. Heusinger CF: Hals-Kiemen-Fisteln von noch nicht beobachteter Form. *Virchows Arch Path Anat Physiol* 29:358–380, 1864.
35. Hilding DA, Ginsberg RD: Pigmentation of the stria vascularis. *Acta Otolaryngol* 84:24–37, 1977.
36. Hilson D: Malformation of ears as sign of malformation of genitourinary tract. *BMJ* 2:785–789, 1957.
37. Hunter AGW: Inheritance of branchial sinuses and preauricular fistulae. *Teratology* 9:225–228, 1974.
38. Johnston MC, Listgarten MA: Observations on the migration, interaction and early differentiation of orofacial structures. In: *Developmental Aspects of Oral Biology,* Slavkin HC, Bavetta LA (eds), Academic Press, New York, 1972, p 53–80.
39. Karmody CS, Feingold M: Autosomal dominant first and second branchial arch syndrome. *Birth Defects* 10(7):31–40, 1974.
40. Kindred JE: Inheritance of a pit in the skin of the left ear. *J Hered* 12:366–367, 1921.
41. Konig R et al: Branchio-oto-renal (BOR) syndrome: variable expression in a five-generation pedigree. *Eur J Pediatr* 153:446–450, 1994.
42. Kumar S et al: Autosomal dominant branchio-oto-renal syndrome—localization of a disease gene to chromosome 8q by linkage in a Dutch family. *Hum Mol Genet* 1:491–495, 1992.
43. Lachiewicz AM et al: Hereditary renal disease and preauricular pits: report of a kindred. *J Pediatr* 106:948–950, 1985.
44. Lipkin DF et al: Hereditary congenital cholesteatoma. *Arch Otolaryngol Head Neck Surg* 112:1097–1100, 1986.
45. Lyall D, Stahl W Jr: Latent cervical cysts, sinuses and fistulas of congenital origin. *Surg Gynecol Obstet* 102:417–434, 1956.
46. Marres HAM et al: The deafness, pre-auricular sinus, external ear anomalies and commissural lip pits syndrome-otological, vestibular and radiological findings. *J Laryngol Otol* 108:13–18, 1994.
47. Martini A et al: Branchio-oto-renal dysplasia and branchio-oto-dysplasia: report of eight new cases. *Am J Otol* 8:116–122, 1987.
48. Martins AG: Lateral cervical and preauricular sinuses: their transmission as dominant characters. *BMJ* 1:255–256, 1961.
49. McDonough ES: On the inheritance of ear pit. *J Hered* 32:169–171, 1941.
50. McKusick VA: *Mendelian Inheritance in Man,* 9th ed. Johns Hopkins University Press, Baltimore, 1990.
51. McLaurin JW et al: Hereditary branchial anomalies and associated hearing impairment. *Laryngoscope* 76:1277–1278, 1966.
52. Meggyessy V, Méhes K: Preauricular pits in Hungary: epidemiologic and clinical observations. *J Craniofac Genet Dev Biol* 2:215–218, 1982.
53. Melnick M: Hereditary hearing loss and ear dysplasia—renal adysplasia syndromes: syndrome delineation and possible pathogenesis. *Birth Defects* 16(7):59–72, 1980.
54. Melnick M, Myrianthopoulos NC: External ear malformations: epidemiology, genetics, and natural history. *Birth Defects* 15(9):22–23, 1979.
55. Melnick M et al: Autosomal dominant branchio-oto-renal dysplasia. *Birth Defects* 11(5):121–128, 1975.
56. Melnick M et al: Familial branchio-oto-renal dysplasia: a new addition to the branchial arch syndromes. *Clin Genet* 9:25–34, 1976.
57. Melnick M et al: Branchio-oto-renal dysplasia and branchio-oto-dysplasia: two distinct autosomal dominant disorders. *Clin Genet* 13:425–442, 1978.
58. Miller JB: Branchial cleft cysts, fistulae and appendages. *Laryngoscope* 67:1123–1193, 1957.
59. Morse MJ et al: The association of renal pelviocaliceal dysmorphism and sensorineural deafness: a new syndrome. *J Urol* 125:625–627, 1981.

60. Muckle TJ: Hereditary branchial defects in a Hampshire family. *BMJ* 1:1297–1299, 1961.

61. Nevin NC: Hereditary deafness associated with branchial fistulae and external ear malformations. *J Laryngol Otol* 91:709–716, 1977.

62. Ng YY et al: Computed tomography of earpits-deafness syndrome. *Br J Radiol* 62:947–949, 1989.

63. Onodi L: Über kongenital Ohrfisteln. *Arch Ohr Nase Kehlk Heilkd* 102:128–136, 1918.

64. Ostri B et al: Temporal bone findings in a family with branchio-oto-renal syndrome (BOR). *Clin Otolaryngol* 16:163–167, 1991.

65. Paget J: Cases of branchial fistulae on the external ears. *Lancet* ii:804, 1877.

66. Paget J: Cases of branchial fistulae in the external ears. *Med Chir Trans* 61:41–50, 1878.

67. Preisch JW et al: Gustatory lacrimation in association with the branchio-oto-renal syndrome. *Clin Genet* 27:506–509, 1985.

68. Quick CA et al: The relationship between cochlea and kidney. *Laryngoscope* 83:1469–1482, 1973.

69. Raspino M et al: The branchio-oto-renal syndrome. *J Laryngol Otol* 102:138–141, 1988.

70. Rickard S et al: Oto-facio-cervical syndrome is a contiguous gene syndrome involving *EYA1*: molecular analysis confirms allelism with BOR syndrome and further narrows the Duane syndrome critical region to 1 cM. *Hum Genet* 108:398–403, 2001.

71. Rollnick BR, Kaye CI: Hemifacial microsomia and the branchio-oto-renal syndrome. *J Craniofac Genet Dev Biol* (Suppl)1:287–295, 1985.

72. Rollnick BR, Kaye CI: Letter to the editor. *Am J Med Genet* 27:233, 1987.

73. Rowley PT: Familial hearing loss associated with branchial fistulas. *Pediatrics* 44:978–985, 1969.

74. Saito R et al: Anomalies of the auditory organ in Potter's syndrome. Histopathological findings in the temporal bone. *Acta Otolaryngol* 108:484–488, 1982.

75. Schull WJ, Furuta M: Persistent gill slits—a dominant trait? *Jpn J Hum Genet* 2:33–34, 1957.

76. Sedgwick CE, Walsh JF: Branchial cysts and fistulas—a study of seventy-five cases relative to clinical aspects and treatment. *Am J Surg* 83:3–8, 1952.

77. Shenoi PM: Wildervanck's syndrome: hereditary malformations of the ear in three generations. *J Laryngol Otol* 86:1121–1135, 1972.

78. Slack RWT, Phelps PD: Familial mixed deafness with branchial arch defects (earpit-deafness syndrome). *Clin Otolaryngol* 10:271–277, 1985.

79. Smith PG et al: Clinical aspects of the branchio-oto-renal syndrome. *Otolaryngol Head Neck Surg* 92:468–475, 1984.

80. Smith RJH et al: Localization of the gene for branchiootorenal syndrome to chromosome 8q. *Genomics* 14:841–844, 1992.

81. Stoll C et al: La dysplasie branchio-oto-renale. *Arch Fr Pediatr* 40:763–766, 1983.

82. Stratakis CA et al: Description of a large kindred with autosomal dominant inheritance of branchial arch anomalies, hearing loss, and ear pits, and exclusion of the branchio-oto-renal (BOR) syndrome gene locus (chromosome 8q13.3). *Am J Med Genet* 79:209–214, 1998.

83. Swenson O: Malformation of the head and neck. In: *Pediatric Surgery*, 3rd ed, Swenson D (ed), Appleton-Century-Crofts, New York, 1969, p 313.

84. Vincent C et al: BOR and BO syndromes are allelic defects of *EYA1*. *Eur J Hum Genet* 5:242–247, 1997.

85. Wheeler CE et al: Branchial anomalies in three generations of one family. *Arch Dermatol* 77:715–719, 1958.

86. Whitney DD: Three generations of ear pits. *J Hered* 30:323–324, 1939.

87. Widdershoven J et al: Renal disorders in the branchio-oto-renal syndrome. *Helv Paediatr Acta* 38:513–522, 1983.

88. Wildervanck LS: Hereditary malformations of the ear in three generations. *Acta Otolaryngol* 54:533–560, 1962.

89. Winter JSD et al: A familial syndrome of renal, genital and middle ear anomalies. *J Pediatr* 72:88–93, 1968.

90. Won KH et al: Genetic hearing loss with preauricular sinus and branchiogenic fistula. *Acta Otolaryngol* 103:676–680, 1977.

91. Worley GA et al: Bilateral congenital cholesteatoma in branchio-oto-renal syndrome. *J Laryngol Otol* 113:841–843, 1999.

92. Yashima T et al: Mutation of the *EYA1* gene in patients with branchio-oto syndrome. *Acta Otolaryngol* 123:279–282, 2003.

Lacrimo-auriculo-dento-digital (LADD) syndrome (cup-shaped ears, anomalies of the lacrimal ducts and teeth, and mixed hearing loss) (Levy-Hollister syndrome)

The lacrimo-auriculo-dento-digital (LADD) syndrome was first delineated in 1973 by Hollister et al. (7) in a report of a Mexican father and five of his eight children. Features included nasolacrimal duct obstruction with chronic dacryocystitis, absent lacrimal puncta, cup-shaped ears, peg-shaped teeth with enamel hypoplasia, various preaxial digital anomalies, clinodactyly, and hearing loss. A single patient described by Levy (11) probably had the same syndrome, leading to an alternate eponym, Levy-Hollister syndrome. A possible earlier example is that of Faber (4). Over 20 cases have been described in the literature (1,2,4,6–16,18).

Physical findings. Almost all affected persons have nasolacrimal duct anomalies, including duct aplasia or hypoplasia, nasolacrimal duct obstruction, absent lacrimal puncta usually associated with chronic epiphora, dacryocystitis, recurrent conjunctivitis, and keratoconjunctivitis. Nasolacrimal duct fistulas were noted by Kreutz and Hoyme (9). Completely absent tearing was found in four individuals and reduced tearing in 40% (16,17). Absence of the parotid glands and Stensen's ducts was observed in one of the two patients described by Shiang and Holmes (14). Various salivary gland anomalies were noted in other patients (11,16,18). Faber (4) described a patient with congenital aplasia of both parotid glands and bilateral hypoplastic thumbs, which may well represent an earlier description of this syndrome, as noted above.

Musculoskeletal system. Digital anomalies are variable and include duplicated terminal phalanx of the thumb, digitalized thumb, triphalangeal thumb, thenar muscle hypoplasia, preaxial polydactyly, exaggerated interdigital cleft between the second and third fingers, syndactyly of the second and third digits, and fifth finger clinodactyly (Fig. 6–7B–D). Metacarpophalangeal profiles show shortness of distal phalanges. Other limb anomalies include shortening of the radius and ulna, radioulnar synostosis, and, in one family, absent radius (9). The multiplicity of radial anomalies led Temtamy and McKusick (15) to suggest that LARD (lacrimo-auriculo-radio-dental) syndrome might be a better acronym. Lower limb anomalies are unusual, but Roodhooft et al. (13) described one patient with a supernumerary "metatarsoid" bone and possible phalangeal duplication of the fifth toe. Bamforth and Kaurah (1) noted broad halluces and anomalies of the first two toenails.

Dental findings. Dental anomalies have included hypodontia and peg-shaped incisors, as well as features consistent with enamel dysplasia of both deciduous and permanent teeth. Tooth discoloration, enamel thinning, excessive wear, and premature decay have often led to full mouth edentulation by adolescence or early adulthood. Hollister et al. (7) suggested that the dysplasia might be due to a mild amelogenesis imperfecta–like defect, probably of the hypocalcification type, but this has not been confirmed by pathologic studies.

Genitourinary system. Hollister et al. (7) reported one family member with unilateral renal agenesis. Shiang and Holmes (14) noted a patient with unilateral small scarred kidney and first-degree hypospadias. Roodhooft et al. (13) described one patient with blunted and dilated renal calyces. Bamforth and Kaurah (1) reported two deaths due to renal agenesis.

External ear. Characteristically, simple cup-shaped ears with a short helix and underdeveloped anthelix have been one of the most consistent features, present in 17 of 20 reported cases. The cup-shaped ears may be unilateral, bilateral, or asymmetrical. Hollister et al. (7) noted unilateral cupped ear, in which the hearing loss was ipsilateral (Fig. 6–7A). Thompson et al. (16) reported a patient with unilateral cupped ear but bilateral hearing loss.

Auditory findings. Mixed conductive and sensorineural hearing loss, either unilateral or bilateral, has frequently been reported. It has ranged in severity from mild to severe. Hearing impairment may be predominantly sensorineural. Stiffness of the conductive apparatus, ascertained by impedance audiometry, suggested otosclerosis or ossicular abnormalities (7). Stapes fixation was reported by Ensink and colleagues (3).

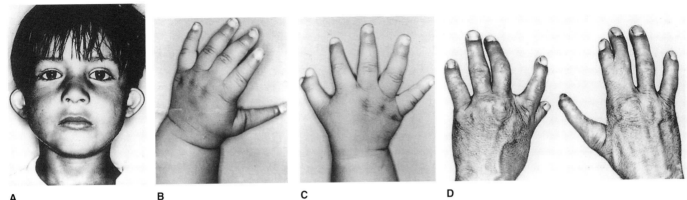

A   B   C   D

Figure 6–7. *Lacrimo-auriculo-dento-digital (LADD) syndrome.* (A) Prominent cup-shaped ears extend at right angles from side of head. Eyes have watery, glistening appearance; on right note an overflow of tears from outer canthus. (B,C) Long, tapering thumbs with large nail, bifid thumb tips with extra ectopic nails, and tapering of second and third digits bilaterally. (D) Right hand has long, tapering thumb with ectopic nail and syndactyly. Left hand has rudimentary thumb fused to index finger, prominent interdigital cleft between second and third fingers, and ulnar deviation. [From DW Hollister et al., *J Pediatr* 83:438, 1973.]

Laboratory findings. Radiographs of the hands showed a wide variation in bony anomalies. Tomograms were unremarkable.

Heredity. The syndrome clearly has autosomal dominant inheritance.

Diagnosis. While each individual feature of the LADD syndrome may occur as an isolated autosomal dominant trait, their combination is unique. The autosomal dominant branchio-oto-renal (BOR) syndrome (5) is similar with hearing loss, malformed pinnae, lacrimal duct stenosis, and renal anomalies. It is distinguished from LADD syndrome by auricular pits, branchial fistulas or cysts, and the absence of dental and digital anomalies. Townes-Brocks syndrome (17), in which there is ear deformity, sensorineural hearing loss, preaxial polydactyly, and imperforate anus, can be distinguished from LADD syndrome by the presence of anomalies of the anus and feet, and the absence of abnormalities of the lacrimal ducts and teeth. Absence of the parotid glands has been associated with lacrimal apparatus malformations in the ectrodactyly–ectodermal dysplasia–clefting (EEC) syndrome (12). Occasionally individuals with LADD syndrome have split-hand malformation (6,10). However, the EEC syndrome can usually be distinguished by the presence of ectodermal defects, renal anomalies, and oral clefting. Hennekam (6) and Lacombe et al. (10) raised the question of whether LADD syndrome and EEC syndrome represent a single causal entity.

Prognosis. Nasolacrimal anomalies may lead to chronic epiphora, dacryocystitis, recurrent conjunctivitis, or keratoconjunctivitis.

Summary. The syndrome is characterized by (*1*) autosomal dominant inheritance; (*2*) almost universal presence of cup-shaped ears; (*3*) nasolacrimal duct obstruction and hypoplasia of lacrimal puncta, with occasional lack of tear formation; (*4*) various preaxial ray/radial anomalies; (*5*) peg-shaped or missing teeth with mild amelogenesis imperfecta; and (*6*) mixed hearing loss with a large sensorineural component.

References

1. Bamforth JS, Kaurah P: Lacrimo-auriculo-dento-digital syndrome: evidence for lower limb involvement and severe congenital renal abnormalities. *Am J Med Genet* 43:932–937, 1992.
2. Calabro A et al: Lacrimo-auriculo-dento-digital (LADD) syndrome. *Eur J Pediatr* 146:536–537, 1987.
3. Ensink RJH, Cremers CWRJ, Brunner HG: Congenital conductive hearing loss in the lacrimoauriculodentodigital syndrome. *Arch Otol Head Neck Surg* 123:97–99, 1997.
4. Faber M: A case of congenital xerostomia. *Acta Paediatr Scand* 30:148–151, 1942.
5. Fraser FC et al: Frequency of the branchio-oto-renal (BOR) syndrome in children with profound loss. *Am J Med Genet* 7:341–349, 1980.
6. Hennekam RCM: LADD syndrome: a distinct entity? *Eur J Pediatr* 146:94–95, 1987.
7. Hollister DW et al: The lacrimo-auriculo-dento-digital syndrome. *J Pediatr* 83:438–444, 1973.
8. Hollister DW et al: Lacrimo-auriculo-dento-digital syndrome. *Birth Defects* 10(5):153–166, 1974.
9. Kreutz JM, Hoyme HE: Levy-Hollister syndrome. *Pediatrics* 82:96–99, 1988.
10. Lacombe D et al: Split hand/split foot deformity and LADD syndrome in a family: overlap between EEC and LADD syndromes. *J Med Genet* 30:700–703, 1993.
11. Levy WJ: Mesoectodermal dysplasia. *Am J Ophthalmol* 63:978–982, 1967.
12. Preus M, Fraser FC: The lobster-claw defect with ectodermal defects, cleft lip-palate, tear duct anomaly and renal anomalies. *Clin Genet* 4:369, 1973.
13. Roodhooft AM et al: Lacrimo-auriculo-dento-digital (LADD) syndrome with renal and foot anomalies. *Clin Genet* 38:228–232, 1990.
14. Shiang EL, Holmes LB: The lacrimo-auriculo-dento-digital syndrome. *Pediatrics* 59:927–930, 1977.
15. Temtamy S, McKusick V: The genetics of hand formation. *Birth Defects* 14(3):98–101, 1978.
16. Thompson E et al: Phenotypic variations in LADD syndrome. *J Med Genet* 22:382–385, 1985.
17. Townes PL, Brocks ER: Hereditary syndrome of imperforate anus with hand, foot and ear anomalies. *J Pediatr* 81:321, 1972.
18. Wiedemann H-R, Drescher J: LADD syndrome: report of new cases and review of the clinical spectrum. *Eur J Pediatr* 144:579–582, 1986.

CHARGE association

The various abnormalities that make up CHARGE association were first described by Hall (38) in 1979. The mnemonic CHARGE (*C*oloboma, *H*eart defects, *A*tresia of choanae, *R*etarded growth and development, *G*enital hypoplasia, *E*ar anomalies and/or deafness) was not proposed until 1981 when Pagon et al. (61) reported an additional 21 patients. Over 150 cases have been reported (1,7–11,13,14,16,22–28,33,34, 38,41,42,45–52,57–63,65,67,72,75,76). Although the most consistent features are still those prefixed by the letters CHARGE, additional abnormalities frequently occur. These include facial palsy, renal abnormalities, orofacial clefts, and tracheoesophageal fistulas. A large series of affected individuals is reported by Tellier and colleagues (75). The reader is directed to two reviews with emphasis on management (15,59).

Craniofacial findings. Choanal atresia is found in 45% of patients (16,24,27,33,38,39,48,51,57,60,61,67,69,72,75), often with bony obstruction of the posterior choanae (16,60). Bilateral choanal atresia frequently causes rapid obstruction of the upper airway after birth, requiring emergency surgery (60), while unilateral obstruction leads to persistent nasal discharge (60). Polyhydramnios is frequently associated with bilateral choanal atresia (38,60,68,75). Characteristically, the face (Fig. 6–8A–D) has a flattened and squared appearance with malar hypoplasia, a bulbous nasal tip with pinched nares, a long philtrum, occasional ptosis or pseudoptosis, and a short neck (11,24,33,38,48,60). Facial asymmetry has been noted even in the absence of facial nerve palsy. Cleft lip and palate (10,11,24,48,57,61,75) or cleft soft palate (8,75) have been found in 15% of patients. Multiple lower lip frenula were noted in one case (24).

Ocular system. Coloboma is the second most common feature of CHARGE association, being present in 75% of patients. It is bilateral or unilateral, affecting the iris, retina, and/or disc. Visual loss varies according to size and location of the coloboma. The "typical" coloboma results from secondary failure of fusion of the choroidal fissure (8,24,61) (Fig. 6–8D). Coloboma is often accompanied by microphthalmia (11,22,33,41,50,57,60,75). Cataracts are occasionally noted in adulthood (24) or in the newborn period (42,50,58). Retinal detachment was found in three members of the family reported by Mitchell et al. (58).

Cardiovascular system. The prevalence of congenital heart disease in CHARGE association has ranged from 60% to 70%. Although

the pattern of congenital heart defects initially appeared to be random (61), a preponderance of conotruncal and aortic arch malformations has recently been recognized (23,34,51). Approximately 40% have a conotruncal anomaly (51), and 36% have an aortic arch anomaly (51). Isolated septal defects are uncommon. This pattern of congenital heart defects differs from that reported in patients with isolated choanal atresia, where ventricular septal defect or patent ductus arteriosus alone or in combination is seen in 17% of patients (35). A pattern of cardiac defects similar to that in CHARGE association has been documented in DiGeorge sequence (21,31,53,68). Other similarities between the CHARGE association and the DiGeorge sequence include ear anomalies, psychomotor retardation, CNS malformations, and clefts of the alveolar ridge, lip, or palate (21,38). Patients with some features of DiGeorge sequence, such as hypocalcemia, T-cell dysfunction, and absence of thymus and/or parathyroids, have been noted in reviews of CHARGE association (26,47,51,61,67,75). These two disorders may share a common error in embryologic development of neural crest.

Central nervous system. Most patients have some degree of retarded development (24,38,39,61). Hall (38) described 17 patients with IQ scores ranging from less than 30 to 78. Pagon et al. (61) reported a similar range of intellectual functioning, with some patients being profoundly retarded and three young adult men who had full IQ scores of

Figure 6–8. *CHARGE association.* (A) Child with CHARGE association, age 5 ears. (B) Teen, age 15 years, with CHARGE association. (C) 18-year-old girl with CHARGE association. (D) Woman, age 47 years, with CHARGE. In all note minor facial asymmetry and squarish face. (E) Colobo-mas of optic nerve, choroid, and retina. Inferior position is typical. (F) Ears from various patients showing variable degrees of abnormal configuration. [(A–D,F) courtesy of Meg Hefner, Columbia, MO; (E) from HM Hittner et al., *J Pediatr Ophthalmol Strabismus* 16:122, 1979.]

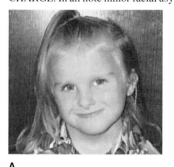

A

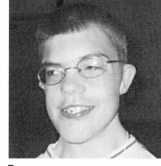

B

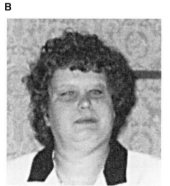

C

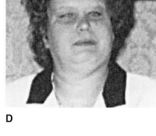

D

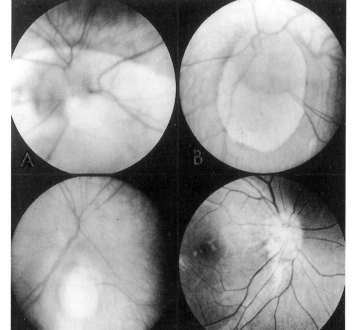

E

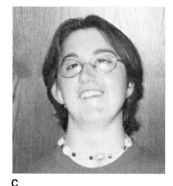
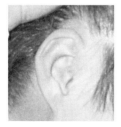

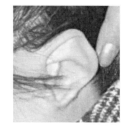

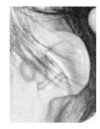

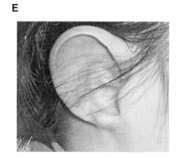

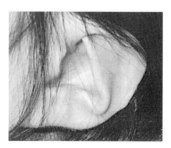

F

70–80 doing well in special education classes. Two patients were reported with normal intellectual function (39). Several others acquired skills that enabled them to function quite well (33). The diagnosis of mental retardation must be made with caution in anyone who has impaired hearing and/or vision. Hearing loss may cause language delay, while blindness impairs motor skills. The combination may produce autistic-like behavior. Elimination of sensory deficits led to improvement in several patients (24). In addition to having intellectual handicap, about 15% of patients are microcephalic (8,24,28,38,42,60,67,75). In some, microcephaly correlates with the presence of mental retardation (60), while in other patients, microcephaly does not correlate with either intellectual handicap or growth retardation (24). Various structural brain anomalies have been described, including cerebellar hypoplasia (41,52), encephalocele (60), absence of septum pellucidum (70), ventriculomegaly (24,52), and hydrocephalus (48). Electroencephalogram (EEG) anomalies (24) including hypsarrythmia (22) have been noted. Various abnormalities of the olfactory system have been described, including absent tracts (39,52), anosmia (24), arhinencephaly (69,73), and Kallmann syndrome (47,61). Hyperreflexia (48,58) and truncal hypotonia (48,58) have been reported. Davenport et al. (24) noted that older patients tend to have a shuffling gait with reduced arm swinging.

Endocrine system. Sixty percent of patients are growth retarded by late infancy (8–10,16,22,24,28,33,38,42,48–51,57–61,67), often despite normal birth weight and birth length (24,60,61). Some authors note spontaneous improvement in height by mid-childhood (60) or normal growth velocity after infancy (39,60). Retarded bone age is common (8,24,60). Formal growth hormone studies are rarely performed, although normal results in two patients (60), and growth hormone deficiency in two patients (9,24) have been reported.

Genital hypoplasia is reported in 40% of patients. It is much easier to recognize in males than in females because of cryptorchidism, micropenis, and hypospadias (24,33,38,51,60,61) (Fig. 6–8E). Labial and/or clitoral hypoplasia (24,70,75) and delayed or absent puberty (9,24,33) are seen. In several patients reduced levels of gonadotropins were confirmed (9,24,33), which suggest hypopituitarism possibly secondary to hypothalamic dysfunction. August et al. (9) described delayed peak thyroid-stimulating hormone (TSH) response to thyrotropin-releasing factor (TRF), while Oley (60) described a reduced response to luteinizing hormone–releasing hormone (LHRH) and human chorionic gonadotropin (HCG). It is interesting to note that cryptorchidism, hypospadias, and micropenis have been linked to intrauterine hypopituitarism (5).

Genitourinary system. Fifteen percent of patients have various renal abnormalities including renal agenesis (48), small kidneys (24,33), rotated kidneys (24,48,60), duplex collecting system (48,60), crossed renal ectopia (60), ectopic renal pelvis (42,60), hydronephrosis (8,41), posterior urethral valves (24), urethral atresia (24), and ureteral reflux (24,33,60).

Musculoskeletal system. Twenty percent have minor skeletal differences, including hypoplastic, asymmetric or bifid vertebrae (41,48,75), reduced number of ribs (41,59,60), reduced number of sternal ossification centers (68), short clavicles (33), congenital dislocation of hips (60), duplicated thumb (27), absent distal phalanges of the fifth digit (24), clinodactyly (58), talipes (28), and atrophy or absence of the muscles of the scapula, arm, and forearm (33). Severe skeletal defects, such as tetraperomelia, are extremely rare (75).

Respiratory and gastrointestinal system. Tracheoesophageal problems are common, although only a few patients have tracheoesophageal fistulas with esophageal atresia (16,24,61). Many patients have difficulty swallowing and feeding, often requiring gastrostomy. The causes, when known, are varied, and include velopharyngeal incompetence (24,60), primary laryngeal cleft (60), intramural cysts of the proximal esophagus (69), and esophageal neuromuscular incoordination (16,27,38,39,41,61). Paralysis of the vocal chords (50,69), imperforate anus (24), posteriorly displaced anus (16), and accessory spleen (72) are rare.

External ear. Abnormalities of the pinnae, with or without hearing loss, are a cardinal feature, and 90% of patients demonstrate a variety of anatomical variants. Most CHARGE ears are short and wide (Fig. 6–8F) (25,27,60,69). Some are cup shaped (57,60,61), thus losing the details of the anthelix, antitragus, concha, and even some detail of the helical fold. A prominent anthelix, with discontinuity between the anthelix and antitragus, and a triangular concha are perhaps the most striking and characteristic features (25,27,69). The anthelix occasionally appears horizontal (11). In the most extreme cases, the anthelix is bent forward, creating the impression that it forms a smooth curve with the superior helical fold. Portions of the helical fold are sometimes missing (25) and look as if they have been snipped off.

Most ears have small or absent lobes (25,27,28,41,60,68). Preauricular tags (41,58) and microtia and atresia of the canal (33,41) are extremely rare. Experimental studies in rodents have shown that early denervation of the facial nerve, which supplies the auricular muscles, may lead to the formation of a simple ear that lacks the usual conchal folds (71). Thus, it is not surprising to find that one-third of patients with the CHARGE association have facial palsy (9,10,14,22,24,33,38,39,41,49–51,60,61,65,69). The more anomalous ear is often present on the side of the facial palsy.

Auditory system. The most detailed study to date (76) reveals hearing loss in approximately 85% of patients. In that study, losses ranged from mild to profound, with 80% having moderately severe loss or worse in the better ear; mixed hearing loss due to ossicular anomalies and/or middle ear effusion was universal. The recurrent otitis media may have resulted from eustachian tube dysfunction secondary to choanal atresia, cleft lip and palate, unilateral facial paralysis, and flattening of the malar eminences. The sensorineural component of the hearing loss ranged from mild to severe or profound. The majority of patients had sloping sensorineural losses, greatest in higher frequencies. In almost every case, sensorineural loss was suspected to be congenital. In many there was evidence of progression. Although mixed hearing loss has been documented by several studies (27,33,60), many authors reported predominantly or exclusively sensorineural hearing loss (16,27,33,57,60,61,79). Rarely, conductive loss was the sole component (60). Thelin et al. (76) described a distinctive "wedge" audiogram secondary to combined middle ear disease and sensorineural loss, which they believed was unique to CHARGE syndrome.

Vestibular system. Computed tomography of the petrosal bones very frequently shows aplasia of the semicircular canals (4,77); indeed, Amiel et al. (7) suggested that temporal bone anomaly be a major diagnostic criteria for CHARGE association. The associated vestibular areflexia may contribute to delays in development and require specific educational interventions (1,4,77).

Radiographic findings. Radiographs confirm the skeletal anomalies and delay in bone age noted above.

Pathology. Evidence for congenital ossicular anomalies has been obtained by direct observation at surgery (65,77). Wright et al. (80) described temporal bone abnormalities in the CHARGE association in great detail, noting absence of the malleus, stapedial footplate, stapedius muscle/tendon and oval window; short bulky incus with a thick, long process and absent lenticular process; and displacement of the facial nerve. One patient also had inner ear anomalies with abnormally short cochlear ducts and a reduced population of ganglion cells. Autopsy in many patients confirmed the neurological, cardiovascular, and renal anomalies noted above.

Heredity. The etiology of the CHARGE association remains unknown, but is likely heterogeneous. There appears to be about a 6% chance of recurrence. Most cases are sporadic but, in at least some instances, CHARGE association appears to be dominantly transmitted.

Support for a high likelihood of new dominant mutations to explain sporadic cases is provided by the finding of increased paternal age (74).

Mitchell et al. (58) described a family in which six individuals from three generations were affected. Ho et al. (42) reported a woman with ocular coloboma, cataracts, and a childhood history of a heart murmur. Her two daughters, by different partners, had coloboma, congenital cataracts, and congenital heart disease. One of the two had slow growth and development. Hittner et al. (41) reported a mother and daughter with colobomatous microphthalmia, heart disease, abnormalities of the external ears, and hearing loss. Pagon et al. (61) reported a 30-year-old woman with colobomatous microphthalmia, patent ductus arteriosus, sensorineural hearing loss, and facial asymmetry whose daughter had coloboma, truncus arteriosus, unilateral cleft lip and palate, and growth retardation. Metlay et al. (57) reported a boy with optic nerve coloboma, congenital heart defects, choanal atresia, growth retardation, abnormal ears, and cleft lip and palate whose mother had coloboma, short stature, and hearing deficit. Collum (20) described a three-generation family in which eight individuals had varying combinations of coloboma, mental retardation, cleft lip and palate, facial asymmetry, and cardiac murmur.

Studies of concordant monozygotic female twins (49,60) support the possibility of monogenic etiology. Autosomal recessive inheritance seems possible in affected siblings with normal parents (10,51,61,62). The normal parents of a child with CHARGE association appear to have a low but not negligible recurrence risk for a similarly affected child. Since the possibility of etiologic diversity in the association remains, teratogens, single-gene disorders, chromosome abnormalities, and other etiologies need to be considered in each family.

Efforts to determine genetic heterogeneity may be hampered by patients with new mutations for the autosomal dominant gene who appear to be "sporadic cases," since lethal congenital anomalies, mental retardation, and infertility, especially in males, may reduce reproductive fitness.

Pathogenesis. Abnormalities in the development, migration, or interaction of cells of the neural crest may contribute to the pathogenesis of the CHARGE association and related complexes such as the DiGeorge sequence (69). Neural crest cells are ectodermal cells that migrate from the neural fold at about the time of neural tube fusion and contribute to the formation of widespread and diverse tissues. The normal flow of neural crest cells into the craniofacial region (43) may be deviated by the nasal and palatal processes into the area of the oronasal membrane contributing to the thickness of the atretic plate of the choanae (40). The branchial arches also arise in part from the neural crest, thus anomalies of the thymus, parathyroid glands, and external and middle ears in the CHARGE association can be explained (21,76,79). Disordered migration of mesenchymal tissue or neural crest cells in the branchial arches may also produce abnormalities of conotruncal septation including tetralogy of Fallot, transposition of the great vessels and truncus arteriosus communis (19), and hypopituitarism and abnormalities of the hypothalamus, leading to retarded growth and hypogenitalism (9).

Diagnosis. Choanal atresia has frequently been shown to be associated with other congenital malformations, particularly congenital heart defects (55,81) and coloboma (30). The combination of congenital heart defect, sensorineural hearing loss, mildly anomalous external ears, velopharyngeal insufficiency, and submucous cleft palate is found in velocardiofacial syndrome. Ocular colobomata have recently been described in this condition (13). Numerous chromosome abnormalities including cat eye syndrome (37), trisomy 22 (17), triploidy (6), long arm deletions of 9 (29), 11 (29), and 13 (78), and partial duplications of 4 (18) and 14 (2) have been reported in patients with colobomata and/or other features of CHARGE association. Dev et al. (26) reported a male infant with CHARGE association and features of the DiGeorge sequence who had a duplication of 1q. Saniaville et al. (66) found subtle chromosome rearrangements using comparative genomic hybridization (CGH) in 2/27 children with CHARGE association. Chromosomal phenocopy should always be excluded before the diagnosis of CHARGE

association is accepted. Several X-linked families, each having some features of the CHARGE association, have been reported (3,32,44,54). Some patients with manifestations of the VATER association (64) (tracheoesophageal fistula, congenital heart disease, and renal malformation) have features that overlap with the CHARGE association. A common teratogen has been considered a possible cause, since many of the features seen in the CHARGE association have also been seen in the thalidomide embryopathy (71), in infants exposed to phenylhydantoin (11) or rubella (56) in utero, and also in infants of diabetic mothers (36).

Prognosis. About 30% to 35% of patients die in the first 3 months of life (38,63). Most of these have the combination of bilateral choanal atresia and complex congenital heart disease. Additional criteria for poor prognosis include male gender, and CNS and/or esophageal malformations (75). In survivors, significant intellectual handicap is common, yet early detection of sensory deficits and appropriate intervention may allow patients to acquire skills that enable them to function quite well (24,33). Hearing loss appears to be progressive, albeit at a slow rate (73). Bauer et al. (12) provide a review of cochlear implantation in children with CHARGE association and note that results were varied, in part because of temporal bone anatomy and in part, an aberrant course of the facial nerve in the occasional patient. Overall prognosis clearly depends on the spectrum of anomalies found.

Summary. The characteristic features of this syndrome include (*1*) occasional autosomal dominant transmission with rare autosomal recessive inheritance, the majority of cases being sporadic; (*2*) various abnormalities of external ear; (*3*) colobomatous microphthalmia; (*4*) congenital heart defects, usually conotruncal; (*5*) choanal atresia; (*6*) retarded growth and development; (*7*) genital hypoplasia, possibly of hypothalamic origin; and (*8*) sensorineural or, more rarely, mixed hearing loss.

References

1. Abadie V et al.: Vestibular anomalies in CHARGE syndrome: investigations on and consequences for postural development. *Eur J Pediatr* 159:569–574, 2000.
2. Abeliovich D et al: 3:1 meiotic disjunction in a mother with a balanced translocation, 46,XX,t(5;14)(p15;q13) resulting in a tertiary trisomy and tertiary monosomy offspring. *Am J Med Genet* 12:83–89, 1982.
3. Abruzzo MA, Erickson RP: Re-evaluation of new X-linked syndrome for evidence of CHARGE syndrome or association. *Am J Med Genet* 34:397–400, 1989.
4. Admiraal RJC, Huygen PLM: Vestibular areflexia as a cause of delayed motor skill development in children with the CHARGE association. *Int J Pediatr Otorhinolaryngol* 39: 205–222, 1997.
5. Allen TD, Griffin JE: Endocrine studies in patients with advanced hypospadias. *J Urol* 131:310–314, 1984.
6. Al Saadi A et al: Triploidy syndrome: a report on two live-born (69,XXY) and one stillborn (69,XXX) infants. *Clin Genet* 9:43–50, 1976.
7. Amiel J et al: Temporal bone anomaly proposed as a major criteria for diagnosis of CHARGE syndrome. *Am J Med Genet* 99:124–127, 2001.
8. Angelman H: Syndrome of coloboma with multiple congenital abnormalities in infancy. *BMJ* 1:1212–1214, 1961.
9. August GP et al: Hypopituitarism and the CHARGE association. *J Pediatr* 103:424–425, 1983.
10. Awrich PD et al: CHARGE association anomalies in siblings. *Am J Hum Genet* 34:80A, 1982.
11. Bartoshesky LE et al: Severe cardiac and ophthalmologic malformations in an infant exposed to diphenylhydantoin in utero. *Pediatrics* 69:202–203, 1982.
12. Bauer PW et al: Cochlear implantation in children with CHARGE association. *Arch Otolaryngol Head Neck Surg* 128:1013–1017, 2002.
13. Beemer FA et al: Letter to the editor: Additional eye findings in a girl with the velo-cardio-facial syndrome. *Am J Med Genet* 24:541–542, 1986.
14. Bergstrom L, Baker BB: Syndromes associated with congenital facial paralysis. *Otolaryngol Head Neck Surg* 89:336–342, 1981.
15. Blake KD et al: CHARGE association: an update and review for the primary pediatrician. *Clin Pediatr* 37:159–174, 1998.
16. Brama I, Engelhard D: Congenital choanal atresia and nerve deafness. *J Laryngol Otol* 3:1223–1228, 1979.
17. Cervenka J et al: Trisomy 22 with "cat eye" anomaly. *J Med Genet* 14:288–290, 1977.

18. Clark CE et al: Brief clinical report: dup(4p15–4pter) in a 19-year-old woman resulting from a maternal 4;14 translocation. *Am J Med Genet* 11:37–42, 1982.
19. Clark EB: Cardiac embryology: its relevance to congenital heart disease. *Am J Dis Child* 140:41–44, 1986.
20. Collum LMT: Uveal colobomata and other anomalies in three generations of one family. *Br J Ophthalmol* 55:458, 1971.
21. Conley ME et al: The spectrum of the DiGeorge syndrome. *J Pediatr* 94:883–890, 1979.
22. Curatolo P et al: Infantile spasms and the CHARGE association. *Dev Med Child Neurol* 25:367–373, 1983.
23. Cyran SE et al: Spectrum of congenital heart disease in CHARGE association. *J Pediatr* 110:576–578, 1987.
24. Davenport SLH et al: The spectrum of clinical features in CHARGE syndrome. *Clin Genet* 29:298–310, 1986.
25. Davenport SLH et al: CHARGE syndrome: part I, External ear anomalies. *Int J Pediatr Otorhinolaryngol* 12:137–143, 1986.
26. Dev VG et al: 1q duplication due to unequal crossover in a patient with CHARGE association and DiGeorge sequence. *Am J Hum Genet* 37:90A, 1985.
27. Dobrowski JM et al: Otorhinolaryngic manifestations of CHARGE association. *Otolaryngol Head Neck Surg* 93:798–803, 1985.
28. Edwards JH et al: Coloboma with multiple congenital anomalies. *BMJ* 2:586–587, 1961.
29. Ferry AP et al: Ocular abnormalities in deletion of the long arm of chromosome 11. *Ann Ophthalmol* 13:1373–1377, 1981.
30. Flake CG, Ferguson CF: Congenital choanal atresia in infants and children. *Ann Otol* 73:458, 1964.
31. Freedom RM et al: Congenital cardiovascular disease and anomalies of the third and fourth pharyngeal pouch. *Circulation* 46:165–171, 1972.
32. Goldberg MF, McKusick VA: X-linked colobomatous microphthalmos and other congenital anomalies. *Am J Ophthalmol* 71:1128–1133, 1971.
33. Goldson E et al: The CHARGE association. How well do they do? *Am J Dis Child* 140:918–921, 1986.
34. Graham HM Jr et al: Cardiac features of the "CHARGE" association: support for involvement of the neural crest. *Proc Greenwood Genet Ctr* 4:81, 1985.
35. Greenwood RD, Deddistt RB: Cardiovascular malformations associated with choanal atresia. *South Med J* 70:195, 1977.
36. Grix A: Malformations in infants of diabetic mothers. *Am J Med Genet* 13:131–137, 1982.
37. Guanti G: The aetiology of cat-eye syndrome reconsidered. *J Med Genet* 18:108–118, 1981.
38. Hall BD: Choanal atresia and associated multiple anomalies. *J Pediatr* 95:395–398, 1979.
39. Harvey AS et al: CHARGE association: clinical features and developmental outcome. *Proc Greenwood Genet Ctr* 9:91, 1990.
40. Hengerer AS, Strome M: Choanal atresia: a new embryologic theory and its influence on surgical management. *Laryngoscope* 92:913–921, 1982.
41. Hittner HM et al: Colobomatous microphthalmia, heart disease, hearing loss, and mental retardation—a syndrome. *J Pediatr Ophthalmol Strabismus* 16:122–128, 1979.
42. Ho CK et al: Ocular colobomata, cardiac defect, and other anomalies: a study of seven cases including two sibs. *J Med Genet* 12:289–293, 1975.
43. Johnston MC, Listgarten MA: Observations on the migration, interaction and early differentiation of orofacial tissues. In: *Developmental Aspects of Oral Biology*, Slavkin HS, Bavetta LA (eds), Academic Press, New York, 1972, pp 53–80.
44. Juberg RC, Marsidi I: A new form of X-linked mental retardation with growth retardation, deafness, and microgenitalism. *Am J Hum Genet* 32:714–722, 1980.
45. Kaplan LC: Choanal atresia and its associated anomalies: further support for the CHARGE association. *Int J Pediatr Otorhinolaryngol* 8:237, 1985.
46. Kaplan LC, Finkelhor B: Psychomotor retardation in CHARGE association. *Proc Greenwood Genet Ctr* 8:202, 1989.
47. Klein VR et al: Choanal atresia and associated anomalies. *Proc Greenwood Genet Ctr* 7:213, 1988.
48. Koletzko B, Majewski F: Congenital anomalies in patients with choanal atresia: CHARGE—association. *Eur J Pediatr* 142:271–275, 1984.
49. Levin DL et al: Concordant aortic arch anomalies in monozygotic twins. *J Pediatr* 83:459–461, 1973.
50. Lillquist K et al: Colobomata of the iris, ciliary body and choroid in an infant with oesophago-tracheal fistula and congenital heart defects. An unknown malformation complex. *Acta Paediatr Scand* 69:427–430, 1980.
51. Lin AE et al: The pattern of cardiovascular malformation in the CHARGE association. *Am J Dis Child* 141:1010–1013, 1987.
52. Lin AE et al: Central nervous system malformations in the CHARGE association. *Am J Med Genet* 37:304–310, 1990.
53. Marmon LM et al: Congenital cardiac anomalies associated with the DiGeorge syndrome: a neonatal experience. *Ann Thor Surg* 38:146–150, 1984.
54. Mattei JP et al: X-linked mental retardation, growth retardation, deafness and microgenitalism. A second familial report. *Clin Genet* 23:70–74, 1983.
55. McGovern FH: The association of congenital choanal atresia and congenital heart disease. *Ann Otol Rhinol Laryngol* 62:394, 1953.
56. Menser MA et al: Congenital rubella: long-term follow-up study. *Am J Dis Child* 118:32–34, 1969.
57. Metlay LA et al: Familial CHARGE syndrome: clinical report with autopsy findings. *Am J Med Genet* 26:577–581, 1987.
58. Mitchell JA et al: Dominant CHARGE association. *Ophthalm Paediatr Genet* 6:31–36, 1985.
59. Oley CA: CHARGE association. In: *Management of Genetic Syndromes*, Cassidy SB, Allanson JE, eds, New York, Wiley-Liss, 2001, pp 71–84.
60. Oley CA et al: A reappraisal of the CHARGE association. *J Med Genet* 25:147–156, 1988.
61. Pagon RA et al: Coloboma, congenital heart disease, and choanal atresia with multiple anomalies: CHARGE association. *J Pediatr* 99:223–227, 1981.
62. Pergament E et al: Microphthalmia, coloboma, cleft palate, ear malformations, ptosis and congenital heart disease: a new malformation syndrome. In: *March of Dimes Birth Defects Conference Abstracts*, 1982, p 233.
63. Primack W, Feingold M: Picture of the month: CHARGE association. *Am J Dis Child* 137:1117–1118, 1983.
64. Quan L, Smith DW: The VATER association: vertebral defects, anal atresia, fistula with esophageal atresia, radial and renal dysplasia: a spectrum of associated defects. *J Pediatr* 82:104–107, 1973.
65. Rapin I, Ruben RJ: Patterns of anomalies in children with malformed ears. *Laryngoscope* 86:1469–1502, 1976.
66. Saniaville D et al: A CGH study of 27 patients with CHARGE association. *Clin Genet* 61:135–138, 2002.
67. Say B et al: The Stickler syndrome (hereditary arthro-ophthalmopathy). *Clin Genet* 12:179, 1977.
68. Shprintzen RJ et al: The velocardiofacial syndrome: a clinical and genetic analysis. *Pediatrics* 67:167–172, 1981.
69. Siebert JR et al: Pathologic features of the CHARGE association: support for involvement of the neural crest. *Teratology* 31:331–336, 1985.
70. Smith DW: *Recognizable Patterns of Human Deformation*. W.B. Saunders, Philadelphia, 1981, pp 137–138.
71. Smithells RW: Defects and disabilities of thalidomide children. *BMJ* 1:269–272, 1973.
72. Stool SE, Kemper BI: Choanal atresia and/or cardiac disease. *Pediatrics* 42:525–528, 1968.
73. Superneau D, Wertelecki W: Choanal atresia, CHARGE association, and limb reduction defects. *Proc Greenwood Genet Ctr* 10:100–101, 1991.
74. Tellier A-L et al: Increased paternal age in CHARGE association. *Clin Genet* 50:548–550, 1996.
75. Tellier A-L et al: CHARGE syndrome: report of 47 cases and review. *Am J Med Genet* 76: 402–409, 1998.
76. Thelin JW et al: CHARGE syndrome. Part II, hearing loss. *Int J Pediatr Otorhinolaryngol* 12:145–163, 1986.
77. Wiener-Vacher SR et al: Vestibular function in children with the CHARGE association. *Arch Otolaryngol Head Neck Surg* 125:342–347, 1999.
78. Wilson L et al: Cytogenetic analysis of a case of "13q-syndrome" (46,XX,del 13) using banding techniques. *J Pediatr Ophthalmol Strabismus* 17:63–67, 1980.
79. Wisniewski L et al: An interstitial deletion of chromosome 9 in a girl with multiple congenital anomalies. *J Med Genet* 14:455–459, 1977.
80. Wright CG et al: Auditory and temporal bone abnormalities in CHARGE association. *Ann Otol Rhinol Laryngol* 95:480–486, 1986.
81. Zagnoer M et al: Choanal atresia and congenital heart disease. *S Afr Med J* 60:815, 1981.

Dysmorphic pinnae, mental retardation, and mixed hearing loss

In 1978, Cantú et al. (1) described a syndrome characterized by mental retardation, malformed low-set ears, and mixed hearing loss in three sibs.

Central nervous system. The IQ was 63 in the boy and 71 in his older sister. The younger girl had normal intelligence.

Auditory system. The oldest sib, a male, had the most significant auricular changes. His right ear was low-set with a hypoplastic crus and deep concha. The left ear exhibited third-degree microtia. A small protuberance of about 0.5 cm in diameter was present in both preauricular regions at the level of the lamina of the supratragal tubercle. The right external auditory canal was hypoplastic (Fig. 6–9). The left external auditory canal was so narrow that the tympanic membrane could not be visualized. A suppurative fistula was present in the left retroauricular region. Two younger female siblings, aged 9 and 4, had similar bilateral symmetrically low-set, small, cupped ears. The boy demonstrated bilateral mixed hearing loss at 60–80 dB. The older girl had pure bilateral conductive loss of 30 dB, while the younger girl had normal audiometry.

Laboratory findings. Polytomographic studies in the boy showed bilateral hypopneumatization. The left malleus and incus appeared fused. Both cochleas were thicker than normal, and the density of the otic capsules was increased. In the older sister, polytomography demonstrated normal pneumatization of the mastoid. The plate of the stapes was abnormally thick on both sides, but more so on one side. There was increased density of the cochlea. Polytomographic studies in the younger girl, despite normal audiometry, showed bilateral thickening of the footplate of the stapes. Since the 9-year-old girl had developed conductive hearing loss after age 6, it is not possible to exclude future hearing impairment in the youngest child.

Heredity. The parents were phenotypically normal but are third cousins of Mexican extraction. Autosomal recessive transmission seems likely.

Diagnosis. These three siblings share many features with the syndrome of dysmorphic pinnae and conductive hearing loss in the Men-

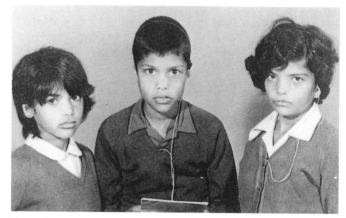

Figure 6–10. *Dysmorphic pinnae, facial palsy, and stapedial anomalies.* Three sibs with conductive hearing loss and stapedial abnormalities; malformations of external ears and variable degrees of facial paralysis evident. [From S Sellars and P Beighton, *Clin Genet* 23:376, 1979.]

nonite sibship described by Mengel et al. (2). In that kindred, however, only conductive hearing loss was diagnosed, and all four males had immature genitalia, with three having hypogonadism.

Prognosis. Hearing loss in this syndrome may not be congenital, as evidenced by the middle child in the sibship. It appears to be progressive.

Summary. Characteristics of this syndrome include (*1*) autosomal recessive inheritance; (*2*) bilateral auricular deformities of varying severity; (*3*) variable degrees of mental retardation; and (*4*) conductive or mixed hearing loss, which is bilateral, progressive, and varies from mild to severe.

References

1. Cantú JM et al: Autosomal recessive sensorineural-conductive deafness, mental retardation, and pinna anomalies. *Hum Genet* 40:231–234, 1978.
2. Mengel MC et al: Conductive hearing loss and malformed lowset ears, as a possible recessive syndrome. *J Med Genet* 6:14–21, 1969.

Dysmorphic pinnae, facial palsy, and stapedial anomalies

In 1983, Sellars and Beighton (5) described a mother and three children (Fig. 6–10) of Indian extraction with auricular, meatal, and stapedial abnormalities, as well as facial palsy.

Physical findings. The middle child, a female, and the mother had bilateral facial paralysis. The younger sister had unilateral facial paralysis. The oldest child, a male, had no evidence of facial weakness.

Auditory system. The boy had bilateral preauricular sinuses and bilateral absence of the upper half of the pinnae with hypoplasia of the left lobule. The right external auditory canal was narrow. The second child had absence of the upper half of both pinnae with narrow external auditory canals and bilateral postauricular sinuses. The younger girl had bilateral preauricular sinuses and absence of the upper helix of the right ear, with narrowing of the external auditory canal. The children's mother, by history, also had bilateral external ear malformations.

Severe to profound bilateral congenital hearing impairment was noted in all sibs. In the boy, audiograms showed a flat 30–40 dB conduction loss on the right and a 50 dB troughed conduction loss on the left. The other two sibs had a 60 dB bilateral conductive loss. The mother is also said to have had profound hearing loss.

Figure 6–9. *Dysmorphic pinnea, mental retardation, and mixed hearing loss.* (A,B) Two sibs showing varying degrees of microtia. Note ear tags. [From JM Cantú et al., *Hum Genet* 40:231, 1978.]

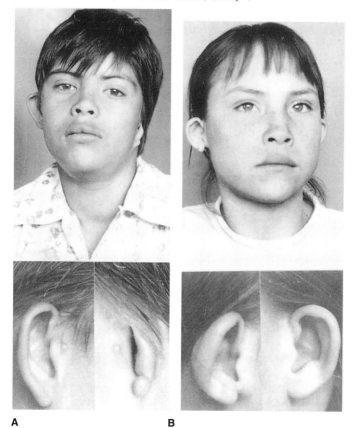

A   B

Pathology. Tympanotomy in the boy revealed absence of the stapes superstructure and a thick, firmly fixed footplate. In the middle child, there was tapering of the long process of the incus with absence of the stapes and its footplate. In the youngest child, the stapes was fixed and there was absence of the lenticular process of the incus.

Heredity. Autosomal dominant inheritance with variable expression is evident.

Diagnosis. External ear malformations are relatively common and usually sporadic, nonsyndromic, and uncomplicated (1). However, about 6% of abnormal auricles are associated with defects of the middle ear (4). Microtia and meatal atresia may have autosomal recessive (3) or autosomal dominant (6) inheritance; external ear abnormalities are also a component of numerous syndromes with widespread skeletal or multisystem involvement. Anderson et al. (2) described dominantly inherited aplasia cutis congenita, ear malformations, facial palsy, and dermal sinuses, but the degree of hearing loss in the various members was not documented.

Prognosis. Hearing loss appears to be profound.

Summary. The syndrome is characterized by (*1*) autosomal dominant inheritance; (*2*) abnormal pinnae, with absence of the upper half of external ear; (*3*) narrowing of external auditory canals; (*4*) pre- or postauricular sinuses; (*5*) unilateral or bilateral facial palsy; and (*6*) stapedial anomalies leading to severe to profound conductive hearing loss.

References

1. Aase JM, Tegtemeier RE: Microtia in New Mexico: evidence for multifactorial causation. *Birth Defects* 13(3A):113–116, 1977.
2. Anderson CE et al: Autosomally dominantly inherited aplasia cutis congenita, ear malformations, right sided facial paresis and dermal sinuses. *Birth Defects* 15(5B):265–270, 1979.
3. Ellwood LC et al: Microtia with meatal atresia in two sibships. *J Med Genet* 5:289–291, 1968.
4. Melnick M, Myrianthopoulos NC: External ear malformation: epidemiology, genetics and natural history. *Birth Defects* 15(9):27–29, 1979.
5. Sellars S, Beighton P: Autosomal dominant inheritance of conductive deafness due to stapedial anomalies, external ear malformations and congenital facial palsy. *Clin Genet* 23:376–379, 1983.
6. Zankl M, Zang KD: Inheritance of microtia and aural atresia in a family with 5 affected members. *Clin Genet* 16:331–334, 1979.

Lop ears, micrognathia, and conductive hearing loss

In 1976, Konigsmark and Gorlin (3) described a mother and son and daughter with lop ears, micrognathia, and mixed, mostly conductive, hearing loss. In 1984, Schweitzer et al. (5) reported a three-generation family with malformed thickened lop auricles, micrognathia, and conductive hearing loss secondary to middle ear ossicular anomalies.

Physical findings. All had class II malocclusion with micrognathia.

Auditory system. The thickened lop auricles had hypertrophic lobes and pinnae. There was no evidence of tags or fistulae. In one family (5), the proband's father, paternal grandfather, two paternal uncles, and one paternal aunt also had similar ears. In the family described by Konigsmark and Gorlin (3), the external canals were markedly narrowed.

In the report of Schweitzer et al. (5), the proband was noted to have a 10 dB speech reception threshold on the right with 100% discrimination, and a maximum conductive hearing loss on the left with a 60 dB speech reception threshold and 100% discrimination. Tympanograms revealed a type C (negative pressure) pattern on the right, with a highly compliant left system. Konigsmark and Gorlin (3) noted a mixed hearing loss, mostly conductive, of 30–60 dB.

Radiographic findings. No abnormalities were found on mastoid or internal auditory canal X-rays or on electronystagmography.

Pathology. Schweitzer et al. (5) described an ossicular chain malformation found on exploratory tympanotomy. The malleus and incus were rudimentary without continuity. The stapedius muscle and tendon were absent and the stapes was rudimentary with a fibrous band connecting the normally mobile footplate to the tympanic membrane. The facial nerve had a dehiscent tympanic segment; the hypotympanum and round window were normal. Konigsmark and Gorlin (3) found fixation of the footplate of the stapes. The posterior crura were 65% of their normal length and were not attached in the footplate. The stapes muscle and tendon were rudimentary.

Heredity. The syndrome has autosomal dominant inheritance.

Diagnosis. This disorder shows some overlap with the autosomal dominant syndrome of thickened ear lobes and incudostapedial abnormalities described by Escher and Hirt (2), and with the autosomal recessive syndrome of dysmorphic pinnae and conductive hearing loss described by Mengel et al. (4). Cantú et al. (1) reported a distinct syndrome with dysmorphic pinnae, mental retardation, and mixed hearing loss inherited as an autosomal recessive trait. In this syndrome, polytomographic studies demonstrated fixed incus and malleus, thickened stapedial footplate, and sclerosis of the otic capsule.

Summary. The characteristic features of the syndrome include (*1*) autosomal dominant transmission; (*2*) malformed, thickened lop auricles; (*3*) micrognathia; and (*4*) conductive hearing loss secondary to middle ear ossicular anomalies.

References

1. Cantú JM et al: Autosomal recessive sensorineural-conductive deafness, mental retardation and pinnae anomalies. *Hum Genet* 40:231–234, 1978.
2. Escher F, Hirt H: Dominant hereditary conductive deafness through lack of incus–stapes junction. *Acta Otolaryngol (Stockh)* 65:25–32, 1968.
3. Konigsmark BW, Gorlin RJ: *Genetic and Metabolic Deafness*. W.B. Saunders, Philadelphia, 1976, p 73.
4. Mengel MC et al: Conductive hearing loss and malformed low-set ears as a possible recessive syndrome. *J Med Genet* 6:14–21, 1969.
5. Schweitzer VG et al: Conductive hearing loss, middle ear ossicular anomalies, malformed thickened lop auricles, and micrognathia: a rare autosomal dominant congenital syndrome. *Am J Otol* 5:387–391, 1984.

Dysmorphic pinnae and conductive hearing loss

In 1969, Mengel et al. (3) reported a syndrome characterized by unilateral or bilateral malformed low-set ears and mild to severe conductive hearing loss. It was found in two sibships in a single kindred of Mennonites in Pennsylvania.

Physical findings. The affected children were smaller than their unaffected sibs.

Central nervous system. Intelligence tests on four of six affected children showed that three were severely retarded, while one was normal.

Cardiovascular system. A moderate systolic blowing murmur at the cardiac apex was found in five of six affected children. No unaffected sibs had heart murmur. Electrocardiograms showed no abnormalities.

Genitorurinary system. Hypogonadism was found in three of four affected males; two of the boys had cryptorchidism.

Auditory system. The pinnae were small in all six affected children, and frequently the helix was folded forward (Fig. 6–11). In one case, the auricle was represented by a small amount of cartilaginous tis-

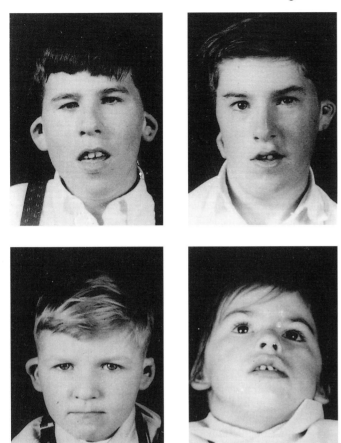

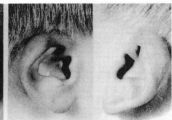

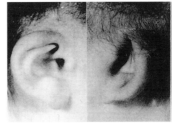

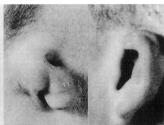

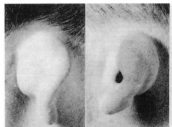

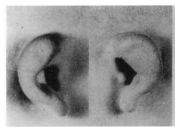

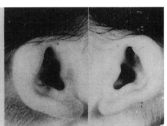

A

B

Figure 6–11. *Dysmorphic pinnae and conductive hearing loss.* (A) Facial view of four affected sibs. (B) Composite photographs showing auricular abnormalities in each of six affected children. Note range of variation of malformation. [From MC Mengel et al., *J Med Genet* 6:14, 1969.]

sue surrounding the external auditory meatus. In four of the six children, one ear was located as much as 4 cm below the other one. Usually, the malpositioned ear showed a greater auricular malformation than the more normally placed ear. In each case, the external auditory canal participated in the malformation, its opening being displaced with the ectopic auricle. There was no atresia of the canal.

Although hearing tests revealed marked variation, all six children had a 70–80 dB hearing loss in at least one ear. In some, the hearing loss was much more marked in one ear than in the other. Audiometric tests showed the impairment to be conductive. Short-increment sensitivity index (SISI) tests, recruitment tests, and tone-decay tests were negative. Pure-tone audiometric results were confirmed by speech reception threshold values.

Vestibular system. Caloric vestibular tests were normal.

Radiographic findings. Skull roentgenograms of two patients were not remarkable. Temporal bone polytomograms of the proband showed ossicular chain abnormalities.

Pathology. Exploratory tympanotomy in one patient showed an ossicular chain anomaly. The malleus was slightly malformed and posteriorly positioned. Both incus and stapes were absent. From the head of the malleus, a small fibrous band passed to the oval window area.

Heredity. The four patients in these two sibships were found to be descendants of a Swiss male who died in 1720. It appears likely that the syndrome has autosomal recessive inheritance.

Diagnosis. The auricular abnormality in this syndrome is similar to that described by Potter (5), Romei (6), and Kessler (2) in several mem-

bers of a family. Apparently, neither hearing loss nor low-set ears was associated with this auricular deformity. Branchio-oto-renal syndrome shows somewhat similar auricular deformities. However, affected persons in the family described by Wildervanck (7) did not have low-set ears, nor was there mental retardation.

The syndrome of dysmorphic pinnae, mental retardation, and mixed hearing loss described by Cantú et al. (1) has some similar features. The parents were third cousins. This family differs in that hearing loss was mixed and the one male in the sibship had no evidence of genital immaturity or hypogonadism.

This condition shares many similarities with CHARGE association—cardiovascular disease, retarded growth and development, hypogonadism, ear anomalies, and hearing loss. However, it lacks the principal features of CHARGE association: coloboma and choanal atresia (4).

Prognosis. The defects are congenital with no evidence of progression.

Summary. Characteristics of this syndrome include (*1*) autosomal recessive inheritance; (*2*) unilateral or bilateral low-set ears; (*3*) unilateral or bilateral malformed pinnae; (*4*) mental retardation in about 50%; (*5*) cardiac murmur; (*6*) hypogonadism in males; and (*7*) mild to severe conductive hearing loss.

References

1. Cantú JM et al: Autosomal recessive sensorineural-conductive deafness, mental retardation, and pinna anomalies. *Hum Genet* 40:231–234, 1978.
2. Kessler L: Beobachtung einer über 6 Generationen einfach-dominant vererbten Mikrotie 1. Grades. *HNO* 15:113–116, 1967.
3. Mengel MC et al: Conductive hearing loss and malformed low-set ears as a possible recessive syndrome. *J Med Genet* 6:14–21, 1969.

4. Pagon RA et al: Coloboma, congenital heart disease, and choanal atresia with multiple anomalies: CHARGE association. *J Pediatr* 99:223–227, 1981.
5. Potter EL: A hereditary ear malformation transmitted through five generations. *J Hered* 28:255, 1937.
6. Romei L: Una famiglia con conformazione del padiglione auricolare del tipo de Potter (cup-shaped ear). *Acta Genet Med (Roma)* 8:483–486, 1959.
7. Wildervanck LS: Hereditary malformations of the ear in three generations. *Acta Otolaryngol (Stockh)* 54:553, 1962.

Familial semicircular canal malformations with external and middle ear abnormalities

Matsunaga and Hirota (2) reported a family (mother and two children) in which lateral semicircular canal (LSC) malformation occurred together with variable external and middle ear abnormalities.

Auditory findings. The daughter had a right preauricular tag, stenotic right auditory canal, and conductive hearing loss on the right. Her brother had a right microtia with atresia of the external auditory canal and mixed hearing loss on the right. Their mother only had mild loss on the right, but she had LSC malformation on the left as demonstrated by computed tomography.

Vestibular system. The children had no vestibular abnormalities; the mother had no caloric response to cold water on the left.

Radiographic findings. All individuals had unilateral LSC malformation as demonstrated by computed tomography.

Heredity. This is likely an autosomal dominant trait with variable expressivity.

Diagnosis. Branchio-oto-renal syndrome and the conditions described by Cantú et al. (1) and Mengel et al. (3) should be excluded.

References

1. Cantú JM et al: Autosomal recessive sensorineural-conductive deafness, mental retardation, and pinna anomalies. *Hum Genet* 40:231–234, 1978.
2. Matsunaga T, Hirota E: Familial lateral semicircular canal malformation with external and middle ear abnormalities. *Am J Med Genet* 116A:360–367, 2003.
3. Mengel MC et al: Conductive hearing loss and malformed low-set ears as a possible recessive syndrome. *J Med Genet* 6:14–21, 1969.

Branchio-oculo-facial (BOF) syndrome (pseudocleft of the upper lip, cleft lip–palate, cervical thymus, and conductive hearing loss)

A syndrome of cervical aplasia cutis congenita, cervical thymus, pseudocleft of the upper lip or cleft lip–palate, congenital nasolacrimal duct obstruction, and conductive hearing loss has been reported by a number of authors (1–13). In 1987, Fujimoto et al. (4) coined the term *branchio-oculo-facial (BOF) syndrome*. Virtually universal, and possibly pathognomonic, are the cervical/infraauricular skin defects. Renal malformations are frequent, while cardiac and CNS defects are rare. Developmental delays, hypotonia, and speech problems are common, although psychomotor performance is generally normal. The reader is referred to an extensive review of the syndrome (9).

Craniofacial findings. The usually sparse scalp hair begins to gray at puberty (1,4,7), and there may be subcutaneous scalp cysts (4). The head is often long and narrow with a high forehead. The nose may be broad and misshapen with a wide bridge and an indented or flattened nasal tip, with short columella. The philtrum is often narrow and prominent with thick fibrous vertical ridges producing a pseudocleft. Other patients have cleft lip and/or palate (1–3,8–14). Paramedian upper lip pits, seen occasionally, correspond to the fusion sites of the median nasal and maxillary prominences (1,4) (Fig. 6–12A).

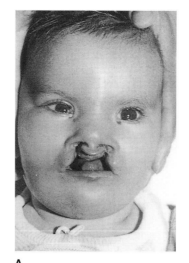

A

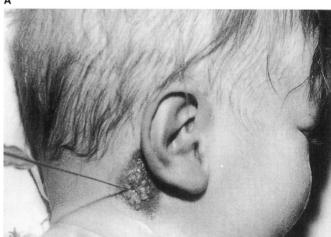

B

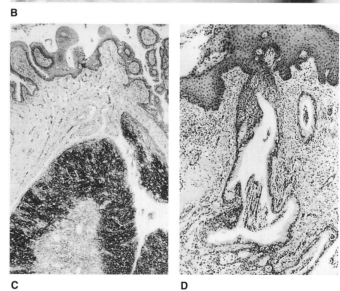

C   D

Figure 6–12. *Branchio-oculo-facial (BOF) syndrome.* (A) Bilateral cleft lip–palate, nasolacrimal obstruction, and almond-shaped upslanting palpebral fissures. (B) Lateral cervical thymus. Child had similar lesion on opposite side. Helix is somewhat hypoplastic. (C) Section taken from neck showing underlying thymus. (D) Section from neck showing mucus-producing epithelia which lined original third pharyngeal pouch. [From W Schweckendiek et al., *Laryngol Rhinol Otol* 56:795, 1977.]

Ocular system. Various eye anomalies have included hypertelorism (4), unilateral microphthalmos (1,4,5), anophthalmos (3,14), myopia (4), cataracts (4,7), strabismus (7), colobomas of iris, choroid, retina, and optic nerve (4,5), and upslanting palpebral fissures (1,4). An almost constant feature is nasolacrimal duct obstruction, which results in dacryocystitis. This in turn leads to thickened lower eyelids (1,2,4,7).

Neck. Bilateral cervical aplasia cutis congenita with thinned epidermis and underlying cervical thymus extending along the sternocleidomastoid muscle is a constant feature (1–14) (Figs. 6–12B,C). These lesions may have a hemangiomatous component or draining sinus fistulae (9). Initially considered atypical, supraauricular defects, with or without draining sinuses, occurring with cervical skin defects or as isolated anomalies, these are now felt to be part of the spectrum (6,9,11,14). Microscopically, a ciliated epithelium representing the pharyngeal epithelium of the third pouch is located between the thymus and the skin (1,8,13,14) (Fig. 6–12D).

Auditory system. The pinnae are posteriorly angulated with a thin helix, prominent anthelix, and upturned lobules (3–7). Pre- and postauricular pits have been documented (4). Conductive hearing loss of mild to moderate degree has been reported (4–7,9).

Heredity. Autosomal dominant inheritance has been demonstrated (1,4,7,9). Marked intrafamilial variability is suggested in this small number of families.

Diagnosis. The BOF syndrome is distinctive, but superficial similarity to other syndromes exists, in particular branchio-oto-renal (BOR) syndrome. Five individuals with BOF have had *EYA1* testing, and no mutations have been found. This result suggests that BOR and BOF syndromes are not allelic (10). Microscopic differential diagnosis would include thymic cyst, ectopic hamartomatous thymoma, and benign lymphoepithelial tumor of the skin (1,3).

Summary. This syndrome is characterized by (*1*) autosomal dominant inheritance; (*2*) cleft lip and/or palate or pseudocleft of the upper lip; (*3*) nasolacrimal duct obstruction; (*4*) prematurely gray hair; (*5*) cervical thymus; (*6*) malformed pinnae; and (*7*) conductive hearing loss.

References

1. Barr RJ et al: Dermal thymus. *Arch Dermatol* 125:1681–1684, 1989.
2. Çivi I et al: Bilateral thymus found in association with unilateral cleft lip and palate. *Plast Reconstr Surg* 83:143–147, 1989.
3. Farmer AW, Maxmen MD: Congenital absence of skin. *Plast Reconstr Surg* 25:291–297, 1960 (case 3).
4. Fujimoto A et al: New autosomal dominant branchio-oculo-facial syndrome. *Am J Med Genet* 27:943–951, 1987.
5. Hall BD et al: A new syndrome of hemangiomatous branchial clefts, lip pseudoclefts, and abnormal facial appearance. *Am J Med Genet* 14:135–138, 1983.
6. Harrison MS: The Treacher Collins-Franceschetti syndrome. *J Laryngol Otol* 71:597–603, 1957 (case R.C.).
7. Lee WK et al: Bilateral branchial cleft sinuses associated with intrauterine and postnatal growth retardation, premature aging and unusual facial appearance: a new syndrome with dominant transmission. *Am J Med Genet* 11:345–352, 1982.
8. Lin AE et al: The branchio-oculo-facial syndrome. *Cleft Palate Craniofac J* 28:96–102, 1991.
9. Lin AE et al: Further delineation of the branchio-oculo-facial syndrome. *Am J Med Genet* 56:42–59, 1995.
10. Lin AE et al: Exclusion of the branchio-oto-renal syndrome locus (*EYA1*) from patients with branchio-oto-facial syndrome. *Am J Med Genet* 91:387–390, 2000.
11. Rosenbaum KN et al: Accessory ectopic cervical thymus with lip pseudoclefts—further confirmation of a new syndrome. In: *Proceedings of the 8th International Congress on Human Genetics*, Abstract 834, October 6–11, 1991, Washington, DC.
12. Schmerler S et al: Long-term evaluation of a child with the branchio-oculofacial syndrome. *Am J Med Genet* 44:177–178, 1992.
13. Schweckendiek W et al: Doppelseitige retro- und subaurikuläre Fisteln mit Ektropium des Fistelgangepithels. *Laryngol Rhinol Otol* 56:795–800, 1977.
14. Tom DWK et al: Inflammatory linear epidermal nevus caused by branchial cleft sinuses in a woman with numerous congenital anomalies. *Pediatr Dermatol* 2:318–321, 1985.

Congenital aural atresia

Microtia/anotia occurs in 1 to 5 per 10,000 births (1,4–7,9,10). In only about 5% of cases does one find atresia without concomitant microtia (7). While atresia may be associated with various syndromes described in this text (Table 6–1), in most cases it is isolated. As an isolated phenomenon, it is more frequently found in males (2 M:1 F), and on the right side (65%).There are racial differences in occurrence rates: in whites the rate is 1:15,000; in Spanish-Americans it is 1:9000; and in Native Americans it is 1:2000 (1,2).

For convenience sake, congenital aural atresia has been divided into three forms based on increasing severity. Type I is characterized by a nearly normal auricle with bony or fibrous atresia of the lateral canal, but normal medial canal and normal middle ear. Type II patients have dysmorphic pinna with partial or total aplasia of the external canal. An atretic plate forms the lateral wall of the middle ear cavity. The malleus and incus are usually deformed or fixed. Type III patients have a severely microtic auricle, and complete bony atresia of the external auditory canal with very small or absent tympanic cavity. The ossicles are rudimentary or missing and the mastoid is not pneumatized.

Type II is the most frequently encountered form. Type III is seen in mandibulofacial dysostosis (3,8).

References

1. Aase J: Microtia—clinical observations. *Birth Defects* 16(4):289–297, 1980.
2. Aase JM, Tegtmeier RE: Microtia in New Mexico. Evidence for multifactorial causation. *Birth Defects* 13(3A):113–116, 1977.
3. Cremers CWRJ et al: Congenital aural atresia. A new subclassification and surgical management. *Clin Otolaryngol* 9:119–127, 1984.
4. Gill NW: Congenital atresia of the ear. A review of the surgical findings in 83 cases. *J Laryngol Otol* 83:551–587, 1960.
5. Grundfast CM, Camilon F: External auditory canal stenosis and partial atresia without associated anomalies. *Ann Otol Rhinol Laryngol* 95:505–508, 1986.
6. Holmes EM: The microtic ear. *Arch Otolaryngol* 49:243–265, 1949.
7. Jafek BW et al: Congenital aural atresia: an analysis of 311 cases. *Trans Am Acad Ophthalmol Otolaryngol* 80:588–596, 1975.
8. Marres EHMA, Cremers CWRJ: Surgical treatment of congenital aural atresia. *Am J Otol* 6:247–249, 1985.
9. Melnick M et al: External ear malformations: epidemiology, genetics and natural history. *Birth Defects* 15(9):1–140, 1979.
10. Sullivan JA et al: Surgical management of congenital atresia of the ear. *J Laryngol Otol* 73:201–222, 1959.

Autosomal dominant aural atresia, microtia, and conductive hearing loss

A number of authors have described familial unilateral or bilateral microtia, aural atresia, and conductive hearing loss (3–5,8). In addition, there have been several cases of sporadic occurrence of meatal atresia, microtia, and hearing loss. It is not possible to know whether these individuals represent autosomal recessive or dominant forms.

Auditory system. Cremers (1) described five families with congenital aural atresia. In some, the auricle anomaly was unilateral, in others, there was bilateral involvement. Orstavik et al. (5) reported extremely variable expression of unilateral accessory auricle so that one cannot completely exclude oculo-auriculo-vertebral spectrum.

J Garza and M Miller (personal communication) noted that the microtia and atresia of the auditory canals were bilateral and symmetrical (Fig. 6–13). Conductive hearing loss was of moderate severity. At surgery, both eardrums were absent, and only half of the incus, half of the malleus, and half of the stapes were present bilaterally. Pfeiffer (7) reported a mother and son with microtia, mostly unilateral. In general, conductive hearing loss has been extremely variable.

Table 6–1. Syndromes with congenital atresia of external auditory canal

Condition	Eponym/Synonym	Inheritance
Mandibulofacial dysostosis	Treacher Collins syndrome	AD
Crouzon syndrome	Craniofacial dysostosis	AD
Oculo-auriculo-vertebral spectrum	Goldenhar syndrome, hemifacial microsomia	Sporadic rare AD
Cleidocranial dysplasia	—	AD
Cryptophthalmia syndrome	Fraser syndrome	AR
Craniometaphyseal dysplasia	—	AD, AR
Branchio-oto-renal syndrome	BOR syndrome, BO syndrome, BOU syndrome	AD
Coxoauricular syndrome	—	AD
Renal and genital anomalies and conductive hearing loss	Winter syndrome	AR
Aural atresia and conductive hearing loss	Hefter-Ganz syndrome	AD
Aural atresia, microtia, hypertelorism, facial clefting, and conductive hearing loss	HMC syndrome, Bixler syndrome	AR
Aural atresia, microtia, and conductive hearing loss	—	AR, AD
Aural atresia, vertical talus, and conductive hearing loss	Rasmussen syndrome	AD
Aural atresia, mental retardation, multiple anomalies, and conductive hearing loss	Cooper-Jabs syndrome	AR
Aural atresia, microtia, aortic arch anomalies, and conductive hearing loss	Kawashima syndrome	AR or XR
Aural atresia, microtia, unusual facies, pseudopapilledema, and mixed hearing loss	Paes-Alves syndrome	AR
Aural atresia, microtia, skin mastocytosis, short stature, and conductive hearing loss	Wolach syndrome	AR?
Chromosome 18 long-arm deletion syndrome	del(18q) syndrome	
Thalidomide embryopathy	—	
Etretinate embryopathy	—	
Fanconi pancytopenia	—	AR
FG syndrome	Opitz-Kaveggia syndrome	XL

AD, autosomal dominant; AR, autosomal recessive; XL, X-linked; XR, X-linked recessive.

Heredity. The occurrence of this syndrome in several generations with male-to-male transmission clearly indicates autosomal dominant inheritance. Expression is extremely variable (1,2) and penetrance in some families is low (2).

Diagnosis. Autosomal recessive aural atresia, microtia, and conductive hearing loss must be excluded. There are several case reports of sporadic and "familial" congenital meatal atresia and microtia (7). It is certainly possible that some of these individuals may have the syndrome. There are several families with microtia, meatal atresia, and conductive hearing loss, but who have other anomalies of the first and second branchial arches such as facial asymmetry, preauricular tags, and

unilateral macrostomia. These individuals may represent the autosomal dominant form of oculo-auriculo-vertebral spectrum (3,4,9).

Prognosis. Hearing loss is congenital and nonprogressive.

Summary. The major characteristics of this syndrome include (*1*) autosomal dominant inheritance; (*2*) unilateral or bilateral microtia; (*3*) unilateral or bilateral aural atresia; and (*4*) congenital moderate to severe conductive hearing loss.

References

1. Cremers CWRJ: Meatal atresia and hearing loss. Autosomal dominant and autosomal recessive inheritance. *Int J Pediatr Otorhinolaryngol* 8:211–213, 1985.
2. Gupta A, Patton MA: Familial microtia with meatal atresia and conductive deafness in five generations. *Am J Med Genet* 59: 238–241, 1995.
3. Guizar-Vázquez J et al: Microtia and meatal atresia in mother and son. *Clin Genet* 14:80–82, 1978.
4. Oliveira CA et al: External and middle ear malformations: autosomal dominant genetic transmission. *Ann Otol Rhinol Laryngol* 98:772–776, 1989.
5. Orstavik KH et al: Right-sided microtia and conductive hearing loss with variable expressivity in three generations. *Clin Genet* 38:117–120, 1990.
6. Patterson JS, Byrne E: Recurrence of microtia in a family: a possible dominant gene? Presented at the 5th Manchester Birth Defects Conference, October 13–16, 1992.
7. Pfeiffer RA: Essai d'une nosologie génétique de l'atresia auris congenita. *J Genet Hum* 30:165–180, 1982.
8. Sanchez-Corona J et al: A distinct dominant form of microtia and conductive hearing loss. *Birth Defects* 18(3B):211–216, 1982.
9. Zankl M, Zang KD: Inheritance of microtia and aural atresia in a family with five affected members. *Clin Genet* 16:331–334, 1979.

Autosomal recessive aural atresia, microtia, and conductive hearing loss

In 1968, Ellwood et al. (3) reported unilateral or bilateral microtia, external auditory canal atresia, and hearing loss in multiple sibships. Konigsmark et al. (7), Dar and Winter (2), and Schmid et al. (9) described additional cases.

Figure 6–13. *Autosomal dominant aural atresia, microtia, and conductive hearing loss.* (A) Mother at age 2 years. (B) Daughter at 2 months of age. [From J Garza and M Miller.]

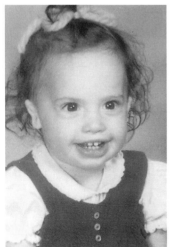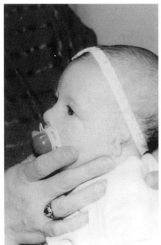

A   B

External ear. In the first family described by Ellwood et al. (3), two of three sibs had similarly anomalous external ears. The auricles were absent, except for a slightly raised soft tissue mass beneath the skin. The external auditory meatus was represented by a small dimple. A further member of the first family, with bilateral anotia and meatal atresia, was described by Dar and Winter (2). Two sibs in the second family reported by Ellwood et al. (3) had severely microtic left ears. These were represented by a small ridge of cartilage beneath the skin, as if the auricle were folded forward. In both sibs, the right pinna was normal except for mild downfolding of the upper portion of the helix. Unilateral meatal atresia was documented. Konigsmark et al. (7) described two male sibs, the older with severe bilateral microtia and meatal atresia, the younger with unilateral microtia and meatal atresia (Fig. 6–14). Schmid et al. (9) also described a family of three sibs with unilateral microtia and meatal atresia.

Auditory system. In the first family of Ellwood et al. (3), audiometric testing performed in one sib at 1 week of age showed a startle reaction only to sounds exceeding 80 dB. The other sibs, at 4 months of age, showed no reaction to strong sound stimuli. In the second sibship, one child had 70 dB hearing loss by air conduction and a 30–50 dB loss by bone conduction, while the other child had normal hearing (3). Konigsmark et al. (7) described one boy with moderate bilateral conductive hearing loss, while his sib had severe sensorineural hearing

Figure 6–14. *Autosomal recessive aural atresia, microtia, and conductive hearing loss.* (A,B) Lateral views showing bilateral microtia and absent external meatal openings. (C,D) Normal right ear but microtic left with a rudiment of cartilage attached superiorly and a small lobule inferiorly. The external auditory canal was absent. [From B Konigsmark et al., *Arch Otolaryngol* 96:105, 1972.]

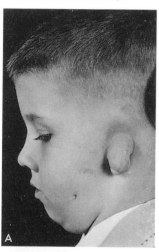
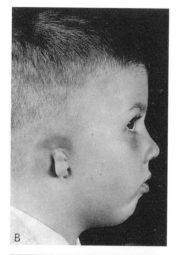
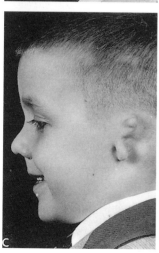
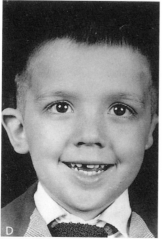

loss in one ear and normal hearing in the other. The three sibs described by Schmid et al. (9) demonstrated high-grade conductive loss. In general, the degree of microtia is roughly correlated with the degree of congenital hearing loss (5,6).

Tomograms revealed abnormalities of the ossicles and middle ear (7) in one child.

Heredity. Both Ellwood et al. (3) and Schmid et al. (9) reported affected sibs born to consanguineous Arab parents. The sister of the father subsequently married the brother of the mother and had an affected child (2). The three sibs reported by Schmid et al. (9) were probably born to fourth cousins. Konigsmark et al. (7) also described sibs. Cremers (1) noted bilateral incomplete bony atresia in sibs in whom there was minimal involvement of the pinnae. Thus, there are several examples of autosomal recessive transmission of this syndrome.

Diagnosis. Autosomal dominant aural atresia, microtia, and conductive hearing loss must be excluded. Case reports of sporadic congenital meatal atresia and microtia are not uncommon (11). Some of these individuals may have the dominant or recessive syndrome. Several families have also been reported (4,8,10,12) with microtia, meatal atresia, and conductive hearing loss but with other features associated with abnormalities in development of the first and second branchial arches such as facial asymmetry, preauricular tags, and lateral extension of the corner of the mouth. Some of these patients must surely represent oculo-auriculo-vertebral spectrum. In these families, both autosomal dominant inheritance with variable expression (unilateral and bilateral involvement) (4,8) and occasional nonpenetrance (12) and autosomal recessive inheritance (10) are represented. It seems unlikely that families reported with additional facial features have the same condition. However, since occasional family members have isolated microtia, meatal atresia, and conductive hearing loss, the distinction between the two conditions remains unclear.

Prognosis. Although two children described by Ellwood et al. (3) died in infancy, the cause of death appears to have been unrelated to the ear defects. The hearing loss is congenital and nonprogressive.

Summary. The major characteristics of this syndrome include (*1*) autosomal recessive inheritance; (*2*) unilateral or bilateral anotia or microtia; (*3*) unilateral or bilateral external meatal atresia; and (*4*) congenital moderate to severe conductive hearing loss.

References

1. Cremers CWRJ: Meatal atresia and hearing loss. Autosomal dominant and autosomal recessive inheritance. *Int J Pediatr Otorhinolaryngol* 8:211–213, 1985.
2. Dar H, Winter ST: Letter to the editor. *J Med Genet* 10:305–306, 1973.
3. Ellwood LC et al: Familial microtia with meatal atresia in two sibships. *J Med Genet* 5:289–291, 1968.
4. Guizar-Vazquez J et al: Microtia and meatal atresia in mother and son. *Clin Genet* 14:80–82, 1978.
5. Jaffe BF: Pinna anomalies associated with congenital conduction hearing loss. *Pediatrics* 57:332–341, 1976.
6. Jahrsdoerfer RA: Congenital atresia of the ear. *Laryngoscope* 88(Suppl 13):1–48, 1978.
7. Konigsmark B et al: Recessive microtia, meatal atresia, and hearing loss. *Arch Otolaryngol* 96:105–109, 1972.
8. Oliveira CA et al: External and middle ear malformations: autosomal dominant genetic transmission. *Ann Otol Rhinol Laryngol* 98:772–776, 1989.
9. Schmid M et al: Familial microtia, meatal atresia, and conductive deafness in three siblings. *Am J Med Genet* 22:327–332, 1985.
10. Strisciuglio P et al: Microtia with meatal atresia and conductive deafness: mild and severe manifestations within the same sibship. *J Med Genet* 23:459–460, 1986.
11. Whetnall E, Fry DB: *The Deaf Child*, Charles C. Thomas, Springfield, IL, 1964, p 96.
12. Zankl M, Zang KD: Inheritance of microtia and aural atresia in a family with five affected members. *Clin Genet* 16:331–334, 1979.

Aural atresia, vertical talus, and conductive hearing loss (Rasmussen syndrome)

In 1979, Rasmussen et al. (3) reported a three-generation kindred in which six members had a syndrome of congenital atresia of the external auditory canal, vertical talus, and ocular hypertelorism. Julia et al. (2) reported an isolated patient.

Craniofacial findings. Facial appearance was normal except for a mild increase in interocular distance (Fig. 6–15A).

Musculoskeletal system. Bilateral clubfeet were found in four of the six affected family members, with vertical talus being demonstrated in two. The isolated patient had vertical talus and hip dislocation.

Auditory system. Congenital bilateral symmetrical and isolated subtotal atresia of the lateral auditory canal with normal pinnae was found in all seven affected patients. The middle ears were found to be normal except for decreased mobility of the malleus in one patient (Fig. 6–15B,C). Conductive hearing loss was estimated to be 45–55 dB.

Heredity. Autosomal dominant inheritance with variable expression seems evident. X-linked dominant inheritance would seem to be excluded by a normal daughter of an affected male.

Diagnosis. This syndrome should be differentiated from aural atresia and conductive hearing loss reported by Hefter and Ganz (1) and Robinow and Jahrsdoerfer (4).

Prognosis. Surgical correction improved the hearing loss. Cognitive development was normal.

Summary. The major characteristics of this syndrome include (*1*) autosomal dominant inheritance; (*2*) bilateral clubfeet and vertical talus; (*3*) atresia of lateral auditory canals with normal pinnae; and (*4*) conductive hearing loss.

References

1. Hefter E, Ganz H: Bericht über vererbte Gehörgansmissbildungen. *HNO* 17:76–78, 1969.
2. Julia S et al: Association of external auditory canal atresia, vertical talus, and hypertelorism: confirmation of Rasmussen syndrome. *Am J Med Genet* 110:179–181, 2002.
3. Rasmussen N et al: Inherited congenital bilateral atresia of the external auditory canal, congenital bilateral vertical talus and increased interocular distance. *Acta Otolaryngol* 88:296–302, 1979.
4. Robinow M, Jahrsdoerfer RA: Autosomal dominant atresia of the auditory canal and conductive deafness. *Am J Med Genet* 4:89–94, 1979.

Aural atresia, mental retardation, multiple congenital anomalies, and conductive hearing loss (Cooper-Jabs syndrome)

In 1987, Cooper and Jabs (1) reported two sibs with bilateral low-set posteriorly angulated ears with marked overlap of the superior helix, atresia of the external auditory canal, and mixed hearing loss in association with cardiovascular, joint, and anal anomalies.

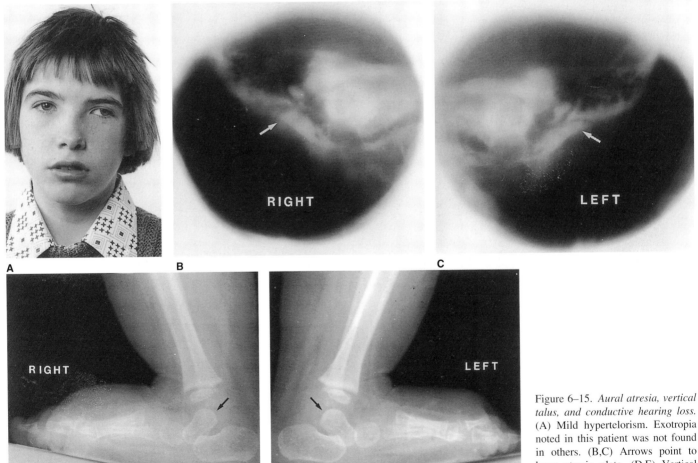

Figure 6–15. *Aural atresia, vertical talus, and conductive hearing loss.* (A) Mild hypertelorism. Exotropia noted in this patient was not found in others. (B,C) Arrows point to bony atresia plate. (D,E) Vertical talus. [From N Rasmussen et al., *Acta Otolaryngol* 88:296, 1979.]

Physical findings. The two sisters had brachycephaly with prominence of the forehead, flattened occiput, and midface hypoplasia (Fig. 6–16). The oldest sibling had arrested hydrocephalus. Height was at the third centile. Both had ventriculoseptal defect, anterior placement of anus, long fifth fingers, proximally placed thumbs, delayed motor and cognitive development, and hypotonia. The older sister exhibited camptodactyly of the interphalangeal joints of the hands, dislocated left hip, talipes calcaneovalgus, and rib anomalies. The youngest sister had hyperextensibility of the hand and wrist joints with talipes equinovarus.

Auditory system. Both sibs had low-set posteriorly rotated ears with marked overlapping of the superior helix. The external auditory canals were atretic.

Audiometry in the older sister revealed the best response at 55–60 dB to speech and at 70 dB to 3000 Hz narrow-band noise. Auditory-evoked potentials were consistent with moderate conductive loss and possible mild sensorineural involvement. When a bone conduction oscillator was placed on the mastoid, there was response to speech at 35–40 dB. Audiography and auditory-evoked potentials in the younger sib revealed bilateral hearing loss, with both conductive and sensorineural components and a response at 70–80 dB.

Polytomograms of the petrous pyramids in the eldest sib revealed atretic external auditory canals, absent tympanic membranes, but normal middle ears. Sclerosis was seen in the periantral triangle.

Heredity. Inheritance is consistent with an autosomal recessive pattern.

Diagnosis. Auditory canal atresia, with or without abnormalities of the pinnae, is estimated to be between 1 and 5 per 20,000 live births (5). Most familial cases of meatal atresia are associated with malformations, especially involving derivatives of the first and second branchial arches (2–4,7,8,10). Several genetic syndromes with aural atresia and multiple-organ involvement have been described (including Saethre-Chotzen syndrome, branchio-oto-renal syndrome, cleidocranial dysplasia, oculodentoosseous syndrome, oto-palato-digital syndrome

type I, Townes-Brocks syndrome, Nager acrofacial dysostosis syndrome, Miller syndrome, velocardiofacial syndrome, and Johanson-Blizzard syndrome). Aural atresia with mental retardation and other malformations may also result from chromosome abnormalities, including trisomy 13, trisomy 18, trisomy 21 (Down syndrome), and del(18q) syndrome. The Cooper-Jabs syndrome most closely resembles Townes-Brocks syndrome (9) and del(18q) syndrome. However, the significant features of these two conditions are lacking. An excellent review of congenital atresia is that of Jahrsdoerfer (6).

Summary. Characteristics of this syndrome include (1) autosomal recessive transmission; (2) bilateral auricular deformities; (3) associated physical findings, including short stature, developmental delay, ventriculoseptal defect, and anterior placement of the anus; (4) atresia of the external auditory meatus; and (5) mixed hearing loss.

References

1. Cooper LF, Jabs EW: Aural atresia associated with multiple congenital anomalies and mental retardation: a new syndrome. *J Pediatr* 110:747–750, 1987.
2. Dar H, Winter ST: Correspondence. *J Med Genet* 10:305, 1973.
3. Ellwood LC et al: Familial microtia with meatal atresia in two sibships. *J Med Genet* 5:289, 1968.
4. Guizar-Vasques J et al: Microtia and meatal atresia in mother and son. *Clin Genet* 14:80–82, 1978.
5. Jafek BW et al: Congenital meatal atresia. *Trans Am Acad Ophthalmol Otolaryngol* 8:588–596, 1975.
6. Jahrsdoerfer RA: Congenital atresia of the ear. *Laryngoscope* 88(Suppl 13):1–48, 1978.
7. Pfeiffer RA: Essai d'une nosologie genetique de l'atresia auris congenita. *J Genet Hum* 30:165–180, 1982.
8. Schmid M et al: Familial microtia, meatal atresia and conductive deafness in three siblings. *Am J Med Genet* 22:327–332, 1985.
9. Townes PL, Brocks ER: Hereditary syndrome of imperforate anus, hand, foot and ear anomalies. *J Pediatr* 81:321–326, 1972.
10. Zankl M, Zang KD: Inheritance of microtia and aural atresia in a family with five affected members. *Clin Genet* 16:331–334, 1979.

Aural atresia, microtia, aortic arch anomalies, and conductive hearing loss

In 1987, Kawashima et al. (5) described three male sibs with a syndrome of microtia, aural atresia, aortic arch anomalies, and conductive hearing loss. Guion-Almeida et al. (4) and Guion-Almeida and Kokitsu-Nakata (3) described two additional patients, both male.

Cardiovascular system. Complex cardiac defects affected all, with septal defects, patent ductus arteriosus, interrupted aortic arch, and other anomalies occurring in various combinations.

Other findings. Micrognathia is a common finding, Hypertelorism is also fairly common. Additional manifestations found in one or two affected boys are high forehead, short nose, cleft palate, and inguinal herniae One boy had left-sided facial paralysis (Fig. 6–17A).

Auditory system. Ears are anomalous, either unilaterally or bilaterally (Fig. 6–17B). Preauricular tags are an occasional finding. When the ear is malformed, the external auditory canal tends to be narrow or atretic. The external auditory canals were atretic. One boy had an auditory brain stem response that was reduced by 60 dB on the left and by 70 dB on the right (5).

Heredity. All affected patients have been male, three of them being siblings. This suggests X-linked recessive inheritance, but autosomal recessive inheritance cannot be ruled out.

Diagnosis. A well-recognized constellation of congenital malformations can be seen in the offspring of mothers who use retinoic acid derivatives during pregnancy. The embryopathy is characterized by anomalies of the head and face, especially small, malformed or miss-

Figure 6–16. *Aural atresia, mental retardation, multiple congenital anomalies, and conductive hearing loss.* One of two sisters with mild prominence of forehead, ocular hypertelorism, and midface hypoplasia. [Courtesy of LF Cooper and EW Jabs, Baltimore, Maryland.]

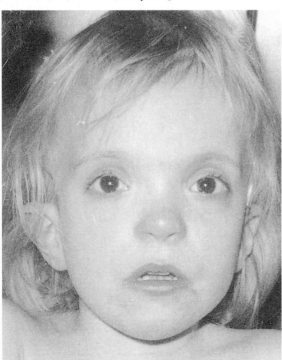

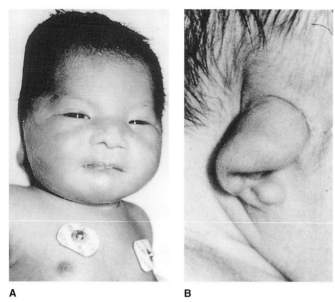

A   **B**

Figure 6–17. *Aural atresia, microtia, aortic arch anomalies, and conductive hearing loss.* (A) High forehead, hypertelorism, short, broad nose. (B) Low-set, small cup-shaped ear. [From H Kawashima et al., *J Pediatr* 111:738, 1987.]

ing ears with micrognathia and cleft palate. Conotruncal defects and aortic arch anomalies, hypoplastic thymus, and CNS anomalies are common (6). Although these three sibs had findings consistent with a diagnosis of isotretinoin embryopathy, their mother had no prenatal history of exposure to isotretinoin. The DiGeorge sequence (1,2) also has ear anomalies and interrupted aortic arch. However, the third sib had normal lymphocyte subsets and serum calcium values. In oculo-auriculo-vertebral spectrum, microtia, preauricular tags, and cardiac defects are also found.

Prognosis. The first two sibs died in the newborn period as a result of congenital heart defects. Progression and extent of hearing loss in the third patient were not reported.

Summary. The characteristic features of this syndrome include (*1*) autosomal or X-linked recessive inheritance; (*2*) malformation of auricles; (*3*) aortic arch anomalies; and (*4*) hearing loss, probably conductive.

References

1. Conley ME et al: The spectrum of the DiGeorge syndrome. *J Pediatr* 94:883–890, 1979.
2. Gorlin RJ et al: *Syndromes of the Head and Neck,* 4th ed. Oxford University Press, New York, 2001, pp 820–822.
3. Guion-Almeida ML, Kokitsu-Nakata NM: Aural atresia, microtia, complex heart defect, and hearing loss syndrome: additional case [letter]. *Am J Med Genet* 117A:83–84, 2003.
4. Guion-Almeida ML et al: A Brazilian boy with aural atresia, microtia, complex heart defect, and hearing loss. *Braz J Dysmorph Speech Hear Disord* 3:21–24, 2000.
5. Kawashima H et al: Syndrome of microtia and aortic arch anomalies resembling isotretinoin embryopathy. *J Pediatr* 111:738–740, 1987.
6. Lammer EJ: Retinoic acid embryopathy. *N Engl J Med* 313:837–841, 1985.

Aural atresia, microtia, hypertelorism, facial clefting, and conductive hearing loss (HMC syndrome, Bixler syndrome)

Hypertelorism, microtia, and cleft lip and palate (HMC syndrome) was described in two sibs by Bixler et al. (3,4), in 1969. In 1976, Schweck-endiek et al. (9) reported identical twins with the same condition, and there have been several isolated case reports (1,2,5,10), one from a con-

sanguineous union (10). Mental retardation was described in half the affected individuals (3,4,9). A so-called Bixler syndrome variant is clearly an example of oculo-auriculo-vertebral spectrum (7).

Physical findings. Most individuals with this condition had growth retardation. Broad nasal root with broadening of the nasal tip, which in extreme cases was bifid (2–4), was common (Fig. 6–18). Almost all patients had ocular hypertelorism. Unilateral or bilateral cleft lip and palate was present in eight of nine individuals, the older twin reported by Schweckendiek et al (9) being the exception. Other facial anomalies included asymmetry, microstomia, and mandibular arch hypoplasia. Mild limb anomalies, including bilateral thenar hypoplasia and shortening of the fifth fingers, were noted in the familial cases (3,4).

Cardiovascular system. Both sisters (3,4) had congenital heart disease with atrial septal defect in the older girl and endocardial cushion defect in the younger. Six other close maternal family members had congenital heart disease, suggesting this may represent an independent genetic defect, since congenital heart disease was not noted in the other cases.

Genitourinary system. Renal anomalies found in several patients included left pelvic kidney (3,4), crossed ectopia of kidney (3,4), unilateral duplication of renal pelvis, and stenosis of ureter (9).

Auditory system. The external ears in the original two sisters (3,4) were markedly abnormal, with bilateral absence of the tragus and anterosuperior helix (Fig. 6–18). One ear was less severely involved in the younger sister. In both, one external auditory meatus was absent, while the other was atretic. Both male twins (9) exhibited right microtia. The second twin had ipsilateral atresia of the external auditory canal.

Figure 6–18. *HMC syndrome.* Frontal views of younger sister (A) and older sister (B). Prominent hypertelorism, broad nasal roots, and repaired cleft lips are evident. (C,D) Lateral facial views of sisters with the HMC syndrome showing microtia in younger sister (C) and older sister (D). Left ears of both sisters show absent external meatuses. [From D Bixler et al., *Am J Dis Child* 118:495, 1969.]

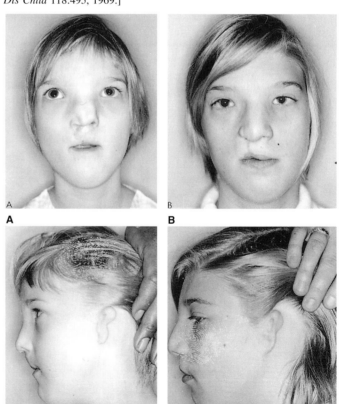

A   **B**

C   **D**

In both twins the left ear was simple without folding of the helix. The boy described by Baraitser (1) had bilaterally malformed pinnae and stenosed external auditory canals. The patient of Fontaine et al. (4) had bilateral dysplasia of the external ears with patent external auditory canals. Patient 2 of the report of Amiel et al. (1) had bilateral anotia.

The two original sisters (3,4) had bilateral conductive hearing loss, whereas one of the twins had unilateral conductive hearing loss (9). Two sporadic patients were too young to assess (2,6). Tomography in one girl revealed bilateral atresia of the external auditory canals with hypoplasia of the left stapes and incus and of the right stapes and malleus. The other girl was thought to have fusion of the ossicles on the left (3,4).

Radiographic findings. Skull radiographs showed a steep mandibular angle, short mandibular ramus, shortened upper facial height, depressed nasal floor, and decreased cranial flexure angle (2,3).

Heredity. Involvement of two of four sibs with normal parents in the original kindred strongly suggests autosomal recessive inheritance.

Diagnosis. In frontonasal malformation, patients have a wide spectrum of anomalies that includes marked hypertelorism, bifid nose, cranium bifidum occultum, and occasionally cleft lip and/or palate (5). Some similar features are found in otopalatodigital I (OPD I) syndrome, including conductive hearing loss, cleft palate, and growth retardation (6). However, the facial and skeletal alterations found in the OPD syndrome are not present in HMC syndrome. Oculo-auriculo-vertebral spectrum commonly has malformations of the pinnae, but cleft lip and palate are relatively uncommon (7%) and severe hypertelorism is not a feature. Motohashi et al. (7) reported a boy with a chromosome abnormality [46,XY,t (1;7)(1q31;7p15)] and features similar to those found in this condition, including hypertelorism, microtia, and cleft palate. However, the child lacked cleft lip and broad/bifid nose and had additional features that included distichiasis, hypoplastic eye lids, and absent lacrimal ducts.

Prognosis. The hearing loss apparently is not progressive. One patient who died in the newborn period succumbed to respiratory complications probably unrelated to the condition (4).

Summary. The characteristic features of this syndrome include (*1*) autosomal recessive inheritance; (*2*) microtia and meatal atresia; (*3*) ocular hypertelorism; (*4*) cleft lip and palate; (*5*) renal anomalies; (*6*) growth retardation; and (*7*) conductive hearing loss.

References

1. Amiel J et al: Hypertelorism-microtia-clefting syndrome (Bixler syndrome): report of two unrelated cases. *Clin Dysmorph* 10:15–18, 2001.
2. Baraitser M: The hypertelorism microtia clefting syndrome. *J Med Genet* 19:387–389, 1982.
3. Bixler D et al: Hypertelorism, microtia and facial clefting: a newly described inherited syndrome. *Am J Dis Child* 118:495–500, 1969.
4. Bixler D et al: Hypertelorism, microtia and facial clefting: a new inherited syndrome. *Birth Defects* 5(2):77–81, 1969.
5. Fontaine G et al: Le syndrome de Bixler ou syndrome HMC (à propos d'une nouvelle observation). *LARC Med* 2:774–776, 1982.
6. Gorlin RJ et al: *Syndromes of the Head and Neck,* 4th ed. Oxford University Press, New York, 2001, pp. 819–820.
7. Ionasescu V, Roberts RJ: Variant of Bixler syndrome. *J Genet Hum* 22:133–138, 1974.
8. Motohashi N et al: Hypertelorism, microtia, cleft palate with a de novo balanced chromosome translocation. *Cong Anom* 25:181–190, 1985.
9. Schweckendiek W et al: HMC syndrome in identical twins. *Hum Genet* 33:315–318, 1976.
10. Verloes A: Hypertelorism-microtia-clefting (HMC) syndrome. *Genet Couns* 5:283–287, 1994.

Aural atresia, microtia, unusual facies, pseudopapilledema, and mixed hearing loss

In 1992, Paes-Alves (2) described three patients in two sibships from a large kindred with a new malformation syndrome. Bertola et al. (1) described an affected young adult.

Clinical findings. All were small (weight <10th centile) at birth. Three of four experienced choking crises during the first year of life. Head circumference was reduced, and the face appeared disproportionately small with micrognathia, retarded and incomplete tooth eruption, dental malocclusion, and a high and narrow palate.

Ocular system. Hypotelorism, blepharophimosis, downslanting palpebral fissures, epicanthal folds, and pseudopapilledema were common. All three Brazilian patients exhibited absence of the superior orbitopalpebral sulcus, although this was not present in the American patient (1).

Integumentary system. Multiple pigmented nevi and café-au-lait spots were noted in two of the four patients.

Musculoskeletal system. Anomalies included short and somewhat webbed fingers, hypoplasia of the thenar, hypothenar, and interdigital areas, bizarre palmar creases, single flexion creases on fingers 2, 3, and/or 5, and palmar keratosis. The feet were small, with unusual form. There was a wide space between the first and second toes, toes 3 and 4 were short, and the calcaneus protruded.

Auditory system. The pinnae were microtic, malformed, and often low-set. Most exhibited atresia of the external auditory meatus. Hearing loss was congenital, bilateral, and mixed, and of moderate severity. Most patients exhibited speech problems.

Heredity. Inheritance was clearly autosomal recessive. The family of three affected individuals was from Bahia, Brazil; the American patient was born to consanguineous parents.

Diagnosis. The syndrome appears quite distinct.

Summary. The characteristics of this syndrome include (*1*) autosomal recessive inheritance; (*2*) microcephaly, maleruption of teeth; (*3*) unusual facies; (*4*) multiple pigmented nevi and café-au-lait spots; (*5*) various digital anomalies; and (*6*) microtia, atresia, and mixed hearing loss.

References

1. Bertola DR et al: Acro-oto-ocular syndrome: further evidence for a new autosomal recessive disorder. *Am J Med Genet* 73:442–446, 1997.
2. Paes-Alves AF et al: Autosomal recessive malformation in syndrome with minor manifestation in the heterozygotes: a preliminary report of a possible new syndrome. *Am J Med Genet* 41:141–152, 1991.

Aural atresia, microtia, skin mastocytosis, short stature, and conductive hearing loss

Wolach et al. (2) described a child, the offspring of consanguineous parents, with microcephaly but normal mentation, upslanting palpebral fissures, hypotonia, feeding problems, short stature, skin mastocytosis, scoliosis, hyperpigmentation of skin of trunk and extremities, hypoplasia of fifth fingers, microtia with atretic external auditory canals, and conductive hearing loss. Hennekam and Beemer (1) described a similarly affected child but with severe mental retardation (Fig. 6–19). Hearing loss was mixed.

Inheritance may possibly be autosomal recessive as the parents were first cousins in the first case (2).

References

1. Hennekam RCM, Beemer FA: Skin mastocytosis, hearing loss with mental retardation. *Clin Dysmorphol* 1:85–88, 1992.
2. Wolach B et al: Skin mastocytosis with short stature, conductive hearing loss and microtia: a new syndrome. *Clin Genet* 37:64–68, 1990.

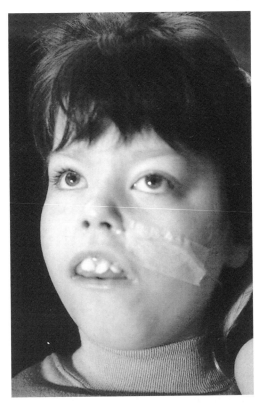

Figure 6–19. *Aural atresia, microtia, skin mastocytosis, short stature, and conductive hearing loss.* Facial appearance of patient. [From RCM Hennekam, FA Beemer, *Clin Dysmorphol* 1:86, 1992.]

Aural atresia and conductive hearing loss (Hefter-Ganz syndrome)

Hefter and Ganz (1) briefly described the combination of meatal atresia and conductive hearing loss in a mother and three of her four children. Robinow and Jahrsdoerfer (2) also reported this combination in a family.

Auditory system. There was such marked bony stenosis of the external auditory meatus that the eardrum was not visible. Conductive hearing loss ranged in the various family members from 10 to 60 dB. Some sibs exhibited mixed hearing loss.

Radiographic findings. The mastoid processes were poorly pneumatized in most of the affected individuals.

Pathology. Surgical examination showed the incus and malleus to be eroded and the stapes and tympanic membrane to be missing. The medial wall of the middle ear was covered with metaplastic epithelium and the floor of the middle ear was fused into a conglomerate mass. In another family member, the entire middle ear cavity was missing.

Heredity. Autosomal dominant inheritance is indicated (1,2).

Prognosis. The more severe the bony meatal atresia, the poorer the surgical results.

Summary. Characteristics include (*1*) autosomal dominant inheritance; (*2*) meatal atresia; and (*3*) hearing loss, largely conductive.

References

1. Hefter E, Ganz H: Bericht über vererbte Gehörgangsmissbildungen. *HNO* 17:76–78, 1969.
2. Robinow M, Jahrsdoerfer RA: Autosomal dominant atresia of the auditory canal and conductive deafness. *Am J Med Genet* 4:89–94, 1979.

Cupped pinnae, microcephaly, mental retardation, and sensorineural hearing loss

In 1987, Kawashima and Tsuji (4) described a mother and son with microcephaly, mild mental retardation, cupped ears, and sensorineural hearing loss. This may be the same disorder as X-linked maxillofacial dysostosis of Toriello et al. (9).

Craniofacial findings. The proband had congenital microcephaly. The face was asymmetric with the left palpebral fissure being narrower than the right. There was prominent glabella and lower lip, and micrognathia. His mother had a head circumference within the normal range (−1.7 SD) and micrognathia but childhood photographs suggested microcephaly (Fig. 6–20).

Central nervous system. At 21 months, the boy's psychomotor development was almost normal (DQ = 85), with mild speech delay. The IQ of the mother at 26 years was measured at 69.

Auditory system. The proband had low-set, cup-shaped pinnae. The mother had low-set, protruding cup-shaped ears with bilateral preauricular tags and attached lobules. The boy had right sensorineural hearing loss. His mother had right sensorineural hearing loss with left mixed loss.

Laboratory findings. Both the boy and his mother had normal karyotypes, EEG, and CT scan. Skull radiographs revealed small cranial vault with asymmetric mandible.

Heredity. Autosomal dominant inheritance appears likely, although X-linked recessive inheritance with heterozygote manifestations in the mother is also a possibility.

Diagnosis. Microcephaly may be inherited or acquired (1), but most cases are sporadic. Genetic microcephaly is estimated to affect between 1/25,000 and 1/50,000 of the population (1). It is more often inherited in an autosomal recessive fashion, although several autosomal dominant microcephalies have been reported. In these latter conditions, microcephaly may be isolated (6) or associated with mental retardation and abnormal facial appearance (3,7), short stature (2), chorioretinal dysplasia (8), and congenital lymphedema (5). None of these is con-

Figure 6–20. *Cupped pinnae, microcephaly, mental retardation, and sensorineural hearing loss.* (A) Proband at 21 months. (B) Mother at 3 years. In both, note cupped ears. [From H Kawashima and N Tsuji, *Clin Genet* 31:303, 1987.]

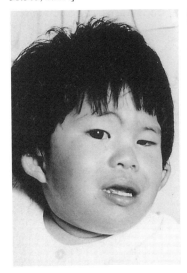
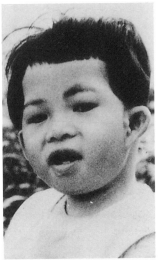

A   B

sistent with the present case. It is possible that this is the same as maxillofacial dysostosis, X-linked.

Prognosis. The hearing loss did not appear to be progressive.

Summary. The characteristic features of this syndrome include (*1*) autosomal dominant inheritance; (*2*) cup-shaped ears with attached lobules, and/or preauricular skin tags; (*3*) microcephaly which may resolve as an adult; (*4*) mild mental retardation; and (*5*) nonprogressive sensorineural hearing loss.

References

1. Böök JA et al: A clinical and genetic study of microcephaly. *Am J Ment Defic* 57:637–660, 1953.
2. Burton BK: Dominant inheritance of microcephaly with short stature. *Clin Genet* 20:25–27, 1981.
3. Haslam RHA, Smith DW: Autosomal dominant microcephaly. *J Pediatr* 95:701–705, 1979.
4. Kawashima H, Tsuji N: Syndrome of microcephaly, deafness/malformed ears, mental retardation, and peculiar facies in a mother and son. *Clin Genet* 31:303–307, 1987.
5. Leung AKC: Dominantly inherited syndrome of microcephaly and congenital lymphedema. *Clin Genet* 26:611–612, 1985.
6. Ramirez ML et al: Silent microcephaly: a distinct autosomal dominant trait. *Clin Genet* 23:281–286, 1983.
7. Rossi LN, Battilana MP: Autosomal dominant microcephaly. *J Pediatr* 101:481–482, 1982.
8. Tenconi R et al: Autosomal dominant microcephaly. *J Pediatr* 102:644, 1983.
9. Toriello HV et al: X-linked syndrome of branchial arch and other defects. *Am J Med Genet* 21:137–142, 1985.

Maxillofacial dysostosis, X-linked

Toriello et al. (7) reported two male sibs and their male first cousin with mild short stature, microcephaly, mild mental retardation, downslanting palpebral fissures due to malar hypoplasia, sparse lateral eyebrows, outstanding pinnae, mild micrognathia, slightly webbed neck, and cryptorchidism (Fig. 6–21). All had mixed hearing loss of sufficient degree to warrant hearing aids. One had stenotic external ear canals. X-linked inheritance seems likely.

Zelante et al. (8) also reported a single affected male. Ensink et al. (2) reported two brothers with similar features. Other examples have also been noted (1,6; S. Boekhorst and HG Brunner, personal communication). It is possible that the mother and son described by Kawashima and Tsuji (3) had X-linked maxillofacial dysostosis. The family reported by Opitz et al. (5) had a very similar physical phenotype, with additional mild brachydactyly, single palmar creases, and subtle interdigital webbing. Deafness was not described. Since the mother's features were as severe as those seen in her four sons, these authors considered autosomal dominant inheritance more likely. There is some resemblance to autosomal dominant maxillofacial dysostosis (4).

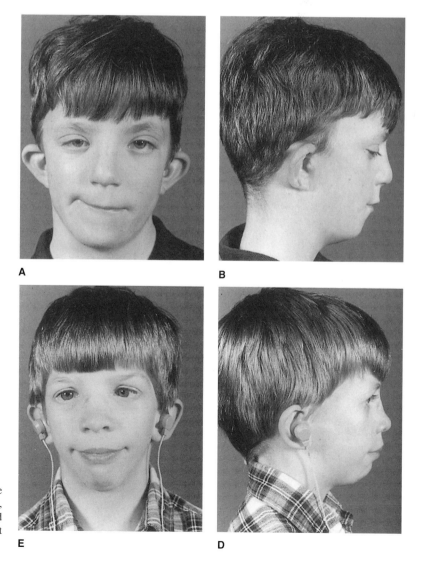

A   B

E   D

Figure 6–21. *Maxillofacial dysostosis, X-linked.* (A–D) Male cousins with microcephaly, downslanting palpebral fissures, sparse eyebrows laterally, outstanding pinnae, hearing loss, mild micrognathia, and slightly webbed neck. [From HV Toriello et al., *Am J Med Genet* 21:137, 1985.]

References

1. Brunner HG et al: Molecular genetics of X-linked hearing impairment. *Ann NY Acad Sci* 630:179–190, 1991.
2. Ensink RJH, Brunner HG, Cremers CWRJ: A new type of maxillofacial dystosis, inherited as an X-linked or autosomal recessive trait. *Genet Couns* 8:285–290, 1997.
3. Kawashima H, Tsuji N: Syndrome of microcephaly, deafness/malformed ears, mental retardation and peculiar facies in a mother and son. *Clin Genet* 31:303–307, 1987.
4. Melnick M, Eastman JR: Autosomal dominant maxillofacial dysostosis. *Birth Defects* 13(3B):39–44, 1977.
5. Opitz JM et al: Acro-facial dysostoses: review and report of a previously undescribed condition: the autosomal or X-linked dominant Catania form of acrofacial dysostosis. *Am J Med Genet* 47:660–678, 1993.
6. Puri RD, Phadke SR: Further delineation of mandibulofacial dysostosis: Toriello type. *Clin Dysmorphol* 11:91–93, 2002.
7. Toriello HV et al: X-linked syndrome of branchial arch and other defects. *Am J Med Genet* 21:137–142, 1985.
8. Zelante L et al: Confirmation of the mandibulofacial dysostosis, Toriello type. *Am J Med Genet* 45:534–535, 1993.

Otofaciocervical syndrome

A family with abnormalities of the external ear, face, and neck was described by Fára et al. (2) in 1967. The father and four of seven children were affected. A sporadic case was reported by Dallapiccola and Mingarelli (1) in 1995. One additional sporadic example is known to us (Allanson, unpublished data). Rajput et al. (4) recently reported an individual with features of branchio-oto-renal syndrome with additional anomalies suggestive of otofaciocervical syndrome, including short neck, sloping shoulders with laterally displaced scapulae, and limited shoulder abduction. Molecular studies have identified a large deletion of the *EYA1* gene region, suggesting that genes lying centromeric to the gene, mutations and intragenic deletions of which lead to branchio-oto-renal syndrome, account for the additional features of otofaciocervical syndrome (5).

Craniofacial findings. The face was long and of an inverted triangular shape, with a relatively broad forehead and narrow mandible (Fig. 6–22A–D). In the family reported (2), lateral cervical fistulas were also present either unilaterally or bilaterally. Lacrimal duct stenosis was noted in the unpublished sporadic case. The palate was highly arched.

Musculoskeletal system. The neck appears long with weak musculature, and the shoulders and clavicles slope downward markedly. The scapulae are located more laterally than normal and show mild winging (Fig. 6–22A–C). A right Sprengel shoulder was noted in the unpublished sporadic case. Most affected persons are short in stature.

Genitourinary system. Unilateral renal agenesis was found in one family member. Intravenous pyelogram (IVP) was normal in the sporadic cases.

Central nervous system. There is mild to moderate hyporeflexia, more marked in the arms than in the legs. Mild intellectual deficit was noted in the family members, but not in the sporadic case.

External ears. The auricles are prominent and have large conchae. Preauricular fistulas are present just in front of the helix (Fig. 6–22E,F). The unpublished sporadic case had a right-sided preauricular fistula and a tag anterior to the left ear.

Auditory system. Otologic examination reveals somewhat atrophic and irregularly thickened tympanic membranes. Audiometric testing of four affected family members showed bilateral conduction hearing loss of 60–70 dB, more marked in low and high frequencies, with 40–50 dB loss in middle frequencies.

Radiographic findings. Radiographs were similar in all affected members of the family. The skull showed narrowing in the middle third of the face, the sella turcica was deep with a slanting clivus, and there was a marked difference in the level of the orbital roof and the cribriform plate (Fig. 6–22G). The temporal pyramids were asymmetric with poor mastoid pneumatization. The clavicles slanted obliquely downward (Fig. 6–22H). Radiographs of the carpal bones showed moderately retarded bone age in three children in the affected family.

In one isolated patient there was spina bifida occulta of the fifth lumbar and first sacral vertebrae. In the other (1), vertebral anomalies and coxa valga were described.

Heredity. The syndrome was observed in a father and in four of his seven children; this is compatible with autosomal dominant inheritance (2).

Diagnosis. The combination of the characteristic facial phenotype, markedly sloping shoulders, auricular abnormalities, and hearing loss appears unique. There is some overlap, however, between this syndrome and the branchio-oto-renal syndrome (3). The latter syndrome lacks anomalies of the shoulder and short stature, while renal anomalies are much more common. Although most individuals with otofaciocervical syndrome (1,2) do not have preauricular tags or lacrimal duct stenosis, the unpublished sporadic patient had both a preauricular tag and lacrimal duct stenosis. The new molecular data of Rickard et al. (5) explain this overlap in phenotype (see branchio-oto-renal syndrome, discussed earlier in this chapter and (3)).

Prognosis. The hearing loss in each of the affected persons was noted in childhood. It is not clear whether the hearing loss was congenital or whether it progressed with age.

Summary. The syndrome is characterized by (*1*) autosomal dominant inheritance; (*2*) prominent auricles with deep conchae; (*3*) preauricular pits; (*4*) lateral cervical fistulas; (*5*) hypoplasia and weakness of the cervical musculature with abnormal range of movement at the shoulders; (*6*) characteristic radiographic abnormalities; and (*7*) moderate to severe conductive hearing loss.

References

1. Dallapicolla B, Mingarelli R: Otofaciocervical syndrome: a sporadic patient supports splitting from the branchio-oto-renal syndrome. *J Med Genet* 32:816–818, 1995.
2. Fára M et al: Dismorphia oto-facio-cervicalis familiaris. *Acta Chir Plast* 9:255–268, 1967.
3. Fraser FC et al: Genetic aspects of the BOR syndrome—branchial fistulas, ear pits, hearing loss and renal anomalies. *Am J Med Genet* 2:241–252, 1978.
4. Rajput K et al: Congenital middle ear cholesteatoma in branchio-oto-renal syndrome. *J Audiol Med* 8:30–37, 1999.
5. Rickard et al: Oto-facio-cervical (OFC) syndrome is a contiguous gene deletion syndrome involving *EYA1*: molecular analysis confirms allelism with BOR syndrome and further narrows the Duane syndrome critical region to 1 cM. *Hum Genet* 108:398–403, 2001

Short stature, hip dislocation, ear malformations, and conductive hearing loss (coxoauricular syndrome)

In 1981, Duca et al. (2) described a mother and three daughters with short stature, minor vertebral and pelvic anomalies, dislocated hips, and hearing loss. They termed this condition the *coxoauricular syndrome*. Two of the daughters had unusual pinnae and hearing impairment.

Musculoskeletal system. All four women had short stature, with reduced lower body segment (Fig. 6–23). In part, the short stature was attributed to congenital dislocation of the hip(s), which was absent in the mother, unilateral in the youngest daughter, and bilateral in the two oldest daughters. There was marked lordosis. The oldest daughter, who had unusually short stature, also had a short wide neck, shield chest

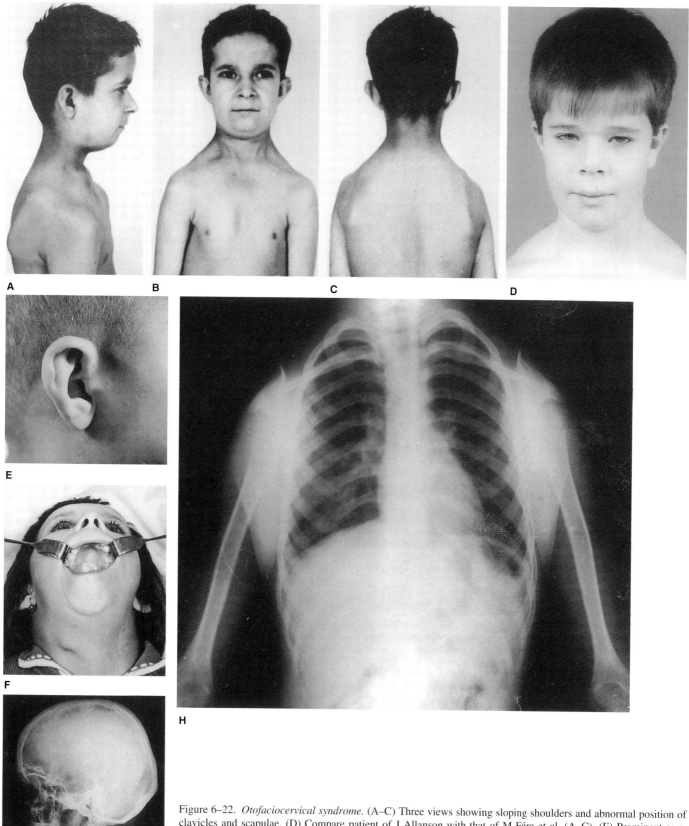

Figure 6–22. *Otofaciocervical syndrome.* (A–C) Three views showing sloping shoulders and abnormal position of clavicles and scapulae. (D) Compare patient of J Allanson with that of M Fára et al. (A–C). (E) Prominent ears, Darwinian tubercle, and fistula at insertions of helix. (F) Highly arched palate; right cervical fistula was present; left cervical fistula had been removed surgically. (G) Lateral view of father's skull showing vertical elongation of head, deep sella turcica, steep clivus, low sphenoid bone, and poor mastoid pneumatization. (H) Radiograph showing depressed position of shoulders. Clavicles are at level of third rib, their outer ends running obliquely downward. The scapulae project at level of axillae. [(A–C), (E–G) from M Fára et al., *Acta Chir Plast (Praha)* 9:255, 1967; (D) courtesy of J Allanson, Ottawa, Ontario, Canada.]

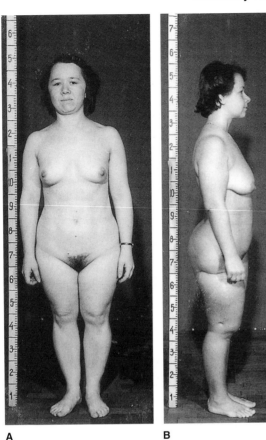
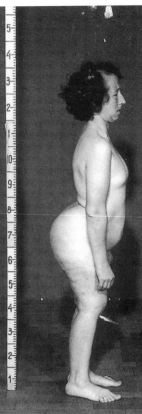

A   B   C   D

Figure 6–23. *Coxoauricular syndrome.* (A–D) Two of four affected individuals showing short stature with reduced lower body segment due to congenital dislocation of hips and marked lordosis. [From D Duca et al., *Am J Med Genet* 8:173, 1981.]

with widely spaced nipples, and cubitus valgus, due to an X chromosome deletion (Turner syndrome).

Auditory system. The mother's right ear was severely microtic, with absence of the external auditory meatus and canal. A daughter had a small right pinna with hypoplasia of helix, anthelix, lobule, tragus, and antitragus. The tragus was replaced by a small pretragal process. The external auditory canal was narrow. On the left, there was severe microtia. Another daughter's right ear was mildly abnormal with overfolding of the helix, hypoplasia of the anthelix, tragus, and antitragus, and stenosis of the external auditory canal.

The mother had unilateral conductive hearing loss (ipsilateral to the microtia). One daughter had bilateral hearing loss, and the other had left-sided hearing loss, contralateral to the pinnal anomalies.

Surgical exploration of the left middle ear in the second daughter revealed hypoplasia of the middle ear, with absence of ossicles and oval window. On the right, there was an almost normal stapes and absent malleus. The inferior long process of the incus was not in contact with the stapes.

Radiographic findings. Vertebral radiographs revealed that all four women had Scheuermann-like spondylosis of the dorsal vertebrae with variable degrees of demineralization, and reduction of height anteriorly with Schmorl's nodules. Pelvic films confirmed dislocation of the hip(s) in the three daughters, with severe deformity of the pelvis and of the head and neck of the femurs, apparent hypoplasia of the pubic and ischial bones, and a periostosis of the superior rim of the iliac wings, which had the appearance of an unfused apophysis of the iliac crest.

Heredity. This syndrome appears to have autosomal dominant transmission. However, X-linked dominant inheritance with hemizygous lethality cannot be excluded since only females were involved.

Diagnosis. Beals (1) described two families with auriculo-osteodysplasia. Twenty-nine affected individuals demonstrated variable combinations of mild to moderate short stature, ear anomalies, principally enlongation and attachment of the lobules, and elbow abnormalities, with hypoplasia of the capitulum and/or dislocation of the radius. One-third of affected females had dislocation of the hips. Beals syndrome can be excluded because of the almost invariable elbow involvement and much milder ear anomalies.

Prognosis. The hearing loss does not appear to be progressive.

Summary. This syndrome is characterized by (*1*) probable autosomal dominant inheritance; (*2*) short stature; (*3*) hip dislocation with minor vertebral anomalies; (*4*) varying degrees of microtia; and (*5*) unilateral or bilateral conductive hearing loss.

References

1. Beals RK: Auriculo-osteodysplasia: a syndrome of multiple osseous dysplasia, ear anomaly, and short stature. *J Bone Joint Surg* 49A:1541, 1967.
2. Duca D et al: A previously unreported, dominantly inherited syndrome of shortness of stature, ear malformations, and hip dislocation: The coxoauricular syndrome—autosomal or X-linked male lethal. *Am J Med Genet* 8:173–180, 1981.

Thickened ear lobes and incudostapedial abnormalities

In 1968, Escher and Hirt (1) described a syndrome characterized by thickened ear lobes, congenitally abnormal incudostapedial joints, and conductive hearing loss. A mother and two affected sons were reported by Wilmot (5). A third family, mother and two daughters, was reported by Kotzot and colleagues (3). R. Engel (Minneapolis, 1986) documented a father and son with thickened ear lobes, medial deviation of the distal thumb, and profound sensorineural hearing loss.

External ear. Thirteen of 14 affected persons in the first kindred had hyperplastic thickened ear lobes (Fig. 6–24A). The rest of the auricle was normal in size and shape (1). In the second family, the changes in the pinnae were less marked (5). The third family had low-set ears, which were small because of reduced size of the upper portion; this is remarkably similar to the configuration in the first family.

Auditory system. Twelve of 14 affected persons reported by Escher and Hirt (1) showed conductive hearing loss. The hearing loss was noted at an early age and was probably congenital, but the severity of the hearing loss was not described, and other audiometric tests were not presented. A 40–60 dB nonprogressive conductive loss was documented by Wilmot (5).

Bilateral tympanotomies were performed on one patient and unilateral tympanotomy on another by Escher and Hirt (1). The ossicular changes were very similar in the three ears observed. The malleus was normal, the long crus of the incus was curved into a long hook, and the head of the stapes was absent (Fig. 6–24B,C). In each case, a fibrous band connected these two ossicles. In the family of Wilmot (5), tympanotomy in the mother showed a shortened long process of the incus. The stapes was mobile but headless and rotated with both crura imbedded in the promontory. Changes in the sons were similar to those observed in the mother. In one son, the footplate was fixed. Similar findings were described in family three (3).

Vestibular system. No vestibular findings were described.

Figure 6–24. *Thickened ear lobes and incudostapedial abnormalities.* (A) Thickened ear lobe. (B) Incus with hook on distal end. (C) Diagram of three surgically treated ears showing missing connection between incus and stapes. [From F Escher and H Hirt, *Acta Otolaryngol* 65:25, 1968.]

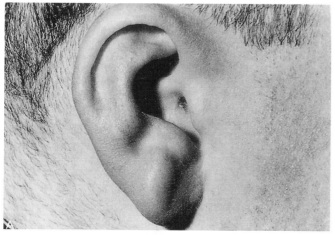

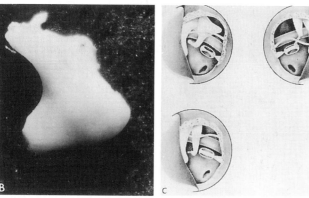

Heredity. Autosomal dominant transmission was evident.

Pathogenesis. It is interesting that although the major portion of the incus arises from the first visceral arch, the long crus arises from the second arch (2). During the sixth to seventh week of fetal life, the joint between the incus and stapes dissolves, with secondary reunion developing about the 23rd week of gestation. It thus appears that the dominant gene causing this abnormality is related to the proper development of this joint during embryogenesis. Wilmot (5) suggested that the anomaly developed prior to the sixth week of fetal development. Hearing loss has been reported in association with absence of the long process of the incus (4).

Diagnosis. The external ear abnormality in this syndrome is only mild, in marked contrast to the moderate and severe auricular deformities seen in other syndromes described in this section. Some patients with this syndrome may have no external ear abnormality. The moderately severe conductive hearing loss differs from otosclerosis in that the syndrome considered here is congenital and apparently nonprogressive. The definitive diagnosis requires examination of middle ear structures.

Prognosis. Prognosis is excellent. The cosmetic defect is minimal, and the hearing loss may be corrected. One child died of complications arising from a congenital heart defect (3). Despite small numbers of individuals with this condition, this seems likely to be unrelated to the syndrome.

Summary. This syndrome is characterized by (*1*) autosomal dominant transmission with complete penetrance; (*2*) hypertrophic ear lobes in most cases; and (*3*) congenital conductive hearing loss due to malformation of the incudostapedial junction.

References

1. Escher F, Hirt H: Dominant hereditary conductive deafness through lack of incus-stapes junction. *Acta Otolaryngol (Stockh)* 65:25–32, 1968.
2. Hanson JR et al: Branchial sources of the auditory ossicles in man. *Arch Otolaryngol* 75:200, 1962.
3. Kotzot D et al: Escher-Hirt syndrome. *Clin Dysmorphol* 6:315–321, 1997.
4. White JW: Conductive deafness due to congenital absence of the long process of the incus. *Clin Proc Wash DC Child Hosp* 20:283–288, 1964.
5. Wilmot TJ: Hereditary conductive deafness due to incus-stapes abnormalities and associated with pinna deformity. *J Laryngol Otol* 84:469–479, 1970.

Wilms tumor, auditory canal stenosis, and conductive hearing loss

Schimmenti et al. (1) reported a family with apparent autosomal dominant inheritance of Wilms tumor and branchial cleft anomalies. A mother and two daughters were affected. The mother had bilateral Wilms tumors resected at 9 months of age, bilateral auditory canal stenosis, right-sided hearing loss, long narrow face, wide mouth, and high arched palate. At the time of the report, the mother had two children (Fig. 6–25). The older, a school-aged girl, had bilateral Wilms tumors resected in the first year of life. The child had auditory canal stenosis, long narrow facies, wide mouth, left-sided cataract, myopia, and strabismus. The younger child, a toddler who had recently undergone resection of bilateral Wilms tumor, had bilateral auditory canal stenosis with limited air conduction, malformed low-set ears, bilateral blepharophimosis and ptosis, microphthalmia, left infranasal coloboma, and absent left superior lacrimal punctum. Development of the mother and both children was normal. Consanguinity of the parents was denied. Chromosomes of all individuals were normal.

References

1. Schimmenti LA et al: Autosomal dominant inheritance of Wilms' tumor and branchial cleft anomalies. A new syndrome. *Am J Hum Genet* (Suppl)53:503, 1993.

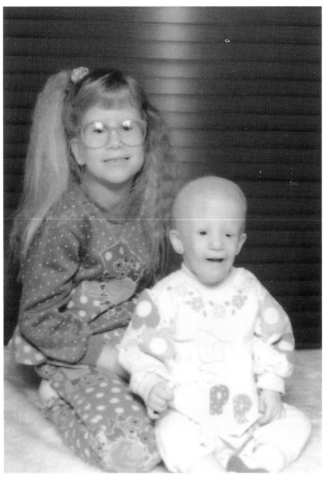

Figure 6–25. *Wilms tumor, auditory canal stenosis, and conductive hearing loss.* Sibs with branchial cleft anomalies and bilateral Wilms tumor. [From Schimmenti LA et al., *Am J Hum Genet* (Suppl) 53:503, 1993.]

Branchio-oto-costal syndrome

Clementi et al. (1) reported three sibs with a distinctive pattern of conductive deafness, bilateral preauricular and commissural lip pits, unilateral branchial sinus, and rib anomalies. The latter consisted of rib hypoplasia with absent ossification of the posterolateral segments of the upper ribs. In one sister, surgical exploration of the ear showed ossicular abnormalities. One brother had sensorineural deafness. The palate was high and narrow leading to dental crowding, with cleft of the soft palate demonstrated in one brother. Delayed language development was described in two of the three sibs. Renal anomalies were excluded in two of the sibs; the third was not evaluated. On the basis of parental consanguinity, lack of clinical variability, and affected males and female, autosomal recessive inheritance seemed likely.

References

1. Clementi M, Mammi I, Tenconi R: Family with branchial arch anomalies, hearing loss, ear and commissural lip pits, and rib anomalies. A new autosomal recessive condition: branchio-oto-costal syndrome. *Am J Med Genet* 68:91–93, 1997.

Marres syndrome

Marres and Cremers (3) reported a large family with variable expression of an autosomal dominant condition with features similar to branchio-oto-renal syndrome. Those features included preauricular sinus with or without a cyst, commissural lip pits, anomalies of the pinna,

and conductive or mixed hearing loss, particularly affecting middle and lower frequencies. The pinnae showed overfolding and thickening of the helix, with reduction of the triangular fossa.

Tympanometry, stapedial reflexes, and surgical exploration, reported in detail in Marres et al. (4), documented ossicular abnormalities. The authors consider this condition to be separate from branchio-oto-renal syndrome on the basis of absence of cervical fistulae and renal anomalies and the presence of commissural pits. Molecular evaluation of the extended family by linkage analysis has provided evidence that this condition is not allelic to *EYA1* at 8q13 (1) but, in fact, is linked to 1q31 (2).

References

1. Kumar S et al: Autosomal-dominant branchio-otic syndrome (BO) is not allelic to the branchio-oto-renal (BOR) gene at 8q13. *Am J Med Genet* 76:395–401, 1998.
2. Kumar S et al: Genome-wide search and genetic localization of a second gene associated with autosomal dominant branchio-oto-renal syndrome: clinical and genetic implications. *Am J Hum Genet* 66:1715–1720, 2000.
3. Marres HAM, Cremers CWRJ: Congenital conductive or mixed deafness, preauricular sinus, external ear anomaly, and commissural lip pits: an autosomal dominant inherited syndrome. *Ann Otol Rhinol Laryngol* 100:928–932, 1991.
4. Marres HAM et al: The deafness, preauricular sinus, external ear anomaly and commissural lip pits syndrome—otological, vestibular and radiological findings. *J Laryngol Otol* 108:13–18, 1994.

Koch-Kumar syndrome

Koch et al. (1) described a three-generation family with the combination of small, dysmorphic auricles, congenital conductive hearing loss,

Figure 6–26. *Gripp syndrome.* (A) Male patient at 19 months, with downslanting palpebral fissures without lower lid coloboma, microtia. (B) Maternal cousin at age 3 years. Note similar phenotype. [From KW Gripp et al., *Am J Med Genet* 101:169, 2001, reprinted by permission of Wiley-Liss, Inc., a subsidiary of John Wiley & Sons, Inc.]

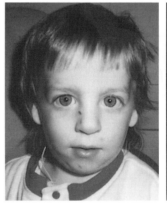
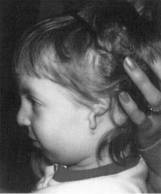

A

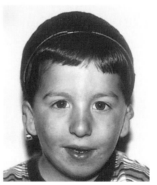
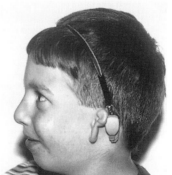

B

and commissural lip pits. The ears were cupped and small. Commmissural lips pits were not present in all affected individuals, but when they were present they were unilateral or bilateral. Hearing loss affected approximately 50% of those considered affected; degree of loss ranged from 25 to 60 dB. One individual had high-frequency sensorineural loss as well. Linkage studies indicated that the gene was not linked to 1q (Marres syndrome) or 8q (BOR), thus suggesting that this is a unique, distinct syndrome. Inheritance is autosomal dominant.

Reference

1. Koch SMP et al: A family with autosomal dominant inherited dysmorphic small auricles, lip pits, and congenital conductive hearing impairment. *Arch Otolaryngol Head Neck Surg* 126:639–644, 2000.

Gripp syndrome

Gripp and colleagues (1) reported two boys, first cousins, with microtia, absent external auditory canals, conductive hearing loss, micrognathia, cleft palate, downslanting palpebral fissures with sparse lower lid lashes, and Diamond-Blackfan anemia (DBA) (Fig. 6–26). Patient 1 demonstrated abnormally formed middle ear structures with normal inner ears. Similar studies were not carried out on patient 2. The sister of patient 2 had hematological findings consistent with DBA, but without evidence of anemia. The mothers of these boys,

who are sisters, show none of these features. Their husbands are healthy and unrelated to their wives or each other. The differential diagnosis of this condition includes Treacher Collins syndrome. *TCOF1* mutation analysis in patient one was negative. Mutations in *RPS19* are described in 25% of persons with DBA—none was identified in either of these boys.

There is a single case report in the literature that shares these features. This female was born with bilateral microtia, slightly downslanting palpebral fissures, sparse eyelashes on the lower lids (without coloboma), cleft palate, and micrognathia, and she presented with DBA at 3 months (2). Analysis of *TCOF1* did not reveal a mutation.

The inheritance pattern in this syndrome is unclear. Since patient 2's sister showed hematological findings in keeping with DBA and no other features, and since both mothers were normal, there may be incomplete penetrance of an autosomal dominant gene. X-linked inheritance seems unlikely given the absence of a shared region of the X chromosome in the two boys and the sister of patient 2. It would not explain the other reported female. Additional cases will be required to further our understanding of genetic cause.

References

1. Gripp KW et al: Bilateral microtia and cleft palate in cousins with Diamond-Blackfan anemia. *Am J Med Genet* 101:268–274, 2001.
2. Hasan R, Inouye S: Diamond-Blackfan anemia associated with Treacher Collins syndrome. *Pediatr Hematol Oncol* 10:261–265, 1993.

Appendix

Other entities with external ear anomalies

Entity	External Ear Finding	Chapter in this Book
Acrocephaly, limb anomalies, short stature, ear malformations with preauricular pits, and mixed hearing loss	Preauricular pits	8 (musculoskeletal)
Rigid mask-like face, ear anomalies, preaxial polydactyly, toe malformations, mixed hearing loss	Microtia	8 (musculoskeletal)
Brachyphalangy, polydactyly, absent tibiae, dysmorphic pinnae, hearing loss	Malformed pinnae with preauricular pits and/or tags	8 (musculoskeletal)
BRESHECK	Large ears	9 (renal
Aplasia cutis–ear malformations	Lop ears	14 (integumentary)

Chapter 7
Genetic Hearing Loss Associated with Eye Disorders
WILLIAM J. KIMBERLING

Usher syndrome is the most commonly occurring disorder in this category. Patients with this syndrome have sensorineural hearing loss and loss of vision due to retinitis pigmentosa. Estimates of its prevalence among profoundly deaf children range from 3% to 8%.

In addition to their association with eye disease and hearing loss, some syndromes discussed in this chapter involve the nervous system while others involve different, sometimes multiple, systems. For example, Refsum syndrome and Alström syndrome could have been assigned to Chapters 12 or 13, Endocrine and Metabolic Disorders. Gordon syndrome is included in Chapter 10 on genetic hearing loss associated with nervous system disorders. The IVIC syndrome might easily have been assigned to Chapter 8, Genetic Hearing Loss Associated with Musculoskeletal Disorders, but it seemed best to include the syndrome here.

Usher syndrome: retinitis pigmentosa, sensorineural hearing loss, and vestibular areflexia

Usher syndrome is characterized by retinitis pigmentosa and sensorineural hearing loss. It is genetically and clinically heterogeneous, thus there are three clinical forms. Type I is characterized by congenital severe to profound hearing loss with development of retinitis pigmentosa by age 10 years and absent vestibular responses. In type II there is usually stable congenital moderate hearing loss in the low frequencies sloping to severe or profound hearing loss in the higher frequencies with onset of retinitis pigmentosa from the mid-teens to early 20's and normal vestibular responses. Type III patients have progressive hearing loss with progressive vestibular involvement and variable severity of retinitis pigmentosa (43,44,75). Thirteen different genes are believed to be involved, of which 6 have been identified (67). Generally, mutations in specific genes seem to be correlated with one of the three specific phenotypes. However, it is now becoming clear that some of these aberrant genes can produce overlapping phenotypes (see Table 7–1 for a summary of the genes and the phenotypes they produce).

Soon after development of the ophthalmoscope, the syndrome was described by Albrecht von Graefe (86) in 1858. He credited the discovery to his cousin, Alfred von Graefe, also an ophthalmologist. In 1861, after systematically examining the deaf population of Berlin, Liebreich (54) reported several affected sibs and parental consanguinity. Usher (80) extensively documented the disorder in 1914 and confirmed autosomal recessive inheritance.

The prevalence of retinitis pigmentosa among congenitally profoundly deaf children has been estimated at 3%–6% (83) and possibly 50% of the deaf–blind population. If one assumes a prevalence of 1/1000 for profound childhood hearing loss, this is in accord with the 2.5–4.5/100,000 population prevalence estimates made in Denmark (55), Sweden (35), Norway (33), Finland (65), Colombia (77), and the United States (18). Conversely, about 18% of retinitis pigmentosa patients in the United States have Usher syndrome (18). Grøndahl and Mjøen (34) found 50% to be type I, 35% to be type II, and 15% to be type III; and Tamayo et al. (77) found 70% to be type I, 25% to be type II, and 5% to be type III. A marked predominance of those with severe congenital hearing loss has generally been reported by other authors (35,60). However, Fishman et al. (29) indicated that type II is not rare.

Usher syndrome appears to be more common in northern Sweden and in the Acadian population of Louisiana.

Ocular system. Initial eye symptoms may appear as early as preschool age in the form of night blindness. Restriction of peripheral vision may be noticed in the early teens and usually becomes pronounced by 20 years of age. Because of the reduction in visual fields, the patient becomes legally blind long before losing the ability to read and communicate visually with sign language. Prior to 30 years of age, central vision is reasonably good in all three types, but it deteriorates slowly, progressing to blindness in about 40% of patients in their fifth decade, in about 60% of those in the sixth decade, and in about 75% in their seventh decade in all types (20,29,30,32,67). Cataracts are a frequent complication that, unless corrected, contribute to the visual loss. Visual loss has considerable interfamilial variability that may be due to background genes, differences between the different genes involved, and/or differences in the nature of the pathologic mutations. Early in life, the fundus may display little in the way of pigmentation and can present in the form of retinitis sine pigmenti. As the patient gets older, ophthalmoscopic examination shows a typical slowly progressive retinitis pigmentosa beginning with granular accumulations of pigment clumping, giving the appearance of bone spicules in the mid-periphery of the fundus with extension toward the periphery (Fig. 7–1A,B). Optic discs become pale and arterioles become narrowed. Visual fields slowly constrict, sometimes accompanied by decreasing visual acuity. The blindness is due to degeneration of rod photoreceptor cells. Mild spontaneous nystagmus has been observed in 20% of type I cases (61).

It is thought that type II has a milder form of retinitis pigmentosa than that of type I (30,31), but the overlap in symptoms is great enough that the severity of the retinitis pigmentosa is usually not sufficient to differentiate the different clinical types. Mutations in some of the Usher related genes have been reported not to cause retinitis pigmentosa. Absence of retinitis pigmentosa associated with *MYO7A* mutation was reported for two cases of nonsyndromic hearing loss from China (56) and one from Tunisia (91); however, some members from the family from Tunisia were later reported to have developed retinitis pigmentosa (96). A study of a series of U.S. families with nonsyndromic recessive hearing loss failed to show any significant contribution of *MYO7A* suggesting most *MYO7A* mutations will be associated with retinitis pigmentosa (7). Mutations in *CDH23* may be associated with isolated retinitis pigmentosa (6,16,17).

Auditory system. The audiologic profiles are distinct for the three types. The hearing loss for most patients with type I is profound. The audiograms in type I are flat, with recordings being only barely perceptible in the very low frequencies (Fig. 7–1C). For type II, there is typically a sloping hearing loss that is most severe at high frequencies but only moderate in the speech range (51,75) (Fig. 7–1D). The hearing loss in type III is progressive, starting at about age 3–5 years. It continues to become a moderate to severe sloping hearing loss at young adulthood and then progresses to a profound loss across all frequencies by the fourth to fifth decade (42,66). As a consequence, type III audiograms resemble those expected for type II when the patient is young but progress into a flat profound loss when the patient is an older adult. The hearing loss in type II can be progressive, but it seldom shows the same steep loss characteristic of type III (81).

Table 7–1. Usher syndrome genes and overlapping syndromes

Usher Type	Gene Locus	Causative Gene, If Known	Other Hearing Loss conditions Caused by Gene Mutation
IA	14q32		
IB	11q13.5	Myosin VIIA (*MYO7A*)	DFNB2, DFNA11
IC	11p15.1	*USHIC* (harmonin)	DFNB18
ID	10q21–22	*CDH23*	DFNB12
IE	21q21		
IF	10q21–22	*PCDH15*	?DFNB23
IG	17q24–q25		?DFNA20, ?DFNA26
IIA	1q41	Usherin	Retinitis pigmentosa without hearing loss
IIB	3p24.2–p23		?DFNB6 (unlikely)
IIC	5q14–q21		
II (unspecified)	Unknown		
IIIA	3q21–25		
III (unspecified)	20q		

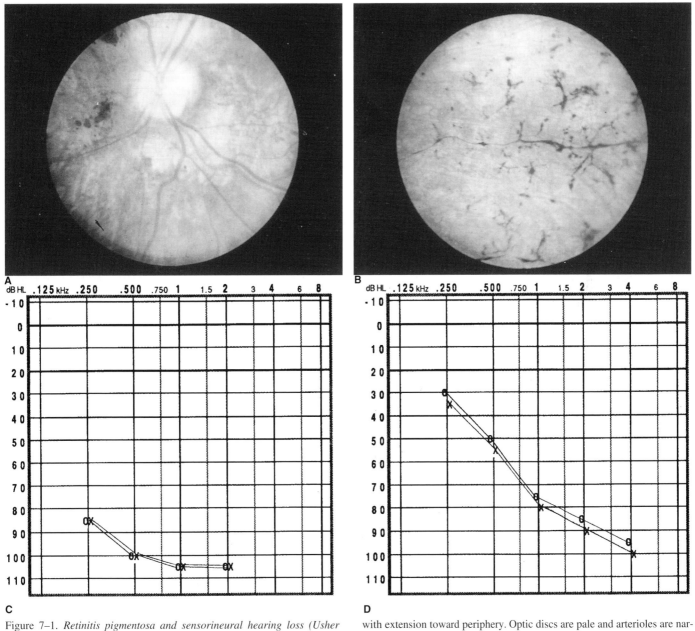

Figure 7–1. *Retinitis pigmentosa and sensorineural hearing loss (Usher syndrome).* (A,B) Fundi views showing granular accumulation of pigment clumping, giving appearance of bone spicules in mid-periphery of fundus with extension toward periphery. Optic discs are pale and arterioles are narrowed. (C) Type I. (D) Type II.

127

Some audiometric differences have been noted between molecular subtypes. Mutations in *MYO7A* appear to almost consistently produce a profound hearing loss, although a progressive loss was reported in two siblings with putative pathologic mutations (57). Hearing loss characteristic of Usher types I, II, and III have been observed with *CDH23* mutations (6).

Vestibular system. Vestibular response to caloric, rotational, and posturographic testing is absent or markedly reduced in type I (35,51,61,83), normal in type II (46,60,61), and appears to be progressively diminished with age in type III (34,47).

Central nervous system. Most patients with Usher syndrome have normal intelligence and normal neurological function. Abnormalities such as ataxia, mental retardation, and psychosis have been described in some patients, especially those with type I, but the frequency and spectrum of abnormalities have not been adequately studied. Peripheral (vestibular) ataxia is observed in most patients with mutations in type I genes. According to Hallgren (35) and Möller et al. (61), type I patients are delayed in walking until 18 months. Later, they may be clumsy at running or riding a bicycle. The gait disturbance is usually noticed in childhood and becomes more broad based with age. As visual loss progresses, gait becomes shuffling or stumbling. Coordination of hands and trunk is normal. Those with type II walk at a normal age and have no gait disturbances. Hallgren (35) first proposed that the ataxia was labyrinthine in origin, and more formal balance/vestibular studies, as well as magnetic resonance imaging (MRI) evaluation of the cerebellum, suggest that there is no central component to the ataxia (61). However, several recent studies have described abnormalities on imaging studies that suggest a central origin. These include cerebellar atrophy on computed tomography (CT) or MRI scans, and high-signal abnormalities in the midbrain on MRI scans (15,49,71,78).

Hallgren (35) observed mental retardation in 41 of 172 affected individuals from a large Swedish family, although it was severe in only 4 persons. Hallgren's study was completed in 1955, before more careful intellectual evaluation of the deaf–blind was common practice, and it is likely that this number was an overestimate. Psychosis was diagnosed in 26 of the 112 persons who could be evaluated. Vernon (83) reported similar frequencies of both mental retardation and psychosis in a much smaller series. Testing was difficult and probably unreliable in many patients because of the associated hearing and visual deficits.

Laboratory findings. Blood and urine analyses and skull radiographic studies have been normal. Electroencephalographic abnormalities have been an inconstant finding (1,65) (see Retinitis pigmentosa, nystagmus, hemiplegic migraine, and sensorineural hearing loss, below). Bazan et al. (8) reported decreased docosahexaenoate (DHA) and arachidonate in plasma phospholipids and Conner (21) reported a similar deficiency of DHA in sperm from patients with type II.

Pathology. In the few studies published, the bony cochlea has been normal. Histologic findings in types I, II, and III have shown degeneration of the hair cells of the organ of Corti and spiral ganglion cells with atrophy of the stria vascularis (9,22,63,72,74,88). The patient of Belal (9) had type II or type III Usher syndrome. Although the patient did not have total hearing loss, on autopsy the hair cells in the basal 15 mm had completely degenerated and the spiral ganglion population was markedly reduced in areas corresponding to the degenerated organ of Corti. Thus, the degree of inner ear pathology appears to be more related to the degree of hearing loss than to the precise classification. One patient described by Wagenaar et al. (88), who was shown to have either Usher 1D or 1F by linkage, demonstrated a cochleosaccular degeneration.

A microtubular abnormality has been suggested by Hunter et al. (38) to explain the irreversible progressive loss of photoreceptors in Usher syndrome; two other studies have reported contradictory results regarding the structural and motility abnormalities in sperm. Conner (21) observed reduced sperm motility in Usher II patients but van Aarem et al. (82) observed no abnormalities in a series of patients with molecularly confirmed cases of Usher IIA.

Heredity. Numerous examples of affected sibs with normal, often consanguineous, parents indicate autosomal recessive inheritance for all three types. Depending upon the specific subtype, carrier rates are estimated to vary between 1/75 and 1/150. Although heterozygotes are stated to exhibit either mild hearing loss or mild retinal findings (25,48,60,70,76), others have not supported this finding (32,74,87).

A putative X-linked recessive family was reported (24) that was later shown to have a mutation in the *USH2A* gene. The gene for type II Usher syndrome has been localized to the distal-most region of the long arm at 1q32 (45,53,92). This gene for Usher type II has been identified and codes for a basement membrane–associated protein termed usherin (27). Several mutations in the *USH2A* gene have been reported (2,10,26,27,52,58,64,94). Genetic heterogeneity is likely since not all families map to that area (68); linkage to 3p (37) and 5q (69) has been demonstrated in addition to the possible existence of a fourth linkage group (68). Type I Usher syndrome is also heterogeneous; seven linkage groups have been observed and four genes identified: *MYO7A* (11q), *CDH23* (10q), *PCDH15* (11q), and *USH1C* (11p). Several mutations have been observed in *MYO7A* (13,23,39,64,90,93), *CDH23* (5,6,16,17,85), *USH1C* (14,84,88,92,97), and *PCDH15* (3,4). The Usher I genes linked to chromosomes 14q (41), 21q (19), and 17q (62) remain to be identified. The gene for Usher type III has been recently identified and several pathologic mutations observed (28,40). The *MYO7A* (11q) form is the most common molecular type in those of European origin with the type I phenotype. The *CDH23* type is probably the second most common form of Usher type I. While the *USH1C* (11p) form is more frequent among Acadians, the other types do not appear to be as frequent. *USH2A* mutations are the most common form of the milder Usher type II phenotype, and one single mutation, the 2299delG, accounts for about 15% of all the mutant alleles in populations of European ancestry. One specific mutation in the *USH3* gene is common in Finland (40); however, Usher type III is found outside that population and one mutation appears to be specific to the Ashkenazi Jewish population (28).

Diagnosis. Most patients with vestibular areflexia, retinopathy, and hearing loss probably have Usher syndrome type I, II, or III. A few patients have had later onset of these symptoms, including the hearing loss, and may have a separate syndrome (see Ataxia, pigmentary retinopathy, and sensorineural hearing loss in Chapter 10) (79). The same combination of manifestations occurs in some patients with mitochondrial encephalomyopathies, including Kearns-Sayre syndrome. Patients with motor and sensory neuropathy, pigmentary retinopathy, and sensorineural hearing loss have clinical signs and magnetoencephalogram (MEG) abnormalities consistent with peripheral neuropathy, which are not observed in patients with type I or II Usher syndrome.

Early diagnosis is extremely important for early entry in a rehabilitative program for the affected child, as well as for genetic counseling of the family. Given the widespread acceptance of newborn hearing screening, the possibility of early diagnosis is very real. Certainly any child with a profound hearing loss who walks after the age of 18 months should be considered a good candidate for Usher type I. Early diagnosis can be made using DNA testing, and *MYO7A* testing is recommended in all children suspected of having Usher type I by virtue of having a profound hearing loss with delayed walking.

In addition to diagnosis by ophthalmoscopy, the retinitis pigmentosa may be diagnosed by electroretinography, electrooculography, visual field tests, and dark adaptation recording (1,61,75). Vestibular function tests should be carried out on every profoundly deaf child.

Diagnosis of the molecular subtypes can be made reliably only by DNA testing. There is currently no direct test of the protein products.

Retinitis pigmentosa as an isolated finding can be inherited as an autosomal recessive, autosomal dominant, or X-linked condition (89), and some degree of sensorineural hearing loss can be found in about 20% of patients (59). A combination of retinitis pigmentosa and hearing loss can be found in several syndromes (see Table 7–2). The association

Table 7–2. Syndromes of pigmentary retinopathy

Condition or system	Syndrome										
	Usher syndrome	Alström syndrome	Edwards syndrome	Laurence-Moon syndrome	Bardet-Biedl syndrome	Leber congenital amaurosis	Gordon syndrome	Hersh syndrome	Young syndrome	Refsum syndrome	Coppeto-Lessell syndrome
Pigmentary retinopathy	Present	Present	Present	Present	Present	Present	Present	Present	Present	Present	Present
Sexual development	Normal	Small testes	Small testes, gynecomastia	Hypogenitalism	Hypogenitalism	Normal	Normal	Hypoplastic genitalia in male	Normal	Normal	Normal
Mental development	Retarded and/or psychotic in 25%	Normal	Retarded	Retarded	Retarded	Variable	Retarded	Retarded	Normal	Normal	Variable
Auditory function	SND	SND	SND	Normal in 95%	Normal in 95%	Variable	SND	SND	SND	SND	SND
Hand anomalies	None	None	None	None	Polydactylyl	None	None	None	None	None	None
Neurologic abnormalities	None	None	Minor pyramidal tract changes	Spastic paraplegia	None	Variable	Progressive quadriparesis	Hypotonia	Migraine	Motor and sensory losses	Dystonia
Glucose metabolism	Normal	Diabetes mellitus	Diabetes mellitus	Normal	Glucose intolerance common	Normal	Normal	Normal	Normal	Normal	Normal
Obesity	Absent	Present	Absent	Absent	Present	Absent	Absent	Absent	Absent	Absent	Absent
Renal disease	None	Chronic nephropathy	None	None	Renal anomalies in 90%	None	None	None	None	None	None
Skin	Normal	Acanthosis nigricans	Acanthosis nigricans	Normal	Normal	Absent	Normal	Normal	Normal	Ichthyosis	Normal

SND, sensorineural deafness. Based in part on JA Edwards et al., *Am J Med* 60:23, 1976 and RH Millay et al., *Am J Ophthalmol* 102:482, 1986.

with autoimmune disease has been noted (22). In Alström syndrome, the patient is obese and may have diabetes mellitus. Individuals with Refsum syndrome have mental deterioration, progressive peripheral neuropathy, and elevated phytanic acid levels. In Bardet-Biedl syndrome there is mental deficiency, obesity, hypogonadism, and polydactyly. In Laurence-Moon syndrome, mental retardation, hypogenitalism, and spastic paraplegia are seen. Patients with Cockayne syndrome are distinguished by their small stature, severe mental deficiency, and so-called "bird-like" face.

Retinitis pigmentosa has been noted in progressive external ophthalmoplegia, retinal pigmentary degeneration, cardiac conduction defects, and mixed hearing loss (Kearns-Sayre syndrome). Mild retinal changes are seen in progressive rod-cone dystrophy, renal dysfunction, and sensorineural hearing loss.

Treatment. Clinical trials on vitamin A supplementation have provided evidence that ingestion of 15,000 IU of vitamin A palmitate slows the progression of the retinitis pigmentosa (11,12). Cochlear implants have been successful in type I patients, but success is generally correlated with early intervention (36,50,73,95). In light of the potential for eventual loss of vision in these patients, early detection and implantations seem advisable. No studies have been reported on the efficacy of the cochlear implant in type III patients or those with Usher type II who have become profoundly deaf.

Prognosis. Many patients are forced to retire from their occupations at age 30–40 years because of advancing failure of vision.

Summary. This syndrome is characterized by (*1*) autosomal recessive inheritance; (*2*) retinitis pigmentosa with childhood visual loss in type I, post-pubertal loss in type II, and variable loss in type III; (*3*) congenital severe sensorineural hearing loss in type I, moderate to severe loss of mostly high tones in type II, and variable hearing loss in type III; and (*4*) absent vestibular response in type I with delayed motor milestones in childhood.

References

1. Abraham FA et al: Usher's syndrome: electrophysiological tests of the visual and auditory systems. *Doc Ophthalmol* 44:435–444, 1977.
2. Adato A et al: Three novel mutations and twelve polymorphisms identified in the *USH2A* gene in Israeli USH2 families. *Hum Mutat* 15:388, 2000.
3. Ahmed ZM et al: Mutations of the protocadherin gene *PCDH15* cause Usher syndrome type 1F. *Am J Hum Genet* 69:25–34, 2001.
4. Alagramam KN et al: Mutations in the novel protocadherin *PCDH15* cause Usher syndrome type 1F. *Hum Mol Genet* 10:1709–1718, 2001.
5. Astuto LM et al: Genetic heterogeneity of Usher syndrome: analysis of 151 families with Usher type I. *Am J Hum Genet* 67:1569–1574, 2000.
6. Astuto LM et al: CDH23 mutation and phenotype heterogeneity: a profile of 107 diverse families with Usher syndrome and nonsyndromic deafness. *Am J Hum Genet* 71:262–275, 2002.
7. Astuto LM et al: Searching for evidence of DFNB2. *Am J Med Genet* 109:291–297, 2002.
8. Bazan NG et al: Decreased content of docosahexaenoate and arachidonate in plasma. *Biochem Biophys Res Commun* 141:600–604, 1995.
9. Belal A: Usher's syndrome (retinitis pigmentosa and deafness): a temporal bone report. *J Laryngol Otol* 89:175–181, 1975.
10. Beneyto MM et al: Prevalence of 2314delG mutation in Spanish patients with Usher syndrome type II (USH2). *Ophthalm Genet* 21:123–128, 2000.
11. Berson EL: Nutrition and retinal degenerations. *Int Ophthalmol Clin* 40:93–111, 2000.
12. Berson EL et al: Vitamin A supplementation for retinitis pigmentosa. *Arch Ophthalmol* 111:1456–1459, 1993.
13. Bharadwaj AK et al: Evaluation of the myosin VIIA gene and visual function in patients with Usher syndrome type I. *Exp Eye Res* 71:173–181, 2000.
14. Bitner-Glindzicz M et al: A recessive contiguous gene deletion causing infantile hyperinsulinism, enteropathy and deafness identifies the Usher type 1C gene. *Nat Genet* 26:56–60, 2000.
15. Bloom TD et al: Usher's syndrome: CNS defects determined by computed tomography. *Retina* 3:108–113, 1983.
16. Bolz H et al: Mutation of *CDH23*, encoding a new member of the cadherin gene family, causes Usher syndrome type 1D. *Nat Genet* 27:108–112, 2001.
17. Bork JM et al: Usher syndrome 1D and nonsyndromic autosomal recessive deafness DFNB12 are caused by allelic mutations of the novel cadherin-like gene *CDH23*. *Am J Hum Genet* 68:26–37, 2001.
18. Boughman JA et al: Usher syndrome: definition and estimate of prevalence from two high risk populations. *J Chron Dis* 36:595–603, 1983.
19. Chaib H et al: A newly identified locus for Usher syndrome type I, USH1E, maps to chromosome 21q21. *Hum Mol Genet* 6:27–31, 1997.
20. Cherry PM: Usher's syndrome. *Ann Ophthalmol* 5:743–752, 1973.
21. Conner RCR: Complicated migraine: a study of permanent neurological and visual defects caused by migraine. *Lancet* 2:1072–1075, 1962.
22. Cowan CL et al: Retinitis pigmentosa associated with hearing loss, thyroid disease, vitiligo, and alopecia areata: retinitis pigmentosa and vitiligo. *Retina* 2:84–88, 1982.
23. Cuevas JM et al: Identification of three novel mutations in the *MYO7A* gene. *Hum Mutat* 14:181, 1999.
24. Davenport SLH et al: Usher syndrome in four hard of hearing siblings. *Pediatrics* 62:578–583, 1978.
25. De Haas EBH et al: Usher's syndrome with special reference to heterozygous manifestations. *Doc Ophthalmol* 28:166–190, 1970.
26. Dreyer B et al: Identification of novel *USH2A* mutations: implications for the structure of USH2A protein. *Eur J Hum Genet* 8:500–506, 2000.
27. Eudy JD et al: Mutation of a gene encoding a protein with extracellular matrix motifs in Usher syndrome type IIa. *Science* 280:1753–1757, 1998.
28. Fields RR et al: Usher syndrome type III: revised genomic structure of the USH3 gene and identification of novel mutations. *Am J Hum Genet* 71:607–617, 2002.
29. Fishman GA: Usher's syndrome: visual loss and variations in clinical expressivity. *Perspect Ophthalmol* 3:97–103, 1979.
30. Fishman GA et al: Usher's syndrome. Ophthalmic and neuro-otologic findings suggesting genetic heterogeneity. *Arch Ophthalmol* 101:1367–1374, 1983.
31. Fishman GA et al: Prevalence of foveal lesions in type 1 and type 2 Usher's syndrome. *Arch Ophthalmol* 113:770–773, 1995.
32. Grøndahl J: Tapeto-retinal degeneration in four Norwegian counties. I. Diagnostic evaluation of 89 probands. *Clin Genet* 29:1–16, 1986.
33. Grøndahl J: Estimation of prognosis and prevalence of retinitis pigmentosa and Usher syndrome in Norway. *Clin Genet* 31:255–264, 1987.
34. Grøndahl J, Mjøen S: Usher syndrome in four Norwegian counties. *Clin Genet* 30:14–28, 1986.
35. Hallgren B: Retinitis pigmentosa combined with congenital deafness; with vestibulo-cerebellar ataxia and neural abnormality in a proportion of cases. *Acta Psychiatr Scand* 138(Suppl):1–101, 1959.
36. Hinderlink JB et al: Results from four cochlear implant patients with Usher's syndrome. *Ann Otol Rhinol Laryngol* 103:285–293, 1994.
37. Hmani M et al: A novel locus for Usher syndrome type II, USH2B, maps to chromosome 3 at p23–24.2. *Eur J Hum Genet* 7:363–367, 1999.
38. Hunter DG et al: Abnormal sperm and photoreceptor axonemes in Usher's syndrome. *Arch Ophthalmol* 104:385–389, 1986.
39. Janecke AR et al: Twelve novel myosin VIIA mutations in 34 patients with Usher syndrome type I: confirmation of genetic heterogeneity. *Hum Mutat* 13:133–140, 1999.
40. Joensuu T et al: Mutations in a novel gene with transmembrane domains underlie Usher syndrome type 3. *Am J Hum Genet* 69:673–684, 2001.
41. Kaplan J et al: A gene for Usher syndrome type I (USH1A) maps to chromosome 14q. *Genomics* 14:979–987, 1992.
42. Karjalainen S et al: Progressive hearing loss in Usher's syndrome. *Ann Otol Rhinol Laryngol* 98:863–866, 1989.
43. Keats BJ, Corey DP: The Usher syndromes. *Am J Med Genet* 89:158–166, 1999.
44. Kimberling WJ, Moller C: Clinical and molecular genetics of Usher syndrome. *J Am Acad Audiol* 6:63–72, 1995.
45. Kimberling WJ et al: Localization of Usher syndrome type II to chromosome 1q. *Genomics* 7:245–249, 1990.
46. Kimberling WJ et al: Linkage of Usher syndrome type I gene (*USH1B*) to the long arm of chromosome 11. *Genomics* 14:988–994, 1992.
47. Kimberling WJ et al: Genetic heterogeneity of Usher syndrome. *Adv Otorhinolaryngol* 56:11–18, 2000.
48. Kloepfer HW et al: The hereditary syndrome of congenital deafness and retinitis pigmentosa. *Laryngoscope* 76:850–862, 1966.
49. Koizumi J et al: CNS changes in Usher's syndrome with mental disorder: CT, MRI and PET findings. *J Neurol Neurosurg Psychiatry* 51:987–990, 1988.
50. Konradsson KS et al: Usher's syndrome and cochlear implant [letter]. *Laryngoscope* 107:406–407, 1997.
51. Kumar A et al: Vestibular and auditory function in Usher's syndrome. *Ann Otol Rhinol Laryngol* 93:600–608, 1984.

52. Leroy BP et al: Spectrum of mutations in *USU2A* in British patients with Usher syndrome type II. *Exp Eye Res* 72:503–509, 2001.

53. Lewis RA et al: Mapping recessive ophthalmic diseases: linkage of the locus for Usher syndrome type II to a DNA marker on chromosome 1q. *Genomics* 7:250–256, 1990.

54. Liebreich R: Abkunft aus Ehen unter Blutsverwandten als grund von Retinitis Pigmentosa. *Dtsch Klin* 13:53–55, 1861.

55. Lindenov H: The etiology of deaf-mutism with special reference to heredity. *Op Ex Domo Biol Hered Hum Univ Hafnienses* 8:1–268, 1945.

56. Liu XZ et al: Mutations in the myosin VIIA gene cause non-syndromic recessive deafness. *Nat Genet* 16:188–190, 1997.

57. Liu XZ et al: Mutations in the myosin VIIA gene cause a wide phenotypic spectrum, including atypical usher syndrome. *Am J Hum Genet* 63:909–912, 1998.

58. Liu XZ et al: A mutation (2314delG) in the Usher syndrome type IIA gene: high prevalence and phenotypic variation. *Am J Hum Genet* 64:1221–1225, 1999.

59. McDonald JM et al: Sensorineural hearing loss in patients with typical retinitis pigmentosa. *Am J Ophthalmol* 105:125–131, 1988.

60. McLeod AC et al: Clinical variation in Usher's syndrome. *Arch Otorhinolaryngol* 94:321–334, 1971.

61. Möller CG et al: Usher syndrome: an otoneurologic study. *Laryngoscope* 99:73–79, 1989.

62. Mustapha M et al: A novel locus for Usher syndrome type I, USH1G, maps to chromosome 17q24-25. *Hum Genet* 110:348–350, 2002.

63. Nager FR: Zur Histologie der Taubstummheit bei Retinitis pigmentosa. *Beitr Pathol* 77:288–303, 1927.

64. Najera C et al: Mutations in myosin VIIA (*MYO7A*) and usherin (*USH2A*) in Spanish patients with usher syndrome types I and II, respectively. *Hum Mutat* 20:76–77, 2002.

65. Nuutila A: Dystrophia retinae pigmentosa–dysacusis syndrome (DRD): a study of the Usher or Hallgren syndrome. *J Genet Hum* 18:57–58, 1970.

66. Pakarinen L et al: Usher's syndrome type 3 in Finland. *Laryngoscope* 105:613–617, 1995.

67. Petit C: Usher syndrome: from genetics to pathogenesis. *Annu Rev Genomics Hum Genet* 2:271–297, 2001.

68. Pieke-Dahl SA et al: Genetic heterogeneity of Usher syndrome type II. *J Med Genet* 30:843–848, 1993.

69. Pieke-Dahl SA et al: Genetic heterogeneity of Usher syndrome type II: localisation to chromosome 5q. *J Med Genet* 37:256–262, 2000.

70. Pinckers A et al: The electrooculogram in heterozygote carriers of Usher syndrome, retinitis pigmentosa, neuronal ceroid lipofuscinosis, senior syndrome and choroideremia. *Ophthalm Genet* 15:25–30, 1994.

71. Schaefer GB et al: Volumetric neuroimaging in Usher syndrome: evidence of global involvement. *Am J Med Genet* 79:1–4, 1998.

72. Shinkawa H, Nadol J: Histopathology of the inner ear in Usher's syndrome as observed by light and electron microscopy. *Ann Otol Rhinol Laryngol* 95:313–318, 1986.

73. Shiomi Y et al: Cortical activity of a patient with Usher's syndrome using a cochlear implant. *Am J Otolaryngol* 18:412–414, 1997.

74. Siebenmann F, Bing R: Über den Labyrinth und Hirnbefund bei einem an retinitis pigmentosa erblindeten Angeboren-taubstummen. *Z Ohrenheilkd* 54:265–280, 1907.

75. Smith RJ et al: Clinical diagnosis of the Usher syndromes. Usher Syndrome Consortium. *Am J Med Genet* 50:32–38, 1994.

76. Sondheimer S et al: Dark adaptation testing in heterozygotes of Usher's syndrome. *Br J Ophthalmol* 63:547–550, 1979.

77. Tamayo ML et al: Usher syndrome: results of a screening program in Colombia. *Clin Genet* 40:304–311, 1991.

78. Tamayo ML et al: Neuroradiology and clinical aspects of Usher syndrome. *Clin Genet* 50:126–132, 1996.

79. Tuck RR, McLeod JG: Retinitis pigmentosa, ataxia, and peripheral neuropathy. *J Neurol Neurosurg Psychiatry* 46:206–213, 1983.

80. Usher CH: On the inheritance of retinitis pigmentosa with notes of cases. *R Lond Ophthalmol Hosp Rev* 19:130–236, 1914.

81. van Aarem A et al: Stable and progressive hearing loss in type 2A Usher's syndrome. *Ann Otol Rhinol Laryngol* 105:962–967, 1996.

82. van Aarem A et al: Semen analysis in the Usher syndrome type 2A. *J Otorhinolaryngol Relat Spec* 61:126–130, 1999.

83. Vernon M: Usher's syndrome: deafness and progressive blindness. Clinical cases, prevention, theory and literature survey. *J Chronic Dis* 22:133–151, 1969.

84. Verpy E et al: A defect in harmonin, a PDZ domain–containing protein expressed in the inner ear sensory hair cells, underlies Usher syndrome type 1C. *Nat Genet* 26:51–55, 2000.

85. von Brederlow B et al: Identification and in vitro expression of novel *CDH23* mutations of patients with Usher syndrome type 1D. *Hum Mutat* 19:268–273, 2002.

86. von Graefe A: Exceptionelles Verhalten des Gesichtsfeldes bei Pigmententartung der Netzhaut. *Von Graefes Arch Klin Exp Ophthalmol* 4:250–253, 1858.

87. Wagenaar M et al: Clinical findings in obligate carriers of type I Usher syndrome. *Am J Med Genet* 59:375–379, 1995.

88. Wagenaar M et al: Histopathologic features of the temporal bone in Usher syndrome type I. *Arch Otolaryngol Head Neck Surg* 126:1018–1023, 2000.

89. Wang Q et al: Update on the molecular genetics of retinitis pigmentosa. *Ophthalm Genet* 22:133–154, 2001.

90. Weil D et al: Defective myosin VIIa gene responsible for Usher syndrome type 1B. *Nature* 374:60–61, 1995.

91. Weil D et al: The autosomal recessive isolated deafness, DFNB2, and the Usher 1B syndrome are allelic defects of the myosin-VIIA gene. *Nat Genet* 16:191–193, 1997.

92. Weston MD et al: A progress report on the localization of Usher syndrome type II to chromosome 1q. *Ann NY Acad Sci* 630:284–287, 1991.

93. Weston MD et al: Myosin VIIA mutation screening in 189 Usher syndrome type 1 patients. *Am J Hum Genet* 59:1074–1083, 1996.

94. Weston MD et al: Genomic structure and identification of novel mutations in *usherin*, the gene responsible for Usher syndrome type IIa. *Am J Hum Genet* 66:1199–1210, 2000.

95. Young NM et al: Cochlear implants in young children with Usher's syndrome. *Ann Otol Rhinol Laryngol* 104:342–345, 1995.

96. Zina ZB et al: From DFNB2 to Usher syndrome: variable expressivity of the same disease. *Am J Med Genet* 101:181–183, 2001.

97. Zwaenepoel I et al: Identification of three novel mutations in the *USH1C* gene and detection of thirty-one polymorphisms used for haplotype analysis. *Hum Mutat* 17:34–41, 2001.

Alström syndrome: pigmentary retinopathy, diabetes mellitus, obesity, and sensorineural hearing loss

In 1959, Alström et al. (1) described a syndrome characterized by atypical retinal degeneration with loss of central vision, adult diabetes mellitus, transient early obesity, normal intelligence, and progressive sensorineural hearing loss. The sibs described by Boenheim (5) in 1929 are possible early examples.

Physical findings. Mild to moderate truncal obesity, a constant feature, appears in children between 2 and 10 years but lessens with age (25) (Fig. 7–2A,B). Maximum adult heights for males and females have been 65 inches (165 cm) and 63 inches (160 cm), respectively (32). Alter and Moshang (2) have suggested that the short stature is based, at least in some cases, on growth hormone deficiency, while advanced bone age and early *normal* growth velocity are related to hyperinsulinism.

Ocular system. Severe photophobia and nystagmus are often the first signs, occurring frequently in infancy (29). Visual loss is progressive; initially there is night blindness which is followed by loss of peripheral vision. Early retinal changes include optic atrophy, marked vascular attenuation, and salt-and-pepper pigment epithelial abnormalities. Later there are diffuse chorioretinal atrophy and large clumping of pigment with loss of central vision. The bone spicule pigmentation of retinitis pigmentosa is not present (25). Severe visual loss within the first decade is characteristic. Posterior subcapsular cataracts of mild to moderate degree appear during the second decade, as may dislocated lenses and glaucoma (1,16,20,25,32,35). The pupils become nonreactive to light late in the first decade or early in the second decade. Electroretinography (ERG) shows profoundly abnormal rod and cone function (1,32,33). Cone dysfunction is manifest by ERG as early as 6 months of age, rod dysfunction by 5 years (24,33).

Integumentary system. Premature baldness in males and scanty hair or cicatricial alopecia in females have been found in about 50% (16,25). Acanthosis nigricans, principally involving the axillae, has been noted in 60% of cases but has been relatively mild (7,13,18,25). This appears to be related to insulin resistance (26).

Central nervous system. Neurologic findings, except for visual and hearing loss, have been normal. Intelligence has been

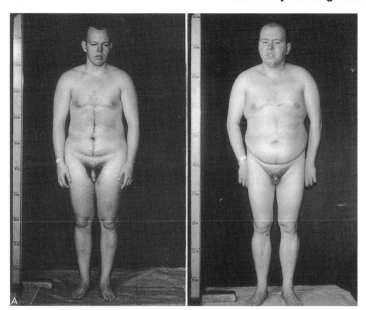
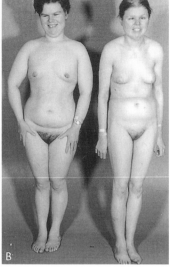
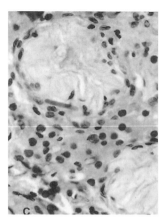
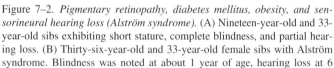

Figure 7–2. *Pigmentary retinopathy, diabetes mellitus, obesity, and sensorineural hearing loss (Alström syndrome).* (A) Nineteen-year-old and 33-year-old sibs exhibiting short stature, complete blindness, and partial hearing loss. (B) Thirty-six-year-old and 33-year-old female sibs with Alström syndrome. Blindness was noted at about 1 year of age, hearing loss at 6 years; partial alopecia began at 20 years of age. Both had difficulties with their menses. Patient at left is wearing a wig. (C) Photomicrograph of testicular specimen showing pale hyalinized tubules. Also note crystalloid of Reinke. [(A,C) from RL Weinstein et al., *N Engl J Med* 281:969, 1969; (B) from JL Goldstein and PJ Fialkow, *Medicine* 52:53, 1973.]

within normal limits in all cases (see Edwards retinopathy syndrome, below).

Endocrine system. Diabetes mellitus has been noted in 75%–80% of cases. Males have small, soft testes with small or normal-sized phalluses. Females have abnormal menstrual history (oligomenorrhea, hypermenorrhea, dysmenorrhea, metromenorrhagia) and sparse axillary and pubic hair but do not have hypogonadism. Neither male nor female patients have produced any offspring. Growth hormone deficiency has been demonstrated (2) and hypothyroidism has been observed in one case (8).

Genitourinary system. Renal dysfunction, the most variable aspect of the syndrome, has been noted in 80% (25). Nephropathy has ranged from mild, exhibiting only impaired glomerular and tubular function manifested by albuminuria, aminoaciduria, and inability to concentrate the urine, to severe, resulting in death (16,25,30). Onset of renal problems may be as early as the second decade (1,16,25).

Musculoskeletal system. Scoliosis (16,20,21,25) in 40% and hyperostosis frontalis interna (15,19,22) have been documented.

Cardiovascular system. Dilated cardiomyopathy can be observed at any age and is an important cause of mortality (14,24,29,34,36). Early signs of heart disease might be detected by EKG as a nonspecific T-wave abnormality (34). In some patients, neonatal presentation of dilated cardiomyopathy may be the presenting sign (W. Reardon, personal communication).

Auditory system. Sensorineural hearing loss is a constant feature. It first becomes evident at about 5 years of age and progresses, becoming moderately severe in the second and third decades (13,36). Békésy, tone-decay, and SISI tests are consistent with a cochlear involvement (16); however, otoacoustic emission (OAE) and brain stem response (ABR) testing, which are critical to proving this assertion, have not been reported.

Vestibular system. No vestibular studies have been reported.

Gastrointestinal system. Hepatic dysfunction and liver cirrhosis have been reported (3,4,27).

Laboratory findings. Diabetes mellitus occurs in 75%–80% of cases (25) with carbohydrate intolerance usually becoming manifest in the third decade (35). Renal impairment is indicated by elevated BUN, albuminuria, nephrogenic or vasopressin-resistant diabetes mellitus, and elevated serum uric acid levels. Hypertriglyceridemia has been found in several cases (25,30,35). Hypercholesterolemia has been reported (37). 17-Ketosteroid levels are decreased and gonadotropin levels are increased in males. Plasma testosterone levels are low. There is insulin resistance but insulin-receptor binding appears to be in the normal range and insulin stimulation of glucose uptake and RNA synthesis is normal (28).

Pathology. Testicular biopsy has shown small hyalinized tubules with occasional Leydig and Sertoli cells and thickening of the lamina propria (36) (Fig. 7–2C). Biopsy of the ovaries of a 16-year-old girl dying of unstated causes showed no abnormalities. Histologic sections of the kidneys have exhibited chronic nephropathy manifested by thickening of glomerular and tubular membranes. Many glomeruli were hyalinized (1,25,32).

Heredity. In all cases, the parents of affected children have been normal. The occurrence of the syndrome in sibs of both sexes and the increased rate of consanguinity are compatible with autosomal recessive inheritance. The gene has been localized to 2p12–13 (10,11,14,23,37) and identified as a large gene called *ALMS1* of unknown function (12,17). There is no linkage evidence for genetic heterogeneity of Alström syndrome (14).

Diagnosis. Laurence-Moon syndrome is characterized by retinitis pigmentosa, mental retardation, hypogenitalism, and spastic paraplegia. Those with Bardet-Biedl syndrome show obesity and retinitis pigmentosa in association with polydactyly, hypogonadism, and mental retardation. Individuals with Alström syndrome do not have mental retardation or polydactyly. Deafness and diabetes mellitus are seen in no more than 5% of patients with Laurence-Moon or Bardet-Biedl syndrome (6,15,31). Furthermore, age of onset of total blindness is before the second decade in Alström syndrome, in contrast to onset in the fourth decade in the Laurence-Moon and Bardet-Biedl syndromes, and the eye findings differ. In Edwards retinopathy syndrome, affected sibs exhibited pigmentary retinopathy, hypogonadism, sensorineural hearing loss, and glucose intolerance, but they were mentally retarded. Burn (6) extensively reviewed the literature prior to 1950. There were several cases that overlapped with Edwards syndrome and Laurence-Moon syndrome (Table 7–2). Codaccione (9) reported the two brothers with infantile diabetes, optic atrophy, hypogonadism, and sensorineural deafness; this may represent a separate syndrome, since there was no evidence of retinitis pigmentosa but there is certainly overlap with DIDMOAD syndrome.

Treatment. Growth hormone replacement was performed in two cases with the result of increased growth velocity as well as a beneficial effect on lipoprotein metabolism (37).

Prognosis. Little hope can be offered to these patients, since vision and hearing deteriorate progressively. Intelligence, however, remains normal. The life span may be shortened by renal dysfunction.

Summary. Characteristics of this syndrome include (*1*) autosomal recessive inheritance; (*2*) onset of atypical retinal degeneration with loss of central vision in infancy; (*3*) onset of diabetes mellitus in childhood; (*4*) transient obesity; (*5*) onset of posterior cortical cataract in second decade; (*6*) onset of nephropathy in the third decade; (*7*) acanthosis nigricans; and (*8*) onset of progressive sensorineural hearing loss in late childhood.

References

1. Alström CH: Retinal degeneration combined with obesity, diabetes mellitus and neurogenous deafness. *Acta Psychiatr Neurol Scand* 34(Suppl 129):1–35. 1959.
2. Alter CA, Moshang T: Growth hormone deficiency in two siblings with Alström syndrome. *Am J Dis Child* 147:97–99, 1993.
3. Awazu M et al: A 27-year-old woman with Alström syndrome who had liver cirrhosis. *Keio J Med* 44:67–73, 1995.
4. Awazu M et al: Hepatic dysfunction in two sibs with Alström syndrome: case report and review of the literature. *Am J Med Genet* 69:13–16, 1997.
5. Boenheim F: Zur Kenntnis der Laurence-Biedlschen Krankheit (cases 3,4). *Endokrinologie* 4:263–273, 1929.
6. Burn RA: Deafness and the Laurence-Moon-Biedl syndrome. *Br J Ophthalmol* 34:65–88, 1950.
7. Chang KW et al: Alström syndrome with hepatic dysfunction: report of one case. *Acta Paediatr Taiwan* 41:270–272, 2000.
8. Charles SJ et al: Alström's syndrome: further evidence of autosomal recessive inheritance and endocrinological dysfunction. *J Med Genet* 27:590–592, 1990.
9. Codaccione JL: Hypotrophie testiculaire primitive chez deux frères atteints de diabete infantile, atrophie optique familial et surdité neurogogène póur l'un. *Ann Endocrinol (Paris)* 30:669–676, 1969.
10. Collin GB et al: Homozygosity mapping at Alström syndrome to chromosome 2p. *Hum Mol Genet* 6:213–219, 1997.
11. Collin GB et al: Alström syndrome: further evidence for linkage to human chromosome 2p13. *Hum Genet* 105:474–479, 1999.
12. Collin GB et al: Mutations in *ALMS1* cause obesity, type 2 diabetes and neurosensory degeneration in Alström syndrome. *Nat Genet* 31:74–78, 2002.
13. Connolly MB et al: Hepatic dysfunction in Alström disease. *Am J Med Genet* 40:421–424, 1991.
14. Deeble VJ et al: The continuing failure to recognise Alström syndrome and further evidence of genetic homogeneity. *J Med Genet* 37:219, 2000.
15. Garstecki DC et al: Speech, language, and hearing problems in the Laurence-Moon-Biedl syndrome. *J Speech Hear Disord* 37:407–413, 1972.
16. Goldstein JL, Fialkow PJ: The Alström syndrome. Report of three cases with further delineation of the clinical, pathophysiological, and genetic aspects of the disorder. *Medicine (Baltimore)* 52:53–71, 1973.
17. Hearn T et al: Mutation of *ALMS1*, a large gene with a tandem repeat encoding 47 amino acids, causes Alström syndrome. *Nat Genet* 31:79–83, 2002.
18. Hung YJ et al: Alström syndrome in two siblings. *J Formos Med Assoc* 100:45–49, 2001.
19. Johnson J: Diabetes, neurogenous deafness and retinal degeneration. *BMJ* 2:646, 1961.
20. Klein D, Ammann F: The syndrome of Laurence-Moon-Bardet-Biedl and allied diseases in Switzerland. Clinical, genetic and epidemiological studies. *J Neurol Sci* 9:479–513, 1969.
21. Kopecky A et al: Alström's syndrome in two sisters [in Czech]. *Cas Lek Cesk* 117:921–923, 1978.
22. Lista GA et al: El sindrome de Alström. *Prensa Med Argent* 59:253–254, 1972.
23. Macari F et al: Refinement of genetic localization of the Alström syndrome on chromosome 2p12–13 by linkage analysis in a North African family. *Hum Genet* 103:658–661, 1998.
24. Michaud JL et al: Natural history of Alström syndrome in early childhood: onset with dilated cardiomyopathy. *J Pediatr* 128:225–229, 1996.
25. Millay RH et al: Ophthalmologic and systemic manifestations of Alström's disease. *Am J Ophthalmol* 102:482–490, 1986.
26. Pfeiffer RA, Pusch R: *Das Syndrom von Alström. Klinische Genetik in der Paediatrie.* Stuttgart: Theime, 1979.
27. Quiros-Tejeira RE et al: Early-onset liver disease complicated with acute liver failure in Alström syndrome. *Am J Med Genet* 101:9–11, 2001.
28. Rudiger HW et al: Impaired insulin-induced RNA synthesis secondary to a genetically defective insulin receptor. *Hum Genet* 69:76–78, 1985.
29. Russell-Eggitt IM et al: Alström syndrome. Report of 22 cases and literature review. *Ophthalmology* 105:1274–1280, 1998.
30. Satman I et al: Evaluation of insulin resistant diabetes mellitus in Alström syndrome: a long-term prospective follow-up of three siblings. *Diabetes Res Clin Pract* 56:189–196, 2002.
31. Schachat AP, Maumenee IH: Bardet-Biedl syndrome and related disorders. *Arch Ophthalmol* 100:285–288, 1982.
32. Sebag J et al: The Alström syndrome: ophthalmic histopathology and retinal ultrastructure. *Br J Ophthalmol* 68:494–501, 1984.
33. Tremblay F et al: Longitudinal study of the early electroretinographic changes in Alström's syndrome. *Am J Ophthalmol* 115:657–665, 1993.
34. Warren SE et al: Late onset dilated cardiomyopathy in a unique familial syndrome of hypogonadism and metabolic abnormalities. *Am Heart J* 114:1522–1524, 1987.
35. Weinstein RL et al: Familial syndrome of primary testicular insufficiency with normal virilization, blindness, deafness and metabolic abnormalities. *N Engl J Med* 281:969–977, 1969.
36. Worthley MI, Zeitz CJ: Case of Alström syndrome with late presentation dilated cardiomyopathy. *Intern Med J* 31:569–570, 2001.
37. Zumsteg U et al: Alström syndrome: confirmation of linkage to chromosome 2p12–13 and phenotypic heterogeneity in three affected sibs. *J Med Genet* 37:E8, 2000.

Edwards retinopathy syndrome: pigmentary retinopathy, diabetes mellitus, hypogonadism, mental retardation, and sensorineural hearing loss

Edwards et al. (2) described four siblings, three males and one female, with pigmentary retinopathy, obesity, diabetes mellitus, hypogonadism, and sensorineural hearing loss. The disorder closely resembles Alström syndrome, but those affected were mentally retarded. Subsequently, a set of male and female sibs (1) were described.

Physical findings. Adult height was below 57 inches in females and below 66 inches in males. Obesity was mild to moderate. Scoliosis was noted in one patient.

Ocular system. As in Alström syndrome, visual impairment, heralded by nystagmus and photophobia, appeared within the first year of life, the children often being blind by age 5 years. Night blindness was absent.

Central nervous system. All affected individuals exhibited mild to moderate (IQ 40–65) mental retardation. Altered peripheral reflexes were found.

Integumentary system. Acanthosis nigricans was evident in all those affected.

Endocrine findings. In females, menarche occurred at a normal time but later there was oligomenorrhea. Affected males had gynecomastia, small testes, and mild subvirilization. Mild to moderate childhood-onset obesity was characteristic. Diabetes mellitus has been found in half the patients. In the first kindred studied (2), one sibling had diabetes mellitus, another had abnormal glucose tolerance, and two had hyperinsulinemia.

Auditory system. Sensorineural hearing loss was noted by 8–10 years and slowly progressed to a 60–75 dB loss (2).

Laboratory findings. Males had elevated plasma luteinizing hormone (LH) and follicle-stimulating hormone (FSH) levels (1,2).

Pathology. Polycystic ovaries were found in one female (1).

Heredity. Inheritance is clearly autosomal recessive.

Diagnosis. Edwards syndrome most closely resembles pigmentary retinopathy, diabetes mellitus, obesity, and sensorineural hearing loss (Alström syndrome), but it differs in having associated psychomotor retardation and lacking cataracts, nephropathy, and baldness (see Table 7–2).

Prognosis. No feature aside from the sensory impairments would be expected to shorten life span.

Summary. Characteristics of this syndrome include (*1*) autosomal recessive inheritance; (*2*) onset in infancy of nystagmus, photophobia, and progressive blindness; (*3*) developmental delay and mild to moderate mental retardation; (*4*) childhood-onset obesity; (*5*) sometimes acanthosis nigricans, diabetes mellitus, and male hypogonadism; and (*6*) onset in late childhood of progressive sensorineural hearing loss.

References:

1. Boor R et al: Familial insulin resistant diabetes associated with acanthosis nigricans, polycystic ovaries, hypogonadism, pigmentary retinopathy, labyrinthine deafness, and mental retardation. *Am J Med Genet* 45:649–653, 1993.
2. Edwards JA et al: A new familial syndrome characterized by pigmentary retinopathy, hypogonadism, mental retardation, nerve deafness and glucose intolerance. *Am J Med* 60:23–32, 1976.

Young syndrome: retinitis pigmentosa, nystagmus, hemiplegic migraine, and sensorineural hearing loss

In 1970, Young et al. (7) reported a syndrome in four members of a family who were affected by hemiplegic migraine and nystagmus. Two of these individuals also had sensorineural hearing loss and retinitis pigmentosa.

Ocular system. Prior to the migraine attack, the altered vision consisted of a sensation of whirling lights, blurred vision, and dark spots in all fields of vision. Upon clearing, this was followed by headache on the side contralateral to the hemiparesis. Jerking nystagmus was permanently present in all affected persons. Night blindness, constricted visual fields, and retinitis pigmentosa were noted in one patient, whereas still another exhibited nystagmus and mild ataxia; neither had migraine or deafness. One patient had bilateral posterior subcapsular cataracts.

Central nervous system. Hemiplegic migraine, a throbbing, vascular headache preceded by sensory and motor phenomena that persisted during and for a brief time after the headache, appeared around the age of 4–5 years in three of four patients and recurred three or more times a year. In the other patient, it first appeared at 10 years of age. Prior to a migraine attack, there was dizziness or light-headedness or a feeling of tightness in one limb. These symptoms occurred simultaneously or in rapid succession and lasted from 15 to 90 minutes. Patients also experienced numbness that began in one hand or foot and spread to half the body, which was followed by severe weakness on the ipsilateral side. This disappeared upon cessation of the headache. The duration of the attacks varied from 12 hours to 5 days. Headache was bilateral in three patients and unilateral in the other patient. During the headache, sensorimotor hemiparesis was present in four individuals, nausea and vomiting were present in three patients, and ataxia and hemiplegia in only one patient. The latter patient had permanent mild ataxia of gait.

Auditory system. Hearing loss was first noted at 4–6 years of age. Bilateral sensorineural hearing loss of 70–80 dB in the frequency ranges of 750–4000 Hz was demonstrated. There was good discrimination bilaterally, no tone decay, and type II Békésy audiograms.

Vestibular system. Vestibular studies were not mentioned.

Laboratory findings. Blood, urine, and cerebrospinal fluid analyses were normal. Electroencephalograms made within 72 hours of the attack of migraine showed a slow-wave abnormality, which subsequently disappeared (Fig. 7–3A,B).

Heredity. This report may simply represent the simultaneous occurrence of two or more disorders in this family, i.e., Usher syndrome, hemiplegic migraine, and familial nystagmus. If the syndrome is unique, it is probably inherited as an autosomal dominant trait with variable expression.

Diagnosis. Retinitis pigmentosa may occur as an isolated finding or may be associated with a plethora of syndromes. Those syndromes in which both hearing loss and retinitis pigmentosa occur are considered in Table 7–2. Retinitis pigmentosa has also been reported in association with migraine (4,5). Connor (4) and Bradshaw and Parsons (3) reviewed the extensive literature on complicated migraine but found no association with hearing loss. The recent finding of the calcium channel gene (*CACNA1A*) causing dominantly inherited familial hemiplegic migraine in addition to vestibular vertigo raises the possibility that certain mutations in such a gene may result in a cochlear defect in addition to migraine and vertigo (1,2). Ohta et al. (6) reported nystagmus and cerebellar manifestations in patients with hemiplegic migraine, but they noted no association with hearing loss.

Prognosis. Life span apparently is not shortened. The visual loss and hearing loss are progressive.

Summary. The characteristics of this syndrome include (*1*) possible autosomal dominant inheritance with variable expressivity; (*2*) retinitis pigmentosa; (*3*) hemiplegic migraine, preceded or accompanied by sensory and motor phenomena; (*4*) jerking nystagmus; and (*5*) severe sensorineural hearing loss.

Figure 7–3. *Retinitis pigmentosa, nystagmus, hemiplegic migraine, and sensorineural hearing loss (Young syndrome).* (A) Electroencephalogram 2 days after attack of migraine with temporary left hemiplegia. Note right hemispheric slow-wave abnormality. (B) Electroencephalogram, taken 10 weeks after a hemiplegic migraine attack, is almost normal. [(A,B) from GF Young et al., *Arch Neurol* 23:201, 1970.]

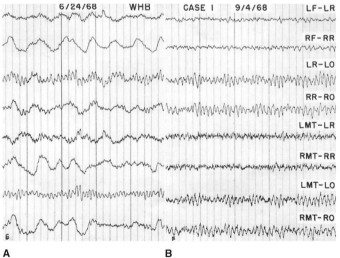

A   B

References

1. Baloh RW: Episodic vertigo: central nervous system causes. *Curr Opin Neurol* 15:17–21, 2002.
2. Baloh RW, Jen JC: Genetics of familial episodic vertigo and ataxia. *Ann NY Acad Sci* 956:338–345, 2002.
3. Bradshaw P, Parsons M: Hemiplegic migraine, a clinical study. *Q J Med* 34:65–85, 1965.
4. Connor RCR: Complicated migraine: a study of permanent neurological and visual defects caused by migraine. *Lancet* 2:1072–1075, 1962.
5. Friedman MW: Occlusion of central retinal vein in migraine. *Arch Ophthalmol* 45:678–682, 1951.
6. Ohta M et al: Familial occurrence of migraine with hemiplegic syndrome and cerebellar manifestations. *Neurology (Minneap)* 17:813–817, 1967.
7. Young GF et al: Familial hemiplegic migraine, retinal degeneration, deafness, and nystagmus. *Arch Neurol* 23:201–209, 1970.

Usher syndrome with vitiligo: retinitis pigmentosa, vitiligo, and sensorineural hearing loss

In 1989, Dereymaeker et al. (4) described the association of retinitis pigmentosa, vitiligo, and sensorineural hearing loss in two unrelated patients. Their first patient presented with severe early-onset sensorineural hearing loss associated with vitiligo and retinitis pigmentosa, both developing late in the second decade. Furthermore, this patient was hypotonic; hypotonia is frequently associated with vestibular areflexia seen with subtypes of Usher type I. The second patient had a bilateral high-frequency sensorineural hearing loss, possibly progressive but distinctly different from the first case, and retinitis pigmentosa with onset in the third decade, vitiligo, and axonal polyneuropathy of the lower limbs. A younger sib had only retinitis pigmentosa and sensorineural hearing loss. The lack of additional findings in the younger sib, plus the fact that the configuration of the audiogram fits one characteristic of Usher type II, suggests that this may have been a case of that syndrome with a chance association of the vitiligo and polyneuropathy.

Gordon (5) reported tapetoretinal degeneration, vitiligo, and sensorineural hearing loss. Alezzandrini (1) also described two unrelated patients: a female who developed retinitis pigmentosa, vitiligo, poliosis, and sensorineural hearing loss after the age of 30 years and a male who exhibited bilateral 30 dB hearing loss after age 20. Cowan et al. (3) reported a female with severe bilateral sensorineural hearing loss from the age of 2 years who developed retinitis pigmentosa in her mid-teens, hypothyroidism in the third decade, and vitiligo and alopecia after the age of 50. Retinitis pigmentosa and sensorineural hearing loss were present in her three sisters, a finding suggesting again that this may be a case of Usher syndrome in combination with an autoimmune disorder. Cernea and Damien (2) reported on a single case of association of vitiligo with RP and hearing loss.

The variability in the severity of the hearing loss suggests that these patients represent examples of different Usher syndrome subtypes with incidental autoimmunity (vitiligo, hypothyroidism, and alopecia). There may be the some relationship of some of the above cases to Vogt-Harada-Koyanagi syndrome.

References

1. Alezzandrini AA: Manifestation unilatérale de dégénérescence tapéto-rétinienne, de vitiligo, de poliose, de cheveux blancs et d'hypoacousie. *Ophthalmologica* 147:409–419, 1964.
2. Cernea P, Damien C: Retinitis pigmentosa, vitiligo and deaf-mutism. Apropos of a case [in French]. *J Fr Ophtalmol* 17:501–503, 1994.
3. Cowan CL et al: Retinitis pigmentosa associated with hearing loss, thyroid disease, vitiligo, and alopecia areata: retinitis pigmentosa and vitiligo. *Retina* 2:84–88, 1982.
4. Dereymaeker AM et al: Retinitis pigmentosa, hearing loss and vitiligo: report of two patients. *Clin Genet* 35:387–389, 1989.
5. Gordon DM: Retinitis pigmentosa "sine pigmento" associated with vitiligo of skin. *Arch Ophthalmol* 50:372–375, 1953.

Hersh syndrome: pigmentary retinopathy, unusual facial phenotype, mental retardation, and sensorineural hearing loss

In 1982, Hersh et al. (1) described male and female sibs with mental retardation, pigmentary retinopathy, unusual facies, and sensorineural hearing loss.

Physical findings. Both sibs were at the fifth percentile for height and weight, but head circumference was essentially normal. Both children had abnormally small feet.

Craniofacial findings. Both patients had frontal bossing with open anterior fontanel. The palpebral fissures were downslanting, especially in the male. Both exhibited midface hypoplasia, flattened nasal bridge, small nose, and low-set pinnae (Fig. 7–4).

Ocular findings. In addition to downslanting palpebral fissures, the male exhibited bilateral esotropia and nystagmus. Funduscopic abnormalities were more marked in the male sib, but both had salt-and-pepper retinal alterations, macular granularity with slight vessel narrowing, and normal optic discs.

Genitourinary findings. The external genitalia of the male were somewhat underdeveloped; penile length was 3.75 cm and testes were undescended.

Neuromuscular findings. Both sibs manifested generalized muscular hypotonia. At 4 years, the male sib was estimated to have a mental age of 12 months, and at 2 years, the female had that of a 9-month-old.

Auditory findings. The male had a 90 dB loss and his sister had a 60–70 dB sensorineural hearing loss. Hearing loss was confirmed by brain stem audiometry.

Vestibular findings. Although no vestibular studies were reported, it seems likely that the vestibular system was involved because of the late age of walking displayed by both children.

Heredity. Inheritance is probably autosomal recessive.

Laboratory findings. Laboratory findings were essentially unremarkable.

Figure 7–4. *Pigmentary retinopathy, unusual facies, mental retardation, and sensorineural hearing loss.* Affected sibs were short with frontal bossing, downslanting palpebral fissures, midface hypoplasia, flat nasal bridge, small nose, and low-set pinnae. [From JH Hersh et al., *Birth Defects* 18(3B): 175, 1982.]

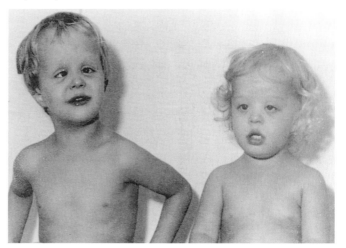

Diagnosis. One must exclude other syndromes of pigmentary retinopathy (see Table 7–2).

Summary. Characteristics of this syndrome include (*1*) autosomal recessive inheritance; (*2*) mental retardation; (*3*) unusual facies; (*4*) pigmentary retinopathy; (*5*) mild hypogonadism; (*6*) hypotonia; and (*7*) marked sensorineural hearing loss.

References

1. Hersh JH et al: Pigmentary retinopathy, hearing loss, mental retardation, and dysmorphism in sibs: a new syndrome? *Birth Defects* 18:175–182, 1982.

Cutis verticis gyrata, retinitis pigmentosa, and sensorineural deafness

Megarbane et al. (1) described two brothers with this combination.

Ocular system. Vision impairment became evident after 10 years of age, with night blindness noted after age 20 years. Ophthalmologic evaluations identified cortical or central and posterior subcapsular cataracts. Electroretinograms were completely flat.

Central nervous system. Mental retardation was present. Microcephaly affected both, and cutis verticis gyrata (scalp folds and furrows) developed around the age of 40 years (Fig. 7–5).

Auditory system. Hearing loss was sensorineural and described as ranging from moderate to profound, and differed between the two ears in each brother. It developed after the age of 20 years.

Heredity. The occurrence of this condition in two brothers suggests autosomal recessive inheritance.

Diagnosis. This condition superficially resembles the Usher syndromes, although the presence of microcephaly and mental retardation should distinguish it from Usher syndrome. Linkage studies ruled out linkage to the USH2A, USH2B, USH2C, and USH3 loci.

Prognosis. Hearing loss and vision loss are progressive. Mental retardation is severe.

Summary. This condition is characterized by (*1*) retinitis pigmentosa after age 20; (*2*) sensorineural hearing loss after age 20; (*3*) microcephaly with adult-onset cutis verticis gyrata; and (*4*) autosomal recessive inheritance.

Reference

1. Megarbane A et al: Microcephaly, cutis verticis gyrata of the scalp, retinitis pigmentosa, cataracts, sensorineural deafness, and mental retardation in two brothers. *Am J Med Genet* 98:244–249, 2001.

Choroideremia and congenital hearing loss with stapes fixation

McCulloch (8) reported several cases of choroideremia, some of which occured in association with deafness. Since then, several cases have been described (1,6,7,10,12,15). The recent discoveries of the juxtaposition of the gene for X-linked choroideremia (CHM; MIM 303100) and mixed hearing loss with stapes fixation and perilymphatic gusher (DFN3 or POU3F4, MIM 304400) have made it evident that the concurrence of the retinal and cochlear symptoms is due to the contiguity of their respective genes on Xq21 (9).

Ocular system. All patients manifested poor night vision from childhood. Chorioretinal atrophy and intraretinal pigmentary clumps without spicule configuration were found in all those affected. The choriocapillaris was absent in the involved areas. Female heterozygotes had milder but distinctive ocular changes (1).

Auditory system. Patients have a congenital and bilateral, mixed (conductive and sensorineural) hearing loss (1,6,9). The *POU3F4* gene involved is the same gene known to cause a perilymphatic gusher that has been observed in many cases with a defective *POU3F4* gene (2,4,14). Some female heterozygotes are reported to have a mild hearing loss (3,14). Reardon et al. (13) performed high-resolution CT scanning of the cochlea in two boys with Xq21 deletions and hearing loss. They found evidence of a bulbous internal auditory meatus that was incompletely separated from the basal bony coil of the cochlea and a dilated facial nerve canal. This was identical to the radiological malformation identified in several families segregating X-linked deafness and known to map to Xq21 (12). Reardon et al. suggested that the phenomenon of perilymphatic gusher may occur in individuals with more extensive clinical findings beyond X-linked hearing loss and could occur in any individual with an Xq21 deletion.

Metabolic findings. Ayazi (1) reported this disorder in combination with obesity, but without any evidence of diabetes mellitus; this family was subsequently found to have a deletion of Xq21 (5,9).

Neurologic findings. Two affected males in one family (9) were intellectually retarded and had an EEG that showed nonspecific slowing without epileptiform discharges. Other cases were similar and have had a deletions comparable to that in Merry's (10) case (7,11,15). The

Figure 7–5. *Cutis verticis gyrata, retinitis pigmentosa, and sensorineural deafness.* (A) Facial phenotype, note hypertelorism, exotropia, and large nose. (B) Anteroposterior and transverse ridges and furrows on the scalp, primarily on the right side. (C) Sloping forehead, hypertelorism, exotropia, large nose. (D) Cutis gyrata. [From A Megarbane et al., *Am J Med Genet* 98:245–246, 2001, reprinted by permission of Wiley-Liss, Inc., a subsidiary of John Wiley & Sons, Inc.]

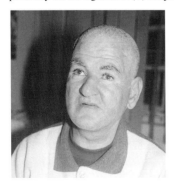
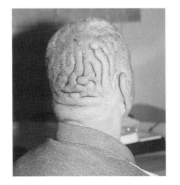
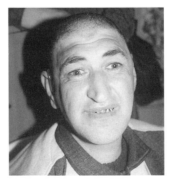
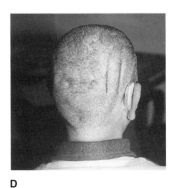

A   B   C   D

association with mental retardation is likely due to the deletion of another contiguous gene distal to DFN3 (7).

Heredity. Inheritance is X-linked and the disorder represents a contiguous gene deletion syndrome involving the choroideremia gene and the gene for mixed hearing loss with perilymphatic gusher. A female with a translocation between Xq21 and chromosome 4 displayed hearing and ocular symptoms that were taken to be an indication that the normal X was preferentially inactivated (6).

Diagnosis. This a contiguous gene deletion syndrome, which includes the gene for X-linked sensorineural hearing loss with gusher association. The diagnosis can be made by showing a deletion either cytogenetically or by FISH.

Summary. Characteristics of this condition include (1) X-linked inheritance with milder expression in female heterozygotes; (2) obesity; (3) choroideremia; and (4) congenital sensorineural or mixed hearing loss.

References

1. Ayazi S: Choroideremia, obesity, and congenital deafness. *Am J Ophthalmol* 92:63–69, 1981.
2. Cremers CW: Audiologic features of the X-linked progressive mixed deafness syndrome with perilymphatic gusher during stapes gusher. *Am J Otol* 6:243–246, 1985.
3. Cremers CW, Huygen PL: Clinical features of female heterozygotes in the X-linked mixed deafness syndrome (with perilymphatic gusher during stapes surgery). *Int J Pediatr Otorhinolaryngol* 6:179–185, 1983.
4. Cremers CW et al: X-linked progressive mixed deafness with perilymphatic gusher during stapes surgery. *Arch Otolaryngol* 111:249–254, 1985.
5. Cremers FP et al: Physical fine mapping of the choroideremia locus using Xq21 deletions associated with complex syndromes. *Genomics* 4:41–46, 1989.
6. Lorda-Sanchez IJ et al: Choroideremia, sensorineural deafness, and primary ovarian failure in a woman with a balanced X-4 translocation. *Ophthalm Genet* 21:185–189, 2000.
7. May M et al: Molecular analysis of four males with mental retardation and deletions of Xq21 places the putative MR region in Xq21.1 between DXS233 and CHM. *Hum Mol Genet* 4:1465–1466, 1995.
8. McCulloch CMRJP: An hereditary and clinical study of choroideremia. *Trans Am Acad Ophthalmol Otolaryngol* 52:160–190, 1948.
9. Merry DE et al: Choroideremia and deafness with stapes fixation: a contiguous gene deletion syndrome in Xq21. *Am J Hum Genet* 45:530–540, 1989.
10. Merry DE et al: DXS165 detects a translocation breakpoint in a woman with choroideremia and a de novo X; 13 translocation. *Genomics* 6:609–615, 1990.
11. Nussbaum RL et al: Isolation of anonymous DNA sequences from within a submicroscopic X chromosomal deletion in a patient with choroideremia, deafness, and mental retardation. *Proc Natl Acad Sci USA* 84:6521–6525, 1987.
12. Phelps PD et al: X-linked deafness, stapes gusher and a distinctive defect of the inner ear. *Neuroradiology* 33:326–330, 1991.
13. Reardon W et al: Phenotypic evidence for a common pathogenesis in X-linked deafness pedigrees and in Xq13–q21 deletion related deafness. *Am J Med Genet* 44:513–517, 1992.
14. Reardon W et al: Neuro-otological function in X-linked hearing loss: a multipedigre assessment and correlation with other clinical parameters. *Acta Otolaryngol* 113:706–714, 1993.
15. Rosenberg T et al: Choroideremia, congenital deafness and mental retardation in a family with an X chromosomal deletion. *Ophthalm Paediatr Genet* 8:139–143, 1987.

Adult Refsum syndrome (ARD, heredopathia atactica polyneuritiformis)

In 1946, Refsum (30) first extensively described a syndrome characterized by retinitis pigmentosa, hypertrophic peripheral neuropathy with both motor and sensory losses, and, at times, sensorineural hearing loss and/or ichthyosis. Phytanic acid accumulation because of defective α-oxidative capacity of phytanic acid was first identified by Klenk and

Kahlke (20) in 1963. An early example is that of Thiébaut et al. (37). Excellent reviews are provided by Refsum and Stokke (32) and Wanders et al. (40). Infantile Refsum syndrome (IRD), while having some similarities with ARD, is phenotypically and genetically distinct.

Physical findings. In most cases, the patient appears normal until the late teen years when failing night vision and unsteadiness of gait become apparent. Progression is slow but continuous so that in the late stages, there are generalized wasting, severe paralysis, and generalized mild ichthyosis (Fig. 7–6A). In undiagnosed, untreated cases, death may result from cardiac complications, mainly arrhythmias due to heart block. The condition may be aggravated by pregnancy (11).

Ocular system. Visual loss is one of the first symptoms of the syndrome. Night blindness, first noted during the second decade, is slowly progressive. Visual fields slowly constrict and there is miosis and hemeralopia. Among 17 patients documented by Skjeldal et al. (35), these were constant features. Examination of the fundi reveals pale discs and mildly increased "salt-and-pepper," less often "bone spicule," retinal pigmentation that is most marked in the macular area and peripheral retina (16). The retinal vessels appear narrower. Posterior and capsular cataracts have been found in about 70% of patients (33,35).

Central nervous system. Anosmia and weakness may be noted in childhood or in early adult years. The weakness especially affects the legs, but eventually also the arms, and with progression results in muscle wasting and paralysis (Fig. 7–6B). During childhood, the distal extremities may exhibit numbness to pinprick and touch. Tendon reflexes may decrease almost to extinction. In a review of 37 patients, Richterich et al. (33), found the following signs in decreasing order: anosmia, paresthesias, pain, and lack of superficial reflexes. Skjeldal et al. (35) and Gibberd et al. (13) noted polyneuropathy (atrophy, sensory disturbances, impaired deep reflexes) in nearly all patients, anosmia in 60%, and ataxia in only 30%.

Cardiovascular system. Twenty-five to eighty percent of two series of Refsum syndrome cases have been found to have heart disease (33,35) consisting of tachycardia, gallop rhythm, cardiac enlargement, and heart failure. Electrocardiographic abnormalities included increased P-Q interval, nodal and auricular extra systoles, and changes in the QRS complex.

Musculoskeletal system. Bony changes were found in 50%–75% of patients and included spondylitis, kyphoscoliosis, hammer toes, and pes cavus, with an occasional shortening of a metapodial bone (21,24,33,35,39) (Fig. 7–6C,D).

Integumentary system. Approximately 50% exhibit ichthyosis, which clinically mimics ichthyosis vulgaris producing a wrinkled appearance of the skin. The scales are light and spare the big flexion areas and the palms and soles (Fig. 7–6E). Palmar creases may be accentuated. However, Davies et al. (7) described severe skin involvement and Puissant et al. (28) noted the occurrence of disseminated xanthomatous dermal nevus cell nevi.

Auditory system. Some degree of sensorineural hearing loss has been documented in about 80% of patients (4,10), with hearing loss often being initially asymmetric. The hearing loss is progressive. It begins in the second or third decade but may not become severe until the fourth decade (8), and especially affects the upper frequencies.

Vestibular system. Caloric vestibular tests have been normal (4).

Pathology. Histologic changes include interstitial polyneuritis and demyelination of the posterior columns of the spinal cord (9). There is marked accumulation of lipid in the meninges. In the cerebral cortex, the blood vessels are surrounded by numerous lipid-laden macrophages. The larger neurons of the central nervous system are somewhat enlarged by lipid granules in their cytoplasm. All peripheral nerves are

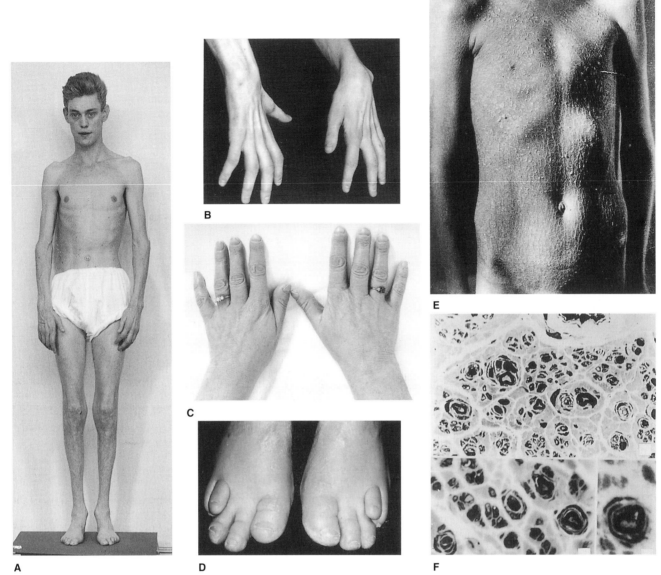

A   **D**   **F**

Figure 7–6. *Adult Refsum syndrome (heredopathia atactica polyneuriti-formis).* (A) Patient showing muscle wasting in lower legs. (B) Atrophy of hand muscles. (C) The hands of a female patient. Notice rather short fingers, very short end phalanges, and broad and short fingernails. Index finger is somewhat longer than middle finger. (D) Short fourth metatarsal. (E) Ichthyosis of skin. (F) Transverse section of nerve showing decreased numbers of myelinated fibers and proliferation of Schwann sheath. [(A,B,E) courtesy of S Refsum, Oslo, Norway; (C) from A Lundberg et al., *Eur Neurol* 8:309, 1972; (F) from M Fardeau and WK Engel, *J Neuropathol Exp Neurol* 28:278, 1969.]

diffusely enlarged. On histologic section, there are reduced numbers of fibrils in each nerve with marked "onion bulb" formation due to proliferation of Schwann cells (6,9,17) (Fig. 7–6F).

Temporal bone study has shown collapse of Reissner's membrane, degeneration of the stria vascularis, atrophy of the organ of Corti, and loss of spiral ganglion cells (15,29). Accumulation of fat in the liver, kidneys, heart, and retina has also been documented (1,6).

Skin biopsy of the ichthyotic areas is usually not striking, showing only a diminished granular layer and mild orthohyperkeratosis. However, lipid stains such as Sudan red exhibit vacuolated keratinocytes that contain multiple lipid droplets in the basal and suprabasal cells. The dermal nevus cell nevi are also vacuolated, preferentially storing phytanic acids. Ultrastructural study shows giant degenerated mitochondria (2).

Pathogenesis. Refsum syndrome is a peroxisomal disorder and involves a defect in the catabolism of phytanic acid. The peroxisomes in

fibroblasts are not reduced in number in the adult form (3), which suggests that the defect does not involve an absence or abnormality of the peroxisomes and is instead due to one or more enzyme deficiencies. Phytanic acid and a methylated fatty acid (3,7,11,15-tetramethylhexadecanoic acid) accumulate in various body tissues because of the failure of degradation of phytanic acid. Since humans cannot synthesize phytanic acid or its free phytol, the source of these substances is dietary. Degradation of these exogenous substances is through α-oxidation, since phytanic acid cannot undergo ordinary β-oxidation (4,5). Steinberg (36) demonstrated that phytanic acid oxidase deficiency does not allow phytanic acid to be degraded to hydroxyphytanic acid. It was subsequently shown that many, but not all, cases are caused by mutations in the gene *PAHX* (PHYH), which codes for peroxisomal oxygenase phytanoyl-CoA 2-hydroxylase. This substance catalyses the initial α-oxidation step in the degradation of phytanic acid (18,19,22). Recently cases not caused by *PAHX* mutations have been shown to be caused by mutations in *PEX7* (peroxin 7 receptor), which maps to

6q22–24. *PEX7* mutations are also responsible for causing rhizomelic chondrodysplasia punctata, a severe condition associated with death in infancy or early childhood (38).

Heredity. Inheritance is autosomal recessive. Most patients have been of Scandinavian origin. Parental consanguinity has been found in about 50% of the cases. Since onset of the disorder is often late, prenatal diagnosis may be academic but it can be done. Heterozygotes can easily be identified either biochemically (33) or by mutation analysis, if *PAHX* or *PEX7* mutation is found. Severity is markedly variable, not only from family to family but between or among sibs (1).

Diagnosis. In Usher syndrome, the retinitis pigmentosa and hearing loss are not associated with hypertrophic peripheral neuropathy. Dejerine-Sottas syndrome is characterized by slowly progressive polyneuropathy and hypertrophic nerves but neither visual nor auditory defects. Kearns-Sayre syndrome can be excluded by absence of night blindness, pupillary abnormalities, peripheral neuritis, and perineural peripheral changes.

Infantile Refsum syndrome is a peroxisomal disorder not associated with cutaneous abnormalities. Other peroxisomal disorders characterized by a deficiency of catalase-containing particles (peroxisomes) are Zellweger syndrome, rhizomelic chondrodysplasia punctata, and infantile adrenoleukodystrophy. All of these peroxisomal disorders together with adult or classic Refsum syndrome exhibit storage of phytanic acid, since they share defective α-oxidation capacity of phytanic acid, which can be demonstrated in skin fibroblast cultures (3,26,27,34).

In Refsum syndrome, there is an increased level (up to 500 mg/dl) of cerebrospinal fluid protein without pleocytosis in 60%. Elevated levels of serum phytanic acid have been considered diagnostic for the disease (normal is ca. 0.2 mg/dl) but patients who live on a diet with low fat content may not have elevated levels (35). Phytanic acid oxidase activity can be demonstrated in cultured skin fibroblasts. The mean and range of normal values are 79 (49–130) pmol/hr/mg of cell protein (35). Patient values have ranged from 2 to 7. This technique is rarely used, however, owing to the low enzyme activity, which requires a large number of fibroblasts for assay. Poulos (25) employed a radioactive phytanic acid as substrate with good success. Molecular approaches to diagnosis may be more cost-effective when the *PAHX* or *PEX7* gene is involved.

Prognosis. The course is variable. Without diet modification and/or plasmapheresis, there is slow progression of the neurologic deficits; complete incapacitation eventually results (12,17,23,31). Among untreated cases, 20% died in the first decade, 30% in the third decade, 20% in the fourth decade, and 10% in the fifth decade of life. Currently, however, with special diet and plasmapheresis, there is a vastly improved outlook for life expectancy. Screening for the syndrome has been carried out (14).

Summary. This syndrome is characterized by (*1*) autosomal recessive inheritance; (*2*) progressive atypical retinitis pigmentosa with constricted visual fields and night blindness; (*3*) mild cerebellar ataxia and nystagmus; (*4*) increased plasma phytanic acid; and (*5*) progressive sensorineural hearing loss in about half of those affected.

References

1. Allen IV et al: Clinicopathological study of Refsum's disease with particular reference to fatal complications. *J Neurol Neurosurg Psychiatry* 41:323–332, 1978.
2. Anton-Lamprecht I, Kahlke W: Zur Ultrastrukturhereditärer Verhornungsstörungen. V. Ichthyosis beim Refsum-Syndrom. *Arch Dermatol Forsch* 250:185–206, 1974.
3. Beard ME et al: Peroxisomes in fibroblasts from skin of Refsum's disease patients. *J Histochem Cytochem* 33:480–484, 1985.
4. Bergsmark J, Djupesland G: Heredopathia atactica polyneuritiformis (Refsum's disease). An audiological examination of two patients. *Eur Neurol* 1:122–130, 1986.
5. Billimoria JD et al: Metabolism of phytanic acid in Refsum's disease. *Lancet* 1:194–196, 1982.
6. Cammermeyer J: Refsum's disease, neuropathological aspects. In: *Handbook of Clinical Neurology*, Vol. 21, Vinken PJ, Gruyn GW (eds), North Holland Publishing Co., Amsterdam, 1975, pp 232–261.
7. Davies MG et al: Epidermal abnormalities in Refsum's disease. *Br J Ophthalmol* 97:401–406, 1977.
8. Djupesland G et al: Phytanic acid storage disease: hearing maintained after 15 years of dietary treatment. *Neurology* 33:237–240, 1983.
9. Fardeau M, Engel WK: Ultrastructural study of a peripheral nerve biopsy in Refsum's disease. *J Neuropathol Exp Neurol* 28:278–294, 1969.
10. Feldmann H: Refsum syndrome, heredopathia atactica polyneuritiformis in the view of the otolaryngologist [in German]. *Laryngol Rhinol Otol (Stuttg)* 60:235–240, 1981.
11. Fryer DG et al: Refsum's disease. *Neurology (Minneap)* 21:162–167, 1971.
12. Gibberd FB et al: Heredopathia atactica polyneuritiformis (Refsum's disease) treated by diet and plasma-exchange. *Lancet* 1:575–578, 1979.
13. Gibberd FB et al: Heredopathia atactica polyneuritiformis: Refsum's disease. *Acta Neurol Scand* 72:1–17, 1985.
14. Goldman JM et al: Screening of patients with retinitis pigmentosa for heredopathia atactica polyneuritiformis (Refsum's disease). *BMJ (Clin Res Ed)* 290:1109–1110, 1985.
15. Hallpike CS: Observations on the structural basis of two rare varieties of hereditary deafness. In: *Myotatic, Kinesthetic and Vestibular Mechanisms*, CIBA Foundation Symposium ed. de Reuch AVS, Knight J (eds), Little Brown, Boston, 1967, pp 284–295.
16. Hansen E et al: Refsum's disease. Eye manifestations in a patient treated with low phytol low phytanic acid diet. *Acta Ophthalmol (Copenh)* 57:899–913, 1979.
17. Hungerbuhler JP et al: Refsum's disease: management by diet and plasmapheresis. *Eur Neurol* 24:153–159, 1985.
18. Jansen GA et al: Refsum disease is caused by mutations in the phytanoyl-CoA hydroxylase gene. *Nat Genet* 17:190–193, 1997.
19. Jansen GA et al: Phytanoyl-coenzyme A hydroxylase deficiency—the enzyme defect in Refsum's disease. *N Engl J Med* 337:133–134, 1997.
20. Klenk E, Kahlke WI: Über das Vorkommen der 3,7,11,15-tetramethyl-hexadecansäure (Phytansäure) in den Cholesterinestern und anderen Lipoidfraktionen der Organe bei einem Krankheitsfall unbekannter Genese (Verdacht auf Heredopathie atactica polyneuritiformis-Refsum-Syndrom). *Hoppe Seylers Z Physiol Chem* 333:133–142, 1963.
21. Lovelock J, Griffiths H: Case report 175: Refsum syndrome. *Skeletal Radiol* 7:214–217, 1981.
22. Mihalik SJ et al: Identification of *PAHX*, a Refsum disease gene. *Nat Genet* 17:185–189, 1997.
23. Moser HW et al: Therapeutic trial of plasmapheresis in Refsum disease and in Fabry disease. *Birth Defects* 16:491–497, 1980.
24. Plant GR et al: Skeletal abnormalities in Refsum's disease (heredopathia atactica polyneuritiformis). *Br J Radiol* 63:537–541, 1990.
25. Poulos A: Diagnosis of Refsum's disease using [1-14C]phytanic acid as substrate. *Clin Genet* 20:247–253, 1981.
26. Poulos A, Sharp P: Plasma and skin fibroblast C26 fatty acids in infantile Refsum's disease. *Neurology* 34:1606–1609, 1984.
27. Poulos A et al: Cerebro-hepato-renal (Zellweger) syndrome, adrenoleukodystrophy, and Refsum's disease: plasma changes and skin fibroblast phytanic acid oxidase. *Hum Genet* 70:172–177, 1985.
28. Puissant A et al: Syndrome de Refsum-Thiebaut avec naevi xanthomateaux disséminés. *Bull Soc Fr Dermatol Syph* 79:462–464, 1972.
29. Rake M, Sanders M: Refsum's disease: a disease of lipid metabolism. *J Neurol Neurosurg Psychiatry* 29:417–421, 1966.
30. Refsum S: Heredopathia atactica polyneuritiformis. *Acta Psychiatr Neurol Scand Suppl* 38:1–303, 1946.
31. Refsum S: Heredopathia atactica polyneuritiformis. Reconsideration. *World Neurol* 1:333–347, 1960.
32. Refsum S, Stokke O: Refsum's disease (heredopathia atactica polyneuritiformis). In: *Neurocutaneous Disease—A Practical Approach*, Gomez M (ed), Butterworth, Boston, 1987, pp 225–235.
33. Richterich R et al: Refsum's disease (heredopathia atactica polyneuritiformis). *Humangenetik* 1:322–336, 1965.
34. Skjeldal OH et al: Phytanic acid oxidase activity in cultured skin fibroblasts. Diagnostic usefulness and limitations. *Scand J Clin Lab Invest* 46:283–287, 1986.
35. Skjeldal OH et al: Clinical and biochemical heterogeneity in conditions with phytanic acid accumulation. *J Neurol Sci* 77:87–96, 1987.
36. Steinberg D: Refsum disease. In: *The Metabolic Basis of Inherited Diseases*, 7th ed., Scriver CR et al. (eds), McGraw-Hill, New York, 1995, pp 2359–2369.
37. Thiébaut F et al: Deux syndromes oto-neuro-oculistiques d'origine congénitale. *Rev Neurol (Paris)* 72:71–75, 1939.

38. Van Den Brink DM et al: Identification of *PEX7* as the second gene involved in Refsum disease. *Am J Hum Genet* 72:471–477, 2003.
39. Wall WJ, Worthington BS: Skeletal changes in Refsum's disease. *Clin Radiol* 30:657–659, 1979.
40. Wanders RJ et al: Refsum disease, peroxisomes and phytanic acid oxidation: a review. *J Neuropathol Exp Neurol* 60:1021–1031, 2001.

Infantile Refsum syndrome

In contrast to adult or classic Refsum syndrome, infantile Refsum syndrome (IRD) or infantile phytanic acid storage disease is characterized by microcephaly, severe developmental delay, hypotonia, hepatomegaly, and dysmorphic facial features. In common with adult Refsum syndrome, there are retinitis pigmentosa, sensorineural hearing loss, and phytanic acid oxidase deficiency. It was first reported by Kahlke et al. (4) in 1974. It has been found to belong to a group of so-called peroxisome biogenesis disorders that includes Zellweger syndrome and neonatal adrenoleukodystrophy (11,13).

Clinical findings. Short stature appears to be a common feature and microcephaly has been noted in 20%–25% of cases. A typical facial appearance, evident in most published cases, is characterized by frontal bossing, epicanthal folds, flat and apparently widened nasal bridge, mild ptosis, and posteriorly rotated pinnae (2,6,8) (Fig. 7–7A). A similar facial phenotype is seen in hyperpipecolic acidemia and neonatal adrenoleukodystrophy. The face at about 1 year somewhat resembles that of 21 trisomy.

A single palmar crease has been noted by a number of investigators (2,6,8).

Ocular system. Retinitis pigmentosa with progressive visual impairment has been a constant feature, as has optic atrophy and narrowed retinal vessels (2,12,14) (Fig. 7–7B). Electroretinograms have shown extinction. Esotropia has been noted in several affected children.

Central nervous system. Microcephaly and mental retardation are marked; in some patients developmental function rarely exceeds the 1-year level. Other abnormalities have included seizures, ataxia, areflexia,

hypotonia, weakness, nystagmus, and anosmia (3,5). Abnormal nerve conduction velocities have been found in some cases (7) but not in others (2,6).

Gastrointestinal system. Hepatomegaly due to portal and intralobular fibrosis is a constant feature. Liver function tests have been abnormal in about 50% (8). These patients have experienced a bleeding diathesis that has been manifest as intracranial hemorrhage (2,7). Steatorrhea in the presence of normal pancreatic function was found by Budden et al. (2).

Musculoskeletal system. Osteopenia has been noted in nearly all cases.

Auditory system. Auditory brain stem evoked response testing has revealed bilateral profound sensorineural hearing loss in all affected individuals.

Laboratory findings. Hypocholesterolemia, with the HDL fraction being especially low, appears to be a common finding (2,4,8). It appears likely that the disturbance of phytanic acid metabolism in this disorder is secondary to a peroxisomal defect that impinges on phytanic acid, pipecolic acid, or very long–chain fatty acid metabolism.

Pathology. Liver biopsy showed accentuated lobular architecture with fibrous bands that link the periportal tracts and progress to micronodular cirrhosis. Ultrastructural changes include marked neutral fat droplets in the cytoplasm. Trilaminar structures, composed of two outer leaflets measuring about 12 nm wide and separated by a clear space of 1–2 nm, lie free or are found adjacent to lysosomes. Similar structures have been found in perivacular cells of the skin. Peroxisomes have been absent (2,8). Similar trilaminar structures have been found in patients with adrenoleukodystrophy.

Pathogenesis. Elevated serum phytanic acid (but less elevated than in classic Refsum syndrome), elevated pipecolic acid, increased very long–chain fatty acids in serum and in cultured fibroblasts, and deficient phytanic acid oxidase have been found in nearly all affected individuals. Peroxisomal function is markedly decreased (2).

Heredity. The hereditary pattern appears to be autosomal recessive. Heterozyotes have had normal values of serum phytanic acid and long-chain fatty acids. The peroxisome biogenesis disorders include Zellweger syndrome (ZS), neonatal adrenoleucodystrophy (NALD), and IRD. Twelve complementation groups have been reported (10). Patients with ZS manifest the severest clinical and biochemical abnormalities, whereas those with NALD and IRD show less severity and the mildest features, respectively. About 65% of the cases with a peroxisome biogenesis disorder have a mutation in the *PEX1* gene, which codes for an AAA ATPase; *PEX2* mutations have also been described (9,13).

Diagnosis. The most common incorrect diagnosis has been Usher syndrome or Leber congenital amaurosis. As indicated in the section on adult Refsum syndrome, infantile Refsum syndrome is similarly characterized by storage of phytanic acid but, in contrast to the adult form, exhibits microcephaly, mental retardation, dysmorphic facial features, and hepatomegaly due to portal and intralobular fibrosis. These findings as well as osteopenia, hypotonia, hypocholesterolemia, hypolipoproteinemia, elevated serum pipecolic acid, phytanic acid oxidase deficiency, and elevated very long–chain fatty acid serum values are shared with other peroxisomal deficiency disorders such as Zellweger syndrome, hyperpipecolic acidemia, and neonatal adrenoleukodystrophy (1).

Summary. This syndrome is characterized by (*1*) autosomal recessive inheritance; (*2*) short stature; (*3*) microcephaly and mental retardation; (*4*) unusual facies; (*5*) retinitis pigmentosa; (*6*) hepatomegaly and abnormal liver function; and (*7*) bilateral profound sensorineural hearing loss.

Figure 7–7. *Infantile Refsum syndrome.* (A) Four-year-old patient with epicanthal folds, flat nasal bridge, and mildly dysmorphic appearance. (B) Retina inferior to disc showing diffuse hypopigmentation, retinal vessel attenuation, and fine granularity from retinal pigmentary dispersion. [Courtesy of RG Weleber, Portland, Oregon.]

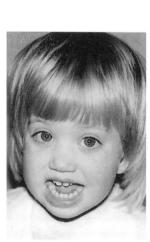
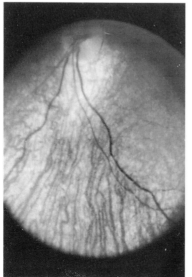

A   B

References

1. Allen IV et al: Clinicopathological study of Refsum's disease with particular reference to fatal complications. *J Neurol Neurosurg Psychiatry* 41:323–332, 1978.
2. Budden SS et al: Dysmorphic syndrome with phytanic acid oxidase deficiency, abnormal very long chain fatty acids, and pipecolic acidemia: studies in four children. *J Pediatr* 108:33–39, 1986.
3. Dubois J et al: MR findings in infantile Refsum disease: case report of two family members. *AJNR Am J Neuroradiol* 12:1159–1160, 1991.
4. Kahlke W et al: Erhöhte Phytansäurespiegel in Plasma und Leber bei einem Kleinkind mit unklarem Hirnschaden. *Klin Wochenschr* 52:651–653, 1974.
5. Naidu S, Moser H: Infantile Refsum disease. *AJNR Am J Neuroradiol* 12:1161–1163, 1991.
6. Poll-Thé BT et al: Infantile Refsum disease: an inherited peroxisomal disorder. Comparison with Zellweger syndrome and neonatal adrenoleukodystrophy. *Eur J Pediatr* 146:477–483, 1987.
7. Poulos A et al: Patterns of Refsum's disease. Phytanic acid oxidase deficiency. *Arch Dis Child* 59:222–229, 1984.
8. Scotto JM et al.: Infantile phytanic acid storage disease, a possible variant of Refsum's disease: three cases, including ultrastructural studies of the liver. *J Inherit Metab Dis* 5:83-90, 1982.
9. Shimozawa N et al: Defective PEX gene products correlate with the protein import, biochemical abnormalities, and phenotypic heterogeneity in peroxisome biogenesis disorders. *J Med Genet* 36:779-781, 1999.
10. Singh AK et al: In situ genetic complementation analysis of cells with generalized peroxisomal dysfunction A. *Hum Hered* 39:298–301, 1989.
11. Tamura S et al: Phenotype–genotype relationships in peroxisome biogenesis disorders of PEX1-defective complementation group 1 are defined by Pex1p–Pex6p interaction. *Biochem J* 357:417–426, 2001.
12. Van dM, V et al: Ophthalmological manifestations of infantile Refsum's disease: apropos of 3 cases [in French]. *Bull Soc Belge Ophtalmol* 250:79–84, 1993.
13. Walter C et al: Disorders of peroxisome biogenesis due to mutations in PEX1: phenotypes and PEX1 protein levels. *Am J Hum Genet* 69:35–48, 2001.
14. Weleber RG et al: Ophthalmic manifestations of infantile phytanic acid storage disease. *Arch Ophthalmol* 102:1317–1321, 1984.

Reinstein syndrome: inverse retinitis pigmentosa, hypogonadism, and sensorineural hearing loss

In 1971, Reinstein and Chalfin (2) reported a syndrome of inverse retinitis pigmentosa, hypogenitalism, and sensorineural hearing loss in one male and two female sibs. Contestabile et al. (1) described a male with inverse retinitis pigmentosa and sensorineural hearing loss who may have had this condition.

Ocular system. Blurring of central vision was first experienced at 20 to 30 years of age (Fig. 7–8A). Over the next 5–10 years, impairment progressed slowly to a stable end point. No impairment of night or color vision was experienced. Fundus changes consisted of a concentration of bone-spicule pigmentation confined to the posterior pole, i.e., surrounding the macula and disc, sometimes in the form of a discrete ring and often with attenuation of retinal vessels and disc pallor. Subadjacent choroidal sclerosis was also found. Discreet mottled macular lesions were noted in all three sibs. Dark adaptation thresholds were elevated, electroretinograms were markedly depressed, and visual fields showed dense central scotomas with peripheral depression (Fig. 7–8B).

Genitourinary system. In the male sib (2), secondary sexual characteristics appeared at 14 years of age. At 60 years the testes were small and soft. The patient denied impotence. The other reported male (1) was not described as having hypogonadism. Neither of two female sibs had spontaneous menarche. Menses, breast development, and pubic hair growth occurred only after hormone therapy.

Auditory system. The male sib noted the onset of a slowly progressive hearing loss from 11 years of age. When over 60 years of age, a moderately severe sensorineural hearing loss was found. At 35 years, a female sib first experienced hearing impairment, which slowly progressed to severe sensorineural loss at frequencies over 2000 Hz. The

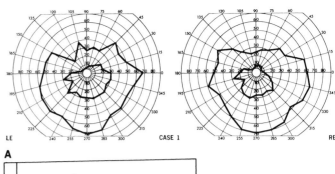

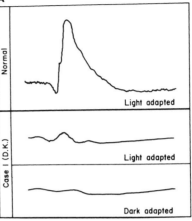

Figure 7–8. *Inverse retinitis pigmentosa, hypogonadism, and sensorineural hearing loss.* (A) Visual fields showing loss of central vision. (B) Electroretinograms showing depressed photic curves and extinguished scotopic curves. [From NM Reinstein and AI Chalfin, *Am J Ophthalmol* 72:332, 1971.]

other female sib initially manifested hearing loss at about 40 years of age and 8 years later had a moderate sensorineural deficit, more marked in higher frequencies. No details regarding onset of hearing loss were provided in the other report (1), although it was noted that loss was more severe for the higher frequencies.

Laboratory findings. No significant findings were reported.

Heredity. The three affected sibs were the product of a consanguineous union. The parents and maternal grandparents were both first cousins of Ashkenazi Jewish extraction. Inheritance appears to be autosomal recessive.

Diagnosis. In contrast to the typical peripheral form of retinitis pigmentosa, which can exist as an isolated finding or as part of several syndromes, inverse retinitis pigmentosa is characterized by absence of night blindness, early loss of central vision, and, frequently, preference for dim rather than bright illumination. Stargardt disease is an autosomal recessive disorder causing a central pigmentary retinopathy but is unassociated with either hypogonadism or hearing loss. Best disease and cone-rod dystrophy also cause a central retinopathy but are dominantly inherited.

Prognosis. Impaired vision, usually appearing in the third decade, progressively deteriorates to severe loss over the next decade.

Summary. Characteristics of this syndrome include (*1*) autosomal recessive inheritance; (*2*) inverse retinitis pigmentosa with absent night blindness, early loss of central vision, and preference for dim illumination; (*3*) hypogonadism; and (*4*) sensorineural hearing loss.

References

1. Contestabile MT et al: Atypical retinitis pigmentosa: a report of three cases. *Ann Ophthalmol* 24:325–334, 1992.

2. Reinstein NM, Chalfin AI: Inverse retinitis pigmentosa, deafness, and hypogenitalism. *Am J Ophthalmol* 72:332–341, 1971.

Miscellaneous disorders of pigmentary retinopathy and sensorineural hearing loss

In this brief section are included two conditions with pigmentary retinopathy that cannot be classified. In one, dental anomalies are the additional manifestation, in the other, peripheral neuropathy occurs.

Bateman et al. (1) reported brothers with clumped pigmentary retinopathy at the periphery that appeared after the first few years of life. Electroretinography showed no rod response and normal cone response. Moderate to severe stable sensorineural hearing loss was evident from before the age of 2 years. One brother had generalized enamel dysplasia, probably due to malabsorption early in life. Inheritance is either autosomal or X-linked recessive.

Bateman et al. (1) also described a patient with retinitis pigmentosa, sensorineural hearing loss, and generalized enamel dysplasia. There was no evidence of night blindness. The patient was not otherwise described. Two other examples of retinitis pigmentosa with hearing loss and enamel dysplasia have been reported (2,3).

Tuck and McLeod (4) described four unrelated patients with retinitis pigmentosa, constricted visual fields, a predominantly sensory neuropathy, cerebellar ataxia, and moderate high-frequency sensorineural hearing loss. Onset of symptoms was before age 20 in two patients and after age 40 in the other two. One patient had low intelligence and extensor plantar responses. Deep tendon reflexes were diminished or absent in three patients. Abnormalities of nerve conduction, predominantly sensory, were noted in all four patients. While Refsum syndrome was suspected, serum phytanic acid levels were normal. Kearns-Sayre syndrome was also excluded.

References

1. Bateman JB et al: Heterogeneity of retinal degeneration and hearing impairment syndromes. *Am J Ophthalmol* 90:755–767, 1980.
2. Innis JW et al: Apparently new syndrome of sensorineural hearing loss, retinal pigment epithelium lesions, and discolored teeth. *Am J Med Genet* 75:13–17, 1998.
3. Pieke-Dahl SA et al: Genetic heterogeneity of Usher syndrome type II: localisation to chromosome 5q. *J Med Genet* 37:256–262, 2000.
4. Tuck RR, McLeod JG: Retinitis pigmentosa, ataxia, and peripheral neuropathy. *J Neurol Neurosurg Psychiatry* 46:206–213, 1983.

Myopia and congenital sensorineural hearing loss

The combination of congenital sensorineural hearing loss, myopia, and low intelligence was described by Eldridge et al. (1) in 1968 in four of seven sibs from an Amish sibship.

Physical findings. Each of the four affected children was well developed with normal stature.

Ocular system. Three sibs exhibited myopia of about 15 diopters, with temporal pallor and a prominent choroidal vascular pattern (Fig. 7–9A).

Central nervous system. Psychometric testing showed retardation. However, this condition may have resulted from sensory deprivation rather than from neurologic disturbance.

Auditory system. Hearing loss in each of the affected children was noted in early childhood. There was no evident progression of the hearing loss. Otologic examinations revealed normal external auditory canals and tympanic membranes. Pure-tone audiometric tests showed a 30–100 dB sensorineural hearing loss, which was more marked in higher frequencies. A SISI test carried out on one child was positive, suggesting a cochlear origin for the hearing loss. Other audiologic tests were not done.

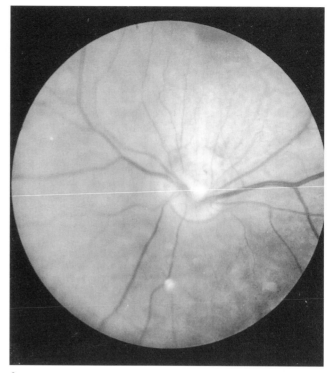

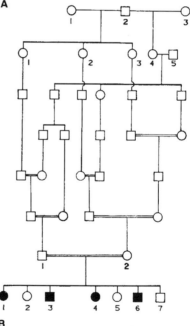

Figure 7–9. *Myopia and congenital sensorineural hearing loss.* (A) Fundus showing temporal pallor and prominent choroidal vascular pattern associated with severe myopia. (B) Pedigree of inbred Amish family showing four affected persons. [From T Eldridge et al., *Arch Otolaryngol* 88:49, 1968.]

Vestibular system. Caloric vestibular tests showed normal vestibular function.

Laboratory findings. Analyses of blood, urine, and cerebrospinal fluid as well as a radiologic survey showed no abnormalities. In a 13-year-old girl an electroencephalogram showed slightly more activity than normal.

Heredity. The pedigree of Eldridge et al. (1) showed four affected in a sibship of seven (Fig. 7–9B). The parents were normal; there was no history of hearing or visual defect in either family. The parents were distantly related, thus making autosomal recessive transmission most likely.

Diagnosis. A family was described by Ohlsson (2) in which three boys in a sibship of seven had sensorineural deafness and severe myopia. Six of the seven sibs, including three with deafness and myopia, had albuminuria or hematuria, as did the mother. Although Ohlsson concluded that the syndrome in this family was different from Alport syndrome because of the milder course of renal disease and severe myopia, we believe that Ohlsson's kindred probably had a variant of Alport syndrome. Myopia of mild degree has been described in Alport syndrome by Sturtz and Burke (3).

Prognosis. There was no evidence of progression of either myopia or hearing loss.

Summary. Characteristics of this syndrome include (*1*) autosomal recessive transmission; (*2*) congenital severe myopia; (*3*) mild intellectual impairment in some affected persons; and (*4*) congenital moderate to severe nonprogressive sensorineural hearing loss.

References

1. Eldridge R et al: Cochlear deafness, myopia, and intellectual impairment in an Amish family. *Arch Otolaryngol* 88:49–54, 1968.
2. Ohlsson L: Congenital renal disease, deafness, and myopia in one family. *Acta Med Scand* 174:77–84, 1963.
3. Sturtz GS, Burke EC: Hereditary hematuria, nephropathia, and deafness. *N Engl J Med* 54:1123–1126, 1956.

Donnai-Barrow syndrome: myopia, hypertelorism, agenesis of corpus callosum, diaphragmatic hernia, exomphalos, and sensorineural hearing loss

In 1993, Donnai and Barrow (3) described two unrelated sets of sibs with hypertelorism, severe myopia, diaphragmatic hernia, omphalocele and/or malrotation of the bowel, and sensorineural hearing loss. Gripp et al. (4), Devriendt et al. (2) and Avunduk et al. (1) have each described similar cases. There are now seven cases reported.

Auditory system. The degree of hearing loss has been reported to range from severe to profound.

Ocular findings. Three cases have been reported to have an inferior iris coloboma (1,3,4). All cases have been reported to have severe myopia. The optic nerve heads were reported to be hyperemic and the retina appeared thin in the case reported by Avunduk et al. (1).

Craniofacial findings. The face exhibited marked hypertelorism, prominent eyes, down-slanted palbebral fissures, and short nose with broad, indented tip. The anterior fontanel may be large. The ears can be malformed and/or posteriorly rotated (Fig. 7–10).

Neurologic findings. Absence of the corpus callosum has been a constant finding. Developmental delay varied from mild to severe.

Other findings. Omphalocele (1,3,4), intestinal malrotation, diaphragmatic hernia (2–4), and agenesis of the diaphragm (4) have been reported.

Heredity. The disorder appears to be autosomal recessive. In two families there were affected sibs (3). Two other cases had consanguineous parents (1,4).

Diagnosis. The facial phenotype is similar to that of DeHauwere syndrome, but that disorder has autosomal dominant inheritance and is not associated with diaphragmatic hernia or exomphalos. In the Holmes-Schepens syndrome (5), the sibs reported had similar facial appearance

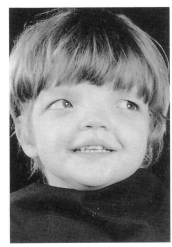 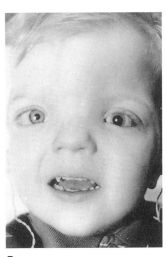

A   **B**

Figure 7–10. *Myopia, hypertelorism, agenesis of corpus callosum, diaphragmatic hernia, exomphalos, and sensorineural hearing loss.* (A,B) Compare facies in two unrelated children. Note hypertelorism, downslanting palpebral fissues, low-set posteriorly rotated ears, and mild mandibular prognathism. Child in (B) had coloboma and retinal detachment. [From D Donnai and M Barrow, *Am J Med Genet*, 47:679, 1993.]

and umbilical hernia (but neither agenesis of the corpus callosum nor diaphragmatic defect) and had a renal defect. The family reported by Devriendt et al. (2) presented with a proteinuria, which led them to postulate that Holmes-Schepens and Donnai-Barrow syndromes were the same.

Summary. Characteristics of this condition include (*1*) autosomal recessive inheritance; (*2*) myopia; (*3*) diaphragmatic hernia; (*4*) omphalocele and/or malrotation of the bowel; (*5*) developmental delay; (*6*) agenesis of the corpus callosum; and (*7*) sensorineural hearing loss.

References

1. Avunduk AM et al: High myopia, hypertelorism, iris coloboma, exomphalos, absent corpus callosum, and sensorineural deafness: report of a case and further evidence for autosomal recessive inheritance. *Acta Ophthalmol Scand* 78:221–222, 2000.
2. Devriendt K et al: Proteinuria in a patient with the diaphragmatic hernia-hypertelorism-myopia-deafness syndrome: further evidence that the facio-oculo-acoustico-renal syndrome represents the same entity. *J Med Genet* 35:70–71, 1998.
3. Donnai D, Barrow M: Diaphragmatic hernia, exomphalos, absent corpus callosum, hypertelorism, myopia, and sensorineural deafness: a newly recognized autosomal recessive disorder? *Am J Med Genet* 47:679–682, 1993.
4. Gripp KW et al: Diaphragmatic hernia-exomphalos-hypertelorism syndrome: a new case and further evidence of autosomal recessive inheritance. *Am J Med Genet* 68:441–444, 1997.
5. Holmes LB, Schepens CL: Syndrome of ocular and facial anomalies, telecanthus, and deafness. *J Pediatr* 81:552–555, 1972.

Holmes-Schepens syndrome: myopia, hypertelorism, and congenital sensorineural hearing loss (facio-oculo-acoustico-renal syndrome)

In 1972, Holmes and Schepens (2) reported a sister and brother with severe myopia, hypertelorism, and congenital sensorineural hearing loss. The same children were reported by Murdoch and Mengel (4) and by Özer (5). Fraser (1) described a single case. Two additional cases were reported by Liberfarb (3) (Fig. 7–11).

Physical findings. Head circumference is large. The brows are prominent with a broad, flat nasal bridge. The anterior fontanel remains open. Height has ranged from the 10th to 25th percentile.

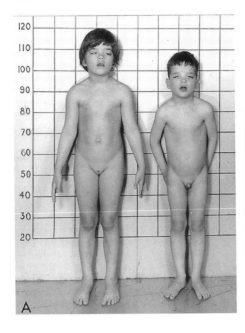

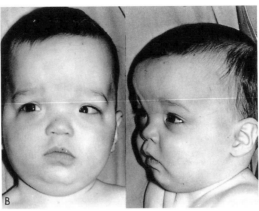

Figure 7–11. *Myopia, hypertelorism, and congenital sensorineural hearing loss (facio-oculo-acoustico-renal syndrome, Holmes-Schepens syndrome).* (A) Sibs with severe congenital hearing loss and severe eye abnormalities and telecanthus. Note flat nasal bridge. (B) Male sib at 7 months of age. Note large head circumference, prominent frontal bone, and ocular hypertelorism. [(A) from FL Özer, *Birth Defects* 10(4):168, 1974; (B) from LB Holmes and CL Schepens, *J Pediatr* 81:552, 1972.]

Ocular system. The sister had congenital myopia in excess of 10 diopters, posterior staphyloma, incompletely developed filtration angle, extensive choroidal atrophy, posterior subcapsular cataracts, iris stroma hypoplasia, and congenital pupillary membrane.

The brother had congenital myopia of 25 diopters, pupillary remnants, nasal synechiae, incompletely developed filtration angle, and unilateral iris coloboma. Retinal detachment occurred at about 4 years of age, followed by cataract development a year later. At 6 years of age, retinal detachment occurred in the other eye. In both children, the inferior lacrimal punctae were laterally displaced. Inner canthal, interpupillary, and outer canthal distances were all greater than normal. There was downslanting of the palpebral fissures.

Central nervous system. Intelligence was normal in the girl. The boy was hyperactive and somewhat mentally retarded.

Auditory system. Both sibs had severe congenital sensorineural hearing loss. No other data were presented.

Vestibular system. No vestibular findings were described.

Other findings. The boy had umbilical hernia, inguinal hernia, and intussusception. Ureteral reflex and dilatation were also described.

Laboratory findings. Albuminuria was found in both sibs. The boy had generalized aminoaciduria. The patients of Fraser (1) exhibited marked proteinuria.

Heredity. The syndrome appears to have autosomal recessive inheritance.

Diagnosis. Myopia has been described in a number of disorders discussed in this section, but the combination of myopia and other symptoms described here appears unique. Although patients with Waardenburg syndrome have increased inner canthal distances and displacement of lacrimal puncta, the rest of the stigmata as well as the inheritance pattern are different.

Prognosis. Retinal detachment occurred in the male sib. Cataracts were present in both sibs. It is not known whether renal complications supervened.

Summary. This syndrome is characterized by (1) autosomal recessive inheritance; (2) hypertelorism and prominent brows; (3) my-

opia, choroidal atrophy, cataract, iris stroma hypoplasia, and possibly retinal detachment; and (4) congenital profound sensorineural hearing loss.

References

1. Fraser GR: *The Causes of Profound Deafness in Childhood.* Johns Hopkins University Press, Baltimore, 1976.
2. Holmes LB, Schepens CL: Syndromes of facial anomalies, telecanthus, and deafness. *J Pediatr* 81:552–555, 1972.
3. Liberfarb R: Facio-oculo-acoustico-renal syndrome. In: *Diseases Affecting the Eye and Kidney,* Regenbogen L, Eliahou HE (eds), Karger, Basel, 1993, pp 377–380.
4. Murdoch JL, Mengel MC: An unusual eye-ear syndrome with renal abnormality. *Birth Defects* 7:136, 1971.
5. Özer FL: A possible "new" syndrome with eye and renal anomalies. *Birth Defects* 10:168, 1974.

Harboyan syndrome: congenital corneal dystrophy and progressive sensorineural hearing loss

Harboyan et al. (2) first reported the combination of congenital corneal dystrophy and progressive sensorineural hearing loss in 2 of 10 sibs from a first-cousin mating and in 1 of 10 sibs from another first-cousin mating by the same father. Other families have subsequently been reported (1,5,7).

Ocular system. Whitish opacities of the cornea with decreased vision were evident from birth (Fig. 7–12A). Ophthalmologic examination of the three patients, ranging in age from 12 to 50 years, showed similar changes. The corneal epithelium was roughened but did not stain. The stroma was thickened, edematous, and homogeneously white. Vision was decreased to 20/200 bilaterally at puberty with marked deterioration with age. A younger woman exhibited increased intraocular pressure, possibly due to increased corneal rigidity. These observations suggest some progressive loss of vision.

Auditory system. Hearing loss has been noticed in the second decade and is slowly progressive.

Vestibular system. Caloric vestibular tests were normal in all three patients.

Laboratory findings. Routine laboratory tests, including levels of urinary mucopolysaccharides, were normal.

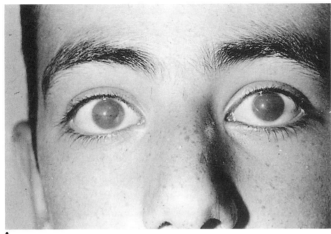

A

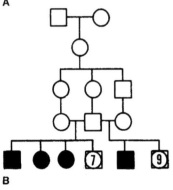

B

Figure 7–12. *Congenital corneal dystrophy and progressive sensorineural hearing loss (Harboyan syndrome).* (A) Note homogeneous white opacification of corneas in 12-year-old male. (B) Modified pedigree showing parental consanguinity. [From G Harboyan et al., *Arch Ophthalmol* 85:27, 1971.]

Heredity. Normal parents, affected sibs, and parental consanguinity indicate autosomal recessive inheritance (Fig. 7–12B). The gene has been localized to 20p13 (1).

Diagnosis. Congenital corneal dystrophy may be an isolated finding that has both autosomal dominant and recessive forms (3). Corneal clouding is a feature of several mucopolysaccharidoses (Hurler, Scheie, Morquio, and Maroteaux-Lamy syndromes). The clinical features of these conditions, however, are quite distinct. In congenital glaucoma, one finds corneal haziness, photophobia, enlarged cornea, increased intraocular pressure, and lacrimation. In Cogan syndrome, there is photophobia and injection of the eyes; the keratitis is deep in the stroma. Tinnitus, severe vertigo, and ultimately marked hearing loss and decreased labyrinthine function are also associated with Cogan syndrome. Congenital syphilitic keratitis must also be excluded.

In Fehr's autosomal recessive corneal dystrophy, the corneal changes become evident during the first decade of life; in the present syndrome the dystrophy is congenital (1,2,5,7). We are aware of only one example of the association of Fehr's corneal dystrophy with congenital neural hearing loss. The patient was the offspring of a consanguineous union (6).

A possible example of Harboyan syndrome are the sibs reported by Scialfa et al. (8). The parents were consanguineous. However, these sibs differed in having mental retardation and clinodactyly of fifth fingers. Another similar family was reported by Kurt et al. (4). but these cases also had a severe myopia and the hearing loss was conductive or mixed but only neurosensory in 1 of 14 cases.

Prognosis. The loss of vision and hearing is slowly progressive.

Summary. Major features of this syndrome include (*1*) autosomal recessive inheritance; (*2*) congenital corneal dystrophy with slow progression; and (*3*) childhood onset of slowly progressive sensorineural hearing loss.

References

1. Abramowicz MJ et al: Corneal dystrophy and perceptive deafness (Harboyan syndrome): CDPD1 maps to 20p13. *J Med Genet* 39:110–112, 2002.
2. Harboyan G et al: Congenital corneal dystrophy. Progressive sensorineural deafness in a family. *Arch Ophthalmol* 85:27–32, 1971.
3. Kirkness CM et al: Congenital hereditary corneal oedema of Maumenee: its clinical features, management, and pathology. *Br J Ophthalmol* 71:130–144, 1987.
4. Kurt E et al: Familial pathologic myopia, corneal dystrophy, and deafness: a new syndrome. *Jpn J Ophthalmol* 45:612–617, 2001.
5. Magli A et al: A further observation of corneal dystrophy and perceptive deafness in two siblings. *Ophthalm Genet* 18:87–91, 1997.
6. Moro F, Ameidi B: Distrófia corneale screziata (o di Fehr) associata a sordita e balbuzie. *Ann Ottalmol Clin Ocul* 83:30–52, 1957.
7. Puga AC et al: Congenital corneal dystrophy and progressive sensorineural hearing loss (Harboyan syndrome). *Am J Med Genet* 80:177–179, 1998.
8. Scialfa A et al: Dystrophie congénitale héréditaire de la cornéa associée à des anomalies extraoculaire diverses. *Ophthalmologica* 171:410–418, 1975.

Hallermann-Doering syndrome: familial band keratopathy, abnormal calcium metabolism, and hearing loss

A syndrome comprising band keratopathy, abnormal calcium metabolism, and hearing loss and occurring in three of five brothers was described by Hallermann and Doering (2) in 1963.

Ocular system. The three brothers exhibited the senile type of band keratopathy. Although the authors did not describe the age of onset of the degeneration, they did not find it in the patients' offspring, none of whom had reached the age of 45.

Auditory system. The three brothers, ranging from 65 to 69 years of age, had a hearing loss, the severity of which was not indicated. Age of onset or possible progression of hearing loss was not mentioned.

Laboratory findings. Metabolic studies showed a normal plasma concentration of calcium. However, the mean transit time of calcium in the metabolically active pool studied with ^{47}Ca was significantly prolonged. They found that the totally available active calcium was increased, whereas its turnover was sluggish and reduced.

Heredity. Three of five sibs had the syndrome. Although the father was not examined, the paternal uncle probably had the same disorder, according to the authors. Children of the affected persons did not exhibit signs of the syndrome, although they may have been too young to display any. Examination and metabolic studies of the parents of the affected individuals would have been valuable. It is possible that the syndrome is autosomal dominant with incomplete penetrance, but it is just as likely that it is autosomal recessive.

The authors mentioned another family in which both parents had hearing deficit. Of 10 children in this family, 1 had band keratopathy and hearing loss, whereas 6 others had hearing loss but no corneal involvement. Three were normal. No metabolic studies were done. The authors suggested that members of this family had the same syndrome.

Diagnosis. Band keratopathy has been described in a father and son. However, no hearing loss was mentioned (1). Band keratopathy with severe sensorineural hearing loss appeared in a 24-year-old female as a presenting sign of hyperparathyroidism (3).

Prognosis. Apparently, this disease appears in the later decades of life and is slowly progressive.

Summary. Characteristics of this syndrome include (*1*) possible autosomal dominant transmission with variable expressivity; (*2*) band keratopathy with onset in later decades; (*3*) abnormal calcium metabolism characterized by prolonged transit time of calcium in the metabolically active pool; and (*4*) hearing loss, otherwise undefined.

References

1. Glees M: Über familiäres Auftreten der primären bandförmigen Hornhautdegeneration. *Klin Monatsbl Augenheilk* 116:185–187, 1950.
2. Hallermann W, Doering P: Primäre bandförmigen Hornhautdegeneration, Schwerhörigkeit und gestörter Calciumumsatz—ein hereditäre Symptomenkomplex. *Ber Dtsch Ophthalmol Ges* 65:285–288, 1963.
3. Petrohelos M et al: Band keratopathy with bilateral deafness as a presenting sign of hyperparathyroidism. *Br J Ophthalmol* 61:494–495, 1977.

Ehlers-Danlos syndrome, type VI (keratoconus/keratoglobus, blue sclerae, loose ligaments, and hearing loss) (EDS VI, ocular form)

The combination of keratoconus or keratoglobus, blue sclerae, loose ligaments, and hearing loss was probably first described by Behr (2) in 1913. Numerous cases have since been reported (1,3–8,10–12,19). It is likely that this disorder is the same as the syndrome of brittle cornea, blue sclerae, and red hair (9,14,16,18). It has been classified as Ehlers-Danlos syndrome, type VI, or the ocular form. Both an *a* and *b* form exist, based on molecular mechanisms.

Physical findings. Affected individuals have muscular hypotonia, ocular manifestations (ocular fragility, retinal detachment, glaucoma, and so on), joint hypermobility, and skin hyperextensibility. Patients are usually of normal stature and body proportions, but some have been described as having a Marfanoid habitus (8,11). Most patients have kyphoscoliosis (Fig. 7–13A–G).

Ocular system. All patients had blue sclerae and nearly all had bilateral keratoconus or keratoglobus, i.e., cone-shaped cornea or globe-shaped cornea, respectively (Fig. 7–13H). The cornea is transparent and thinned, especially peripherally.

Gradual and progressive visual impairment began after puberty with perforation of the thinned cornea (*a sine qua non* of keratoconus and keratoglobus) and traumatic cataract. Corneal perforation occurred in at least 50% (3,6). Microcornea, retinal detachment, and glaucoma have also been described (7,19).

Musculoskeletal system. Kyphoscoliosis is a nearly constant finding.

Hyperextensible joints are present in nearly all cases, which may have resulted in falls with resultant fractures in a few cases (3) (Fig. 7–13I). Hernias are relatively common, with umbilical and inguinal both described (11,12,15).

Oral findings. Dental alterations termed "dentinogenesis imperfecta" have been reported but not documented.

Vascular system. Cardiovascular complications are frequent, including aortic regurgitation and mitral valve prolapse (9) and arterial rupture (17,19).

Auditory system. In one patient of Greenfield et al. (6), mixed hearing loss was found. Progressive unilateral hearing loss began at 10 years of age, followed by contralateral loss at 27 years of age. At 30 years, bilateral otosclerosis was established. In the other sib, progressive bilateral hearing loss began at 14 years of age. In the two brothers studied by Behr (2), one had bilateral hearing loss not otherwise characterized. Sensorineural loss at higher frequencies was described by Biglan et al. (3) (Fig. 7–13J). Lamba et al. (12) described bilateral conductive hearing loss. Hyams et al. (9) described hearing loss that was probably conductive.

Vestibular system. Vestibular tests were not mentioned.

Laboratory findings. The diagnosis can be confirmed by determination of hydroxylysine levels in hydrolyzed dermis and/or ascertainment of reduced enzyme activity in cultured fibroblasts (17). The ration of lysyl pyridinoline to hydroxylysyl pyridinoline in urine is also altered, and can be used as a diagnostic test (17).

Heredity. The disorder clearly has autosomal recessive inheritance. Parental consanguinity has been demonstrated. The cause of one form of EDS VI is mutation of the gene for lysyl hydroxylase (*PLOD*), which maps to 1p36.3–p36.2 (10). However, not all cases of EDS VI have lysyl hydroxylase deficiency, so there is clearly heterogeneity within this condition (4).

Diagnosis. Severe myopia and loose joints are also seen in Stickler syndrome. Blue sclerae can occur in a number of connective tissue disorders—osteogenesis imperfecta, Marfan syndrome, Hallermann-Streiff syndrome, and incontinentia pigmenti. However, there should be no difficulty in excluding these conditions on clinical grounds. Keratoconus is usually an isolated finding, but there are several kindreds in which transmission has been autosomal dominant or autosomal recessive (13). Keratoconus has also been reported in association with oculodentoosseous dysplasia, and occasionally with osteogenesis imperfecta and Rieger syndrome.

Prognosis. The outlook for these patients is generally good. The syndrome is not life threatening, but the hearing loss is progressive. The keratoconus may cause rupture of the cornea with resultant complications.

Summary. The characteristics of the syndrome include (*1*) autosomal recessive inheritance; (*2*) keratoconus or keratoglobus with thin, fragile cornea; (*3*) blue sclerae; (*4*) loose ligaments; and (*5*) mixed hearing loss.

References

1. Badtke G: Über eine eigenartigen Fall von Keratokonus und blauen Skleren bei Geschwistern. *Klin Monatsbl Augenheilkd* 106:585–592, 1941.
2. Behr C: Beitrage zur Aetiologie des Keratokonus. *Klin Monatsbl Augenheilkd* 51:281–286, 1913.
3. Biglan AW et al: Keratoglobus and blue sclerae. *Am J Ophthalmol* 83:225–233, 1979.
4. Cadle RG et al: Phenotypic Ehlers-Danlos, type VI with normal lysyl hydroxylase activity and macrocephaly. *Am J Hum Genet* 37:A48, 1985.
5. Farag TI, Schimke RN: Ehlers-Danlos syndrome: a new oculo-scoliotic type with associated polyneuropathy? *Clin Genet* 35:121–124, 1989.
6. Greenfield G et al: Blue sclerae and keratoconus: key features of a distinct heritable disorder of connective tissue. *Clin Genet* 4:8–16, 1973.
7. Heikkinen J et al: Duplication of seven exons in the lysyl hydroxylase gene is associated with longer forms of a repetitive sequence within the gene and is a common cause for the type VI variant of Ehlers-Danlos syndrome. *Am J Hum Genet* 60:48–56, 1997.
8. Heim P et al: Ehlers-Danlos syndrome type VI (EDS VI): problems of diagnosis and management. *Acta Paediatr* 87:708–711, 1998.
9. Hyams SW et al: Blue sclerae and keratoglobus. Ocular signs of a systemic connective tissue disorder. *Br J Ophthalmol* 53:53–58, 1969.
10. Hyland J et al: A homozygous stop codon in the lysyl hydroxylase gene in two siblings with Ehlers-Danlos syndrome type VI. *Nat Genet* 2:228–231, 1992.
11. Jarisch A et al: Sibs affected with both Ehlers-Danlos syndrome type VI and cystic fibrosis. *Am J Med Genet* 78:455–460, 1998.
12. Lamba PA et al: Blue sclerae with keratoglobus. *Orient Arch Ophthalmol* 9:123–126, 1971.
13. *Online Mendelian Inheritance in Man,* OMIM (TM). Johns Hopkins University, Baltimore, MD. MIM Number 148300. World Wide Web URL: http://www.ncbi.nlm.nih.gov/omim/.
14. Royce PM et al: Brittle cornea syndrome: an heritable connective tissue disorder distinct from Ehlers-Danlos syndrome type VI and fragilitas oculi, with spontaneous perforation of the eye, blue sclerae, red hair and normal collagen lysyl hydroxylation. *Eur J Pediatr* 149:465–469, 1990.
15. Sigurdson E et al: The Ehlers-Danlos syndrome and colonic perforation: report of a case and physiologic assessment of underlying motility disorder. *Dis Colon Rectum* 28:962–966, 1985.

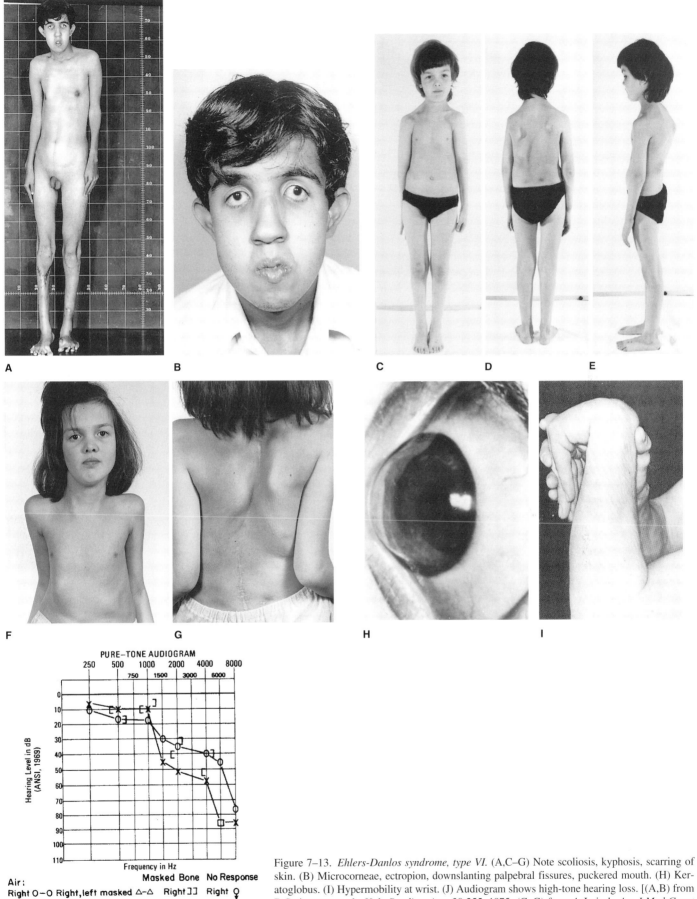

Figure 7–13. *Ehlers-Danlos syndrome, type VI.* (A,C–G) Note scoliosis, kyphosis, scarring of skin. (B) Microcorneae, ectropion, downslanting palpebral fissures, puckered mouth. (H) Keratoglobus. (I) Hypermobility at wrist. (J) Audiogram shows high-tone hearing loss. [(A,B) from B Steinmann et al., *Helv Paediatr Acta* 30:255, 1975; (C–G) from A Jarisch, *Am J Med Genet* 78:455, 1998, reprinted by permission of Wiley-Liss, Inc., a subsidiary of John Wiley & Sons, Inc.; (H–I) from AW Biglan et al., *Am J Ophthalmol* 83:255, 1979.]

16. Stein R et al: Brittle cornea. A familial trait associated with blue sclera. *Am J Ophthalmol* 66:67–69, 1968.
17. Steinmann B et al: The Ehlers-Danlos syndrome. In: *Connective Tissue and Its Heritable Disorders: Molecular, Genetic, and Medical Aspects*, Royce PM, Steinmann B (eds), Wiley-Liss, New York, 1993, pp 351–407.
18. Ticho U et al: Brittle cornea, blue sclerae and red hair syndrome (the brittle cornea syndrome). *Br J Ophthalmol* 64:175–177, 1980.
19. Wenstrup RJ et al: Ehlers-Danlos syndrome type VI: clinical manifestations of collagen lysyl hydroxylase deficiency. *J Pediatr* 115:405–409, 1989.

Ramos-Arroyo-Saksena syndrome: corneal anesthesia, retinal abnormalities, mental retardation, unusual face, and sensorineural hearing loss

In 1987, Ramos-Arroyo et al. (1) and Saksena et al. (2) described the same male and female sibs with hypesthetic corneas, absence of retinal pigment, persistent patent ductus arteriosus, moderate mental retardation, unusual facies, and sensorineural hearing loss. Their mother had similar facial phenotype, retinal changes, and mild to moderate sensorineural hearing loss. A second family was described by Wong et al. (3).

Clinical findings. The children in the initial family exhibited failure to thrive, slim body build, and short stature; their mother, apart from failure to thrive, had a similar appearance.

Craniofacial findings. The face was reported to be broad, flat, and square, with frontal bossing, upslanting palpebral fissures, medial eyebrow flare, mild hypertelorism, depressed nasal root and bridge, and midfacial hypoplasia. The ramus was prominent and the chin wide (2) (Fig. 7–14A).

Ocular system. Corneal anesthesia with secondary neurotrophic corneal keratitis, increased tear production, and corneal erosions were present. On fundoscopic examination, absence of the peripapillary choriocapillaris and retinal pigment epithelium was noted (Fig. 7–14B). There was poor visual acuity.

Central nervous system. The intelligent quotients in the female and male sibs reported by Ramos-Arroyo et al. (1) were estimated at 44 and 50, respectively, and speech was impaired.

Cardiovascular system. Persistent patent ductus arteriosus was present in two cases (3). One patient had difficulty swallowing (3).

Auditory findings. Mild to severe sensorineural hearing loss has been observed.

Heredity. The pattern seen in both families suggests autosomal dominant inheritance.

Summary. Characteristic findings include (*1*) autosomal dominant inheritance; (*2*) corneal anesthesia; (*3*) absence of retinal pigment epithelium; (*4*) moderate mental retardation; (*5*) unusual facies; and (*6*) moderate to severe sensorineural hearing loss.

References

1. Ramos-Arroyo MA et al: Congenital corneal anesthesia with retinal abnormalities, deafness, unusual facies, persistent ductus arteriosus, and mental retardation: a new syndrome? *Am J Med Genet* 26:345–354, 1987.
2. Saksena SS et al: Craniofacial pattern profile (CFPP) evaluation of facial dysmorphology in a familial syndrome with corneal anesthesia and multiple congenital anomalies. *Am J Phys Anthropol* 74:465–471, 1987.
3. Wong VA et al: Congenital trigeminal anesthesia in two siblings and their long-term follow-up. *Am J Ophthalmol* 129:96–98, 2000.

DeHauwere syndrome: iris dysplasia, hypertelorism, psychomotor retardation, and sensorineural hearing loss

In 1973, DeHauwere et al. (1) described a syndrome of mesodermal dysgenesis of the iris, hypertelorism, telecanthus, sensorineural hearing loss, psychomotor retardation, and hypotonia in two generations. A similar disorder was reported by von Noorden and Baller (2).

Physical findings. Height was below the third percentile with head circumference at or below the tenth percentile.

Ocular system. Hypoplasia of the iris stroma, abnormally prominent line of Schwalbe, adhesions between the iris and posterior surface of the cornea, and pear-shaped pupils (Rieger anomaly) have been constant features. Ocular hypertelorism and strabismus were marked (Fig. 7–15A–C).

Central nervous system. Psychomotor retardation was common. In the children, milestones were reached late. The adult had an IQ of 75.

Musculoskeletal system. Hypotonia and hyperlaxity of joints with dislocation of the hips were documented in all patients.

Auditory system. Mild sensorineural hearing loss was noted in each patient.

Vestibular system. Vestibular studies were not mentioned.

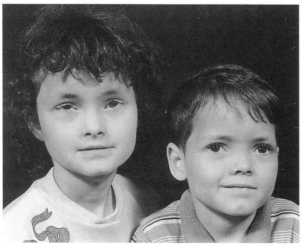

A

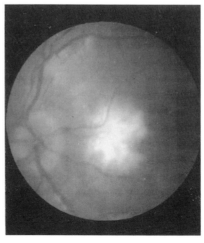

B

Figure 7–14. *Corneal anesthesia, retinal abnormalities, mental retardation, unusual facies, and sensorineural hearing loss.* (A) Both sibs have frontal bossing, mild hypertelorism, with depressed nasal root. Female sib has had tarsorrhaphies. (B) Nonprogressive absence of choriocapillaris retinal pigment epithelium nasal to optic disc. [Courtesy of MA Ramos-Arroyo, Pamplona, Spain.]

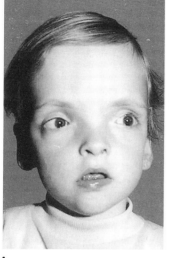
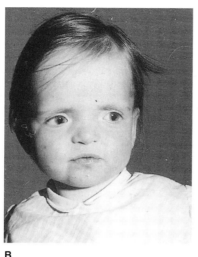
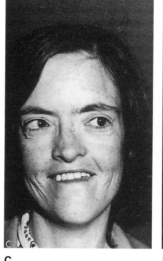
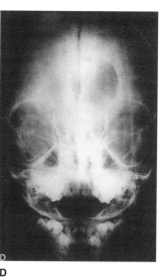

A   B   C   D

Figure 7–15. *Iris dysplasia, hypertelorism, psychomotor retardation, and sensorineural hearing loss.* (A–C) Note irregular pupils and orbital hypertelorism in a mother and her two children. A similarly affected child had died. (D) Pneumoencephalogram showing hypertelorism, dilated and asymmetric lateral ventricles, and indication of a fifth ventricle. [From RC DeHauwere et al., *J Pediatr* 82:679, 1973.]

Laboratory findings. Radiologic findings included retarded bone age, ocular hypertelorism, coxa valga, and hip dislocation. Pneumoencephalographic studies revealed dilated ventricles (Fig. 7–15D).

Routine laboratory studies of urine, serum, and cerebrospinal fluid were unremarkable, as were electroencephalographic, electromyographic, and nerve conduction studies.

Pathology. No pathologic studies were conducted.

Heredity. The syndrome has dominant inheritance. X-linkage cannot be excluded since there has been no male-to-male transmission.

Diagnosis. One must exclude Rieger syndrome, which comprises autosomal dominant inheritance of Rieger anomaly, maxillary hypoplasia, and hypodontia.

Prognosis. Prognosis depends largely on the degree of psychomotor retardation, since none of the other components cause severe disability.

Summary. Characteristics of this syndrome include (*1*) autosomal dominant inheritance; (*2*) Rieger mesodermal dysgenesis of the iris; (*3*) hypertelorism; (*4*) psychomotor retardation; (*5*) hypotonia with joint hypermobility; (*6*) dilated cerebral ventricles; and (*7*) mild sensorineural hearing loss.

References

1. De Hauwere RC et al: Iris dysplasia, orbital hypertelorism, and psychomotor retardation: a dominantly inherited developmental syndrome. *J Pediatr* 82:679–681, 1973.
2. von Noorden GK, Baller BS: The chamber angle in split-pupil. *Arch Ophthalmol* 70:598–602, 1963.

Axenfeld-Rieger anomaly, cardiac malformations, and sensorineural hearing loss

This is an autosomal dominant condition first described by Cunningham et al. (1) and later Grosso et al. (2). Affected individuals have in various combinations ocular anterior chamber anomalies, cardiac malformations, and hearing loss.

Ocular system. Affected individuals have variable manifestations of the Axenfeld-Rieger anomaly, which affects the anterior chamber of the eye, particularly angle structures. Findings can include prominent and anteriorly displaced Schwalbe line, iridocorneal synechiae, iris hypoplasia, or corectopia. Secondary glaucoma is a common manifestation.

Auditory system. When present, hearing loss was sensorineural and had its onset in late childhood through early adulthood.

Cardiac findings. Cardiac defects were only occasionally present, but included atrial septal defect and mitral valve and/or tricuspid valve insufficiency.

Heredity. Inheritance is clearly autosomal dominant.

Diagnosis. This condition closely resembles Rieger syndrome, but cardiac defects and sensorineural hearing loss do not occur in that condition.

Prognosis. Most individuals had a normal life span.

Summary. This condition consists of (*1*) Axenfeld-Rieger anomaly; (*2*) cardiac defects; (*3*) postnatal onset sensorineural hearing loss; and (*4*) autosomal dominant inheritance.

References

1. Cunningham ET Jr. et al: Familial Axenfeld-Rieger anomaly, atrial septal defect, and sensorineural hearing loss: a possible new genetic syndrome. *Arch Ophthalmol* 116:78–82, 1998.
2. Grosso S et al: Familial Axenfeld-Rieger anomaly, cardiac malformations, and sensorineural hearing loss: a provisionally unique genetic syndrome? *Am J Med Genet* 111:182–186, 2002.

Abruzzo-Erickson syndrome: ocular coloboma, cleft palate, short stature, hypospadias, and mixed hearing loss

In 1977, Abruzzo and Erickson (1) described a syndrome of cleft palate, coloboma of the eye, hypospadias, short stature, radial synostosis, and mixed hearing loss in two male sibs and their mother's brother.

Physical findings. Stature was below the third centile in all three. Adult height in the maternal uncle was 5 feet.

Craniofacial findings. The face tended to be flat with the pinnae being long and soft. Cleft palate was present in both sibs and a submucous cleft palate in the uncle.

Ocular system. Colobomas of the iris, choroid, and retina were found in both sibs.

Musculoskeletal system. Radial synostosis was noted in the uncle and in one sib. There was wide spacing between the second and third metacarpals and some ulnar deviation of index fingers.

Genitourinary system. Hypospadias of varying degree was present in all three affected individuals. Cryptorchidism was noted in the uncle. A horseshoe kidney was found in one sib.

Auditory system. Sensorineural hearing loss was noted at 20 years of age in the uncle. It was progressive and resulted in severe loss at 34 years. Both sibs had 10–25 dB sensorineural loss and a greater conductive loss attributed to many middle ear infections secondary to cleft palate.

Heredity. The observation of three affected males with minor stigmata in carrier females suggests X-linked inheritance.

Diagnosis. Several of the stigmata are found in CHARGE association (3). Abruzzo and Erickson (2) have argued that, because their patients did not have choanal atresia, retarded development, or genital hypoplasia, they did not have familial CHARGE association.

Summary. Characteristics of this syndrome have included (*1*) probable X-linked inheritance; (*2*) coloboma of iris, choroid and retina; (*3*) cleft palate; (*4*) short stature; (*5*) radial synostosis; (*6*) hypospadias; and (*7*) sensorineural hearing loss.

References

1. Abruzzo MA, Erickson RP: A new syndrome of cleft palate associated with coloboma, hypospadias, deafness, short stature, and radial synostosis. *J Med Genet* 14:76–80, 1977.
2. Abruzzo MA, Erickson RP: Re-evaluation of new X-linked syndrome for evidence of CHARGE syndrome or association. *Am J Med Genet* 34:397–400, 1989.
3. Tellier AL et al: CHARGE syndrome: report of 47 cases and review. *Am J Med Genet* 76:402–409, 1998.

Aniridia and sensorineural hearing loss

Courteney-Harris and Mills (1) reported a father and daughter with bilateral aniridia and sensorineural hearing loss. Another daughter had only hearing loss, which suggests a possibility that the aniridia and hearing loss were unrelated. The father had nonprogressive 35–60 dB sensorineural loss since childhood. Similar findings were noted in both daughters. Aniridia and hearing loss have been reported as a component in a rare disorder involving Wilms tumor and nephropathy (2,3). Aniridia is almost always (if not always) caused by mutations in *PAX6* (4), and mutations in this gene should be sought in other individuals with the combination of aniridia/hearing loss.

References

1. Courteney-Harris RG, Mills RP: Aniridia and deafness: an inherited disorder. *J Laryngol Otol* 104:419–420, 1990.
2. de Chadarevian JP et al: Aniridia/glaucoma and Wilms tumor in a sibship with renal tubular acidosis and sensory nerve deafness. *Am J Med Genet Suppl* 3:323–328, 1987.
3. Mayer UM: Peters' anomaly and combination with other malformations (series of 16 patients). *Ophthalm Paediatr Genet* 13:131–135, 1992.
4. Prosser J, van Heyningen V: *PAX6* mutations reviewed. *Hum Mutat* 11:93–108, 1998.

Jan syndrome: congenital total color blindness, cataracts, hyperinsulinism, and sensorineural hearing loss

Jan et al. (4) reported congenital total color blindness, cataracts, hyperinsulinism, and sensorineural hearing loss in sisters. Both sibs exhibited truncal adiposity. Newell and Diddie (10) described color blindness, mental retardation, euthyroid goiter, and sensorineural hearing loss in three sibs.

Ocular system. Hyperopia, marked photophobia, and vertical pendular to jerky nystagmus were found in the first years of life. Visual fields showed peripheral constriction, especially nasally. The retina became diffusely stippled with fine pigment at 15 years. Posterior subcapsular central fluffy cataracts were noted at about the same time (4). No mention of cataracts was made by Newell and Diddie (10). Color vision assessment showed complete absence of color discrimination.

Auditory system. Bilateral nonprogressive mild to severe sensorineural hearing loss was found. The sibs reported by Jan et al. (4) had mild to moderate loss at 5–6 years of age, whereas Newell and Diddie's cases had a hearing loss that was severe and congenital (10).

Vestibular findings. Caloric irrigation indicated a defect in one sister reported by Jan et al. (4), but documentation was not extensive.

Laboratory findings. Hyperinsulinism was found in both sisters by Jan et al. (4). Urinary 17-ketosteroid levels were elevated. High plasma thyroid levels were noted by Newell and Diddie (10).

Heredity. Autosomal recessive inheritance appears likely.

Diagnosis. Total color blindness is a rare autosomal recessive disorder due to at least two genes, *CNGA32* (5) and *CNGB3* (6), both of which are found in association with photophobia, nystagmus, and vision loss. The optic discs are pale. However, the hearing loss and other findings in the syndrome under discussion are not typically present (9). Andersen (1) described the co-occurrence of total color blindness and sensorineural hearing loss but it appears coincidental. Ferguson (2) and Macgregor and Harrison (8) reported total color blindness in four sibs: two had hypertension and all had hearing loss but "otosclerosis" was stated to run in the family. Progressive total color blindness, liver degeneration, endocrine dysfunction, and sensorineural hearing loss has been found with hearing loss in six females from two sibships in a consanguineous family and in an isolated male (3,7).

Summary. Characteristics of this syndrome include (*1*) autosomal recessive inheritance; (*2*) total color blindness; (*3*) retinal pigmentation; (*4*) cataracts; (*5*) hyperinsulinism; (*6*) possibly mild mental retardation; and (*7*) nonprogressive mild to severe sensorineural hearing loss.

References

1. Andersen SR: On congenital total colour blindness coexisting with heredolabyrinthine deafness. *Acta Ophthalmol* 24:99–112, 1946.
2. Ferguson JWMA: Four cases of congenital total color-blindness, with otosclerosis and hypertension as associated hereditary abnormalities. *Trans Ophthalm Soc UK* 69:249–263, 1949.
3. Hansen E et al: A familial syndrome of progressive cone dystrophy, degenerative liver disease, endocrine dysfunction and hearing defect. I. Ophthalmological findings. *Acta Ophthalmol (Copenh)* 54:129–144, 1976.
4. Jan JE et al: Familial congenital monochromatism, cataracts, and sensorineural deafness. *Am J Dis Child* 130:1349–1350, 1976.
5. Kohl S et al: Total colour blindness is caused by mutations in the gene encoding the alpha-subunit of the cone photoreceptor cGMP-gated cation channel. *Nat Genet* 19:257–259, 1998.
6. Kohl S et al: Mutations in the *CNGB3* gene encoding the beta-subunit of the cone photoreceptor cGMP-gated channel are responsible for achromatopsia (ACHM3) linked to chromosome 8q21. *Hum Mol Genet* 9:2107–2116, 2000.

7. Larsen IF et al: Familial syndrome of progressive cone dystrophy, degenerative liver disease and endocrine dysfunction. II. Clinical and metabolic studies. *Clin Genet* 13:176–189, 1978.
8. Macgregor AG, Harrison RR: Congenital total colour blindness associated with otosclerosis. *Ann Eugen* 15:219–233, 1950.
9. Madsen PH: Total achromatopsia in two brothers. *Acta Ophthalmol (Copenh)* 45:587–593, 1967.
10. Newell FW, Diddie KR: Typische Monochromasie, angeborene Taubheit und Resistenz gegenüber der intrazellulären Wirkung des Thyreoideahormons. *Klin Monatsbl Augenheilkd* 171:731–734, 1977.

Hansen syndrome: progressive cone dystrophy, liver degeneration, endocrine dysfunction, and sensorineural hearing loss

Hansen et al. (2), Larsen et al. (3) and Berg et al. (1) described two families with a syndrome of total color blindness (progressive cone dystrophy), liver degeneration, endocrine system dysfunction, and sensorineural hearing loss in seven patients.

Endocrine findings. Some of the affected individuals had children; two probably were infertile, and three had repeated spontaneous abortions. Primary hypothyroidism was found in two patients and another two had low normal thyroid function with protracted thyrotropin releasing hormone response, suggesting a hypothalamic disorder. Enlarged sella turcica was found in three, and in one of these, an empty sella was demonstrated by surgery. Two patients had a defect in ACTH reserve. Maturity-onset diabetes of the young was found in three patients, and a fourth had borderline glucose tolerance. Hypertension was observed in the patients who were diabetic.

Ocular system. Vision is reduced from early childhood. Photophobia and better visual performance in twilight than in daylight were observed. Initially there was some ability to see colors, but from around the age of puberty, only grayish tones were seen and a magnifying glass was needed to read. Vision deteriorated further, and at the end of the second decade, the patients were nearly blind with total achromatopsia with a scotopic spectral sensitivity pattern.

The fundi appeared atrophic with no pigmentation. The vessels were attenuated and disc pallor was seen. The least affected patient had moderately reduced color vision within a small central area and a rod response only in the more peripheral parts.

Hepatic system. Four patients had liver degeneration, elevated transaminase, nonspecific parenchymal degeneration, fatty infiltration, and isolated liver cell necrosis on biopsy.

Auditory system. All except the youngest patient had at least moderate sensorineural hearing loss, which was cochlear and progressive. The hearing loss in one patient, however, appeared to be congenital and sensorineural.

Laboratory findings. Elevated creatinine phosphokinase was noted.

Heredity. Inheritance appears to be autosomal recessive. In the first kindred, there were six affected females in two highly inbred sibships. The second family had one affected male (1).

Diagnosis. There is overlap with the syndrome of congenital total color blindness, cataracts, hyperinsulinism, and sensorineural hearing loss, which also has autosomal recessive inheritance. One must also exclude progressive rod-cone dystrophy, renal dysfunction, and sensorineural hearing loss.

Summary. Characteristics of this syndrome include (*1*) autosomal recessive inheritance; (*2*) progressive total color blindness; (*3*) liver degeneration; (*4*) endocrine dysfunction (sterility, hypothyroidism, diabetes); and (*5*) sensorineural hearing loss.

References

1. Berg K et al: Familial syndrome of progressive cone dystrophy, degenerative liver disease, and endocrine dysfunction. III. Genetic studies. *Clin Genet* 13:190–200, 1978.
2. Hansen E et al: A familial syndrome of progressive cone dystrophy, degenerative liver disease, endocrine dysfunction and hearing defect. I. Ophthalmological findings. *Acta Ophthalmol (Copenh)* 54:129–144, 1976.
3. Larsen IF et al: Familial syndrome of progressive cone dystrophy, degenerative liver disease and endocrine dysfunction. II. Clinical and metabolic studies. *Clin Genet* 13:176–189, 1978.

Beighton syndrome: rod-cone dystrophy, renal dysfunction, and sensorineural hearing loss

Beighton et al. (1) described a syndrome comprising progressive rod-cone dystrophy, renal dysfunction, and sensorineural hearing loss in 14 children from 9 Afrikaner families in South Africa. Each of the children was initially misdiagnosed as having retinitis pigmentosa or Usher syndrome. This disorder has so far been found only in the Afrikaner population.

Auditory system. A progressive hearing loss was present with onset in the first decade and progression to profound hearing loss in the second decade in at least two cases.

Vestibular system. Cold water calorics produced no response in one case and minimal response in another, raising the possibility of some vestibular involvement.

Visual system. A rod-cone dystrophy, rather than retinitis pigmentosa, is an appropriate description of the retinal findings. Contrary to what is usually seen in retinitis pigmentosa and the Usher syndromes, there is a significant macular component as evidenced by an early loss of central vision, hypopigmentation of the retinal epithelium, and minimal bone spicules. Childhood cataracts were a complicating factor in 4 of 14 cases.

Neurologic findings. Intelligence was reported to be normal.

Renal system. The Fanconi nephrosis, manifest first by albuminuria by the age of 6 years, leads to rachitic skeletal changes within the first decade and, ultimately, kidney failure. Growth retardation and malalignment of weight-bearing bones are the main skeletal manifestations of this disorder.

Heredity. Inheritance is autosomal recessive.

Differential Diagnosis. Usher syndrome was the initial diagnosis in several cases; however, Usher syndrome has a slightly different retinal phenotype and has no associated renal complications. Alström syndrome is associated with renal dysplasia but typically has associated obesity and diabetes. Retinitis pigmentosa with renal disease and skeletal changes is seen in Mainzer-Saldino syndrome, but no hearing loss was noted (3). Renal dysplasia-retinal dysplasia has been noted in one case of Loken-Senior syndrome (2).

Prognosis. The condition is seriously handicapping. Children with this disorder face a triple handicap: profound hearing loss, blindness, and skeletal problems secondary to the Fanconi nephrosis. There was significant mortality noted in the original series of patients, as evidenced by the report that 8 of 14 children died between the ages of 3 and 20 years, mostly from renal failure. With early recognition and management, this risk can be expected to decline.

Treatment. Management will involve the medical treatment of the renal complication and orthopedic correction of the skeletal problems. Kidney transplantation is an option. Cochlear implants may be considered once the hearing loss has progressed to the severe to profound stage. Visual symptoms may be partially helped by the use of low vision aids; because of the early onset of the cataracts, cataract surgery may be considered at an earlier age than typical for most patients with retinitis pigmentosa.

References

1. Beighton P et al: Rod-cone dystrophy, sensorineural deafness, and renal dysfunction: an autosomal recessive syndrome? *Am J Med Genet* 47:832–836, 1993.
2. Kobayashi Y et al: Renal retinal dysplasia with diffuse glomerular cysts. *Nephron* 39:201–205, 1985.
3. Mainzer F et al: Familial nephropathy associated with retinitis pigmentosa, cerebellar ataxia and skeletal abnormalities. *Am J Med* 49:556–562, 1970.

IVIC syndrome: ophthalmoplegia, radial ray hypoplasia, thrombocytopenia, and congenital mixed hearing loss (oculo-oto-radial syndrome)

Arias et al. (1) reported a syndrome of radial ray hypoplasia, external ophthalmoplegia, thrombocytopenia, and congenital mixed hearing loss. Nineteen members in five generations were affected. The term *IVIC syndrome* used by Arias et al. (1) is derived from the Institute Venezolano de Investigaciones Cientificas. Another family with three affected in two generations was observed (9), as was a third with an affected mother and son (2). Elcioglu and Berry (3) observed a family with at least seven affected family members, including a pair of identical twin highly discordant with regard to severity. Neri and Sammito (7) suggested the alternative name oculo-oto-radial syndrome.

Musculoskeletal system. The upper extremity was chiefly affected. Radial ray defects varied from an almost normal thumb to sessile thumb to triphalangeal thumb to a severely malformed arm. Bilateral hypoplasia or distal displacement of the thumbs was the most common alteration, and hypoplasia of thenar muscles was a constant feature.

Radiographically, there was delayed growth in the forearms, clavicles, calvaria, and spine. The thumb, when present, had a long, slender metacarpal and short distal phalanx. The sesamoid bone of the first metacarpal was always absent. The radial carpal bones were always hypoplastic, and they were fused in 40%. Most patients had limitation of movement at elbows, wrists, and interphalangeal joints. Vertebral and femoral length were reduced. Other anomalies included proximal fusion of radius and ulna and immaturity of distal epiphyses of radius and ulna.

Ocular system. Ophthalmoplegia was a common feature. Extraocular muscles were involved, producing strabismus. Medial and lateral recti were most often and most severely affected but all extraocular muscles could be affected. Asymmetric ophthalmoplegia was noted in 40%.

Other findings. About 10% of patients exhibited imperforate anus. Dermatoglyphic alterations included a high a–b ridge count, distally placed or absent t triradius, and increased pattern frequency in the second interdigital area. Incomplete right bundle branch block was found in 7 of 19 affected members.

Auditory system. Bilateral congenital mixed loss, either partial or total, was evident, with high-frequency loss being most common.

Laboratory findings. Mild thrombocytopenia and leukocytosis were present before age 50.

Heredity. Autosomal dominant inheritance is clearly evident. Penetrance was complete but there is variable expression (3). Arias et al. (1) traced the disorder in his family from the Canary Islands to Venezuela.

Diagnosis. IVIC syndrome most overlaps with Okihiro syndrome, in which radial ray defects, ophthalmoplegia, and hearing loss occur (4,6). Anal atresia has also been described in Okihiro syndrome (5,8). Whereas the cause of Okihiro syndrome is known to be *SALL4* mutation (5), the cause of IVIC is unknown. Other conditions that may resemble IVIC are the lacrimo-auriculo-dento-digital (LADD) syndrome and Townes-Brocks syndrome. Thrombocytopenia is associated with absent radii in the TAR syndrome, but hearing loss is not a feature of that disorder.

Summary. Characteristics of this syndrome include (*1*) autosomal dominant inheritance; (*2*) radial ray hypoplasia; (*3*) external ophthalmoplegia; (*4*) thrombocytopenia; and (*5*) congenital mixed hearing loss.

References

1. Arias S et al: The IVIC syndrome: a new autosomal dominant complex pleiotropic syndrome with radial ray hypoplasia, hearing impairment, external ophthalmoplegia and thrombocytopenia. *Am J Med Genet* 6:25–59, 1980.
2. Czeizel A et al: IVIC syndrome: report of a third family. *Am J Med Genet* 33:282–283, 1989.
3. Elcioglu N, Berry AC: Monozygotic twins discordant for the oculo-oto-radial syndrome (IVIC syndrome). *Genet Counsel* 8:201–206, 1997.
4. Hayes A et al: The Okihiro syndrome of Duane anomaly, radial ray abnormalities, and deafness. *Am J Med Genet* 22:273–280, 1985.
5. Kohlhase J et al: Okihiro syndrome is caused by *SALL4* mutations. *Hum Mol Genet* 11:2979–2987, 2002.
6. MacDermot KD, Winter RM: Radial ray defect and Duane anomaly: report of a family with autosomal dominant transmission. *Am J Med Genet* 27:313–319, 1987.
7. Neri G, Sammito V: Re: IVIC syndrome report by Czeizel et al. [Letter]. *Am J Med Genet* 33:284, 1989.
8. Reardon W et al: Mutations in *SALL4* on chromosome 20 cause Okihiro syndrome. Presented at the 10th Manchester Birth Defects Conference, 2002.
9. Sammito V et al: IVIC syndrome: report of a second family. *Am J Med Genet* 29:875–881, 1988.

Cataracts and progressive sensorineural hearing loss

In 1982, Nadol and Burgess (3), described a four-generation kindred with cochleosaccular degeneration and cataracts affecting 15 members. Another family of eight affected members in four generations was reported by Guala et al. (1).

Ocular system. The cataracts in some members were congenital; in others they appeared in childhood. In still others, cataracts appeared in the fourth decade. Involvement was asymmetric.

Auditory system. The sensorineural hearing loss appeared during the first to fourth decade and was progressive, resulting in total hearing loss in midlife.

Vestibular findings. A few patients exhibited a staggering gait.

Pathology. Histopathologic sections of the temporal bones revealed severe cochleosaccular degeneration (1,3) (Fig. 7–16A,B).

Heredity. Autosomal dominant inheritance is clearly evident (1,2) (Fig. 7–16C). Lalwani et al. (2) mapped a locus for nonsyndromic dominant deafness causing cochleosaccular degeneration to chromosome 22. Whether the two families cited here are variants of this DFNA17 remains to be explored.

Diagnosis. Cataracts, both congenital and those appearing later in life, have inordinate numbers of syndromal associations. However, this binary combination of cataracts and hearing loss appears distinct.

Summary. Characteristics include (*1*) autosomal dominant inheritance; (*2*) cataracts with variable onset; and (*3*) progressive sensorineural hearing loss.

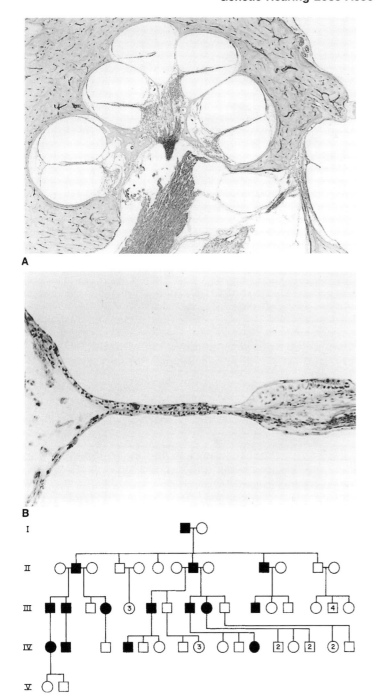

Figure 7–16. *Cataracts and progressive sensorineural hearing loss.* (A) Midmodiolar section of right cochlea of proband. Otic capsule is normal. There is reduction of spiral ganglion cells (SG) in basal turn. Organ of Corti demonstrates total loss of hair cells and has been reduced to flattened layer of epithelial cells on basilar membrane. Saccule macula (S) also demonstrates severe degeneration. Original magnification, ×19. (B) Higher-power magnification of organ of Corti of basal turn. There are no remaining hair cells or supporting cells. Cochlear duct is collapsed and Reissner's membrane lies against spiral limbus (SL), tectorial membrane (TM), and flattened squamous epithelial cells on basilar membrane. There is a reduced number of cochlear neurons. Original magnification, ×230. (C) Pedigree of family exhibiting autosomal dominant inheritance. Affected individuals with congenital cataracts and progressive hearing loss are indicated by blackened profiles. [From JB Nadol Jr and B Burgess. *Laryngoscope* 92:1028, 1982.]

References

1. Guala A et al: A syndrome of progressive sensorineural deafness and cataract inherited as an autosomal dominant trait. *Clin Genet* 41:293–295, 1992.
2. Lalwani AK et al: A new locus for nonsyndromic hereditary hearing impairment, DFNA17, maps to chromosome 22 and represents a gene for cochleosaccular degeneration. *Am J Hum Genet* 64:318–323, 1999.
3. Nadol JB Jr, Burgess B: Cochleosaccular degeneration of the inner ear and progressive cataracts inherited as an autosomal dominant trait. *Laryngoscope* 92:1028–1037, 1982.

Nucci syndrome: congenital cataracts, hypercholesterolemia, spasticity of lower limbs, and sensorineural hearing loss

In 1990, Nucci and Mets (2) described 4-year-old and 8-year-old brothers with congenital nuclear cataracts, hypercholesterolemia, spasticity of lower limbs, possible mild mental retardation, and sensorineural hearing loss. A second possible case was described by Guillen-Navarro but this case was not reported to have hypercholesterolemia and had patchy hypopigmented areas and atretic ear canals (1).

The case reported by Nucci and Mets (2) showed a 25 dB loss at 500 Hz but precipitous falling off to 100 dB at 4000 Hz.

Inheritance may be autosomal or X-linked recessive. The case reported by Guillen-Navarro (1) had consanguineous parents, suggesting an autosomal recessive etiology.

References

1. Guillen-Navarro E et al: A new form of complicated hereditary spastic paraplegia with cataracts, atretic ear canals and hypopigmentation. *Clin Neurol Neurosurg* 100:64–67, 1998.
2. Nucci P, Mets MB: Cataract, hearing loss and hypercholesterolemia. *Acta Ophthalmol (Copenh)* 68:739–742, 1990.

Schaap syndrome: congenital cataracts, hypogonadism, hypertrichosis, and hearing loss

Schaap et al. (2) reported three male sibs with the combination of mild mental retardation, congenital cataract, sensorineural hearing loss, hypogonadism, hypertrichosis, and short stature. The parents were consanguineous, which suggests autosomal recessive inheritance for this entity. All had congenital cataracts, which were described as being lamellar in two. Hearing loss was sensorineural, but it is unknown if the loss was congenital or not. It was diagnosed by age 2 years in one boy, 6 years in another, and at an unknown age in the third. All three had short stature, hypogonadism, and hypertrichosis affecting the back, shoulders, arms, and legs. Although mental retardation was present, it was described as mild in all three. There are some resemblances to Begeer syndrome (1) and CAHMR (CAtaracts, Hypertrichosis, and Mental Retardation) syndrome (3), but cataracts occurred at an earlier age in those with Begeer syndrome, and hearing loss and hypogonadism were not described for CAHMR syndrome.

References

1. Begeer JH et al: Two sisters with mental retardation, cataract, ataxia, progressive hearing loss, and polyneuropathy. *J Med Genet* 28:884–885, 1991.
2. Schaap C et al: Three mildly retarded siblings with congenital cataracts, sensorineural deafness, hypogonadism, hypertrichosis and short stature: a new syndrome? *Clin Dysmorphol* 4:283–288, 1995.
3. Temtamy SA, Sinbawy AHH: Cataract, hypertrichosis and mental retardation (CAHMR): a new autosomal recessive syndrome. *Am J Med Genet* 41:432–433, 1995.

Oculo-facio-cardio-dental (OFCD) syndrome

Hayward (2) described a woman with canine gigantism and radiculomegaly who also had congenital cataracts. Marashi and Gorlin (3,4) described three individuals with this condition, and suggested it comprised a specific syndrome. Other cases have been described by Wilkie et al. (7), Obwegeser and Gorlin (5), Aalfs et al. (1), and Schulze et al. (6), who also provided a good review of this condition. Facial phenotype consisted of long narrow face, ptosis, high nasal bridge with broad nasal tip, and long philtrum (Fig. 7–17A,B). Other manifestations included congenital cataract, microphthalmia, mild cardiac defects, and occasional short stature. The dental anomalies are striking, in that there were radiculomegaly, oligodontia, delayed dentition, and abnormal enamel. Two of the 12 described individuals have had mild sensorineural hearing loss (1). The gene maps to Xp11.2-p21.2 and is allelic with Lenz microphthalmia (Gorlin, personal communication, 2003).

References

1. Aalfs CM et al: Cataracts, radiculomegaly, septal heart defects and hearing loss in two unrelated females with normal intelligence and similar facial appearance: confirmation of a syndrome? *Clin Dysmorphol* 5:93–103, 1996.
2. Hayward JR: Cuspid gigantism. *Oral Surg Oral Med Oral Pathol* 49:500–501, 1980.
3. Marashi AH, Gorlin RJ: Cataracts and radiculomegaly of canines. *Oral Surg Oral Med Oral Pathol* 70:802–803, 1990.
4. Marashi AH, Gorlin RJ: Radiculomegaly of canine teeth and congenital cataracts: confirmation of a syndrome. *Am J Med Genet* 42:143, 1992.
5. Obwegeser HI, Gorlin RJ: Oculo-facio-cardio-dental (OFCD) syndrome. *Clin Dysmorphol* 6:281–283, 1997.
6. Schulze BRB et al: Rare dental abnormalities seen in oculo-facio-cardio-dental (OFCD) syndrome: three new cases and review of nine patients. *Am J Med Genet* 82:429–438, 1999.
7. Wilkie AOM et al: Congenital cataract, microphthalmia and septal heart defect in two generations: a new syndrome? *Clin Dysmorphol* 2:114–119, 1992.

Cataracts, sensorineural hearing loss, Down syndrome–like facial appearance, short stature, and mental retardation

Gripp et al. (1) described two unrelated patients with a strikingly similar phenotype and suggested they had a provisionally unique syndrome.

Ocular findings. Both individuals had congenital cataracts.

Central nervous system. Both patients had mental retardation, one with autistic features. Seizures affected one individual.

Facial findings. The face was described as Down syndrome–like. Facial profile was flat, with upslanting palpebral fissures, small nose, and small mouth.

Figure 7–17. *OFCD syndrome.* (A,B) Twenty-one-year-old female with congenital microphthalmia and cataract. The nose is pointed. [Courtesy of RCM Hennekam. Amsterdam, The Netherlands.]

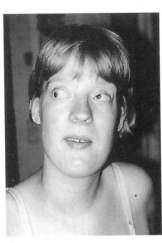 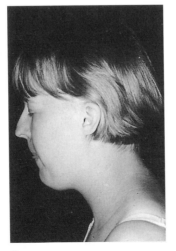

A   B

Auditory system. Hearing loss developed during late infancy, and was mixed in one child and sensorineural in the other child.

Other findings. Both individuals had short stature (<5th centile). One child had idiopathic chondrolysis, whereas the other had bilateral radioulnar synostosis. One child also had a diaphragmatic hernia and pericardial effusion, whereas the other had inguinal hernia and hydrocele.

Heredity. The mode of inheritance is unknown; both were isolated cases.

Prognosis. Prognosis is unknown. The older individual was 15 years old at the time of the report.

Summary. This condition includes (*1*) congenital cataracts; (*2*) Down syndrome–like face; (*3*) short stature; (*4*) postnatal-onset hearing loss; (*5*) mental retardation; and (*6*) occasional other anomalies.

Reference

Gripp KW et al: Apparently new syndrome of congenital cataracts, sensorineural deafness, Down syndrome–like facial appearance, short stature, and mental retardation. *Am J Med Genet* 61:382–386, 1996.

Congenital cataracts, subluxation of radial heads, unusual face, and sensorineural hearing loss

Waterson (personal communication, 1990) reported a male with bilateral congenital cataracts, a somewhat flattened face, short columella, bilaterally subluxed radial heads, and severe bilateral sensorineural hearing loss.

Ohdo syndrome: mental retardation, congenital heart disease, blepharophimosis/ptosis, hypoplastic teeth, and hearing loss

In 1986, Ohdo et al. (9) reported a syndrome of blepharophimosis, blepharoptosis, hypoplastic teeth, mental retardation, and hearing loss in two sibs and their first cousin. Similar examples were later observed (1,3,6,8,10).

Craniofacial findings. The face is characterized by blepharophimosis, blepharoptosis, amblyopia, wide and depressed nasal bridge, long flat philtrum, thin vermilion, small ears, microstomia, and hypoplastic teeth (Fig. 7–18).

Central nervous system. Mental retardation was found in most cases, with IQs ranging from 37 to 56.

Other findings. Variable features have included congenital heart anomalies (10), cryptorchidism (1,6,10), hypothyroidism (J Clayton-Smith, personal communication), hyperextensible joints, postaxial polydactyly (3), and clinodactyly of fifth fingers (1,6,10), hypotonia (1,6,10), café-au-lait spots (1,6), proteinuria (1,9,10), and circumferential skin rings around the penis (J Clayton-Smith, personal communication).

Auditory system. Auricular stenosis (1,9) and small pinnae (9,10) have been observed. Hearing loss was a constant but not well-documented feature (1,6,9,10).

Heredity. Ohdo et al. (9) reported two affected siblings and a cousin and suggested recessive inheritance; other cases were sporadic except for the report of an affected mother and child (8), which indicates that the inheritance is possibly dominant with reduced penetrance.

Diagnosis. While chromosomal duplication syndromes such as dup(10q) and dup(20p) show clinical overlap with Ohdo syndrome, the most compelling overlap is with the condition known as Young-Simp-

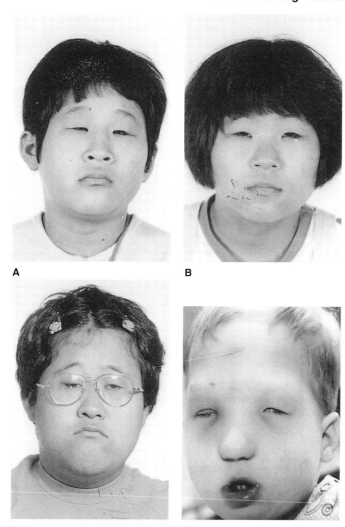

A B

C D

Figure 7–18. *Blepharophimosis-ptosis, mental retaration, congenital heart disease, hypoplastic teeth, and hearing loss (Ohdo syndrome).* (A–C) Two sibs and their first cousin with blepharophimosis, blepharoptosis, wide and depressed nasal bridge, and microstomia. (D) Similarly affected child. [(A–C) from S Ohdo et al., *J Med Genet* 23:242, 1986; (D) From LG Biesecker, *J Med Genet* 28:131, 1991.]

son syndrome (11). In this disorder, blepharophimosis and microcephaly occur in association with a bulbous nose, congenital heart defects, mental retardation, and hypothyroidism. Because there have been patients with overlapping phenotypes (3,7), it has been suggested these are the same condition (4). Other entities to consider in the differential diagnosis include Dubowitz syndrome, Michels syndrome, Marden-Walker syndrome, Tsukahara syndrome, and fetal alcohol syndrome (3). Buntinx and Majewski (2) reported a patient with blepharophimosis, iris coloboma, postaxial polydactyly, agenesis of corpus callosum, hydroureter, developmental delay, and hearing loss. Biesecker (1) has elegantly discussed the differential diagnosis. Also to be considered in diagnosis is blepharophimosis-ptosis epicanthus inversus syndrome (BPES), the gene for which has been mapped to 3q22 (5).

Summary. The characteristics of this disorder include (*1*) possible autosomal recessive inheritance; (*2*) blepharophimosis-ptosis; (*3*) mental retardation; (*4*) dysmorphic pinnae with auricular stenosis; and (*5*) hearing loss, possibly conductive.

References

1. Biesecker LG: The Ohdo blepharophimosis syndrome: a third case. *J Med Genet* 28:131–134, 1991.
2. Buntinx I, Majewski F: Blepharophimosis, iris coloboma, microgenia, hearing loss, postaxial polydactyly, aplasia of corpus callosum, hydroureter, and developmental delay. *Am J Med Genet* 36:273–274, 1990.
3. Clayton-Smith J et al: A distinctive blepharophimosis syndrome. Presented at the 5th Manchester Birth Defects Conference, 1992.
4. Holder-Espinasse M et al: Mental retardation and blepharophimosis in two patients: overlapping features between Young-Simpson and Ohdo syndrome. Presented at the 10th Manchester Birth Defects Conference, 2002.
5. Jewett T et al: Blepharophimosis, ptosis, and epicanthus inversus syndrome (BPES) associated with interstitial deletion of band 3q22: review and gene assignment to the interface of band 3q22.3 and 3q23. *Am J Med Genet* 47:1147–1150, 1993.
6. Maat-Kievit A et al: Two additional cases of the Ohdo blepharophimosis syndrome. *Am J Med Genet* 47:901–906, 1993.
7. Marques-de-Faria AP et al: A boy with mental retardation, blepharophimosis and hypothyroidism: a diagnostic dilemma between Young-Simpson and Ohdo syndrome. *Clin Dysmorphol* 9:199–204, 2000.
8. Mhanni AA et al: Vertical transmission of the Ohdo blepharophimosis syndrome. *Am J Med Genet* 77:144–148, 1998.
9. Ohdo S et al: Mental retardation associated with congenital heart disease, blepharophimosis, blepharoptosis, and hypoplastic teeth. *J Med Genet* 23:242–244, 1986.
10. Say B, Barber N: Mental retardation with blepharophimosis. *J Med Genet* 24:511, 1987.
11. Young ID, Simpson K: Unknown syndrome: abnormal facies, congenital heart defects, hypothyroidism and severe retardation. *J Med Genet* 24:715–716, 1987.

Michels syndrome: blepharophimosis/ptosis, inverse epicanthus, cleft lip–palate, mental retardation, and mixed hearing loss (oculopalatoskeletal syndrome)

Michels et al. (6) described four sibs with the eyelid triad of blepharophimosis, blepharoptosis, and inverse epicanthus with limitation of upward gaze, hypertelorism, cleft lip and palate, various skeletal anomalies, mild mental retardation, and mixed hearing loss. An additional nine cases in five families have been reported (1–3,8,10).

Ocular system. All individuals had blepharophimosis, ptosis, and inverse epicanthus as well as hypertelorism (Fig. 7–19). Bilateral wedge-shaped corneal stromal opacities were present superiorly and extended over the pupil with adhesions extending from the opacity to the iris. All patients exhibited limitation of upward gaze.

Oral findings. Oromandibular anomalies ranged from cleft lip–palate to abnormal palate to malocclusion (2,6,8).

Central nervous system. Deep tendon reflexes were hyperactive with bilateral ankle clonus. Intelligence quotients ranged from 60 to 80 (1,3,6,8).

Musculoskeletal system. Clinodactyly was reported in one case (2). Michels et al. observed short fifth fingers with a single flexion crease, bilaterally (6). Spina bifida occulta was found in two of the four sibs. Two exhibited flattened occiput with poor development of the squamosal portion of the occipital bone. Early closure of the lambdoidal suture was found in two sibs.

Auditory system. Bilateral moderate to severe conductive hearing loss was observed in Michels family (6).

Other findings. Short stature (2) and/or growth retardation (6) appears to be a consistent finding. Laryngomalacia has been reported in one case (8).

Heredity. All cases have appeared either sporadically or in multiply affected sibships; one case had consanguineous parents (3). Inheritance is clearly autosomal recessive. A gene for blepharophimosis-ptosis and epicanthus inversus (BPES) syndrome has been mapped to chromosome 3q22 (5).

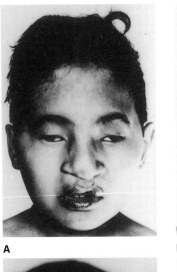
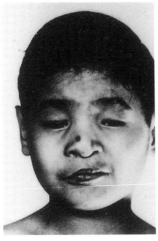

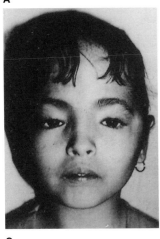
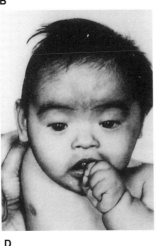

A   **B**

C   **D**

Figure 7–19. *Blepharophimosis-ptosis, inverse epicanthus, cleft lip–palate, mental retardation, and mixed hearing loss (Michels syndrome).* (A–D) Blepharoptosis, blepharophimosis, and epicanthus inversus. Note repaired cleft lip in upper two patients. [From VV Michels et al., *J Pediatr* 93:444, 1978.]

Diagnosis. The syndrome should clearly be separated from BPES not associated with other anomalies. Jackson and Barr (4) reported two female sibs with blepharophimosis-ptosis, partial subluxation of the radial head, narrowing of ear canals, and destruction of middle ear, resulting in moderately severe conductive hearing loss. There was slightly below-normal intelligence but no mention of cleft lip–palate. Ohdo et al. (9) described female sibs and a female paternal cousin with blepharophimosis-ptosis, mental retardation, and hearing loss. The syndrome reported by Mutchinick (7) has some overlapping features.

Summary. Characteristics of this condition include (*1*) autosomal recessive inheritance; (*2*) blepharophimosis-ptosis; (*3*) inverse epicanthus; (*4*) mental retardation; (*5*) cleft lip and palate; and (*6*) mixed hearing loss.

References

1. Cunniff C, Jones KL: Craniosynostosis and lid anomalies: report of a girl with Michels syndrome. *Am J Med Genet* 37:28–30, 1990.
2. De La Paz MA et al: A sibship with unusual anomalies of the eye and skeleton (Michels' syndrome). *Am J Ophthalmol* 112:572–580, 1991.
3. Guion-Almeida ML, Rodini ES: Michels syndrome in a Brazilian girl born to consanguineous parents. *Am J Med Genet* 57:377–379, 1995.
4. Jackson LG, Barr MA: Conductive deafness with ptosis and skeletal malformations in sibs: a probably autosomal recessive disorder. *Birth Defects* 14:199–204, 1978.
5. Jewett T et al: Blepharophimosis, ptosis, and epicanthus inversus syndrome (BPES) associated with interstitial deletion of band 3q22: review and gene

assignment to the interface of band 3q22.3 and 3q23. *Am J Med Genet* 47:1147–1150, 1993.
6. Michels VV et al: A clefting syndrome with ocular anterior chamber defect and lid anomalies. *J Pediatr* 93:44–46, 1978.
7. Mutchinick O: A syndrome of mental and physical retardation, speech disorders, and peculiar facies in two sisters. *J Med Genet* 9:60–63, 1972.
8. Nowaczyk MJ, Sutcliffe TL: Blepharophimosis, minor facial anomalies, genital anomalies, and mental retardation: report of two sibs with a unique syndrome. *Am J Med Genet* 87:78–81, 1999.
9. Ohdo S et al: Mental retardation associated with congenital heart disease, blepharophimosis, blepharoptosis, and hypoplastic teeth. *J Med Genet* 23:242–244, 1986.
10. Perez-Caballero MC et al: Blepharophimosis, ptosis and epicanthus inversus syndrome plus sensorineural deafness [in Spanish]. *An Esp Pediatr* 51:530–532, 1999.

Cryptophthalmos syndrome (Fraser syndrome)

In 1872, Zehender (28) described a condition that consists of extension of the skin of the forehead to completely cover one or both eyes, total or partial soft tissue syndactyly of fingers and/or toes, coloboma of nasal alae, abnormal hairline, various urogenital abnormalities, and mixed hearing loss. The condition has also been called Fraser syndrome (7). Over 100 cases have been reported under a variety of names. There have been several excellent reviews (6,9,12,23–26).

Craniofacial findings. The face is asymmetric in about 10% of patients. In the case of renal agenesis, there is a Potter sequence phenotype (4,9). Abnormality of the nose is seen in about 85% of patients. It is usually broad with a low nasal bridge and a midline groove extending to the nasal tip. Alar defects or colobomata may be unilateral or bilateral, and frequently there is associated nasal asymmetry (Fig. 7–20A).

Ocular system. It should be emphasized that cryptophthalmos is not a constant feature (13,19), being found in 85% of cases, and is bilateral in only 53% (24). The eyebrows may be completely or partially missing (25,29). The globes can be seen and felt beneath the skin, which extends from the forehead to cover the eye(s). Exposure to strong light may induce reflex wrinkling of the skin resulting from contraction of the orbicularis muscles. With unilateral cryptophthalmos, the opposite eye may exhibit upper lid coloboma, microphthalmia, or epibulbar

Figure 7–20. *Cryptophthalmos syndrome (Fraser syndrome).* (A) Cryptophthalmos in a Greenlandic boy of normal intelligence. He had unilateral renal aplasia and hypospadias. (B,C) Variable soft tissue syndactyly of fingers and toes. [(A) from M Warburg, *Birth Defects* 7(3):136, 1971; (B,C) from ND Dinno et al., *Clin Pediatr* 13:219, 1974.]

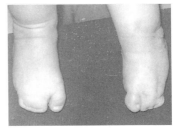

B

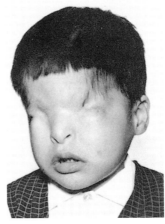

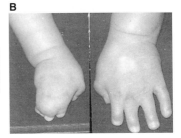

A   **C**

dermoid. The anterior segment is very dysplastic with a thin cornea fused to overlying skin. Angle structure abnormalities and lens anomalies (aphakia, calcified displaced lens) are also found (1,24,25). Lashes, meibomian glands, puncta, and lacrimal glands are absent (4). The posterior segment is relatively intact. In about 25%, a tongue of hair extends from the forehead into the area normally occupied by the eye.

Genitourinary system. Abnormal genitalia are found in about 80% of patients. Male genital anomalies include cryptorchidism (31.5%), micropenis (15%), hypospadias (9%), hypoplastic scrotum and/or atypical scrotal raphe (9%), and other, less frequent, anomalies including phimosis and chordee. Female genital anomalies include clitoromegaly (36%), uterine anomalies (17%), labial anomalies (hypoplasia, absence, or fusion) (17%), vaginal agenesis, atresia, or aplasia (12%), and rectovaginal or perineal fistula (9%). Ambiguous genitalia affect 17% (24). Greenberg et al. (11) reported gonadal dysgenesis and gonadoblastoma. Renal agenesis occurs with high frequency and may be unilateral (22%) or bilateral (23%). Abnormality of the ureters and/or bladder is found in 15%–18% (24). Cystic dysplasia of the kidneys affects another 12%.

Central nervous system. Mental retardation has been found in about half of those whose intelligence has been documented (24). Cerebral malformations include hydrocephalus, encephalocele, polymicrogyria, holoprosencephaly, periventricular leukomalacia, gliosis, and low brain weight (24).

Musculoskeletal system. Marked soft tissue syndactyly of the fingers and/or toes has been present in about 60%. The changes resemble those of Apert syndrome (25) (Fig. 7–20B,C).

Other skeletal defects, occurring in about 70%, have included small orbits, skull asymmetry, deformed optic foramina, absent sphenoid wing, lucent parietal defects, and diastema of the pubic symphysis. Other low-frequency skeletal changes have been summarized by Thomas et al. (26) and Slavotinek and Tifft (24). Omphalocele or umbilical hernia has been found in about 10%–15% (9).

Oral findings. Cleft lip and/or cleft palate and ankyloglossia have been noted in about 10% (9). Malocclusion is common. Laryngeal stenosis or atresia is also common, occurring in 30% (24).

Miscellaneous findings. Anal anomalies, including imperforate anus, anal atresia, and anal stenosis affect 27% of patients (24).

Auditory system. The pinnae are small (16%) and poorly modeled, low-set, or posteriorly rotated in at least 50% of cases. In about 5%, the skin of the upper part of the helix is continuous with that of the scalp. In 18%, the external auditory canals are narrowed or completely stenotic in the outer third to outer half. However, in many individuals the internal canal is normal (9,12,26). The stenosis may be present bilaterally, even though the cryptophthalmos is unilateral (23). Ossicles are malformed, resulting in mixed, mostly conductive hearing loss (12).

Vestibular system. No studies have been reported.

Laboratory findings. Radiographic studies have shown calcification of the lens, parietofrontal flattening, parietal lacunae, basal encephalocele, widening of the pubic symphysis, urogenital anomalies, and bowel malrotation (10,15).

Pathology. Several detailed pathologic studies have been carried out (2,16,26).

Heredity. The syndrome has autosomal recessive inheritance. Parental consanguinity has been present in about 25% (24). Among 86 cases, 48 were familial and 38 were sporadic (26). The syndrome has been reported in monozygous twins (21). Prevalence is estimated at 11/100,000 (17). The gene (*FRAS1*) maps to 4q21 which controls an extracellular matrix protein (18,27).

Diagnosis. This disorder is usually so striking that other conditions would not be considered. In an analysis of 86 cases, Thomas et al. (26) developed major and minor criteria. Slavotinek and Tifft (24) more recently reviewed 117 published cases and discussed the proposed diagnostic criteria. On the basis of both reviews, the major criteria should include cryptophthalmos, syndactyly, abnormal genitalia, and a history of the syndrome in a sibling. Slavotinek and Tifft suggested adding a tongue of hair extending from the scalp to the eyebrow as another important manifestation. Minor criteria should include a host of anomalies of the nose (particularly the nasal coloboma), ears, and larynx; umbilical hernia or low-set umbilicus; renal agenesis; and gastrointestinal abnormalities. Diagnosis is based on the presence of two or more major criteria and one minor criterion, or one major criterion and four or more minor criteria according to the Thomas et al. (26) schema.

Prenatal diagnosis has been accomplished using fetoscopy and ultrasound (2,5,8,9).

Prognosis. About 50% of patients survive for a year or more, 25% are stillborn, and 20% die within the first year of life, with most deaths occurring within the first week of life. In those that survive, surgical correction of partial cryptophthalmos has been attempted with partial success (3,14,20,22). Death has usually been associated with renal agenesis and/or laryngeal stenosis (9).

Summary. Cryptophthalmos syndrome is characterized by (*1*) autosomal recessive inheritance; (*2*) unilateral or more often bilateral extension of skin of the forehead to completely cover the eye or eyes; (*3*) variable soft tissue syndactyly of fingers and/or toes; (*4*) coloboma of nasal alae; (*5*) various urogenital anomalies; and (*6*) mixed hearing loss and atresia of external auditory canals.

References

1. Barry DR, Shortland-Webb WR: A case of cryptophthalmos syndrome. *Ophthalmologica* 180:234–240, 1980.
2. Boyd PA et al: Fraser syndrome (cryptophthalmos-syndactyly syndrome): a review of eleven cases with postmortem findings. *Am J Med Genet* 31:159–168, 1988.
3. Brazier DJ et al: Cryptophthalmos: surgical treatment of the congenital symblepharon variant. *Br J Ophthalmol* 70:391–395, 1986.
4. Codére F et al: Cryptophthalmos syndrome with bilateral renal agenesis. *Am J Ophthalmol* 91:737–792, 1982.
5. Feldman E et al: Microphthalmia—prenatal ultrasonic diagnosis. *Prenat Diagn* 5:205–207, 1985.
6. François J: Syndrome malformatif avec cryptophtalmie. *Acta Genet Med (Roma)* 18:18–50, 1969.
7. Fraser CR: Our genetic "load." A review of some aspects of genetical variation. *Ann Hum Genet* 25:387–415, 1962.
8. Fryns JP et al: Diagnostic echographic findings in cryptophthalmos syndrome (Fraser syndrome). *Prenat Diagn* 17:282–286, 1997.
9. Gattuso J et al: The clinical spectrum of the Fraser syndrome: report of three new cases and review. *J Med Genet* 24:549–555, 1987.
10. Goldhammer Y, Smith JL: Cryptophthalmos syndrome with basal encephaloceles. *Am J Ophthalmol* 80:146–149, 1975.
11. Greenberg F et al: Gonadal dysgenesis and gonadoblastoma in situ in a female with Fraser (cryptophthalmos) syndrome. *J Pediatr* 108:952–954, 1986.
12. Ide CH, Wollschlaeger PB: Multiple congenital abnormalities associated with cryptophthalmia. *Arch Ophthalmol* 81:640–644, 1969.
13. Koenig R, Spranger J: Cryptophthalmos-syndactyly syndrome without cryptophthalmos. *Clin Genet* 29:413–416, 1986.
14. Konrad G et al: Bilateraler vollständiger Kryptophthalmus. *Klin Monatsbl Augenheilkd* 190:121–124, 1987.
15. Levine RS et al: The cryptophthalmos syndrome. *AJR Am J Roentgenol* 143:375–376, 1984.
16. Lurie IW, Cherstvoy ED: Renal agenesis as a diagnostic feature of the cryptophthalmos-syndactyly syndrome. *Clin Genet* 25:528–532, 1984.
17. Martinez-Frias ML et al: Sindrome de Fraser: frecuencia en nuestro medio y aspectos clinico-epidemiologicos de una serie consecutiva de casos. *An Esp Pediatr* 48:634–638, 1998.
18. McGregor L et al: Fraser syndrome and mouse blebbed phenotype caused by mutations in the FRAS1/Fras1 encoding a putative extracellular matrix protein. *Nat Genet* 34:209–214, 2003.
19. Meinecke P: Cryptophthalmos-syndactyly syndrome without cryptophthalmos. *Clin Genet* 30:527–528, 1986.

20. Monima WG, Biermann B: Cryptophthalmos: symptoms and treatment of a rare deformity. *J Maxillofac Surg* 5:208–210, 1977.
21. Mortimer G et al: Fraser syndrome presenting as monozygotic twins with bilateral renal agenesis. *J Med Genet* 22:76–78, 1985.
22. Ohtsuka H et al: Bilateral cryptophthalmos with multiple associated congenital malformations. *Ann Plast Surg* 15:448–453, 1985.
23. Schönenberg H: Kryptophthalmus-Syndrom. *Klin Padiatr* 185:165–172, 1973.
24. Slavotinek AM, Tifft CJ: Fraser syndrome and cryptophthalmos: review of the diagnostic criteria and evidence for phenotypic modules in complex malformation syndromes. *J Med Genet* 39:623–633, 2002.
25. Sugar HS: The cryptophthalmos-syndactyly syndrome. *Am J Ophthalmol* 66:897–899, 1968.
26. Thomas IT et al: Isolated and syndromic cryptophthalmos. *Am J Med Genet* 25:85–98, 1986.
27. Vrontou S et al: *Fra1* deficiency results in cryptophthalmos renal agenesis and blebbed phenotype in mice. *Nat Genet* 34:209–214, 2003.
28. Zehender W: Eine Missgeburt mit hautüberwachsenen Augen oder Kryptophthalmus. *Klin Monatsbl Augenheilkd* 10:225–234, 1872.
29. Zinn S: Cryptophthalmia. *Am J Ophthalmol* 40:219–223, 1955.

Ocular albinism and sensorineural hearing loss

Winship et al. (1) described a large Afrikaner family in which seven males had this combination inherited as an X-linked recessive trait.

Ocular system. The irides are pale blue and retinal pigment reduced. There is marked horizontal nystagmus. Vision is severely impaired. Fundoscopic examination revealed patchy hypopigmentation and pigment clumping with large choroidal vessels on a background of pallor. There was a fine network of thin vessels at the periphery (Fig. 7–21A). Female heterozygotes had neither nystagmus nor visual impairment, but fundoscopic changes were variable, in some cases being similar to those of affected males.

Auditory system. Hearing loss is sensorineural and progressive. Onset is in the fourth or fifth decade. In some males hearing loss was severe; in others, only high-frequency loss was present (Fig. 7–21B). Female heterozygotes had no hearing loss.

Heredity. Inheritance is clearly X-linked recessive.

Diagnosis. This condition can be distinguished from other forms of ocular albinism by the presence of hearing loss. X-linked albinism–deafness includes patchy skin hypo- or hyperpigmentation and does not include eye findings in the phenotype. Linkage of this condition to Xp22.3 was established (2) and, because one form of ocular albinism also maps to this region, it was suggested that the two disorders are allelic or that this condition is a contiguous gene deletion syndrome.

Prognosis. Individuals end up blind and deaf by late middle age.

Summary. This condition is characterized by (1) ocular albinism; (2) onset of sensorineural hearing loss after the third decade; and (3) X-linked recessive inheritance.

Reference

1. Winship I et al: X-linked inheritance of ocular albinism with late-onset sensorineural deafness. *Am J Med Genet* 19:797–803, 1984.
2. Winship IM et al: X-linked ocular albinism and sensorineural deafness: linkage to Xp22.3. *Genomics* 18:444–445, 1993.

Norrie syndrome (oculoacousticocerebral dysplasia)

Norrie syndrome, the most important cause of congenital bilateral retinal detachment, was probably first described by Fernandez-Santos (14) in 1905 and by Heine (22) in 1925. In 1927, Norrie (35) reported the condition in two affected families. Warburg (59–65,67), who carried out extensive studies, first suggested X-linked recessive inheritance and

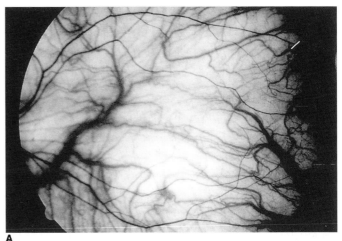

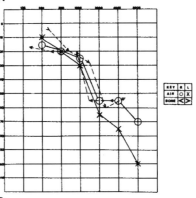

Figure 7–21. *Ocular albinism and sensorineural hearing loss.* (A) Fundus photograph of affected male showing changes typical of ocular albinism. (B) Audiogram of affected male demonstrating high-tone sensorineural hearing loss. [From I Winship et al., *Am J Med Genet* 19:797, 1984.]

noted the frequent association with hearing loss and dementia. For an excellent description of historical development of the syndrome see Warburg (62,65).

Auditory system. About 35% of patients manifest progressive sensorineural hearing loss that develops after 10 years of age (range 4 months to 45 years) (27,38,54,62). Hearing loss (38,59,60) has varied from 20 to 100 dB and is more often symmetric. A flat hearing loss or a slope toward higher frequencies has been found in 17 of 20 ears (39) (Fig. 7–22C,D). The hearing loss is of cochlear origin with no involvement of the brain stem as measured by electrocochleography and brain stem evoked responses (40). Békésy threshhold testing and pure-tone audiograms of known female heterozygotes demonstrated dips in about 40% (37), a finding that was not replicated by the same group (39).

Histopathologic study of cochlea has revealed atrophy of the stria vascularis and degeneration of hair cells and cochlear neurons. Connective tissue proliferation was noted in the spiral ganglion (34).

Ocular system. There is congenital or progressive blindness during infancy because of retinal dysplasia, which leads to retinal detachment, pseudotumorous proliferation, and bulbar atrophy. During the first few days of life, this presents as falciform folds of the retina, leukocoria, hemorrhagic retinal detachments, shallow anterior chambers, posterior synechiae, and elongated ciliary processes. The corneas are usually clear at birth (16). During preschool years, secondary cataract develops, the corneas become opaque (band degeneration), and the eyes begin to shrink (phthisis bulbi) (Fig. 7–22A,B). There may be significant pain. By the age of 10 years, progression of eye changes ceases

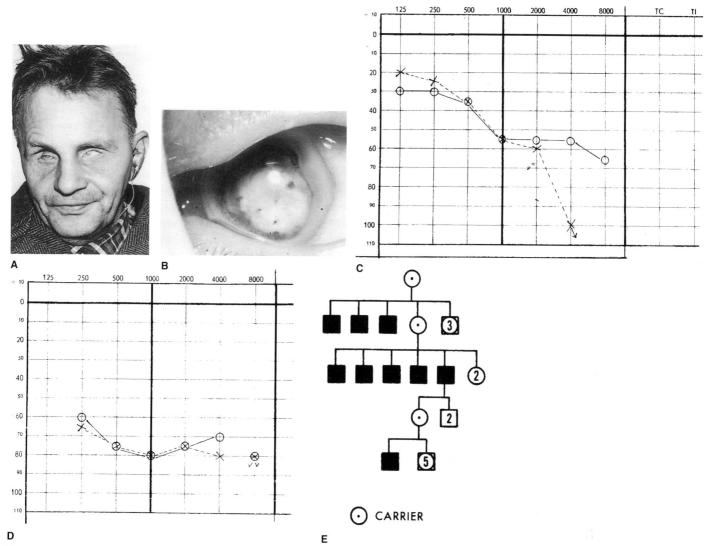

Figure 7–22. *Norrie syndrome (oculoacousticocerebral dysplasia)*. (A) Eyes are deep-set and phthisic. The corneas are hazy. (B) Eye of 2-year-old boy with clear cornea, cataract, and pigmentation in the anterior chamber. (C,D) Audiograms of patients with Norrie syndrome, showing moderate to severe bilateral hearing loss. (E) Pedigree of affected family showing X-linked inheritance. [(A,C–E) from M Warburg, *Acta Ophthalmol (Kbh)* (Suppl) 89:1, 1966; (B) from LB Holmes, *J Pediatr* 79:89, 1971.]

(6,54). Females occasionally manifest ocular symptoms showing some degree of pathology in both eyes (49,53,68). In one case, there was unilateral involvement resulting in phthisis bulbi in a female carrier (68).

Central nervous system. About 35% of patients exhibit severe progressive mental retardation. About 25% manifest psychosis; 30% are only mildly retarded, and 35% are normal. Among the severely retarded, deterioration begins after the first few years of life. In milder cases, later deterioration may occur, with some individuals requiring institutionalization in the fifth or sixth decade (15,44,65), particularly if they have hearing loss. Some middle-aged men retain excellent mental health. Seizures have been observed in a few families (62,65,68).

Laboratory findings. Electroencephalographic studies show marked diffuse abnormalities with distinct spikes.

Pathology. When phthisis has occurred, the eyeball is small with a dome-shaped cornea. A vascular membrane often covers the anterior surface of the iris. The lens is cataractous. The vitreous cavity is filled with glial fibers and vascular scar tissue with proliferation of retinal pigment epithelium. The inner layer of the retina is absent except for malformed retinal rosettes, i.e., retinal dysplasia. The choroid is ede-matous with engorged blood vessels. Sections of the optic nerve show myelinated fibers only in the periphery with connective tissue occupying the rest of the nerve (34). The optic tracts are small, even, thread-like, consisting mostly of glia. The lateral geniculate bodies are about half the normal size. The medial surface of the occipital lobe is smaller than normal (1,25,33,44,58,65).

Heredity. Norrie syndrome has X-linked recessive inheritance with complete penetrance in males (Fig. 7–22E). The syndrome has been reported over widely spread geographical areas and in different races (27). Phillips et al. (44) calculated the mutation rate to be about 3.9×10^{-6}.

By 1985, Gal et al. (17), Bleeker-Wagemakers et al. (4), and de la Chapelle et al. (11) had located the gene on the proximal short arm of the X chromosome at about Xp11.3 and were able to first determine carrier status and then provide a method of prenatal diagnosis (10,19,70). Pettenati et al. (43) noted a four-generation family of Norrie syndrome patients with inversion in the area of the gene. Gal et al. (18) and others (2,5,8,9,12,13,28) further demonstrated that the gene deletion, if wider, results in severe mental retardation, microcephaly, hypogonadism, growth retardation, and increased susceptibility to infections. In some patients with Norrie syndrome, the monoamine oxidase A and B genes are deleted as well (12,30,50–52).

The gene involved has been identified and named *NDP*. It is located at Xp11.3 and encodes a protein called norrin consisting of 133 amino acids (3). The exact function of the NDP protein remains unknown. Norrin may play a role in regulating neural differentiation (8,32,55), but recent evidence indicates that norrin is a secreted protein that forms disulfide-bonded oligomers within the extracellular matrix (42).

Both missense and nonsense mutations have been observed in the *NDP* gene; these mutations produce a variety of different, though related, phenotypes: Norrie disease, X-linked and sporadic exudative vitreoretinopathy, retinopathy of maturity, and Coats disease (7,20, 21,23,24,26,29,31,36,41,46–48,50,56,57,68,69). The genotype–phenotype correlation remains unclear.

Diagnosis. Diagnosis is based on histopathology of the eye when available, family history, and molecular studies of the *NDP* gene. Patients with juvenile retinoschisis have much better vision than do patients with Norrie syndrome. Persistent hyperplastic vitreous, falciform folds, retinoblastoma, retinal detachment, toxoplasmosis, retrolental fibroplasia, and trauma with massive retinal fibrosis must be excluded, and X-linked congenital cataract and X-linked microphthalmia may require differentiation (66,68). Intrauterine diagnosis has been made in the third trimester of pregnancy by ultrasonography (45).

Prognosis. All affected persons become blind. The moderate to severe sensorineural hearing loss does not appear to be progressive. Infantile psychosis is progressive with affected children appearing mentally normal for only the first 1 or 2 years of life. In middle-aged males, psychosis and hallucinations have been seen.

Summary. The major characteristics of this syndrome include (*1*) X-linked recessive transmission; (*2*) eye changes, including retinal glial proliferation, complicated cataract, and phthisis; (*3*) mild to severe mental deficiency in about two-thirds of the cases; and (*4*) mild to severe sensorineural hearing loss in about one-third of the patients.

References

 1. Apple DJ et al: Ocular histopathology of Norrie's disease. *Am J Ophthalmol* 78:196–203, 1974.
 2. Bergen AA et al: Detection of a new submicroscopic Norrie disease deletion interval with a novel DNA probe isolated by differential Alu PCR fingerprint cloning. *Cytogenet Cell Genet* 62:231–235, 1993.
 3. Berger W et al: Mutations in the candidate gene for Norrie disease. *Hum Mol Genet* 1:461–465, 1992.
 4. Bleeker-Wagemakers LM et al: Close linkage between Norrie disease, a cloned DNA sequence from the proximal short arm, and the centromere of the X chromosome. *Hum Genet* 71:211–113, 1983.
 5. Bleeker-Wagemakers LM et al: Norrie disease as part of a complex syndrome explained by a submicroscopic deletion of the X chromosome. *Opthalm Paediatr Genet* 9:137–142, 1988.
 6. Brini A et al: Maladie de Norrie. *Ann Ocul (Paris)* 205:1–16, 1972.
 7. Caballero M et al: Two novel mutations in the Norrie disease gene associated with the classical ocular phenotype. *Ophthalm Genet* 17:187–191, 1996.
 8. Chen ZY et al: Norrie diease gene characterization of deletions and possible function. *Genomics* 16:533–535, 1993.
 9. Collins FA et al: Clinical, biochemical, and neuropsychiatric evaluation of a patient with a contiguous gene syndrome due to a microdeletion Xp11.3 including the Norrie disease locus and monoamine oxidase (MAOA and MAOB) genes. *Am J Med Genet* 42:127–134, 1992.
10. Curtis D et al: Carrier detection and prenatal diagnosis in Norrie disease. *Prenat Diagn* 9:735–740, 1989.
11. de la Chapelle A et al: Norrie disease caused by a gene deletion allowing carrier detection and prenatal diagnosis. *Clin Genet* 28:317–320, 1985.
12. Diergaarde PJ et al: Physical fine-mapping of a deletion spanning the Norrie gene. *Hum Genet* 84:22–26, 1989.
13. Donnai D et al: Norrie disease resulting from a gene deletion: clinical features and DNA studies. *J Med Genet* 25:73–78, 1988.
14. Fernandez-Santos J: Total congenital detachment of the retina in two brothers. *Ann Ocul* 34:338–340, 1905.
15. Forssman H: Mental deficiency and pseudoglioma, a syndrome inherited as an X-linked recessive. *Am J Ment Defic* 64:984–987, 1960.
16. Fradkin AH: Norrie's disease. Congenital progressive oculo-acoustico-cerebral degeneration. *Am J Ophthalmol* 72:947–948, 1971.
17. Gal A et al: Norrie's disease: close linkage with genetic markers from the proximal short arm of the X chromosome. *Clin Genet* 27:282–283, 1985.
18. Gal A et al: Submicroscopic interstitial deletion of the X chromosome explains a complex genetic syndrome dominated by Norrie disease. *Cytogenet Cell Genet* 42:219–224, 1986.
19. Gal A et al: Prenatal exclusion of Norrie disease with flanking DNA markers. *Am J Med Genet* 31:449–453, 1988.
20. Haider MZ et al: Missense mutations in Norrie disease gene are not associated with advanced stages of retinopathy of prematurity in Kuwaiti Arabs. *Biol Neonate* 77:88–91, 2000.
21. Haider MZ et al: Retinopathy of prematurity: mutations in the Norrie disease gene and the risk of progression to advanced stages. *Pediatr Int* 43:120–123, 2001.
22. Heine L: Über das familiäre Auftreten von Pseudoglioma congenitum bei zwei Brüdern. *Z Augenheilkd* 56:155–164, 1925.
23. Hiraoka M et al: Insertion and deletion mutations in the dinucleotide repeat region of the Norrie disease gene in patients with advanced retinopathy of prematurity. *J Hum Genet* 46:178–181, 2001.
24. Hiraoka M et al: X-linked juvenile retinoschisis: mutations at the retinoschisis and Norrie disease gene loci? *J Hum Genet* 46:53–56, 2001.
25. Jacklin HN: Falciform fold, retinal detachment, and Norrie's disease. *Am J Opthalmol* 90:76–80, 1980.
26. Johnson K et al: X-linked exudative vitreoretinpathy caused by an arginine to leucine substitution (R121L) in the Norrie disease protein. *Clin Genet* 50:113–115, 1996.
27. Johnston SS et al: Norrie's disease. *Birth Defects* 18:729–738, 1982.
28. Joy JE et al: Abnormal protein in the cerebrospinal fluid of patients with a submicroscopic X-chromosomal deletion associated with Norrie disease. Preliminary report. *Appl Theor Electrophor* 2:3–5, 1991.
29. Kellner U et al: Ocular phenotypes associated with two mutations (R121W, C126X) in the Norrie disease gene. *Ophthalm Genet* 17:67–74, 1996.
30. Levy ER et al: Localization of human monoamine oxidase-A gene to Xp11.23–11.4 by in situ hybridization: implications for Norrie disease. *Genomics* 5:368–370, 1989.
31. Meire FM et al: Isolated Norrie disease in a female caused by a balanced translocation t(X;6). *Ophthalm Genet* 19:203–207, 1998.
32. Meitinger T et al: Molecular modeling of the Norrie disease protein predicts a cystine knot growth factor tertiary structure. *Nat Genet* 5:376–380, 1993.
33. Moreira-Filho CA, Neustein I: A presumptive new variant of Norrie's disease. *J Med Genet* 16:125–128, 1979.
34. Nadol JB Jr et al: Histopathology of the ears, eyes, and brain in Norrie's disease (oculoacousticocerebral degeneration). *Am J Otolaryngol* 11:112–124, 1990.
35. Norrie G: Causes of blindness in children. Twenty-five years' experience of Danish institues for the blind. *Ann Ophthalmol (Copenh)* 5:357–386, 1927.
36. Ott S et al: A novel mutation in the Norrie disease gene. *J AAPOS* 4:125–126, 2000.
37. Parving A: Reliability of Bekesy threshold tracing in identification of carriers of genes for an X-linked disease with deafness. *Acta Otolaryngol* 85:40–44, 1978.
38. Parving A: Hearing disorder in Norrie's syndrome. *Adv Audiol* 3:52–57, 1985.
39. Parving A, Schwartz M: Audiometric tests in gene carriers of Norrie's disease. *Int J Pediatr Otorhinolaryngol* 21:103–111, 1991.
40. Parving A et al: Electrophysiological study of Norrie's disease. An X-linked recessive trait with hearing loss. *Audiology* 17:293–298, 1978.
41. Pendergast SD et al: Study of the Norrie disease gene in 2 patients with bilateral persistent hyperplastic primary vitreous. *Arch Ophthalmol* 116:381–382, 1999.
42. Perez-Vilar J, Hill RL: Norrie disease protein (norrin) forms disulfide-linked oligomers associated with the extracellular matrix. *J Biol Chem* 272:33410–33415, 1997.
43. Pettenati MJ et al: Inversion (X)(p11.4q22) associated with Norrie disease in a four-generation family. *Am J Med Genet* 45:577–580, 1993.
44. Phillips CI et al: Probably Norrie's disease due to mutation: two sporadic sibships of two males each: a necropsy of one case, and, given Norrie's disease, a calculation of the gene mutation frequency. *Br J Ophthalmol* 70:305–313, 1986.
45. Redmond RM et al: In utero diagnosis of Norrie disease by ultrasonography. *Ophthalm Paediatr Genet* 14:1–3, 1993.
46. Rehm HL et al: Norrie disease gene mutation in a large Costa Rican kindred with a novel phenotype including venous insufficiency. *Hum Mutat* 9:402–408, 1997.
47. Shastry BS: Identification of a recurrent missense mutation in the Norrie disease gene associated with a simplex case of exudative vitreoretinopathy. *Biochem Biophys Res Commun* 246:35–38, 1998.

48. Shastry BS et al: Identification of novel missense mutations in the Norrie disease gene associated with one X-linked and four sporadic cases of familial exudative vitreoretinopathy. *Hum Mutat* 9:396–401, 1997.

49. Shastry BS et al: Norrie disease and exudative vitreoretinopathy in families with affected female carriers. *Eur J Ophthalmol* 9:238–242, 1999.

50. Sims KB et al: Monoamine oxidase deficiency in males with an X chromosome deletion. *Neurology* 2:1069–1076, 1989.

51. Sims KB et al: Norrie disease gene is distinct from the monoamine oxidase genes. *Am J Hum Genet* 45:424–434, 1989.

52. Sims KB et al: The Norrie disease gene maps to a 150 kb region on chromosome Xp11.3. *Hum Mol Genet* 1:83–89, 1992.

53. Sims KB et al: Norrie disease in a family with a manifesting female carrier. *Arch Ophthalmol* 115:517–519, 1997.

54. Skevas A et al: Norrie-Wardburg syndrome. *Laryngorhinootologie* 7:534–536, 1992.

55. Strasberg P et al: A novel mutation in the Norrie disease gene predicted to disrupt the cystine knot growth factor motif. *Hum Mol Genet* 4:2179–2180, 1995.

56. Talks SJ et al: De novo mutations in the 5′ regulatory region of the Norrie disease gene in retinopathy of prematurity. *J Med Genet* 38:E46, 2001.

57. Torrente I et al: Two new mutations (A105T and C110G) in the *norrin* gene in two Italian families with Norrie disease and familial exudative vitreoretinopathy. *Am J Med Genet* 72:242–244, 1997.

58. Townes PL, Roca PD: Norrie's disease (hereditary oculo-acoustic-cerebral degeneration). Report of a United States family. *Am J Ophthalmol* 76:797–803, 1973.

59. Warburg M: Norrie's disease. A new hereditary pseudotumor of the retina. *Ann Ophthalmol (Kbh)* 39:757–772, 1961.

60. Warburg M: Norrie's disease. Atrophia bulbosum hereditarium. *Acta Ophthalmol (Copenh)* 41:134–146, 1963.

61. Warburg M: Norrie's disease. *Trans Ophthalmol Soc UK* 85:391–408, 1965.

62. Warburg M: Norrie's disease. A congenital progressive oculo-acoustico-cerebral degeneration. *Acta Ophthalmol (Copenh) Suppl* 89:1–147, 1966.

63. Warburg M: Norrie's disease. *J Ment Defic Res* 12:247–251, 1968.

64. Warburg M: Norrie's disease. *Birth Defects* 7:117–124, 1971.

65. Warburg M: Norrie's disease—differential diagnosis and treatment. *Acta Ophthalmol (Copenh)* 53:217–236, 1975.

66. Warburg M: Retinal malformations. Aetiological heterogeneity and morphological similarities in congenital retinal non-attachment and falciform folds. *Trans Ophthalmol Soc UK* 99:272–283, 1979.

67. Warburg M et al: Norrie's disease: delineation of carriers among daughters of obligate carriers by linkage analysis. *Trans Ophthalmol Soc UK* 105(pt 1):88–93, 1986.

68. Yamada K et al: Two Thai families with Norrie disease (ND): association of two novel missense mutations with severe ND phenotype, seizures, and a manifesting carrier. *Am J Med Genet* 100:52–55, 2001.

69. Zaremba J et al: Intrafamilial variability of the ocular phenotype in a Polish family with a missense mutation (A63D) in the Norrie disease gene. *Ophthalm Genet* 19:157–164, 1998.

70. Zhu DP et al: Microdeletion in the X-chromosome and prenatal diagnosis in a family with Norrie disease. *Am J Med Genet* 33:181–183, 1989.

Gernet syndrome: optic atrophy and severe sensorineural hearing loss

In 1963, Gernet (5) described a mother and daughter with congenital sensorineural hearing loss and progressively decreasing vision due to optic atrophy first noted in childhood. Since then, there have been a number of cases reported that, because of inter- and intrafamilial variability, cannot be clearly separated into distinct categories (1,2,4,7–10). While there may be genetic heterogeneity, the resolution of how many and which genes are involved must await molecular genetic analysis.

Ocular system. The onset of visual loss has varied from the first to the third decade. The optic atrophy is progressive and has varied in severity in the oldest affected members of the various kindreds from 20/40 to 20/200 (9) (Fig. 7–23). There is considerable intrafamilial variability. A protan-deutan color defect has been present in nearly all affected individuals.

Central nervous system. Cranial nerve functions except for hearing and visual loss have been normal. Strength, sensation, reflexes, and coordination tests have been normal.

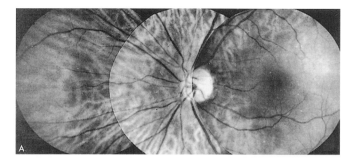

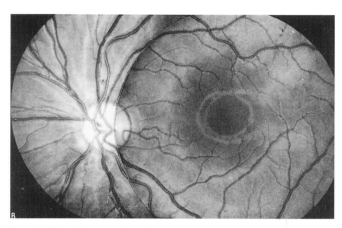

Figure 7–23. *Optic atrophy and severe sensorineural hearing loss (Gernet syndrome).* (A) Fundus showing optic nerve atrophy, normal macular reflex, and retinal periphery. (B) Fundus with optic nerve atrophy. [From BW Konigsmark et al., *Arch Opthalmol* 91:99, 1974.]

Auditory system. Sensorineural hearing loss has been severe and congenital or infantile in most cases (2,4,5,7) but has been moderate to severe with onset in the first or second decade in two families (1,6,9).

Temporal bone tomograms have been normal. Normal conduction velocity and latency times have been found with stimulation of various peripheral nerves.

Vestibular system. Opticokinetic responses and caloric vestibular tests have been normal (8).

Heredity. Inheritance is clearly autosomal dominant.

Diagnosis. Optic atrophy by itself may have autosomal dominant inheritance. In some patients there may be mild to moderate sensorineural loss. Among a group of 31 patients with dominant optic atrophy, Hoyt (6) found 8 with hearing loss, and 17 had blue-yellow and 8 had red-green dyschromatopsia. The hearing loss had considerable intrafamilial variability and appeared later in life than did the optic atrophy.

Several syndromes include hearing loss and optic atrophy (Table 7–3). In the syndrome of optic atrophy, ataxia, and progressive sensorineural hearing loss (Sylvester syndrome), the hearing deficit is only moderate and slowly progressive. In the syndrome considered here, there was no evidence of ataxia. The syndrome of optic atrophy, polyneuropathy, and sensorineural hearing loss has autosomal recessive inheritance and includes a slowly progressive distal weakness. In the diabetes insipidus, diabetes mellitus, optic atrophy, and deafness (DIDMOAD) syndrome, the hearing deficit progresses slowly over the first three decades of life, eventually resulting in severe hearing loss; in the present syndrome the hearing loss is congenital.

Opticocochleodentate degeneration clearly differs from the present syndrome because of its recessive transmission, infantile onset of progressive spastic quadriplegia, and progressive hearing and mental dete-

Table 7–3. Syndromes with optic trophy and sensorineural hearing loss

Syndrome	Inheritance	Visual Loss Onset, Severity	Hearing Loss Onset, Severity	Associated Findings	Chapter in this Book
Optic atrophy, congenital SND (Gernet syndrome)	AD	Childhood or midlife, moderate loss	Congenital, moderate or severe loss	None	7 (eye)
Optic atrohy, ataxia, SND (Sylvester syndrome)	AD	First decade, progressive loss	First decade, moderate loss	Ataxia	10 (neurological)
Optic atrophy, polyneuropathy, SND (Rosenberg-Chutorian syndrome)	SR	Second decade, moderate loss	First decade, moderate to severe loss	Motor and sensory neuropathy	10 (neurological)
Optic atrophy, diabetes mellitus, diabetes insipidus (DIDMOAD)	AR	First decade, severe loss	First decade, mild to moderate loss	Nystagmus, diminished reflexes	12 (endocrine)
Optico-cochleo-dentate degeneration (Muller-Zeman syndrome)	AR	Infancy	Infancy	Quadriplegia, mental deterioration, death in childhood	10 (neurological)
Optic atrophy, dementia, SND (Jensen syndrome)	XR	Second or third decade, moderate to severe loss	First decade, severe loss	Dementia	7 (eye)
Optic atrophy, dementia, SND (Mohr-Tranebjaerg syndrome)	XR	Teen years	Early childhood	Dementia	7 (eye)
Optic atrophy, ptosis, ophthalmoplegia, dystaxia, myopathy (Treft syndrome)	AD	First decade, moderate to marked loss	First or second decade, mild to severe loss	Ptosis	10 (neurological)
Optic atrophy, polyneuropathy SND (Jecquier-Deonna syndrome)	AR	Late first decade or early second decade	Late first decade or early second decade	Motor and sensory loss, postural Scheuermann disease	10 (neurological)
Optic atrophy, motor and sensory neuropathy, SND (Iwashita)	AR	Second decade	Second decade	Motor and sensory neuropathy	10 (neurological)
Optic atrophy, brachytelephalangy, SND (Berk-Tabatznik syndrome)	Unknown	Congenital	Congenital	Brachytelephalangy, short stature, cervical kyphosis, spastic quadriplegia	10 (neurological)
Optic atrophy, dysphagia, esotropia, SND (Schmidley syndrome)	XR	Infancy or early childhood	Infancy, progressive	Esotropia, dysphagia	10 (neurological)
Optic atrophy, ataxia, SND (Dobyns syndrome)	AR or XR	Early childhood	Early childhood	Motor and sensory neuropathy	10 (neurological)
Optic atrophy, mental retardation, pigmentary retinopathy, SND (Gordon syndrome)	AR	Early childhood	Early childhood	Pigmentary retinopathy, spastic quadriplegia, mental retardation	10 (neurological)
Optic atrophy, adrenocortical deficiency, hepatosplenomegaly, pigmentary retinopathy, SND (Dyck syndrome)	AR or XR	Infancy	Infancy	Adrenocortical deficiency, hepatosplenomegaly, pigmentary retinoapthy	10 (neurological)
Optic atrophy, motor and sensory neuropathy, SND (Hagemoser syndrome)	AD	Childhood	Childhood	Motor and sensory neuropathy	10 (neurological)
Optic atrophy, dementia, hypotonia, quadriplegia, SND (Seitelberger disease)	AR	Early childhood	Late childhood	Dementia, hypotonia, spastic quadriplegia	10 (neurological)
Alström syndrome	AR	First decade, severe loss	First decade, severe, progressive loss	Pigmentary retinopathy, diabetes mellitus, obesity	7 (eye)
Optic atrophy and deafness (Ozden syndrome)	AD	First decade	First decade		7 (eye)
Cockayne syndrome	AR	First decade	First decade	Growth failure, mental retardation, skin photosensitivity	10 (neurological)
Fatal X-linked ataxia with deafness and loss of vision (Arts syndrome)	XR	First few years	Congenital	Ataxia, hypotonia, loss of milestones	10 (neurological)
Cerebellar ataxia, pes cavus, optic atrophy, SND (Capos syndrome)	AD or mitochondrial	Childhood	Childhood	Ataxia, pes cavus	10 (neurological)
Spinocerebellar ataxia with blindness and deafness (SCABD)	AR	Teens	Teens	Cochlear degeneration	10 (neurological)
Gustavson syndrome	XR	?Congenital	?Congenital	Microcephaly, death by early childhood	10 (neurological)

AD, autosomal dominant; AR, autosomal recessive; SND, sensorineural deafness; XR, X-linked recessive.

rioration. The syndrome of optic atrophy, dementia, and sensorineural loss is X-linked. Leber's optic atrophy, certainly a genetically heterogeneous condition, is occasionally (ca. 8%) associated with neural hearing loss (3). One can also find optic atrophy with progressive hearing loss in Kearns-Sayre syndrome and with the Mohr-Tranebjaerg syndrome.

Prognosis. Vision decreases progressively from midlife. The hearing loss is congenital, severe, and nonprogressive.

Summary. Characteristics of this syndrome include (*1*) autosomal dominant transmission; (*2*) progressive optic atrophy; and (*3*) congenital, generally severe, sensorineural hearing loss.

References

1. Amemiya T, Honda A: A family with optic atrophy and congenital hearing loss. *Ophthalmic Genet* 15:87–93, 1994.
2. Deutman AF, Baarsma GS: Optic atrophy and deaf mutism, dominantly inherited. *Docum Ophthalmol Proc Ser* 17:145–154, 1978.
3. de Weerdt CJ, Went LN: Neurological studies in families with Leber's optic atrophy. *Acta Neurol Scand* 47:541–554, 1971.
4. Fraser GR: *The Causes of Profound Deafness in Childhood*, 1st ed. London: Bathen Tindall, 1976.
5. Gernet HH: Hereditäre Opticusatrophie in Kombination mit Taubheit. *Ber Dtsch Ophthalmol Ges* 65:545–547, 1963.
6. Hoyt CS: Autosomal dominant optic atrophy. A spectrum of disability. *Ophthalmology* 87:245–251, 1980.
7. Kollarits CR et al: The autosomal dominant syndrome of progressive optic atrophy and congenital deafness. *Am J Ophthalmol* 87:789–792, 1979.
8. Konigsmark BW et al: Dominant congenital deafness and progressive optic nerve atrophy. Occurrence in four generations of a family. *Arch Ophthalmol* 91:99–103, 1974.
9. Mets MB, Mhoon E: Probable autosomal dominant optic atrophy with hearing loss. *Ophthalm Paediatr Genet* 5:85–89, 1985.
10. Michal S et al: Atrophic optique hérédo-familiale dominante associée à surdimutité. *Ann Oculist* 201:431–435, 1968.

Jensen syndrome: optic atrophy, dementia, and sensorineural hearing loss

In 1981, Jensen (1) first reported the association of optic atrophy, dementia, and profound sensorineural hearing loss in three males, a boy and two maternal uncles in a Danish family. In 1987, Jensen et al. (2) wrote a follow-up report.

Auditory system. Hearing was considered normal during the first year, but hearing loss was noticed soon after (1–2 years) and progressed rapidly to severe bilateral sensorineural loss. Audiometry results suggested cochlear origin.

Vestibular system. No mention was made of vestibular testing.

Ocular system. Visual loss began in the teen years (14–19 years), at which time the fundi appeared normal. It then progressed to severe visual impairment with pale, atrophic optic discs over the following decade. The youngest affected patient was asymptomatic at 10 years and had normal fundi. However, visual evoked potential testing suggested a subclinical demyelinating optic nerve lesion.

Central nervous system. Mental changes such as organic psychosis began in the 20's and 30's. These progressed to an organic dementia associated with severe mental deterioration, motor disability, and death by about 40 years.

Laboratory findings. No helpful laboratory studies were reported.

Pathology. Autopsy in one patient showed extensive calcifications, located in all parts of the brain, which affected all structures including meninges, vessels, and neurons. Other changes included diffuse and focal atrophy of brain tissue, especially depletion of neurons within the cerebral cortex and severe demyelination of the optic chiasma. No abnormalities were seen in other organs.

Heredity. Two brothers and their nephew were affected. Neither their sister (mother of the affected nephew) nor their mother had any symptoms. Thus, inheritance is X-linked recessive (Fig. 7–24). Recently Tranebjaerg et al. (3) found a mutation in the *DDP* gene at Xq22, thus Jensen syndrome is allelic to Mohr-Tranebjaerg syndrome.

Diagnosis. Optic atrophy and hearing loss occur together in many other disorders, but all have additional manifestations. Examples include Cockayne syndrome, opticocochleodentate degeneration, and ataxia, optic atrophy, and sensorineural hearing loss (autosomal dominant or recessive).

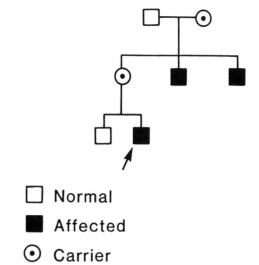

□ Normal
■ Affected
⊙ Carrier

Figure 7–24. *Optic atrophy, dementia, and sensorineural hearing loss (Jensen syndrome).* Pedigree of family shows X-linked recessive inheritance. [From PKA Jensen, *Am J Med Genet* 9:55, 1981.]

Prognosis. This disorder is associated with severe neurological disability and death by about 40 years.

Summary. This disorder is characterized by (*1*) X-linked recessive inheritance; (*2*) optic atrophy; (*3*) dementia; and (*4*) profound sensorineural hearing loss.

References

1. Jensen PK: Nerve deafness: optic nerve atrophy, and dementia: a new X-linked recessive syndrome? *Am J Med Genet* 9:55–60, 1981.
2. Jensen PK et al: The syndrome of opticoacoustic nerve atrophy with dementia [letter]. *Am J Med Genet* 28:517–518, 1987.
3. Tranebjaerg L et al: Jensen syndrome is allelic to Mohr-Tranebjaerg syndrome and both are caused by stop mutations in the DDP gene [abstract]. *Am J Hum Genet* 61:A349, 1997.

Berk-Tabatznik syndrome: congenital optic atrophy, brachytelephalangy, and sensorineural hearing loss

In 1961, Berk and Tabatznik (1) reported a 16-year-old female with congenital optic atrophy, cervical kyphosis, and hypoplasia of distal phalanges. Hartwell et al. (2) reported a 7-year-old with similar features but who also had hearing loss.

Clinical findings. Short stature was evident in both patients. One patient had midfacial hypoplasia with depressed nasal root and bridge and epicanthal folds.

Ocular findings. Visual impairment due to congenital optic atrophy was present in both.

Musculoskeletal system. The terminal phalanges were hypoplastic in both patients.

Central nervous system. Spastic quadriparesis was present in both patients. In one patient (1) there was cervical kyphosis. However, both had cervical vertebral wedging.

Auditory system. Profound sensorineural hearing loss was noted by Hartwell et al. (2).

Vestibular system. Vestibular tests were not described.

Heredity. Inheritance is unknown. Both patients represented sporadic occurrences in several large normal sibships.

Diagnosis. To be excluded is opticocochleodentate degeneration, but that is much more severe, with death occurring in childhood.

Summary. Characteristics of this syndrome include (*1*) unknown inheritance; (*2*) congenital optic atrophy; (*3*) cervical kyphosis; (*4*) spastic quadriparesis; (*5*) brachytelephalangy; (*6*) short stature; and (*7*) sensorineural hearing loss.

References

1. Berk ME, Tabatznik BZ: Cervical kyphosis from posterior hemivertebrae with brachyphalangy and congenital optic atrophy. *J Bone Joint Surg* 43B:77–86, 1961.
2. Hartwell EA et al: Congenital optic atrophy and brachytelephalangy: the Berk-Tabatznik syndrome. *Am J Med Genet* 29:383–389, 1988.

Ozden optic atrophy and deafness

Ozden et al. (*1*) described the combination of optic atrophy and deafness in a large Turkish family. Linkage studies excluded linkage to nonsyndromic optic atrophy.

Ocular system. Optic atrophy leading to visual loss had its onset in the first decade. Blepharochalasis was an additional ocular finding.

Auditory system. Hearing loss was sensorineural, with onset in the first decade. It varied in severity, ranging from profound to moderate. In those with moderate hearing loss, the low frequencies were more severely affected.

Heredity. Inheritance is clearly autosomal dominant.

Diagnosis. This condition resembles other conditions with optic atrophy and hearing loss, but can be distinguished by age of onset for both hearing loss and optic atrophy, as well as lack of additional findings.

Prognosis. Both hearing loss and vision loss were progressive. Cognitive development appeared unimpaired.

Summary. This condition has (*1*) optic atrophy, (*2*) sensorineural hearing loss, (*3*) autosomal dominant inheritance.

Reference

Ozden S et al: Progressive autosomal dominant optic atrophy and sensorineural hearing loss in a Turkish family. *Ophthalm Genet* 23:29–36, 2002.

Mohr-Tranebjaerg syndrome (DFN1): X-linked optic atrophy, spastic paraplegia, dystonia, and auditory neuropathy

A type of X-linked early-onset sensorineural hearing loss was originally described in a large kindred by Mohr and Mageroy (*5*) in 1960. This disorder was originally considered to be nonsyndromic. In a follow-up report of the same family, Tranebjaerg et al. (*7*) restudied and extensively characterized 16 affected members. Older affected males in the family showed progressive neural degeneration affecting both the brain and eyes.

Auditory system. Hearing impairment is the first presenting symptom in affected males. The hearing was normal until about age 1.5 to 3 years, and some speech did develop. Hearing loss was then rapidly progressive, reaching a severe to profound stage by early teenage years. The hearing loss typically involved all frequencies equally. Speech intelligibility decreases commensurate with the decline of hearing acuity. The findings of involvement of the spiral ligament (*4*) suggest that the hearing loss is an auditory neuropathy. Study of a family with three affected males (R. Varga, personal communication) showed that the youngest affected male had otoacoustic emmissions in the presence of

a severe to profound hearing loss. A CT scan of the temporal bone was not remarkable. Female heterozygotes were reported to have a mild progressive hearing loss.

Vestibular system. Vestibular studies in one patient were reported to be normal.

Ophthalmologic findings. Visual problems began during the teenage years, first with the onset of photophobia. Visual acuity was markedly decreased by the mid-30's and males complained about the lack of effect of stronger glasses. With only one exception, ERGs were reported to be normal. The visual abnormalities were suggestive of the involvement of a central visual pathway. One affected male had an abnormal ERG showing retinal abnormality involving both the rods and cones; the findings in only this patient were compatible with central choroidal dystrophy.

Central nervous system. Personality disturbance can be severe. Affected males are irritable and have aggressive outbursts and have paranoid symptoms. All the older affected males had dysphagia. Electromyelogram and muscle biopsy results revealed a mild peripheral neuropathy in some males. Cerebral CT scans in males over the age of 40 showed generalized cerebral atrophy. Dystonia and/or spasticity were present in most patients.

Laboratory findings. Temporal bone radiographs, electroencephalographic studies, and cerebrospinal fluid and urine analysis were normal.

Pathology. In a 66-year-old patient with a 151delT mutation the dystonia/deafness peptide 1 (*DDP1*) gene, the organ of Corti, spiral ligament, and the stria vascularis were unaffected (*4*). Rather, there was an almost complete loss of spiral ganglion cells. The vestibular hair cells were preserved. These findings suggest that the hearing loss is probably an auditory neuropathy. Neuropathologic examination also revealed atrophy of the cerebrum and a complete absence of optic nerve neurons. The retina was interpreted to be normal for the age of the case studied (*4*).

Heredity. Only males have been affected and transmission is clearly X-linked. The gene is on the long arm of the X chromosome near Xq22 (*1,7*). The gene involved has been identified as a mitochondrial associated autosomal gene, *Tim8-13*, coding for a protein involved in intermembrane protein transport in mitochondria (*6,8*). Several cases have been reported with mutations in the *DDP1* gene (*2,3,8,9,10*).

Diagnosis. Causes of childhood hearing loss such as meningitis and viral infections should be ruled out. A careful history to determine whether there is any evidence of progression of hearing loss in childhood is important in separating X-linked congenital sensorineural hearing loss, which is often not progressive, from this disorder, which shows progression in childhood. To be excluded are autosomal recessive dystonia, pigmentary retinopathy, and sensorineural hearing loss (Coppeto-Lessell syndrome); dystonia and sensorineural hearing loss (Scribanu-Kennedy syndrome); and spastic quadriparesis, dementia, mental retardation, optic atrophy, pigmentary retinopathy, and sensorineural hearing loss (Gordon syndrome). CONTIG syndromes involving the *DDP* gene are possible. Three unrelated males with deafness and agammaglobulinemia were observed to have an X chromosomal deletion involving the Bruton tyrosine kinase (Btk) and the *DDP* gene.

Prognosis. Individuals have progressive hearing loss, and the neurologic symptoms worsen with time.

Summary. Characteristics of this type of hearing loss include (*1*) X-linked inheritance; (*2*) blindness; (*3*) spastic paraplegia and dystonia; (*4*) mental retardation; and (*5*) moderate sensorineural hearing loss in early childhood with essentially complete loss of hearing by school age.

References

1. Bach I et al: Physical fine mapping of genes underlying X-linked deafness and non fra (X)-X-linked mental retardation at Xq21. *Hum Genet* 89:620–624, 1992.
2. Hayes MW et al: X-linked dystonia-deafness syndrome. *Mov Disord* 13:303–308, 1998.
3. Jin H et al: A novel X-linked gene, *DDP*, shows mutations in families with deafness (DFN-1), dystonia, mental deficiency and blindness. *Nat Genet* 14:177–180, 1996.
4. Merchant SN et al: Temporal bone histopathologic and genetic studies in Mohr-Tranebjaerg syndrome (DFN-1). *Otol Neurotol* 22:506–511, 2001.
5. Mohr J, Mageroy K: Sex-linked deafness of a possibly new gene type. *Acta Genet (Basel)* 10:54–62, 1960.
6. Paschen SA et al: The role of the TIM8-13 complex in the import of TIM23 into mitochondria. *EMBO J* 19:6392–6400, 2000.
7. Tranebjaerg L et al: A new X-linked recessive deafness syndrome with blindness, dystonia, fractures, and mental deficiency is linked to Xq22. *J Med Genet* 32:257–263, 1995.
8. Tranebjaerg L et al: A de novo missense mutation in a critical domain of the X-linked *DDP* gene causes the typical deafness-dystonia-optic atrophy syndrome. *Eur J Hum Genet* 8:464–467, 2000.
9. Trandebjaerg L et al: X-linked recessive deafness-dystonia syndrome (Mohr-Tranebjaerg syndrome). *Adv Otorhinolaryngol* 56:176–180, 2000.
10. Ujike H et al: A family with X-linked dystonia-deafness syndrome with novel mutation of the DDP gene. *Arch Neurol* 58:1004–1007, 2001.

Appendix

Other conditions that include eye abnormalities*

Entity	Eye Finding	Chapter in this Book
CHARGE association	Coloboma	6 (external ear)
Marshall syndrome	Myopia, cataracts	8 (musculoskeletal)
Oculodentoosseous dysplasia	Microcornea	8 (musculoskeletal)
Chondrodysplasia, Khaldi	Retinitis pigmentosa	8 (musculoskeletal)
Stickler syndrome	Myopia	8 (musculoskeletal)
Hypoplastic thumbs, coloboma of choroid, cataracts, developmental delay, and sensorineural HL	Choroid coloboma, cataracts	8 (musculoskeletal)
Sorsby syndrome	Macular colobomas	8 (musculoskeletal)
Dysplasia of capital femoral epiphyses, severe myopia, and sensorineural HL	Severe myopia	8 (musculoskeletal)
Spondyloepiphyseal dysplasia, myopia, and sensorineural HL	Severe myopia	8 (musculoskeletal)
Multiple epiphyseal dysplasia, myopia, conductive HL	Severe myopia	8 (musculoskeletal)
Horizontal gaze palsy, scoliosis, and sensorineural HL	Horizontal gaze palsy	8 (musculoskeletal)
Metaphyseal dysplasia, retinal pigmentary changes, and sensorineural HL	Retinal pigmentary changes	8 (musculoskeletal)
Bowed tibiae, dislocated elbows, scoliosis, microcephaly, cataract, and sensorineural HL	Cataract	8 (musculoskeletal)
Fine-Lubinsky syndrome	Cataracts	8 (musculoskeletal)
SHORT syndrome	Rieger anomaly	8 (musculoskeletal)
Renal rickets, retinitis pigmentosa, and progressive sensorineural HL	Retinitis pigmentosa	9 (renal)
Renal failure, cataracts, recurrent infections, and conductive HL	Cataracts	9 (renal)
Renal-coloboma syndrome	Coloboma	9 (renal)
BRESHECK	Microphthalmia	9 (renal)
Stromgren syndrome	Cataracts	10 (neurologic)
Begeer syndrome	Cataracts	10 (neurologic)
Flynn-Aird syndrome	Cataracts, pigmentary retinopathy	10 (neurologic)
Hallgren syndrome	Pigmentary retinopathy	10 (neurologic)
Gordon syndrome	Pigmentary retinopathy	10 (neurologic)
Campbell-Clifton syndrome	Chorioretinitis	10 (neurologic)
N syndrome	Nystagmus, visual impairment	10 (neurologic)
Oculopalatocerebral dwarfism	Persistent hyperplastic primary vitreous	10 (neurologic)
Coppetto-Lessell syndrome	Pigmentary retinopathy	10 (neurologic)
Nathalie syndrome	Cataracts	10 (neurologic)
Borud syndrome	Pigmentary retinopathy	10 (neurologic)
Deafness, congenital heart defects, and posterior embryotoxon	Posterior embryotoxon	11 (cardiac)
CHIME	Retinal colobomas	14 (integumentary)
Sensorineural HL, retinal pigment epithelium lesions, and discolored teeth	Retinal pigment epithelium lesions	15 (oral and dental)

*See also Table 7–3.
HL, hearing loss.

Chapter 8
Genetic Hearing Loss Associated with Musculoskeletal Disorders
ROBERT J. GORLIN

The musculoskeletal disorders described in this chapter have been organized under the following headings: craniotubular bone disorders, chondrodysplasias, craniosynostoses, acral-orofacial syndromes, other skeletal disorders, and miscellaneous musculoskeletal disorders. Some conditions with skeletal components such as Treacher Collins syndrome, Nager syndrome and Genée-Wiedemann syndrome appear in Chapter 6.

Craniotubular Bone Disorders

Craniometaphyseal dysplasia

Craniometaphyseal dysplasia was erroneously reported in the early literature as Pyle disease. It is characterized by an unusual face and club-shaped metaphyseal flaring of long bones. Autosomal dominant and recessive inheritance patterns have been observed. Extreme variability in the dominant form does not allow for differentiation from the recessive form, whereas the latter appears to be somewhat less variable. Although some recessive cases appear to be more severe than dominant examples, in a sporadic case it is not possible to clinically distinguish between the two forms (18,40). About 80 cases have been reported. The basic defect is altered bone turnover (21,32,33).

Clinical findings. Usually within the first year of life, the root of the nose begins to broaden and an elevated wing of bone gradually extends bilaterally over the nasal bridge to the zygomas. Increasing bony sclerosis narrows the nasal lumen, leading to obstruction, with resultant open mouth (2,23) (Fig. 8–1A–D,I,J).

In 30–50% of patients, narrowing of the cranial foramina causes peripheral facial nerve paralysis, hearing loss, headache, or vertigo (2,5,16). Hypertelorism is a constant feature. Nystagmus is common. Rarely, there is visual loss because of optic atrophy (13,16). This suggests bony encroachment on the optic foramina. The alveolar ridges may be thickened. Occasionally there is delayed eruption of permanent teeth.

Auditory system. Bony alterations in the temporal bone and pyramid produce mixed hearing loss that becomes evident in childhood in about one-half the cases. It is slowly progressive until there is moderate to severe (30–90 dB) loss by the fourth decade (2,5,14,16). However, in one report, conductive loss was present before 1 year of age (28).

Radiographic findings. Hyperostosis and sclerosis involve the frontal and occipital portions of the calvaria, skull base, and, less often, mandible. There is increased bone deposit on the walls of the paranasal sinuses and underpneumatization of mastoid cells. Most marked is frontonasal hyperostosis (Fig. 8–1E). The ribs are widened and dense (Fig. 8–1F). Long bones have club-shaped metaphyseal flare (Erlenmeyer flask–shaped) and exhibit decreased density. The changes are far milder than those seen in Pyle disease and may be minimal during the first years of life. Cortical hyperostosis of diaphyses is noted in the young, but disappears with age. Short tubular bones exhibit the same changes as those noted in long bones (Fig. 8–1G,H).

Heredity. Autosomal dominant (1–33) and autosomal recessive (34–47) forms have been observed. The autosomal dominant form has been mapped to 5p15.2–p14.1 (6,19,21), while the recessive type has been located at 6q21–q22 (37). The dominant form is caused by mutations in the multipass transmembrane protein, ANKH, which is involved in the transport of intracellular pyrophosphate into extracellular matrix. The mutated protein has a dominant negative effect on the function of ANKH since reduced levels of pyrophosphate in bone matrix cause increased mineralization (21,32).

Diagnosis. While one cannot differentiate between dominant or recessive inheritance in the isolated patient, separation from those with Pyle disease and craniodiaphyseal dysplasia is usually clinically easy. However, Reardon et al. (44) pointed out the difficulty of diagnosis in some cases. Treatment has been discussed (5,6,10).

Summary. Characteristics include (*1*) autosomal dominant and autosomal recessive forms; (*2*) hyperostosis and sclerosis of calvaria, skull base, and sometimes mandible; (*3*) long bones and short bones with mild metaphyseal flare; (*4*) occasional facial palsy; and (*5*) mixed hearing loss.

References (Craniometaphyseal dysplasia, dominant)

1. Beighton P: Craniometaphyseal dysplasia (CMD), autosomal dominant form. *J Med Genet* 32:370–374, 1995.
2. Beighton P et al: Craniometaphyseal dysplasia: Variability of expression within a large family. *Clin Genet* 15:252–258, 1979.
3. Bricker SL et al: Dominant craniometaphyseal dysplasia. *Dentomaxillofac Radiol* 12:95–100, 1983.
4. Carlson DH, Harris GBC: Craniometaphyseal dysplasia: a family with three documented cases. *Radiology* 103:147–151, 1972.
5. Carnevale A et al: Autosomal dominant craniometaphyseal dysplasia: Clinical variability. *Clin Genet* 23:17–22, 1983.
6. Chandler D et al: Refinement of the chromosome 5p locus for craniometaphyseal dysplasia. *Hum Genet* 108:394–397, 2001.
7. Colavita N et al: Cranio-metaphyseal dysplasia. *Australas Radiol* 32:257–262, 1988.
8. Cole DEC, Cohen MM Jr: A new look at craniometaphyseal dysplasia. *J Pediatr* 112:577–579, 1988.
9. Cooper JC: Craniometaphyseal dysplasia. A case report and review of the literature. *Br J Oral Surg* 12:196–204, 1974.
10. Fanconi S et al: Craniometaphyseal dysplasia with increased bone turnover and secondary hyperparathyroidism: therapeutic effect of calcitonin. *J Pediatr* 112:587–590, 1988.
11. Guibaud P et al: La dysplasie cranio-métaphysaire. *Pédiatrie* 28:149–161, 1973.
12. Holt JF: The evolution of cranio-metaphyseal dysplasia. *Ann Radiol* 9:209–224, 1966.
13. Jend HH et al: Cranio-metaphyseal stratiform dysplasia—conventional radiography and CT findings. *Eur J Radiol* 1:261–265, 1981.
14. Keitzer G, Paparella MM: Otolaryngological disorders in craniometaphyseal dysplasia. *Laryngoscope* 79:921–941, 1969.
15. Key LL et al: Treatment of craniometaphyseal dysplasia with calcitriol. *J Pediatr* 112:583–586, 1988.
16. Kletzer GR et al: Otolaryngologic features of craniometaphyseal dysplasia. *Otolaryngol Head Neck Surg* 96:548–553, 1989 (same case as ref. 18).
17. Martin FW: Craniometaphyseal dysplasia. *J Laryngol Otol* 91:159–169, 1977.
18. Morgan DW et al: Hearing loss due to cranio-metaphyseal dysplasia. *J Laryngol Otol* 104:807–808, 1990.

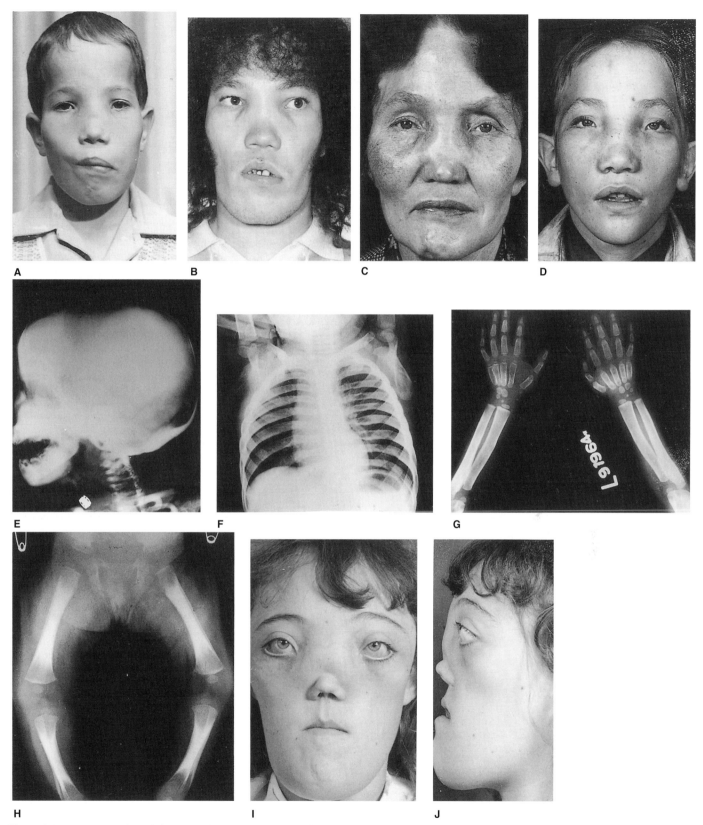

Figure 8–1. *Craniometaphyseal dysplasia, dominant.* (A) Facial features showing hypertelorism, broad nasal bridge, enlarged paranasal area, and left facial paralysis. (B) Same person at age 24. (C,D) Note similar paranasal enlargement in mother and son. (E) Note square-shaped skull and deposit of bone in paranasal area. (F) Note wide ribs. (G) Poor modeling of long bones and bones of hand. (H) Typical metaphyseal radilucency and condensation of diaphyses. *Craniometaphyseal dysplasia, recessive.* (I,J) Head appears rather large with extremely broad and flat nasal body. Paranasal masses and mandibular prognathism are due to bony involvement. [(F,G) from DR Millard Jr et al., *Am J Surg* 113:615, 1967.]

19. Nürnberg P et al: The gene for autosomal dominant craniometaphyseal dysplasia maps to chromosomal 5p and is distinct from the growth hormone–receptor gene. *Am J Hum Genet* 61:918–923, 1997.

20. Puliafito CA et al: Optic atrophy and visual loss in craniometaphyseal dysplasia. *Am J Ophthalmol* 92:696–701, 1981.

21. Reichenberger E et al: Autosomal dominant craniometaphyseal dysplasia is caused by mutations in the transmembrane protein ANK. *Am J Hum Genet* 68:1321–1326, 2001.

22. Richards A: Craniometaphyseal and craniodiaphyseal dysplasia: head and neck manifestations and management. *J Laryngol Otol* 110:328–338, 1996.

23. Rimoin DL et al: Cranio-metaphyseal dysplasia (Pyle's disease): autosomal dominant inheritance in a large kindred. *Birth Defects* 5(4):96–104, 1969.

24. Schaefer B et al: Dominantly inherited craniodiaphyseal dysplasia: a new craniotubular dysplasia. *Clin Genet* 30:381–391, 1986.

25. Schröder C et al: Craniometaphysäre Dysplasie—characterische Röntgenbefunde. *Klin Pädiatr* 204:174–176, 1992.

26. Schwahn B et al: Autosomal dominant craniometaphyseal dysplasia. *Monatsschr Kinderheilkd* 144:1073–1077, 1996.

27. Shea J et al: Cranio-metaphyseal dysplasia: the first successful surgical treatment for associated hearing loss. *Laryngoscope* 91:1369–1374, 1981.

28. Sheppard WM et al. Craniometaphyseal dysplasia: a case report and review of medical and surgical management. *Int J Pediatr Otorhinolaryngol* 67:71–77, 2003.

29. Spiro PC et al: Radiology of the autosomal dominant form of craniometaphyseal dysplasia. *S Afr Med J* 49:839–842, 1975.

30. Spitzer W, Steinhauser EW: Die kraniometaphysäre Dysplasie. *Dtsch Zahnärtzl Z* 36:96–100, 1981.

31. Taylor DB, Sprague P: Dominant craniometaphyseal dysplasia—a family study over five generations. *Australas Radiol* 33:87–89, 1989.

32. Tinschert S, Braun HL: Craniometaphyseal dysplasia in six generations of a German kindred. *Am J Med Genet* 77:175–181, 1998.

33. Yamamoto T et al: Bone marrow derived osteoclast-like cells from a patient with craniometaphyseal dysplasia lack expression of osteoclast-reactive vacuolar proton pump. *J Clin Invest* 91:362–367, 1993.

References (Craniometaphyseal dysplasia, recessive)

34. Boltshauser E et al: Cerebromedullary compression in recessive craniometaphyseal dysplasia. *Neuroradiology* 38:193–195, 1996.

35. Elçioglu N, Hall CM: Temporal aspects in craniometaphyseal dysplasia, autosomal recessive type. *Am J Med Genet* 76:245–251, 1998.

36. Graf K: Die Bedeutung des Pyle-Syndroms (Leontiasis ossea) für die Oto-Rhino-Laryngologie. *Z Laryngol Rhinol* 44:438–445, 1965.

37. Iughetti P et al: Mapping of the autosomal recessive (AR) craniometaphyseal dysplasia locus to chromosome region 6q21–22 and confirmation of genetic heterogeneity for mild Arsponsylocostal dysplasia. *Am J Med Genet* 95:482–491, 2000.

38. Jackson WP et al: Metaphyseal dysplasia, epiphyseal dysplasia, diaphyseal dysplasia and related constitutions. *Arch Intern Med* 94:871–885, 1957.

39. Lehmann ECH: Familial osteodystrophy of the skull and face. *J Bone Joint Surg* 39B:313–315, 1957.

40. Lievre JA, Fischgold H: Leontiasis ossea chez l'enfant (osteopetrose partielle probable). *Presse Med* 64:763–765, 1956.

41. Millard DR et al: Craniofacial surgery in craniometaphyseal dysplasia. *Am J Surg* 113:615–621, 1967.

42. Nicolo A, Briani S: La displasia craniometafisaria. *Ann Radiol Diagn* 39:185–202, 1966.

43. Penchaszadeh VB et al: Autosomal recessive craniometaphyseal dysplasia. *Am J Med Genet* 5:43–55, 1980.

44. Reardon W et al: Sibs with mental retardation, supraorbital sclerosis and metaphyseal dysplasia: frontometaphyseal dysplasia, craniometaphyseal dysplasia, or a new syndrome? *J Med Genet* 28:622–626, 1991.

45. Ross MW, Altman DH: Familial metaphyseal dysplasia: review of the clinical and radiological features of Pyle's disease. *Clin Pediatr* 6:143–149, 1967.

46. Sommer F: Eine besondere Form einer generalisierten Hyperostose mit Leontiasis ossea faciei et cranii. *Radiol Clin (Basel)* 23:65–75, 1954.

47. Wemmer V, Böttger E: Die kraniometaphysäre Dysplasie (Jackson). *Roefo* 128:66–69, 1978.

Craniodiaphyseal dysplasia

In 1958, Joseph et al. (7) first used the term *craniodiaphyseal dysplasia* to designate a severe bone disorder characterized by massive generalized hyperostosis and sclerosis, involving in particular the skull and facial bones (1–16,18–20). The patient described by Schaefer et al. (17)

really had craniometaphyseal dysplasia of the dominant type. The movie *Mask* concerned a patient with craniodiaphyseal dysplasia. About 15 patients have been reported.

Clinical features. Facial and cranial thickening, distortion, and enlargement are severe. Nasal obstruction and recurrent upper respiratory infection appear within the first few years or even the first few months of life (12). Head circumference is increased. Marked bony thickening, hypertelorism, nasal flattening, occlusion of lacrimal ducts, and severe dental malocclusion generally follow. Bilateral choanal stenosis can be demonstrated within the first few years. All patients have severe hypertelorism, lacrimal duct obstruction resulting from bony overgrowth, and diminished visual acuity or blindness as a result of optic atrophy (Fig. 8–2A). Compression of nearly all cranial nerves results from bony overgrowth. This relentless process is associated with headache, progressive mental retardation, and seizures.

Developmental milestones including speech are delayed (5,11,14,18). Often there is lack of sexual maturation. Stature has been retarded in several cases (5,10,18), and early death has occurred in about 50%.

Musculoskeletal system. Radiographically, the skull and facial bones as well as the mandible are severely sclerotic and hyperostotic. The paranasal sinuses and mastoids do not develop (Fig. 8–2B–D). Progression of the disease is documented by Tucker et al. (20). There is moderate thickening and marked sclerosis of the ribs and clavicles. The long tubular bones do not exhibit metaphyseal flare, but rather have a policeman's nightstick shape and show diaphyseal endostosis. The short tubular bones of the hands and feet, particularly the first metapodial, exhibit cylinderization. A few investigators have found elevated levels of serum alkaline phosphatase, but normal levels of calcium and phosphorus (1,6–8,19). The bone trabeculae are thick and have very wide uncalcified osteoid seams (1,12).

Auditory system. Hearing loss, at first conductive but becoming mixed, has been described in almost all cases, but extensive documentation has been sparse. Halliday (5) reported sensorineural hearing deficit.

Heredity. Inheritance is confusing. Male and female sibs were reported by de Souza (3). The parents of Halliday's (5) patients were consanguineous. This would suggest autosomal recessive inheritance. However, Brueton and Winter (2) opined that the sibs described by de Souza (3) really had van Buchem disease. The rest of the cases were isolated examples.

Diagnosis. To be excluded would be Camurati-Engelmann disease, craniometaphyseal dysplasia, van Buchem disease, and sclerosteosis.

Summary. Characteristics include (*1*) unknown inheritance; (*2*) massive enlargement and sclerosis of cranial and facial bones, ribs, and clavicles; (*3*) cylinderization of long bones and diaphyseal endostosis; (*4*) bony overgrowth of cranial foramina resulting in blindness and deafness; (*5*) elevated levels of alkaline phosphatase; and (*6*) mixed hearing loss.

References

1. Bonucci E et al: Histologic, microradiographic and electron microscopic investigations of bone tissue in a case of craniodiaphyseal dysplasia. *Virchow Arch A Pathol Anat Histopathol* 373:167–175, 1977.

2. Brueton LA, Winter RM: Craniodiaphyseal dysplasia. *J Med Genet* 27:701–706, 1990.

3. de Souza O: Leontiasis ossea. *Porto Allegre (Brazil) Faculdade de Med Dos Cursos* 13:47–54, 1927.

4. Fosmoe RJ et al: van Buchem's disease (hyperostosis corticalistata familiaris). *Radiology* 90:771–774, 1968.

5. Halliday J: A rare case of bone dysplasia. *Br J Surg* 37:52–63, 1949–1950.

6. Itakagi Y et al: A case of craniodiaphyseal dysplasia. *No To Hattatsu* 21:69–73, 1989.

7. Joseph R et al: Dysplasia cranio-diaphysaire progressive: ses relations avec la dysplasie diaphysaire progressive de Camurati-Engelmann. *Ann Radiol* 1:477–490, 1958.

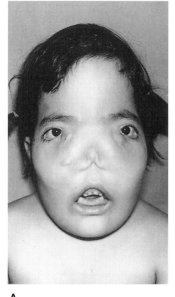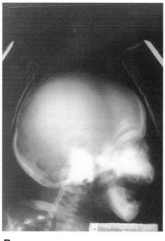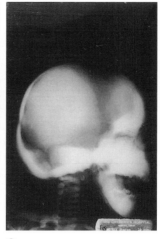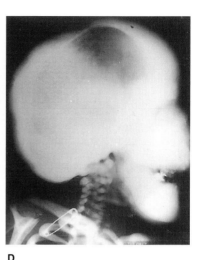

A   B   C   D

Figure 8–2. *Craniodiaphyseal dysplasia.* (A) Five-year-old showing marked enlargement of cranium, facial bones, and mandible. Note severe ocular hypertelorism and dental malocclusion. (B–D) Lateral skull radiographs at 3½ months (left), 18 months (center), and 5 years (right) showing progression of hyperostosis involving cranium, facial bones, mandible, and proximal cervical spine. There is no development of paranasal sinuses and mastoids. [(A–D) from RI Macpherson, *J Can Assoc Radiol* 25:22, 1974.]

8. Kaitila I et al: Craniodiaphyseal dysplasia. *Birth Defects* 11(6):359–361, 1975.
9. Kirkpatrick DB et al: The craniotubular bone modeling disorders: a neurosurgical introduction to rare skeletal dysplasias with cranial nerve compression. *Surg Neurol* 7:221–232, 1977 (same case as ref. 8).
10. Levy MH, Kozlowski K: Cranio-diaphyseal dysplasia. *Australas Radiol* 31:431–435, 1987.
11. Macpherson RI: Craniodiaphyseal dysplasia, a disease or group of diseases? *J Can Assoc Radiol* 25:22–23, 1974 (case 1).
12. McHugh DA et al: Nasolacrimal obstruction and facial bone histopathology in craniodiaphyseal dysplasia. *Br J Ophthalmol* 78:501–503, 1994.
13. McKeating JB, Kershaw CR: Craniodiaphyseal dysplasia. *J R Nav Med Serv* 73:81–93, 1987.
14. Menichini G et al: Singolare caso di malattia iperostosica del tipo displasia cranio-diafisaria. *Minerva Pediatr* 29:1485–1489, 1977.
15. Richards A: Craniometaphyseal and craniodiaphyseal dysplasia. Head and neck manifestations and management. *J Laryngol Otol* 110:328–338, 1961.
16. Scarfo GB et al: Idrocephalo associato a displasia cranio-diafisaria. *Radiol Med* 65:249–252, 1979.
17. Schaefer B et al: Dominantly inherited craniodiaphyseal dysplasia. A new craniotubular dysplasia. *Clin Genet* 30:381–391, 1986.
18. Stransky E et al: On Paget's disease with leontiasis ossea and hypothyreosis starting in early childhood. *Ann Paediatr* 199:393–408, 1962.
19. Thurnau GR et al: Management and outcome of two pregnancies in a woman with craniodiaphyseal dysplasia. *Am J Perinatol* 8:56–61, 1991.
20. Tucker AS et al: Craniodiaphyseal dysplasia: evolution over a five-year period. *Skeletal Radiol* 1:47–53, 1976.

Frontometaphyseal dysplasia

In 1969, Gorlin and Cohen (8) separated frontometaphyseal dysplasia from other craniotubular dysplasias. Frontometaphyseal dysplasia is characterized by pronounced bony supraorbital ridges, mixed hearing loss, and generalized skeletal dysplasia. About 30 cases have been subsequently described by numerous authors (1–23, 25–28).

Craniofacial findings. The marked supraorbital ridge, wide nasal bridge, downward slanting palpebral fissures, and small pointed chin give the patient a striking appearance (Fig. 8–3A). Enlargement of the supraorbital ridge becomes evident before puberty (4). Missing permanent teeth and retained deciduous teeth (1,4,8) may occur. Most patients have malocclusion. Congenital glottic and subglottic stenoses may occur (5,17).

Musculoskeletal system. There is both primary and secondary wasting of hand muscles (Fig. 8–3B). Dorsiflexion of the wrist and extension of the elbows are reduced, with pronation and supination being extremely limited. Flexion deformities of the fingers and ulnar deviation of the wrist are progressive. Finger mobility is essentially limited to the metacarpophalangeal joints. The thumbs tend to be broad. Hammer toes have also been noted. Scoliosis, which is usually mild, is a fairly common manifestation (21). However, Morava et al. (21) described two families in which scoliosis was severe and progressive.

Radiographic findings. Radiographic findings include a thick, torus-like frontal ridge, absence of frontal sinuses, "Hershey kiss" or "top-of-the-mosque" defects of supraorbital rims, arched superior borders of maxillary sinuses, short maxilla, elongated cranial base, and antegonial notching of the mandible with marked hypoplasia of the angle and condyloid process (1,8,10,13,15) (Fig. 8–3C). A mandibular spur has been reported as characteristic (7).

The foramen magnum is greatly enlarged, and numerous vertebral anomalies have been noted; for example, the odontoid process is located too far anteriorly, the atlas has no posterior arch, and the lumbar vertebrae are flattened. There are fusion of the second and third cervical vertebrae, and subluxation of the third and fourth vertebrae. The shoulders may be highly positioned. Scoliosis may be marked with resultant shortening of the trunk (18,19,23,25). Restrictive chest bellows disease has been recorded (8,18). The long bones manifest increased density in the diaphyseal region, with lack of modeling in the metaphyseal area producing an Erlenmeyer flask deformity. The legs may be laterally bowed. Marked flaring of the iliac bones and coxa valga are noted, as well as fused and eroded carpal bones, wide elongated middle phalanges, and increased interpediculate distances in the lumbar region of the spine (4,8,11,15) (Fig. 8–3D,E). The ribs and vertebrae are irregularly contoured (10) and the lower ribs are "coat hanger" in form. A characteristic metacarpophalangeal profile has been suggested (11).

Auditory system. Progressive mixed hearing loss has been reported (1,8,28,29).

Vestibular system. Arenberg et al. (1) described marked hypofunction on caloric testing.

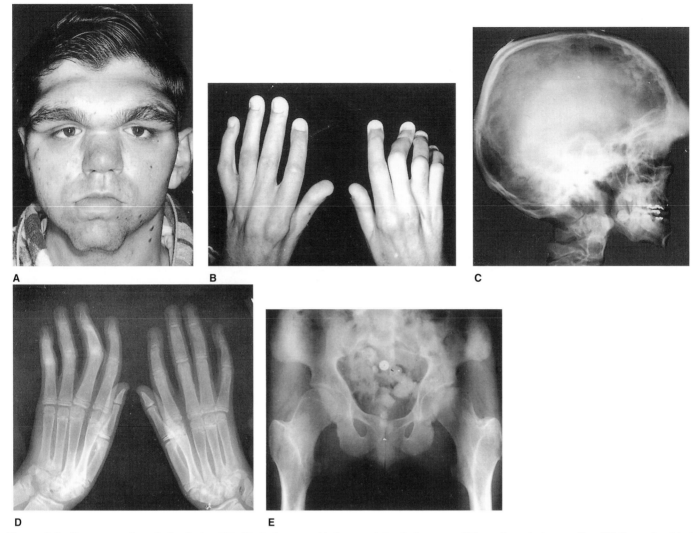

Figure 8–3. *Frontometaphyseal dysplasia.* (A) Marked supraorbital ridge, wide nasal bridge, and small pointed chin give patient a striking appearance. (B) Wasting of interosseous muscles of hands, ulnar deviation of fingers. (C) Radiograph showing supraorbital torus, hypoplasia and dysplasia or mandible, and cervical anomalies. (D) Generalized lack of modeling of long bones. (E) Marked flaring of iliac bones, widened femoral necks. [(A,D) from RJ Gorlin and MM Cohen Jr, *Am J Dis Child* 118:487, 1969.]

Other findings. Urinary tract anomalies (hydroureter, hydronephrosis, renal duplication) (5,7,13,14,24) and obstructive airway disease (1,5,8) are probably relatively common complications. Mitral valve prolapse has been reported (22) as well as atrial septal defects, pulmonary stenosis, and tricuspid atresia (1,4,7). Bands of soft tissue extending from the medial edge of the scapula to the vertebral column have been noted (26). Hirsutism of the buttocks and thighs is common. Several patients had cryptorchidism (1,7).

Heredity. Inheritance is X-linked with variable expression in carrier females (1,2,6,7,9,11). Although some authors have suggested autosomal dominant inheritance (3,14), there has been no male-to-male transmission. Verloes et al. (27), Superti-Furga and Gimelli (25), and Morava et al. (21) opined and Robertson et al. (24) proved that frontometaphyseal dysplasia, Melnick-Needles syndrome, and otopalatodigital I and II syndromes are allelic variants. The filamin A (actin-binding) (FLNA) gene at Xq28 is mutated (24).

Diagnosis. Frontometaphyseal dysplasia is easily distinguished from craniometaphyseal dysplasia and craniodiaphyseal dysplasia. Pronounced supraorbital ridges are found in otopalatodigital syndrome, type I, and to some degree in Melnick-Needles syndrome. Diagnosis may be difficult in the neonate. It rests on increased bone density, rib configuration, widened metaphyses, and externally rotated iliac bones (7).

Summary. Characteristics of this syndrome include (*1*) X-linked inheritance; (*2*) characteristic facial phenotype marked by pronounced supraorbital ridges and pointed chin; (*3*) wasting of arm and leg muscles with flexion deformity of joints; (*4*) characteristic skeletal changes; and (*5*) mixed but mostly conductive hearing loss.

References

1. Arenberg JK et al: Otolaryngologic manifestations of frontometaphyseal dysplasia. The Gorlin-Holt syndrome. *Arch Otolaryngol* 99:52–58, 1974.
2. Balestrazzi P: Hérédite liée au sexe dans la dysplasia fronto-metaphysaire. *J Génét Hum* 33:419–425, 1985.
3. Beighton P, Hamersma H: Frontometaphyseal dysplasia: autosomal dominant or X-linked. *J Med Genet* 17:53–56, 1980.
4. Danks DM et al: Fronto-metaphyseal dysplasia. *Am J Dis Child* 123:254–258, 1972.
5. Fitzsimmons JS et al: Fronto-metaphyseal dysplasia: further delineation of the clinical syndrome. *Clin Genet* 22:195–205, 1982.
6. Franceschini P et al: Esophageal atresia with distal tracheoesophageal fistula in a patient with frontometaphyseal dysplasia. *Am J Med Genet* 73:10–14, 1997.
7. Glass RBJ, Rosenbaum KN: Frontometaphyseal dysplasia: neonatal radiographic diagnosis. *Am J Med Genet* 57:1–5, 1995.
8. Gorlin RJ, Cohen MM Jr. Frontometaphyseal dysplasia: a new syndrome. *Am J Dis Child* 118:487–494, 1969.

9. Gorlin RJ, Winter RB: Frontometaphyseal dysplasia—evidence for X-linked inheritance. *Am J Med Genet* 5:81–84, 1980.

10. Holt JF et al: Frontometaphyseal dysplasia. *Radiol Clin North Am* 10:225–243, 1972.

11. Jend-Rossman I et al: Frontometaphyseal dysplasia: symptoms and possible mode of inheritance. *J Oral Maxillofac Surg* 42:743–748, 1984.

12. Jervis GA, Jenkins EC: Frontometaphyseal dysplasia. *Syndrome Ident* 3:18–19, 1975.

13. Kanemura T et al: Frontometaphyseal dysplasia with congenital urinary tract malformations. *Clin Genet* 16:399–404, 1979.

14. Kassner EG et al: Frontometaphyseal dysplasia: evidence for autosomal dominant inheritance. *AJR Am J Roentgenol* 127:927–933, 1976.

15. Kleinsorge H, Böttger E: Das Gorlin-Cohen-Syndrom (fronto-metaphysäre Dysplasie). *Roefo* 127:451–458, 1977.

16. Kung DS, Sloane GM: Cranioplasty in frontometaphyseal dysplasia. *Plast Reconstr Surg* 102:1144–1146, 1998.

17. Leggett JM: Laryngo-tracheal stenosis in frontometaphyseal dysplasia. *J Laryngol Otol* 102:74–78, 1988.

18. Lipson E et al: Restrictive chest bellows disease and frontometaphyseal dysplasia. *Chest* 103:1264–1265, 1993.

19. Medlar RC, Crawford AH: Frontometaphyseal dysplasia presenting as scoliosis: a report of a family with four cases. *J Bone Joint Surg Am* 60:392–394, 1978.

20. Mersten A et al: Cranio-metaphyseal dysplasia. *Radiol Diagn* 21:70–74, 1980.

21. Morava E et al.: Clinical and genetic heterogeneity in frontometaphyseal dysplasia: severe progressive scoliosis in two families. *Am J Med Genet* 116A:272–277, 2003.

22. Park JM et al: Mitral valve prolapse in a patient with frontometaphyseal dysplasia. *Clin Paediatr* 25:469–471, 1986.

23. Reardon W et al: Sibs with mental retardation, supraorbital sclerosis and metaphyseal dysplasia: frontometaphyseal dysplasia, craniometaphyseal dysplasia, or a new syndrome? *J Med Genet* 28:662–626, 1991.

24. Robertson SP et al: Localized mutations in the gene encoding the cytoskeletal protein filamin A cause diverse malformations in humans. *Nat Genet* 33:487–491, 2003.

25. Superti-Furga A, Bimelli F: Fronto-metaphyseal dysplasia and the oto-palato-digital syndrome. *Dysmorphol Clin Genet* 1:2–5, 1987.

26. Ullrich E et al: Frontometaphyseal dysplasia: report of two familial cases. *Australas Radiol* 23:265–271, 1979.

27. Verloes A et al: Fronto-otopalatodigital osteodysplasia: clinical evidence for a single entity encompassing Melnick-Needles syndrome, otopalatodigital syndromes types 1 and 2, and frontometaphyseal dysplasia. *Am J Med Genet* 90:407–422, 2000.

28. Walker BA: A craniodiaphyseal dysplasia or craniometaphyseal dysplasia, ? type. *Birth Defects* 5(4):298–300, 1969.

Progressive diaphyseal dysplasia (Camurati-Engelmann disease)

First reported independently in the 1920s by Camurati (4) and Engelmann (10), progressive diaphyseal dysplasia is a sclerotic and hyperostotic disorder of bone (23,24). More than 200 cases have been reported. The prevalence has been estimated to be lower than 1 in 1,000,000 live births (32,33).

Clinical findings. The most common clinical findings include delayed ambulation, bone pain, generalized neuromuscular weakness, thin musculature with disproportionately long limbs, bowed tibiae, broadly based waddling gait, and flat feet (Fig. 8–4A,B). This condition can be manifest as early as the third to fifth years of life, although the mean age is about 15–20 years (11,12,40). There may be genua vara, genua valga, lumbar lordosis, or scoliosis. Less often there is hepatosplenomegaly. Secondary sexual development is poor. Some patients exhibit frontal bossing, exophthalmos, papilledema, epiphora, optic atrophy, and headache (13,22,28,29,37). Sense of taste and smell may be lost (16).

Radiographic findings. There is symmetric irregular spindle-shaped, sclerotic cortical thickening of the mid-diaphyses of long tubular bones and narrowing of medullary cavities. With age, the process extends proximally and distally toward the metaphyses, which are rarely involved. The epiphyses are not affected. The base of the skull and calvaria are sclerotic in 70% of cases. The mandible is sclerotic in 25% and occasionally is significantly enlarged. The cervical vertebrae, clavicles, pelvic bones, hand and foot bones, and ribs are affected in about

Figure 8–4. *Progressive diaphyseal dysplasia (Camurati-Engelmann disease).* (A) Ten-year-old boy exhibiting general asthenic appearance, poor muscle mass, pronation of feet, and characteristic long limbs. (B) Note less marked phenotypic changes in 10-year-old girl. (C) Diagrammatic illustration of bony involvement. (D) CAT scan showing hyperostosis of facial bones; note thickness of anterior maxillary wall. [(A) from RS Sparkes and CB Graham Jr, *J Med Genet* 9:73, 1972; (B) courtesy of H-R Wiedemann, Kiel, Germany; (D) from PN Demas and GC Sotereanos. *Oral Surg Oral Med Oral Pathol* 68:686, 1989.]

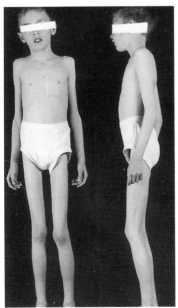
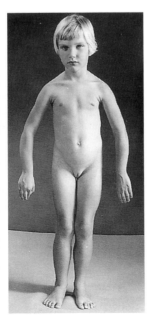
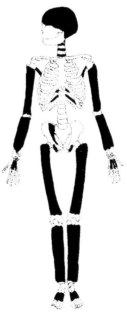
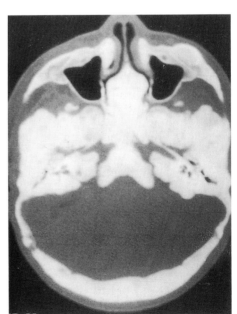

A   **B**   **C**   **D**

20% (28,31,39) (Fig. 8–4C,D). It may be related to Ribbing disease (26).

Auditory system. Mixed hearing loss based on stenosis has been noted in 5%–7% (1,5,7–10,16,17,25,27,28,36,38,39). Sparkes and Graham (36) recorded slit-like internal auditory canals.

Vestibular system. Vestibular disturbances can be noted (8,16, 20,38).

Laboratory findings. Serum alkaline phosphatase, urinary hydroxyproline, and erythrocyte sedimentation rate may be elevated (11,14,35). Anemia is relatively frequent. The scintigraphic changes are striking and not always correlated with radiographic changes (15).

Heredity. Inheritance is autosomal dominant with considerable variation in expression. Anticipation has been reported (33). New mutations account for about 50% of cases (28). The gene has been mapped to 19q13.2–q13.3 (11,18), and has been identified as transforming growth factor beta-1 (*TGFB1*) (19,21,30). Although it had been suggested that this is a homogeneous condition (1,6) recently two girls with a Camurati-Engelmann phenotype were found to have no mutations in *TGFB1* (30). The reporting authors referred to this condition as Camurati-Engelmann II (30).

Diagnosis. Diaphyseal sclerosis can be seen in craniometaphyseal dysplasia. Infantile cortical hyperostosis is distributed asymmetrically and regresses early. In van Buchem disease, the width of tubular bones is not increased, and mandibular enlargement is great. Carnitine levels may be low (3). Surely the child reported by Sennaroğlu et al. (34) has diaphyseal dysplasia.

Summary. The characteristics of this condition include (*1*) autosomal dominant inheritance; (*2*) sclerosis and hyperostosis of skull and long bones; (*3*) weakness and reduction in muscle mass; (*4*) leg pain and abnormal gait; and (*5*) mixed hearing loss and vestibular disturbances.

References

1. Applegate LJ et al: MR of multiple cranial neuropathies in a patient with Camurati-Engelmann disease. *AJNR Am J Neuroradiol* 12:557–559, 1990.
2. Belinda A et al: Genetic heterogeneity of the Camurati-Engelmann disease. *Clin Genet* 58:150–152, 2000.
3. Bye AME et al: Progressive diaphyseal dysplasia and a low muscle carnitine. *Pediatr Radiol* 18:340, 1988.
4. Camurati M: Di un raro di osteite simmetrica ereditaria degli arti inferiori. *Clin Organi Mov* 6:622–665, 1922.
5. Clybouw C et al: Camurati-Engelmann disease: contribution of bone scintigraphy to the genetic counseling. *Genet Couns* 5:195–198, 1994.
6. Cormier-Daire V et al: Genetic homogeneity of the Camurati-Engelmann disease. *Clin Genet* 58:150–152, 2000.
7. Crisp AJ, Brenton DP: Engelmann's disease of bone—a systemic disorder? *Ann Rheum Dis* 41:183–188, 1982.
8. Dannenmaier B, Weber B: Beobachtungen zum Camurati-Engelmann-Syndrom. *Roefo* 151:175–178, 1989.
9. Demas PN, Sotereanos GC: Facial skeletal manifestations of Engelmann's disease. *Oral Surg Oral Med Oral Pathol Endod* 68:686–690, 1989.
10. Engelmann G: Ein Fall von Osteopathia hyperostotica (sclerosis) multiplex infantiles. *Fortschr Roentgenol* 39:1011–1116, 1929.
11. Ghadami M et al: Genetic mapping of the Camurati-Engelmann disease locus to chromosome 9q13.1–q13.3. *Am J Hum Genet* 66:143–147, 2000.
12. Ghosal SP et al: Diaphyseal dysplasia associated with anemia. *J Pediatr* 113:49–57, 1988.
13. Grey AC et al: Engelmann's disease: a 45-year follow-up. *J Bone Joint Surg Br* 78:488–491, 1996.
14. Gümrük F et al: Ghosal haemato-diaphyseal dysplasia: a new disorder. *Eur J Pediatr* 152:218–221, 1993.
15. Hanson W, Parnes LS: Vestibular nerve compression in Camurati-Engelmann disease. *Ann Otol Rhinol Laryngol* 104:823–825, 1995.
16. Hellier WPL, Brookes GB: Vestibular nerve dysfunction and decompression in Engelmann's disease. *J Laryngol Otol* 110:462–465, 1996.
17. Huygen PLM et al: Camurati-Engelmann disease presenting as 'juvenile otosclerosis'. *Int J Pediatr Otolaryngol* 37:129–141, 1996.
18. Janssens K et al: Localisation of the gene causing diaphyseal dysplasia Camurati-Engelmann to chromosome 19q13. *J Med Genet* 37:245–249, 2000.
19. Janssens K et al: Mutations in the gene encoding the latency-associated peptide of TFG-β1 cause Camurati-Engelmann disease. *Nat Genet* 26:273–274, 2000.
20. Kaftari JK et al: Progressive diaphyseal dysplasia (Camurati-Engelmann): radiologic follow-up and CT findings. *Radiology* 164:777–782, 1987.
21. Kinoshita A et al: Domain-specific mutations in *TGFB1* result in Camurati-Engelmann disease. *Nat Genet* 26:19–20, 2000.
22. Kuhlencordt F et al: Diaphysäre Dysplasie (Camurati-Engelmann-Syndrom) mit fortschreitendem Visusverlust. *Dtsch Med Wochenschr* 106:617–621, 1981.
23. Kumar B et al: Progressive diaphyseal dysplasia (Engelmann's disease): scintigraphic radiographic-clinical correlations. *Radiology* 140:87–92, 1981.
24. Labat ML et al: Monocytic origin of fibroblasts: spontaneous transformation of blood monocytes into neo-fibroblastic structures in osteomyelosclerosis and Engelmann's disease. *Biomed Pharmacother* 45:289–299, 1991.
25. Lenarz T, Gülzow J: Neuroootologische Frühsymptome der Camurati-Engelmann-Krankheit. *Laryngol Rhinol Otol* 62:463–467, 1983.
26. Makita Y et al: Intrafamilial phenotypic variability in Engelmann disease (ED): Are ED and Ribbing disease the same entity? *Am J Med Genet* 91:153–156, 2000.
27. Miyamoto RT et al: Neurotologic manifestations of the osteopetroses. *Arch Otolaryngol* 106:210–214, 1980 (cases 2,3).
28. Morse PH et al: Ocular findings in hereditary diaphyseal dysplasia (Engelmann's disease). *Am J Ophthalmol* 68:100–104, 1969.
29. Naveh Y et al: Progressive diaphyseal dysplasia: genetics and clinical and radiologic manifestations. *Pediatrics* 74:399–405, 1984.
30. Nishimura G et al: Camurati-Engelmann disease type II: progressive diaphyseal dysplasia with striations of the bones. *J Med Genet* 107:5–11, 2002.
31. Ramon Y, Buchner A: Camurati-Engelmann's disease affecting the jaws. *Oral Surg* 22:592–599, 1966.
32. Saraiva JM: Progressive diaphyseal dysplasia: a three generation family with markedly variable expressivity. *Am J Med Genet* 71:348–352, 1997.
33. Saraiva JM: Anticipation in progressive diaphyseal dysplasia. *J Med Genet* 37:394–395, 2000.
34. Sennaroğlu L et al: Otological findings in idiopathic hyperphosphatasia. *J Laryngol Otol* 113:158–160, 1999.
35. Smith R et al: Clinical and biochemical studies in Engelmann's disease (progressive diaphyseal dysplasia). *Q J Med* 46:273–294, 1977.
36. Sparkes RS, Graham CB: Camurati-Engelmann disease. *J Med Genet* 9:73–85, 1972.
37. Tucker AS et al: Craniodiaphyseal dysplasia: evolution over a five-year period. *Skeletal Radiol* 1:47–55, 1976.
38. Van Dalsem VF et al: Progressive diaphyseal dysplasia. *J Bone Joint Surg Am* 61:596–598, 1979.
39. Wilhelm KR et al: Die Wertigkeit verschiedener radiologischer Untersuchungsverfahren in der Verlaufskontrolle der Camurati-Engelmannschen Krankheit. *Fortschr Roentgenstr* 147:278–282, 1987.
40. Yoshioka H et al: Muscular changes in Engelmann's disease. *Arch Dis Child* 55:716–719, 1980.

Osteopetrosis

Osteopetrosis is a group of disorders characterized by failure of resorption of the primary spongiosa by osteoclasts, resulting in increased osseous density in which cortical and cancellous bone cannot be distinguished radiographically. Histologically, there is an increased number of osteoclasts (38,50).

Osteopetrosis has been traditionally divided into two groups: congenital or malignant autosomal recessive type and adult or benign autosomal dominant form. However, there is likely further genetic heterogeneity: (*a*) severe autosomal recessive osteopetrosis (Albers-Schönberg disease or precocious type); (*b*) mild autosomal recessive osteopetrosis (intermediate type); (*c*) autosomal recessive osteopetrosis with renal tubular acidosis (carbonic anhydrase II deficiency); and (*d*) benign autosomal dominant osteopetrosis (delayed types). Still other forms likely exist. All forms appear to be due to defects in osteoclastic resorption (25).

The auditory system is affected primarily in Albers-Schönberg disease and in the autosomal dominant forms. Hearing loss occurs less often in autosomal recessive osteopetrosis with renal tubular acidosis and in mild autosomal recessive osteopetrosis. For full explication, consult Gorlin et al. (28) and Greenspan (29).

Severe autosomal recessive osteopetrosis (Albers-Schönberg disease)

Severe autosomal recessive osteopetrosis is characterized by increased density of nearly all bones and the complications that occur from failure of resorption of the primary spongiosa and its resultant complications: anemia, hepatosplenomegaly, blindness, hearing loss, facial paralysis, and osteomyelitis. The involved bones are expanded, splayed, and dense, with the epiphysis, metaphysis, and diaphysis being involved to a similar degree. The cortical and cancellous bones are indistinguishable radiographically. Pathogenesis is extensively discussed by Reeves et al. (48) and Lajeunesse et al. (36). Over 500 cases have been reported. Bollerslev (11) estimated that the frequency is 1 in 20,000 births in Denmark.

Clinical findings. All tubular bones may be involved, but growth is usually normal. The skull is thickened and dense, mainly at its base, but the calvaria and paranasal sinuses are poorly aerated, and the facial bones appear denser than normal (23,24,44,45) (Fig. 8–5A). Especially revealing are magnetic resonance imaging (MRI) studies (19).

Neurologic findings. Defective vision and nystagmus are extremely common and are the first findings at a median age of 2 months (1,16,27) (Fig. 8–5B). Optic atrophy eventuating from pressure of bone on optic veins is a relatively common complication. Facial paralysis re-sults from the pressure of dense bone on the foramen of the seventh cranial nerve (6,37). Mental retardation occurs in about 20% (32).

Musculoskeletal findings. The bones are extremely dense but not distorted in form (Fig. 8–5C). The epiphyses, metaphyses, and diaphyses are similarly involved. The cortical and cancellous bones are indistinguishable (43). Fractures are common (Fig. 8–5D).

Oral findings. Osteomyelitis of the jaws seems to be a significant complication of dental extraction, presumably the result of a deficient blood supply (21,53). It may lead to extraoral fistulas. Primary molars and all permanent teeth are greatly distorted and remain totally or partially embedded in basal bone (9). Ankylosis of cementum to bone has been described (63). The teeth appear to be secondarily affected by failure of bone resorption and/or osteomyelitis (20).

Hematopoietic findings. Although the liver and spleen are normal at birth, in over 50% of the cases they enlarge in childhood because of extramedullary hematopoiesis. Hemolytic anemia and thrombocytopenia are found and generalized lymphadenopathy has been noted in about 20%.

Auditory system. Between 25% and 50% of patients have moderate mixed sensorineural and conductive hearing loss beginning in childhood (5,31,41). In general, investigators have not reported detailed au-

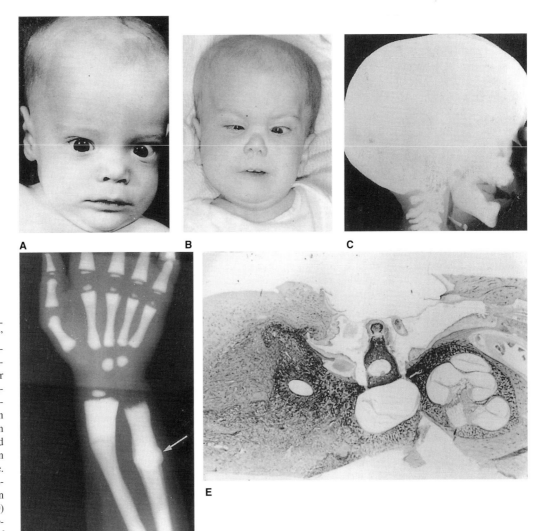

Figure 8–5. *Osteopetrosis.* (A) A 3-month-old infant exhibiting "squared" head form, hepatosplenomegaly, blindness, and anemia. (B) Note similar facies and severe strabismus in another child who is blind. (C,D) Marked increased density of all bones. Note fractures of radius and ulna. (E) Section showing striking differences between lighter-staining periosteal bone and darker-staining osteopetrotic bone in endochondral layer of otic capsule. Abnormal bone obliterates area of mastoid antrum. [(A) from RD Thompson et al., *J Oral Surg* 27:63, 1969; (D) from EN Myers and S Stool, *Arch Otolaryngol* 89:460, 1969; (E) courtesy of EN Myers, Pittsburgh, Pennsylvania.]

diometric findings. In about half the cases there is a history of otitis media (62). In the mild recessive form of osteopetrosis, about 40% have significant hearing loss (28).

Ossicular chain involvement was described by Myers and Stool (41) with ring-shaped stapes, but was normal in the case of Suga and Lindsay (55). Bony exostoses were also noted (55).

Temporal bone changes have been described in a child with moderate hearing loss (41). The middle ear cavity was smaller than normal; there was marked hypertrophy of the mucosa and small incomplete fallopian canals. A portion of the facial nerve was herniated into the middle ear. Abnormal otosclerotic bone, evident throughout the temporal bone, covered the periosteal and endosteal layers of the otic capsule. The ossicles, which were composed of otosclerotic bone, lacked medullary cavities. The stapes was thickened, preserving its fetal shape through lack of remodeling. The organ of Corti, vestibular labyrinth, and the spiral ganglion were normal. The round window membrane was markedly thickened. There was no pneumatization of mastoid cells, these areas being filled with chondrocytes and osteoblasts (Fig. 8–5E).

Heredity. Autosomal recessive inheritance with frequent occurrence in sibs and parental consanguinity has been demonstrated by many investigators. One causative gene has been mapped to 11q13 (30) and has been identified as the TCIRG1 osteoblast-specific unit of the vacuolar protein pump (26,33). Mutations in the *CLCN7* gene, which usually causes one form of autosomal dominant osteopetrosis, have also been found in individuals with autosomal recessive osteopetrosis (18,34). In one family, affected individuals were homozygous for *CLCN7* mutations whereas the heterozygous parents were unaffected (18). The authors postulated that dominant-negative mutations caused autosomal dominant osteopetrosis, whereas heterozygosity for loss-of-function mutations was not associated with a clinical phenotype.

Diagnosis. A lethal form of osteopetrosis was reported in two sibs by El Khazen et al. (22). There were in utero fractures, hip dislocation, hydrocephaly, and hypoplasia of the cerebellum. No osteoclasts were found.

Prognosis. Jagadha et al. (31) described neuronal storage disease in infantile osteopetrosis as a recessive disorder. They cited several other cases. These infants exhibited hearing loss. Rees et al. (47) noted the same condition in twins. The recessive form may even be recognized in utero or at birth (43). Severe anemia, jaundice, hepatosplenomegaly, and failure to thrive characterize the neonatal form. There is also reduced host defense (48). The infant may be stillborn or survive only a few months (63). Bone marrow transplantation has been carried out but without great success (27).

Summary. The major characteristics of this condition are (*1*) autosomal recessive inheritance; (*2*) osteosclerosis with involvement of all bones of the skeleton; (*3*) facial palsy and visual loss; and (*4*) mild to moderate mixed hearing loss.

Benign autosomal dominant osteopetrosis

The dominant forms of osteopetrosis are more common than the recessive forms and are not associated with anemia, hepatosplenomegaly, blindness, or mental retardation. At least 40% of patients are asymptomatic, being diagnosed radiologically (32). The rest present because of backache, headache, or, rarely, trigeminal neuralgia (11,60).

The dominant forms usually become manifest somewhat later in life than autosomal recessive types (10,12,13). Type I is rarely associated with fractures following minor trauma (32,35,56), whereas fractures occur in about 60% of those with type II (8). The condition appears silently within the first few years of life, being manifest by increased radiopacity of the skull. It is frequently discovered by routine X-rays of the chest. Density is most marked at the diaphyseal ends of long bones, gradually extending to the epiphyses and to the marrow cavity (32).

Clinical findings. The calvaria is thick and sclerotic in type I, the cranial base in type II (see Table 8–1). Osteomyelitis of the mandible occurs in about 10%–20% of patients, as do cranial nerve palsies of II, III, and VII (17,32,38). In type I, there is more often involvement of cranial nerve V while in type II, cranial nerve VII is more frequently affected. There is no endplate sclerosis of vertebral bodies, and no "bone-within-bone" appearance in the ilia in type I, as there is in type II (10,13,14). There is usually some lack of remodeling, particularly in the femur and tibia in both types. Elevated serum acid phosphatase (32,50) has been noted in type II. Fifth nerve involvement is essentially limited to type I—the seventh nerve far more often in type II.

Auditory system. Most patients with type I and about half of those with type II manifest conductive hearing loss (11,14,32). Narrowing of the internal auditory meatus (11,39) is significantly more severe in type I. Milroy and Michaels (39) described the temporal bone in a type I patient. The ossicles were enlarged with fixation of the stapes. Miyamoto et al. (40) described a five-generation family with osteopetrosis and facial palsy. Hearing was normal in the proband but there was sclerosis of the temporal bones.

Heredity. In one family, linkage with a locus at 1p21, near M-CSF, was found (57). However, Cleiren et al. (18) found mutations in the *CLCN7* gene in this family; since *CLCN7* maps to 16p13.3, linkage to 1p21 was obviously ruled out. Although autosomal dominant osteopetrosis may be heterogeneous on the basis of clinical grounds (3,7,59), no convincing evidence for a gene locus other than *CLCN7* at 16p13.3 has been presented.

Diagnosis. Generalized increase in bone density also accompanies pycnodysostosis and sclerosteosis. Hearing loss in intermediate osteopetrosis is rare (4).

Summary. Characteristics include (*a*) autosomal dominant inheritance; (*b*) increased radiopacity of the entire skeleton; (*c*) basically asymptomatic course; (*d*) rare osteomyelitis; and (*e*) conductive hearing loss in about 20%.

Autosomal recessive osteopetrosis with renal tubular acidosis (carbonic anhydrase II deficiency)

At least 30 patients have been reported with severe osteopetrosis, short stature, mild to severe mental retardation, basal ganglia calcification, visual impairment, mixed renal tubular acidosis, hepatosplenomegaly, extramedullary hemopoiesis, pancytopenia, and sensorineural hearing loss (2,15,46,51,56,61).

Inheritance is autosomal recessive and is more common in Arabs (28). The molecular basis for the defective carbonic anhydrase II has been ascertained (49,51,54,58). The gene has been mapped to 8q22 (42,49,52).

Summary. The syndrome is characterized by (*1*) autosomal recessive inheritance; (*2*) osteopetrosis; (*3*) mental retardation; (*4*) renal tubular acidosis; (*5*) defective carbonic anhydrase II; and (*6*) sensorineural hearing loss.

Table 8–1. Autosomal dominant osteopetrosis

Changes	Type I	Type II
Skull	Thick vault	Dense base
Spine	± Sclerosis	"Sandwich" vertebrae
Pelvis	No subcrestal sclerosis	Subcrestal sclerosis
Serum acid phosphatase	Normal	Elevated
Osteoclasts	Reduced in size and number	Increased in size, number, and number of nuclei
Fractures	Few %	60%

References

1. Ainsworth JR et al: Visual loss in infantile osteopetrosis. *J Pediatr Ophthalmol Strabismus* 30:201–203, 1993.
2. Aramaki S et al: Carbonic anhydrase deficiency in three unrelated Japanese patients. *J Inherit Metab Dis* 16:982–990, 1993.
3. Andersen PE Jr, Bollerslev J: Heterogeneity of autosomal dominant osteopetrosis. *Radiology* 164:223–224, 1987.
4. Beighton P et al: Osteopetrosis in South Africa. *S Afr Med J* 55:659–665, 1979.
5. Bejaoui M et al: La forme recessive de l'osteopetrose. *Arch Fr Pédiatr* 49:629–631, 1992.
6. Benecke JE: Facial nerve dysfunction in osteopetrosis. *Laryngoscope* 103:494–497, 1993.
7. Benichou OD et al: Further evidence for genetic heterogeneity within type II autosomal dominant osteopetrosis. *J Bone Miner Res* 15:1900–1904, 2000.
8. Benichou OD et al: Type II autosomal dominant osteopetrosis (Albers-Schönberg disease): clinical and radiological manifestations in 42 patients. *Bone* 26:87–93, 2000.
9. Bjorvatn K et al: Oral aspects of osteopetrosis. *Scand J Dent Res* 87:245–252, 1979.
10. Bollerslev J: Osteopetrosis. A genetic and epidemiological study. *Clin Genet* 31:86–90, 1987.
11. Bollerslev J: Autosomal dominant osteopetrosis. Bone metabolism and epidemiologic, clinical and hormonal aspects. *Endocrinol Rev* 10:45–67, 1989.
12. Bollerslev J, Mosekilde L: Autosomal dominant osteopetrosis. *Clin Orthop Rel Res* 294: 45–51, 1993.
13. Bollerslev J et al: Autosomal dominant osteopetrosis. *J Laryngol Otol* 101:1088–1091, 1987.
14. Bollerslev J et al: Autosomal dominant osteopetrosis. An otoneurological investigation of the two radiological types. *Laryngoscope* 98:411–413, 1988.
15. Bourke E et al: Renal tubular acidosis and osteopetrosis in sibs. *Nephron* 28:268–272, 1981.
16. Charles JM, Key D: Developmental spectrum of children with congenital osteopetrosis. *J Pediatr* 132:371–374, 1998.
17. Chindia ML et al: Osteopetrosis presenting as paroxysmal trigeminal neuralgia. *Int J Oral Maxillofac Surg* 20:198–200, 1991.
18. Cleiren E et al: Albers-Schonberg disease (autosomal dominant osteopetrosis, type II) results from mutations in the *ClCN7* chloride channel gene. *Hum Mol Genet* 10:2861–2867, 2001.
19. Curé JK et al: Cranial MR imaging of osteopetrosis. *AJNR Am J Neuroradiol* 21:1110–1115, 2000.
20. Droz-Deprez D et al: Infantile osteopetrosis. A case report on dental findings. *J Oral Pathol Med* 21:422–425, 1992.
21. Dyson DP: Osteomyelitis of the jaws in Albers-Schönberg disease. *Br J Oral Surg* 7:178–187, 1970.
22. El Khazen N et al: Lethal osteopetrosis with multiple fractures in utero. *Am J Med Genet* 23:811–819, 1986.
23. Elster AD et al: Cranial imaging in autosomal recessive osteopetrosis. I. Facial bones and calvarium. *Radiology* 183:129–135, 1992.
24. Elster AD et al: Cranial imaging in autosomal recessive osteopetrosis. II. Skull base and brain. *Radiology* 183:137–144, 1992.
25. El Tawil T, Stoker DT: Benign osteopetrosis: a review of 42 cases showing two different patterns. *Skeletal Radiol* 22:587–593, 1993.
26. Frattini A et al: Defects in TCIRG subunit of the vacuolar proton pump are responsible for a subset of human autosomal recessive osteopetrosis. *Nat Genet* 25:343–346, 2000.
27. Gerritsen EJA et al: Autosomal recessive osteopetrosis: variability of findings at diagnosis and during the natural course. *Pediatrics* 93:247–253, 1994.
28. Gorlin RJ et al: *Syndromes of the Head and Neck*, 4th ed. Oxford University Press, New York, 2001.
29. Greenspan A: Sclerosing bone dysplasias in a target-site approach. *Skeletal Radiol* 20:561–583, 1991.
30. Heaney C et al: Human autosomal recessive osteopetrosis maps to 11q13, a position predicted by comparative mapping of the murine osteosclerosis (*os*) mutation. *Hum Mol Genet* 7:1407–1410, 1998.
31. Jagadha V et al: The association of infantile osteopetrosis and neuronal storage disease in two brothers. *Acta Neuropathol* 75:233–240, 1988.
32. Johnston CC et al: Osteopetrosis: a clinical, genetic, metabolic and morphologic study of the dominantly inherited benign form. *Medicine* 47:149–167, 1968.
33. Kornak U et al: Mutations in the α2 subunit of the vacuolar H$^+$-ATPase cause infantile malignant osteopetrosis. *Hum Mol Genet* 9:2059–2063, 2000.
34. Kornak U et al: Loss of the ClC-7 chloride channel leads to osteopetrosis in mice and men. *Cell* 104:205–215, 2001.
35. Kuhlencordt F et al: Die Osteopetrosis Albers-Schönberg. *Ergeb Inn Med Kinderheilk* 39:135–160, 1977.
36. Lajeunesse D et al: Demonstration of an osteoclast defect in two cases of human malignant osteopetrosis. *J Clin Invest* 98:1835–1842, 1996.
37. Lehman RAW et al: Neurological complications of infantile osteopetrosis. *Ann Neurol* 2:378–384, 1977.
38. Milgram JW, Jasty M: Osteopetrosis. A morphological study of twenty-one cases. *J Bone Joint Surg Am* 64:912–929, 1982.
39. Milroy CM, Michaels L: Temporal bone pathology of the adult-type osteopetrosis. *Arch Otolaryngol Head Neck Surg* 116:79–84, 1990.
40. Miyamoto RT et al: Neurotological manifestations of the osteopetroses. *Arch Otolaryngol* 106:210–214, 1980 [case 1 is part of family reported by Welford et al. (35)].
41. Myers EN, Stool S: The temporal bone in osteopetrosis. *Arch Otolaryngol* 89:460–469, 1969.
42. Naikai H et al: The gene for human carbonic anhydrase II (*CA2*) is located at chromosome 8q22. *Cytogenet Cell Genet* 44:234–235, 1987.
43. Oğur G et al: Prenatal diagnosis of autosomal recessive osteopetrosis, infantile type, by X-ray evaluation. *Prenat Diagn* 15:477–481, 1995.
44. Patel PJ et al: Osteopetrosis: brain ultrasound and computed tomography findings. *Eur J Pediatr* 151:827–828, 1992.
45. Paulose KO et al: Osteopetrosis (marble bone disease)—agenesis of paranasal sinuses. *J Laryngol Otol* 102:1047–1051, 1988.
46. Rajeh SA et al: The syndrome of osteopetrosis, renal acidosis and cerebral calcification in two sisters. *Neuropediatrics* 19:162–165, 1988.
47. Rees H et al: The association of neuro-axonal dystrophy and osteopetrosis: a rare autosomal recessive disorder. *Pediatr Neurosurg* 22:321–327, 1995.
48. Reeves J et al: The pathogenesis of infantile malignant osteopetrosis. Bone mineral metabolism and complications in five infants. *Metab Bone Dis Res* 3:135–142, 1981.
49. Roth DE et al: Molecular basis of human carbonic anhydrase II deficiency. *Proc Natl Acad Sci USA* 89:1804–1808, 1992.
50. Shapiro F et al: Human osteopetrosis. A histologic, ultrastructural and biochemical study. *J Bone Joint Surg Am* 62:384–399, 1980.
51. Sly WS et al: Carbonic anhydrase II deficiency in 12 families with the autosomal recessive syndrome of osteopetrosis with renal tubular acidosis and cerebral calcification. *N Engl J Med* 313:139–145, 1985.
52. Soda H et al: A point mutation in exon 3 (his107-tyr) in two unrelated Japanese patients with carbonic anhydrase deficiency with central nervous system involvement. *Hum Genet* 97:435–437, 1996.
53. Steiner M et al: Osteomyelitis of the mandible associated with osteopetrosis. *J Oral Maxillofac Surg* 41:395–405, 1983.
54. Strisgiulio P et al: Variable clinical presentation of carbonic anhydrase deficiency. Evidence for genetic heterogeneity? *Eur J Pediatr* 149:337–340, 1990.
55. Suga F, Lindsay JR: Temporal bone histopathology of osteopetrosis. *Ann Otol Rhinol Laryngol* 85:15–24, 1976.
56. Svoboda PJ et al: Albers-Schönberg disease complicated with periodontal disease. *J Periodontol* 54:592–597, 1983.
57. Van Hul W et al: Localization of a gene for autosomal dominant osteopetrosis (Albers-Schönberg disease) to chromosome 1p21. *Am J Hum Genet* 61:363–370, 1997.
58. Vanta PJ et al: Carbonic anhydrase II deficiency syndrome in a Belgian family is caused by a point mutation at an invariant histidine residue (107 His-Tyr): Complete structure of the normal human *CAII* gene. *Am J Hum Genet* 49:1082–1090, 1991.
59. Walpole IR et al: Autosomal dominant osteopetrosis type II with "malignant" presentation: further support for heterogeneity? *Clin Genet* 38:257–263, 1990.
60. Welford NT: Facial paralysis associated with osteopetrosis (marble bones): report of a case of the syndrome occurring in five generations of the same family. *J Pediatr* 55:67–72, 1959.
61. Whyte MP et al: Osteopetrosis, renal tubular acidosis, and basal ganglia calcification in three sisters. *Am J Med* 69:64–74, 1980.
62. Wilson CJ, Vellodi A: Autosomal recessive osteopetrosis: diagnosis, management, and outcome. *Arch Dis Child* 83:449–452, 2000.
63. Younai F et al: Osteopetrosis: a case report including gross and microscopic findings in the mandible at autopsy. *Oral Surg* 65:214–221, 1988.

Dysosteosclerosis

Dysosteosclerosis is characterized by disproportionately short and bent tubular bones with thickening of the skull (1–20).

Craniofacial findings. The anterior fontanel tends to remain open. There is frontal and biparietal bossing and narrow chin. Oligodontia and poorly calcified teeth with late eruption as well as natal teeth have been described (4,9,11,18). Osteomyelitis of the mandible has been reported (11).

Musculoskeletal system. The patient is short and there is a tendency to bone fractures (8,16,17). The limbs are disproportionately shortened in comparison to the trunk and somewhat bowed. Pectus carinatum has been noted in several patients. Histopathology of the growth plates has been described (7).

Radiographic findings. Radiographically, the calvaria and skull base are thickened. There is sclerosis of the orbital roofs, absent paranasal sinuses, and constriction of the foramina (Fig. 8–6A). The clavicles, scapulae, and ribs are sclerotic and irregular. The vertebral bodies are flattened (platyspondylic) and irregularly dense. Long tubular bones are bent in the region of the shortened, thickened diaphyses. The metaphyses are bottle-shaped. The epiphyses and metaphyses are sclerotic, but the submetaphyseal areas are clear and their trabecular structure is coarse and irregular (Fig. 8–6B). Short tubular bones exhibit similar changes (Fig. 8–6C). Pectus may be seen. Iliac bones are hypoplastic and sclerotic.

Central nervous system. During early childhood, there may be cranial nerve involvement resulting in optic atrophy, abducens palsy, and facial paralysis. Some degree of spasticity and exaggerated reflexes have been evident (2,3,6,8,14). A few patients have manifested progressive mental retardation. Intracerebral calcifications have been reported in one case (1).

Other findings. Macular atrophy of the skin has been found in several patients (2,3,13,14,18). The fingernails are flattened.

Auditory system. Progressive otosclerosis has been a feature in several cases (1,8).

Heredity. Affected sibs (2,3,10,17) and parental consanguinity (2,3,5,14,20) indicate autosomal recessive inheritance. There also appears to be an X-linked recessive form (13).

Summary. Characteristics include (*1*) autosomal recessive inheritance; (*2*) short stature; (*3*) bent tubular bones that are thickened and sclerotic; (*4*) platyspondyly; (*5*) delayed closure of skull foramina; (*6*) macular atrophy of skin; and (*7*) variable progressive otosclerosis.

References

1. Chitayat D et al: Skeletal dysplasia, intracerebral calcifications, optic atrophy, hearing impairment, and mental retardation: nosology of dysosteosclerosis. *Am J Med Genet* 43:517–523, 1992.
2. Ellis RWB: Osteopetrosis. *Proc R Soc Med* 27:1563–1571, 1933–4.
3. Field CE: Albers-Schönberg disease: an atypical case. *Proc R Soc Med* 32:320–324, 1938–9.
4. Fryns JP et al: Dysosteosclerosis in a mentally retarded boy. *Acta Paediatr Belg* 33:53–56, 1980.
5. Houston CS et al: Dysosteosclerosis. *AJR Am J Roentgenol* 130:988–991, 1978.
6. John E et al: Dysosteosclerosis. *Australas Radiol* 40:345–347, 1996.
7. Kaitila I, Rimoin DL: Histologic heterogeneity in the hyperostotic bone dysplasias. *Birth Defects* 12(6):71–79, 1976.
8. Kirkpatrick DB et al: The craniotubular bone modeling disorders: a neurological introduction to rare skeletal dysplasias with cranial nerve compression. *Surg Neurol* 7:221–232, 1977.
9. Leisti J et al: Dysosteosclerosis. *Birth Defects* 11(6):349–351, 1975.
10. Nema HV: Craniometaphyseal dysplasia. *Br J Ophthalmol* 58:107–109, 1974.
11. Packota GV et al: Osteomyelitis of the mandible in a patient with dysosteosclerosis. *Oral Surg Oral Med Oral Pathol Endod* 71:145–147, 1993 [same patient as in (3)].
12. Parascandolo S et al: Su un caso clinico di displasia cranio-metaphisaria. *Min Stomatol* 34:671–675, 1985.
13. Pascual-Castroviejo I et al: X-linked dysosteosclerosis. *Eur J Pediatr* 126:127–138, 1977.
14. Roy C et al: Un nouveau syndrome osseux avec anomalies cutanées et troubles neurologiques. *Arch Fr Pédiatr* 25:893–905, 1968.
15. Sener RN et al: Dysosteosclerosis. Clinicoradiologic findings including brain MRI. *Comput Med Imaging Graph* 21:355–357, 1997.
16. Spranger J et al: Die Dysosteosclerose—eine Sonderform der generalisierten Osteosklerose. *Fortschr Röntgenstr* 109:504–512, 1968.
17. Stehr L: Pathogenese und Klinik der Osteosklerosen. *Arch Orthop Unfall Chir* 41:156–182, 1942.
18. Temtamy SA et al: Metaphyseal dysplasia, anetoderma and optic atrophy: an autosomal recessive syndrome. *Birth Defects* 10(12):61–71, 1974.
19. Utz W: Manifestation der Dysosteosklerose im Kieferbereich. *Dtsch Zahnärztl Z* 25:48–50, 1970.
20. Venturto V et al: A case of autosomal recessive form of cranio-metaphyseal dysplasia with unusual features and with bone fragility. *Australas Radiol* 31:79–81, 1987.

Figure 8–6. *Dysosteosclerosis.* (A) Sclerosis of cranial vault and base of skull with underpneumatization in 10-year-old boy. (B) Sclerosis of diaphyses, epiphyses, and adjacent metaphyseal regions; undermodeling and shortening of femora with wide, radiolucent metaphyseal flare; bowing of femora. (C) Epimetaphyseal sclerosis with submetaphyseal radiolucency of short tubular bones; undermodeling with metaphyseal flare; sclerosis of carpal bones and epimetaphyseal parts of radius and ulna. [From RJ Gorlin et al., *Birth Defects* 5(4):79, 1969.]

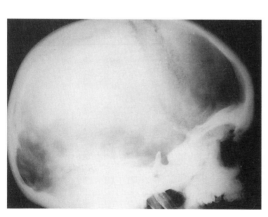

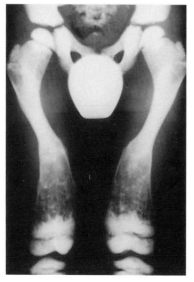

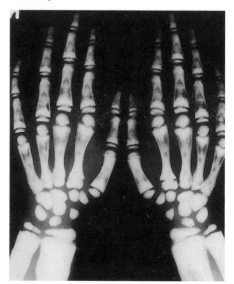

A   B   C

Sclerosteosis

Sclerosteosis was described as early as 1929 by Hirsch (16). Several other reports of the disorder (13) antedate Hansen's (15) definition of sclerosteosis. The disorder is characterized by generalized osteosclerosis with hyperostosis of the calvaria, mandible, clavicles, and pelvis, rather different from that observed in van Buchem disease. In sclerosteosis, usually there are syndactyly and other abnormalities of the digits. The disorder appears to be one of osteoblast hyperactivity (18). About 90 cases have been described. Hamersma et al. (14) provide a good review of the natural history of this disorder.

Craniofacial findings. The typical face, evident by the age of 5 years, is characterized by frontal prominence, hypertelorism, and broad flat nasal root (Fig. 8–7A–C). The mandible is prognathic, broadened, and squared, and dental malocclusion is frequent. The face may be distorted with relative midfacial hypoplasia. Head circumference is enlarged. Facial nerve paralysis, transient in infancy, is common in adulthood. Characteristically, it is unilateral for many years. There is increased intracranial pressure in 80% (4,7,18). Ataxia has been reported (18). Exophthalmos, optic atrophy, reduced visual fields, convergent strabismus, nystagmus, chronic headache, and decreased sensory function of the trigeminal nerve have been described in adults (10,11). Visual loss occurs in 30%. Only rarely, however, is there total blindness. Several patients have died suddenly from impaction of the medulla in the foramen magnum (4,12).

Musculoskeletal system. Final height attainment is over 180 cm in 70% of patients. In about 80%, there is asymmetric partial or complete cutaneous syndactyly of the index and middle fingers. There may be radial deviation of the distal phalanx of the index fingers (Fig. 8–7D). The nails on the involved digits are hypoplastic in 80%. Height may be correlated with syndactyly.

Radiographic findings. Radiographically, the calvaria becomes thickened and sclerotic in infancy, gradually increasing until about age 30. The base is dense and the foramina obliterated. The mandible is massive, prognathic, often asymmetric, and with an obtuse angle. The clavicles and ribs are broadened and dense because of cortical thickening. The scapulae, pelvis, and vertebral endplates and pedicles are uniformly sclerotic. The tubular bones, in addition to increased density, exhibit a lack of diaphyseal modeling. The index finger may have no middle phalanx or only a small triangular bone (delta phalanx) producing radial deviation (Fig. 8–7E). Bony syndactyly may involve the second and third fingers (5).

Auditory system. Bilateral sensorineural, mixed, or conductive hearing loss—a constant feature of the disorder—may appear early in infancy, during childhood, or late in adolescence (10,11). Nager and Hamersma (17) found that mixed hearing loss appears in childhood in most cases. Beighton and Hamersma (3) described fixed ossicles.

Heredity. Inheritance is autosomal recessive. Most patients have been South African of Dutch ancestry (3,6,7,13). Prevalence has been estimated to be about 1/60,000 in Afrikaners (2). Sclerosteosis has also been seen in many other parts of the world (9,13,19,20). The gene maps to 17q12–q21, the same region as that for van Buchem disease (1). However, they are not allelic (8). Sclerosteosis is due to loss of *SOST*

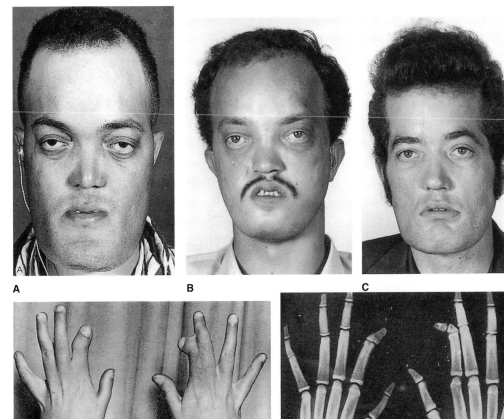

Figure 8–7. *Sclerosteosis.* (A) There is marked mandibular growth following puberty; mandible assumes square form. Mixed hearing loss, facial palsy, headache, exophthalmos, and blindness are common complications. (B) Exophthalmos and facial palsy. Lips cannot close over teeth. (C) Grossly enlarged cranial vault and mandible. Expressionless facies is due to seventh nerve involvement. (D) Soft tissue syndactyly of second and third fingers was present bilaterally. Third and fourth fingers were partly fused unilaterally. (E) Radiograph shows hypoplasia or absence of middle phalanx of second digit together with radial deviation of terminal phalanx. [(A) courtesy of CJ Witkop Jr, Minneapolis, Minnesota; (B,C) from H Hamersma, *Laryngoscope* 80:1518, 1970; (D,E) courtesy of AS Truswell, *J Bone Joint Surg* 40B:208, 1958.]

product, but van Buchem disease is not (8). Heterozygotes exhibit increased calvarial width and density (1; P Beighton, personal communication, 1989).

Diagnosis. Patients with van Buchem disease tend to be of normal height and never have involvement of digits. As noted above, most are of Dutch ancestry. Sclerosteosis tends to be more severe in its manifestations. Hearing loss (90%) and raised intracranial pressure (80%) are more common than in those with van Buchem disease. Beighton et al. (7), having examined 80 Afrikaners with sclerosteosis in South Africa and 15 patients with van Buchem, have extensively discussed similarities and differences.

Summary. Characteristics include (1) autosomal recessive inheritance; (2) generalized osteosclerosis with hyperostosis of calvaria, mandible, clavicles, and pelvis; (3) syndactyly of the second and third fingers; (4) increased height; (5) increased intracranial pressure; (6) cranial nerve dysfunction; and (7) mixed hearing loss.

References

1. Balemans W et al: Localization of the gene for sclerosteosis to the van Buchem disease-gene region on chromosome 17q12–q21. *Am J Hum Genet* 64:1661–1669, 1999.
2. Beighton P: Sclerosteosis. *J Med Genet* 25:200–203,1988.
3. Beighton P, Hamersma H: Sclerosteosis in South Africa. *S Afr Med J* 55:783–788, 1979.
4. Beighton P et al: The clinical features of sclerosteosis: a review of the manifestations in twenty-five affected individuals. *Ann Intern Med* 84:393–397, 1976.
5. Beighton P et al: The radiology of sclerosteosis. *Br J Radiol* 49:934–939, 1976.
6. Beighton P et al: Sclerosteosis—an autosomal recessive disorder. *Clin Genet* 11:1–7, 1977.
7. Beighton P et al: The syndromic status of sclerosteosis and van Buchem disease. *Clin Genet* 25:175–181, 1984.
8. Brunkow ME et al: Bone dysplasia sclerosteosis results from loss of SOST gene product, a novel cystine knot-containing protein. *Am J Hum Genet* 68:577–589, 2001.
9. Bueno M et al: Sclerosteosis in a Spanish male: first report in a person of Mediterranean origin. *J Med Genet* 31:976–977, 1994.
10. Dort JC et al: The fallopian canal and facial nerve in sclerosteosis of the temporal bone. *Am J Otol* 11:320–325, 1990.
11. Duplessis JJ: Sclerosteosis: neurosurgical experience with 14 cases. *J Neurosurg* 78:388–392, 1993.
12. Epstein S et al: Endocrine function in sclerosteosis. *S Afr Med J* 55:1105–1110, 1979.
13. Gorlin RJ et al: *Syndromes of the Head and Neck*, 4th ed. Oxford University Press, New York, 2001.
14. Hamersma H et al: The natural history of sclerosteosis. *Clin Genet* 63:192–197, 2003.
15. Hansen HG: Sklerosteose. In: *Handbuch der Kinderheilkunde*, Vol 6, Opitz H, Schmid F (eds), Springer-Verlag, Berlin, 1967, pp 351–355.
16. Hirsch IS: Generalized osteitis fibrosa. *Radiology* 13:44–84, 1929.
17. Nager GT, Hamersma H: Sclerosteosis involving the temporal bone: clinical and radiologic aspects. *Am J Otolaryngol* 4:1–17, 1983 and 7:1–16, 1986.
18. Stein SA et al: Sclerosteosis: neurogenic and pathophysiologic analysis of an American kinship. *Neurology* 33:267–277, 1983.
19. Sugiura Y, Yasuhara T: Sclerosteosis. *J Bone Joint Surg Am* 57:273–276, 1975.
20. Tacconi P et al: Sclerosteosis: report in a black African man. *Clin Genet* 53:497–501, 1998.

van Buchem disease

van Buchem disease (generalized cortical hyperostosis) is characterized by osteosclerosis of skull, mandible, clavicles, and ribs and by hyperplasia of diaphyseal cortex of long and short bones. The most extensive monograph is that of van Buchem in 1976 (15). About 25 patients have been documented.

Craniofacial findings. Facial changes develop slowly but usually become apparent before the second decade. A most striking finding is a wide and thickened mandible, suggesting acromegaly (Fig. 8–8A). Rarely, skull circumference is enlarged. Occasionally, there is mild exophthalmos. Patients experience headache, unilateral or rarely bilateral facial paralysis, and optic atrophy. Facial palsy may be the initial finding (6).

Musculoskeletal system. Radiographic changes include thickening of the calvaria and increased density of the skull base (Fig. 8–8B,C). The body of the mandible is greatly enlarged in all measurements; the angle is obtuse. The long tubular bones exhibit diaphyseal thickening and are roughly textured (Fig. 8–8D). The cortical hyperostosis is predominantly endosteal in character. In severe cases, the medullary cavity is occluded. The transverse diameter of the diaphysis is normal or increased. Elevated serum alkaline phosphatase has been noted in most cases.

Auditory system. Among 15 patients described by van Buchem (15), 13 had hearing loss. Gradual impairment of hearing began at about 15 years of age. One patient had severe hearing loss by age 38 years. Of seven patients described by Van der Wouden (16), all had bilateral symmetric hearing loss. Some cases showed sensorineural hearing loss, whereas others manifested mixed hearing loss. Speech audiometry often demonstrated loss of discrimination. Tone-decay and SISI tests were positive in some cases.

Heredity. The disorder has autosomal recessive inheritance (1–4,6,8,12–18). Most examples have been in South Africans of Dutch ancestry. The disorder maps to 17q12–q21 (17), the same region as sclerosteosis, but they are not allelic. Recently Staehling-Hampton et al. (11) found a 52 kb deletion in patients with van Buchem disease; although this region corresponds to no known gene, because of this region's position between the *SOST* and *MEOX1* (a gene which is involved in the development of the axial skeleton), a possible dysregulatory effect of this deletion was postulated.

Diagnosis. The patient described by Dixon et al. (5) has a separate disorder. We have observed the same condition in sibs and coined the term *pseudo–van Buchem disease* (Fig. 8–8E,F). Autosomal dominant osteosclerosis (7) is clearly separated from van Buchem disease, with which it is sometimes erroneously confused in the literature. In this condition, there are no neurological complications (such as hearing loss), and no exophthalmos, hypertelorism, or elevated alkaline phosphatase. Sclerosteosis, earlier thought to be allelic to van Buchem disease, has been demonstrated not to be, although it maps to the same area of chromosome 17q (3). Endosteal hyperostosis, Worth type, has been mistaken for van Buchem disease (10).

Summary. Characteristics include (1) autosomal recessive inheritance; (2) hyperostosis and osteosclerosis of the skeleton; and (3) mixed hearing loss.

References

1. Beighton P et al: The syndromic status of sclerosteosis and van Buchem disease. *Clin Genet* 25:175–181, 1984.
2. Bettini R et al: Endosteal hyperostosis with recessive transmission (van Buchem disease). A case report. *Recenti Prog Med* 82:24–28, 1991.
3. Brunkow ME et al: Bone dysplasia sclerosteosis results from loss of the SOST gene product, a novel cystine knot-containing protein. *Am J Hum Genet* 68:577–589, 2001.
4. Cook JV et al: Van Buchem disease with classical radiological features and appearances on cranial computed tomography. *Br J Radiol* 62:74–77, 1989.
5. Dixon JM et al: Two cases of van Buchem's disease. *J Neurol Neurosurg Psychiatry* 45:913–918, 1982.
6. Fryns JP, van den Berghe H: Facial paralysis at the age of 2 months as a first clinical sign of van Buchem disease (endosteal hyperostosis). *Eur J Pediatr* 147:99–100, 1988.
7. Gorlin RJ, Glass L: Autosomal dominant osteosclerosis. *Radiology* 125:547–548, 1977.
8. Jacobs P: van Buchem disease. *Postgrad Med J* 53:497–505, 1977.
9. Sala O: ORL importance of some aspects of osteopetrosis. *Boll Mal Orecch* 71:577–592, 1953.

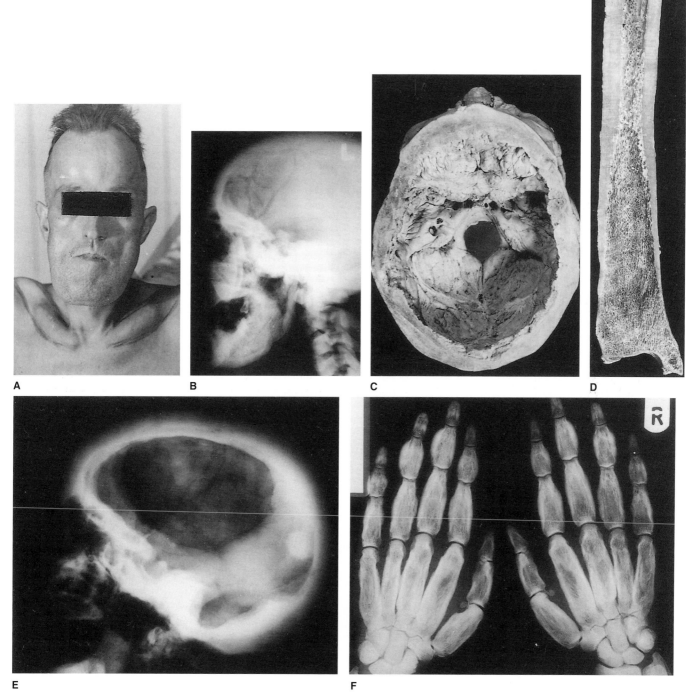

Figure 8–8. *van Buchem disease.* (A) Broad chin, thick clavicles. (B) Thickening of skull and mandible. (C) Base of skull formed of thickened sclerotic bone without diploë. Note multiple excrescences. (D) Thickening of diaphysis of tibia. *Pseudo–von Buchem disease.* (E) Marked thickening of calvaria and skull base. (F) Note marked predominantly diaphyseal, cortical thickening of metacarpals and phalanges to a far greater degree than in classic van Buchem patients. [(A–D) from FS van Buchem et al., *Am J Med* 33:387, 1962; (E,F) from JM Dixon et al., *J Neurol Neurosurg Psychiatry* 45:913, 1982.]

10. Schendel SA: Van Buchem disease: surgical treatment of the mandible. *Ann Plast Surg* 20:462–467, 1988.

11. Staehling-Hampton K et al: A 52-kb deletion in the *SOST–MEOX1* intergenic region on 17q12–q22 is associated with van Buchem disease in the Dutch population. *Am J Med Genet* 110:144–152, 2002.

12. Toledo F et al: Hiperostosis endosteal (enfermedad de Van Buchem). *Radiologia* 24:49–52, 1982.

13. van Buchem FSP et al: Hyperostosis corticalis generalisata familiaris. *Acta Radiol* 44:109–114, 1955.

14. van Buchem FSP et al: Hyperostosis corticalis generalisata: report of seven cases. *Am J Med* 33:387–397, 1962.

15. van Buchem FSP et al: *Hyperostosis Corticalis Generalisata Familiaris (van Buchem's Disease).* American Elsevier, New York, 1976.

16. Van der Wouden A: Deafness caused by hyperostosis corticalis generalisata. *Pract Otorhinolaryngol* 30:91–92, 1968.

17. Van Hul W et al: Van Buchem disease (hyperostosis corticalis generalisata) maps to chromosome 17q12–q21. *Am J Hum Genet* 62:391–393, 1998.

18. Veth RPH et al: Van Buchem disease and aneurysmal bone cyst. *Arch Orthop Trauma Surg* 104:65–68, 1985.

Hyperphosphatasemia

Hyperphosphatasemia (juvenile Paget disease) is characterized by swelling of the limbs during early infancy, followed by fracture and bending with enlargement of the calvaria (13). A good review is that of Spindler et al. (22).

Clinical findings. Hyperphosphatasemia is characterized by fever, bone pain, and swelling of extremities during the first year of life (8). Later, enlargement of the calvaria and often numerous fractures and bending of the bones of the extremities occur, particularly anterior bowing of legs and general broadening of diaphyseal areas of tubular bones (28) (Fig. 8–9A,B). However, healing is normal. Headache and hypertension are frequent (16,17). Cardiomegaly has been described (15). The sclerae may be blue (12). Intelligence is normal. Hearing is commonly diminished and angioid streaking of the retina has been reported (12,17,25). The skin exhibits pseudoxanthoma elasticum (7,10,14,17,20).

Musculoskeletal system. Histologically, there is intensive metaplastic fibrous bone formation as well as increased osteoblastic and osteoclastic activity, very similar to that seen in Paget disease but without typical mosaic or regression lines (26). Since chondral ossification is not markedly disturbed (epiphyses are normally formed and the joints are not involved), growth is not seriously diminished. Muscle weakness, which retards walking, running, and jumping, is frequent. Multiple osteogenic sarcoma of the skull has been reported in one case (18).

Radiographic findings. Examination of the skull reveals changes ("cotton ball patches") remarkably like those seen in Paget disease (Fig. 8–9C). There is flattening of vertebral bodies. Long bones exhibit bending, overcylinderization, and generalized cortical widening. Bone trabeculation is coarse and bone density diminished (Fig. 8–9D,E). Short bones are involved to a lesser degree, mostly on the endosteal side (4,19). The facial bones, except in the patient reported by Marshall (16), have not been involved. Scintigraphic changes are striking (15). Teeth are shed early due to root resorption (12).

Auditory system. Progressive mixed 60–80 dB hearing loss has been evident from the fourth to the 14th year of life (25). The ear canals are narrowed. Eyring and Eisenberg (12) described high-frequency sensorineural hearing loss. Mitsudo (17) noted diminished hearing bilaterally.

Laboratory findings. The blood picture is generally normal, although anemia was described in Swoboda's patients (24). Serum alkaline phosphatase (normal ≤25) may exceed 500 King-Armstrong units (KAU) (17). Serum acid phosphatase (normal 1.5–3.5 KAU) as well as urinary hydroxyproline and leucine aminopeptidase (6) are elevated.

Heredity. The condition has autosomal recessive inheritance (3,11,12,15,21,22,24,25). In two unrelated Navajo patients, Whyte et al. (27) and Cundy et al. (5) found mutations in *TNFRSF11B*. About half of the patients have been of Puerto Rican origin (1,2,9,12,24,26).

Diagnosis. Dominant benign hyperphosphatasemia must be excluded.

Summary. Characteristics include (*1*) autosomal recessive inheritance; (*2*) fever, bone pain, and swelling during early years; (*3*) enlarge-

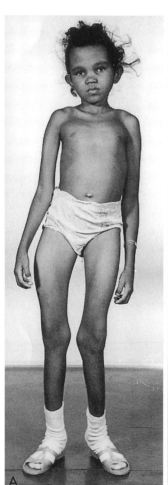
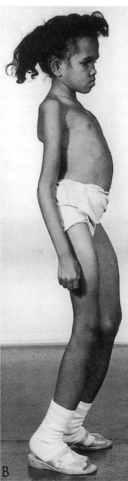
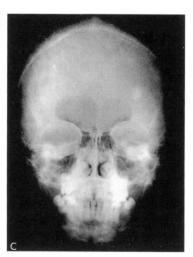
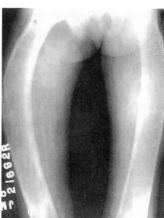
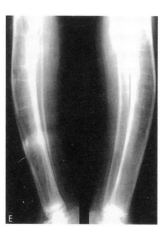

Figure 8–9. *Hyperphosphatasemia.* (A,B) An 11-year-old child with enlargement of skull, high forehead, wide face, and bowing of lower extremities. (C–E) Calvaria greatly thickened and exhibiting patches of increased density. Long bones of lower extremities are expanded and bowed. [From H Bakwin et al., *AJR Am J Roentgenol* 91:609, 1964.]

ment of the calvaria; (4) frequent pseudoxanthoma elasticum; (5) radiographic changes similar to those of Paget disease; (6) elevated serum alkaline and acid phosphatase; and (7) progressive mixed hearing loss.

References

1. Bakwin H, Eiger MS: Fragile bones and macrocranium. *J Pediatr* 49:558–564, 1956.
2. Bakwin H et al: Familial osteoectasia with macrocranium. *AJR Am J Roentgenol* 91:609–617, 1964.
3. Blanco O et al: Familial idiopathic hyperphosphatasia. *J Bone Joint Surg Br* 59:421–427, 1977.
4. Caffey J: *Caffey's Pediatric X-ray Diagnosis*, 8th ed. Year Book Medical Publishers, Chicago, 1985, p 651.
5. Cundy T et al: A mutation in the gene TNFRSF11B encoding osteoprostegerin causes an indiopathic hyperphosphatasia phenotype. *Hum Mol Genet* 11:2119-2127, 2002.
6. Desai MP et al: Chronic idiopathic hyperphosphatasia in an Indian child. *Am J Dis Child* 126:626–628, 1973.
7. Döhler JR et al: Idiopathic hyperphosphatasia with dermal pigmentation—a 20 year follow-up. *J Bone Joint Surg Br* 68:305–310, 1986.
8. Dunn V et al: Familial hyperphosphatasemia: diagnosis in early infancy and response to human thyrocalcitonin therapy. *AJR Am J Roentgenol* 132:541–545, 1979.
9. Einhorn TA et al: Hyperphosphatasemia in an adult. Clinical, roentgenographic, and histomorphometric findings and comparison to classical Paget's disease. *Clin Orthop* 204:253–260, 1986.
10. Eng AM, Bryant J: Clinical pathologic observations in pseudoxanthoma elasticum. *Int J Dermatol* 14:585–605, 1975.
11. Eroglu M, Taneli NN: Congenital hyperphosphatasia (juvenile Paget's disease)—eleven years follow-up of three sisters. *Ann Radiol (Paris)* 20:145–150, 1977.
12. Eyring EJ, Eisenberg E: Congenital hyperphosphatasia. *J Bone Joint Surg Am* 50:1099–1117, 1968.
13. Fanconi G et al: Osteochalasia desmalis familiaris. *Helv Paediatr Acta* 19:279–295, 1964.
14. Fretzin DF: Pseudoxanthoma elasticum in hyperphosphatasia. *Arch Dermatol* 111:271–272, 1975.
15. Iancu TC et al: Chronic familial hyperphosphatasemia. *Radiology* 129:669–676, 1978.
16. Marshall WC: A case of progressive osteopathy with hyperphosphatasia. *Proc R Soc Med* 55:238–239, 1962.
17. Mitsudo SM: Chronic idiopathic hyperphosphatasia associated with pseudoxanthoma elasticum. *J Bone Joint Surg Am* 53:303–314, 1971.
18. Nehrlich AG et al: Multifocal osteogenic sarcoma of the skull in a patient who had congenital hyperphosphatasemic skeletal dysplasia. *J Bone Joint Surg Am* 74:1090–1095, 1992.
19. Saraf SK, Gupta SK: Juvenile Paget's disease. *Australas Radiol* 33:189–191, 1989.
20. Saxe N, Beighton P: Cutaneous manifestations of osteoectasia. *Clin Exp Dermatol* 7:605–609, 1982.
21. Singer F et al: Hereditary hyperphosphatasia: 20-year follow-up and response to disodium editronate. *J Bone Mineral Res* 9:733–738, 1994 [follow-up cases reported by Thompson et al. (26)].
22. Spindler A et al: Chronic idiopathic hyperphosphatasemia: report of a case treated with pamidronate and a review of the literature. *J Rheum* 19:642–645, 1992.
23. Stemmermann GN: A histologic and histochemical study of familialosteoectasia. *Am J Pathol* 48:641–651, 1966.
24. Swoboda W: Hyperostosis corticalis deformans juvenilis: ungewöhnliche generalistierte Osteopathie bei zwei Geschwistern. *Helv Paediatr Acta* 13:292–312, 1958.
25. Thompson RC et al: Hereditary hyperphosphatasia: studies in three siblings. *Am J Med* 47:209–219, 1969.
26. Whalen JP et al: Calcitonin treatment in hereditary bone dysplasia with hyperphosphatasemia: a radiographic and histologic study of the bone. *AJR Am J Roentgenol* 129:29–35, 1977.
27. Whyte MP et al: Osteoprotegerin deficiency and juvenile Paget's disease. *N Engl J Med* 347:175–184, 2002.
28. Woodhouse N et al: Paget's disease in a 5-year-old: acute response to human calcitonin. *BMJ* 4:267–268, 1972.

Oculodentoosseous dysplasia (oculodentodigital syndrome)

Oculodentoosseous dysplasia was described in part as early as 1920 by Lohmann (28), and later by others (3,30,37). The syndrome characterized by narrow nose with hypoplastic alae and thin nostrils, microcornea with iris anomalies, syndactyly and/or camptodactyly of postaxial fingers, hypoplasia or aplasia of middle phalanx of fifth fingers and toes, and enamel hypoplasia was first fully described by Meyer-Schwickerath et al. (29) in 1957. About 150 cases have been reported to date.

Craniofacial findings. Short narrow palpebral fissures, epicanthal folds, and long thin nose with prominent nasal bridge and hypoplastic alae nasi produce a characteristic physiognomy (Fig. 8–10A). Head circumference may be somewhat reduced (27,39,46), and hyperostosis of the skull has been reported (9,36,39). The pinnae may be abnormally modeled and/or outstanding. Dry, lusterless hair that fails to grow to normal length has been noted in 30% of patients (18,27,29,36,46,47).

Nervous system. Spastic paraplegia, sometimes progressive (2,4,5,8,16,19,21,31–33,42,44), cerebral white matter anomalies (16,19,21,22,43), basal ganglia calcification (1,4), ataxia (39), neurogenic bladder disturbances (32,33,43), and learning disabilities (25,32,33) have been noted.

Ocular system. Striking eye changes consist of short narrow palpebral apertures, microcornea (6–9 mm in diameter), and epicanthal folds in childhood (10,12,14,26) (Fig. 8–10A). The oft-quoted findings of hypertelorism and microphthalmia are spurious (12,14), except in a possible recessive form (see Diagnosis). The pupil may be eccentric. The iris may consist of fine porous spongy tissue. Between the frill and the pupillary rim are crypts and lacunae, and the iris frill may overlie the pupillary rim. Remnants of the pupillary membrane may be present along the iris margin rather than across the pupil (9,11,18,29). A number of patients have exhibited strabismus or secondary glaucoma (12,25,37,45,49). There may be an increase in the number of disc vessels (25). Persistent hyperplastic primary vitreous has been noted occasionally (20,48). It has been suggested that this is characteristic of the "recessive" form of the disorder (48) (vide infra). Radiographically, orbital hypotelorism has been demonstrated in 40% (14).

Oral findings. Generalized enamel hypoplasia has been noted by a number of investigators (11,13,39,40,46) (Fig. 8–10B). The alveolar ridge of the mandible may be wider than normal (7,18,25,38,50). Cleft lip–palate (13,15,31,32,50) and microdontia (13,22,50) have been observed by several authors (13,15,31,50).

Musculoskeletal system. Most patients have a gracile build. Camptodactyly of the fifth or, less often, of the fourth fingers is a common finding. Clinically, the fifth finger appears to be shortened. Bilateral syndactyly of the fourth and fifth fingers (rarely the third) with ulnar clinodactyly and syndactyly of the third and fourth toes are often present (37,39) (Fig. 8–10C).

Radiographically, the middle phalanx of the fifth finger is cuboid or deltoid or occasionally absent (47) (Fig. 8–10D). The feet, clinically normal, exhibit aplasia or hypoplasia of the middle phalanx of one or more toes (Fig. 8–10E). In at least one case there was postaxial hexadactyly of toes (26). Lack of modeling of the metaphyseal area of the long bones is relatively common (9,10,13,18,27,38).

Auditory system. Conductive hearing loss has been described in a number of patients (13,15,24,39,47), in part because of recurrent otitis media.

Heredity. The syndrome has autosomal dominant inheritance (10,30,34,36,39). New mutations represent approximately 50% of cases (39). Jones et al. (24) found advanced age in fathers of isolated patients with the disorder. Although affected sibs with normal parents have been described (11,15), these cases can be attributed to the variable expressivity of the disorder (31,33,39,43). Anticipation has been suggested (10,25,31,43). The gene has been mapped to 6q22–q23 (5,17), and has been identified as the connexin-43 (*GJA1*) gene (35). Perhaps the gene for type III syndactyly maps to the same area (35,41). There may, however, be genetic heterogeneity (see Diagnosis) (48).

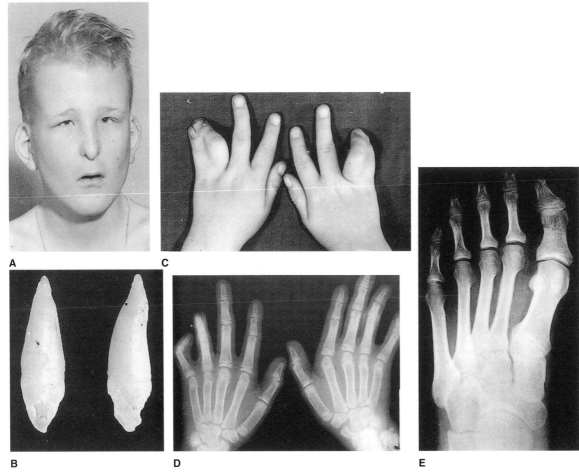

Figure 8–10. *Oculodentoosseous dyplasia (oculodentodigital syndrome).*
(A) Characteristic facies showing microcornea and lack of nasal alar flare.
(B) Note marked hypoplasia of enamel. (C) Soft tissue syndactyly and ulnar deviation of the fourth and fifth digits. (D) Note poor modeling of metacarpals, abbreviated middle phalanx of fifth finger, and camptodactyly of left fifth finger. There is a mild cone-shaped epiphysis of distal thumb phalanx. (E) Note missing middle phalanges of toes. [(A) from RJ Gorlin et al., *J Pediatr* 63:69, 1963; (C) from SH Reisner et al., *Am J Dis Child* 118:600, 1969.]

Diagnosis. A child with many similar stigmata, but with rudimentary dry and brittle nails, was described by Whitwell (51). Two related males reported by Beighton et al. (4) exhibited marked cranial hyperostosis, massive mandibular overgrowth, gross clavicular widening, blindness, microphthalmia, calcification of basal ganglia, cataracts, cleft lip–palate, and spastic quadriplegia. Perhaps this represents an autosomal recessive form. Brueton et al. (6) raised the question of heterogeneity regarding the finding of type III syndactyly.

Although the eye anomalies appear to be similar to those observed in Rieger syndrome, there is neither microcornea nor enamel hypoplasia in the latter, although tooth formation is suppressed. Microcornea in combination with glaucoma, epicanthal folds, absent frontal sinuses, and hyperkeratosis of the palms may exhibit autosomal dominant inheritance (23).

Summary. The syndrome is characterized by (*1*) autosomal dominant inheritance; (*2*) typical face showing thin nose with hypoplastic alae; (*3*) microcornea; (*4*) enamel hypoplasia; (*5*) bilateral camptodactyly and often syndactyly of the fourth and fifth fingers; (*6*) poor modeling of metaphyseal areas of long bones; and (*7*) conductive hearing loss.

References

1. Barnard A et al: Intracranial calcification in oculodento-osseous dysplasia. *S Afr Med J* 59:758–762, 1981.
2. Battisti C et al: Oculo-dento-digital syndrome (Gorlin syndrome): clinical and genetic report of a new family. *Acta Neurol (Napoli)* 14:103–110, 1992.
3. Bauer KH: Homoitransplantation von Epidermis bei eineiigenen Zwillingen. *Bruns Beitr Klin Chir* 141:442–447, 1927.
4. Beighton P et al: Oculo-dento-osseous dysplasia: heterogeneity or variable expression? *Clin Genet* 16:169–177, 1979.
5. Boyadjiev SA et al: Linkage analysis narrows the critical region for oculodentodigital dysplasia on chromosome 6q22–q23. *Genomics* 58:34–40, 1999.
6. Brueton LA et al: Oculodentodigital dysplasia and type III syndactyly: separate genetic entities or disease spectrum? *J Med Genet* 27:169–175, 1990.
7. Cowan A: Leontiasis ossea. *Oral Surg* 12:983–989, 1959.
8. Cox DR et al: Neurological abnormalities in oculodentodigital dysplasia: a new clinical finding. *Clin Res* 26:193, 1978.
9. David JEA, Palmer PES: Familial metaphyseal dysplasia. *J Bone Joint Surg Br* 40:87–93, 1958.
10. Dudgeon J, Chisolm JA: Oculo-dento-digital dysplasia. *Trans Ophthalmol Soc UK* 94:203–210, 1974.
11. Eidelman E et al: Orodigitofacial dysostosis and oculodentodigital dysplasia. *Oral Surg* 21:311–319, 1967.
12. Fára M, Gorlin RJ: The question of hypertelorism in oculodentoosseous dysplasia. *Am J Med Genet* 10:101–102, 1981.
13. Fára M et al: Oculodentodigital dysplasia. *Acta Chir Plast* 19:110–122, 1977.
14. Farman AG et al: Oculodentodigital dysplasia. *Br Dent J* 142:405–408, 1977.
15. Gillespie FD: Hereditary dysplasia oculodentodigitalis. *Arch Ophthalmol* 71:187–192, 1964.
16. Ginsberg LE et al: Oculodental digital dysplasia: neuroimaging in a kindred. *Neuroradiology* 38:84–86, 1996.
17. Gladwin A et al: Localization of a gene for oculodentodigital syndrome to human chromosome 6q22–q24. *Hum Mol Genet* 6:123–127, 1997.
18. Gorlin RJ et al: Oculodentodigital dysplasia. *J Pediatr* 63:69–75, 1963.

19. Grubbs RE et al: Central nervous system abnormalities in oculodentodigital dysplasia syndrome. *Am J Med Genet* 55:A82, 1994.
20. Gutierrez Diaz A et al: Oculodentodigital dysplasia. *Ophthalmol Paediatr Genet* 1:227–232, 1982.
21. Gutmann DH et al: Oculodentodigital dysplasia syndrome associated with abnormal cerebral white matter. *Am J Med Genet* 41:18–20, 1991.
22. Haines JO, Rogers SC: Oculodento-digital dysplasia: a rare syndrome. *Br J Radiol* 48:932–936, 1975.
23. Holmes LB, Walton DS: Hereditary microcornea, glaucoma and absent frontal sinuses. *J Pediatr* 74:968–972, 1969.
24. Jones KL et al: Older paternal age and fresh gene mutation: Data on additional disorders. *J Pediatr* 86:84–88, 1975.
25. Judisch GF et al: Oculodentodigital dysplasia. *Arch Ophthalmol* 97:878–884, 1979.
26. Kadrnka-Lovrencic M et al: Die oculo-dento-digitale Dysplasie (das Meyer-Schwickerath-Syndrom). *Monatsschr Kinderheilkd* 121:595–599, 1973.
27. Kurlander GJ et al: Roentgen differentiation of the oculodentodigital syndrome and the Hallermann-Streiff syndrome of infancy. *Radiology* 86:77–85, 1966.
28. Lohmann W: Beitrag zur Kenntnis des reinen Mikrophthalmus. *Arch Augenheilkd* 86:136–141, 1920.
29. Meyer-Schwickerath G et al: Mikrophthalmussyndrom. *Klin Monatsbl Augenheilkd* 131:18–30, 1957.
30. Mohr OL: Dominant acrocephalosyndactyly. *Hereditas* 25:193–203, 1939.
31. Nivelon-Chevallier A et al: Dysplasia oculo-dento-digitale. *J Génét Hum* 29:171–179, 1981.
32. Norton KK et al: Oculodentodigital dysplasia with cerebral white matter abnormalities in a two-generation family. *Am J Med Genet* 57:458–461, 1995.
33. Opjordsmoen S, Nyberg-Hansen R: Hereditary spastic paraplegia with neurogenic bladder disturbances and syndactylia. *Acta Neurol Scand* 61:35–41, 1980.
34. Patton MA: Oculodentoosseous syndrome. *J Med Genet* 22:386–389, 1985.
35. Paznekas WA et al: Connexin 43 (GJA1) mutation cause the pleiotropic phenotype of oculodentodigital dysplasia. *Am J Hum Genet* 72:408–418, 2003.
36. Pfeiffer RA et al: Oculo-dento-digitale Dysplasie. *Klin Monatsbl Augenheilkd* 152:247–262, 1968.
37. Pitter J, Svejda J: Über den Einfluss der Röntgenstrahlen auf die Entstehung von Missbildungen der menschlichen Frucht. *Ophthalmologia* 123:386–393, 1952.
38. Rajic DS, de Veber LL: Hereditary oculodentoosseous dysplasia. *Ann Radiol* 9:224–231, 1966.
39. Reisner SH et al: Oculodentodigital dysplasia syndrome. *Am J Dis Child* 118:600–607, 1969.
40. Scheutzel P: Oculodentodigital syndrome: report of a case. *Dentomaxillofac Radiol* 20:175–178, 1991.
41. Schrander-Stumpel CTRM et al: Type III syndactyly and oculodentodigital dysplasia: a clinical spectrum. *Genet Couns* 4:271–276, 1993.
42. Schrander-Stumpel CTRM et al: Central nervous system abnormalities in oculodentodigital dysplasia. *Genet Couns* 7:233–235, 1996.
43. Shapiro RE et al: Evidence for genetic anticipation in the oculodentodigital syndrome. *Am J Med Genet* 71:36–41, 1997.
44. Stanislaw CL et al: Oculodentodigital dysplasia with cerebral white matter abnormalities. *Proc Greenwood Genet Ctr* 17:20–24, 1998.
45. Sugar HS: Oculodentodigital dysplasia syndrome with angle-closure glaucoma. *Am J Ophthalmol* 86:36–38, 1978.
46. Sugar HS et al: The oculo-dento-digital dysplasia syndrome. *Am J Ophthalmol* 61:1448–1451, 1966.
47. Thodén CJ et al: Oculodentodigital dysplasia syndrome. *Acta Paediatr Scand* 66:635–638, 1977.
48. Traboulsi EI: Persistent hyperplastic primary vitreous and recessive oculodento-osseous dysplasia. *Am J Med Genet* 24:95–100, 1986.
49. Traboulsi EI, Parks MM: Glaucoma in oculodentoosseous dysplasia. *Am J Ophthalmol* 105:310–313, 1990.
50. Weintraub DM et al: A family with oculodentodigital dysplasia. *Cleft Palate J* 12:323–329, 1975.
51. Whitwell GPB: A case of ectodermal defect associated with hypertelorism. *Br J Dermatol* 43:648–652, 1931.

Osteopathia striata with cranial sclerosis

Osteopathia striata, or striated skeleton, with cranial sclerosis was first described by Voorhoeve (27) in 1924. About 50 cases have been described. The syndrome has been extensively reviewed (8,14,28).

Craniofacial findings. The cranium is biparietally enlarged, occurring in some patients even from birth. Adult head circumference is often 60–65 cm. There is frontal bossing and the face appears somewhat squared. Nasal obstruction may be evident in infancy (12). The nasal bridge is broad and the eyes appear wide-set (23,24). Visual fields may be reduced (4). A few patients have exhibited facial palsy (15) or other cranial nerve deficits (13,28).

Musculoskeletal findings. Radiographically there is hyperostosis of the cranial vault with marked increase in density of the cranial base (17,21,26) (Fig. 8–11A). This may be progressive in childhood. The sinuses may be obscured and the mastoid air cells diminished. The anterior fontanel closes late (5). The ribs and medial clavicles are somewhat broad. The long bones and iliac wings appear to have linear striations, hence the name *osteopathia striata* (Fig. 8–11B). Occasionally, there is generalized increased bone density. Scoliosis is present in at least 15% (12). Spina bifida occulta in the lumbar region is common (12). Fractures have been reported in one case (19).

Mental retardation. Mild, rarely moderate, mental retardation has been found in about 20% of cases (1,12).

Cardiac anomalies. Atrial and/or ventricular septal defects have been documented (4,14,16,20,22,25).

Oral findings. Cleft palate or bifid uvula occurs in about 40% (1,5,15,18,23). Abbreviated tooth roots or unerupted teeth have been described (7,10).

Auditory system. Progressive hearing loss, found in about 50%, is usually mixed, variable in severity, and often involves the low frequencies as well as high frequencies (1,12,20,21,23). The external auditory canal has been stenosed in a few cases, as has the eustachian canal (20). Small middle ear cavity and abnormal ossicle fixation have been demonstrated (20) (Fig. 8–11C,D).

Heredity. Although autosomal dominant inheritance was favored earlier (1,5,6,8,12), the ratio of females to males (2.5F:1M) (9) and the lack of male-to-male transmission clearly suggest X-linked dominant inheritance (2,3,13,22).

Diagnosis. Other bone dysplasias such as osteopoikilosis, autosomal dominant osteopetrosis, sclerosteosis, pycnodysostosis, and craniometaphyseal dysplasia must be excluded. Osteopathia striata may be found in a number of syndromes (11).

Summary. Characteristics include (*1*) X-linked dominant inheritance; (*2*) enlarged head circumference; (*3*) long bones radiographically appearing combed; (*4*) increased density of skull base; (*5*) mild mental retardation in 30%; (*6*) cleft palate in 50%; and (*7*) mixed hearing loss in 50%.

References

1. Bass HN et al: Osteopathia striata syndrome: clinical, genetic and radiologic considerations. *Clin Pediatr* 19:369–373, 1980.
2. Behninger C, Rott HD: Osteopathia striata with cranial sclerosis: literature reappraisal argues for X-linked inheritance. *Genet Couns* 11:157–167, 2000.
3. Bueno AL et al: Severe malformations in males from families with osteopathia striata and cranial sclerosis. *Clin Genet* 54:400–405, 1999.
4. Clementi M et al: Is visual field reduction a component manifestation of osteopathia striata with cranial sclerosis? *Am J Med Genet* 46:724–726, 1993.
5. Cortina H et al: Familial osteopathia striata with cranial condensation. *Pediatr Radiol* 11:87–90, 1981.
6. Currarino G, Friedmann JM: Severe craniofacial sclerosis with multiple anomalies in a boy and his mother. *Pediatr Radiol* 16:441–443, 1986.
7. Daley TD et al: Osteopathia striata, short stature, cataracts and microdontia. *Oral Surg Oral Med Oral Pathol Endod* 81:356–360, 1996.
8. de Keyser J et al: Osteopathia striata with cranial sclerosis. *Clin Neurol* 84:41–48, 1983.
9. Gay BB et al: Osteopathia striata with cranial sclerosis. *Pediatr Radiol* 24:56–60, 1994.

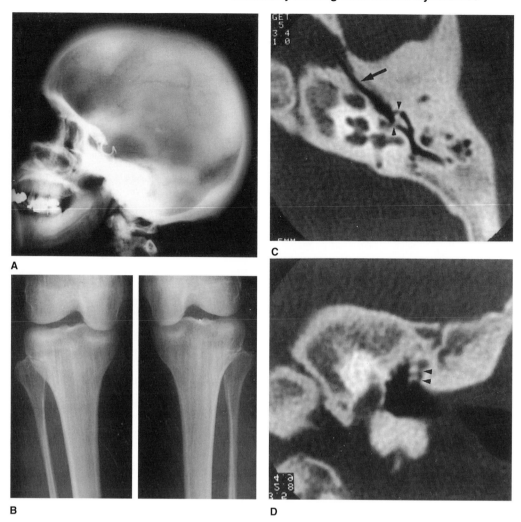

Figure 8–11. *Osteopathia striata.* (A) Marked increase in density and thickness of cranial base, cranial vault, and facial bones. (B) Osteopathia striata well visualized in proximal tibial metaphyses. (C,D) Axial and coronal CT scans of temporal bone showing thickened sclerotic bone with small mastoid antrum and middle ear cavity. Ossicles are abnormally fixed. Eustachian canal is narrow. Auditory canals are patent. [(A,B) from G Currarino and JM Friedman, *Pediatr Radiol* 16:441, 1986; (C,D) from GT Odrezin and N Krasikov, *Am J Neuroradiol* 14:72, 1993.]

10. Goodmann JR, Robertson CV: Osteopathia striata: a case report. *Int J Paediatr Dent* 3:151–156, 1993.
11. Hoeffel JC et al: L'osteopathie striée. *Ann Pédiatr* 40:285–290, 1993.
12. Horan FT, Beighton PH: Osteopathia striata with cranial sclerosis: an autosomal dominant entity. *Clin Genet* 13:201–206, 1978.
13. Keymolen K et al: How to counsel in osteopathia striata with cranial sclerosis. *Genet Couns* 8:207–211, 1997.
14. König R et al: Osteopathia striata with cranial sclerosis: variable expressivity in a four generation pedigree. *Am J Med Genet* 63:69–73, 1996.
15. Kornreich L et al: Osteopathia striata, cranial sclerosis with cleft palate and facial nerve palsy. *Eur J Pediatr* 147:101–103, 1988.
16. Lazar CM et al: Osteopathia striata with cranial sclerosis. *J Bone Miner Res* 14:152–153, 1999.
17. Mohan V et al: Osteopathia striata with cranial sclerosis. *Australas Radiol* 34:249–252, 1990.
18. Nakamura T et al: Osteopathia striata with cranial sclerosis affecting three family members. *Skeletal Radiol* 14:267–269, 1985.
19. Nakamura T et al: Unclassified sclerosing bone dysplasia with osteopathia striata, cranial sclerosis, metaphyseal undermodeling, and bone fragility. *Am J Med Genet* 76:389–394, 1998.
20. Odrezin GT, Krazikov N: CT scan of the temporal bone in a patient with osteopathia striata and cranial sclerosis. *AJNR Am J Neuroradiol* 14:72–75, 1993.
21. Paulsen K: Otologisch Befunde bei der Hyperostosis generalisata (Uehlinger-Syndrom). *Z Laryngol Rhinol Otol* 46:815–824, 1967.
22. Pellegrino JE et al: Further clinical delineation and increased morbidity in males with osteopathia striata with cranial sclerosis: an X-linked disorder? *Am J Med Genet* 30:159–165, 1997.
23. Piechowiak H et al: Cranial sclerosis with striated bone disease (osteopathia striata). *Klin Pädiatr* 198:418–424, 1986.
24. Robinow M, Unger F: Syndrome of osteopathia striata, macrocephaly, and cranial sclerosis. *Am J Dis Child* 138:821–823, 1984.
25. Savarirayan R et al: Osteopathia striata with cranial sclerosis: highly variable phenotypic expression within a family. *Clin Genet* 52:199–205, 1997.
26. Schnyder PA: Osseous changes of osteopathia striata associated with cranial sclerosis. *Skeletal Radiol* 5:19–22, 1980.
27. Voorhoeve N: L'image radiologique non encore décrite d'une anomalie du squelette. *Acta Radiol* 3:407–427, 1924.
28. Winter RM et al: Osteopathia striata with cranial sclerosis: highly variable expression within a family including cleft palate in two neonatal cases. *Clin Genet* 18:462–474, 1980.

Chondrodysplasias

Achondroplasia

Achondroplasia is a rhizomelic form of short-limbed dwarfism associated with enlarged head, depressed nasal bridge, short stubby trident hands, lordotic lumbar spine, prominent buttocks, and protuberant abdomen. The reader is referred to the following references for comprehensive coverage: general review (14,15,29); histology (27,33,35); radiology (23,24); and cephalometrics (10).

Growth curves have been described by Horton et al. (19). Final adult height is 130 cm for males and 123 cm for females. Mean adult weights are 55 kg for males and 46 kg for females (20). There is a tendency toward obesity (17).

Reproductive fitness is considerably reduced among those with achondroplasia because of social difficulties in finding mates. This is changing, however, with the advent of Little People groups. In addition, obstetrical problems of achondroplastic women (prematurity and the necessity for cesarean deliveries due to cephalopelvic disproportion) reduce the number of offspring.

Craniofacial findings. The head is enlarged, with frontal bossing and low nasal bridge (Fig. 8–12A). Occasionally, these features are not present at birth, but disproportionate growth of the head occurs during the first year of life and then parallels the normal curve (8,24,29).

Central nervous system. Intelligence is almost always normal, although acquisition of motor skills may be delayed because of the large head and short extremities (8,45). Head control may not occur until 3 to 4 months and affected children may not walk until 24 to 36 months. Ultimately, however, development is normal (21).

Significant hydrocephaly (stepwise increase in the head growth slope) with neurologic signs and symptoms has occurred in a few instances (8,32,42), and most evidence to date seems to favor communicating hydrocephaly (13,22,32). The narrow spinal canal predisposes to neurologic complications with age (34). Compression of the cord and nerve rootlets results from osteophytes, prolapsed intervertebral discs, or deformed vertebral bodies.

Musculoskeletal system. Enlarged calvaria and basilar kyphosis are constant features. In contrast to the normal anterior cranial base, the posterior cranial base length is shorter than normal. The foramen magnum is small. The maxilla is hypoplastic, resulting in midface deficiency and relative mandibular prognathism (10). The frontal and occipital bones may be prominent (23,24). Partial occipitalization of the first cervical vertebra occurs in most cases.

The interpediculate distances progressively narrow from the upper to the lower lumbar spine, the pedicles are shortened in anteroposterior diameter, the posterior aspect of the vertebral bodies is concave, and the bony spinal canal diameters are decreased, particularly in the lumbar region. Anterior wedging of vertebral bodies (particularly in the region of the thoracolumbar junction) with resultant kyphosis may be prominent (23,24). Kyphosis occurs in about 20% of cases and scoliosis in 7% (44).

The pelvis is broad and short. Narrowing of the pelvic inlet prevents vaginal delivery in pregnant achondroplastic females. The superior acetabular margins are oriented horizontally, and the sacrosciatic notches are narrowed (Fig. 8–12B) (15,16). Legs are frequently bowed because of lax knee ligaments.

Limb bones are shortened in a rhizomelic pattern, which is more prominent in the upper extremities. There is incomplete extension at the elbows. The fingers cannot be approximated (Fig. 8–12C). Genua vara are found in 15% (44). The fibula is overly long at the ankle compared to the tibia, leading in some cases to varus foot deformity.

Auditory system. Glass et al. (11) noted that 97% of 88 patients reported a history of ear infection and/or hearing loss and 72% had a hearing loss of 22 dB or greater. Similar findings have been noted by Hall (15) and Brinkmann et al. (5). In a detailed audiologic study of 28 patients, Glass et al. (12) found that 13 had conductive hearing loss in at least one ear. Both type B tympanograms, indicative of an immobile tympanic membrane, and type C tympanograms, indicative of eustachian tube dysfunction, were recorded in different patients. Sensorineural hearing loss was found in 7 of 28 patients. Progressive otosclerosis was documented by Carlin et al. (6). Temporal bone changes

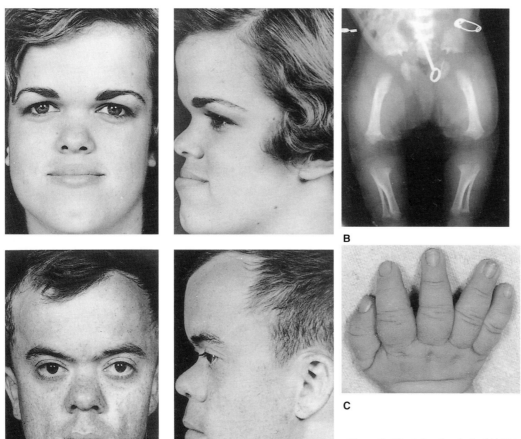

B

C

Figure 8–12. *Achondroplasia.* (A) Note frontal bossing, depressed nasal bridge, and relative mandibular prognathism in two patients. (B) Characteristic radiographic changes in newborn. Note small pelvic bones with narrow, slit-like sacrosciatic notches and shortened long bones of extremities with characteristic alterations. (C) Inability to approximate terminal digits.

A

have been found, but they do not correlate with the hearing loss (7,35). Stura et al. (39) studied 18 patients and found 10 with hearing loss, 7 conductive and 3 sensorineural. Berkowitz et al. (2) and others (14,26,36) noted increased otitis media with resultant hearing loss.

Heredity. The frequency of achondroplasia has been estimated as ranging between 1/16,000 and 1/35,000 live births (38). More than 80% of recorded cases of achondroplasia are sporadic, representing new mutations. Increased paternal age at time of conception is associated with sporadic cases (30). Among familial cases, autosomal dominant inheritance can be demonstrated. Homozygosity, which is lethal, has been reported in a few instances in which both parents have achondroplasia (29). Several authors (4,18,31,37) have described affected sibs born to clinically unaffected parents. Henderson et al (18) demonstrated germline mosaicism in the apparently unaffected mother of their patients. Mettler and Fraser (28) estimate the recurrence risk to a sibling of a child with achondroplasia and unaffected parents as .02%. Achondroplasia, mapping to 4p16.3 (25,41), represents mutations in *FGFR3* (3,9,40,43). Wilkin et al. (43) noted that the mutation always occurs on the male chromosome.

Diagnosis. In infancy, achondroplasia should be distinguished from the various types of achondrogenesis and thanatophoric dysplasia (9). Other chondrodystrophies such as Ellis–van Creveld syndrome, metatropic dysplasia, diastrophic dysplasia, asphyxiating thoracic dystrophy, hypochondroplasia, and pseudoachondroplasia should be ruled out (14). Prenatal diagnosis of both heterozygous and homozygous achondroplasia has been carried out (1).

Summary. Characteristics include (*1*) autosomal dominant inheritance, although about 80% of cases represent new mutations; (*2*) short-limbed dwarfism; (*3*) enlarged head; (*4*) short trident hands; (*5*) lordotic spine; (*6*) typical skeletal changes; and (*7*) frequent hearing loss.

References

1. Bellus GA et al: First trimester prenatal diagnosis in couple at risk for homozygous achondroplasia. *Lancet* 2:1511–1512, 1994.
2. Berkowitz RG et al: Middle ear disease in childhood achondroplasia. *Ear Nose Throat J* 70:305–308, 1991.
3. Bonaventure J et al: Common mutations in the *FGFR3* gene account for achondroplasia, hypochondroplasia, and thanatophoric dwarfism. *Am J Med Genet* 63:148–154, 1996.
4. Bowen P: Achondroplasia in two sisters with normal parents. *Birth Defects* 10(12):31–36, 1974.
5. Brinkmann G et al: Cognitive skills in achondroplasia. *Am J Med Genet* 47:800–804, 1993.
6. Carlin ME et al: Does achondroplasia predispose to otosclerosis? Presented at the March of Dimes Clinical Genetics Conferences, Baltimore, Maryland, July 10–13, 1988.
7. Cobb SR et al: Computed tomography of the temporal bone in achondroplasia. *AJNR Am J Neuroradiol* 9:1195–1199, 1988.
8. Cohen ME et al: Neurological abnormalities in achondroplastic children. *J Pediatr* 71:367–376, 1967.
9. Cohen MM Jr: Achondroplasia, hypochondroplasia, and thanatophoric dysplasia: clinically related skeletal dysplasias that are also related at the molecular level. *Int J Oral Maxillofac Surg* 27:451–455, 1998.
10. Cohen MM Jr et al: A morphometric analysis of the craniofacial configuration in achondroplasia. *J Craniofac Genet Dev Biol* (Suppl)1:139–165, 1985.
11. Glass L et al: Speech, hearing and craniofacial morphology in patients with achondroplasia. Unpublished data, 1980.
12. Glass L et al: Audiologic findings of patients with achondroplasia. *Int J Pediatr Otorhinolaryngol* 3:129–135, 1981.
13. Gordon N: The neurological complications of achondroplasia. *Brain Dev* 22:3–7, 2000.
14. Gorlin RJ et al: *Syndromes of the Head and Neck*, 4th ed. Oxford University Press, New York, 2001.
15. Hall JG: The natural history of achondroplasia. *Basic Life Sci* 48:3–9, 1988.
16. Hecht JT, Butler IJ: Neurologic morbidity associated with achondroplasia. *J Child Neurol* 5:84–97, 1990.
17. Hecht JT et al: Obesity and achondroplasia. *Am J Med Genet* 31:597–602, 1988.
18. Henderson S et al: Germline and somatic mosaicism in achondroplasia. *J Med Genet* 37:956–958, 2000.
19. Horton WA et al: Standard growth curves for achondroplasia. *J Pediatr* 93:435–438, 1978.
20. Hunter AGW et al: Standard weight for height curves in achondroplasia. *Am J Med Genet* 62:255–261, 1996.
21. Hunter AGW et al: Medical complications of achondroplasia: a multicentre patient review. *J Med Genet* 35:705–712, 1998.
22. James AE et al: Hydrocephalus in achondroplasia studied by cisternography. *Pediatrics* 49:46–49, 1972.
23. Langer LO Jr et al: Achondroplasia. *AJR Am J Roentgenol* 100:12–26, 1967.
24. Langer LO Jr et al: Achondroplasia. Clinical radiologic features with comment on genetic implications. *Clin Pediatr* 7:474–485, 1968.
25. LeMerrer M et al: A gene for achondroplasia/hypochondroplasia maps to chromosome 4p. *Nat Genet* 6:318–321, 1994.
26. Mahomed NN et al: Functional health status of adults with achondroplasia. *Am J Med Genet* 78:30–35, 1998.
27. Maynard JA et al: Histochemistry and ultrastructure of the growth plate in achondroplasia. *J Bone Joint Surg Am* 63:969–979, 1981.
28. Mettler G, Fraser FC: Recurrence risk for sibs of children with "sporadic" achondroplasia. *Am J Med Genet* 90:250–251, 2000.
29. Nicoletti B et al (eds): *Human Achondroplasia. A Multidisciplinary Approach. First International Symposium on Human Achondroplasia, 1986, Rome, Italy*. Plenum Press, New York, 1988.
30. Orioli IM et al: Effect of paternal age in achondroplasia, thanatophoric dysplasia and osteogenesis imperfecta. *Am J Med Genet* 59:209–217, 1995.
31. Philip N et al: Achondroplasia in sibs of normal patients. *J Med Genet* 25:857–859, 1988.
32. Pierre-Kahn A et al: Hydrocephalus and achondroplasia: a study of 24 observations. *Childs Brain* 7:205–219, 1980.
33. Ponseti IV: Skeletal growth in achondroplasia. *J Bone Joint Surg Am* 52:701–716, 1970.
34. Reid CS et al: Cervicomedullary compression in young patients with achondroplasia: value of comprehensive neurologic and respiratory evaluation. *J Pediatr* 110:522–530, 1987.
35. Rimoin DL: Histopathology and ultrastructure of cartilage in the chondrodystrophies. *Birth Defects* 10(9):1–18, 1974.
36. Shohat M et al: Hearing loss and temporal bone structure in achondroplasia. *Am J Med Genet* 45:548–551, 1993.
37. Sobetzko D et al: Achondroplasia with the *FGFR3* 11389 → a (6380R) mutation in two sibs sharing a 4p haplotype derived from their unaffected father. *J Med Genet* 37:958–939, 2000.
38. Stoll C et al: Birth prevalence rates of skeletal dysplasias. *Clin Genet* 35:88–92, 1989.
39. Stura M et al: Problemi audiologici negli acondroplasici. *Minerva Pediatr* 39:499–501, 1987.
40. Superti-Furga A et al: A glycine 375 to cystein substitution in the transmembrane domain of FGFR3 in a newborn with achondroplasia. *Eur J Pediatr* 154:215–219, 1995.
41. Velinor M et al: The gene for achondroplasia maps to the telomeric region of chromosome 4p. *Nat Genet* 6:314–317, 1994.
42. Wassman ER Jr, Rimoin DL: Cervicomedullary compression with achondroplasia. *J Pediatr* 113:411, 1988.
43. Wilkin DJ et al: Mutations in fibroblast growth-factor receptor 3 in sporadic cases of achondroplasia occur exclusively on the paternally derived chromosome. *Am J Hum Genet* 63:711–716, 1998.
44. Wynne-Davies R et al: Achondroplasia and hypochondroplasia: Clinical variations and spinal stenosis. *J Bone Joint Surg Br* 63:508–515, 1981.
45. Yamada HK et al: Neurologic manifestations of pediatric achondroplasia. *J Neurosurg* 54:49–57, 1981.

Campomelic syndrome

Campomelic syndrome is characterized by macrocephaly, small face, micrognathia, and bent femora and tibiae. It was first recognized as an entity by Spranger et al. (35) and Maroteaux et al. (22) in the 1970s. Birth prevalence has been estimated to be from 1/100,000 to as high as 1.6/10,000 (27). At least 200 cases have been reported.

In about 50% of the cases, the child is either stillborn or dies within a few hours. Nearly all have succumbed by 10 months of age. However, a few have lived for many years (14). Mental retardation is evident in nearly all those that survive (14). At least 85% exhibit respiratory distress as a result of small thoracic cage, narrow larynx, hypoplastic trachea, and, possibly, central nervous system (CNS)-based hypotonia. Polyhydramnios, beginning at about 32 weeks, is common.

Craniofacial findings. Frequent features are macrocephaly, dolichocephaly, large anterior fontanel and sutures, disproportionately small face, short narrow palpebral fissures, apparent hypertelorism, flat nasal bridge, low-set ears with soft pinnae, small nose with anteverted nostrils, long philtrum, small mouth, retroglossia, micrognathia, and short neck with redundant skin (24) (Fig. 8–13A). Cleft palate is present in at least 65%–80% (4).

Musculoskeletal system. The long bones of the lower extremities are bent, but to varied degrees. The genesis of bowing and shortening of the lower limbs has been discussed by Lazjuk, et al. (17) and Pazzaglia and Beluffi (30). Cases without campomelio have been documented (7,9,11,20,26). The bones of the upper extremities are mildly bowed in 20%–25%. The elbows may be dislocated. Pretibial skin dimples over the most convex site are found in about 90%. Talipes equinovarus is a very common feature. There is often a wide space between the hallux and the second toe.

Radiographic findings. Changes include tall narrow orbits (70%–90%), hypoplastic bladeless scapulae (90%), small bell-shaped chest (80%), nonmineralized sternum (80%), slender ribs (60%–85%), 11 ribs (55%–70%), slender trachea (70%), flattened and/or hypoplastic vertebral bodies (particularly cervical) with nonmineralized pedicles (80%), and kyphoscoliosis (70%). Bowed shortened tibiae and femora, hypoplastic fibulae, narrow iliac wings with increased acetabular angles, late developing pubic bones, vertical and widely spaced ischia, and dislocated hips are almost constant findings (Fig. 8–13B). The proximal tibial and distal femoral epiphyses are absent in 85%. The talus is nonmineralized in 80%. The hands exhibit clinodactyly, brachydactyly, and small middle phalanges in 70% (5).

Other findings. Autopsy findings have shown absence or hypoplasia of olfactory tracts or bulbs (25%), hydrocephalus (10%–25%), variable congenital heart anomalies [VSD, ASD, PDA, tetralogy of Fallot, stenosis of aortic isthmus (20%–30%)], deficiency of laryngeal and tracheobronchial cartilages (30%–40%), and hydroureter and hydronephrosis (20%–30%) (33). Renal hypoplasia is also found. Sex reversal is frequent but not always complete; some patients have ambiguous genitalia (2–4,8,16,23,25,29).

Figure 8–13. *Campomelic syndrome.* (A) Note large head, short neck, and marked angulation of bones of lower leg. (B) Radiograph showing bending of femora, tibiae, and fibulae. [(A) from HJ Mellows et al., *Clin Genet* 18:137, 1980.]

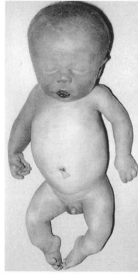
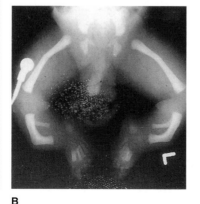

A   **B**

Auditory system. Hearing loss is found in all those that survive (10,14,37,39). For those with an early demise, autopsy has shown malformed ossicles, hypoplastic cochlea and semicircular canals, large epitympanic space, aberrant course of facial nerve, and lack of cartilage cells in the otic capsule (39).

Heredity. Inheritance, originally thought to be autosomal recessive (6,12), is actually autosomal dominant (18). The male:female phenotypic ratio is 1:3 and many females have a 46,XY karyotype with sex reversal, as noted above; such infants are H-Y antigen negative (29,31). The chromosomal sex ratio is, of course, 1:1. The occurrence in sibs can be explained by gonadal mosaicism (34). Cases of translocation or inversion led to the mapping of the gene to 17q24.3–q25 (21,26). Mutations of *SOX9* gene, an SRY-related sex-determining gene, have been described. SOX9 is a transcription factor expressed during chondrogenesis together with COL2A1 and during gonadal development. Campomelic dysplasia without campomelia is also due to mutations in *SOX9* (1,9,25,28).

Diagnosis. Kozlowski et al. (15) describe several disorders with bent bones, and Hall and Spranger (13) list nearly 30 conditions with congenital bowing of long bones. Kyphomelic dysplasia, Stüve-Wiedemann syndrome, Schwarz-Jampel syndrome, type 2, and a number of conditions discussed elsewhere (10,12,13,19,32,36,38,40) need to be ruled out. The disorder has been diagnosed prenatally (5,10,41).

Summary. Characteristics include (1) autosomal dominant inheritance; (2) relatively frequent sex reversal; (3) frequent lethality; (4) bent femora and tibiae; and (5) conductive hearing loss in survivors.

References

1. Bell DM et al: SOX9 directly regulates the type II collagen gene. *Nat Genet* 16:174–178, 1997.
2. Bricarelli F et al: Sex reversed XY females with campomelic dysplasia are H-Y negative. *Hum Genet* 57:15–22, 1981.
3. Cameron FJ et al: A novel germ line mutation in the *SOX9* causes familial campomelic dysplasia and sex reversal. *Hum Mol Genet* 5:1625–1630, 1996.
4. Cooke CT et al: Campomelic dysplasia with sex reversal: morphological and cytogenetic studies of a case. *Pathology* 17:526–529, 1985.
5. Cordone M et al: In utero ultrasonographic features of campomelic dysplasia. *Prenat Diagn* 9:745–750, 1989.
6. Cremin BJ et al: Autosomal recessive inheritance in camptomelic dwarfism. *Lancet* 1:488–489, 1973.
7. Decsi T, Botykai A: Campomelic dysplasia without campomelia. *Pädiatr Pädol* 27:29–30, 1992.
8. Foster JAW et al: Campomelic dysplasia and autosomal sex reversal caused by mutations in an SRY-related gene. *Nature* 372:525–530, 1994.
9. Freidrich U et al: Campomelic dysplasia without overt campomelia. *Clin Dysmorphol* 1:172–178, 1992.
10. Gillerot Y et al: Campomelic syndrome: manifestations in a 20-week fetus and case history of a five-year-old child. *Am J Med Genet* 34:589–592, 1989.
11. Glass RBJ, Rosenbaum KN: Acampomelic campomelic dysplasia: further radiographic variations. *Am J Med Genet* 69:29–32, 1997.
12. Hall BD, Spranger JW: Familial congenital bowing with short bones. *Radiology* 132:611–614, 1979.
13. Hall BD, Spranger JW: Congenital bowing of the long bones: a review and phenotype analysis of 13 undiagnosed cases. *Eur J Pediatr* 133:131–138, 1980.
14. Houston CS et al: The campomelic syndrome: a review, report of 17 cases and follow-up on the currently 17-year-old boy first reported by Maroteaux in 1971. *Am J Med Genet* 15:3–28, 1983.
15. Kozlowski K et al: Syndromes of congenital bowing of the long bones. *Pediatr Radiol* 7:40–48, 1979.
16. Kwok C et al: Mutations in *SOX9*, the gene responsible for campomelic dysplasia and autosomal sex reversal. *Am J Hum Genet* 57:1028–1036, 1995.
17. Lazjuk GI et al: Campomelic syndromes. Concepts of the bowing and shortening in the lower limbs. *Teratology* 35:1–8, 1987.
18. Lynch SA et al: Campomelic dysplasia: evidence of autosomal dominant inheritance. *J Med Genet* 30:683–686, 1993.
19. MacLean RN et al: Skeletal dysplasia with short angulated femora (kyphomelic dysplasia). *Am J Med Genet* 14:373–380, 1983.
20. Macpherson RI et al: Acampomelic-campomelic dysplasia. *Pediatr Radiol* 20:90–93, 1989.

21. Mansour S et al: A clinical and genetic study of campomelic dysplasia. *J Med Genet* 32:415–20, 1995.
22. Maroteaux P et al: Le syndrome campomelique. *Presse Méd* 22:1157–1162, 1971.
23. Meyer J et al: Mutational analysis of the *SOX9* gene in campomelic dysplasia and autosomal sex reversal: lack of genotype/phenotype correlations. *Hum Mol Genet* 6:91–98, 1997.
24. Mintz SM, Adibfar A: Management of maxillofacial deformity in a patient with campomelic dysplasia. *J Oral Maxillofac Surg* 52:618–623, 1994.
25. Morais da Silva S et al: SOX9 expression during gonadal development implies a conserved role for the gene in testis differentiation in mammals and birds. *Nat Genet* 14:62–68, 1996.
26. Ninomiya S et al: Acampomelic campomelic syndrome and sex reversal associated with de novo t(12;17) translocation. *Am J Med Genet* 56:31–34, 1995.
27. Norman EK et al: Campomelic dysplasia—an underdiagnosed condition? *Eur J Pediatr* 152:331–333, 1993.
28. Olney PN et al: Campomelic syndrome and deletion of *SOX9*. *Am J Med Genet* 84:20–24, 1999.
29. Pauli RM, Pagon RA: Abnormalities of sexual differentiation in campomelic dwarfs. *Clin Genet* 18:223–225, 1980.
30. Pazzaglia UE, Beluffi G: Radiology and histopathology of the bent limbs in campomelic dysplasia. Implications in the aetiology of the disease and review of theories. *Pediatr Radiol* 17:50–55, 1987.
31. Puck SM et al: Absence of H-Y antigen in an XY female with campomelic dysplasia. *Hum Genet* 57:23–27, 1981.
32. Rezza E et al: Familial congenital bowing with thick bones and metaphyseal changes, a distinct entity. *Pediatr Radiol* 14:323–327, 1984.
33. Ruan L et al: Campomelic syndrome-laryngotracheomalacia treated with single stage laryngotracheal reconstruction. *Int J Pediatr Otorhinolaryngol* 37:277–282, 1996.
34. Shafai T, Schwartz L: Camptomelic dwarfism in siblings. *J Pediatr* 89:512–513, 1976.
35. Spranger JW et al: Increasing frequency of a syndrome of multiple osseous defects. *Lancet* 2:716, 1970.
36. Stüve A, Wiedemann H-R: Angeborene Verbiegungen langer Röhrenknochen–eine Geschwisterbeobachtung. *Z Kinderheilkd* 111:184–192, 1971.
37. Takahashi H et al: Temporal bone histopathological findings in campomelic dysplasia. *J Laryngol Otol* 106:361–365, 1992.
38. Temple IK et al: Kyphomelic dysplasia. *J Med Genet* 26:457–468, 1989.
39. Tokita N et al: The campomelic syndrome. Temporal bone histopathologic features and otolaryngologic manifestations. *Arch Otolaryngol* 105:449–454, 1979.
40. Viljoen D, Beighton P: Kyphomelic dysplasia: further delineation of the phenotype. *Dysmorphol Clin Genet* 1(4):136–141, 1988.
41. Winter R et al: Prenatal diagnosis of campomelic dysplasia by ultrasonography. *Prenat Diagn* 5:1–8, 1985.

Spondyloepiphyseal dysplasia congenita

Spondyloepiphyseal dysplasia (SED) congenita was first described by Spranger and Wiedemann in 1966 (14). The prevalence is approximately 1/100,000 (16,19). SED congenita is etiologically heterogeneous (5,8,11,13,16,17), but the classic form is discussed here. A defect in type II collagen is responsible (1,11,15) (see Heredity).

Clinical findings. Short stature leads to a final height attainment of 84–128 cm (6). There is disproportionate shortness of the neck and trunk and coxa vara. The head appears to sit upon the trunk and is often held in retroflexion (Fig. 8–14A). General anesthesia may be a problem (12). The extremities are proportionately shortened but the hands and feet are normal. The chest is small and bell-shaped and the abdomen is protuberant. Respiratory complications are relatively rare (4). Stiffness, limitation at the hips, and waddling gait are evident. Most patients exhibit pectus carinatum, moderate thoracic kyphoscoliosis, and, in particular, lumbar lordosis. Talipes varus occurs in about 10%–15%. Nonprogressive myopia of 5 diopters or greater has been documented in about half of the children. In those with high myopia, vitreoretinal degeneration is encountered and vitreous synersis is apparently present in all patients. Retinal detachment, in spite of earlier reports (7,14), is rare (19). Cleft palate occurs in about 15%–20% (17,19). Mental deficiency has been rarely documented (3).

Radiographic findings. In the affected infant, the vertebral bodies appear ovoid in lateral view (Fig. 8–14B,C). The odontoid is usually hypoplastic and may dislocate (9). As the child matures, there is platyspondyly with posterior wedging of vertebral bodies. Mild to moderate metaphyseal alterations are noted in long bones of infants (Fig. 8–14D). Ossification is retarded in the sternum, pubic bones, distal femoral and proximal tibial epiphyses, talus, and calcaneus (Fig. 8–14E). The iliac bones are hypoplastic. The upper femoral epiphyses are small and deformed, late to develop, and in coxa vara position (Fig. 8–14F) (10,14).

Auditory system. Moderately severe (30–60 dB) sensorineural hearing loss, especially marked in the high tones, has been reported in about 30% (3).

Heredity. Inheritance is autosomal dominant (14). It has been grouped with Kniest dysplasia, Stickler syndrome, hypochondrogenesis, and a number of other disorders as one of type II collagenopathy. Mutations of *COL2A1* gene have been found (1). The gene maps to 12q13.11–q13.2 (2,18).

Diagnosis. Morquio syndrome is characterized by growth deficiency and skeletal deformity, becoming apparent during the second year of life. There is corneal clouding, keratosulfaturia, and autosomal recessive inheritance. Heterogeneous forms of SED congenita are discussed by Gorlin et al (3).

Summary. Characteristics include (*1*) autosomal dominant inheritance; (*2*) short stature; (*3*) short neck; (*4*) bell-shaped chest; (*5*) myopia; (*6*) cleft palate in 15%–20%; (*7*) recognizable dysplastic bone changes; and (*8*) moderately severe sensorineural hearing loss in 30%.

References

1. Anderson IJ et al: Spondyloepiphyseal dysplasia congenita: genetic linkage to type II collagen (COL2AI). *Am J Hum Genet* 46:896–901, 1993.
2. Cole WG et al: The clinical features of spondyloepiphyseal dysplasia congenita resulting from the substitution of glycine 997 by serine in the alpha1(II) chain of type II collagen. *J Med Genet* 30:27–35, 1993.
3. Gorlin RJ et al: *Syndromes of the Head and Neck*, 4th ed. Oxford University Press, New York, 2001.
4. Harding CO et al: Respiratory complications in children with spondyloepiphyseal dysplasia congenita. *Pediatr Pulmonol* 9:49–54, 1990.
5. Harrod MJE et al: Genetic heterogeneity in spondyloepiphyseal dysplasia congenita. *Am J Med Genet* 18:311–320, 1984.
6. Horton WA et al: Growth curves for height for diastrophic dysplasia, spondyloepiphyseal dysplasia congenita, and pseudoachondroplasia. *Am J Dis Child* 136:316–319, 1982.
7. Ikegawa S et al: Retinal detachment in spondyloepiphyseal dysplasia congenita. *J Pediatr Orthop* 13:791–792, 1993.
8. Kozlowski K et al: Dysplasia spondylo-epiphysealis congenita Spranger-Wiedemann: a critical analysis. *Australas Radiol* 21:260–280,1977.
9. LeDoux MS et al: Stabilization of the cervical spine in spondyloepiphyseal dysplasia congenita. *Neurosurgery* 28:580–583, 1991.
10. Maroteaux P et al: Spondylo-epiphyseal dysplasia congenita. *Pediatr Radiol* 10:250, 1981.
11. Murray TG et al: Spondyloepiphyseal dysplasia congenita: light and electron microscopic studies of the eye. *Arch Ophthalmol* 103:407–411, 1985.
12. Rodney GE et al: Spondyloepiphyseal dysplasia congenita. *Anaesthesia* 46:648–650, 1991.
13. Spranger JW, Maroteaux P: Genetic heterogeneity of spondyloepiphyseal dysplasia congenita? *Am J Med Genet* 14:601–602, 1983.
14. Spranger J, Wiedemann H-R: Dysplasia spondyloepiphysaria congenita. *Helv Paediatr Acta* 21:598–611, 1966.
15. Spranger J et al: The type II collagenopathies: a spectrum of chondrodysplasias. *Eur J Pediatr* 153:56–65, 1994.
16. Stoll C et al: Birth prevalence rates of skeletal dysplasia. *Clin Genet* 35:88–92, 1989.
17. Sugiura Y et al: Spondyloepiphyseal dysplasia congenita. *Int Orthoped* 2:47–51, 1978.
18. Tiller GE et al: An RNA-splicing mutation in the type II collagen gene (*COL2AI*) in a family with spondyloepiphyseal dysplasia congenita. *Am J Hum Genet* 56:388–395, 1995.

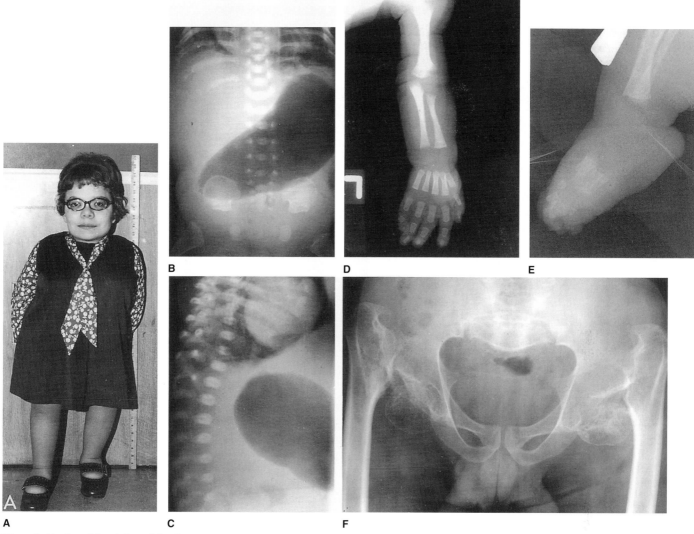

Figure 8–14. *Spondyloepiphyseal dysplasia congenita.* (A) Adult with short stature, severe myopia, retinal detachment, scoliosis, and sensorineural hearing loss. Patient had severe coxa vara, which produced a waddling gait. (B,C) Radiographs of newborn showing ovoid vertebral bodies, shortened ilia, and absence of pubic bone. (D) Radiograph of newborn showing abbreviation of humerus. (E) Absent talus and calcaneus in newborn. (F) Note femoral heads in acetabular area.

19. Wynne-Davies R, Hall C: Two clinical variants of spondylo-epiphyseal dysplasia congenita. *J Bone Joint Surg Br* 64:435–441, 1982.

Kniest dysplasia (metatropic dysplasia, type II)

In 1952, Kniest (9) described a form of generalized spondyloepimetaphyseal bone dysplasia with short-trunk dwarfism and scoliosis. Twenty-five years later, Kniest and Leiber (10) reviewed the condition. Spranger et al. (21) discussed the career of Kniest.

Clinical findings. The face is round, with the midface flat and the nasal bridge depressed, giving the eyes a somewhat exophthalmic appearance (Fig. 8–15A). The nostrils may appear anteverted. The neck is usually short. The head appears to sit on the thorax. At birth, cleft palate (present in about 40% of patients), clubfoot, and prominent knees may be noted (2,4–6,10,18,19). Lordosis and/or dorsal kyphosis and tibial bowing usually develop within the first few years of life (Fig. 8–15B). The neck may be unstable (15). The child may not sit and walk until 2 and 3 years, respectively. By that time, most joints become progressively enlarged and stiff and the gait is waddling. Movement at the metacarpophalangeal joint is normal, but the child cannot make a fist. The fifth fingers are generally not involved. The palms may have a violaceous hue. The elbows, wrists, and knees become particularly enlarged, and flexion and extension of most joints become progressively reduced (16). The feet are flat and outturned. Hernia is frequent. Adult height ranges between 105 and 145 cm.

Ocular system. Severe myopia and lattice degeneration with or without retinal detachment and/or cataract formation have been present in about 40% of cases (2,8,14,18).

Musculoskeletal system. Radiographically, the neurocranium is large in comparison with the facial skeleton. The anterior fontanel is late to close. The cranial base angle is flattened and the sella turcica is anteriorly displaced. The odontoid is short and wide (4,5,8). Platyspondyly, particularly of the upper thoracic part of the spine, is severe. The vertebrae exhibit vertical clefts. The long bones are somewhat short, slightly bowed, and have flared metaphyses. The epiphyses are large, irregular, and punctate. The hands show epiphyseal and carpal retardation with generalized osteopenia. Later, the carpal bones assume bizarre shapes and sizes. The iliac bones are small, particularly in relation to the large capital femoral epiphysis and proximal femoral metaphysis (Fig. 8–15C). The pubic rami are poorly ossified. The femoral

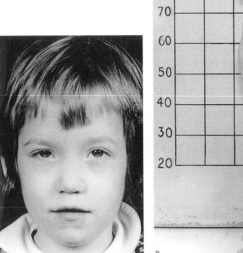
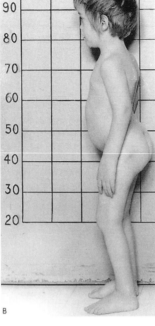
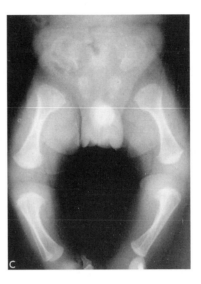

Figure 8–15. *Kniest dysplasia (metatropic dysplasia, type II).* (A) The nasal bridge is depressed. (B) Lumbar lordosis with dorsal kyphosis develops within first few years of life. Joints become enlarged and stiff and result in waddling gait. (C) Radiograph showing shortened long bones with enlarged metaphyses. The iliac wings are broad and reduced in height, especially in relation to the large capital femoral epiphysis and proximal femoral metaphysis. Note delayed appearance of epiphyses. [(A,B) from DC Siggers et al., *Birth Defects* 10(9):193, 1974; (C) from FN Silverman, *Birth Defects* 5(4):45, 1969.]

capital epiphyses form late, the necks are wide and short with a poorly ossified central area, and there may be coxa vara. The trochanter is prominent (11,12). Prenatal diagnosis has been accomplished by ultrasound (1), but difficulty has been experienced (7).

Auditory system. Conductive and/or sensorineural hearing loss is a frequent finding and may develop before puberty (5). Recurrent otitis media and respiratory infections are common (6).

Pathology. Histopathologic examination of bones has shown that the disorganized growth plates contain large chondrocytes that lie in a very loosely woven matrix containing numerous empty spaces ("Swiss cheese cartilage") (2,17). The chondrocytes have Schiff-positive inclusions. This represents type II procollagen (5). Ultrastructural studies of cartilage cells have shown dilated cisternae of rough with accumulated protein. There is vacuolar degeneration of extralacunar matrix in the area of the resting cartilage adjacent to the growth plate. Keratan sulfaturia has been found (4,8). Electromicroscopic studies have been carried out (5).

Heredity. Most patients have been isolated examples, but several authors (8,13,20) have noted the disorder in two generations. Identical twins have been described (6). Mutations in *COL2A1* gene located at 12q13.11–q13.2 have been found (3,20,22,23). These mutations cause incorporation of shortened chains into the collagen fibrils resulting in malalignment of cross-linking sites.

Diagnosis. Dyssegmental dysplasia, type Rolland-Desbuquois, and Burton syndrome (6) should be excluded.

Summary. Characteristics include (*1*) autosomal dominant inheritance, most cases being isolated; (*2*) disproportionate short stature; (*3*) round flattened face with short neck; (*4*) enlarged stiff joints; (*5*) myopia; (*6*) spondyloepimetaphyseal bone dysplasia; (*7*) cleft palate; and (*8*) mixed hearing loss.

References

1. Browley B et al: The prenatal sonographic features of Kniest syndrome. *J Ultrasound Med* 10:705–707, 1991.
2. Chen H et al: Kniest dysplasia: neonatal death with necropsy. *Am J Med Genet* 6:171–178, 1980.
3. Freisinger P et al: Type II collagenopathies: are there additional family members? *Am J Med Genet* 63:137–143, 1996.
4. Friede H et al: Craniofacial and mucopolysaccharide abnormalities in Kniest dysplasia. *J Craniofac Genet Dev Biol* 5:267–276, 1985.
5. Gilbert-Barness E et al: Kniest dysplasia: radiologic, histopathological, and scanning electromicroscopic findings. *Am J Med Genet* 63:34–45, 1996.
6. Gorlin RJ et al: *Syndromes of the Head and Neck*, 4th ed. Oxford University Press, New York, 2001.
7. Kerleroux J et al: The difficulty of prenatal diagnosis of Kniest syndrome. A propos of a case mimicking spondylo-epiphyseal dysplasia congenita. *J Gynecol Obstet Biol Reprod* 23:69–74, 1994.
8. Kim HJ et al: Kniest syndrome with dominant inheritance and mucopolysacchariduria. *Am J Med Genet* 27:755–764, 1975.
9. Kniest W: Zur Abgrenzung der Dysostosis enchondralis von der Chondrodystrophie. *Z Kinderheilkd* 70:633–640, 1952.
10. Kniest W, Leiber B: Kniest-Syndrom. *Monatsschr Kinderheilkd* 125:970–973, 1977.
11. Kozlowski K et al: Metatropic dwarfism and its variants. *Australas Radiol* 20:367–385, 1976.
12. Lachman RS et al: The Kniest syndrome. *AJR Am J Roentgenol* 123:805–814, 1975.
13. Maroteaux P, Spranger J: La maladie de Kniest. *Arch Fr Pédiatr* 30:735–750, 1973.
14. Maumenee I, Traboulsi EI: The ocular findings in Kniest dysplasia. *Am J Ophthalmol* 100:155–160, 1985.
15. Merrill KD, Schmidt TL: Occipitoatlantal instability in a child with Kniest syndrome. *J Pediatr Orthop* 9:338–340, 1989.
16. Oestreich AE, Prenger EC: MR demonstrates cartilaginous megaepiphyses of the hips in Kniest dysplasia of the young child. *Pediatr Radiol* 22:302–303, 1992.
17. Rimoin DL et al: Chondro-osseous pathology in the chondrodystrophies. *Clin Orthop* 114:137–152, 1976.
18. Silengo MC et al: Kniest disease with Pierre Robin syndrome and hydrocephalus. *Pediatr Radiol* 13:106–109, 1983.
19. Spranger J, Maroteaux P: Kniest disease. *Birth Defects* 10(12):50–56, 1974.
20. Spranger J et al: Kniest dysplasia is caused by dominant collagen 2 (*COL2A1*) mutations: Parental somatic mosaicism manifesting as Stickler phenotype and mild SED. *Pediatr Radiol* 24:431–435, 1994.
21. Spranger J et al: Kniest dysplasia: Dr W. Kniest, his patient, the molecular defect. *Am J Med Genet* 69:79–84, 1997.
22. Wilkin DJ et al: Small deletions in the type II collagen triple helix produce Kniest dysplasia. *Am J Med Genet* 85:105–112, 1999.
23. Winterpacht A et al: Kniest and Stickler dysplasia phenotypes caused by collagen type II gene (*COL2A1*) defect. *Nat Genet* 3:323–326, 1993.

Other Chondrodysplasias

Metaphyseal chondrodysplasia, type Rimoin-McAlister

In 1971, Rimoin and McAlister (3) reported three male sibs with short-limbed dwarfism, metaphyseal dysostosis, mild mental retardation, and conductive hearing loss.

Physical findings. Short stature, due to abbreviated limbs, was striking in all three sibs. Height was below the third centile and birth weight and length were normal. Head circumference was large (Fig. 8–16A).

Musculoskeletal system. Short stature in one sib was first noted by school authorities at registration for primary school. At that time, his 3-year-old and 1-year-old brothers were also noted to be short. Pains in the knees and genua vara were noted in late childhood in two children. Another child had unilateral genu valgum. The feet and hands were short and broad, and the fingers were loose-jointed. Scoliosis and/or lumbar lordosis were noted in two of three sibs.

Radiographically, changes were limited essentially to the metaphyses of long bones, including those of hands and feet (Fig. 8–16B). The skull was large relative to height. The vertebrae appeared proportionally small in all dimensions but were not deformed. Increased lumbar lordosis was evident in the two older brothers, one of whom had rotary scoliosis. The ribs were short and widened anteriorly and showed cupping and irregularity of the costochondral margins. Premature sternal fusion was noted. The vertical and transverse diameters of the iliac bones were decreased; the iliac wings were narrowed and their lateral margins were angulated. All long tubular bones were markedly shortened (Fig. 8–16C). The femoral neck was remarkably short, resulting in severe coxa vara (Fig. 8–16D). The greater trochanters appeared relatively

prominent. The lower limbs were bowed, and the fibula was longer than the tibia, especially distally.

The most severe changes were in the metaphyses, which were widened and irregular and had broad zones of irregular dense calcification and focal radiolucent areas. The epiphyses tended to fuse early but asymmetrically. The glenoid fossae were flattened and there was loss of the normal humeral neck angle. The distal ulnae were shortened and deformed relative to the radii. The hands and feet were short and broad. The short tubular bones of the hands were also severely abbreviated and showed marked epiphyseal-metaphyseal flaring. The phalanges were wide and, with the exception of the second and fifth distal phalanges, showed early epiphyseal fusion.

Central nervous system. IQ in the three children was estimated at about 70–80.

Ocular system. Two of three sibs wore glasses. Two had hyperopia and alternating esotropia; the other had strabismus. Anterior polar cataract was found in one.

Auditory system. Hearing difficulties were first observed at adolescence, bilateral moderate conductive hearing loss being found in the three sibs. Recurrent ear infections were noted in all three. Polytomography of the mastoid areas revealed bilateral low placement of ossicles as well as striking upward angulation of internal auditory canals.

Heredity. Autosomal or X-linked recessive inheritance is likely.

Diagnosis. Metaphyseal dysostosis sui generis is very heterogeneous. For differential diagnosis of the many other types of chondrodystrophy with metaphyseal dysostosis, the reader should consult Spranger et al. (4).

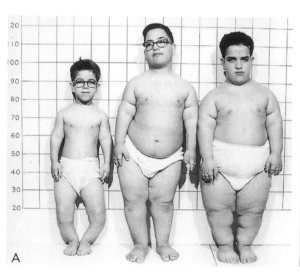
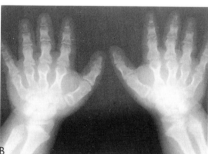
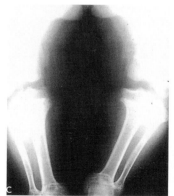
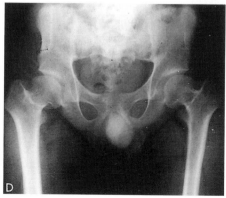

Figure 8–16. *Metaphyseal chondrodysplasia, type Rimoin-McAlister.* (A) Three brothers with short-limbed dwarfism. Note genua valga in two of the sibs. (B) Radiograph of hands showing shortened tubular bones with widened metaphyses and cone-shaped epiphyses. Note metaphyseal flaring and irregularity of radius and ulna. (C) Fibulae are relatively long distally with genua vara. Note shortening and minimal epiphyseal deformity. Metaphyses are irregular and flared. (D) Iliac wings are narrow and pelvic inlet is flattened. Note coxa vara. [(A) from DL Rimoin and WH McAlister, *Birth Defects* 7(4):116, 1971; (B–D) courtesy of DL Rimoin, Torrance, California.]

Chondrodysplasia, type Temtamy

In 1974, Temtamy et al. (5) reported a syndrome of recurrent bone fractures, short stature, failure to thrive, leukoderma, and hearing loss.

Physical findings. Failure to gain weight was noted from birth. The face was characterized by square bulging forehead, small eyes, and scanty eyebrows and eyelashes. Leukodermic patches of feathery appearance developed over the extensor surfaces of the upper and lower limbs and on the chest. Recurrent fractures of long bones following minor trauma appeared after walking commenced. The degree of bone deformity was variable, but stature was considerably shorter than the third centile.

Radiographic findings. The lower ends of long bones were widened and splayed with coarse trabeculation and pseudocyst formation. The metaphyseal margins sometimes showed irregularity; epiphyses had prominent trabecular patterning. Skeletal defects were variable in degree.

Auditory system. One of the three affected sibs reported by Temtamy et al. (5) had severe congenital hearing loss.

Heredity. Inheritance was autosomal recessive.

Diagnosis. To be ruled out are the various forms of osteogenesis imperfecta and osteogenesis imperfecta–like disorders discussed by Gorlin et al. (1).

Chondrodysplasia, type Khaldi

In 1989, Khaldi et al. (2) described a Tunisian family in which three children had an unusual osteochondroplasia, retinitis pigmentosa, and sensorineural hearing loss. An additional sib had sensorineural hearing loss but no bone dysplasia.

Musculoskeletal findings. Growth retardation was marked. Marked scoliosis and lumbar lordosis were noted from the age of 2 years (Fig. 8–17A,B). Ambulation was extremely difficult. Radiographically, there were osteoporosis, scoliosis, tall vertebral bodies, retarded bone age, dislocation of the hips, and dysplasia of the femoral heads (Fig. 8–17C,D).

Retinitis pigmentosa and marked sensorineural hearing loss were evident before the age of 2 years.

Heredity. The parents were first cousins. Inheritance is probably autosomal recessive.

References

1. Gorlin RJ et al: *Syndromes of the Head and Neck*, 4th ed. Oxford University Press, New York, 2001.
2. Khaldi F et al: Nanisme ostéochondrodysplastique, familial associé à une surdité et une hérédo-dégénérescence tapéto-rétinienne. *Arch Fr Pédiatr* 46:429–432, 1989.
3. Rimoin DL, McAlister WH: Metaphyseal dysostosis, conductive hearing loss, and mental retardation: a recessively inherited syndrome. *Birth Defects* 7(4):116–122, 1971.
4. Spranger JW et al: *Bone Dysplasias: An Atlas of Constitutional Disorders of Skeletal Development*. W.B. Saunders, Philadelphia, 1974.
5. Temtamy SA et al: A "new" bone dysplasia with autosomal recessive inheritance. *Birth Defects* 10(10):165–170, 1974.

Craniosynostoses

Apert syndrome

Apert syndrome is characterized by craniosynostosis, midfacial malformations, and symmetric syndactyly of the hands and feet, minimally involving digits 2, 3, and 4 (7). Apert (1) is credited with the discovery of the syndrome in 1906. The most exhaustive publications are those of Cohen and MacLean (7), Cohen and Kreiborg (3–6), Kreiborg and Cohen (14), and Kreiborg et al. (15,16). More than 300 cases have been reported to date.

Cohen et al. (8) calculated a birth prevalence of 15.5/1,000,000 based on 57 cases. They estimated that Apert syndrome accounted for about 4.5% of all cases of craniosynostosis.

Craniofacial findings. During infancy, there is a complete, widely gaping midline calvarial defect that extends almost from the root of the nose to the posterior fontanel via the metopic and sagittal areas and the anterior fontanel. The defect is widely patent during infancy and only gradually fills in completely during the second to third year of life. Bony islands form within the calvarial defect, grow, and coalesce until the gap is completely covered by bone. The coronal suture is fused at birth. The lambdoid suture appears to be a true suture that forms interdigitations visible on radiographs and on dry skulls, occasionally associated with wormian bones (16).

Hyperacrobrachycephaly is commonly observed, and the occiput is flattened. The forehead is steep, and during infancy a horizontal groove that disappears with age may be present above the supraorbital ridges. The cranial base is malformed and often asymmetric. The anterior cranial fossa is very short. Shallow orbits and, frequently, orbital hypertelorism are associated. The sella is enlarged, and the clivus and anterior cranial fossa are very short. The lesser sphenoidal wings slope upwardly and laterally. The greater wings of the sphenoid are protruded. The cranial base angle is variable, but platybasia occurs most commonly. Cloverleaf skull may be observed on occasion (7).

The middle third of the face is retruded and commonly hypoplastic, resulting in relative mandibular prognathism. The nasal bridge is depressed, and the nose is beaked and humped (Fig. 8–18A,B) (7).

Hypertelorism, proptosis, downslanting palpebral fissures, and, frequently, strabismus are observed (7). Albinoid findings have also been noted. Iris transillumination and depigmentation of fundus are associated with absent or diffuse foveal reflexes. Unlike classical oculocutaneous albinism, however, visual acuity is not severely impaired, and pendular nystagmus is not observed. In some patients, light hair color and pale skin are also noted (20). Optic atrophy occurs occasionally and, rarely, luxation of eye globes, congenital glaucoma, keratoconus, and ectopia lentis have been reported (7).

The ears are frequently low-set and are sometimes asymmetrically placed in frontal view.

Oral manifestations have been studied in a large series by Kreiborg and Cohen (14); findings are summarized in Table 8–2. In the relaxed state, the lips frequently assume a trapezoidal configuration because of the markedly reduced anterior upper face height. The palate is highly arched and constricted and usually has a median furrow. Lateral palatal swellings are present, which increase in size with age. These swellings have been shown to have excess mucopolysaccharide content, predominantly hyaluronic acid and, to a lesser extent, sulfated mucopolysaccharides (26). Cleft soft palate or bifid uvula is observed in 76% of cases. The hard palate is shorter than normal, but the soft palate is both longer and thicker than normal (22,23). Alterations in nasopharyngeal architecture consist of reduction in pharyngeal height, width, and depth (23).

Musculoskeletal system. A mid-digital hand mass minimally involving the second, third, and fourth fingers is always observed (7) (Fig. 8–18C). Associated synonychia is variable in degree. The first and fifth fingers may be joined to the mid-digital hand mass or may be separate. When the thumb is free, it is broad and often deviates radially. Some degree of brachydactyly involving all five fingers is usually present. The interphalangeal joints become stiff by 4 years of age (7).

Radiographically, the first metacarpal is normal. The proximal phalanx of the thumb is short, frequently narrow, and sometimes delta-shaped. The distal phalanx of the thumb is enlarged and trapezoidal in form. In approximately half the cases, only the distal phalanx is present in the thumb. The proximal ends of the fourth and fifth metacarpals

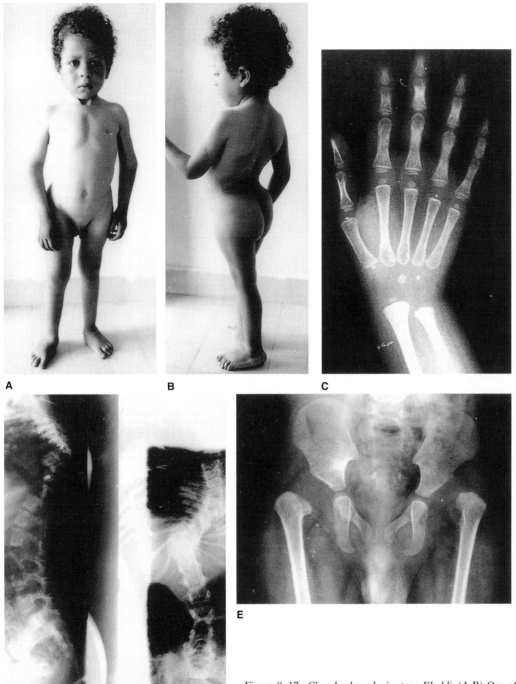

A B C

D E

Figure 8–17. *Chondrodysoplasia, type Khaldi.* (A,B) One of three children with osteodysplasia, retinitis pigmentosa, and sensorineural hearing loss. Note scoliosis and lumbar lordosis. (C) Long thin bones, osteoporosis, retarded bone age. (D) Tall vertebral bodies, rotatory scoliosis. (E) Dislocated hips, dysplastic femoral heads. [From F Khaldi et al., *Arch Fr Pédiatr* 46:429, 1989.]

are frequently fused. Symphalangism of the proximal interphalangeal joints occurs by 4–6 years of age. The distal interphalangeal joints are less frequently fused.

In the feet, syndactyly involves the second, third, and fourth toes (Fig. 8–18D). The first and fifth toes are sometimes free and sometimes joined by soft tissue union to the second and fourth toes, respectively. Toenails may be separate or partially continuous. The great toes are broad, and hallux varus is commonly observed (7).

The distal phalanx of the great toe is enlarged and trapezoidal (Fig. 8–18E). The proximal phalanx of the great toe is malformed, and the second phalanges of the second to fifth toes are often absent. The first metatarsal is broad, shortened in some instances, and may exhibit par-

tial duplication. Symphalangism, fusion of tarsal bones, six metatarsals, and other bony abnormalities may be observed in the feet (7).

Progressive calcification and fusion of the bones of hands, feet, and cervical spine occur with age in all Apert syndrome patients. Fusion of proximal interphalangeal joints is evident by 4–6 years, the fingers becoming gradually stiff.

Growth. At birth, length, weight, and head circumference tend to be above the 50th centile. Birth measurements are explained by megalencephaly, dramatically shortened cranial base, fusion of the coronal suture, and the wide calvarial midline defect, which result in a tall, wide, and large head (6) (Fig. 8–18F).

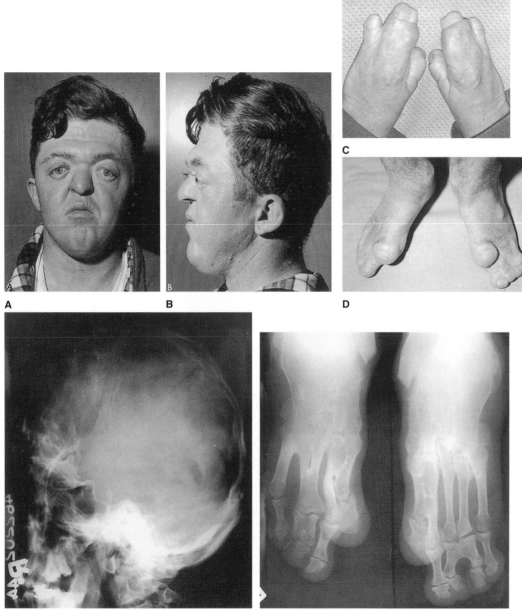

Figure 8–18. *Apert syndrome.* (A,B) Typical facies exhibiting brachycephaly, exorbitism, and midface hypoplasia. (C,D) Extensive syndactyly of both hands and feet. (E) Brachycephaly with coronal synostosis. (F) Note short halluces and synostosis of metatarsals and phalanges. [(A–D) courtesy of JM Opitz, Helena, Montana.]

The growth pattern in infancy and childhood consists of a gradual decrease in height so that most values fall between the 5th and 50th centiles. From adolescence to adulthood, the decrease in centiles becomes more pronounced. This two-step deceleration in height results primarily from rhizomelic shortening of lower limbs, and is more exaggerated in females than in males (6).

Central nervous system. A significant proportion of patients are mentally retarded (3,21). Lefebvre et al. (17) assessed 20 children with a full battery of psychometric tests. Mean IQ was 73.6 with a range of 52–89. Patton et al. (21) found that approximately half of their patients had an IQ greater than 70, although none had an IQ above 100 (n = 29). Only 7% had IQs lower than 35. Patients with normal intelligence and above average intelligence have been observed, however (10).

Cohen and Kreiborg (3) observed that nonprogressive ventriculomegaly is very common.

Other findings. Progressive generalized bony dysplasia and ankylosis with progressive limitation of motion particularly at the shoulders and to a lesser extent at the elbows have been observed (5,12). Krei-

borg et al. (15) found cervical fusions in 68% of their Apert sample (n = 68). C_5–C_6 involvement occurred most commonly. Single fusions were found in 37% and multiple fusions in 31%.

Acne vulgaris with unusual extension to the forearms may be seen in more than 70% (n = 19) of patients at adolescence and thereafter. Frank comedones and pustules occurring on the face, chest, back, and upper arms and hyperseborrhea have been documented (7,25).

Auditory system. Because of frequent mental retardation, the relatively mild congenital conductive hearing loss associated with the syndrome is sometimes ignored, although otologic and audiologic records are now routinely kept in most large craniofacial centers. Gould and Caldarelli (11) studied otologic and audiologic records in 17 patients. Serous otitis media and its sequelae were common. Stapedial footplate fixation was noted in one patient, and a dehiscent jugular bulb was seen in two cases. Bergstrom et al. (2) reported four patients with conductive hearing loss. Fixation of the stapedial footplate was found in one. Phillips and Miyamoto (24) reported three cases of conductive hearing loss with one having ankylosis of the stapedial footplate. Lindsay et al. (19) reviewed the temporal bone histologically; the stapedial footplate

Table 8–2. Apert syndrome—oral manifestations

Feature	Sample size (*n*)	Percentage
Palate		
Cleft soft palate[1]	75	41
Bifid uvula	75	35
Byzantine arch palate	68	94
Dentition		
Severely delayed eruption	19	68
Ectopic eruption[2]	54	50
Shovel-shaped incisors	56	30
Occlusion		
First molar occlusion		
Normal occlusion	53	19
Distal occlusion	53	13
Mesial occlusion	53	68
Mandibular overjet	53	81
Anterior openbite	51	73
Posterior crossbite		
Unilateral	51	22
Bilateral	51	63
Midline deviation	21	57
Maxillary crowding	23	96
Mandibular crowding	23	87

[1]Posterior part of bony palate may be notched.
[2]Maxillary molars, maxillary incisors, and maxillary premolars, in that order.
From S Kreiborg and MM Cohen Jr, *J Craniofac Genet Dev Biol* 11:7, 1992.

showed cartilaginous fixation, an incompletely developed annular ligament, and an enlarged subarcuate fossa.

Heredity. Cohen and Kreiborg (4), reviewing nine familial instances, noted autosomal dominant inheritance. In a study of 94 Apert pedigrees, Cohen and Kreiborg (3) found 93 sporadic cases, 1 familial instance, and an equal number of affected males and females. Erickson and Cohen (9) showed increased paternal age in sporadic cases. Rarity of familial instances was explained by reduced genetic fitness. Severe malformations and mental deficiency, found in many cases, greatly diminish desirability as mates.

The syndrome is due to mutations in fibroblast growth factor receptor 2 (FGFR2) at 10q23 (27). New mutations come from the male (10).

Diagnosis. Apert syndrome should be distinguished from Pfeiffer syndrome, Saethre-Chotzen syndrome, Jackson-Weiss syndrome, Crouzon syndrome, and Carpenter syndrome.

Prenatal diagnosis. Prenatal diagnosis of Apert syndrome has been reported (13,18).

Summary. Characteristics include (*1*) autosomal dominant inheritance (although nearly all cases are sporadic, representing new mutations); (*2*) craniosynostosis, resulting in hyperacrobrachycephaly; (*3*) soft tissue syndactyly and progressive synostosis of hands and feet; (*4*) midfacial hypoplasia; (*5*) hypertelorism; (*6*) frequent mental retardation; and (*7*) mild congenital conductive hearing loss.

References

1. Apert E: De l'acrocéphalosyndactylie. *Bull Soc Méd Paris* 23:1310–1330, 1906.
2. Bergstrom L et al: Otologic manifestations of acrocephalosyndactyly. *Arch Otolaryngol* 96:117–123, 1972.
3. Cohen MM Jr, Kreiborg S: The central nervous system in the Apert syndrome. *Am J Med Genet* 35:36–45, 1990.
4. Cohen MM Jr, Kreiborg S: Genetic and family study of the Apert syndrome. *J Craniofac Genet Dev Biol* 11:7–17, 1991.
5. Cohen MM Jr, Kreiborg S: Skeletal abnormalities in the Apert syndrome. *Am J Med Genet* 47:624–632, 1993.
6. Cohen MM Jr, Kreiborg S: A clinical study of the craniofacial features in Apert syndrome. *Int J Oral Maxillofac Surg* 25:45–53, 1996.
7. Cohen MM Jr, MacLean RE: *Craniosynostosis: Diagnosis, Evaluation, and Management*, 2nd ed. Oxford University Press, New York, 2000.
8. Cohen MM Jr et al: Birth prevalence study of the Apert syndrome. *Am J Med Genet* 42:655–659, 1992.
9. Erickson JD, Cohen MM Jr: A study of parental age effects on the occurrence of fresh mutations for the Apert syndrome. *Ann Hum Genet (London)* 38:89–96, 1974.
10. Gorlin RJ et al: *Syndromes of the Head and Neck,* 4th ed. Oxford University Press, New York, 2001.
11. Gould HJ, Caldarelli DD: Hearing and otopathology in Apert syndrome. *Arch Otolaryngol* 108:347–349, 1982.
12. Harris V et al: Progressive generalized bony dysplasia in Apert syndrome. *Birth Defects* 14(6B):175, 1977.
13. Hill LM et al: The ultrasound detection of Apert syndrome. *J Ultrasound Med* 6:601–604, 1987.
14. Kreiborg S, Cohen MM Jr: The oral manifestations of Apert syndrome. *J Craniofac Genet Dev Biol* 12:41–48, 1992.
15. Kreiborg S et al: Cervical spine in the Apert syndrome. *Am J Med Genet* 43:704–708, 1992.
16. Kreiborg S et al: Comparative 3-dimensional analysis of CT-scans of the calvaria and cranial base in Apert and Crouzon syndromes. *J Craniofac Maxillofac Surg* 21:181–188, 1993.
17. Lefebvre A et al: A psychiatric profile before and after reconstructive surgery in children with Apert's syndrome. *Br J Plast Surg* 39:510–513, 1986.
18. Leonard CO et al: Prenatal fetoscopic diagnosis of the Apert syndrome. *Am J Med Genet* 11:5–9, 1982.
19. Lindsay JR et al: Acrocephalosyndactyly (Apert's syndrome): temporal bone findings. *Ann Otol Rhinol Laryngol* 84:174–178, 1975.
20. Margolis S et al: Depigmentation of hair, skin, and eyes associated with the Apert syndrome. *Birth Defects* 14(6B):341–360, 1978.
21. Patton MA et al: Intellectual development in Apert's syndrome: a long-term follow-up of 29 patients. *Am J Med Genet* 25:164–167, 1988.
22. Peterson SJ, Pruzansky S: Palatal anomalies in the syndromes of Apert and Crouzon. *Cleft Palate J* 11:394–403, 1974.
23. Peterson-Falzone SJ et al: Nasopharyngeal dysmorphology in the syndromes of Apert and Crouzon. *Cleft Palate J* 18:237–250, 1981.
24. Phillips SG, Miyamoto RT: Congenital conductive hearing loss in Apert syndrome. *Otolaryngol Head Neck Surg* 95:429–433, 1986.
25. Solomon LM et al: Pilosebaceous abnormalities in Apert type acrocephalosyndactyly. *Birth Defects* 7(8):193–195, 1971.
26. Solomon LM et al: Apert syndrome and palatal mucopolysaccharides. *Teratology* 8:287–292, 1973.
27. Wilkie AOM et al: Apert syndrome results from localized mutations of *FGFR2* and is allelic to Crouzon syndrome. *Nat Genet* 9:1650–172, 1995.

Crouzon syndrome (craniofacial dysostosis)

Crouzon syndrome, characterized by craniosynostosis, maxillary hypoplasia, shallow orbits, and ocular proptosis, was first described by Crouzon (10) in 1912, and 86 published cases were reviewed by Atkinson (3) by 1937. Numerous other publications have since appeared, the most complete study being the monograph of Kreiborg (17) in which he analyzed 61 cases. Cohen and MacLean (8) provided an exhaustive review in 2000.

Variability in expression characterizes Crouzon syndrome. Nowhere is this more apparent than in the pedigree reported by Shiller (30). The proband, the most severely affected member of the family, presented with cloverleaf skull. Several sibs manifested classic Crouzon syndrome. The affected mother and various other members of the family exhibited ocular proptosis and midface deficiency without craniosynostosis.

Craniofacial findings. Cranial malformation in Crouzon syndrome depends on the order and rate of progression of sutural synostosis. Brachycephaly is most commonly observed, but scaphocephaly, trigonocephaly, and, as already indicated, cloverleaf skull may be observed. The calvaria and base of infants with Crouzon syndrome are discussed by Kreiborg et al. (22). Craniosynostosis commonly begins very early and is usually complete by 2–3 years of age. The pattern is entirely different from that observed in Apert syndrome. Occasionally, no sutural involvement may be noted. Shallow orbits with ocular proptosis are an essential diagnostic feature. Diagnosis may be evident at birth or during the first year of life. On occasion, the phenotypic features of Crouzon syndrome may be absent and evolve gradually during the first few years of life. Various sutures may be prematurely synostosed, and multiple sutural involvement is found eventually in most cases. Increased digital markings on skull radiographs are common (8,17). An extensive anthropometric study of the skull and face of 61 patients was carried out by Kolar et al. (16).

Ocular proptosis, a constant feature, is secondary to shallow orbits and results in a high frequency of exposure conjunctivitis or keratitis (Fig. 8–19). Luxation of eyeglobes has been observed occasionally. Exotropia is an extremely common finding (8,17). Poor vision occurs in approximately 46%, with optic atrophy found in 22% and blindness in 7% (17). Low-frequency findings include nystagmus, iris coloboma, aniridia, anisocoria, corectopia, microcornea, megalocornea, keratoconus, cataract, ectopia lentis, blue sclera, and glaucoma (3,8,17).

Approximately 50% of patients have lateral palatal swellings but in only a few instances are they large enough to produce the median palatal pseudocleft appearance found so frequently in Apert syndrome (17,24). Cleft lip and cleft palate rarely occur (17). Because of maxillary hypoplasia in Crouzon syndrome, the anteroposterior dimension of the maxillary dental arch is shortened. Dental arch width is also reduced, and the constricted arch gives the appearance of highly arched palate, although palatal height is normal by measurement. Unilateral or bilateral posterior crossbite is evident in two-thirds of Crouzon syndrome patients. Crowding of maxillary teeth is common, and ectopic eruption of maxillary first molars occurs in approximately 47%. Anterior openbite, mandibular overjet, and crowding of mandibular anterior teeth are also commonly observed (18,21). Aplasia of single teeth (or rarely more), shovel-shaped maxillary incisors, and abnormal premolar morphology have been observed with the same low frequency found in the general population (17,24,25).

Central nervous system. In Kreiborg's (17) material, frequent headaches were found in 29% of patients. Seizures occurred in 12%, and marked mental deficiency was found in only 3%. The association of progressive hydrocephaly is rare (8,14).

Other findings. Deviation of the nasal septum was observed in 33% of Kreiborg's series (17). Calcification of the stylohyoid ligament was especially common, being found in 88%. Cervical fusion occurred in 25%, with single fusions in 20% and multiple fusions in only 5%. C_2–C_3 involvement was extremely common (2,17). Minor anomalies of the hand bones have been noted (1). Cartilaginous sleeve abnormalities of the trachea have occurred in some instances (11,12,28).

Acanthosis nigricans has been observed in association with Crouzon-like syndrome by Suslak (31), Reddy (26), and Breitbart et al. (6). This has been termed "Crouzono-dermo-skeletal dysplasia." It maps to 4p16.3 and not to 10q23, the locus for Crouzon syndrome (vide infra, see Heredity) (8,15).

Cementomas were observed in the patient reported by Suslak (31). This has since been confirmed.

Auditory system. Conductive hearing loss was found in 55% ($n = 49$) and atresia of the external auditory canals in 13% ($n = 53$) in Kreiborg's series (17). Corey et al. (9) noted similar figures. On tomographic study, Schurmans and Hariga (29), observed deformity of the acoustic meatus. Radiographs have shown well-developed labyrinths. The elegant tomographic studies by Terrahe (32) of the temporal bones showed outward rotation of petrous pyramids secondary to cranial base dysplasia and resulting in obliquity of the ear canals, atypical course of facial nerve, and hyperostosis. Terrahe emphasized that the primary changes were ossicular fixation with intratympanic bony masses, ossicular anomalies, and closure of the oval window.

Temporal bone study has shown stenosis or atresia of the external auditory canal as well as absence of the drum, deformity of the stapes and bony fusion to the promontory, ankylosis of the malleus to the outer wall of the epitympanum, distortion, and narrowing of the middle ear and mastoid air spaces. Baldwin (5) also found the periosteal portion of the labyrinth to be underdeveloped. The malleus and incus were ankylosed to the lateral wall of the epitympanic recess, and the crura of the stapes were oblique to the footplate with the incudostapedial joint in contact with the promontory. Either the round window or the oval window or both were narrower than normal. The tympanic membrane was missing.

Vestibular system. Aubrey (4) described a normal vestibular system.

Heredity. Crouzon syndrome has autosomal dominant transmission with variable expression (3,10,17,20). In Atkinson's review (3), 67% of the cases were familial and 33% were sporadic, representing fresh mutations. In Kreiborg's monograph (17), 44% were familial and 56% occurred sporadically. Over 30 mutations have been found in the *FGFR2* gene on 10q23. Spontaneous mutations are of paternal origin (13,15). Rollnick et al. (27), Kreiborg and Cohen (19), and Navarette et al. (23) reported examples of germinal mosaicism. In Kreiborg's (17) study, increased paternal age at the time of conception was a statistically significant factor in new mutations. Birth prevalence is 15.5/1,000,000. Its occurrence among all cases of craniosynostosis is 4.5%. Direct and indirect estimates of birth prevalence give similar results (7).

Diagnosis. Crouzon syndrome should be distinguished from simple craniosynostosis, Crouzono-dermo-skeletal syndrome, Apert syndrome, Pfeiffer syndrome, Saethre-Chotzen syndrome, and Jackson-Weiss syndrome.

Summary. Characteristics include (*1*) autosomal dominant inheritance; (*2*) premature variable craniosynostosis; (*3*) ocular hypertelorism, midface hypoplasia, and ocular proptosis; (*4*) relative mandibular prognathism; (*5*) atresia of auditory canals in about 15%; and (*6*) conductive hearing loss in about 50%.

Figure 8–19. *Crouzon syndrome (craniofacial dysostosis).* (A,B) Note mild ocular hypertelorism, proptosis of globes, and midfacial hypoplasia with relative mandibular prognathism. [Courtesy of P Tessier, Paris, France.]

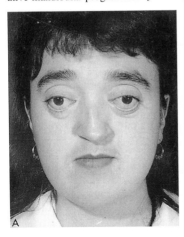 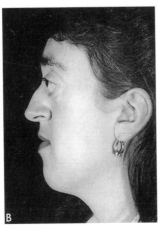

References

1. Anderson PJ et al: Hand anomalies in Crouzon syndrome. *Skeletal Radiol* 26:113–115, 1997.
2. Anderson PJ et al: The cervical spine in Crouzon syndrome. *Spine* 22:402–405, 1997.
3. Atkinson FRB: Hereditary craniofacial dysostosis, or Crouzon's disease. *Med Press Circular* 195:118–124, 1937.
4. Aubrey M: Examen otologique de 10 cas de dysostose cranio-faciale de Crouzon. *Rev Neurol* 63:302–305, 1935.
5. Baldwin JL: Dysostosis craniofacialis of Crouzon. *Laryngoscope* 78:1660–1676, 1968.

6. Breitbart AS et al: Crouzon's syndrome associated with acanthosis nigricans. Ramifications for the craniofacial surgeon. *Ann Plast Surg* 22:310–315, 1989.

7. Cohen MM Jr, Kreiborg S: Birth prevalence studies of the Crouzon syndrome: comparison of direct and indirect methods. *Clin Genet* 41:12–15, 1992.

8. Cohen MM Jr, MacLean RE: *Craniosynostosis: Diagnosis, Evaluation, and Management*, 2nd ed. Oxford University Press, New York, 2000.

9. Corey JP et al: Otopathology in cranial facial dysostosis. *Am J Otol* 8:14–17, 1987.

10. Crouzon O: Dysostose cranio-faciale héréditaire. *Bull Soc Méd Hôp Paris* 33:545–555, 1912.

11. Davis S et al: Tracheal cartilagenous sleeve. *Pediatr Pathol* 12;349–364, 1992.

12. Devine P et al: Completely cartilaginous trachea in a child with Crouzon syndrome. *Am J Dis Child* 138:140–143, 1984.

13. Glaser RL et al: Paternal origin of *FGF22* mutations in sporadic cases of Crouzon and Pfeiffer syndrome. *Am J Hum Genet* 66:768–777, 2000.

14. Golabi M et al: Radiographic abnormalities of Crouzon syndrome. A survey of 23 cases. *Proc Greenwood Genet Ctr* 3:102, 1984.

15. Jabs E et al: Jackson-Weiss and Crouzon syndromes are allelic with mutations in fibroblast growth factor receptor 2. *Nat Genet* 3:275–279, 1995.

16. Kolar JC et al: Patterns of dysmorphology in Crouzon syndrome: an anthropometric study. *Cleft Palate J* 25:235–244, 1988.

17. Kreiborg S: Crouzon syndrome. *Scand J Plast Reconstr Surg Suppl* 18:1–198, 1981.

18. Kreiborg S: Craniofacial growth in plagiocephaly and Crouzon syndrome. *Scand J Plast Reconstr Surg* 15:187–197, 1981.

19. Kreiborg S, Cohen MM Jr: Germinal mosaicism in Crouzon syndrome. *Hum Genet* 84:487–488, 1990.

20. Kreiborg S: Variable expressivity of Crouzon's syndrome within a family. *Scand J Dent Res* 85:175–184, 1977.

21. Kreiborg S, Pruzansky S: Craniofacial growth in premature craniofacial synostosis. *Scand J Plast Reconstr Surg* 15:171–186, 1981.

22. Kreiborg S et al: Comparative 3-dimensional analysis of CT-scans of the calvaria and cranial base in Apert and Crouzon syndromes. *J Craniofac Maxillofac Surg* 21:181–188, 1993.

23. Navarette C et al: Germinal mosaicism in Crouzon syndrome. *Clin Genet* 40:29–34, 1991.

24. Peterson SJ, Pruzansky S: Palatal anomalies in the syndromes of Apert and Crouzon. *Cleft Palate J* 11:394–403, 1974.

25. Peterson-Falzone SJ et al: Nasopharyngeal dysmorphology in the syndromes of Apert and Crouzon. *Cleft Palate J* 18:237–250, 1981.

26. Reddy BSN: An unusual association of acanthosis nigricans and Crouzon's disease. *J Dermatol* 12:85–90, 1985.

27. Rollnick BR et al: Germinal mosaicism in Crouzon syndrome. *Clin Genet* 33:145–150, 1988.

28. Sagehashi N: An infant with Crouzon syndrome with a cartilaginous trachea and a human tail. *J Craniomaxillofac Surg* 20:21–23, 1992.

29. Schurmans P, Hariga J: Dysostose crâniofaciale familiale et malformations nerveuses associées. *Acta Neurol Belg* 63:794–820, 1963.

30. Shiller JG: Craniofacial dysostosis of Crouzon: a case report and pedigree with emphasis on heredity. *Pediatrics* 23:107–112, 1959.

31. Suslak E: Crouzon's craniofacial dysostosis, periapical cemental dysplasia, and acanthosis nigricans: the pleiotropic effect of a single gene? Presented at the Society of Craniofacial Genetics, Denver, June 17, 1984.

32. Terrahe K: Das Gehörorgan bie den kraniofazialen Missbildungssyndromen nach Crouzon und Apert. *Z Laryngol Rhinol* 50:794–802, 1971.

Pfeiffer syndrome

In 1964, Pfeiffer (23) described a syndrome consisting of craniosynostosis, broad thumbs, broad great toes, and variable partial soft tissue syndactyly of the hands in eight affected individuals in three generations. There have been several fine reviews (3,4,19,24,25,27).

Sporadic examples of Pfeiffer syndrome have been reported (3–5,14). The most exhaustive reviews are those of Cohen (3,4). Cohen and MacLean (4) discussed three subtypes of Pfeiffer syndrome with prognostic significance. These are summarized in Table 8–3. These do not correspond to mutations in different genes, but are divisions based on clinical grounds.

Craniofacial findings. The skull in type 1 is usually turribrachycephalic. Craniofacial asymmetry may be present in some instances. Cloverleaf skull is a hallmark of type 2. Maxillary hypoplasia and relative mandibular prognathism are observed. The nasal bridge is depressed. Hypertelorism, downslanting palpebral fissures, ocular proptosis, and strabismus are common (4,16,29). The nose may be beaked (Fig. 8–20A,B). The palate is highly arched, the alveolar ridges are broad, and teeth are crowded (4). Some affected individuals are fair and have prominent veins. Natal teeth may be seen in type 3 (1).

Central nervous system. In type 1 Pfeiffer syndrome, intelligence is usually normal (4,16,23), but mental deficiency has been observed in a number of cases (4). Progressive hydrocephalus, distortive ventriculomegaly, Arnold-Chiari malformation, and seizures have been noted (18,29). Association with cloverleaf skull anomaly is seen in type 2 (9,12,33). Although children with type 3 usually have early demise (3,4), Robin et al. (27) described seven children with type 3 and survival into childhood who had moderate to no intellectual impairment. All cases of type 2 or 3 to date have been sporadic, and none has occurred within an affected family. Various other anomalies, not usually found with the usual form of Pfeiffer syndrome, may be observed in Pfeiffer cloverleaf patients. Mental development is generally poor, and early demise during infancy is common, even when extensive craniofacial surgery is performed (4).

Hands and feet. The thumbs and great toes are usually broad and usually with varus deformity (10,11,23) (Fig. 8–20C). Mild soft tissue syndactyly may especially involve digits 2 and 3 and sometimes digits 3 and 4 of both hands and feet (4,23). Partial soft tissue syndactyly between toes 1 and 2 has also been reported (4,35). Brachydactyly may be observed and, in some cases, syndactyly is absent (4). Clinodactyly has also been noted (4,29).

Brachymesophalangy of both hands and feet is frequently present. Middle phalanges may be absent in some cases. The distal phalanx of the great toe is broad, and the proximal phalanx malformed. The first metatarsal is broad, may be shortened, and may be partially duplicated in some instances (4,16,23).

Accessory epiphyses in the first and second metatarsals and double ossification centers in the proximal phalanx of the great toe have been

Table 8–3. Clinical subtypes of Pfeiffer syndrome

Type	Major characteristics	Other anomalies	Life span	Inheritance pattern
Type 1	Craniosynostosis, midface deficiency, broad thumbs, broad great toes, brachydactyly, variable syndactyly	Various low-frequency anomalies (e.g., cervical vertebral anomalies)	Compatible with life	Autosomal dominant
Type 2	Cloverleaf skull, severe ocular proptosis, broad thumbs, broad great toes, brachydactyly, variable syndactyly	Elbow ankylosis/synostosis,[1] clusters of unusual anomalies	Usually early demise	Sporadic to date
Type 3	Craniosynostosis, severe ocular proptosis, broad thumbs, broad great toes, brachydactyly, variable syndactyly	Clusters of unusual anomalies	Usually early demise	Sporadic to date

[1]Early ankylosis is characteristic of type 2 but may also be observed with some frequency in type 3 and occasionally in type 1.
From MM Cohen Jr, *Am J Med Genet* 45:300, 1993.

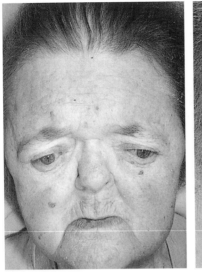
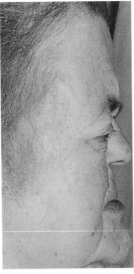

A   B

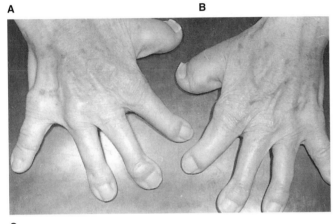

C

Figure 8–20. *Pfeiffer syndrome.* (A,B) Hypertelorism, downslanting palpebral fissures, and midface deficiency. (C) Broad radially deviated thumbs, brachydactyly, and clinodactyly of terminal phalanges.

reported. Partial duplication of the great toe may be observed occasionally. Symphalangism of both hands and feet has been reported. Fusion of carpals and tarsals, in some instances involving the proximal ends of the metacarpals and metatarsals, respectively, has also been noted (4,16,35).

Other findings. Fused cervical vertebrae and lumbar vertebrae have been described (20). Shortened humerus, cubitus valgus, radiohumeral and radioulnar synostosis, abnormalities of the pelvis, coxa valga, and talipes calcaneovarus have been reported occasionally (4,16,29). Low-frequency abnormalities have included pyloric stenosis, umbilical hernia, malpositioned anus at the scrotal base, bifid scrotum, widely spaced nipples, ptosis of eyelids, corectopia, scleralization of the cornea, optic nerve hypoplasia, choanal atresia, preauricular tag, bifid uvula, supernumerary teeth, gingival hypertrophy, and craniolacunae noted on 30 CT (4,16,29,34).

Auditory system. Hearing loss has been noted in some cases (6,15,16). Fixation of the ossicular chain has included fusion of the incus to the epitympanum and ankylosis of the stapes (5). The auditory canals have been absent in one Pfeiffer cloverleaf case (4).

Heredity. Pedigrees consistent with autosomal dominant transmission were noted by several authors (16,26,29,35). Penetrance has been complete, and expressivity has been markedly variable, particularly with

respect to the presence or absence of soft tissue syndactyly (30). Rarely, the thumbs are normal (2,28). Pfeiffer syndrome is heterogeneous, with mutations in *FGFR1* (21) and *FGFR2* (13,32) described. *FGFR2* mutations can also cause Pfeiffer syndromes 2 (24,31) and 3 (8) and Crouzon and Jackson-Weiss syndromes (17). New mutations are usually paternal in origin (7).

Diagnosis. Pfeiffer syndrome should be distinguished from Apert syndrome, Crouzon syndrome, Saethre-Chotzen syndrome, and Jackson-Weiss syndrome.

Summary. Characteristics include (*1*) autosomal dominant inheritance; (*2*) craniosynostosis; (*3*) broad thumbs and great toes; (*4*) variable syndactyly; and (*5*) occasional conductive hearing loss.

References

1. Alvarez MP et al: Natal molars in Pfeiffer syndrome type 3. *J Clin Pediatr Dent* 18:21–24, 1993.
2. Baraitser M et al: Pitfalls of genetic counseling in Pfeiffer syndrome. *J Med Genet* 17:250–256, 1980.
3. Cohen MM Jr: Pfeiffer syndrome update, clinical subtypes, and guidelines for differential diagnosis. *Am J Med Genet* 45:300–307, 1993.
4. Cohen MM Jr, MacLean RE: *Craniosynostosis: Diagnosis, Evaluation, and Management,* 2nd ed. Oxford University Press, New York, 2000.
5. Cornejo-Roldan LR et al: Analysis of the mutational spectrum of the *FGFR2* gene in Pfeiffer syndrome. *Hum Genet* 104:425–431, 1999.
6. Cremers CWRJ: Hearing loss in Pfeiffer's syndrome. *Int J Pediatr Otorhinolaryngol* 3:343–353, 1987.
7. Glaser R et al: Paternal origin of *FGFR2* mutations in sporadic cases of Crouzon syndrome and Pfeiffer syndrome. *Am J Hum Genet* 66:768–777, 2000.
8. Gripp KW et al: The phenotype of the fibroblast growth factor receptor 2 Ser 351 Cys mutation: Pfeiffer syndrome type 3. *Am J Med Genet* 78:356–360, 1998.
9. Hodach RJ et al: Studies of malformation syndromes in man. XXXVI: the Pfeiffer syndrome, association with Kleeblattschädel and multiple visceral anomalies. Case report and review. *Z Kinderheilkd* 119:87–103, 1975.
10. Kerr NC et al: Brief clinical report: type 3 Pfeiffer syndrome with normal thumbs. *Am J Med Genet* 66:138–143, 1996.
11. Kreiborg S, Cohen MM Jr: A severe case of Pfeiffer syndrome associated with stub thumb on the maternal side of the family. *J Craniofac Genet Dev Biol* 13:73–75, 1993.
12. Kroczek RA et al: Cloverleaf skull associated with Pfeiffer syndrome: pathology and management. *Eur J Pediatr* 145:442–445, 1986.
13. Lajeunie E et al: *FGFR2* mutations in Pfeiffer syndrome. *Nat Genet* 9:108, 1995.
14. Lenz W: Zur Diagnose und Ätiologie der Akrocephalosyndaktylie. *Z Kinderheilkd* 79:546–558, 1957.
15. Manns KJ, Bopp KP: Dysostosis craniofacialis Crouzon mit digitaler Anomalie. *Med Klin* 60:1899–1903, 1971.
16. Martsolf JT et al: Pfeiffer syndrome. *Am J Dis Child* 121:257–262, 1971.
17. Meyers GA et al: *FGFR2* exon IIIa and IIIc mutations in Crouzon, Jackson-Weiss, and Pfeiffer syndromes: evidence for missense changes, insertions, and a deletion due to alternative RNA splicing. *Am J Hum Genet* 58:491–498, 1996.
18. Moore MH, Hanieh A: Hydrocephalus in Pfeiffer syndrome. *J Clin Neurosci* 1:202–204, 1994.
19. Moore MH et al: Pfeiffer syndrome: a clinical review. *Cleft Palate Craniofac J* 32:62–70, 1995.
20. Moore MH et al: Spinal anomalies in Pfeiffer syndrome. *Cleft Palate Craniofac J* 32:251–254, 1995.
21. Muenke M et al: A common mutation in the fibroblast growth factor receptor 1 gene in Pfeiffer syndrome. *Nat Genet* 8:269–274, 1994.
22. Passos-Bueno MR et al: Pfeiffer mutation in an Apert patient: how wide is the spectrum of variability due to mutations in the *FGFR2* gene? *Am J Med Genet* 71:243–247, 1997.
23. Pfeiffer RA: Dominant erbliche Akrocephalosyndaktylie. *Z Kinderheilkd* 90:301–320, 1964.
24. Plomp AS et al: Pfeiffer syndrome type 2: further delineation and review of the literature. *Am J Med Genet* 75:245–251, 1998.
25. Rasmussen SA, Frias JL: Mild expression of the Pfeiffer syndrome. *Clin Genet* 33:5–10, 1988.
26. Robin NH et al: Linkage of Pfeiffer syndrome to chromosome 8 centromere and evidence for genetic heterogeneity. *Hum Mol Genet* 3:2153–2158, 1994.

27. Robin NH et al: Favorable prognosis for children with Pfeiffer syndrome types 2 and 3: implications for classification. *Am J Med Genet* 75:240–244, 1998.

28. Rutland P et al: Identical mutations in the *FGFR2* gene cause both Pfeiffer and Crouzon phenotypes. *Nat Genet* 9:173–176, 1995.

29. Saldino RM et al: Familial acrocephalosyndactyly (Pfeiffer syndrome). *AJR Am J Roentgenol* 116:609–622, 1972.

30. Sanchez JM, De Negrotti TC: Variable expression in Pfeiffer syndrome. *J Med Genet* 18:73–75, 1981.

31. Schaefer F et al: Novel mutation in the *FGFR2* gene at the same codon as the Crouzon syndrome mutations in a severe Pfeiffer syndrome type 2 case. *Am J Med Genet* 75:252–255, 1998.

32. Schell U et al: Mutations in *FGFR1* and *FGFR2* cause familial and sporadic Pfeiffer syndrome. *Hum Mol Genet* 4:323–328, 1995.

33. Soekarman D et al: Pfeiffer acrocephalosyndactyly syndrome in mother and son with cloverleaf skull anomaly in the child. *Genet Couns* 3:217–220, 1992.

34. Steinberger D et al: Mutation of *FGFR2* (cys278phe) in craniolacunia and pansynostosis. *J Med Genet* 36:499–500, 1999.

35. Zippel H, Schuler KH: Dominant vererbte Akrozephalosyndaktylie (ACS). *Fortschr Röntgenstr* 110:2340–2345, 1969.

Saethre-Chotzen syndrome

Saethre-Chotzen syndrome is characterized by a broad and variable pattern of malformations, including craniosynostosis, low-set frontal hairline, facial asymmetry, ptosis of eyelids, deviated nasal septum, brachydactyly, partial cutaneous syndactyly (especially of the second and third fingers), and various skeletal anomalies.

First recognized as an entity by Saethre (28) in 1931 and by Chotzen (5) in 1932, many authors have since reported affected families and sporadic cases (1,2,4,10,13,15,17,22,23,30). The most extensive discussions of early cases have been published by Pantke et al. (20), Cohen (6,7), and Cohen and MacLean (8).

Craniofacial findings. Craniosynostosis is a facultative rather than an obligatory abnormality. When present, the time of onset and degree of craniosynostosis are quite variable. Brachycephaly or acrocephaly with coronal sutural synostosis is frequently observed, and involvement is often asymmetric, producing plagiocephaly and facial asymmetry. Trigonocephaly has also been observed (15). Frontal bossing, parietal bossing, and flattened occiput have been reported in various cases. Large late-closing fontanels, large parietal foramina, ossification defects of the calvaria, and enlargement of the sella turcica have also been recorded. Calvarial hyperostosis was noted (1,5,6,13,15,20).

Low-set frontal hairline is commonly observed. Ptosis of eyelids, hypertelorism, and strabismus are common (Fig. 8–21). Occasionally, the forehead may be protuberant in association with metopic synostosis and hypotelorism (9). Blepharophimosis is evident in some cases. Tear duct stenosis may be a feature. Low-frequency findings have included epicanthic folds, optic atrophy, downslanting palpebral fissures, irregular eyelid margins, and sparse eyebrows medially with heavy eyebrows laterally (5,6,13,20).

The nasofrontal angle may be flattened in some instances. Maxillary hypoplasia with relative mandibular prognathism may be evident. The midface may be broad and flat in some cases. The nose is often beaked, and deviation of the nasal septum is common (6,13,20).

Oral anomalies include narrow or highly arched palate, occasional cleft palate, malocclusion, supernumerary teeth, enamel hypoplasia, and other dental defects (6,13,20).

Central nervous system. Intelligence is usually normal (20), but mild to moderate mental retardation has been observed in a number of cases (5). Significant learning difficulties have been observed in those with deletions (16). Neonatal seizures, epilepsy, and schizophrenia have also been noted (5,28).

Musculoskeletal system. Some degree of brachydactyly may be observed (6,20). Partial cutaneous syndactyly is present in some instances, most frequently between the second and third fingers, but sometimes extending from the second to fourth fingers (8,20,28) (Fig. 8–21D,E). Clinodactyly, especially of the fifth finger, has been found occasionally (1,13). The distal phalanges may be hypoplastic, and,

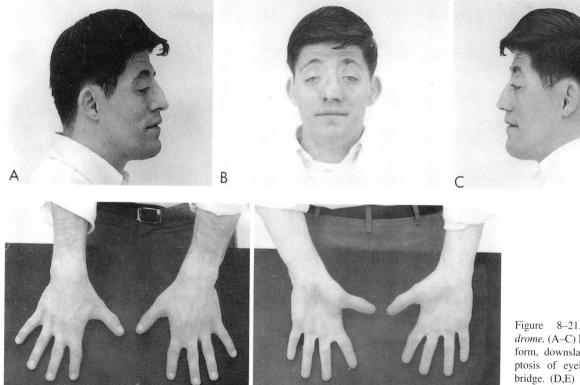

Figure 8–21. *Saethre-Chotzen syndrome.* (A–C) Note brachycephalic head form, downslanting palpebral fissures, ptosis of eyelids, and unusual nasal bridge. (D,E) Webbing between index and middle fingers. [From S Kreiborg et al., *Teratology* 6:287, 1972.]

rarely, finger-like thumbs have been noted (13). Radiographic changes in the hands have been discussed by Anderson et al (2). Dermatoglyphic findings have included single palmar creases, distally placed axial triradii, an increased frequency of thenar and hypothenar patterns, an increased frequency of fingertip arch patterns, and low total ridge count (1,13,20).

Partial cutaneous syndactyly between the second and third toes, but occasionally involving other toes, has been reported (5,28). Broad great toes and hallux valgus have been noted in some instances (13,20,28).

Other findings. Short stature has been documented in some instances (13,20). Defects of the cervical and lumbar spine have been reported by several authors (5,20,28). Other findings have included cryptorchidism, renal anomalies, and congenital cardiac defects (1,8).

Auditory system. The ears may be low-set, small, posteriorly angulated, or have folded helices or prominent antihelical crura. Pantke et al. (20) reported that 15% of Saethre-Chotzen patients had mild conductive hearing loss—in some cases, unilaterally. They noted further that 11 of 22 published individuals in which audiometric examinations were carried out exhibited hearing defects. In most cases, the type and/or degree of hearing loss was not specified. However, Chotzen (5) and Ensink et al. (12) noted conductive hearing loss of moderate degree. Dolivo and Gillieron (10) reported mixed hearing loss.

Heredity. Autosomal dominant inheritance is evident with a high degree of penetrance and variable expressivity (6,7,19). Incomplete penetrance was documented by Carter et al. (4). Mutations in the *TWIST* gene localized to 7p21.2 (3,11,14,24–26) have been found. The *TWIST* gene codes for a transcription factor. A few examples of translocation have been noted (24,27,29). There may be heterogeneity (18,21). A good review of the present molecular status is that of Zackai and Stolle (31).

Diagnosis. Saethre-Chotzen syndrome is frequently confused with simple craniosynostosis. It should also be distinguished from Crouzon syndrome, Pfeiffer syndrome, Apert syndrome, muenke syndrome, and Jackson-Weiss syndrome. Because syndactyly is not an obligatory anomaly of the Saethre-Chotzen syndrome, a sporadic case without this finding can present difficulties in diagnosis.

Summary. Characteristics includes (*1*) autosomal dominant inheritance; (*2*) variable craniosynostosis; (*3*) eyelid ptosis; (*4*) facial asymmetry; (*5*) straight nasofrontal angle; (*6*) brachydactyly and occasional mild syndactyly; and (*7*) occasional conductive hearing loss.

References

1. Aase JM, Smith DW: Facial asymmetry and abnormalities of palms and ears: a dominantly inherited developmental syndrome. *J Pediatr* 76:928–930, 1970.
2. Anderson PJ et al: The hands in Saethre-Chotzen syndrome. *J Craniofac Genet Dev Biol* 16:228–233, 1996.
3. Brueton LA et al: The mapping of a gene for craniosynostosis: evidence for linkage of the Saethre-Chotzen syndrome to distal chromosome 7p. *J Med Genet* 29:681–685, 1992.
4. Carter CO et al: A family study of craniosynostosis, with probable recognition of a distinct syndrome. *J Med Genet* 19:280–285, 1982.
5. Chotzen F: Eine eigenartige familiäre Entwicklungsstörung (Akrocephalosyndaktylie, Dysostosis craniofacialis und Hypertelorismus). *Monatsschr Kinderheilkd* 55:97–122, 1932.
6. Cohen MM Jr: An etiologic and nosologic overview of craniosynostosis syndromes. *Birth Defects* 11(2):137–189, 1975.
7. Cohen MM Jr: Craniosynostosis and syndromes with craniosynostosis: incidence, genetics, penetrance, variability, and new syndrome updating. *Birth Defects* 15(5B):85–89, 1979.
8. Cohen MM Jr, MacLean RE: *Craniosynostosis: Diagnosis, Evaluation, and Management,* 2nd ed. Oxford University Press, New York, 2000.
9. Cristofori G, Filippi G: Saethre-Chotzen syndrome with trigonocephaly. *Am J Med Genet* 44:611–614, 1992.
10. Dolivo G, Gillieron JD: Une famille de "Crouzon-fruste" ou "pseudo-Crouzon." *J Genet Hum* 4:88–101, 1955.
11. El Ghouzzi V et al: Saethre-Chotzen mutations cause TWIST protein degradation or impaired nuclear location. *Hum Mol Genet* 9:813–819, 2000.
12. Ensink RJH et al: Clinical records. Hearing loss in the Saethre-Chotzen syndrome. *J Laryngol Otol* 110:952–957, 1996.
13. Friedman JM et al: Saethre-Chotzen syndrome: a broad and variable pattern of skeletal malformations. *J Pediatr* 91:929–933, 1977.
14. Howard TD et al: Mutations in TWIST, a basic helix-loop-helix transcription factor, in Saethre-Chotzen syndrome. *Nat Genet* 15:36–41, 1997.
15. Hunter AGW et al: Case report: trigonocephaly and associated minor anomalies in mother and son. *J Med Genet* 13:77–79, 1976.
16. Johnson D et al: A comprehensive screen for *TWIST* mutations in patients with craniosynostosis identifies a new microdeletion syndrome of chromosome band 7p21.1. *Am J Hum Genet* 63:1282–1293, 1998.
17. Kreiborg S et al: The Saethre-Chotzen syndrome. *Teratology* 6:287–294, 1972.
18. Ma HW et al: Possible genetic heterogeneity in the Saethre-Chotzen syndrome. *Hum Genet* 98:228–232, 1996.
19. Niemann-Seyde SC et al: Saethre-Chotzen syndrome (ACS III) in four generations. *Clin Genet* 40:271–276, 1991.
20. Pantke OA et al: The Saethre-Chotzen syndrome. *Birth Defects* 11(2):190–225, 1975.
21. Paznekas WA et al: Genetic heterogeneity of Saethre-Chotzen syndrome, due to *TWIST* and *FGFR* mutations. *Am J Hum Genet* 62:1370–1380, 1998.
22. Pruzansky S et al: Roentgencephalometric studies of the premature craniofacial synostoses: report of a family with the Saethre-Chotzen syndrome. *Birth Defects* 11(2):226–237, 1975.
23. Reardon W, Winter RM: Saethre-Chotzen syndrome. *J Med Genet* 31:393–396, 1994.
24. Reardon W et al: Cytogenetic evidence that the Saethre-Chotzen gene maps to 7p21.2. *Am J Med Genet* 47:633–636, 1993.
25. Reid CS et al: Saethre-Chotzen syndrome with familial translocation at chromosome 7p22. *Am J Med Genet* 47:637–639, 1993.
26. Rose CSP et al: Localization of the genetic locus for Saethre-Chotzen syndrome to a 6 cM region of chromosome 7 using four cases with apparently balanced translocations at 7p21.2. *Hum Mol Genet* 3:1405–1408, 1994.
27. Rose CSP et al: The *TWIST* gene, although not disrupted in Saethre-Chotzen patients with apparently balanced translocations of 7p21, is mutated in familial and sporadic cases. *Hum Mol Genet* 6:1369–1373, 1997.
28. Saethre H: Ein Beitrag zum Turmschädelproblem (Pathogenese, Erblichkeit und Symptomologie). *Dtsch Z Nervenheilkd* 117:533–555, 1931.
29. Wilkie AOM et al: Saethre-Chotzen syndrome associated with balanced translocations involving 7p21: three further families. *J Med Genet* 32:174–180, 1995.
30. Young I, Harper PS: An unusual form of familial acrocephalosyndactyly. *J Med Genet* 19:286–288, 1982.
31. Zackai EH, Stolle CA: A new twist: some patients with Saethre-Chotzen syndrome have a microdeletion syndrome. *Am J Hum Genet* 63:1277–1281, 1998.

Chemotactic defect, craniosynostosis, short stature, and sensorineural hearing loss (Thong syndrome)

Thong et al. (3) and Thong and Simpson (2) reported a brother and sister with recurrent infections and proportionate stature below the third centile. The brother had sensorineural hearing loss. The female sib manifested coronal synostosis, an anteriorly placed ectopic anus, and congenital glaucoma, while her brother exhibited sensorineural hearing loss and an osteogenic sarcoma. Both had a narrow face, a long nose, and a small chin. Etzioni et al. (1) described a child stated to have Saethre-Chotzen syndrome with defective neutrophil chemotaxis. Perhaps they have the same disorder. There is also overlap with acrocraniofacial dysostosis.

References

1. Etzioni A et al: Saethre-Chotzen syndrome associated with defective neutrophil chemotaxis. *Acta Paediatr Scand* 79:375–379, 1990.
2. Thong YH, Simpson DA: The syndrome of abnormal neutrophil chemotaxis, unusual facies, proportionate small stature, and sensorineural deaf-mutism. *Acta Paediatr Scand* 70:575, 1981.
3. Thong YH et al: Abnormal neutrophil chemotaxis in a syndrome of unusual facies, proportionate short stature, and sensorineural deafness-mutism. *Acta Paediatr Scand* 67:383–388, 1978.

Auralcephalosyndactyly

In 1988, Kurczynski and Casperson (1) reported an autosomal dominantly inherited syndrome consisting of craniosynostosis involving the coronal suture, unusual ears shaped like question marks, and cutaneous syndactyly of the fourth and fifth toes. Legius et al. (2) questioned whether auralcephalosyndactyly was a newly recognized syndrome or a variant of Saethre-Chotzen syndrome. In our opinion, auralcephalosyndactly is a distinct entity, although the two patients reported by Legius et al. (2) represent cases of Saethre-Chotzen syndrome.

Auditory system. The family reported by Kurczynski and Casperson (1) had conductive hearing loss.

References

1. Kurczynski TW, Casperson SM: Auralcephalosyndactyly: a new hereditary craniosynostosis syndrome. *J Med Genet* 25:491–493, 1988.
2. Legius E et al: Auralcephalosyndactyly: A new craniosynostosis syndrome or a variant of the Saethre-Chotzen syndrome? *J Med Genet* 26:522–524, 1989.

Acrocephaly, limb anomalies, short stature, ear malformations with preauricular pits, and mixed hearing loss (acro-cranio-facial dysostosis)

In 1988, Kaplan et al. (5) reported two sisters with abnormal auricles and preauricular pits, mixed hearing loss, craniofacial anomalies with craniosynostosis, cleft palate, and digital anomalies.

Craniofacial findings. The first girl had hypertelorism, broad nose with high bridge and small nares, cleft palate, and micrognathia (Fig. 8–22,A,B). The second girl had acrocephaly, with tall flat forehead, wide sagittal sutures, horizontal groove above the eyebrows, and delayed closure of the anterior fontanel. She had telecanthus with downslanting palpebral fissures, marked proptosis, and ptosis. The nasal bridge was broad and beaked in profile, with anteverted nares and choanal stenosis. There was bony obstruction of the nasolacrimal duct. The philtrum was short with thickened lips. The palate had a narrow midline cleft, and there was micrognathia. Both had low-set ears with preauricular pits (Fig. 8–22A,B). The second girl had thick and overturned helices with a prominent crus of the anthelix. The external auditory canals were narrow.

Musculoskeletal system. The first child had short broad tips of thumbs, and fingers with small nails (Fig. 8–22C) and proximally placed moderately rotated halluces with relatively long second toes (Fig. 8–22D). The second child had bulbous finger tips with flat wide nails. Both great toes were proximally placed and narrow. There was bilateral metatarsus adductus.

Other findings. Both children had short stature. The first child had atrial and ventricular septal defects and transposition of great vessels. The second child had pectus excavatum and small inverted nipples. She had global developmental delay, particularly in motor function and language.

Auditory system. Auditory evoked responses in the second girl showed moderately severe, nonprogressive, bilateral sensorineural and conductive hearing loss from 8 months of age. Normal interwave latencies suggested normal brain stem conduction.

Laboratory findings. Tomography of the middle and inner ears in the second child, at 2 years and 4 months of age, showed bilaterally normal cochleas, but a malformed right malleus and incus with an underdeveloped left incus and stapes. Ultrasound studies and computed tomography (CT) scan of the brain were normal. Voiding cystourethrography demonstrated bilateral vesicoureteric reflux.

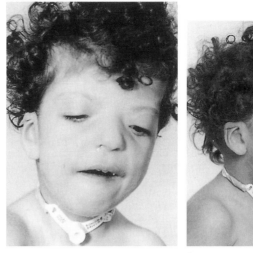
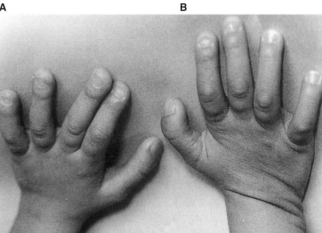
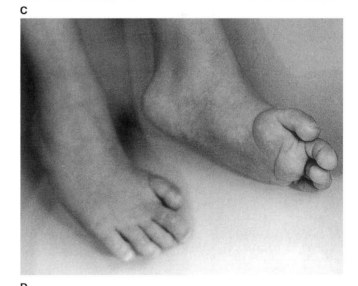

Figure 8–22. *Acro-cranio-facial dysostosis.* (A,B) One of two sisters with acrocephaly, hypertelorism, shallow orbits, ptosis, downslanting palpebral fissures, dysmorphic pinnae, cleft palate, and pectus excavatum. (C) Long thumbs, with single interphalangeal joint. (D) Rotated, abbreviated, and proximally placed halluces. [(A,B) from P Kaplan, *Am J Med Genet* 29:95, 1988; (C,D) courtesy of P Kaplan, Philadelphia, Pennsylvania.]

Radiographic findings. X-rays revealed multiple skeletal anomalies. In the first child there were 11 pairs of ribs, wide interpedicular distance of the lumbar spine, and small iliac wings. The thumbs, index, and fifth fingers had short metacarpals and distal phalanges. The first metatarsals were very short, and there was hypoplasia of the distal phalanges of the great toes. Other toes had immature middle and distal phalanges.

In the second girl, acrocephaly due to coronal synostosis was evident. The mandibular angle was increased, with a notch in the body of the mandible, underlying the tooth bud of the first molar (antegonial notching). There was widening of the interpedicular distance of the lumbar spine and increased height of vertebral bodies with posterior scalloping. The iliac wings flared with narrow supra-acetabular regions, small and steep acetabula, and bilateral coxa valga. The distal phalanges of the thumbs and first metacarpals were markedly short. There was partial duplication of the distal phalanx of the thumbs, and the metacarpophalangeal profile was abnormal. In both feet there was severe hypoplasia of the first ray, with a very small, abnormally shaped triangular first metatarsal. There was severe hypoplasia of the distal phalanges. Bone age corresponded to chronological age.

Heredity. These two girls were the only children of consanguineous parents. The mother, her sister, and three brothers had preauricular pits. Autosomal recessive inheritance is likely.

Diagnosis. The two sisters described here have a syndrome easily recognizable by 25 weeks gestation. Although differing in inheritance pattern, it has many similarities to the autosomal dominant acrofacial dysostosis syndrome reported by Reynolds et al (6). Craniosynostosis was not evident in Reynolds's family, and limb anomalies were less severe than in these two sisters.

Similar craniofacial anomalies are found in the autosomal recessive postaxial acrofacial dysostosis (Genée-Wiedemann) (3). However, these sisters did not have postaxial hypoplasia or polydactyly, or abnormalities of the middle phalanges.

Kaplan's patients also share many features with two oto-palato-digital syndrome (1,4), including external and bony ear anomalies, hypertelorism or telecanthus, cleft palate and micrognathia, proximally placed and abnormally shaped first digits of the hands and feet with short distal phalanges, conductive and sensorineural hearing loss, short stature, and psychomotor retardation. However, there are differences phenotypically, radiologically, and in the mode of inheritance. There are also similarities to Saethre-Chotzen syndrome and Pfeiffer syndrome. These patients did not have polydactyly or syndactyly, and radiologically the metacarpophalangeal pattern profile was very different from those seen in Saethre-Chotzen syndrome and Pfeiffer syndrome (2).

Prognosis. The hearing loss in this syndrome showed no evidence of progression.

Summary. The characteristics of this syndrome include (1) autosomal recessive transmission; (2) malformation of the auricles with narrow external auditory canals; (3) characteristic craniofacial anomalies, short stature, and developmental delay; and (4) moderately severe, nonprogressive, sensorineural and conductive hearing loss.

References
1. Brewster TG et al: Oto-palato-digital syndrome, type II—an X-linked skeletal dysplasia. *Am J Med Genet* 20:249–254, 1985.
2. Escobar V, Bixler D: The acrocephalosyndactyly syndromes: a metacarpophalangeal pattern profile analysis. *Clin Genet* 11:295–305, 1977.
3. Genée E: Une forme extensive de dysostose mandibulofaciale. *J Génét Hum* 17:42–52, 1969.
4. Gorlin RJ et al: *Syndromes of the Head and Neck*, 4th ed. Oxford University Press, New York, 2001.
5. Kaplan P et al: A new acro-cranio-facial dysostosis syndrome in sisters. *Am J Med Genet* 29:95–106, 1988.
6. Reynolds JF et al: A new autosomal dominant acrofacial dysostosis syndrome. *Am J Med Genet* (Suppl)2:143–150, 1986.

Aural-digital-anal syndrome

The aural-digital-anal syndrome consists of bifid and/or triphalangeal thumbs and either imperforate or anteriorly-placed anus. Coronal synostosis appears to be a variable feature. The syndrome was stated to have autosomal dominant inheritance (1), but we wonder whether these cases are examples of Townes-Brocks syndrome. There is also overlap with the syndrome of chemotactic defect, craniosynostosis, short stature, and sensorineural hearing loss.

Auditory system. Affected individuals have sensorineural hearing loss.

Reference
1. Sheffield LJ et al: Auro-digital-anal syndrome. *Pathology* 13:175–176, 1980.

Fryns craniosynostosis syndrome

In 1990, Fryns et al. (1) reported a mother and son with craniosynostosis affecting the coronal and metopic sutures; asymmetric long face with high, narrow forehead; short upper lip; and highly arched palate. Inheritance may be autosomal dominant.

Auditory system. Sensorineural hearing loss of 35–45 dB in the low and middle frequencies was present in both mother and son.

Reference
1. Fryns JP et al: Craniosynostosis and low middle frequency perceptive deafness in mother and son. A distinct entity? *Genet Couns* 1:63–66, 1990.

Gorlin-Chaudhry-Moss syndrome

In 1960, Gorlin et al. (1) described a syndrome in two female sibs that consists of craniosynostosis, midface hypoplasia, hypertrichosis, and anomalies of the eyes, teeth, heart, and external genitalia. There was no parental consanguinity. Autosomal recessive inheritance seemed likely. Other sporadic cases have been reported by Ippel et al. (2) and Preis et al. (3), who suggested this condition may be the same as Saethre-Chotzen syndrome. The condition should also be distinguished from Crouzon syndrome.

The original sibs were short and of stocky build. Both held their heads in mild anteflexion when walking. Pronounced midface hypoplasia and depressed supraorbital ridges were observed but were more pronounced in the older sib. Hypertrichosis of the scalp, arms, legs, and back was noted. The scalp hairline was lower than normal. Downslanting palpebral fissures, inability to fully open or close the eyes, upper eyelid colobomas, microphthalmia, and hyperopia were reported. The younger sib had unilateral persistence of the iridopupillary membrane (Fig. 8–23).

Oral anomalies consisted of class III malocclusion, highly arched narrow palate, hypodontia, microdontia, and abnormally shaped teeth. Other findings included patent ductus arteriosus, pronounced hypoplasia of the labia majora, and umbilical hernia.

Radiographic examination of the skull revealed premature synostosis of the coronal suture, brachycephaly, hypoplastic maxillary and nasal bones, hypertelorism, lordosis of the petrous ridges, clival hypoplasia, and elevation of the lesser sphenoidal wings.

Auditory system. Bilateral conductive hearing deficit was a feature in both sibs.

References
1. Gorlin RJ et al: Craniofacial dysostosis, patent ductus arteriosus, hypertrichosis, hypoplasia of labia majora, dental and eye anomalies. *J Pediatr* 56:778–785, 1960.
2. Ippel P et al: Craniofacial dysostosis, hypertrichosis, genital hypoplasia, ocular, dental, and digital defects. Confirmation of the Gorlin-Chaudhry-Moss syndrome. *Am J Med Genet* 44:518–522, 1992.

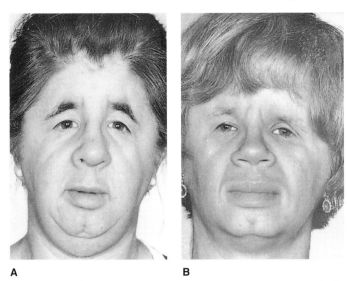

A   **B**

Figure 8–23. *Gorlin-Chaudhry-Moss syndrome.* (A,B) Note hypertrichosis, severe midface hypoplasia, eyelid ptosis, downslanting palpebral fissures, and chin dimples.

3. Preis S et al.: Gorlin-Chaudhry-Moss or Saethre-Chotzen syndrome? *Clin Genet* 47:267–269, 1995.

Hersh craniosynostosis syndrome

In 1986, Hersh et al. (1) described a syndrome in a brother and sister consisting of coronal synostosis in the brother, dolichocephaly without synostosis in the sister, and shared features including hypertelorism, flat nasal bridge, broad nasal tip, micrognathia, and sparse curly hair. There

was no evidence of syndactyly. Intellectual abilities and language skills were normal in the sister. The brother had low–average nonverbal intelligence with significant language delay and autistic-like behavior. Consanguinity was evident; the parents were first cousins. Thus, autosomal recessive inheritance seems likely.

Auditory system. The brother and sister both had sensorineural hearing deficit.

Reference

1. Hersh JH et al: Craniosynostosis, sensorineural hearing loss and craniofacial abnormalities in siblings. *Proc Greenwood Genet Ctr* 5:186, 1986.

Acral-Orofacial Syndromes

Oral-facial-digital syndrome, type I

Oral-facial-digital syndrome, type I (OFD I), first defined by Papillon-Léage and Psaume (24) in 1954, is characterized by hyperplastic frenula, multilobulated tongue, hypoplasia of nasal alar cartilages, median pseudocleft of upper lip, asymmetric cleft palate, various malformations of digits, and mild mental retardation. More than 250 cases have been recorded and there are several extensive reviews (13,16,20,21,29). Birth prevalence of about 1/50,000 has been suggested (33).

Craniofacial findings. The face is remarkably distinctive. Frontal bossing has been documented in 30% of patients. Usually there is euryopia, but in about 35%, dystopia canthorum is evident (19). Some aquiline thinning of the nose, due at least in part to hypoplasia of alar cartilages, and a pseudocleft in the midline of the upper lip are present in about 35% (Fig. 8–24A). The upper lip is usually short, and the nasal root is broad. One nostril may be smaller than the other, and there may

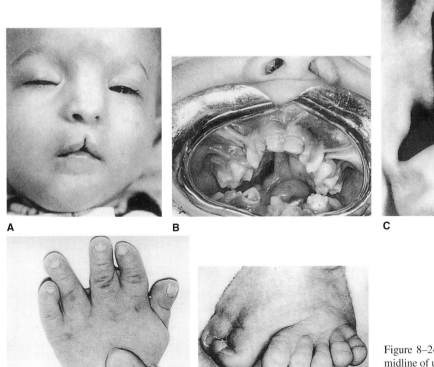

A   **B**   **C**

D   **E**

Figure 8–24. *Oral-facial-digital syndrome, type I.* (A) Pseudocleft of midline of upper lip. (B) Numerous hypertrophic frenula traversing mucobuccal folds. Asymmetric palatal cleft. (C) Transient milia. (D) Brachydactylyl and clinodactyly. (E) Pre- and postaxial polydactyly.

be flattening of the nasal tip (24). Because of zygomatic hypoplasia, the midfacial region is flattened in about 25% (21).

Oral manifestations. Most striking are the "clefts" associated with hyperplasia of frenula. There is often (in about 45% of Caucasians) a small midline "cleft" in the upper lip extending through the vermilion border. African-Americans rarely have upper midline labial clefts (26). Upon retraction of the short upper lip, a wide, thickened, or hyperplastic reduplicated frenum is seen to be associated with the pseudocleft. This, in part, eradicates the mucobuccal fold in the area. Because of these bands, complete retraction of the lip is often not possible. Thick frenula are seen in virtually all patients (13,19) (Fig. 8–24B).

The palate is cleft laterally, with deep bilateral grooves extending medially from the maxillary buccal frenula, dividing the palate into an anterior segment (containing incisors and canines) and two lateral palatal processes containing the premolars and molars. The soft palate is completely and asymmetrically cleft in at least 80% (13,21). In some persons, a large bony ridge extends from the alveolar crest medially to the midline in the canine-premolar area, somewhat resembling a misplaced torus.

Numerous thick fibrous bands are evident in the lower mucobuccal fold in 75% of cases. Cleft tongue with two lobes is seen in 30% and with three or more lobes in 45%. On the ventral surface of the tongue, between the tongue halves or lobules, a small whitish hamartomatous mass is noted in about 70% (19,21). This mass consists of fibrous connective tissue, salivary gland tissue, fat, a few striated or smooth muscle fibers, and, rarely, cartilage (21). Ankyloglossia or tongue-tie of a diffuse nature is found in at least 30% (19,21).

Malposition of the maxillary canine teeth, supernumerary maxillary deciduous canines and premolars, and infraocclusion are common. Supernumerary secondary canines, often separated by the clefts, are noted in about 20%. The canine crown form is often T-shaped. Aplasia of mandibular lateral incisors occurs in about 50% and appears to be predicated on the effect of the fibrous bands on developing tooth germs. The mandible is small or hypoplastic with a short ramus.

Integumentary system. Commonly there are evanescent milia of the face and ears (Fig. 8–24C). These usually disappear before the third year of life (28). About 65% have dryness, brittleness, and/or alopecia of scalp hair following Blaschko lines (6,17,25). A preponderance of whorls has been noted on dermatoglyphic study (8,25).

Skeletal system. Malformations of the fingers, seen in 50%–70% of patients, include clinodactyly, syndactyly, and brachydactyly of digits 2–5 (Fig. 8–24D) (8,19,25,28,29,31). Toe malformations, noted in 25%, include unilateral hallucal polysyndactyly, syndactyly, and brachydactyly (Fig. 8–24E). Bilateral polydactyly of halluces has been documented on one occasion (30). The hallux is often bent in a fibular direction, with brachydactyly and hypoplasia of the second to fifth toes. Occasionally, there is a postminimus finger or toe.

The nasion-sella-basion (cranial base) angle is increased, being about 144 degrees and exceeding the normal value of 131 degrees (SD = 4.5 degrees) by almost 3 SD (1,7,16,29) in about one-half the patients.

Radiographic examination shows the short tubular bones of the hands and feet to be irregularly short and thick. Irregular reticular pattern of radiolucency and/or spicule-like formation is observed in metacarpals and, especially, phalanges (34). Some patients have cone-shaped epiphyses in the fingers. Irregularities of long bones have also been noted (30).

Urinary system. Adult-onset bilateral polycystic kidneys, usually asymptomatic, have been reported in about 50% (5,9,19,33). In one instance (30), the kidneys were normal at 1 year; reevaluation at 11 years demonstrated bilateral polycystic kidneys. Others have found progressive renal insufficiency (4,23). We are suspicious that the infants reported to have prenatal onset polycystic kidney disease had a different disorder (22).

Central nervous system. Mild mental retardation is seen in about 40% (19,21). The IQ usually ranges from 70 to 90. Various CNS alterations have been described including hydrocephaly, hydranencephaly, pachygyria, arachnoid cysts, porencephaly, and partial agenesis of corpus callosum (5,16,18,19,28,32). These and other anomalies have been reviewed by Wood et al. (34) and Baraton (3).

Auditory system. Conductive hearing loss has been noted in some cases (8).

Laboratory aids. CAT scan and/or nuclear magnetic imaging (NMI) can be employed for brain and kidney abnormalities. Prenatal diagnosis has been made (27).

Heredity. The syndrome has X-linked dominant inheritance although 75% of cases are sporadic. It is limited to females and lethal in males (8,13,16). It has been described in a 47,XXY Klinefelter male (33). Another male has been reported (15). The gene has been mapped to Xp22.2–Xp22.3 (10,11,14) and escapes inactivation (12). It has been identified as the *CXORF5* gene (12). In the most perplexing pedigree of Vaillaud et al (31,32), the disorder appears to have been transmitted through unaffected males, a genetic pattern also noted in craniofrontonasal dysplasia.

Diagnosis. OFD I should be distinguished from OFD II and OFD IV (2). Hallucal polydactyly is a feature of many syndromes. Labiogingival frenula may be observed in Opitz trigonocephaly (C) syndrome and attachment of the lip to the gingiva is found in Ellis–van Creveld syndrome.

Summary. Characteristics include (*1*) X-linked dominant inheritance, lethal in the male; (*2*) pseudocleft in the midline of the upper lip; (*3*) mild mental retardation in about 40%; (*4*) bifid, trifid, or tetrafid tongue with hamartomata; (*5*) asymmetric cleft palate; (*6*) hyperplastic frenula, which divide the alveolar ridge; (*7*) various hand anomalies including brachydactyly, clinodactyly, and occasionally polydactyly; (*8*) adult polycystic disease of kidneys; and (*9*) occasional decreased hearing.

References

1. Aduss H, Pruzansky S: Postnatal craniofacial development in children with the OFD syndrome. *Arch Oral Biol* 9:193–203, 1954.
2. Annerén G et al: Oro-facio-digital syndromes I and II: radiological methods for diagnosis and the clinical variations. *Clin Genet* 26:178–186, 1984.
3. Baraton J: Les malformations cérébrales dans le syndrome oro-facio-digital de Papillon-Léage et Psaume. *J Radiol Électrol* 58:103–110, 1977.
4. Coll E et al: Sporadic orofaciodigital syndrome type I presenting as end-stage renal disease. *Nephrol Dial Transplant* 12:1040–1042, 1997.
5. Connacher AA et al: Orofaciodigital syndrome type I associated with polycystic kidneys and agenesis of the corpus callosum. *J Med Genet* 24:116–122, 1987.
6. del C Boente M et al: A mosaic pattern of alopecia in the oral-facial-digital syndrome type I (Papillon-Léage and Psaume syndrome). *Pediatr Dermatol* 16:367–370, 1999.
7. Dodge JA, Kernohan DC: Oral-facial-digital syndrome. *Arch Dis Child* 42:214–219, 1967.
8. Doege TC et al: Mental retardation and dermatoglyphics in a family with the oral-facial-digital syndrome. *Am J Dis Child* 116:615–622, 1968.
9. Donnai D et al: Familial orofaciodigital syndrome I presenting as adult polycystic kidney disease. *J Med Genet* 24:84–87, 1987.
10. Feather SA et al: The oral-facial-digital syndrome type 1 (OFD1), a cause of polycystic kidney disease and associated malformations, maps to Xp22.2–Xp22.3. *Hum Mol Genet* 6:1163–1167, 1997.
11. Fenton OM, Watt-Smith SR: The spectrum of the oral-facial-digital syndrome. *Br J Plast Surg* 38:532–539, 1985.
12. Ferrante MI et al: Identification of the gene for oral-facial-digital type I syndrome. *Am J Hum Genet* 68:569–576, 2001.
13. Fuhrmann W et al: Das oro-facio-digitale Syndrom. *Humangenetik* 2:133–164, 1966.
14. Gedeon AK et al: Gene localization for oral-facial-digital syndrome type 1 (OFD 1: MIM 311200) proximal to DXS85. *Am J Med Genet* 82:352–354, 1999.

15. Goodship J et al: A male with type I orofaciodigital syndrome. *J Med Genet* 28:691–694, 1991.
16. Gorlin RJ, Psaume J: Orodigitofacial dysostosis: a new syndrome. A study of 22 cases. *J Pediatr* 61:520–530, 1962.
17. Happle R et al: Wie verlaufen die Blaschko-linien am behaarten Kopf? *Hautarzt* 35:366–369, 1984.
18. Leâo MJ, Ribiero-Silva ML: Orodigitofacial syndrome type I in a patient with severe CNS defects. *Pediatr Neurol* 13:247–251, 1995.
19. Majewski F et al: Das oro-facio-digitale Syndrom. *Z Kinderheilkd* 112:89–112, 1972.
20. Martinot VL et al: Orodigitofacial syndromes types I and II: clinical and surgical studies. *Cleft Palate Craniofac J* 31:401–408, 1994.
21. Melnick M, Shields ED: Orofaciodigital syndrome, type I: a phenotypic and genetic analysis. *Oral Surg* 40:599–610, 1975.
22. Nishimura G et al: Fetal polycystic disease in oro-facio-digital syndrome type I. *Pediatr Radiol* 29:506–508, 1999.
23. Odent S et al: Central nervous system malformations and early end-stage renal disease in oro-facio-digital syndrome type I: a review. *Am J Med Genet* 75:389–394, 1998.
24. Papillon-Léage (Mme), Psaume J: Une malformation héréditaire de la musqueuse buccale et freins anormaux. *Rev Stomatol (Paris)* 55:209–227, 1954.
25. Reinwein H et al: Untersuchungen an einer Familie mit oral-facial-digital Syndrom. *Humangenetik* 2:165–177, 1966.
26. Salinas CF et al: Variability of expression of the orofaciodigital syndrome type I in black females. *Am J Med Genet* 38:574–582, 1991.
27. Shipp TD et al: Prenatal diagnosis of oral-facial-digital syndrome, type I. *J Ultrasound Med* 19:491–494, 2000.
28. Solomon L et al: Pilosebaceous dysplasia in the OFD syndrome. *Arch Dermatol* 102:598–602, 1970.
29. Stahl A, Fuhrmann W: Oro-facio-digitales Syndrom. *Dtsch Med Wochenschr* 92:1224–1228, 1968.
30. Stapleton FB et al: Cystic kidneys in a patient with oral-facial-digital syndrome, type I. *Am J Kidney Dis* 1:288–293, 1982.
31. Vaillaud JC et al: Le syndrome oro-facio-digital. Etude clinique et génétique à propos de 10 cas dans une màme famille. *Rev Pediatr* 4:383–392, 1968.
32. Vissian L, Vaillaud JC: Le syndrome oro-facio-digital. *Ann Dermatol Syphiligr (Paris)* 99:5–20, 1972.
33. Wahrman J et al: The oral-facial-digital syndrome: a male lethal condition in a boy with 47/XXY chromosome. *Pediatrics* 37:817–821, 1966.
34. Wood BP et al: Cerebral abnormalities in the oral-facial-digital syndrome. *Pediatr Radiol* 3:130–136, 1975.

Oral-facial-digital syndrome, type IV (Baraitser-Burn syndrome)

Oral-facial-digital syndrome, type IV (OFD IV) consists of oral, facial, and digital anomalies together with tibial dysplasia and/or mesomelia. About 25 cases have been reported (1–15).

Orofacial findings. Facial anomalies have included broad nasal root (11,13), broad nasal tip (5,6,12), hypertelorism or telecanthus (2,11,13), micrognathia (2,12,13), hypoplastic mandible (2), and low-set ears (2,6) (Fig. 8–25A). Numerous oral anomalies are present, including cleft lip (5,6,13), cleft or highly arched palate (2,5,6,9,12), bifid uvula (12), cleft or hypoplastic maxillary and/or mandibular alveolar ridge (2,6,12,13), oral frenulae (9), and lingual hamartoma (2,5,9,12,13). Dental anomalies are also common and generally include absent and supernumerary teeth (5,6,11–13). Goldstein and Medina (6) further described the teeth as being small and exhibiting abnormal crown and root morphology (hypertaurodontism and talonism). Absent or hypoplastic epiglottis has been found (9,13).

Central nervous system. Although intelligence has been reported as normal in several cases (11), most patients have been mentally retarded (2,4,5). We have also seen a child with OFD IV with retardation secondary to porencephaly.

Musculoskeletal system. Digital anomalies were varied, but generally present. Both pre- and postaxial polydactyly of the hands have been described (6,9); syndactyly (5,12), clinodactyly (6,11,13), and brachydactyly (11–13) can also occur (Fig. 8–25B). Preaxial poly-

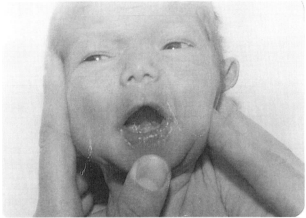

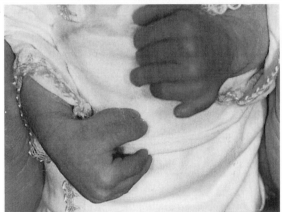

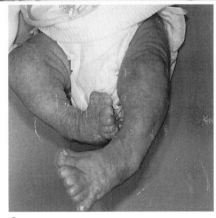

C

Figure 8–25. *OFD IV.* (A) Median pseudocleft lip and lobulated tongue, (B) bilaterally bifid thumb and polysyndactyly, (C) mesomelic shortening of the lower limb. (From Tuysuz B et al, *Genet Couns* 10:189–192, 1999. Reprinted with permission of JP Fryns, ed.)

dactyly of the feet was described as well as both pre- and postaxial polydactyly (9,13) (Fig. 8–25C).

Talipes equinovarus has also been reported (2,9,12). Mesomelia of varying degrees is present in most cases, and often the tibia is noted to be dysplastic. Several authors (2,12) observed the tibia to be short with midshaft bowing. Büttner and Eysholdt (3) and Fenton and Watt-Smith (5) reported the tibia as being pseudoarthrotic. Other tibial anomalies include proximal metaphyseal or epiphyseal flattening (2,6,12) and/or metaphyseal flaring (7,9). Forearms can also be short (11) and stature, when noted, is below the third centile (6,11,12).

The chest is sometimes small and pectus carinatum or excavatum has been noted (12–14).

Auditory system. Conductive hearing loss occurs in some patients (2,6,9,12).

Heredity. Inheritance is autosomal recessive, as affected sibs and parental consanguinity have been reported (2,6).

Diagnosis. OFD IV should be distinguished from OFD I and particularly from OFD II.

Summary. Characteristics include (*1*) autosomal recessive inheritance; (*2*) bifid tongue with hamartomata; (*3*) mild mental retardation; (*4*) various digital anomalies; (*5*) shortened tibiae; and (*6*) occasional conductive hearing loss.

References

1. Baraitser M et al: A female infant with features of Mohr and Majewski syndromes: variable expression, a genetic compound, or a distinct entity? *J Med Genet* 20:65–67, 1983.
2. Burn J et al: Orofacial digital syndrome with mesomelic limb shortening. *J Med Genet* 21:189–192, 1984.
3. Büttner A, Eysholdt KG: Die angeborenen Verbiegungen und Pseudoarthrosen des Unterschenkels (case 14). *Ergeb Chir Orthoped* 36:165–222, 1950.
4. Digilio MC et al: Joint dislocation and cerebral anomalies are consistently associated with oral-facial-digital syndrome type IV. *Clin Genet* 48:156–159, 1995.
5. Fenton OM, Watt-Smith SR: The spectrum of the oral-facial-digital syndrome. *Br J Plast Surg* 38:532–539, 1985.
6. Goldstein E, Medina JL: Mohr syndrome or OFD II: report of two cases. *J Am Dent Assoc* 89:377–382, 1974.
7. Meinecke P, Hayek H: Orofaciodigital syndrome type IV (Mohr-Majewski syndrome) with severe expression expanding the known spectrum of anomalies. *J Med Genet* 27:200–202, 1990.
8. Moerman P, Fryns JP: Oral-facial-digital syndrome type IV (Mohr-Majewski syndrome): a fetopathological study. *Genet Couns* 9:39–43, 1998.
9. Nevin NC, Thomas PS: Orofaciodigital syndrome type IV: report of a patient. *Am J Med Genet* 32:151–154, 1989.
10. Nevin NC et al: Orofaciodigital syndrome type IV. *Am J Med Genet* 43:902–904, 1992.
11. Shaw M et al: Oral facial digital syndrome—case report and review of the literature. *Br J Oral Surg* 19:142–147, 1981.
12. Sugarman GI: Orofacial defects and polysyndactyly. Syndrome identification case report 91. *J Clin Dysmorphol* 1:16–19, 1983.
13. Temtamy S, McKusick VA: The genetics of hand malformations. *Birth Defects* 14(3):434, 1978.
14. Toriello HV et al: Six patients with oral-facial-digital syndrome IV: the case for heterogeneity. *Am J Med Genet* 69:250–260, 1997.
15. Wolf H: Mediane Oberlippenspalte mit Persistenz des Frenulum tectolabiale. *Dtsch Zahnärztl Z* 7:373–379, 1952.

Oral-facial-digital syndrome, type VI (Váradi syndrome)

Oral-facial-digital syndrome, type VI (OFD VI) is characterized by hypertelorism, cleft lip/palate, hyperplastic frenulae, lingual or sublingual lumps, mental retardation, postaxial polydactyly, and a central Y-shaped metacarpal. There are numerous cases in the literature, some of which have been erroneously categorized as OFD II or Joubert syndrome with polydactyly (1,8).

Musculoskeletal system. Digital anomalies include postaxial polydactyly (rarely preaxial), clinodactyly, and syndactyly of the hands. Most striking is a central Y-shaped metacarpal (9) (Fig. 8–26). The feet usually have postaxial polydactyly.

Central nervous system. Various cerebellar defects are accompanied by severe mental retardation and absent or hypoplastic cerebellar vermis as well as variants of Dandy-Walker malformation (3). Hypothalamic hamartoma has been noted (14). Recurrent episodes of tachypnea and hyperpnea are common. Postnatal growth retardation, hypotonia, and gait disturbance are found.

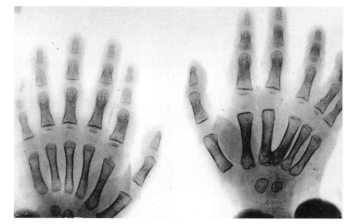

Figure 8–26. *Oral-facial-digital syndrome, type VI.* Note hexadactyly. Hand on the right shows characteristic proximal fusion of central metacarpals.

Auditory system. Several children had conductive hearing loss (6,10,11).

Heredity. Inheritance is autosomal recessive (4,5,7,10,16).

Diagnosis. Other oral-facial-digital syndromes must be excluded as well as hydrolethalus and Pallister-Hall syndrome (2,12,15). Until molecular separation of these many entities has been accomplished, they will remain a puzzle (13,15).

Summary. Characteristics include (*1*) autosomal recessive inheritance; (*2*) bifid or trifid tongue with hamartomata; (*3*) cleft palate; (*4*) digital anomalies with central Y-shaped metacarpal; (*5*) various cerebellar defects; and (*6*) occasional conductive hearing loss.

References

1. Annerén G et al: Oro-facio-digital syndromes I and II: radiologic methods for diagnosis and the clinical variations. *Clin Genet* 26:178–186, 1984.
2. Bankier A, Rose CM: Váradi syndrome or Opitz trigonocephaly: overlapping manifestations of two cousins. *Am J Med Genet* 53:85–86, 1994.
3. Doss BJ et al: Neuropathologic findings in a case of OFDS type VI (Váradi syndrome). *Am J Med Genet* 77:38–42, 1998.
4. Egger J et al: Joubert-Boltshauser syndrome with polydactyly in siblings. *J Neurol Neurosurg Psychiatry* 45:737–739, 1982.
5. Genčík A, Genčíkova A: Mohr syndrome in two sibs. *J Génét Hum* 31:307–315, 1983.
6. Gustavson KH et al: Syndrome characterized by lingual malformation, polydactyly, tachypnea, and psychomotor retardation (Mohr syndrome). *Clin Genet* 2:261–266, 1971 (same as patient 3 in ref. 1).
7. Haumont D, Pelc SC: The Mohr syndrome: are there two variants? *Clin Genet* 24:41–46, 1983.
8. Hooft C, Jongbloet P: Syndrome oro-digito-facial chez deux freres. *Arch Fr Pédiatr* 21:729–740, 1964.
9. Hsieh Y-C, Hou J-W: Oral-facial-digital syndrome with Y-shaped fourth metacarpals and endocardial cushion defect. *Am J Med Genet* 86:278–281, 1999.
10. Mattei JF, Aymé S: Syndrome of polydactyly, cleft lip, lingual hamartomas, renal hypoplasia, hearing loss, and psychomotor retardation: variant of the Mohr syndrome or a new syndrome? *J Med Genet* 20:433–435, 1983.
11. Muenke M et al: Oral-facial-digital syndrome type VI (Váradi syndrome): further clinical delineation. *Am J Med Genet* 35:360–369, 1990.
12. Muenke M et al: On lumping and splitting: a fetus with clinical findings of the oral-facial-digital syndrome, type VI, the hydrolethalus syndrome, and the Pallister-Hall syndrome. *Am J Med Genet* 41:548–556, 1991.
13. Neri G et al: Oral-facial-skeletal syndromes. *Am J Med Genet* 59:365–368, 1995.
14. Stephan MJ et al: Hypothalamic hamartoma in oral-facial-digital syndrome type VI (Váradi syndrome). *Am J Med Genet* 51:131–136, 1994.
15. Toriello HV: Heterogeneity and variability in the oral-facial-digital syndromes. *Am J Med Genet Suppl* 4:149–159, 1988.
16. Váradi V et al: Syndrome of polydactyly, cleft lip/palate or lingual lump, and psychomotor retardation in endogamic gypsies. *J Med Genet* 17:119–122, 1980.

Otopalatodigital syndrome, type I

Otopalatodigital syndrome, type I (OPD I) is characterized by distinctive facial appearance, conductive hearing loss, short stature, cleft palate, and generalized bone dysplasia (4,23). Verloes et al. (24) and Superti-Furga (21) opined that OPD I, frontometaphyseal dysplasia, and Melnick-Needles syndromes are variants of a single disorder. This has since been verified (20).

Craniofacial and orofacial findings. The face in males is characteristic (4,5,14,15) (Fig. 8–27A). An overhanging brow, prominent supraorbital ridges, and downslanting palpebral fissures are noted. Hypertelorism and broad nasal root give the patient a so-called pugilistic appearance. Slight notching may be noted at the junction between the medial third and lateral two-thirds of the upper eyelid margin in some affected males (6). The corners of the mouth are often downturned (Fig. 8–27B). Facial features in affected females are more variable and usually more mild than those in affected males. The most constant features in affected females are overhanging brow, hyperteloric appearance, prominent lateral supraorbital ridges, depressed nasal bridge, and flat midface (6,25). Cleft palate has been seen in all affected males except one (16); it has not been found in affected females.

Central nervous system. Most male patients have low normal intelligence, with intelligence quotients ranging between 75 and 90. Speech development is slow.

Musculoskeletal system. Skeletal growth is retarded; all male patients are below the tenth centile and may be below the third centile for height (6). The trunk is small, and there is pectus excavatum (4). Limited elbow extension and wrist supination have been noted in several patients, some of whom have subluxation of radial heads (4,12,23). Hands and feet are striking (4). Thumbs and halluces are spatulate and especially abbreviated. Clefting between the hallux and the other toes is exaggerated (Fig. 8–27C). The toes and fingers are irregular in form and direction of curvature. The second and third fingers may deviate to the ulnar side, while the fifth finger often bends to the radial side. Affected females are not unusually short; although only mild abnormalities may be observed in the hands, the feet usually have more obvious abnormalities (6).

Radiographic alterations are marked. Frontal and occipital bossing and thickening give the skull a mushroom-like appearance. The skull base is thick, the facial bones are hypoplastic, and the paranasal sinuses and mastoids are poorly pneumatized. The nasion-sella-basion angle is about 116 degrees (normal mean = 132 degrees), and the mandibular plane angle is increased. The mandible is small and the mandibular an-gle is more obtuse than normal (6,12). The clivus, or basisphenoid, lies further posteriorly than normal in relation to the cervical spine. These changes are essentially limited to affected males.

Iliac bones are small, with decreased flare. Coxa valga is a common finding. The lower tibia is laterally bowed. Failure of fusion of several vertebral arches is common.

Distinctive changes in hands of males include shortening of radial side of middle phalanx of fifth finger, clinodactyly, short distal phalanx of thumb (which during development has a cone-shaped epiphysis), accessory ossification center in second metacarpal, teardrop-shaped trapezium, transverse capitate, and trapezium–scaphoid fusion (6,12,17,18,22). Females may have greater multangular–scaphoid fusion.

In affected males, radiologic abnormalities in the feet include short phalanges and metatarsals of great toes. The second and third metatarsals are long and abnormally shaped because of their fusion with the cuneiform bones. The fifth metatarsal may be prominent, with an extra ossification center. Tarsal fusions are common, and males usually have two ossification centers in the navicular bone.

Auditory system. Mental retardation and slow speech development may be related to the conductive hearing loss that, in the few patients tested, ranged from 30 to 90 dB. However, not all patients have hearing loss (16). Abnormally shaped middle ear ossicles and small external auditory canals have been found (1–4,8,11,13,16,23).

Heredity. Inheritance is X-linked with variable heterozygote expression (7,8,11,14). The gene has been located at Xq28 (2,9) and identified as the filamin A (*FLNA*) gene (20). There is therefore allelism among OPDI, OPD II, frontometaphyseal dysplasia and Melnick-Needles syndrome (10,19,20,21,24).

Diagnosis. Larsen syndrome shares a number of features, such as cleft palate and joint dislocations, with the OPD I syndrome. However, patients with Larsen syndrome have a different facial appearance, multiple carpal bones, a juxtacalcaneal bone, and false flexion creases of the fingers. Larsen syndrome is also X-linked but far more severe in its skeletal manifestations. Acro-cranio-facial dysostosis is also more marked in its expression. The patients described as having X-linked cleft palate in one study (25) are examples of OPD, type I.

Summary. The characteristics of this condition include (*1*) X-linked inheritance with expression in many female heterozygotes; (*2*) characteristic face having large supraorbital ridges, broad nasal bridge, and downslanting palpebral fissures; (*3*) cleft palate; (*4*) subluxation of radial heads; (*5*) wide space between abbreviated halluces and the other toes; (*6*) other radiographic changes; and (*7*) conductive hearing loss.

Figure 8–27. *Otopalatodigital syndrome, type I.* (A) Three affected sibs flanked by their two normal male sibs. (B) Broad nasal base gives patients a pugilistic appearance. (C) Feet of three sibs showing short halluces and exaggerated separation between first and second toes, syndactyly, and clinodactyly of lesser toes. [From BA Dudding et al., *Am J Dis Child* 113:214, 1967.]

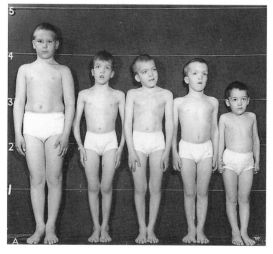

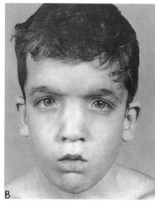

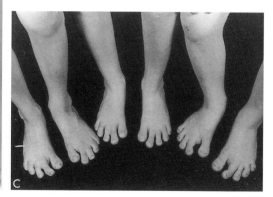

References

1. Aase JM: Oto-palato-digital syndrome. *Birth Defects* 5(3):43–44, 1969.
2. Biancalana V et al: Oto-palato-digital syndrome type I. Further evidence for assignment of the locus to Xq28. *Hum Genet* 88:228–230, 1991.
3. Buran DJ, Duvall AJ III: The oto-palato-digital (OPD) syndrome. *Arch Otolaryngol* 85:394–399, 1967 (same cases reported in refs. 4, 7, 8, and 12).
4. Dudding BA et al: The oto-palato-digital syndrome. A new symptom-complex consisting of deafness, dwarfism, cleft palate, characteristic facies, and a generalized bone dysplasia. *Am J Dis Child* 113:214–221, 1967 (same cases reported in refs. 3, 7, 8, and 12).
5. Fryns JP et al: The otopalatodigital syndrome. *Acta Paediatr Belg* 31:159–163, 1978.
6. Gall JC Jr et al: Oto-palato-digital syndrome: comparison of clinical and radiographic manifestations in males and females. *Am J Hum Genet* 24:24–36, 1972 (same cases reported in ref. 25).
7. Gorlin RJ: Discussion on oto-palato-digital syndrome. *Birth Defects* 5(3):45–47, 1969 (same cases reported in refs. 3, 4, 8, and 12).
8. Gorlin RJ et al: The oto-palato-digital (OPD) syndrome in females. *Oral Surg* 35:218–224, 1973. (Same cases reported in refs. 3, 4, 7, and 12).
9. Hoar D et al: Tentative assignment of gene for oto-palato-digital syndrome to distal Xq(Xq26–q28). *Am J Med Genet* 42:170–172, 1992.
10. Horn D et al: Oto-palato-digital syndrome with features of type I and II in brothers. *Genet Couns* 6:233–240, 1995.
11. Ichimura K, Hoshino T: Otological findings in oto-palato-digital syndrome. *Jiibinkoka* 53:287–293, 1981.
12. Langer LO Jr: The roentgenologic features of the oto-palato-digital (OPD) syndrome. *AJR Am J Roentgenol* 100:63–70, 1967 (same cases reported in refs. 3, 4, 7, and 8).
13. Nager GT, Char F: The otopalatodigital (OPD) syndrome: (conductive deafness, cleft palate and anomaly of digits). *Birth Defects* 7(7):273–274, 1971.
14. Pazzaglia VE, Giampiero B: Oto-palato-digital syndrome in four generations of a large family. *Clin Genet* 30:338–344, 1986.
15. Plenier V et al: Le syndrome oto-palato-digital. A propos de trois cas feminins. *Rev Stomatol Chir Maxillofac* 84:322–329, 1983.
16. Podoshin L et al: The oto-palato-digital syndrome. *J Laryngol Otol* 90:407–411, 1976.
17. Poznanski AK et al: The hand in the oto-palato-digital syndrome. *Ann Radiol* 16:203–209, 1973.
18. Poznanski AK et al: Otopalatodigital syndrome: radiologic findings in the hand and foot. *Birth Defects* 10(5):125–149, 1974.
19. Robertson SP et al: Linkage of otopalatodigital syndrome type 2 (OPD2) to distal Xq28: evidence of allelism with OPD1. *Am J Hum Genet* 69:223–227, 2001.
20. Robertson SP et al: Localized mutations in the gene encoding the cyto-skeletal protein filamin A cause diverse malformations in humans. *Nat Genet* 33:487–491, 2003.
21. Superti-Furga A: Otopalatodigital syndrome, and frontometaphyseal dysplasia, splitters and lumpers, and paternity of ideas. *Am J Med Genet* 95:86, 2000.
22. Takato T et al: Otopalatodigital syndrome. *Ann Plast Surg* 14:371–374, 1985.
23. Taybi H: Generalized skeletal dysplasia with multiple anomalies. A note on Pyle's disease. *AJR Am J Roentgenol* 88:450–457, 1962.
24. Verloes A et al: Fronto-otopalatodigital osteodysplasia: clinical evidence for a single entity encompassing Melnick-Needles syndrome, otopalatodigital syndrome types 1 and 2, and frontometaphyseal dysplasia. *Am J Med Genet* 90:407–422, 2000.
25. Weinstein ED, Cohen MM: Sex-linked cleft palate. Report of a family and review of 77 kindreds. *J Med Genet* 3:17–22, 1966 (same cases reported in ref. 6).

Otopalatodigital syndrome, type II

Otopalatodigital syndrome, type II (OPD II), delineated by Fitch et al. (6) in 1976, is characterized by short stature, unusual facial phenotype, cleft palate, and multiple skeletal anomalies. Skeletal manifestations are far more severe in this syndrome than they are in OPD I. About 30 cases have been reported to date.

Craniofacial findings. Hypertelorism, frontal bossing, broad nasal bridge, downslanting palpebral fissures, midface hypoplasia, low-set ears, and marked mandibular micrognathia are observed (2,4,16) (Fig. 8–28A). Carrier females may have midfacial abnormalities (2,4,16), but others appear quite normal (11,15). Cleft palate is found in affected

Figure 8–28. *Otopalatodigital syndrome, type II.* (A) Hypertelorism, downslanting palpebral fissures, midface hypoplasia, dislocated radial heads, knock knees, and rockerbottom feet. (B) Radiographic changes include curvature of humerus and radius, anomalies of metacarpals and phalanges, small first metacarpal, large proximal phalanges, hip dislocation, curvature of femora, hypoplastic fibulae, advanced bone age, curvature of tibia, absence of ossification of first metatarsals and its phalanges, and short fifth metatarsal. (C) Anomalies of metacarpals and phalanges. Note extra bone between proximal phalanx and metacarpal on fifth finger, enlarged epiphyses, capitate-hamate complex. (D) Hypoplastic first and fifth toes. [(A,D) from K Kozlowski, *Pediatr Radiol* 6:97, 1977; (B,C) from M André et al., *J Pediatr* 98:747, 1981.]

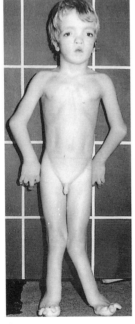
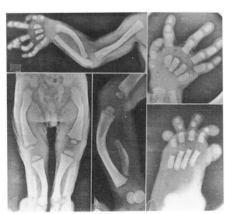
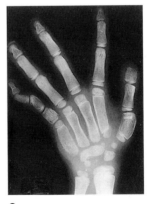
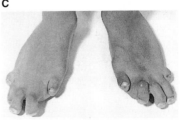

A   B   D

males. Bifid uvula has been noted in a carrier female (6). In some instances, frank Robin sequence may be present (2).

Central nervous system. Psychomotor development and intelligence appear normal in some patients (7), whereas others are mentally retarded (8). Hydrocephalus has been noted (7,18,20).

Musculoskeletal system. The anterior fontanel may be large (6). The base of the skull is sclerotic (6). Clavicles are thin and wavy. The thorax is small, and there may be pectus excavatum. Ribs are wide posteriorly and anteriorly, while narrow in their middle portions. Vertebrae are flattened. The humeri, radii, femora, and tibiae are bowed; curving of long bones may disappear early in life (7) (Fig. 8–28B,C). Radial heads may be dislocated. Fibulae are small or absent. Ilia are hypoplastic. Thumbs are broad and short, as are the great toes (Fig. 8–28D). Fingers are held in a flexed, overlapping position. Tubular bones of hands and feet are deformed and bones of the wrists and ankles are hypoplastic and malformed. Rocker-bottom feet may be present (2,4,9). Carrier females may have abnormalities of the hands and feet (6,16).

Other findings. Omphalocele (13,17,20), hydronephrosis, hydroureter, and chordee (7,20) have been noted.

Auditory system. Hearing loss has been described (7–9); one patient (7) had aseptic meningitis twice during the first year of life. Bilateral conductive hearing loss was described in a carrier female (2); malformed ossicles were noted at surgery. The 2-year-old male reported by Shi (16) likely had OPD II (H Schucknecht, personal communication, 1985). Histologic studies of his temporal bone revealed malformed ossicles and abnormalities of the bony labyrinth.

Heredity. Inheritance is X-linked recessive.

Laboratory aids. Prenatal diagnosis has been done by ultrasound (13,19). Both membranous bone formation and bone remodeling are defective (15).

Diagnosis. This syndrome should be distinguished from OPD syndrome, type I, Larsen syndrome, boomerang dysplasia, atelosteogenesis I and II, campomelic dysplasia, lethal Melnick-Needles syndrome, and trisomy 18 (1,3,5,10,14). There is similarity to acro-coxo-melic dysplasia, an autosomal recessive disorder described by Plauchu et al. (12).

Prognosis. Death has occurred, usually because of respiratory infection, within the first 5 months of life in at least 12 cases (2,6,16,20); another patient died of similar causes at age 2 years (16). Those who survive have short stature.

Summary. Characteristics include (*1*) X-linked inheritance with mild expression in female heterozygotes; (*2*) short stature; (*3*) unusual face; (*4*) cleft palate; (*5*) skeletal dysplasia; and (*6*) conductive hearing loss in some patients.

References

1. Alembik Y et al: On the phenotypic overlap between "severe" oto-palato-digital type II syndrome and Larsen syndrome. Variable manifestation of a single autosomal dominant gene. *Genet Couns* 8:133–137, 1997.
2. André M et al: Abnormal facies, cleft palate, and generalized dysostosis: a lethal X-linked syndrome. *J Pediatr* 98:747–752, 1981.
3. Blanchet P et al: Multiple congenital anomalies associated with an oto-palato-digital syndrome type II. *Genet Couns* 4:289–294, 1993.
4. Brewster TG et al: Oto-palato-digital syndrome, type II—an X-linked skeletal dysplasia. *Am J Med Genet* 20:249–254, 1985.
5. Corona-Rivera JR et al: Infant with manifestations of oto-palato-digital syndrome type II and of Melnick-Needles syndrome. *Am J Med Genet* 85:79–81, 1999.
6. Fitch N et al: A familial syndrome of cranial, facial, oral, and limb abnormalities. *Clin Genet* 10:226–231, 1976.
7. Fitch N et al: The oto-palato-digital syndrome, proposed type II. *Am J Med Genet* 15:655–664, 1983.
8. Kaplan J, Maroteaux P: Syndrome oto-palato-digital de type II. *Ann Génét* 27:79–82, 1984.
9. Kozlowski K et al: Oto-palato-digital syndrome with severe X-ray changes in two half-brothers. *Pediatr Radiol* 6:97–102, 1977.
10. Nishimura G et al: Atypical skeletal changes in otopalatodigital syndrome type II: phenotypic overlap among otopalatodigital syndrome type II, boomerang dysplasia, atelosteogenesis type I and type II and lethal male phenotype of Melnick-Needles syndrome. *Am J Med Genet* 73:132–138, 1997.
11. Ogata T et al: Oto-palato-digital syndrome, type II: evidence for defective intramembranous ossification. *Am J Med Genet* 36:226–231, 1990.
12. Plauchu H et al: Le nanisme acro-coxo-mésomélique: variété nouvelle de nanisme récessif autosomique. *Ann Génét* 27:83–87, 1984.
13. Ricanda D et al: Prenatal diagnosis of oto-palato-digital syndrome, type II: the diagnostic problem of a bone dysplasia with multiple malformations. *Am J Hum Genet* (Suppl) 49:176, 1991.
14. Robertson S et al: Are Melnick-Needles syndrome and oto-palato-digital syndrome type II allelic? Observations in a four-generation kindred. *Am J Med Genet* 71:341–347, 1997.
15. Savarirayan R et al: Oto-palato-digital syndrome, type II: report of three cases with further delineation of the chondro-osseous morphology. *Am J Med Genet* 95:193–200, 2000.
16. Shi S-R: Temporal bone findings in a case of otopalatodigital syndrome. *Arch Otolaryngol* 11:119–121, 1985.
17. Stillman S et al: Otopalatodigital syndrome and omphalocele. *Dysmorphol Clin Genet* 5:2–10, 1991.
18. Stratton R, Bluestone D: Oto-palato-digital syndrome type II with X-linked cerebellar hypoplasia/hydrocephalus. *Am J Med Genet* 41:169–172, 1991.
19. Vigneron J et al: Le syndrome oto-palato-digital de type II. Diagnostique prénatal par echographie. *J Génét Hum* 35:69, 1987.
20. Young K et al: Otopalatodigital syndrome type II associated with omphalocele: Report of three cases. *Am J Med Genet* 45:481–487, 1993.

EEC syndrome (ectrodactyly–ectodermal dysplasia–clefting syndrome)

The first report of the syndrome of ectrodactyly of the hands and feet, nasolacrimal duct obstruction, and cleft lip–palate was likely that of Eckoldt and Martens (13) in 1804. Another early description was by Cruveilhier (12). In excess of 250 cases have since been reported (18,48,53).

Craniofacial findings. Facial features include dacryocystitis, keratoconjunctivitis, tearing, photophobia, and cleft lip (Fig. 8–29A). Scalp hair, lashes, and eyebrows are nearly always sparse (4,15,39).

Limbs. Ectrodactyly involves all four extremities in 60% of cases (18). However, 40% have asymmetric anomalies (Fig. 8–29B,C). Other patients have been described without ectrodactyly (16). Occasionally, soft tissue syndactyly, especially of the toes, occurs (6,41).

Eyes. Absent lacrimal punctas, noted in about 90% of patients, are associated with tearing, blepharitis, dacryocystitis, keratoconjunctivitis, and photophobia (3,7,15,23,24,25,28,34,41,50,54,60). Corneal ulcers and scarring (7,15,41) result. The number of meibomian orifices is reduced (36,41).

Skin, hair, and nails. Hypopigmentation of skin and hair has been noted in most white patients (1,4,7,15,41), but black patients have normal pigmentation. The scalp hair has a silvery blond sheen and may be coarse and dry in 80% (Fig. 8–29D). Scalp hair, eyebrows, and lashes are sparse in 20% (7,15,41,50,54). Nails are dysplastic in 80% (4,23,41,54). Absent or sparse sebaceous glands have been observed on skin biopsy (41). About 10% have many pigmented nevi (7,15,41), and widespread comedone nevi have been described (28).

Central nervous system. Microcephaly and mental retardation have been reported in about 10% (4,15,18,41,50), but there may have been an ascertainment bias.

Genitourinary system. Kidney and ureter malformations (duplication of the kidney, collecting system and ureter, absent kidney, small

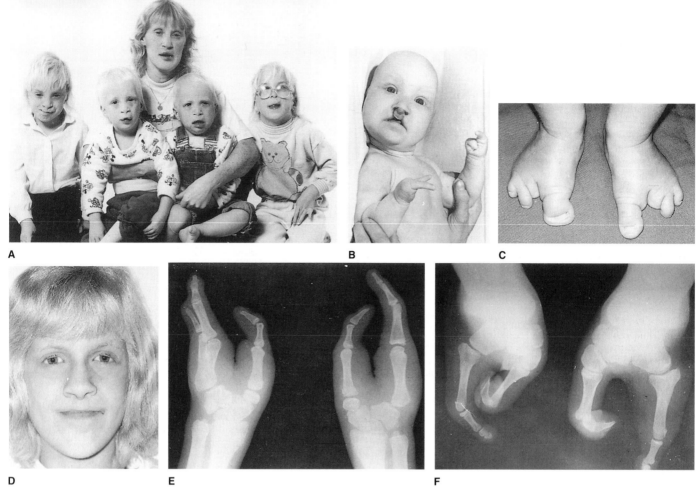

Figure 8–29. *EEC syndrome (ectrodactyly-ectodermal dysplasia-clefting syndrome).* (A) Affected mother with four affected children. (B) Note deficiency of hair, ectrodactyly, and cleft lip. (C) Ectrodactyly of feet. (D) Older child with repaired bilateral cleft lip and Dynel-like alteration of hair. Note thickening of upper eyelids. (E,F) Ectrodactyly of hands and feet. [(B) from RA Rüdiger et al., *Am J Dis Child* 120:160, 1970.]

dysplastic kidney, hydronephrosis, and hydroureter) have been reported in at least 45% (4,15,22,23,26,30,31,37,49,56), as has hypospadias (46). Cryptorchidism (21) and prune belly (22) have been noted, as has rectal atresia (32).

Laryngologic manifestations. Breathy voice has been observed in some patients. Laryngoscopic examination showed no visible form of incomplete closure along the vocal folds, although the folds were dry, suggesting that reduction in lubrication resulted in an incomplete seal between the folds during phonation. Spectrographic analysis showed abnormal voice quality (43). Choanal atresia has been noted (10,57).

Oral manifestations. Cleft lip–palate, often bilateral, is found in about 60%–75% of patients (4,7,9,15,23,28,40,41,50,54). In possibly 10%, cleft palate without cleft lip was noted (47,49). Clefting is absent in other patients (9,28,41). Congenitally missing permanent teeth and coniform teeth (28) are common. Anodontia has been the sole manifestation in one patient (11). Enamel dysplasia (4,54) has been noted. Xerostomia (41), requiring large amounts of water while eating, and enamel dysplasia may contribute to high dental caries rate. Parotid duct atresia has been documented (41). A deep anteroposterior furrow in the midline of the dorsum of the tongue has also been described, as well as candidal cheilitis and candidal perleche (41) presumably as secondary phenomena.

Auditory system. Conductive hearing loss has been documented in about 30% (7,9,23,29,54,56,61). Bystrom et al. (7) described mod-

erate conductive loss and Swallow et al (54) described moderate low-frequency conductive deafness. Wildervanck (61) described 40–100 dB sensorineural hearing loss in brothers with the syndrome. Tolmie et al. (56) noted severe congenital hearing loss in a father and son and reported cochlear malformation with rostral dilatation and abnormal vestibule. Bystrom et al. (7) noted absence of the incus.

Vestibular system. A caloric vestibular test in one patient showed marked depression of the vestibular response and minimal nystagmus produced by cold water (61).

Heredity. About 50% of cases represent sporadic examples of the disorder (4,6,15,23,39–41,50,51,54). In the other 50%, transmission of the disorder from an affected parent to one or more children has been observed (9,18,33,42,47,51,59,62); others have reported affected sibs born to presumably normal parents (18). There is also considerable variation in expression among affected members of the same kindred (33,51). Penetrance is somewhat less than 80% (18). The syndrome has autosomal dominant inheritance with low penetrance and variable expressivity (55). One ectrodactyly locus (EEC1) is at 7q11.2 (17,20,45). A second gene (EEC2) has mapped to 19p13–q13, a third to 10q24, and a fourth (EEC3) to 3q27 (2,18). This last gene is *p63*, in which missense mutations are responsible for most cases of the syndrome. However, only 85% of EEC patients exhibit the mutations (2,8). Many conditions (Rapp-Hodgkin, ECP, Hay-Wells, ADULT syndromes) are allelic (18,38,44).

Radiographic findings. Missing middle rays are evident (Fig. 8–28E,F).

Diagnosis. Ectrodactyly may be an isolated finding or may occur with or without more severe limb reduction defects in a variety of different syndromes. Ectrodactyly syndromes have been reviewed by Schroer (52). The LADD syndrome must be excluded (27). Although lacrimal duct obstruction occurs in 1%–2% of the general population, it occurs in about 10% of cleft lip–palate cases (18). The differential diagnosis of EEC syndrome and conditions with cleft lip–palate, limb reduction defects, and ectodermal dysplasia (Rapp-Hodgkin, Hay-Wells, ECP, ADULT, etc., syndromes) has been addressed in detail by Gorlin et al. (18) and Fosko et al. (14). However, Moerman and Fryns (35) described Rapp-Hodgkin syndrome in a woman and EEC in her daughter, suggesting that at least some of these conditions represent variable expression of the same entity. Raas-Rothschild et al. (46) described short stature, asymmetric ectrodactyly, short webbed neck, posteriorly rotated low-set pinnae, epicanthic folds, oligodontia, mental retardation, and sensorineural hearing loss. Prenatal diagnosis has been accomplished (5). Van Bokhoven et al. (58) described a syndrome with mammary hypoplasia, ectrodactyly, ectodermal anomalies, and cleft palate, which was mapped to 3q27. Allelism with ulnar-mammary syndrome was also excluded.

Summary. Characteristics of this condition include (1) sporadicity but, in some cases, autosomal dominant inheritance with incomplete penetrance; (2) variable ectrodactyly of hands and feet; (3) absence of lacrimal puncta; (4) cleft lip–palate; (5) variable pigment dilution of hair; (6) conductive hearing loss in 30%; and (7) possible vestibular abnormalities.

References

1. Annerén G et al: Ectrodactyly–ectodermal dysplasia–clefting syndrome. The clinical variations and prenatal diagnosis. *Clin Genet* 40:257–262, 1991.
2. Barrow LL et al: Analysis of the *p63* gene in classic EEC syndrome, related syndromes and nonsyndromic orofacial clefts. *Am J Hum Genet* 67: Abst 602, 2000.
3. Baum JL, Bull MJ: Ocular manifestations of the ectrodactyly, ectodermal dysplasia, cleft lip–palate syndrome. *Am J Ophthalmol* 78:211–216, 1974.
4. Bixler D et al: The ectrodactyly–ectodermal dysplasia–clefting (EEC) syndrome. *Clin Genet* 3:43–51, 1971.
5. Bronshtein M, Gershoni-Baruch R: Prenatal transvaginal diagnosis of the ectrodactyly ectodermal dysplasia, cleft palate (EEC) syndrome. *Prenat Diagn* 13:519–522, 1993.
6. Buss PW et al: Twenty-four cases of the EEC syndrome: clinical presentation and management. *J Med Genet* 32:716–723, 1995.
7. Bystrom EB et al: The syndrome of ectrodactyly, ectodermal dysplasia and clefting (EEC). *J Oral Surg* 33:192–198, 1975.
8. Celli J et al: Heterozygous germline mutations in the p53 homolog p63 are the cause of EEC syndrome. *Cell* 99:143–153, 1999.
9. Chiang TP, Robinson GC: Ectrodactyly, ectodermal dysplasia, and cleft lip/palate syndrome: the importance of dental anomalies. *J Dent Child* 41:38–42, 1974.
10. Christodoulou J et al: Choanal atresia as a feature of ectrodactyly–ectodermal dysplasia–clefting (EEC) syndrome. *J Med Genet* 26:586–589, 1989.
11. Chrzanowska KH et al: Anodontia as a sole clinical sign of the ectrodactyly–ectodermal dysplasia–cleft lip (EEC) syndrome. *Genet Couns* 1:67–73, 1990.
12. Cruveilhier J: *Anatomie Pathologique du Corps Humaine. Maladies des Extremities*, Vol. II, part 38. S. Bailliere, Paris, 1829–1842.
13. Eckoldt JG, Martens FH: *Über eine sehr Komplicierte Hasenscharte.* Steinacker, Leipzig, 1804.
14. Fosko SW et al: Ectodermal dysplasias associated with clefting: significance of scalp dermatitis. *J Am Acad Dermatol* 27:249–256, 1992.
15. Fried K: Ectrodactyly–ectodermal dysplasia–clefting (EEC) syndrome. *Clin Genet* 3:396–400, 1972.
16. Fryns JP et al: EEC syndrome without ectrodactyly: report of two new families. *J Med Genet* 27:165–168, 1990.
17. Fukushima Y et al: The breakpoints of the EEC syndrome (ectrodactyly, ectodermal dysplasia and cleft lip/palate) confirmed to 7q21.21 and 9p12 by fluorescence in situ hybridization. *Clin Genet* 44:50, 1993.
18. Gorlin RJ et al: *Syndromes of the Head and Neck*, 4th ed. Oxford University Press, New York, 2001.
19. Gurrieri F et al: A split hand–split foot (*SHFM3*) gene is located at 10q24–25. *Am J Med Genet* 62:427–436, 1996.
20. Hasegawa T et al: EEC syndrome with balanced reciprocal translocation between 7q11.21 and 9p2 (or 7p11.2 and 9q12) in 3 generations. *Clin Genet* 40:202–206, 1991.
21. Hecht F: Updating a diagnosis: the EEC/EECUT syndrome. *Am J Dis Child* 139:1185, 1985.
22. Ivarrson S et al: Coexisting ectrodactyly–ectodermal dysplasia–clefting (EEC) and prune belly syndromes. *Acta Radiol Diagn* 23:287–292, 1982.
23. Kaiser-Kupfer M: Ectrodactyly, ectodermal dysplasia and clefting syndrome. *Am J Ophthalmol* 76:992–998, 1973.
24. Knudtzon J, Aarskog D: Growth hormone deficiency associated with ectrodactyly–ectodermal dysplasia–clefting syndrome and isolated absent septum pellucidum. *Pediatrics* 79:410–412, 1987.
25. Koniszewski G et al: Augenbeteiligung bei ektodermaler Dysplasia. *Klin Monatsbl Augenheilkd* 190:519–523, 1987.
26. Küster W: Further reports of urinary tract involvement in EEC syndrome. *Am J Dis Child* 140:411, 1986.
27. Lacombe D et al: Split hand/foot deformity and LADD syndrome in a family: overlap between the EEC and LADD syndromes. *J Med Genet* 30:700–703, 1992.
28. Leibowitz MR, Jenkins T: A newly recognized feature of ectrodactyly, ectodermal dysplasia, clefting (EEC) syndrome: comedone naevus. *Dermatologica* 169:80–85, 1984.
29. Lewis MB, Pashayan HM: Ectrodactyly, cleft lip and palate in two half sibs. *J Med Genet* 18:394–396, 1981.
30. London R et al: Urinary tract involvement in EEC syndrome. *Am J Dis Child* 139:1191–1193, 1985.
31. Maas SM et al: EEC syndrome and genitourinary anomalies: an update. *Am J Med Genet* 63:472–478, 1996.
32. Majewski F, Goecke T: Rectal atresia as rare manifestation in EEC syndrome. *Am J Med Genet* 63:190–192, 1996.
33. Majewski F, Küster W: EEC syndrome sine? *Clin Genet* 33:69–72, 1988.
34. McNab AA et al: The EEC syndrome and its ocular manifestations. *Br J Ophthalmol* 73:261–264, 1989.
35. Moerman P, Fryns JP: Ectodermal dysplasia, Rapp-Hodgkin type in a mother and severe ectrodactyly–ectodermal dysplasia–clefting syndrome (EEC) in her child. *Am J Med Genet* 63:479–481, 1996.
36. Mondino BT et al: Absent meibomian glands in the ectrodactyly–ectodermal dysplasia–clefting syndrome. *Am J Ophthalmol* 97:496–501, 1984.
37. Nardi AC et al: Urinary tract involvement in EEC syndrome: a clinical study in 25 Brazilian patients. *Am J Med Genet* 44:803–806, 1992.
38. Opitz JM et al: The ECP syndrome, another autosomal dominant cause of monodactylous ectrodactyly. *Eur J Pediatr* 133:217–220, 1980.
39. Parent P et al: Le syndrome EEC. *Ann Pédiatr* 34:293–300, 1987.
40. Parkash H et al: Ectrodactyly, ectodermal dysplasia, cleft lip and palate (EEC)—a rare syndrome. *Int J Pediatr* 50:337–340, 1983.
41. Pashayan HM et al: The EEC syndrome. *Birth Defects* 10(7):105–127, 1974.
42. Penchaszadeh VB, De Negrotti TC: Ectrodactyly–ectodermal dysplasia–clefting (EEC) syndrome, dominant inheritance and variable expression. *J Med Genet* 13:281–284, 1976.
43. Peterson-Falzone SJ et al: Abnormal laryngeal vocal quality in ectodermal dysplasia. *Arch Otolaryngol* 107:300–304, 1981.
44. Propping P, Zerres K: ADULT-syndrome: an autosomal-dominant disorder with pigment anomalies, ectrodactyly, nail dysplasia and hypodontia. *Am J Med Genet* 45:642–648, 1993.
45. Qumsiyeh MB: EEC syndrome (ectrodactyly, ectodermal dysplasia, and cleft lip/palate) is on 7q11.2–q21.3. *Clin Genet* 42:101, 1992.
46. Raas-Rothschild A et al: Newly recognized ectrodactyly/deafness syndrome. *J Craniofac Genet Dev Biol* 9:121–127, 1989.
47. Rodini ES, Richieri-Costa A: EEC syndrome: report on 20 new patients. Clinical and genetic considerations. *Am J Med Genet* 37:42–53, 1990.
48. Roelfsma NM, Cobben JM: The EEC syndrome: a literature study. *Clin Dysmorphol* 5:115–127, 1996.
49. Rollnick BR, Hoo JJ: Genitourinary anomalies are a component manifestation in the ectodermal dysplasia, ectrodactyly, cleft lip/palate (EEC) syndrome. *Am J Med Genet* 29:131–136, 1988.
50. Rüdiger RA et al: Association of ectrodactyly, ectodermal dysplasia and cleft lip–palate: the EEC syndrome. *Am J Dis Child* 120:160–163, 1970.
51. Schmidt R, Nitowsky HM: Split hand and foot deformity and the syndrome of ectrodactyly, ectodermal dysplasia, and clefting (EEC). A report of five patients. *Hum Genet* 39:15–25, 1977.
52. Schroer RJ: Split-hand/split-foot. *Proc Greenwood Genet Ctr* 5:65–75, 1986.
53. Seno H et al: Ectrodactyly, ectodermal dysplasia, and cleft lip syndrome. *Scand J Plast Reconstr Hand Surg* 30:227–230, 1996.
54. Swallow JN et al: Ectrodactyly, ectodermal dysplasia and cleft lip and cleft palate (EEC syndrome). *Br J Dermatol* 89(Suppl 9):54–56, 1973.

55. Tse K et al: Dilemmas in counselling: the EEC syndrome. *J Med Genet* 27:752–755, 1990.
56. Tolmie JL et al: Autosomal dominant ectrodactyly and deafness. Presented at the 5th Manchester Birth Defects Conference, October 13–16, 1992.
57. Tucker K, Lipson A: Choanal atresia as a feature of ectrodactyly–ectodermal dysplasia–clefting (EEC) syndrome. *J Med Genet* 27:213, 1990.
58. Van Bokhoven H et al: Limb mammary syndrome: a new genetic disorder with mammary hypoplasia, ectrodactyly, and other hand/foot anomalies maps to human chromosome 3q27. *Am J Hum Genet* 64:538–546, 1999.
59. Wallis CE: Ectrodactyly (split-hand/split-foot) and ectodermal dysplasia with normal lip and palate in a four generation kindred. *Clin Genet* 34:252–257, 1988.
60. Wiedemann H-R, Dibbern H: EEC-Syndrom. *Med Welt* 31:1862–1863, 1980.
61. Wildervanck LS: Perceptive deafness associated with split-hand and -foot, a new syndrome? *Acta Genet (Basel)* 13:161–169, 1963.
62. Zlotogora J: On the inheritance of the split hand/split foot malformation. *Am J Med Genet* 53:29–32, 1994.

Split hand/split foot with sensorineural deafness

Tackels-Horne et al (3) described two families with the combination of split hand/split foot malformations (SHFM) and sensorineural hearing loss. None had ectodermal defects. The presentation was variable, with some family members having only hearing loss and others having only limb defects. The inheritance was autosomal dominant, and the gene was mapped to 7q21. Others have also described families with split hand/split foot anomalies and hearing loss, with deletion of or translocation involving 7q21. Although linkage studies weren't done, the family reported by Tolmie et al. (4) may be another example of this condition, as are others described in the previous section on EEC syndrome. Haberlandt et al. (1) reported on a child with deletion 7q21.1–q21.3. In addition to unilateral split foot, the boy had minor facial anomalies (hypertelorism, small nose, micrognathia, submucous cleft palate), hypopigmented retina, hypodontia, sparse light hair, pale skin, and hearing loss, with MRI demonstrating Mondini malformation of the inner ear. Ignatius et al. (2) described a child with a complex chromosome rearrangement involving 7q21.3 who had SFHM of all limbs, congenital hearing loss, submucous cleft palate, microcephaly, and mental retardation. The variation in phenotypes among these individuals is likely attributable to deletion of contiguous genes in the individuals with chromosome anomalies.

References

1. Haberlandt E et al: Split hand/split foot malformation associated with sensorineural deafness, inner and middle ear malformation, hypodontia, congenital vertical talus, and deletion of eight microsatellite markers in 7q21.1–q21.3. *J Med Genet* 38:405–409, 2001.
2. Ignatius J et al: Split hand/split foot malformation, deafness, and mental retardation with a complex cytogenetic rearrangement involving 7q21.3. *J Med Genet* 33:507–510, 1996.
3. Tackels-Horne D et al: Split hand/split foot malformation with hearing loss: first report of families linked to the SHFM1 locus in 7q21. *Clin Genet* 59:28–36, 2001.

4. Tolmie JL et al: Autosomal dominant ectrodactyly and deafness. Presented at the 5th Manchester Birth Defects Conference, October 13–16, 1992.

Glossopalatine fusion, micrognathia, digital anomalies, stenotic ear canals, and conductive hearing loss

Jorgenson (2) described a female infant with marked micrognathia and fusion of an extremely small tongue to the hard palate. The terminal phalanx of each thumb was hypoplastic and all fingernails were hyperconvex.

The pinnae were cup-shaped and intruded at their lower edges. The lobes were small. Small fleshy tags were found on the left side of the face. The external ear canals were stenotic. The conductive hearing loss was assumed to be largely attributable to stenotic canals.

Although glossopalatine ankylosis and digital hypoplasia is a well-recognized syndrome, we are unaware of stenotic ear canals being associated (1). There was overlap with oculo-auriculo-vertebral spectrum.

References

1. Gorlin RJ et al: *Syndromes of the Head and Neck*, 4th ed. Oxford University Press, New York, 2001, p. 830.
2. Jorgenson RJ: Case report 97: tongue fusion, micrognathia and digital defects. *J Clin Dysmorphol* 1(2):8–9, 1983.

Other Skeletal Disorders

The osteogenesis imperfectas

Osteogenesis imperfecta (OI) is a heterogeneous group of heritable disorders of type I collagen metabolism characterized by bone fragility. Associated features in some affected individuals include blue sclerae, opalescent teeth with characteristic radiologic features, hearing loss, deformity of the long bones and spine, and joint hyperextensibility. Clinical and genetic studies delineate at least four major syndrome groups (56), although all of these syndromes are heterogeneous at the clinical, radiographic, and molecular levels (2–10,13,23–25,31,55,56,58,64,65). In a recent review, Cole and Cohen (16) indicated that more than 80 different mutations of the *COL1A1* and *COL1A2* genes have been identified in OI patients to date. All pedigrees of OI with hearing loss are linked to the *COL1A1* gene on chromosome 17q21.31 (66). *COL1A2* maps to 7q22.1. Mutations result in the substitution of another amino acid for glycine in the triple helix, rendering the collagen unstable and deficient in amount. The estimated prevalence of all types combined is about 0.5/10,000 births (63). Extensive reviews are those of Smith et al. (61), van der Harten et al. (69), and Gorlin et al. (24).

The four major types (57) are summarized briefly in Table 8–4. In the text that follows, only type I is discussed in detail. Type III is briefly considered and the auditory findings in type IV are mentioned.

Life expectancy has been discussed in the various types (43).

Table 8–4. Osteogenesis imperfecta

Type	Key features	Inheritance	Molecular cause
I	Significant variability in number and severity of fractures, even within families, blue sclerae	AD	Mutations in *COL1A1* or *COL1A2*, most often functional null mutations
II	Prenatal-onset bone fragility with several congenital of fractures, early death	Most AD mutations; AR very rarely	Mutations in *COL1A1* or *COL1A2*
III	Moderately severe to severe bone fragility, prenatal onset of fractures, blue sclerae	AR	One family in which child was homozygous for *COL1A2* mutation; parents both had OI I
IV	Mild to moderate bone fragility, with light blue sclerae in infancy and normal or or near-normal scleral color in adulthood; dentinogenesis in some	AD	Mutations in *COL1A1* (infrequent) or *COL1A2*

AD, autosomal dominant; AR, autosomal recessive; OI, osteogenesis imperfecta.

The general aspects of the osteogenesis imperfectas are then addressed under the headings of Heredity, Diagnosis, and Summary.

Type I

Craniofacial findings. The gray-blue sclerae may be striking. A triangular face is frequently noted (41), as is temporal bulging (57). The maxilla may be hypoplastic with a relative mandibular prognathism (Fig. 8–30A).

Oral manifestations. Heterogeneity based on the presence or absence of dental abnormalities has been noted (31,40,52). Paterson et al. (40) recognized that two groups of families with OI type I can be distinguished: a group with normal teeth (type IA) and a group with specific dental abnormalities (type IB). In patients with dental abnormalities, deciduous and permanent teeth are opalescent, and amber or blue-gray on eruption (32). On radiographic examination, there is increased constriction at the coronal–radicular junctions, and pulps become obliterated with secondary dentin. However, pulps may be wider than normal during early development (32). Roots are thinner and shorter than normal (52). Extensive discussion of dental abnormalities is available at the clinical and basic levels (21,24,31–35,39,52).

Ocular system. Blue sclerae are characteristic and color is consistent within families, although the degree of blueness varies from one family to another (60). Disordered molecular organization and other basic ocular defects are discussed elsewhere (20,30,32).

Central nervous system. Results of CT scans have been normal (68), and ventricles are normal in size. Pozo et al. (46) reported advanced basilar impression resulting in ventricular dilatation, multiple neurological disturbances in the foramen magnum compression syndrome, and death from acute brain stem compression, but this is rare. Half of the 56 patients studied by Reite and Solomons (48) had abnormal electroencephalograms, although their patients represented a heterogeneous group.

Cardiovascular system. The frequency of symptomatic cardiovascular anomalies is low (47,70). Hortop et al. (26) reported nonprogressive aortic root dilatation in about 12%. In one study, 9% had asymptomatic mitral valve prolapse; 24% of males but only 4% of females had asymptomatic aortic root dilatation. Aortic regurgitation has been observed in patients after the third decade, as has mitral regurgitation (24). Aortic aneurysm and dissection do not occur. Mitral valve leaflets were thin in half the patients reported by White et al. (70). Microscopic findings in the valves include myxoid degeneration and atrophy and, in the aorta, cystic medial necrosis.

Musculoskeletal manifestations. Birth weights and birth lengths are generally normal. Short stature is of postnatal onset and usually mild, but by adulthood, one-half of the affected patients are less than the third centile for height (57).

Head size is usually large (53,66,68). Wormian bones, platybasia, and occipitalization of upper cervical vertebrae are common (41,57).

Multiple fractures occur in about 90% (57). There is considerable variability within and between families in the age of onset and frequency of fractures. Reduction in fracture frequency at puberty has been noted, followed by increase in fracture frequency in women after menopause. Long bone deformity consists of bowing and angulation (57). About 20% of adults have kyphosis or scoliosis, which may be progressive (57). Trunk shortening has also been described (4). Osteopenia may be minimal and undetectable on skeletal radiographs. There is increased susceptibility to osteosarcoma (16).

Paterson et al. (40) found a significantly higher fracture rate between ages 5 and 20 years in patients with type I OI and opalescent teeth (type IB) than in those with type I who had normal teeth (type IA). They also found that individuals with type IB were more likely to have had a fracture at birth, to have higher fracture frequency, and to have height below the second centile. Patients with normal teeth were more likely than patients with opalescent teeth to have prolonged fracture-free periods during childhood. These two groups, however, were similar in frequency of joint hyperextensibility, bruising, hearing impairment, and joint dislocation (41).

Other abnormalities. Hernias and excessive sweating have been reported (41). Easy bruisability is a feature in over 75% of patients (41).

Auditory system. Hearing loss, rarely detected before 10 years of age, usually begins with a conductive loss in the late second or early third decade (49). With age, mixed, but especially sensorineural, hearing loss is progressive (7,18,22,44,49,51,54,62). Riedner et al. (49) noted that by the fifth decade, half of all patients had hearing loss, whereas by the seventh decade, all individuals had hearing loss, although the number of older individuals tested was small. Cox and Simmons (18) reported similar findings. Garretsen (22) and Garretsen and

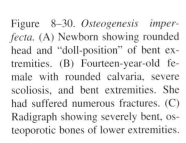
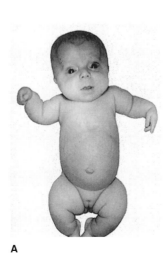
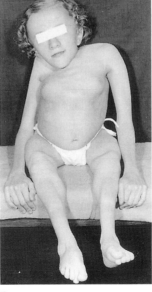
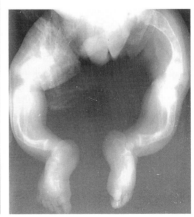

Figure 8–30. *Osteogenesis imperfecta.* (A) Newborn showing rounded head and "doll-position" of bent extremities. (B) Fourteen-year-old female with rounded calvaria, severe scoliosis, and bent extremities. She had suffered numerous fractures. (C) Radiograph showing severely bent, osteoporotic bones of lower extremities. **A**

B

C

Cremers (23), studying 142 patients, found that 50% had a hearing loss of greater than 30 dB. There is a loss of about 1 dB/year from 500 to 4000 Hz. Shapiro et al. (53) reported audiologic abnormalities in a heterogeneous group of patients: 50% younger than 30 years of age and 95% over 30 had hearing loss. Half of all patients examined had sensorineural loss. Conductive loss in this syndrome has been attributed to ossicular immobility at the stapes footplate (9,19,43,49,51). Fracture of the stapedial crura and atrophy of the stapes may also contribute to loss of hearing acuity (37,49). Ross et al. (50) suggested that both OI and otosclerosis lead to similar labyrinthine bony alterations based on different etiologies or on whether they coexist, otosclerosis being part of OI. Nager (38) reached similar conclusions.

Berger et al. (6) and others (1,7,9,27,51,54,72) noted both deficient and abnormal ossification in the otic capsule, bony walls of the middle ear, and ossicles. Fractures or microfractures were found in the crura of the stapes, handle of malleus, and otic capsule. Hemorrhage into the inner ear was found by several investigators (1,6,7,27).

Vestibular function. In one study (29), over half of the patients had vertigo. Some, but not all, had abnormal electronystagmography and/or basilar impression.

Type III

Type III osteogenesis imperfecta is characterized as progressively deforming with normal sclerae. Head size is disproportionately large compared to the rest of the body, but the ossification defect in the skull is not as severe as that in OI, type II. Frontal and temporal bossing contribute to the triangular facial appearance (Fig. 8–30B).

Fractures are present at birth in more than half of the infants. All have numerous fractures by 1–2 years of age. Long bones are subject to multiple fractures and bowing (Fig. 8–30B,C). The limbs are not as short or as deformed as in OI, type II. In the first few years, metaphyses develop increasing density and irregularity, which progress so that by the end of the first decade, metaphyses and epiphyseal zones are replaced by whorls of radiodensity. Progressive and marked vertebral flattening with "codfish" changes are also observed. Trunk shortening is common and severe kyphoscoliosis may develop, most patients becoming markedly handicapped.

Auditory system. Although hearing loss has been said to occur infrequently (57), audiologic findings have not been well documented in patients with unequivocal type III. However, it is our experience, based on about 100 patients, that 5% or less have conductive hearing loss.

Type IV (A,B)

Osteogenesis imperfecta type IV is phenotypically similar to type I, but the sclerae are more often light blue or gray, rather than strikingly blue as they are in type I. Additional manifestations include increased incidence of bruising, nosebleeds, excessive sweating, and joint hypermobility (40).

Auditory system. In patients over 30, the frequency of hearing impairment (30%) is less than that in osteogenesis imperfecta type I (45). Kuurila et al. (28) found conductive hearing loss in 4.4% of those younger than 17 years.

Heredity. Probably all types of OI have autosomal dominant inheritance (65,71). Those previously thought to have autosomal recessive inheritance probably represent gonadal mosaicism (11,12). Somatic cell mutations have also been shown (17).

Diagnosis. A large number of osteogenesis-like syndromes distinguishable from the major types listed in Table 8–4 are known (3–5,8,14,15,20,24,36,45–47), and these have been discussed exten-

sively by Gorlin et al. (24). Prenatal diagnosis has been accomplished (67).

Summary. Characteristics of this syndrome include (*1*) autosomal dominant inheritance; (*2*) increased bone fragility; (*3*) osteoporosis; (*4*) various other anomalies, depending on the specific type of osteogenesis imperfecta; and (*5*) hearing loss, generally mixed.

References

1. Altmann F, Kornfeld M: Osteogenesis imperfecta and otosclerosis. New investigations. *Ann Otol Rhinol Laryngol* 76:89–104, 1967.
2. Andersen PE, Hauge M: Osteogenesis imperfecta: a genetic, radiological, and epidemiological study. *Clin Genet* 36:250–255, 1989.
3. Beighton P: Familial dentinogenesis imperfecta, blue sclerae, and wormian bones without fractures: another type of osteogenesis imperfecta? *J Med Genet* 88:124–128, 1985.
4. Beighton P et al: Skeletal complications in osteogenesis imperfecta. A review of 153 South African patients. *S Afr Med J* 64:565–568, 1983.
5. Beighton P et al: The ocular form of osteogenesis imperfecta: a new autosomal recessive syndrome. *Clin Genet* 28:69–74, 1985.
6. Berger G et al: Histopathology of the temporal bone in osteogenesis imperfecta: a report of 5 cases. *Laryngoscope* 95:193–199, 1985.
7. Bergstrom L: Osteogenesis imperfecta: otologic and maxillofacial aspects. *Laryngoscope* 87(Suppl 6):1–42, 1977.
8. Brady AF, Patton MA: Osteogenesis imperfecta with arthrogryposis multiplex congenita (Bruck syndrome)—evidence for possible autosomal recessive inheritance. *Clin Dysmorphol* 6:329–336, 1997.
9. Brosnan M et al: Surgery and histopathology of the stapes in osteogenesis imperfecta tarda. A report of 10 cases. *Arch Otolaryngol* 103:294–298, 1977.
10. Byers PH: Disorders of collagen metabolism. In: *Metabolic Basis of Inherited Disease*, 7th ed., Scriver CR, Beaudet AL, Sly SW, Valle D (eds), McGraw-Hill, New York, 1995, pp. 4029–4077.
11. Byers PH et al: Osteogenesis imperfecta: translation of mutation to phenotype. *J Med Genet* 28:433–442, 1991.
12. Cohen-Solal L et al: Dominant mutations in familial lethal and severe osteogenesis imperfecta. *Hum Genet* 87:297–301, 1991.
13. Cohn DH et al: Recurrence of lethal osteogenesis imperfecta due to parental mosaicism for a dominant mutation in a human type I collagen gene (*COL1A1*). *Am J Hum Genet* 46:591–601, 1990.
14. Colavita N et al: Calvarial doughnut lesions with osteoporosis, multiple fractures, dentinogenesis imperfecta and tumorous changes in the jaws. *Australas Radiol* 28:226–231, 1984.
15. Cole DEC, Carpenter TO: Bone fragility, craniosynostosis, ocular proptosis, hydrocephalus, and distinctive facial features: a newly recognized type of osteogenesis imperfecta. *J Pediatr* 110:76–80, 1987.
16. Cole DEC, Cohen MM Jr: Osteogenesis imperfecta: an update. *J Pediatr* 119:73–74, 1991.
17. Constantinou-Deltas CD et al: Somatic cell mosaicism: another source of phenotypic heterogeneity in nuclear families with osteogenesis imperfecta. *Am J Med Genet* 45:246–251, 1993.
18. Cox JR, Simmons CL: Osteogenesis imperfecta and associated hearing loss in five kindreds. *S Med J* 75:1222–1226, 1982.
19. Cremers CWRJ, Garretsen AJM: Stapes surgery in osteogenesis imperfecta. *Am J Otol* 10:474–476, 1989.
20. Frontali M: Osteoporosis-pseudoglioma syndrome: report of three affected sibs and an overview. *Am J Med Genet* 22:35–47, 1985.
21. Gage JP et al: Dentine is biochemically abnormal in osteogenesis imperfecta. *Clin Sci* 70:339–346, 1986.
22. Garretsen TJTM: Osteogenesis Imperfecta Type I. Otological and Clinical Genetic Aspects. PhD Thesis, Catholic University, Nijmegen, The Netherlands, 1992.
23. Garretsen TJTM, Cremers CWRJ: Clinical and genetic aspects in autosomal dominant inherited osteogenesis imperfecta type I. *Ann NY Acad Sci* 630:240–248, 1991.
24. Gorlin RJ et al: *Syndromes of the Head and Neck*, 4th ed. Oxford University Press, New York, 2001.
25. Hollister DW: Molecular basis of osteogenesis imperfecta. *Curr Probl Dermatol* 17:76–94, 1987.
26. Hortop J et al: Cardiovascular involvement in osteogenesis imperfecta. *Circulation* 73:54–61, 1986.
27. Igarashi M et al: Inner ear pathology in osteogenesis imperfecta congenita. *J Laryngol Otol* 94:697–705, 1980.
28. Kuurila K et al: Hearing loss in children with osteogenesis imperfecta. *Eur J Pediatr* 159:515–519, 2000.
29. Kuurila K et al: Vestibular dysfunction in adult patients with osteogenesis imperfecta. *Am J Med Genet* 120A:350–358, 2003.

30. Lanting PJH et al: Decreased scattering coefficient of blue sclerae. *Clin Genet* 27:187–190, 1985.
31. Levin LS et al: Scanning electron microscopy of teeth in autosomal dominant osteogenesis imperfecta: support for genetic heterogeneity. *Am J Med Genet* 5:189–199, 1980.
32. Levin LS et al: The dentition in the osteogenesis imperfecta syndromes. *Clin Orthop Rel Res* 159:64–74, 1981.
33. Lukinmaa P-L et al: Dental findings in osteogenesis imperfecta: I. Occurrence and expression of type I dentinogenesis imperfecta. *J Craniofac Genet Dev Biol* 7:115–125, 1987.
34. Lukinmaa P-L et al: Dental findings in osteogenesis imperfecta: II. Dysplastic and other developmental defects. *J Craniofac Genet Dev Biol* 7:127–135, 1987.
35. Lund AM et al: Dental manifestations of osteogenesis imperfecta and abnormalities of collagen I metabolism. *J Craniofac Genet Dev Biol* 18:30–37, 1998.
36. McLean JR et al: The Grant syndrome. Persistent wormian bones, blue sclerae, mandibular hypoplasia, shallow glenoid fossae and campomelia—an autosomal dominant trait. *Clin Genet* 29:523–529, 1986.
37. Müller E: Die Schwerhörigkeit bei Osteogenesis imperfecta. *Laryngol Rhinol* 53:805–809, 1974.
38. Nager GT: Osteogenesis imperfecta of the temporal bone and its relation to otosclerosis. *Ann Otorhinolaryngol* 97:585–593, 1988.
39. Nuytinck L et al: Osteogenesis imperfecta phenotypes resulting from serine for glycine substitutions in the alpha2 (I) collagen chain. *Eur J Hum Genet* 5:161–167 1997.
40. Paterson CR et al: Osteogenesis imperfecta type I. *J Med Genet* 20:203–205, 1983.
41. Paterson CR et al: Osteogenesis imperfecta with dominant inheritance and normal sclerae. *J Bone Joint Surg Br* 65:35–39, 1983.
42. Paterson CR et al: Clinical and radiological features of osteogenesis imperfecta type IV. *Acta Paediatr Scand* 76:548–552, 1987.
43. Paterson CR et al: Life expectancy in osteogenesis imperfecta. *BMJ* 312:351–353, 1996.
44. Pederson U: Hearing loss in patients with osteogenesis imperfecta. *Scand Audiol* 13:67–74, 1984.
45. Pederson U: Osteogenesis imperfecta. Clinical features. Hearing loss and stapedectomy. *Acta Otolaryngol Suppl* 145:1–36, 1985.
46. Pozo JL et al: Basilar impression in osteogenesis imperfecta. A report of three cases in one family. *J Bone Joint Surg Br* 66:233–238, 1984.
47. Pyeritz RE: Heritable disorders of connective tissue. In: *Genetics of Cardiovascular Disease*, Pierpont ME, Moller JH (eds), Marinus Nijhoff Publishing, Boston, 1986, pp 265–303.
48. Reite M, Solomons C: The EEG in osteogenesis imperfecta. *Clin Electroencephalog* 11:16–21, 1980.
49. Riedner ED et al: Hearing patterns in dominant osteogenesis imperfecta. *Arch Otolaryngol* 106:737–740, 1980.
50. Ross UH et al: Osteogenesis imperfecta: clinical symptoms and update findings in computed tomography and tympano-cochlear scintigraphy. *Acta Otolaryngol (Stockh)* 113:620–624, 1993.
51. Sando I et al: Osteogenesis imperfecta tarda and otosclerosis. A temporal bone report. *Ann Otol Rhinol Laryngol* 90:199–203, 1981.
52. Schwartz S, Tsipouras P: Oral findings in osteogenesis imperfecta. *Oral Surg Oral Med Oral Pathol Endod* 57:161–167, 1984.
53. Shapiro JR et al: Hearing and middle ear function in osteogenesis imperfecta. *JAMA* 247:2120–2126, 1982.
54. Shea JJ, Postma DS: Findings and long-term surgical results in the hearing loss of osteogenesis imperfecta. *Arch Otolaryngol* 108:467–470, 1982.
55. Sillence DO: Osteogenesis imperfecta. An expanding panorama of variants. *Clin Orthop* 159:11–25, 1981.
56. Sillence DO et al: Clinical variability in osteogenesis imperfecta—variable expressivity or genetic heterogeneity. *Birth Defects* 15(5B):113–129, 1979.
57. Sillence DO et al: Genetic heterogeneity in osteogenesis imperfecta. *J Med Genet* 16:101–116, 1979.
58. Sillence DO et al: Osteogenesis imperfecta type II. Delineation of the phenotype with reference to genetic heterogeneity. *Am J Med Genet* 17:407–423, 1984.
59. Sillence DO et al: Osteogenesis imperfecta type III. Delineation of the phenotype with reference to genetic heterogeneity. *Am J Med Genet* 23:821–832, 1986.
60. Sillence DO et al: Natural history of blue sclerae in osteogenesis imperfecta. *Am J Med Genet* 45:183–186, 1993.
61. Smith R et al: *The Brittle Bone Syndrome. Osteogenesis Imperfecta.* Butterworths, London, 1983.
62. Stewart EJ, O'Reilly BF: A clinical and audiological investigation of osteogenesis imperfecta. *Clin Otolaryngol* 14:509–514, 1989.
63. Stoll C et al: Birth prevalence rates of skeletal dysplasias. *Clin Genet* 35:88–92, 1989.
64. Stolz MR et al: Osteogenesis imperfecta. *Perspect Clin Orthoped* 242:120–136, 1989.
65. Sykes B: Linkage analysis in dominantly inherited osteogenesis imperfecta. *Am J Med Genet* 45:212–216, 1993.
66. Sykes B et al: Consistent linkage of dominantly inherited osteogenesis imperfecta to the type I collagen loci: COL1A1 and COL1A2. *Am J Hum Genet* 46:293–307, 1990.
67. Thompson EM: Non-invasive prenatal diagnosis of osteogenesis imperfecta. *Am J Med Genet* 45:201–206, 1993.
68. Tsipouras P: Osteogenesis imperfecta. In: *Heritable Disorders of Connective Tissue*, 5th ed., Beighton P (ed), C.V. Mosby, St. Louis, 1993, pp 281–314.
69. van der Harten H et al: Perinatal lethal osteogenesis imperfecta. Radiologic pathologic evaluation of seven prenatally diagnosed cases. *Pediatr Pathol* 8:233–252, 1988.
70. White NJ et al: Cardiovascular abnormalities in osteogenesis imperfecta. *Am Heart J* 106:1416–1420, 1983.
71. Willing MC et al: Molecular heterogeneity in osteogenesis imperfecta type I. *Am J Med Genet* 45:223–227, 1993.
72. Zajtchuk JT, Lindsay JR: Osteogenesis imperfecta congenita and tarda. A temporal bone report. *Ann Otol Rhinol Laryngol* 84:350–358, 1975.

Paget disease of bone (osteitis deformans)

In 1876, Paget (28) described osteitis deformans, which begins in middle age and is characterized by changes in shape, size, and direction of involved bones. It subsumes familial progressive osteolysis that appears to have earlier onset and more aggressive behavior (1). Usually the disorder symmetrically affects the skull and bones of the lower extremities (11). The bones enlarge and soften, and those that are weight-bearing yield and become curved and misshapen. With extensive cranial and vertebral changes, neurologic signs and symptoms often appear. Paget disease of bone is common, occurring with an incidence of about 4.5% in the United States and Latin America (33). Beethoven may have had the condition (26).

During the early stages of the disorder, there is an increase in osteoblastic activity and osteoclastic bone resorption accompanied by defects in calcification of the newly formed bone matrix, which is not adequately remodeled according to the lines of stress (23). Paget disease exhibits both qualitative and quantitative abnormalities of bone formation. The osteoclasts have many more nuclei than normal and tend to be larger and more irregular in size and shape (29).

Craniofacial findings. Clinical alterations begin in the fifth decade with progressive skull enlargement and frontal bossing. The maxilla becomes especially enlarged (Fig. 8–31A,B). There is tortuosity of the terminal branches of the temporal artery in about 70% of the cases (Fig. 8–31C).

Musculoskeletal system. The onset of bony changes is insidious and progresses slowly. When symptoms are a feature, bone pain has been noted in about 50% of the cases. The bones most strikingly involved are the sacrum, pelvis, lumbar vertebrae, femur, and skull. The cranium may gradually enlarge, and the patient may become aware of the disorder when his or her hat no longer fits. About 15% have involvement of the maxilla or, rarely, the mandible. Kyphosis and bowing of the leg bones result in shortened stature. The involved bones are more susceptible to fracture, but they usually heal well. Sarcomatous changes occur in 1%–3%. One may also rarely find true giant cell tumor of bone.

Radiographic findings. The early stage of osteitis deformans is osteoclastic. In later stages, the affected bones assume a "cotton-wool" appearance as a result of formation of premature, coarse-fibered bone in discontinuous trabeculae that gradually are replaced by thick trabeculae with a mosaic pattern (Fig. 8–31D,E). Radiographs show increased size of affected bones, coarse trabeculation, and bowing of the extremities. Most frequently involved are the skull, tibiae, pelvis, vertebrae, and femora.

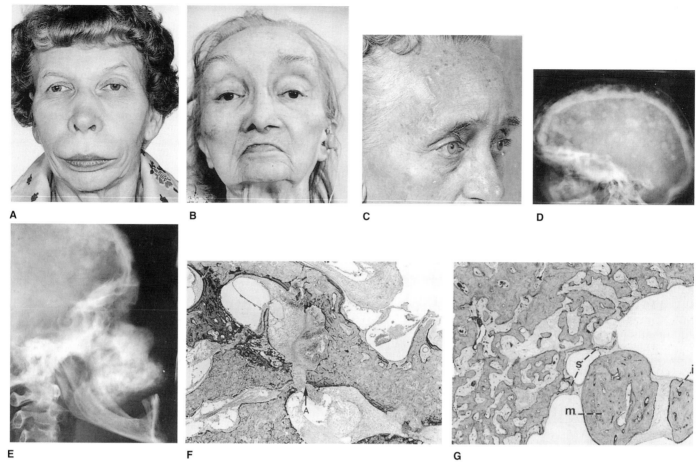

Figure 8–31. *Paget disease of bone (osteitis deformans).* (A,B) Facies of two older individuals with long-standing history of head enlargement and deformity with concomitant hearing loss. (C) Increased tortuosity and enlargement of anterior branch of superficial temporal artery. (D) "Cotton-wool" appearance of skull as well as thickening of calvaria. (E) Note similar changes in maxillary ara of second patient. (F) Photomicrograph of cochlear duct of patient with Paget's disease. Labyrinthine capsule is extensively replaced by Paget bone. Note dilated duct, absorption of walls of posterior canal, fibrosis in middle ear, scala tympani, and posterior canal. Also note fracture from posterior canal ampulla to scali tympani and round window niche. (G) Temporal bone section showing Pagetic projections (s) arising from epitympanic wall and lying in close proximity to head of malleus (m) and incus (i). [(B) from SM Gage et al., *Oral Surg* 20:616, 1965; (C,G) from DG Davies, *Acta Otolaryngol (Suppl)* 242:1, 1968; (F) from JR Lindsay and RH Lehman, *Laryngoscope* 79:213, 1969.]

Pathology. The skull is enlarged, and the calvaria is markedly thickened and shows narrowing of the diploë. Recently affected long bones may show sharp lines of demarcation between involved areas and the normal cortex. This suggests that Paget disease begins focally and spreads gradually.

Histologic sections reveal a characteristic mosaic bone pattern. This results from resorption of older, calcified bone and deposition of the new osteoid layers, thereby altering the original architecture. This alteration is associated with fibrosis and increased vascularity of marrow spaces.

Central nervous system. Neuromuscular disturbances, such as sensory-motor, reflex, gait, or central nervous system changes, are common. About 20% of those with skull involvement experience tinnitus and/or vertigo. In advanced disease, headache, especially occipital, is an almost constant feature (6,8). Occasionally there is involvement of the optic nerve, and, following collapse of an osteoporotic vertebra, there is compression of the spinal cord. Optic atrophy due to compression of the nerves in the optic foramina is a rare complication.

Auditory system. Patients may have narrowing and/or tortuosity of the external auditory meatus (6,36). Marked involvement of the auditory system more often accompanies advanced skull changes. In a review of 400 cases, Goldstein et al. (9) noted hearing impairment in

only 5% of the cases. Davies (6), by contrast, found hearing loss in 40%. The hearing loss may be conductive, sensorineural, or mixed (4,12,21). Among 99 patients, Fowler (8) found that hearing loss was the initial symptom in 3 and a major symptom in 41. Tinnitus was present in 10 and vertigo in 23. Harner et al (12) reviewed 463 patients and noted that most had mixed loss. While sensorineural loss was common, it did not seem to be part of the disease process. Tinnitus and vertigo were noted in 20%. Many investigators (3,4,36) found mixed deafness most frequently. Audiometric tests did not suggest evidence of a retrocochlear focus of the disease to account for the sensorineural component. Petasnick (30), however, found sensorineural loss to be more common. In a study of 41 patients, Lenarz et al. (21) found conductive hearing loss in 20% and sensorineural hearing loss in all.

Davies (6) noted that most patients have conductive loss in the low frequencies—the air–bone gap being greatest at 500 Hz. SISI scores were low at low frequencies but were high at high frequencies (above 1000 Hz) (4).

Tomography has shown demineralization of the petrous pyramid. About 60% of patients manifest partial or complete demineralization of the cochlea, whereas approximately 50% exhibit changes in the rest of the otic capsule. Thickening of the footplate of the stapes is evident in about 25%. Over 65% of patients with conductive loss have no radiographic changes in the middle ear (30).

Vestibular system. Among 28 patients complaining of vertigo, Davies (6) found a diminished caloric reaction in only two individuals. Others who have found decreased caloric response include Clemis et al. (4), Harner et al. (12), and Simmons (34). In the three cases we studied, one patient had no response to caloric stimulation, whereas the other two were normal.

Temporal bone findings. There have been several reports of histopathologic changes in the temporal bones (6,10,22,25,31,32,37). The earliest changes include increased remodeling of bone surrounding vascular channels near the labyrinthine capsule and finally encroaching upon the endosteum of the membranous labyrinth (10,31) (Fig. 8–31F,G). There is a variable degree of degeneration of sensory cells of the saccular and utricular maculae and cristae of the semicircular canals. In the organ of Corti there is degeneration of the stria vascularis and hair cells, edema of the tectorial membrane, and dilation of the cochlear duct. Kornfield's (18) study of seven temporal bones affected with osteitis deformans showed that when the innermost portion of the capsule was affected, there was thickening of the stria adjacent to the thickenings and formation of intravascular concrements. There were also occasional findings of microaneurysms. Few authors (2) found compression of the auditory nerve in the internal auditory meatus. Thus, the pathologic changes appear to originate from encroachment on the labyrinthine capsule by the altered bone and possibly by the attendant vascular changes. Lenarz et al. (21) noted hair cell damage in 80%, with over 30% having a retrocochlear lesion, depending on the degree of deformity of the temporal bone. Khetarpar and Schuknecht (16) did not find ossicular fixation in 26 temporal bones. They concluded that hearing loss was due to changes in bone density, mass, and form.

Laboratory findings. Serum alkaline phosphatase levels are greatly elevated. In about 10% of patients, the urinary calcium level is high. Serum calcium and phosphorus levels are normal (17).

Etiology. Paget disease has autosomal dominant inheritance with incomplete penetrance and variable expressivity (7,20,24). About 40% have affected first-degree relatives (5).

The disorder is heterogeneous, some cases (see Familial expansile osteolysis) being caused by mutation in *TNFRSF11A* gene (PDB2) on chromosome 18q21.2, which encodes RANK, a protein essential in osteoclast formation (5). Other gene loci are PDB1 on 6p, PDB3 on 5q35, and PDB4 on 5q31 (13–15,19,27,35,38). Recently the sequestosome 1 (*SQSTM1*) gene was mapped to the PDB3 critical region, and is thus responsible for some familial, as well as some sporadic cases of Paget's disease.

Summary. Characteristics include (*1*) autosomal dominant inheritance with incomplete penetrance and variable expression; (*2*) onset in middle age; (*3*) macrocephaly; (*4*) bending of weight-bearing bones; (*5*) involvement of sacrum, pelvis, vertebrae, long bones, and skull; (*6*) neurologic deficits and/or spinal cord compression; (*7*) elevated alkaline phosphatase; and (*8*) mixed hearing loss.

References

1. Adams DA et al: Otological manifestations of a new familial polyostotic bone dysplasia. *J Laryngol Otol* 105:80–84, 1991.
2. Applebaum EL, Clemis JD: Temporal bone histopathology of Paget's disease with sensorineural hearing loss and narrowing of the internal auditory canal. *Laryngoscope* 87:1753–1759, 1977.
3. Baraka ME: Rate of progression of hearing loss in Paget's disease. *J Laryngol Otol* 98:573–575, 1984.
4. Clemis JD et al: The clinical diagnosis of Paget's disease of the temporal bone. *Ann Otol Rhinol Laryngol* 76:611–623, 1967.
5. Cody JD et al: Genetic linkage of Paget's disease of the bone to chromosome 18q. *Am J Hum Genet* 61:1117–1122, 1997.
6. Davies DG: Paget's disease of the temporal bone. A clinical and histopathological survey. *Acta Otolaryngol (Stockh) Suppl* 242:1–47, 1968.
7. Evens RG, Bartter FC: The hereditary aspects of Paget's disease: (osteitis deformans). *JAMA* 205:900–902, 1968.
8. Fowler EP Jr: Nerve deafness from noninflammatory lesions. *Trans Am Otol Soc* 27:381–392, 1937.
9. Goldstein H et al: Paget's disease of the bones (osteitis deformans), with report of seven additional cases. *Med Times* 54:194–200, 1926.
10. Gussen R: Early Paget's disease of the labyrinthine capsule. *Arch Otolaryngol* 91:341–345, 1970.
11. Hamdy RC: Clinical features and pharmacologic treatment of Paget's disease. *Endocrinol Metab Clin North Am* 24:421–436, 1995.
12. Harner SG et al: Paget's disease and hearing loss. *Otolaryngology* 86:869–874, 1978.
13. Haslam SI et al: Paget's disease of bone: evidence for a susceptibility locus on chromosome 18q and for genetic heterogeneity. *J Bone Miner Res* 13:911–917, 1998.
14. Hocking LJ et al: Domain-specific mutations in sequestosome 1 (SQSTM1) cause familial and sporadic Paget disease. *Hum Mol Genet* 11:2735–2739, 2002.
15. Hughes AE et al: Mutations in *TNFRSF11A*, affecting the signal peptide of RANK, cause familial expansile osteolysis. *Nat Genet* 24:45–48, 2000.
16. Khetarpar U, Schuknecht HF: In search of pathologic correlates for hearing loss and vertigo in Paget's disease. A clinical and histopathologic study of 26 temporal bones. *Ann Otol Rhinol Laryngol* (Suppl)145:1–16, 1990.
17. Klein RM, Norman A: Diagnostic procedures for Paget's disease: radiologic, pathologic and laboratory testing. *Endocrinol Metab Clin North Am* 24:437–450, 1995.
18. Kornfield M: Pathological changes in the stria vascularis in Paget's disease. *Pract Otorhinolaryngol* 29:406–432, 1967.
19. Laurin N et al: Paget disease of bone: mapping at locus at 5q35–qter and 5q31. *Am J Hum Genet* 69:528–543, 2001.
20. Leach RJ et al: Genetics of endocrine disease: the genetics of Paget's disease of the bone. *Endocrinol Metab Clin North Am* 86:24–28, 2001.
21. Lenarz T et al: Hörstörungen bei Morbus Paget. *Laryngol Rhinol Otol* 65:213–217, 1986.
22. Lindsay JR, Suga F: Paget's disease and sensorineural deafness. Temporal bone histopathology of Paget's disease. *Laryngoscope* 86:1029–1042, 1976.
23. Mills BG: Bone resorbing cells and human clinical conditions. In: *Bone, Vol II. The Osteoclast*, Hall BK (ed), CRC Press, Boca Raton, 1991, pp 175–252.
24. Morales-Piga AA et al: Frequency and characteristics of familial aggregation in Paget disease of bone. *J Bone Miner Res* 10:663–670, 1995.
25. Nager GT: Paget's disease of the temporal bone. *Ann Otol Suppl* 22:1–32, 1975.
26. Naiken VS: Did Beethoven have Paget's disease of bone? *Ann Intern Med* 74:995–999, 1971.
27. Nance MA et al: Heterogeneity in Paget's disease of the bone. *Am J Med Genet* 92:303–307, 2000.
28. Paget J: On a form of chronic inflammation of bones (osteitis deformans). *Proc R Med Chir Soc (Lond)* 8:127–128, 1876.
29. Parfitt AM: Bone-forming cells in clinical conditions. In: *Bone, Vol. I. The Osteoblast and Osteocyte*, Hall BK (ed), Telford Press, Caldwell, NJ, 1990, pp 351–429.
30. Petasnick JP: Tomography of the temporal bone in Paget's disease. *AJR Am J Roentgenol* 105:838–843, 1969.
31. Proops D et al: Paget's disease and the temporal bone—a clinical and histopathological review of six temporal bones. *J Otolaryngol* 14:20–29, 1985.
32. Ramsay HAW, Linthicum FH: Cochlear histopathology in Paget's disease. *Am J Otolaryngol* 14:60–61, 1993.
33. Schajowicz F et al: Metastases of carcinoma in the Pagetic bone. A report of two cases. *Clin Orthop* 228:290–296, 1988.
34. Simmons FB: Patients with bilateral loss of caloric response. *Ann Otol Rhinol Laryngol* 82:175–178, 1973.
35. Siris ES: Epidemiological aspects of Paget disease: family history and relationship to other medical conditions. *Semin Arthritis Rheum* 23:222–225, 1994.
36. Sparrow NL, Duvall AJ: Hearing loss and Paget's disease. *J Laryngol* 81:601–611, 1967.
37. Tamari M: Histopathologic changes of the temporal bone in Paget's disease. *Ann Otol* 51:170–208, 1942.
38. Wu RK et al: Familial incidence of Paget's disease and secondary osteogenic sarcoma: a report of three cases from a single family. *Clin Orthop Rel Res* 265:306–309, 1991.

Familial expansile osteolysis

Osterberg et al. (9), in 1988, and Barr et al. (2) and Wallace et al. (11), in 1989, described a family of 42 affected individuals in five generations from Northern Ireland with an apparently unique disorder of bone, similar to Paget disease.

Musculoskeletal system. From late adolescence to middle age, bone pain of variable severity, site, and length of duration was experienced. The skeleton was both generally and focally involved (Fig. 8–32A,B). About 90% of the lesions occurred in the appendicular skele-

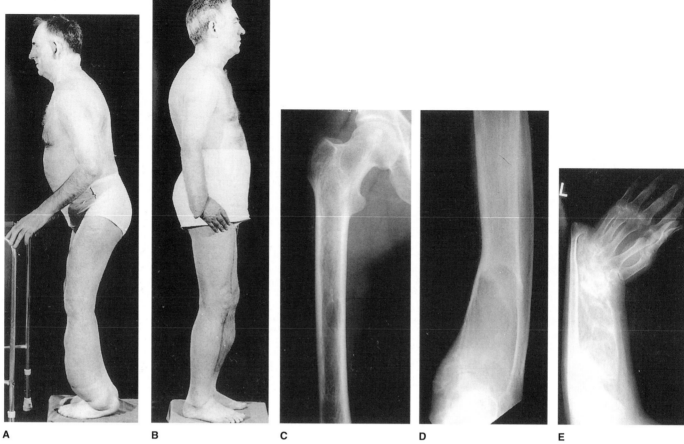

A   **B**   **C**   **D**   **E**

Figure 8–32. *Familial expansile osteolysis.* (A) Lower limb deformity. (B) Deformity of left radius, right tibia and fibula, and left tibia. (C–E) Early, intermediate, and late stage. [From PH Osterberg et al., *J Bone Joint Surg* 70B:225, 1988.]

ton. The long bones, particularly the humerus, radius, ulna, and tibia, were abnormally modeled with a disordered trabecular ("fish-net") pattern. In addition, focal lesions characterized by gradual expansion with cortical thinning, loss of trabeculae, and expansion of bone were evident (Fig. 8–32C–E). The axial skeleton was essentially normal (3,10). Fracture occurred in a number of affected individuals.

Dental system. There was premature loss of teeth with bizarre and extensive resorption of the roots in the cervical region and at the root apices (8).

Auditory system. Hearing loss was evident prior to the age of 10 years. Initially conductive (20–30 dB loss), it progressed to mixed hearing loss (40–45 dB) in older members. High-frequency loss was most marked (1). There was often a well-marked notch at 2000 Hz. Speech discrimination was 80% or better. Exploration showed that the long process of the incus was absent, thin, or replaced by fibrous connective tissue (5). The stapes was fixed in some cases. Microscopically, a large amount of woven bone was present.

Laboratory findings. Laboratory findings included variably elevated serum alkaline phosphatase levels and increased urinary hydroxyproline excretion.

Heredity. Autosomal dominant inheritance was clearly evident. Linkage to 18q21.1–q22 has been established (6), making it allelic to one form of Paget disease. Mutations in the gene *TNFRSF11A* cause the syndrome (7). The gene is related to the signal peptide RANK, in the PDB2 region which is required in osteoclast formation.

Diagnosis. Differential diagnosis would include Paget disease, polyostotic fibrous dysplasia, and Gorham disease. Microscopically, there is resemblance to classic Paget disease.

References

1. Adams DA et al: Otological manifestations of a new familial polyostotic bone disorder. *J Laryngol Otol* 105:80–84, 1991.
2. Barr RJ et al: Idiopathic multicentric osteolysis: report of two new cases and a review of the literature. *Am J Med Genet* 32:556, 1989.
3. Crone MD et al: The radiographic features of familial expansile osteolysis. *Skeletal Radiol* 19:245–250, 1990.
4. Dickson GR et al: Familial expansile osteolysis: a morphological, histomorphometric, and serological study. *Bone* 12:331–338, 1991.
5. Esselman GH et al: Conductive hearing loss caused by hereditary incus necrosis: a study of familial expansile osteolysis. *Otolaryngol Head Neck Surg* 114:639–641, 1996.
6. Hughes AE et al: Genetic linkage of familial expansile osteolysis to chromosome 18q. *Hum Mol Genet* 3:359–362, 1994.
7. Hughes AE et al: Mutations in *TNFRSF11A*, affecting the signal peptide of RANK, cause familial expansile osteolysis. *Nat Genet* 24:45–48, 2000.
8. Mitchell CA et al: Dental abnormalities associated with familial expansile osteolysis: a clinical and radiologic study. *Oral Surg Oral Med Oral Pathol Oral Radiol* 70:301–307, 1990.
9. Osterberg PH et al: Familial expansile osteolysis. *J Bone Joint Surg Br* 70:255–260, 1988.
10. Pai GS, Macpherson RI: Idiopathic multicentric osteolysis: report of two new cases and a review of the literature. *Am J Med Genet* 29:929–936,1988.
11. Wallace RGH et al: Familial expansile osteolysis. *Clin Orthop Rel Res* 248:265–277, 1989.

Fibrodysplasia ossificans progressiva

Fibrodysplasia ossificans progressiva (FOP) is a rare connective tissue disorder with progressive ectopic ossification of tendons, ligaments, facial and skeletal muscles, malformed halluces and thumbs, hearing loss, and baldness. Progressive disability due to ectopic calcification is erratic, but severe restriction of movement eventually occurs and is especially evident in the shoulders and spine (2,9). The condition was first recorded by Guy Patin in 1692 (31). The term *myositis ossificans progressiva* is said to have been assigned by von Dusch in 1868 (2). Since connective tissue is primarily affected, especially aponeuroses, fasciae, and tendons, the term *myositis* is no longer appropriate. In 1918, Rosenstirn (35) analyzed 200 cases. By 1982, an excess of 550 examples had been noted (8). An additional 150 cases have been recorded (16,18,19,29,30,32,36,37,39). Many large series of patients have been followed (2,9,34,42).

Clinical findings. Clinical features include malformation of hallux, hearing loss, baldness, and rarely mental deficiency. Other skeletal abnormalities include short thumbs due to short first metacarpals; clinodactyly of the fifth fingers; short broad femoral necks; abnormal cervical vertebrae with small bodies, large pedicles, and large spinous processes; progressive bony ankylosis of cervical spine; and, occasionally, exostoses of proximal tibiae (9,34) (Fig. 8–33A–C). Regular CT scanning is necessary (22). The radiographic spectrum of abnormalities has been reviewed elsewhere (12,41) (Fig. 8–33D).

Ectopic ossification is progressive and begins in early childhood. The site of onset is most commonly the neck or paraspinal region and less commonly the head or limbs (5). When new lumps appear, reddening of overlying skin may occur and pain may sometimes be present. Certain areas within the connective tissue are prone to ossification, especially paraspinal muscles, limb girdle muscles, and muscles of mastication. Involvement of joint capsules, ligaments, and plantar fasciae is common. MRI is indicated (4). In FOP patients, various factors are known to precipitate ectopic ossification, such as muscle trauma, biopsy, surgical procedures to excise ectopic bone, intramuscular injections, careless venipuncture, and dental

treatment (2,9,23,24,34,38). All patients eventually develop restriction of movement and physical handicap. Episodes of ossification and subsequent disability are characteristically erratic. The disorder is known to have long periods of inactivity. Although ectopic ossification is most marked prior to puberty, new lumps may occur during the sixth and seventh decades. Ectopic calcification has the most severe effect on axial connective tissues, and limb involvement is most marked proximally (6,9). Chest wall fixation may lead to diminished pulmonary reserve, and most patients eventually die from respiratory failure (10).

Baldness occurs in approximately 25% of all patients. The diffuse type, when present, becomes evident in middle age and the majority of those affected are female. It appears to be a primary feature of FOP, although it might conceivably represent a secondary effect of nutritional deficiency based on inability to open the jaws. Mental deficiency is found only as a low-frequency abnormality (3,9). Good reviews are those of Buyse et al. (3) and Connor (7).

Auditory system. Hearing loss has been reported in at least 25% of patients (3,17,27,34,40). Approximately 65% have conductive hearing loss and 35% sensorineural hearing loss. In some cases, hearing loss is noted in early childhood, whereas in others, it occurs in late childhood.

Pathogenesis. Fibrodysplasia ossificans progressiva is a distinctive histopathologic entity that can be differentiated from other soft tissue lesions that ossify, such as myositis ossificans, extraosseous osteosarcoma, and osseous metaplasia (21). Early FOP is characterized by multifocal, interconnecting nodules of spindle-shaped, fibroblast-like cells in a distinctive connective tissue matrix with bone spicules occupying the central area. Foci of chondroid differentiation may sometimes be observed. Lesions evolve to become mature lamellar bone with adipose and hematopoietic tissue in the cancellous spaces; the rim of fibroblast-like cells is no longer evident. Such pathologic features suggest that the spindle-shaped cells, like periosteum, are precursors of the osseous tissue found in FOP lesions. Detailed pathogenetic and biochemical aspects have been discussed elsewhere (2,20,28,40).

Figure 8–33. *Fibrodysplasia ossificans progressiva.* (A) Progressive disability with severe restriction of movement in shoulders and spine. (B) Short fixed thumb secondary to short first metacarpal. Note calcification at wrist. (C) Short first metatarsal results in short hallux. (D) Note short first metacarpal and fusion with proximal phalanx.

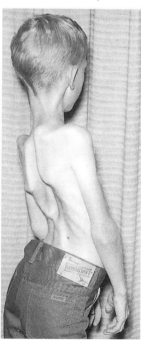
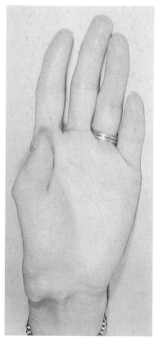
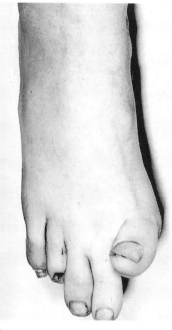
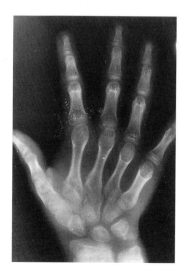

A   B   C   D

Heredity. At least 95% of cases are sporadic (2,42). Autosomal dominant inheritance is based on several instances of parent-to-child and male-to-male transmission (8,11,13,17,20) and on concordant monozygotic twins (14,43). However, most cases arise as new mutations. Genetic fitness due to disability is close to zero. A significant paternal age effect for new mutations has been demonstrated in three separate studies (8,33,42). At least two genes can be responsible. One gene maps to 4q27-31 (15), and based on the finding of a 42 base pair deletion in the *Noggin* (*NOG*) gene in a patient with FOP, *NOG* was thought to be the causative gene (25). However, Xu et al. (44) did not find any *NOG* mutations in over 30 patients with FOP, so *NOG* is less likely of a candidate gene in this region. Other families map to 17q21–q22 (26). Kaplan et al. (20) noted similarity in mutation in the FOP gene and those in *dpp* (decapentaplegic) in fruit flies. There is strong homology with the *BMP* gene (bone morphogenetic protein), especially *BMP4*.

Diagnosis. Delayed diagnosis is commonplace in patients with FOP even though they have characteristic skeletal malformations. Common misdiagnoses are hallux valgus, diaphyseal aclasia, Klippel-Feil anomaly, and various forms of arthrogryposis. Swellings, depending upon their site, may be mistaken for lymphadenopathy, sarcoma, or even mumps. A number of entities have similarities to FOP including osseous metaplasia, extraskeletal osteosarcoma (1), myositis ossificans (especially with a previous history of trauma), and bone formation occurring with pilomatrixoma (12).

Summary. Characteristics include (*1*) autosomal dominant inheritance, although most cases are sporadic; (*2*) progressive ectopic calcification leading to severe restriction of movement; (*3*) malformation of hallux and reduction of digits; (*4*) baldness; and (*5*) hearing loss, both conductive and sensorineural.

References

1. Allan CJ, Soule EH: Osteogenic sarcoma of the somatic soft tissues—clinicopathologic study of 26 cases and review of the literature. *Cancer* 27:1121–1132, 1971.
2. Beighton P: Fibrodysplasia ossificans progressiva. In: *McKusick's Heritable Disorders of Connective Tissue*, 5th ed., Beighton P (ed), C.V. Mosby, St. Louis, 1993, pp 501–518.
3. Buyse G et al: Fibrodysplasia ossificans progressiva: still turning to wood after 300 years? *Eur J Pediatr* 154:694–699, 1996.
4. Caron KH et al: MR imaging of early fibrodysplasia ossificans progressiva. *J Comput Assist Tomogr* 14:318–321, 1990.
5. Chichareon V et al: Fibrodysplasia ossificans progressiva and associated osteochondroma of the coronoid process in a child. *Plast Reconstr Surg* 103:1238–1243, 1999.
6. Cohen RB et al: The natural history of heterotopic ossification in patients who have fibrodysplasia ossificans progressiva. A study of forty-four patients. *J Bone Joint Surg Am* 75:215–219, 1993.
7. Connor JM: Fibrodysplasia ossificans progressiva: lessons from rare maladies. *N Engl J Med* 335:591–593, 1996.
8. Connor JM, Evans DAP: Genetic aspects of fibrodysplasia ossificans progressiva. *J Med Genet* 19:35–39, 1982.
9. Connor JM, Evans DAP: Fibrodysplasia ossificans progressiva: the clinical features and natural history of 34 patients. *J Bone Joint Surg Br* 64:76–83, 1982.
10. Connor JM et al: Cardiopulmonary function in fibrodysplasia ossificans progressiva. *Thorax* 36:419–423, 1981.
11. Connor JM et al: A three generation family with fibrodysplasia ossificans progressiva. *J Med Genet* 30:687–689, 1993.
12. Cremin B et al: The radiological spectrum of fibrodysplasia ossificans progressiva. *Clin Radiol* 33:499–508, 1982.
13. Debeney-Bruyerre C et al: Myositis ossificans progressiva: five generations where the disease was exclusively limited to the jaws. *Int J Oral Maxillofac Surg* 27:299–302, 1998.
14. Eaton WL et al: Early myositis ossificans progressiva occurring in homozygotic twins. A clinical and pathologic study. *J Pediatr* 50:591–598, 1957.
15. Feldman G et al: Fibrodysplasia ossificans progressiva, a heritable disorder of severe heterotopic ossification maps to human chromosome 4q27–31. *Am J Hum Genet* 66:128–135, 2000.
16. Heifetz SA et al: Myositis (fasciitis) ossificans in an infant. *Pediatr Pathol* 12:223–229, 1992.
17. Janoff HB et al: Mild expression of fibrodysplasia ossificans progressiva: a report of 3 cases. *J Rheumatol* 22:976–978, 1995.
18. Janoff HB et al: Fibrodysplasia ossificans progressiva in two half sisters: evidence for maternal mosaicism. *Am J Med Genet* 61:320–324, 1996.
19. Jouve JL et al: Myositis ossificans: report of seven cases in children. *J Pediatr Ophthalmol Strabismus* 6:33–41, 1997.
20. Kaplan FS et al: Genetic transmission of fibrodysplasia ossificans progressiva. *J Bone Joint Surg Am* 75:1214–1220, 1993.
21. Kaplan FS et al: The histopathology of fibrodysplasia ossificans progressiva. *J Bone Joint Surg Am* 75:320–330, 1993.
22. Kransdorf MJ et al: Myositis ossificans: MR appearance with radiologic–pathologic correlation. *AJR Am J Roentgenol* 157:1243–1248, 1991.
23. Lanchoney TF et al: Permanent heterotopic ossification at the injection site after diphtheria-tetanus-pertussis immunizations in children who have fibrodysplasia ossificans progressiva. *J Pediatr* 126:762–763, 1995.
24. Luchetti W et al: Severe restriction in jaw movement after routine injection of local anesthetics in patients with fibrodysplasia ossificans progressiva. *Oral Surg Oral Med Oral Pathol Oral Radiol Endod* 81:21–25, 1996.
25. Lucotte G et al: A de novo heterozygous deletion of 42 base-pairs in the *noggin* gene of fibrodysplasia ossificans progressiva, a heritable disorder of severe heterotopic ossification, maps to chromosome 4q27–31. *Am J Hum Genet* 66:128–135, 2000.
26. Lucotte G et al: Localization of gene for fibrodysplasia ossificans progressive (FOP) to 17q21–22. *Genet Couns* 11:329–334, 2000.
27. Ludman H et al: Deafness in myositis ossificans progressiva. *J Laryngol Otol* 82:57–63, 1968.
28. Miller RL et al: Studies on alkaline phosphatase activity in cultured cells from a patient with fibrodysplasia ossificans progressiva. *Lab Invest* 37:254–259, 1977.
29. Nuovo MA et al: Myositis ossificans with atypical clinical, radiographic, or pathologic findings: a review of 23 cases. *Skeletal Radiol* 21:87–101, 1992.
30. Nussbaum BL et al: Fibrodysplasia ossificans progressiva: report of a case with guidelines for pediatric dental and anesthetic management. *J Dent Child* 63:448–450, 1996.
31. Patin G: Lettres choisies de feu Monsieur Guy Patin. Letter of 27 August 1648 written to AF. Cologne: Laurens, 1:28, 1692.
32. Rocke DM et al: Age- and joint-specific risk of initial heterotopic ossification in patients who have fibrodysplasia ossificans progressiva. *Clin Orthop* 301:243–248, 1994.
33. Rogers JG, Chase GA: Paternal age effect in fibrodysplasia ossificans progressiva. *J Med Genet* 16:147–148, 1979.
34. Rogers JG, Geho WB: Fibrodysplasia ossificans progressiva. *J Bone Joint Surg Am* 61:909–914, 1979.
35. Rosenstirn J: A contribution to the study of myositis ossificans progressiva. *Ann Surg* 68:485–520, 591–637, 1918.
36. Shafritz AB et al: Overexpression of an osteogenic morphogen in fibrodysplasia ossificans progressiva. *N Engl J Med* 335:555–561, 1996.
37. Shah PB et al: Spinal deformity in patients who have fibrodysplasia ossificans progressiva. *J Bone Joint Surg Am* 76:1442–1450, 1994.
38. Shipton EA et al: Anaesthesia in myositis ossificans progressiva: a case report and clinical review. *S Afr Med J* 67:26–28, 1985.
39. Smith R et al: Fibrodysplasia (myositis) ossificans progressiva: clinicopathological features and natural history. *Q J Med* 89:445–456, 1996.
40. Sörensen MS: Fibrodysplasia ossificans progressiva and hearing loss. *Int J Pediatr Otorhinolaryngol* 14:79–82, 1987.
41. Thickman D et al: Fibrodysplasia ossificans progressiva. *AJR Am J Roentgenol* 139:935–941, 1982.
42. Tünte W et al: Zur Genetik der Myositis ossificans progressiva. *Humangenetik* 4:320–351, 1967.
43. Vastine JA et al: Myositis ossificans progressiva in homozygotic twins. *AJR Am J Roentgenol* 59:204–212, 1948.
44. Xu M-Q et al: Linkage exclusion and mutational analysis of the *noggin* gene in patients with fibrodysplasia ossificans progressiva (FOP). *Clin Genet* 58:291–298, 2000.

Stickler syndromes (hereditary arthroophthalmopathy)

The syndrome of flat midface, cleft palate, high myopia with retinal detachment and cataracts, hearing loss, and arthropathy with generally mild spondyloepiphyseal dysplasia was described by Stickler and coworkers (32,33) in 1965–1967. It is now known as Stickler 1 syndrome and constitutes 25%, of Stickler syndromes. A combination of eye findings, hearing loss, cleft palate, marfanoid build, and bone changes are found. The binary combination of eye changes and cleft palate was described both earlier and later by a large number of authors. Excellent reviews are those of Temple (34) and Snead and Yates (26).

Stickler syndrome 2, representing another 25%, is characterized by midface hypoplasia, anteverted nostrils, small mandible, sensorineural

(40%) or mixed (30%) hearing loss, and joint pain (50%). Height is not reduced. There is mild myopia (16,28). Phenotypically, this form is similar to, or possibly identical to, Marshall syndrome, the latter probably having an in-frame deletion near the 3' end of the gene. The so-called Weissenbacher-Zweymüller phenotype, present during infancy, is also seen in Kniest syndrome (8,9,24).

Craniofacial findings. The craniofacial spectrum ranges from an essentially normal face (15%–25%) to midfacial flattening due to short maxilla, prominent eyes, epicanthal folds, depressed nasal bridge, long philtrum, and small chin (Fig. 8–34A). The face becomes less distinctive with age. Cleft palate, submucous cleft palate, and abnormal palatal mobility have been reported in 20% of cases (7) (Fig. 8–34B). About 30% of infants with Robin sequence have Stickler syndrome (12,22,23).

Ocular system. In type 1, myopia of 8–18 diopters is found in 75%–80% of patients, usually earlier than 6 years of of age. It is possibly congenital and stable. Before the 20th year, paravascular pigmented lattice degeneration or retinal detachment is observed in 70%, often bilaterally. If untreated, this leads to blindness. Associated eye findings are astigmatism (60%), wedge and fleck-type curved cortical cataracts (45%), strabismus (30%), and open-angle glaucoma (10%). Detachment occurs in 60%. Eye findings have been extensively discussed (4,10,15,17,25).

Musculoskeletal system. Some patients have a marfanoid body habitus, but at least 25% are below the third centile in height. In childhood, joint hypermobility is common. The joints may be enlarged, often hyperextensible (35%), and sometimes painful and warm with use, becoming stiff with rest (Fig. 8–34C,D). Talipes equinovarus may occur.

Radiographic findings. In infancy, there is rhizomelic shortening of limbs, metaphyseal widening, and vertebral coronal clefts. During childhood, mild spondyloepiphyseal dysplasia (multiple epiphyseal ossification disturbances, moderate flattening of vertebral bodies) and

diminution of the width of the shaft of tubular bones are noted (Fig. 8–34E). Scoliosis has been evident in 10%. The pelvic bones are hypoplastic, the femoral necks being poorly modeled and plump (Fig. 8–34F). There is progressive early joint degeneration in 30%, beginning in the third or fourth decade (13). The skeletal features observed radiographically and the clinical joint involvement are not always present in Stickler syndrome (19,30). Short cranial base and hypoplastic midface have been borne out by cephalometric study (22).

Other findings. Mitral valve prolapse has been found in almost 50% in some surveys (14) but not in others (26).

Auditory system. Progressive sensorineural high-tone hearing loss has been noted in 60% of type 1 patients (19,29,32,34,39). In type 2, sensorineural hearing loss occurs in 90%.

Heredity. Inheritance for both types is clearly autosomal dominant with considerable variable expression. Mutations in the collagen (*COL2A1*) gene for Stickler syndrome type 1 is at 12q13.11 (2,3,11,27). Virtually all mutations involve premature stop codons (1,21).

Type XI collagen, a heterotrimer composed of α1(XI), α2(XI), and α1 (II) chains, copolymerizes with type II collagen and probably regulates fibril thickness. Mutations of the *COL11A1* gene that maps to 1q21 lead to type 2 Stickler syndrome and/or Marshall syndrome (20,26,31). Nonocular Stickler syndromes are known as OSMED. There are dominant and recessive forms resulting from mutations in *COL11A2*, which are discussed in the subsequent section. In OSMED, the midface is smaller, height is reduced, epiphyses are enlarged, and eye involvement is missing (5,18,35). There may well be further heterogeneity (6,16,36–38).

Diagnosis. All patients with Robin sequence, especially with autosomal dominant history, should be examined periodically for severe myopia to prevent ocular complications of the Stickler syndrome. Other disorders with some degree of overlap include Wagner syndrome, Marshall syndrome, Kniest dysplasia, SED congenita, SPONASTRIME

Figure 8–34. *Stickler syndrome.* (A) Round face with midface hypoplasia. (B) Submucous palatal cleft and bifid uvula. (C,D) Enlargement of elbows and knees. (E) Note especially flattening of the ends of metacarpals and radii. (F) Degenerative changes at hip. [(A) from J Hall, *Birth Defects* 10(8):157, 1974.]

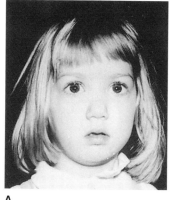
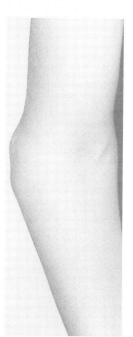
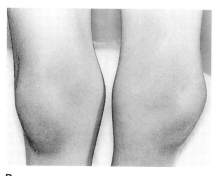
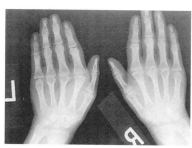
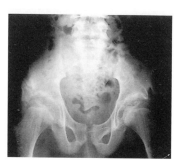
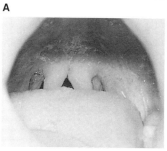

A

B

C

D

E

F

dysplasia, and OSMED, both dominant and recessive. Knobloch syndrome, a recessive disorder, consists of retinal detachment and occipital exencephaloceles.

Summary. Characteristics include (*1*) autosomal dominant inheritance; (*2*) ossification disturbances, including epiphyseal abnormalities; diaphyseal narrowing, and platyspondyly; (*3*) joint hypermobility; (*4*) hypoplastic midface; (*5*) severe myopia and often retinal detachment; (*6*) occasionally cleft palate; and (*7*) mixed hearing loss.

References

1. Ahmad NN et al: A second mutation in the type II procollagen gene (*COL2A1*) causing Stickler syndrome (arthroophthalmopathy) is also a premature termination codon. *Am J Hum Genet* 52:39–45, 1993.
2. Ahmad NN et al: Stickler syndrome: a mutation in the nonhelical 3 end of the type II procollagen gene. *Arch Ophthalmol* 113:1454–1457, 1995.
3. Ballo R et al: Stickler-like syndrome due to a dominant negative mutation in the *COL2A1* gene. *Am J Med Genet* 80:6–11, 1998.
4. Blair NP et al: Hereditary progressive arthro-ophthalmopathy of Stickler. *Am J Ophthalmol* 88:876–888, 1979.
5. Brunner HG et al: A Stickler syndrome is linked to chromosome 6 near the *COL11A2* gene. *Hum Mol Genet* 3:1561–1564, 1994.
6. Fryer AE et al: Exclusion of *COL2A1* as a candidate gene in a family with Wagner-Stickler syndrome. *J Med Genet* 27:91–93, 1990.
7. Hall JG, Herrod H: The Stickler syndrome presenting as a dominantly inherited cleft palate and blindness. *J Med Genet* 12:397–404, 1975.
8. Haller JO et al: The Weissenbacher-Zweymüller syndrome of micrognathia and rhizomelic chondrodysplasia at birth with subsequent normal growth. *AJR Am J Roentgenol* 125:936–943, 1975.
9. Kelly TE et al: The Weissenbacher-Zweymüller syndrome: possible neonatal expression of the Stickler syndrome. *Am J Med Genet* 11:113–119, 1982.
10. Knobloch WH: Inherited hyaloideo-retinopathy and skeletal dysplasia. *Trans Am Ophthalmol Soc* 73:417–429, 1975.
11. Knowlton RG et al: Genetic linkage analysis of hereditary arthro-ophthalmopathy (Stickler syndrome) and the type II procollagen gene. *Am J Hum Genet* 45:681–688, 1989.
12. Kreidler JF et al: Robin-Syndrom mit Oberkiefer-und Nasenhypoplasie—eine erbliche Missbildungskombination? *Fortschr Kiefer Gesichtschir* 21:262–266, 1976.
13. Lewkonia RM: The arthropathy of hereditary arthroophthalmopathy (Stickler syndrome). *J Rheumatol* 19:1271–1275, 1992.
14. Liberfarb RM, Goldblatt A: Prevalence of mitral valve prolapse in the Stickler syndrome. *Am J Med Genet* 24:387–392, 1986.
15. Liberfarb RM et al: The Wagner-Stickler syndrome: a study of 22 families. *J Pediatr* 99:394–399, 1981.
16. Martin S et al: Stickler syndrome: further mutations in *COL11A1* and evidence for additional locus heterogeneity. *Eur J Hum Genet* 7:807–814, 1999.
17. Nielsen CE: Stickler's syndrome. *Acta Ophthalmol* 59:286–295, 1981.
18. Pihlajamaa T et al: A heterozygous glycine substitution in the *COL11A2* gene in the original patient with the Weissenberger-Zweymüller syndrome (heterozygous OSMED) proves its identity with the non-ocular Stickler syndrome. *Am J Med Genet* 80:115–120, 1998.
19. Popkin JS, Polomeno RC: Stickler's syndrome (hereditary progressive arthro-ophthalmopathy). *Can Med Assoc J* 111:1071–1076, 1974.
20. Richards AJ et al: A family with Stickler syndrome type 2 has a mutation in the *COL11A1* gene resulting in the substitution of glycine 97 by valine in alpha-1(XI) collagen. *Hum Mol Genet* 5:1339–1343, 1996.
21. Ritvaniemi P et al: A fourth example suggests that premature termination codons in the *COL2A1* gene are a common cause of the Stickler syndrome. *Genomics* 17:218–221, 1993.
22. Saksena SS et al: Stickler syndrome: a cephalometric study of the face. *J Craniofac Genet Dev Biol* 3:19–28, 1983.
23. Schreiner RL et al: Stickler syndrome in a pedigree of Pierre Robin syndrome. *Am J Dis Child* 126:86–90, 1973.
24. Scribanu N et al: The Weissenbacher-Zweymüller phenotype in the neonatal period as an expression in the continuum of manifestations of the hereditary arthroophthalmopathies. *Ophthalmol Paediatr Genet* 8:159–162, 1987.
25. Seery CM et al: Distinctive cataract in the Stickler syndrome. *Am J Ophthalmol* 110:143–148, 1990.
26. Snead MP, Yates JR: Clinical and molecular genetics of Stickler syndrome. *J Med Genet* 36:353–359, 1999.
27. Snead MP et al: Stickler syndrome: correlation between vitreoretinal phenotypes and linkage to *COL2A1*. *Eye* 8:609–614, 1994.
28. Snead MP et al: Stickler syndrome type 2 and linkage to the *COL11A1* gene. *Ann NY Acad Sci* 785:331–332, 1996.
29. Spallone A: Stickler's syndrome: a study of 12 families. *Br J Ophthalmol* 71:504–509, 1987.
30. Spranger J: Arthro-ophthalmopathia hereditaria. *Ann Radiol (Paris)* 11:359–364, 1968.
31. Spranger J: The type XI collagenopathies. *Pediatr Radiol* 28:745–750, 1998.
32. Stickler GB, Pugh DG: Hereditary progressive arthro-ophthalmopathy. II. Additional observation on vertebral anomalies, a hearing defect and a report of a similar case. *Mayo Clin Proc* 42:495–500, 1967.
33. Stickler GB et al: Hereditary progressive arthroophthalmopathy. *Mayo Clin Proc* 40:433–455, 1968.
34. Temple IK: Stickler's syndrome. *J Med Genet* 26:119–126, 1989.
35. Vikkula M et al: Autosomal dominant and recessive osteochondrodysplasia associated with *COL11A2* locus. *Cell* 80:431–437, 1995.
36. Vintiner GM et al: Genetic and clinical heterogeneity of Stickler syndrome. *Am J Med Genet* 41:44–48, 1991.
37. Weaver EJ et al: Linkage analysis of the type II collagen gene (*COL2A1*) and hereditary arthroophthalmopathy (AOM) in three large families. *Cytogenet Cell Genet* 51:1103, 1989.
38. Wilkin DJ et al: Correlation of linkage data with phenotype in eight families with Stickler syndrome. *Am J Med Genet* 80:121–127, 1998.
39. Zlotogora J et al: Variability of Stickler syndrome. *Am J Med Genet* 42:337–339, 1992.

Myopia, congenital and juvenile cataracts, saddle nose, and sensorineural hearing loss (Marshall syndrome)

Seven members in four generations of a family studied by Marshall (9) in 1958 had short stature, hypoplastic nasal bones, congenital and juvenile cataracts, myopia with vitreoretinal degeneration, and sensorineural hearing loss. Other kindreds have been reported (8,11,12,16–18,21,23–25). There has been considerable debate concerning the identity of this disorder with type 2 Stickler syndrome, a condition that has marked overlap (6,13,20,24,26). Aymé and Preus (3) suggested on objective criteria that they were separate conditions.

Craniofacial findings. The facial appearance, produced by the markedly small nose with sunken nasal bridge, anteverted nostrils, and hypoplastic or flattened midface, is striking (Fig. 8–35).

Ocular system. Failing vision usually occurs in the second decade of life, but may occur within the first 6 months (9,16). Posterior polar cortical and subcapsular opacities that were spontaneously resorbed were noted in the second, third, and fourth decades by Ruppert et al. (16). Although the mother reported by Zellweger et al. (25) had cataracts since 15 years of age, her children had not yet developed cataracts at 7–11 years of age. Severe myopia (10 diopters or more) was also evident from birth, as was fluid vitreous. Retinal detachment may be noted (9,16). In three individuals with *COL11A1* mutations a vitreous type 2 phenotype occured. In this phenotype, there are sparse, irregularly thickened bundles of fibers in the vitreous cavity (20). However, Parentin et al. (14) found type 1 vitreous phenotype in one family with a suspected *COL11A1* mutation.

Auditory system. Affected family members reported some hearing loss in childhood (9). This loss progresses and eventually hearing aids are required. Audiometric tests show about 50 dB mixed or mostly sensorineural hearing loss. Ruppert et al. (16) found severe hearing loss as early as 9 months of age in one child; at 6 years it did not appear to be progressive. A moderate high-tone sensorineural loss was noted in the father, and there were normal vestibular findings. Griffith et al. (7) did not observe any cochlear bony defect nor any middle ear defect on CT.

Radiographic findings. These include hypoplastic nasal bones, hypoplastic maxilla, absent frontal sinuses, and thickening of the outer table of the skull. O'Donnell et al. (12) noted intracranial calcifications, beaked or bullet-shaped vertebrae in children, markedly concave vertebral margins in adults, small irregular pelvis with delayed closure of pubic and ischial bones, coxa valga, mild bowing of radius and ulna, and somewhat irregular epiphyses of extremities.

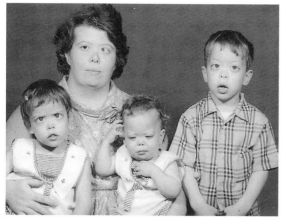
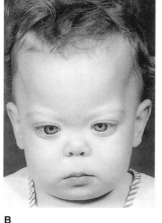
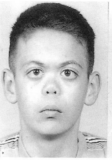
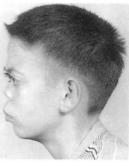

A   **B**   **C**

Figure 8–35. *Myopia, cataracts, saddle nose, and sensorineural hearing loss (Marshall syndrome).* (A) Similar face in a mother and three of her affected children. (B) Face of child seen in (A). (C) Face shows small nose, depressed nasal bridge, and anteverted nostrils. Note that both eyes may be seen from the side. [(A,B) from H Zellweger et al., *J Pediatr* 84:868, 1975; (C) from D Marshall, *Am J Ophthalmol* 45:143, 1958.]

Heredity. The disorder, occurring in several generations, is clearly dominant. Griffith et al. (6) demonstrated a splicing defect at the *COL11A1* locus at 1p21, which has been confirmed by others (2,15). The genes involved in Stickler syndrome are *COL2A1* (4), *COL11A1* (10), and *COL11A2* (1,5,19). Annunen et al. (2) suggested that the nature of the mutation in the *COL11A1* gene determined whether the phenotype would be that of Marshall, Stickler, or an overlap syndrome.

Diagnosis. Saddle-nose defect may be seen in congenital syphilis, acrodysostosis, Stickler syndromes, chondrodysplasia punctata, coumarin embryopathy, and OSMED (22). Myopia may occur as an isolated finding, as an autosomal dominant or recessive trait, or as a component of numerous syndromes such as X-linked myopia and external ophthalmoplegia, spondyloepiphyseal dysplasia congenita, Stickler syndrome, and Wagner syndrome.

Summary. Characteristics include (*1*) autosomal dominant inheritance; (*2*) myopia; (*3*) congenital and juvenile cataracts; (*4*) saddle nose; and (*5*) sensorineural hearing loss.

References

1. Admiraal RJ et al.: Hearing loss in the nonocular Stickler syndrome caused by a *Coll1A2* mutation. *Laryngoscope* 110:457–461, 2000.
2. Annunen S et al: Splicing mutations of 54-bp exons in the *COL11A1* gene cause Marshall syndrome, but other mutations cause overlapping Marshall/Stickler phenotypes. *Am J Hum Genet* 65:974–983, 1999.
3. Aymé S, Preus M: The Marshall and Stickler syndromes: objective rejection of lumping. *J Med Genet* 21:34–38, 1984.
4. Ballo R et al: Stickler-like syndrome due to a dominant negative mutation in the *COL2A1* gene. *Am J Med Genet* 80:6–11, 1998.
5. Brunner HG et al: A Stickler syndrome gene is linked to chromosome 6 near the *Coll1A2* gene. *Hum Mol Genet* 3:1561–1564, 1994.
6. Griffith AJ et al: Marshall syndrome associated with a splicing defect at the COL11A1 locus. *Am J Hum Genet* 62:816–823, 1998.
7. Griffith AJ et al: Audiovestibular phenotype associated with a *COL11A1* mutation in Marshall syndrome. *Arch Otolaryngol Head Neck Surg* 126:891–894, 2000.
8. Günzel H et al: Marshall-Syndrom. Klinisch-genetische Untersuchungen über eine Familie mit 8 Merkmalträgern. *Kinderarztl Prax* 56:25–31, 1988.
9. Marshall D: Ectodermal dysplasia. Report of kindred with ocular abnormalities and hearing defects. *Am J Ophthalmol* 45:143–156, 1958.
10. Martin S et al: Stickler syndrome: further mutations in *coll1A1* and evidence for additional locus heterogeneity. *Eur J Hum Genet* 7:807–814, 1999.
11. Nguyen J et al: Syndrome de Marshall. *Arch Fr Pediatr* 45:49–51, 1988.
12. O'Donnell JJ et al: Generalized osseous abnormalities in Marshall's syndrome. *Birth Defects* 12(5):299–314, 1976.
13. Opitz JM, Lowry RB: Lincoln vs Douglas again: comments on the papers by Curry et al, Greenberg et al, and Gelmont et al. *Am J Med Genet* 26:69–71, 1987.
14. Parentin F et al: Stickler syndrome and vitreoretinal degeneration: correlation between locus mutation and vitreous phenotype. Apropos of a case. *Graefes Arch Clin Exp Ophthalmol* 239:316–319, 2001.
15. Richards AJ et al: A family with Stickler syndrome type 2 has a mutation in the *COL11A1* gene resulting in the substitution of glycine 97 by valine in alpha-1(XI) collagen. *Hum Mol Genet* 5:1339–1343, 1996.
16. Ruppert ES et al: Hereditary hearing loss with saddle-nose and myopia. *Arch Otolaryngol* 92:95–98, 1970.
17. Shanske AL et al: The Marshall syndrome: report of a new family and review of the literature. *Am J Med Genet* 70:52–57, 1997.
18. Shanske AL et al: Marshall syndrome and a defect at the COL11A1 locus. *Am J Hum Genet* 63:1558–1559, 1998.
19. Sirko-Osadsa DA et al: Stickler syndrome without eye involvement is caused by mutations in *COL11A2*, the gene encoding the alpha2(XI) chain of type XI collagen. *J Pediatr* 132:368–371, 1998.
20. Snead MP, Yates JR: Clinical and molecular genetics of Stickler syndrome. *J Med Genet* 36:353–359, 1999.
21. Stratton RF et al: Marshall syndrome. *Am J Med Genet* 41:35–38, 1991.
22. Van Steensel MAM et al: Oto-spondylo-megaepiphyseal dysplasia (OSMED): clinical description of three patients homozygous for a missense mutation in the *COL11A2* gene. *Am J Med Genet* 70:315–323, 1997.
23. Warman ML et al: Reply to Shanske et al. *Am J Hum Genet* 63:1559–1561, 1998.
24. Winter RM et al: The Weissenbacher-Zweymüller, Stickler and Marshall syndromes. Further evidence for their identity. *Am J Med Genet* 16:189–199, 1983.
25. Zellweger H et al: The Marshall syndrome: report of a new family. *J Pediatr* 84:868–871, 1974.
26. Zlotogora J et al: Variability of Stickler syndrome. *Am J Med Genet* 42:337–339, 1992.

Short stature, low nasal bridge, cleft palate, and sensorineural hearing loss (OSMED, oto-spondylo-megaepiphyseal dysplasia)

Several authors (1–16) described a condition resembling Stickler syndrome but without eye findings. Giedion et al. (3) and Gorlin et al. (4) used the terms *oto-spondylo-megaepiphyseal dysplasia* (OSMED) and *megaepiphyseal dwarfism*, respectively, to apply to the disorder. The same condition was reported by Insley and Astley (4) and Nance and Sweeney (10). About 20 cases have been documented.

Feeding difficulties noted during the neonatal period and infancy are characterized by enteritis and recurrent respiratory problems (bronchitis, pneumonia, etc.) and enteritis. They may recur throughout life.

Craniofacial findings. The nose is very small with anteverted nostrils and the nasal bridge is severely depressed (Fig. 8–36A–D). High myopia is not seen because there is no COL11A2 in the vitreous (13).

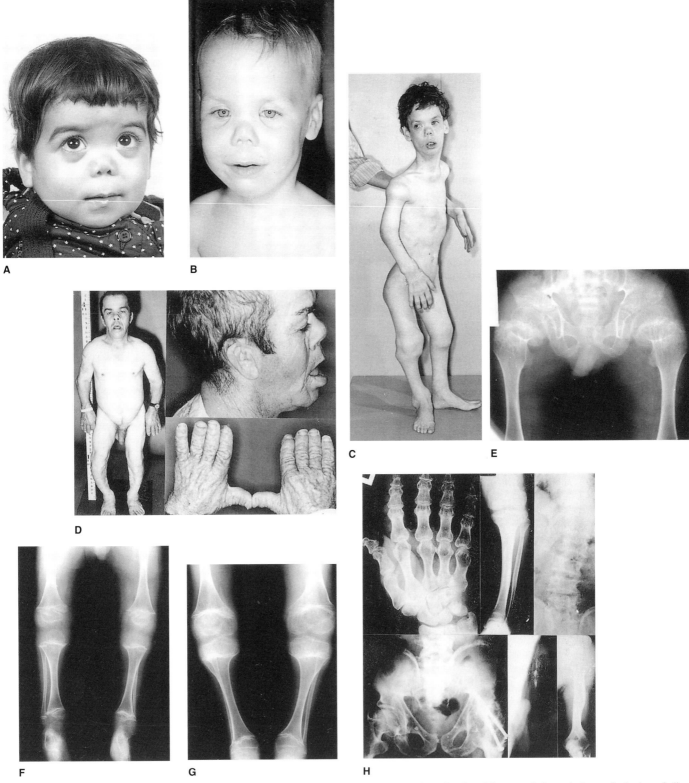

Figure 8–36. *Short stature, low nasal bridge, cleft palate, and sensorineural hearing loss.* (A–C) Small nose with anteverted nostrils and severe nasal bridge depression. Enlargement of joints. Legs are relatively short and broad. (D–F) Note grossly enlarged epiphyses of long bones. (D) Adult male with short stature, large head, saddle nose, deformed pinnae, limitation of elbow extension, stubby fingers, and thick leathery skin. Patient also had cleft palate. [(C) from P Miny, *Am J Med Genet* 21:317, 1985; (D,H) From WE Nance and A Sweeney, *Birth Defects* 6(4):25, 1970.]

The midface is hypoplastic. Cleft palate has been observed in about 65% of cases.

Musculoskeletal system. The limbs are short. The hands are short with stubby fingers. The metacarpophalangeal joints have reduced mobility, and the fifth metacarpals are often short. In later life, the joints become enlarged and painful, and there is lumbar lordosis. Radiographically the leg bones are relatively short and broad (dumbbell form) with mild metaphyseal flaring. The epiphyses are enlarged (Fig. 8–36E–H). Coronal clefts of the spine are seen in infancy. During childhood, platyspondyly with anterior wedging and squared iliac wings become evident. Wide flat epiphyses, metaphyseal flaring, large fused carpal bones (50%), and short metacarpals are seen in adults. The tarsal bones are large in 50%. Osteoarthritis is manifested in early adulthood.

Auditory system. Moderate to severe nonprogressive sensorineural or rarely mixed hearing loss has been documented in most cases.

Heredity. Both homozogous and heterozygous forms have been described. Autosomal recessive inheritance is indicated by parental consanguinity and multiple affected sibs (5,9,14). Homozogosity for a missense mutation in the *COL11A2* gene on 6p21.3 has been demonstrated (8,13–15). The original patient with Weissenbacher-Zweymüller syndrome has been shown to have heterozygous OSMED (nonocular Stickler) syndrome (2,12,15).

Diagnosis. The homozygous recessive form should be distinguished from types 1 and 2 Stickler syndrome and from the dominantly inherited heterozygous nonocular form due to a *COL11A2* splice site mutation at 6p21 (2,15). Both OSMED and Stickler syndromes have midface hypoplasia, epiphyseal dysplasia, and hearing loss that are more marked in OSMED. Myopia and vitreoretinal degeneration are not seen in OSMED.

Summary. Characteristics include (*1*) autosomal recessive inheritance; (*2*) short stature; (*3*) large epiphyses; (*4*) low nasal bridge; (*5*) hypoplastic midface; (*6*) myopia; (*7*) cleft palate; and (*8*) mild to moderate sensorineural hearing loss.

References

1. Al Gazali LI, Lytle W: Otospondylomegaepiphyseal dysplasia: report of three sibs and review of the literature. *Clin Dysmorphol* 3:46–54, 1994.
2. Brunner HG et al: A Stickler syndrome is linked to chromosome 6 near the *COL11A2* gene. *Hum Mol Genet* 3:1561–1564, 1994.
3. Giedion A et al: Oto-spondylo-megaepiphyseal dysplasia (OSMED). *Helv Paediatr Acta* 37:361–380, 1982.
4. Gorlin RJ et al: Megepiphyseal dwarfism. *J Pediatr* 83:633–635, 1973.
5. Insley J, Astley R: A bone dysplasia with deafness. *Br J Radiol* 47:244–251, 1974 (case A).
6. Johnston KM et al: Otospondylo-megaepiphyseal dysplasia (OSMED): differential diagnosis and report of a new case. *Proc Greenwood Genet Ctr* 6:155–156, 1987.
7. Kääriäinen H et al: Bone dysplasia, midface hypoplasia, and deafness: three new patients and review of the literature. *Am J Med Genet* 46:223–227, 1993.
8. Melkoniemi M et al: Autosomal recessive disorder otospondylomegaepiphyseal dysplasia is associated with loss-of-function mutations in the *COL11A2* gene. *Am J Hum Genet* 66:368–377, 2000.
9. Miny P, Lenz W: Autosomal recessive deafness with skeletal dysplasia and facial appearance of Marshall syndrome. *Am J Med Genet* 21:317–324, 1985.
10. Nance WE, Sweeney A: A recessively inherited chondrodystrophy. *Birth Defects* 6(4):25–27, 1970.
11. Pihlajamaa T et al: Heterozygous glycine substitution in Weissenbacher-Zweymüller syndrome demonstrates its identity with heterozygous OSMED (nonocular Stickler syndrome). *Am J Med Genet* 80:115–120, 1998.
12. Rosser EM et al: Nance-Sweeney chondrodysplasia—a further case? *Clin Dysmorphol* 5:207–212, 1996.
13. Spranger J: The type XI collagenopathies. *Pediatr Radiol* 28:748–750, 1998.
14. Van Steensel MAM et al: Oto-spondylo-megaepiphyseal dysplasia (OSMED): clinical description of three patients homozygous for a missense mutation in the *COL11A2* gene. *Am J Med Genet* 70:315–323, 1997.
15. Vikkula M et al: Autosomal dominant and recessive osteochondrodysplasies associated with the COL11A2 locus. *Cell* 80:431–437, 1995.
16. Winter RM et al: The Weissenbacher-Zweymüller, Stickler, and Marshall syndrome: further evidence for their identity. *Am J Med Genet* 16:189–199, 1983 (patient 2).

Hajdu-Cheney syndrome (acroosteolysis, type VI)

The Hajdu-Cheney syndrome, first described by Hajdu and Kauntze (16) in 1948, consists of dissolution of terminal phalanges, dolichocephaly with marked occipital prominence, premature loss of teeth, short stature, and occasional hearing loss. In 1965, Cheney (7) reported familial occurrence. About 50 patients have been described (1–46). Crifasi et al. (8) and Brennan and Pauli (4) provide useful reviews.

Clinical findings. Patients have been generally healthy except for recurrent upper respiratory infections or asthma (2,10,37,41).

Craniofacial findings. The head appears disproportionately large. The hair is low on the forehead and nape. The scalp hair and eyebrows are thick or bushy and coarse with synophrys (19,41,42). The outer supraorbital ridges are often enlarged. There may be mild exophthalmos and hypertelorism. The midface is somewhat hypoplastic and the philtrum is long. The lower third of the face is shortened, in large part due to premature loss of teeth. The mouth tends to be small. The chin usually recedes and the neck is often short (Fig. 8–37A). The ears are low-set.

Ocular system. Myopia, epicanthal folds, nystagmus, reduced visual fields, abducens palsy, disc pallor, morning glory pupil, and optic atrophy have been found (1,2,14,16,19,41,43).

Integumentary system. Generalized hirsutism is relatively frequent (37,39,41,42,44). The skin may be somewhat more elastic than normal. The nails are often wider than they are long and may become coarse and curved (2,11). Prominent sweat pores in axillae, groin, and neck have been noted (1). Nishimura et al. (28) described the skin as being coarse and scaly.

Central nervous system. A serious complication results from impaction of the cerebellum into the foramen magnum (16,19,22,25,33, 37,43). This can cause occipital headache, hydrocephaly, and progressive neurologic deterioration with involvement of cranial nerves (anosmia, trigeminal neuralgia, gruff or low-pitched voice, paralyzed palate, anesthesia of pharynx), cerebellar dysfunction, and syringomyelia (2,14,16,17,19,22,25,27,33,37,38,41–43).

Musculoskeletal system. Progressive basilar invagination, dolichocephaly, and unusual protuberance of the squamous portion of the occipital bone (bathrocephaly) are striking (23,26). Widening of the metopic, coronal, and lambdoidal sutures with multiple wormian bones and depression at the anterior fontanel are evident in most patients (Fig. 8–37B). The frontal sinuses are absent and the maxillary antra underdeveloped. The sella turcica is enlarged, elongated (J-shaped), and wide open with slender clinoids. The anterior nasal spine resorbs (39). The mandibular condyles are positioned anterior to the glenoid fossae, and there may be resorption of the condylar heads (2) or mandibular rami. The mandibular chin button is often missing.

Adult height ranges from 140 to 157 cm but decreases with age. This is due to progressive kyphosis and/or scoliosis, marked osteoporosis, and compression of thoracic vertebrae (11). There is associated pain due in part to compression fractures of the spine (6,7,16). Extension and flexion of the neck are often limited. The superior and inferior surfaces of the vertebrae are concave, assuming a so-called fish-bone shape (43). The cervical spine is often straighter than normal (5,39). Syringomyelia has been reported (1,28).

Intervertebral discs may appear denser than the vertebral bodies. Shortening and clubbing because of resorption of the distal portion of fingers and toes (but primarily fingers) begin around the third or fourth year of life. In severe cases, the middle phalanges can be involved

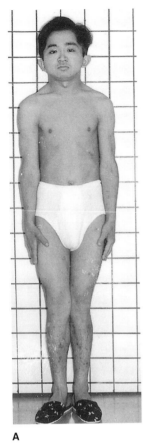
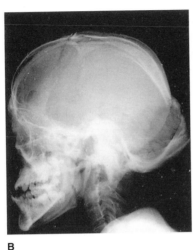
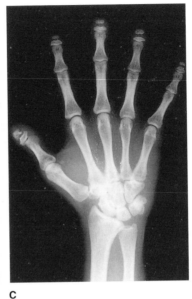

A   B   C

Figure 8–37. *Hajdu-Cheney syndrome.* (A) A somewhat square-appearing face. Eyebrows appear bushy. Terminal phalanges are short with somewhat disproportionate body build. Lower third of face is shortened. (B) Dolichocephaly with unusual protuberance of squamous portion of occipital bone and basilar invagination. Note numerous wormian bones. (C) Note lytic alteration in all terminal phalanges. [From J Kawamura et al., *Neuroradiology* 21: 295, 1981.]

(7,10,11,35) (Fig. 8–37C). The terminal portion of the thumb is especially abbreviated (7,39). All joints are somewhat hyperflexible, especially the interphalangeal joints of the hands (3–6,9,19,33,35,37,41,44). Genua valga are frequent. Long bones, metacarpals, and metatarsals often fracture (5,7,10,29,33,35) with the metaphyseal area of metapodial bones tending to undergo dissolution. There is narrowing of metacarpophalangeal and/or metatarsophalangeal spaces and dissolution of the radial heads (29). The radial head may be dislocated. The tibiae and fibulae may be curved. Clubfeet and umbilical and/or inguinal hernia have been noted (30,36).

Genitourinary findings. Renal cortical cysts, urinary reflux, hypogonadism, and cryptorchidism have been reported. The cysts may lead to hypertension and early renal failure (4,21).

Other findings. Ventral septal defect, PDA (1,3,8,21,37,39,44), and malrotation of the gut have been documented (21,31).

Oral findings. Early loss of teeth due to periodontal disease with marked resorption of the alveolar ridges within 6 months after loss of teeth is a constant feature. Permanent teeth are often impacted (2,6,7,33,39,40,43). Malocclusion is a constant feature. Molar roots may be resorbed. Cleft palate, cleft uvula, and velopharyngeal incompetence have been mentioned (5,22,33,37,41).

Auditory findings. Conductive (7,8,10,18,19,21–23) and mild to moderate sensorineural (11,14,20) hearing loss have been noted in a number of cases.

Heredity. The syndrome has autosomal dominant inheritance with markedly variable expressivity (6,9,15,19) but the vast majority of patients have been isolated examples.

Diagnosis. The term *acroosteolysis* is nonspecific, being used to refer to dissolution of the terminal phalanges of the hands and feet in a

large number of disorders: pycnodysostosis, progeria, mandibuloacral dysplasia, epidermolysis bullosa, Murray-Puretić-Drescher syndrome, Winchester syndrome, Gorham disease, François syndrome, syringomyelia, leprosy, tertiary syphilis, psoriasis, trauma, dominant acroosteolysis, neurogenic ulcerative acropathy, a nephrotic syndrome, manual exposure to polyvinyl chloride, and a host of other disorders (11,24). The serpentine fibula syndrome appears to be allelic with Hajdu-Cheney syndrome (12,13,32,34).

Prognosis. The outlook may be serious, depending on the severity of neurologic damage due to basilar invagination (33,37,43).

The disappearance of the alveolar processes due to premature tooth loss makes for difficulty in prosthodontic rehabilitation.

Summary. Characteristics include (*1*) autosomal dominant inheritance; (*2*) dissolution of terminal phalanges; (*3*) dolichocephaly with occipital prominence; (*4*) short stature; (*5*) premature loss of teeth; and (*6*) conductive or sensorineural hearing loss.

References

1. Adés LC et al: Hydrocephalus in Hajdu-Cheney syndrome. *J Med Genet* 30:175–178, 1993.
2. Allen CM et al: The acro-osteolysis (Hajdu-Cheney) syndrome: review of the literature and report of a case. *J Periodontol* 55:224–229, 1984.
3. Blery M et al: Acro-ostéolyse d'Hajdu-Cheney et anéurysme calcifié sur canal artériel redux. *Ann Radiol* 27:27–30, 1984.
4. Brennan AM, Pauli RM: Hajdu-Cheney syndrome: evolution of phenotype and clinical problems. *Am J Med Genet* 100:292–310, 2001.
5. Brown DM et al: The acro-osteolysis syndrome: morphologic and biochemical studies. *J Pediatr* 88:573–580, 1976.
6. Chawla S: Cranio-skeletal dysplasia with acro-osteolysis. *Br J Radiol* 37:702–705, 1964.
7. Cheney WD: Acro-osteolysis. *AJR Am J Roentgenol* 94:595–607, 1965.
8. Crifasi PA et al: Severe Hajdu-Cheney syndrome with upper airway obstruction. *Am J Med Genet* 70:261–266, 1997.
9. Diren HB et al: The Hajdu-Cheney syndrome: a case report and review of the literature. *Pediatr Radiol* 20:568–569, 1990.

10. Dorst JP, McKusick VA: Acroosteolysis (Cheney syndrome). *Birth Defects* 5(3):215–217, 1969.

11. Elias AN et al: Hereditary osteodysplasia with acro-osteolysis (the Hajdu-Cheney syndrome). *Am J Med* 65:627–636, 1978.

12. Exner GG: Serpentine fibula-polycystic kidney syndrome. *Eur J Pediatr* 147:544–546, 1988.

13. Fryns JP: Serpentine fibula syndrome: a variant clinical presentation of Hajdu-Cheney syndrome? *Clin Dysmorphol* 6:287–288, 1997.

14. Fryns JP et al: Vocal cord paralysis and cystic kidney disease in Hajdu-Cheney syndrome. *Clin Genet* 51:271–274, 1997.

15. Grant S et al: Acro-osteolysis (Hajdu-Cheney syndrome). *Oral Surg Oral Path Oral Med* 80:666–668, 1995.

16. Hajdu N, Kauntze R: Cranio-skeletal dysplasia. *Br J Radiol* 21:42–48, 1948.

17. Herrmann J et al: Arthro-dento-osteo-dysplasia (Hajdu-Cheney syndrome). *Z Kinderheilkd* 114:93–110, 1973.

18. Hersovici D et al: Cervical instability as an unusual manifestation of Hajdu-Cheney syndrome of acroosteolysis. *Clin Orthop* 255:111–116, 1990.

19. Iwaya T et al: Hajdu-Cheney syndrome. *Arch Orthop Trauma Surg* 95:293–302, 1979.

20. Kaler SG et al: Hajdu-Cheney syndrome associated with severe cardiac valvular and conduction disease. *Dysmorphol Clin Genet* 4:43–47, 1990.

21. Kaplan P et al: Cystic kidney disease in Hajdu-Cheney syndrome. *Am J Med Genet* 56:25–30, 1995.

22. Kawamura J et al: Hajdu-Cheney syndrome: report of a non-familial case. *Neuroradiology* 21:295–301, 1981.

23. Kawamura J et al: Hajdu-Cheney syndrome: MR imaging. *Neuroradiology* 33:441–442, 1991.

24. Kozlowski K et al: Acroosteolysis: problems of diagnosis—report of four cases. *Pediatr Radiol* 8:79–86, 1979.

25. Matisonn A, Zaidy F: Familial acro-osteolysis. *S Afr Med J* 47:2060–2063, 1973.

26. Muller G et al: Acro-osteolysis (Hajdu-Cheney syndrome). *Acta Radiol* 35:201, 1994.

27. Niijma KH et al: Familial osteodysplasia associated with trigeminal neuralgia: a case report. *Neurosurgery* 15:562–565, 1984.

28. Nishimura G et al: Syringohydromyelia in Hajdu-Cheney syndrome. *Pediatr Radiol* 26:59–61, 1996.

29. Nunziata V et al: High turnover osteoporosis in acro-osteolysis (Hajdu-Cheney syndrome). *J Endocrinol Invest* 13:251–255, 1990.

30. O'Reilly MA, Shaw DG: Hajdu-Cheney syndrome. *Ann Rheum Dis* 53:276–279, 1994.

31. Pelligrini V, Widdowson DJ: CT findings in Hajdu-Cheney syndrome. *Pediatr Radiol* 21:304, 1991.

32. Ramos FJ et al: Further evidence that the Hajdu-Cheney syndrome and the "serpentine fibula–polycystic kidney syndrome" are a single entity. *Am J Med Genet* 78:474–481, 1998.

33. Rosenmann E et al: Sporadic idiopathic acro-osteolysis with cranioskeletal dysplasia, polycystic kidneys and glomerulonephritis: a case of the Hajdu-Cheney syndrome. *Pediatr Radiol* 6:116–120, 1977.

34. Rosser EM et al: Serpentine fibular syndrome: expansion of the phenotype with three affected siblings. *Clin Dysmorphol* 5:105–113, 1996.

35. Shaw DG: Acro-osteolysis and bone fragility. *Br J Radiol* 42:934–936, 1969.

36. Siklar Z et al: Hajdu-Cheney syndrome with growth hormone deficiency and neuropathy. *J Pediatr Endocrinol Metab* 13:951–954, 2000.

37. Silverman FN et al: Acro-osteolysis (Hajdu-Cheney syndrome). *Birth Defects* 10(12):106–123, 1974 (case 1 same as refs. 16 and 45; case 2 same as ref. 15).

38. Tanimoto A et al: Syringomyelia associated with Hajdu-Cheney syndrome: case report. *Neurosurgery* 39:400–403, 1996.

39. Van den Houten BR et al: The Hajdu-Cheney syndrome: a review of the literature and report of 3 cases. *Int J Oral Surg* 14:113–125, 1985.

40. Vanek J: Idiopathische Osteolyse von Hajdu-Cheney. *Roefo* 128:75–79, 1978.

41. Weleber RG, Beals RK: The Hajdu-Cheney syndrome: report of two cases and review of the literature. *J Pediatr* 88:243–249, 1976.

42. Wendel U, Kemperdick H: Idiopathische Osteolyse vom Typ Hajdu-Cheney. *Monatsschr Kinderheilkd* 127:581–584, 1979.

43. Williams B: Foramen magnum impaction in a case of acro-osteolysis. *Br J Surg* 64:70–73, 1977.

44. Zahran M et al: Arthro-osteo-renal dysplasia. *Acta Radiol Diagn* 25:39–43, 1984.

45. Zeman J et al: Hajdu-Cheney syndrome in a 3 1/2 year old girl. *Australas Radiol* 38:228–230, 1994.

46. Zugibe FT et al: Arthrodentoosteodysplasia: a genetic acroosteolysis syndrome. *Birth Defects* 10(5):145–152, 1974.

Hemifacial microsomia, external auditory canal atresia, deafness, Müllerian anomalies, and acro-osteolysis

Brady et al. (1) reported a large inbred family in which several individuals had the above combination. The hearing loss was sensorineural, conductive, or mixed. Müllerian anomalies included absent uterus and vagina in one and abnormal uterus in another. In addition to mild acro-osteolysis, the digits had loss of tissue but with extension of the nail bed over the finger pulp. Cognitive function was normal. Inheritance was thought to be autosomal recessive.

Reference

1. Brady AF et al: Hemifacial microsomia, external auditory canal atresia, deafness and Müllerian anomalies associated with acro-osteolysis: a new autosomal recessive syndrome? *Clin Dysmorphol* 11:155–161, 2002.

Keutel syndrome (calcification of cartilages, brachytelephalangy, multiple peripheral pulmonary stenoses, and mixed hearing loss)

In 1971–1972, Keutel et al. (9,10) reported a syndrome of multiple peripheral pulmonary stenoses, brachytelephalangy, diffuse calcification and/or ossification of cartilages, and mixed hearing loss in two sibs. About 12 patients have been documented to date (2,5,6,9–11,15,16,19).

Clinical findings. Recurrent bronchitis, chronic sinusitis, and otitis media have occurred in nearly all the patients (11). Stature has been at or below the 25th centile in all, and below the third centile in a few (5,11,15). Increased miscarriage has been noted (6).

Craniofacial findings. The face is somewhat flattened with a small depressed nose, small alae nasi, and mild midface hypoplasia, becoming more pronounced with age (Fig. 8–38A). The pinnae are somewhat enlarged and prominent; and pale, stiff, and hard in consistency. Calcification of the auricular cartilages becomes evident within the first 3 years of life and is progressive (Fig. 8–38B,C).

Central nervous system. Some patients have normal intelligence (2,9,10), whereas others have been mildly retarded (5,6,16).

Musculoskeletal system. Variable shortening of the terminal phalanges of hands (brachytelephalangy) has been a constant finding. The halluces also tend to be short.

Radiographic findings. Radiographic studies show calcification of the pinnae (Fig. 8–38B,C), cartilaginous portions of ribs, and laryngotracheal, bronchial, and nasal cartilages (Fig. 8–38D,E). The mastoid processes are abnormally dense. Variable shortening of the terminal phalanges of the fingers and halluces and premature fusion of the epiphyses of these phalanges are evident (Fig. 8–38F).

Peripheral pulmonary stenosis and pulmonary artery hypoplasia have been observed in at least 50% (5,10–12,18). Angiocardiography has revealed systolic pressure elevation in the right ventricle and in the main pulmonary artery and lowered diastolic pressure in the pulmonary vein together with a systolic pressure gradient—a picture compatible with multiple peripheral pulmonary stenoses.

Cardiovascular system. Peripheral pulmonary stenosis and pulmonary artery hypoplasia have been found in at least 50% of patients (5,9–11,17,18).

Auditory system. Hearing loss is noted prior to admission to school. Sensorineural, mixed, or conductive hearing loss of 30–75 dB, being greater at higher frequencies, has been found in nearly all affected individuals (2,5,9–11,15,16,19). The conductive component is probably related to recurrent middle ear infections.

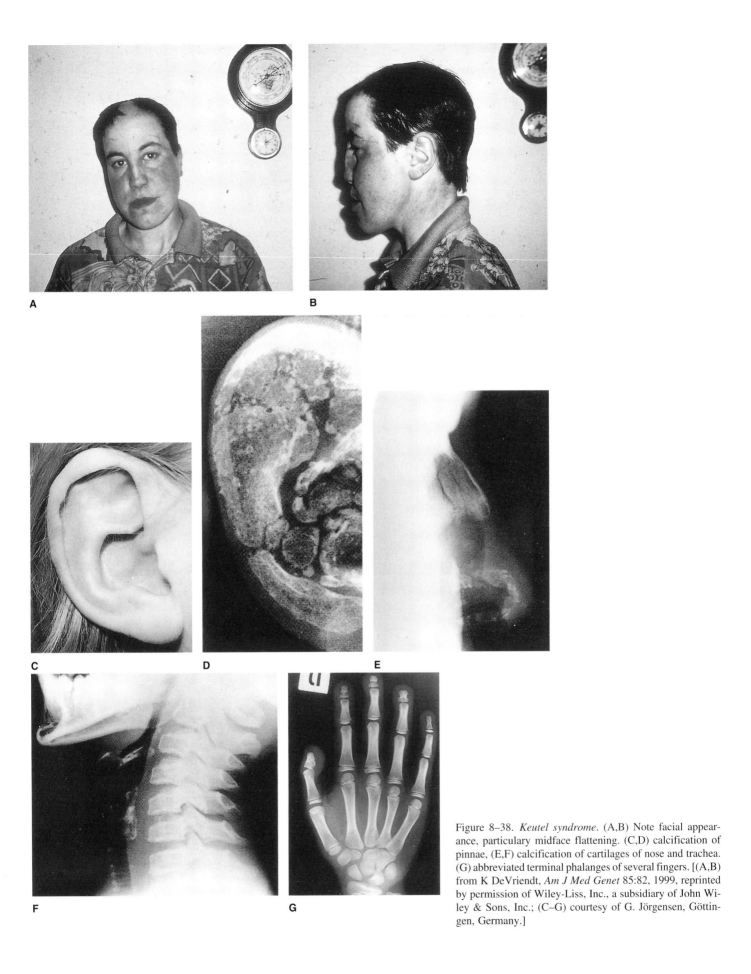

Figure 8–38. *Keutel syndrome.* (A,B) Note facial appearance, particulary midface flattening. (C,D) calcification of pinnae, (E,F) calcification of cartilages of nose and trachea. (G) abbreviated terminal phalanges of several fingers. [(A,B) from K DeVriendt, *Am J Med Genet* 85:82, 1999, reprinted by permission of Wiley-Liss, Inc., a subsidiary of John Wiley & Sons, Inc.; (C–G) courtesy of G. Jörgensen, Göttingen, Germany.]

Vestibular system. Normal caloric response has been noted (10).

Pathology. Meier et al. (13) described autopsy findings in one of the originally reported sibs. New findings included tracheobronchial stenosis, and concentric calcifications affecting the pulmonary, coronary, hepatic, renal, meningeal, and cerebral arteries.

Heredity. Affected sibs (10,11) and parental consanguinity (2,3,10,11) clearly indicate autosomal recessive inheritance. The gene has been mapped to 12p12.3–p13.1, with mutations in the gene encoding human matrix Gla protein (*MGP*) (14).

Diagnosis. Multiple pulmonary stenoses and associated hearing loss have been reported (1). Gyllenswärd et al. (8) noted "malformation of the external ears" in two patients with multiple peripheral pulmonary stenoses, but further definition was not made. Multiple peripheral pulmonary stenoses can be seen in combination with supravalvular aortic stenosis and in Williams syndrome (7).

Calcification and/or ossification of the auricular cartilage can follow frostbite, physical trauma, perichondritis, and can occur in diastrophic dysplasia (4,7,11). Auricular ossification has also been reported as a dominant trait (12).

Summary. Characteristics include (*1*) autosomal recessive inheritance; (*2*) brachytelephalangy; (*3*) calcification and/or ossification of cartilages of nose, auricles, trachea, bronchi, and ribs; (*4*) multiple peripheral pulmonary stenoses; (*5*) recurrent otitis media, sinusitis, and bronchitis; and (*6*) mixed hearing loss.

References

1. Arvidsson H et al: Supravalvular stenoses of the pulmonary arteries: report of eleven cases. *Acta Radiol (Stockh)* 56:466–480, 1961 (case 10).
2. Cormode EJ et al: Keutel syndrome: clinical report and literature review. *Am J Med Genet* 24:289–294, 1986.
3. Devriendt K et al: Follow-up of an adult with Keutel syndrome. *Am J Med Genet* 85:82–83, 1999.
4. Di Bartolomeo JR: The petrified auricle. Comments on ossification, calcification, and exostosis of the external ear. *Laryngoscope* 95:566–576, 1985.
5. Fryns JP et al: Calcification of cartilages, brachytelephalangy and peripheral pulmonary stenosis: confirmation of the Keutel syndrome. *Eur J Pediatr* 142:201–203, 1984.
6. Gilbert B, Lacombe D: Keutel syndrome and miscarriages. *Am J Med Genet* 83:209–211, 1999.
7. Gorlin RJ et al: *Syndromes of the Head and Neck*, 4th ed. Oxford University Press, New York, 2001.
8. Gyllenswärd A et al: Congenital multiple peripheral stenoses of the pulmonary artery. *Pediatrics* 19:399–410, 1957.
9. Keutel J et al: Ein neues autosomal-rezessiv vererbbares Syndrom. *Dtsch Med Wochenschr* 96:1676–1681, 1971.
10. Keutel J et al: A new autosomal recessive syndrome: peripheral pulmonary stenoses, brachytelephalangism, neural hearing loss, and abnormal cartilage calcifications/ossifications. *Birth Defects* 8(5):60–68, 1972.
11. Khosroshahi HE et al: Keutel syndrome: a report of four cases. *Eur J Pediatr* 149:188–191, 1989.
12. Kirsch R: Vererbbare Verknöcherung der Ohrmuschel. *Z Laryngol Rhinol Otol* 32:729–734, 1953.
13. Meier M et al: Tracheobronchial stenosis in Keutel syndrome. *Eur Respir J* 17:566–569, 2001.
14. Munroe PB et al: Mutations in the gene encoding the human Gla protein cause Keutel syndrome. *Nat Genet* 21:142–144, 1999.
15. Say B et al: Unusual calcium deposition in cartilage associated with short stature and peculiar facial features. *Pediatr Radiol* 1:127–129, 1973.
16. Teebi AS et al: Keutel syndrome: further characterization and review. *Am J Med Genet* 78:182–187, 1998.
17. Walbaum R: Les brachydactylies. *J Génét Hum* 31:167–181, 1983.
18. Walbaum R et al: Le syndrome de Keutel. *Pédiatrie* 30:313–314, 1975.
19. Ziereisen F et al: The Keutel syndrome. *Pediatr Radiol* 23:314–315, 1993.

Proximal symphalangism and conductive hearing loss

Proximal symphalangism and carpal and tarsal bone coalition with conductive hearing loss because of fixation of the footplate of the stapes to the round window have been described by many authors (1,3,5–21). Although the digital anomaly existed in the Talbot family of England for several centuries ("Talbot fingers"), the contention that John Talbot, the first Earl of Shrewsbury (1388?–1453), had the disorder has been discounted after close scrutiny of the evidence. John Talbot was made famous by Shakespeare (Henry VI, Part I, Act IV) (4).

Ocular system. Strabismus has been a feature in some cases (6,18).

Musculoskeletal system. The fingers are quite striking; little or no movement is possible in the proximal interphalangeal joints, usually from birth. The skin over the affected joint area is shiny and without hair or wrinkles (Fig. 8–39A,B). In some cases, middle phalanges are shorter and wider than normal. If there is multiple finger involvement, all digits ulnar to the most radially affected digit have the same fusion anomaly. Neither the thumb nor the metacarpophalangeal joints are involved, although there are shortening and flattening of the distal head of the first metacarpal in about 25% of the cases. Some degree of clinodactyly of the little finger is not uncommon.

Clinically, the feet often show a prominence on the medial side at the level of the distal end of the navicular bone. Another prominence is usually seen at the base of the fifth metatarsal.

Tarsal coalition results in decreased movement at the subtaloid and metatarsal joints. The feet are usually flat and the ankles broad. The ability to invert and evert the foot is reduced. In some individuals the gait is almost normal; in others the patient walks on the external border of the feet or, occasionally, on the toes.

Radiographic findings. By adolescence (in some children much earlier), the hands show complete bony fusion of the proximal interphalangeal joints of the little finger and less complete fusion of this joint in the more radially situated fingers. The middle phalanges may be normal, short and massive, or even hypoplastic. Infrequently, there is distal interphalangeal fusion. In some cases, the fifth fingers appear to consist of a hypoplastic middle phalanx fused with the terminal phalanx. The first metacarpal is shortened, and its proximal end is coniform or fused with the adjacent carpus. Epiphyses of the major metacarpals may be somewhat flattened. Carpal bones may show anomalies, including malsegmentation of the triquetrum and partial fusion to both lunate and hamate (7,8,12,16–18) (Fig. 8–39C). Talonavicular fusion is a virtually constant finding (Fig. 8–39D). Less common fusions, including metatarsal and calcaneocuboid, have been described. In the toes, the most common abnormality is fusion of the distal interphalangeal joints; a less common abnormality is proximal fusion. In the kindred reported by Spoendlin (15), carpal and tarsal synostosis was marked, but symphalangism was not present.

Auditory system. The mother and daughter described by Vesell (19) had a 10–60 dB bilateral conductive hearing loss between the frequencies of 500 and 2000 Hz. Both had hearing loss from childhood, the hearing loss probably being congenital. Many individuals in the family described by Strasburger et al. (17) had profound conduction loss. Conductive hearing loss was noted during the first year of life. Tympanotomy revealed bony fusion between the stapes and the petrous portion of the temporal bone. Gorlin et al. (8) and Wayoff (20) also described total ankylosis of the stapes. Cremers et al. (3) reported the histology of the stapes, finding osseous fusion of the footplate with the thickened bone at the oval window niche (Fig. 8–39E).

Heredity. Inheritance is clearly autosomal dominant with variable expression (1,3,5–21). There is linkage to 17q21–q22 (11). Noggin (*NOG*) mutations have been demonstrated (2,7). The condition is allelic with facio-audio-symphalangism (vide infra).

Diagnosis. Proximal symphalangism may occur as an isolated autosomal dominant trait. There are numerous reports, reviewed by several authors, of the association of symphalangism with fusion of the carpus and tarsus. However, in no cases, other than those cited, was hearing loss found (5,9,21). Proximal symphalangism may also occur in dias-

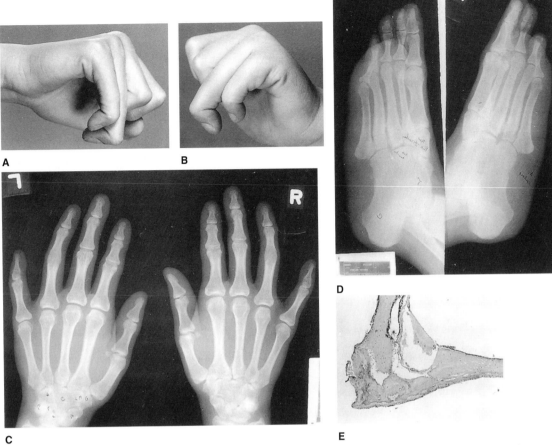

Figure 8–39. *Progressive symphalangism and conductive hearing loss.* (A,B) Typical hand alterations with inability to flex proximal joints in fourth and fifth fingers due to fusion. (C) Note symphalangism in fourth and fifth fingers bilaterally. Fusion in fifth fingers has produced the appearance of only two bones. Also note extensive carpal bone fusion. (D) Extensive talocalcaneal fusion. (E) Stapes. Note thickened posterior part of footplate and fractured part of annular ligament. [(A,B) courtesy of CWRJ Cremers, Nijmegen, The Netherlands; (E) from CWRJ Cremers et al., *Arch Otolaryngol* 111:765, 1985.]

trophic dysplasia and metatropic dysplasia, but these conditions are easily distinguished from the syndrome under discussion here.

Symphalangism and conductive hearing loss must be differentiated from facio-audio-symphalangism with which it is allelic. This disorder also has autosomal dominant inheritance, but is distinguished by characteristic facial phenotype, involvement of other parts of the skeletal system, and frequent association with aplasia or hypoplasia of the fingers or toes.

Summary. The characteristics of the disorder include (*1*) autosomal dominant inheritance; (*2*) progressive proximal fusion of interphalangeal joints of the fingers; (*3*) carpal and tarsal bone fusion; and (*4*) conductive hearing loss.

References

1. Baschek V: Stapes fixation und Symphalangie, ein autosomal dominant erbliches Krankheitsbild. *Laryngol Rhinol Otol* 57:299–304, 1978.
2. Brown DJ et al: Autosomal dominant stapes ankylosis with broad thumbs and toes, hyperopia, and skeletal anomalies is caused by heterozygous nonsense and frameshift mutations in *NOG*, the gene encoding Noggin. *Am J Hum Genet* 71:618–624, 2002.
3. Cremers C et al: Proximal symphalangia and stapes ankylosis. *Arch Otolaryngol* 111:765–767, 1985.
4. Elkington SG, Huntsman RG: The Talbot fingers. A study in symphalangism. *BMJ* 1:407–411, 1967.
5. Geelhoed GW et al: Symphalangism and tarsal coalitions. A hereditary syndrome. A report on two families. *J Bone Joint Surg Br* 51:278–289, 1969.
6. Gloede JF, Stenger HH: Symphalangismus, Strabismus und Mittelohrmissbildungen. *Humangenetik* 22:23–32, 1974.
7. Gong Y et al: Heterogeneous mutations in the gene encoding noggin affect human joint morphogenesis. *Nat Genet* 21:302–304, 1999.
8. Gorlin RJ et al: Stapes fixation and proximal symphalangism. *Z Kinderheilkd* 108:12–16, 1970.
9. Harle TS, Stevenson JR: Hereditary symphalangism associated with carpal and tarsal fusions. *Radiology* 89:91–94, 1967.
10. Murakami Y: Nievergelt-Pearlman syndrome with impairment of hearing. *J Bone Joint Surg Br* 57: 367–372, 1975.
11. Pierson M et al: Symphalangisme et maladie des synostoses multiples: etude de deux familles. *J Génét Hum* 30:351–358, 1982.
12. Polymeropoulos MH et al: Localization of the gene (*SYM1*) for proximal symphalangism to human chromosome 17q21–q22. *Genomics* 27:225–229, 1995.
13. Schulthes GV: Isolierte Stapesankylose als Teilsymptom eines hereditären Missbildungssyndroms. *Laryngol Rhinol Otol* 53:643–647, 1974.
14. Sorri M et al: A family with conductive hearing loss and proximal symphalangism. *Adv Audiol* 3:58–65, 1985.
15. Spoendlin H: Congenital stapes ankylosis and fusion of carpal and tarsal bones as a dominant hereditary syndrome. *Arch Oto Rhino Laryngol* 206:173–179, 1974.
16. Stenger HH, Gloede JF: Symphalangismus und Stapesankylose. *Arch Klin Exp Ohren Nasen Kehlkopfheilkd* 202:632–634, 1972.
17. Strasburger AK et al: Symphalangism: genetic and clinical aspects. *Bull Johns Hopkins Hosp* 117:108–127, 1965.
18. Vase P et al: Congenital stapes fixation, symphalangism and syndactylia. *Acta Otolaryngol* 80:394–398, 1975.
19. Vesell ES: Symphalangism, strabismus, and hearing loss in mother and daughter. *N Engl J Med* 263:839–842, 1960.
20. Wayoff MR: Congenital stapes fixation and multiple synostosis. *Int Cong Ser* 509:156–162, 1979.

21. Wildervanck LS et al: Proximal symphalangism of fingers associated with fusion of os naviculare and talus and occurrence of two accessory bones in the feet (os paranaviculare and os tibiale externum) in a European-Indonesian-Chinese family. *Acta Genet (Basel)* 17:166–177, 1967.

Facio-audio-symphalangism

Maroteaux et al. (10), in 1972, and Herrmann (4), in 1974, reported kindreds with multiple synostoses and conductive hearing loss. The face is characteristic and symphalangism of the fingers and toes occurs together with other skeletal anomalies. Several papers on the subject have appeared (1,2,4,6,13,14,16,17,19). Less certain are other cases in which facial features (7,11,12) or hearing loss (9,15) were not mentioned. The case of Tsuruta et al. (19) is unusual. The question of whether multiple synostoses without facial and audiological abnormalities should be treated differently is discussed by Sugiura and Inagaki (18). The reader should refer to Heredity (below). Besides facio-audio-symphalangism, the term *WL syndrome* has been used (4,5).

Physical findings. Features of the syndrome are summarized in Table 8–5. The nose is long and thin and has minimal alar flare—i.e., it is hemicylindrical (Fig. 8–40A–C). Even though the patient is of normal height, proportions appear abnormal. The gait is waddling; the patient often walks on the outer border of the feet without resting on the heels.

Musculoskeletal system. The upper arms are short. There is cubitus valgus with dislocation of the head of the radius and limitation of pronation, supination, and extension at the elbow.

The fingers are short. There is absence of creases over all proximal interphalangeal joints of fingers and over the fifth, or less often the fourth, distal interphalangeal finger joints. One or more fingernails and/or toenails may be hypoplastic. One or more terminal portions of fingers (rarely the third) and/or toes may be missing (Fig. 8–40D). The fifth finger may exhibit clinodactyly (Fig. 8–40E). The hallux is often short; there may be an increase in the space between the hallux and the rest of the toes.

The hands and feet are most severely affected. Starting in childhood, there is progressive coalition of the lesser multangular-capitate-hamate and triquetral bones, short and broad first metacarpal, progressive prox-imal symphalangism of the second, third, fourth, and fifth digits, and progressive distal symphalangism of the fifth and often the fourth digits. One or more distal phalanges may be hypoplastic and one or more metacarpals and proximal phalanges may be overtubulated (Fig. 8–40F–I).

The forefoot is short and shows coalition of the talus and navicular bone, fusion between second and third cuneiforms, and coalition between both the first two cuneiforms and the tarsometatarsal joints (Fig. 8–40J). There are progressive hallux valgus and proximal symphalangism of the second, third, and fourth digits, and hypoplastic or absent middle and distal phalanges of the fourth and/or fifth digits. The first metatarsal is often short and, like the other metatarsals, may be overtubulated.

The metaphyses of long bones are broad and irregular. The diaphyses may be somewhat bowed. Radiohumeral synostosis, malformed distal humerus and proximal radius, and subluxation of the radial head are common findings (Fig. 8–40K).

Spinal anomalies include hypoplastic spinal processes of cervical vertebrae, fused arches, stenoses, and osteolytic defects in the anterior superior portions of the lower thoracic and upper lumbar vertebrae (2). The patient of Pfeiffer et al (16) had block fusion of C_2–C_3, C_5–C_7, and T_4–T_{10}.

Other findings. Single palmar creases are a common finding. The absence of some digital triradii and the presence of two palmar axial triradii have been observed (10). Strabismus has been noted (4).

Auditory system. Progressive conductive hearing loss is characteristic (4–6,10). A patient of Pfeiffer et al. (16) had minor sensorineural impairment. Ankylosis of the stapedial footplate and malformation of the stapes and the incus have been recorded (4,10,15).

Heredity. Autosomal dominant inheritance is evident. The gene, *noggin,* has been mapped to 17q21–q22 (3,8). This makes this syndrome and proximal symphalangism and conductive hearing loss allelic.

Diagnosis. Symphalangism and conductive hearing loss can be excluded since facial appearance is not altered. Furthermore, the skeletal findings are limited to the hands and feet and aplasia/hypoplasia of the terminal phalanges and nails does not occur.

Table 8–5. Facioaudiosymphalangism—clinical findings

Findings	Frequency[1]	Findings	Frequency
Craniofacial		*Lower Extremities*	
Conductive hearing loss	F	Short legs	I
Broad, hemicylindrical nose	F	Pes planovalgus	I
Narrow upper lip	F	Short foot	F
Internal strabismus	I	Short hallux	F
		Increased gap between hallux and second toe	I
Spinal Anomalies	I	Cutaneous syndactyly 2,3	F
		Absent distal phalanges	F
		Correspondingly absent/hypoplastic toenail	F
Upper Extremities		Proximal symphalangism 2,3,4	F
Short arms	I		
Dislocated radial head	F	*Musculoskeletal*	
Cubitus valgus	F		
Brachydactyly	F	Good muscle development	I
Clinodactyly	I	Prominent chondrocostal junction	F
Symphalangism 2,3,4	F	Pectus excavatum	F
Cutaneous syndactyly 2,3,4	F	Short sternum	I
Hypoplastic/aplastic middle phalanx	F	Anteriorly positioned shoulders	I
Hypoplastic/aplastic distal phalanx	F		
Correspondingly aplastic/hypoplastic nail	F		
Absence of creases over PIP	F		
Absence of creases over DIP	I		

[1]Based on review of 14 cases by SA Hurvitz et al. (4). DIP, distal interphalangeal; F, present in more than 50% of cases; I, present in less than 50% of cases; PIP, proximal interphalangeal.

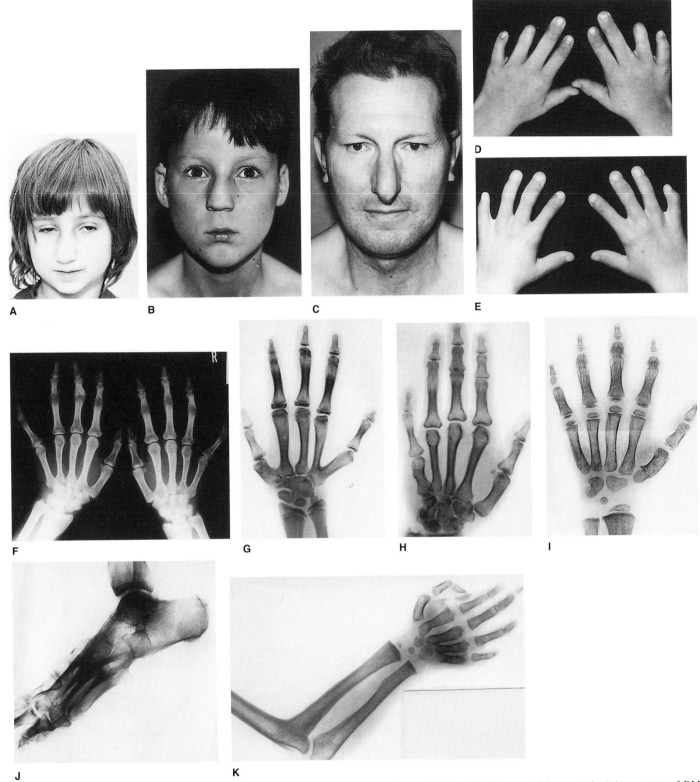

Figure 8–40. *Facio-audio-symphalangism.* (A–C) Long and thin nose with minimal alar flare. (D) Failure of development of terminal portion of fourth digits and absence of proximal flexion creases of fingers. (E) Clinodactyly, brachydactyly, syndactyly, and absence of digital creases indicating the symphalangism. (F–I) Radiographs of hands of individuals from several kindred showing variable symphalangism. Note fusions of carpal bones, proximal fusion of metacarpals 4–5, and abbreviated fifth metacarpal. (J) Talonav-
iculocalcaneal fusion. (K) Humeroradial synostosis. [(A) courtesy of RM Goodman, Tel Hashomer, Israel; (B,D) from J Herrmann, *Birth Defects* 10(5):23, 1974; (C,E) from P Maroteaux et al., *Nouv Presse Med* 1:3041, 1972; (F) from Y Sugiura and Y Inagaki, *Jpn Hum Genet* 26:31, 1981; (G,H,J) from Y Murakami, *J Bone Joint Surg* 57B:367, 1975; (I,K) from P Maroteaux, *Nouv Presse Med* 1:3041, 1972.]

Summary. Characteristics include (*1*) autosomal dominant inheritance; (*2*) unusual face, marked by long, thin hemicylindrical nose; (*3*) unusual gait; (*4*) cubitus valgus; (*5*) progressive symphalangism and carpal and tarsal fusion; and (*6*) progressive conductive hearing loss.

References

1. Da-Silva EO et al: Multiple synostosis syndrome: study of a large Brazilian kindred. *Am J Med Genet* 18:237–247, 1984.
2. Edwards MJ et al: Herrmann multiple synostosis syndrome with neurological complications caused by spinal canal stenosis. *Am J Med Genet* 95:118–122, 2000.
3. Gong Y et al: Heterozygous mutations in the gene encoding noggin affect human joint morphogenesis. *Nat Genet* 21:302–304, 1999.
4. Herrmann J: Symphalangism and brachydactyly syndromes. Report of the WL symphalangism-brachydactyly syndrome. *Birth Defects* 10(5):23–54, 1974.
5. Higashi K, Inoue S: Conductive deafness, symphalangism, and facial abnormalities: the WL syndrome in a Japanese family. *Am J Med Genet* 16:105–109, 1983.
6. Hurvitz SA et al: The facio-audio-symphalangism syndrome—report of a case and review of the literature. *Clin Genet* 28:61–68, 1985.
7. Kassner EG et al: Symphalangism with metacarpophalangeal fusions and elbow abnormalities. *Pediatr Radiol* 4:103–107, 1976.
8. Krakow D et al: Localization of a multiple synostoses syndrome disease gene to chromosome 17q21–22. *Am J Hum Genet* 63:121–124, 1998.
9. Lambert LA: Congenital humeroradial synostotic anomalies. *Pediatrics* 31:573–577, 1947.
10. Maroteaux P et al: La maladie des synostosis multiples. *Nouv Presse Méd* 1:3041–3047, 1972.
11. Murakami Y: Nievergelt-Pearlman syndrome with impairment of hearing. *J Bone Joint Surg Br* 57:367–372, 1975.
12. Nixon JR: The multiple synostoses syndrome. *Clin Orthop* 135:48–51, 1978.
13. Pedersen JC et al: Multiple synostosis syndrome. *Eur J Pediatr* 134:273–275, 1980.
14. Perme CM et al: Case report 857. *Skeletal Radiol* 23:468–470, 1994.
15. Pfeiffer RA: Associated deformities of the head and hands. *Birth Defects* 5(3):18–34, 1969.
16. Pfeiffer RA et al: An autosomal dominant facio-audio-symphalangism syndrome with Klippel-Feil anomaly: a new variant of multiple synostoses. *Genet Couns* 1:133–140, 1990.
17. Poisson D et al: Maladie des synostoses multiples. *Arch Fr Pediatr* 40:35–37, 1983.
18. Sugiura Y, Inagaki Y: Symphalangism associated with synostosis of carpus and/or tarsus. *Jpn J Hum Genet* 26:31–45, 1981.
19. Tsuruta T et al: A case of multiple synostoses syndrome. *Jpn J Hum Genet* 25:55–61, 1980.

Otofacioosseous-gonadal syndrome

Da-Silva et al. (1) described a sibship with a provisionally unique syndrome likely inherited as an autosomal recessive condition. The face was characterized by brachycephaly, prominent forehead, downslanting palpebral fissures, low nasal root, rounded nasal tip with hypoplastic alae nasi, and low-set ears. Sensorineural hearing loss was present. Skeletal anomalies included wormian bones, narrow thorax, genu valgum, carpal fusion, and clubfoot. Cryptorchidism, inguinal hernia, and short stature with delayed bone age also occurred.

Reference

1. da-Silva EO et al: Oto-facio-osseous-gonadal syndrome: a new form of syndromic deafness? *Clin Genet* 52:51–55, 1997.

Facio-auriculo-radial dysplasia

In 1974, Stoll et al. (8) described a syndrome characterized by dysmorphic facial appearnce, asymmetric radial dysplasia, malformations of the external ear, and conductive hearing loss. Harding et al. (4) documented another family and used the term "facio-auriculo-radial dysplasia."

Craniofacial findings. In the first family (8), the father had a long prominent philtrum. The nose was somewhat bulbous with a flattened bridge, and there was midface hypoplasia. His son had a similar appearance (Fig. 8–41A,B). In the second family (4), the mother had mild maxillary hypoplasia. The daughter had a long philtrum, short nose, and midfacial regression.

Musculoskeletal system. Both families presented with striking abnormalities of the upper limbs. In the first family (8), the father had bilateral humeral hypoplasia and absent radii. Thumbs and index fingers were absent. There were three carpal and metacarpal bones (Fig. 8–41C). On the right, two metacarpal bones articulated with a single digit. On the left, there were an additional proximal and middle phalanx. His son had a similar left arm, but three digits were present on the right hand. In the second family, the mother had marked anomaly of both upper limbs, which was more severe on the left (4) (Fig. 8–41D). On the right, the thumb and thenar eminence were absent. There was flexion contracture of the index finger and radial clubbing of the hand. On the left, dislocation of the shoulder was noted. The forearm was considerably

Figure 8–41. *Facio-auriculo-radial dysplasia.* (A,B) Father and son with severely abbreviated upper limbs. (C) Severe mesomelic dysplasia with marked hypoplasia of thumb. (D) Marked reduction of digits and carpal bones on preaxial side. Note absent radius. [(A,B,D) from C Stoll et al., *Arch Fr Pediatr* 31:669, 1974; (C) courtesy of AC Harding, London, England.]

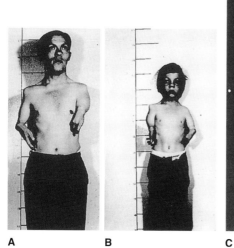
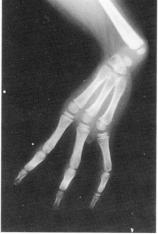
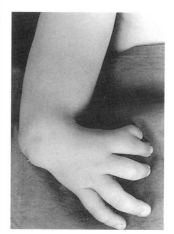

A   B   C   D

shortened, and thumb, index finger, and thenar eminence were absent. Her sister had a rudimentary thumb on the left. The daughter had bilateral reduction anomalies of the forearms, more marked on the left, with bilateral radial clubbing. Both thumbs were rudimentary and arose from the axial border of the index fingers. There was fixed flexion of the right fourth and fifth fingers, and the left second and fourth fingers. Genu varum was noted. Both mother and daughter had short stature with height below the third centile. Short stature was not reported in the first family (8).

Cardiovascular system. Stoll et al. (8) found the father and son to have sinus arrhythmia and considered this to be part of the syndrome. However, electrocardiograms did not appear unusual. Sinus arrhythmia was marked in the son. Normal electrocardiograms were obtained in the second family (4).

External ear. In one family (8), both father and son had similar malformations of the pinnae. The left ear was simple and prominent with an attached lobule and narrowing of the external auditory canal. The right ear had a prominent anthelix. In the family described by Harding et al. (4), the mother had normal external ears, while her daughter had a small cupped right pinna with marked overfolding of the helix.

Auditory system. In the first family (8), both father and son had left-sided conductive hearing loss. In the second family (4), the mother's hearing was normal. Her daughter had considerable hearing loss, more marked on the right. She reacted to moderately high-level intensity test sounds and localized the source reasonably well. Audiometry was impossible because of poor cooperation. The mother's sister, not examined, was said to have partial hearing loss in one ear. Absence of the stapes and oval window was found on surgery (8).

Laboratory findings. Skeletal radiographs in the second family (4) revealed anomalies in the spine and lower limbs. The mother had bilateral hypoplastic fibulae with proximal shortening and a defect in the neural arch of the fifth lumbar vertebra. Her daughter had long clavicles with lateral upward convexities similar to those seen in Holt-Oram syndrome. The lumbar vertebral bodies were fused anteriorly and there was mild posterior wedging.

Heredity. Autosomal dominant inheritance with variable expression was demonstrated.

Diagnosis. The most important syndrome in which auriculofacial malformations and radial dysplasia occur are lacrimo-auriculo-dento-digital (LADD) syndrome (5) and Nager acrofacial dysostosis (7). Isolated defects of the radius or radial ray are found in 1/30,000 live births (1). Carroll and Louis (2) found that 77% of 53 patients with radial dysplasia had associated anomalies of other organ systems. Radial defects have also been observed in sporadic cases of oculo-auriculo-vertebral spectrum (3,6). Also to be excluded is IVIC syndrome in which thrombocytopenia and ophthalmoplegia can occur.

Summary. The syndrome is characterized by (*1*) autosomal dominant inheritance; (*2*) variable abnormalities of external ear; (*3*) midface hypoplasia with a long philtrum and bulbous nose; (*4*) variable abnormalities of radius or radial ray; and (*5*) unilateral or bilateral conductive hearing loss.

References

1. Birch-Jensen A: *Congenital Deformities of the Upper Extremities.* Munksgaard, Copenhagen, 1949.
2. Carroll RE, Louis DS: Anomalies associated with radial dysplasia. *J Pediatr* 84:409–411, 1974.
3. Gorlin RJ et al: Oculo-auriculo-vertebral spectrum. In: *Syndromes of the Head and Neck*, 4th ed., Oxford University Press, New York, 2001, pp. 790–797.
4. Harding AE et al: Autosomal dominant asymmetric radial dysplasia, dysmorphic facies, and conductive hearing loss (facioauriculoradial dysplasia). *J Med Genet* 19:110–115, 1982.
5. Hollister DW et al: The lacrimo-auricular-dento-digital syndrome. *J Pediatr* 83:438–444, 1973.
6. Mandelcorn MS: Goldenhar's syndrome and phocomelia. Case report and etiologic considerations. *Am J Ophthalmol* 72:618–621, 1971.
7. Nager FR, de Reynier JP: Das Gehörorgan bei den angeborenen Kopfmissbildungen. *Pract Otorhinolaryngol (Basel)* 10(Suppl 2):1–128, 1948.
8. Stoll C et al: L'association phocomélie-ectrodactylie, malformations des oreilles avec surdité, arythmie sinusale. *Arch Fr Pédiatr* 31:669–680, 1974.

Hypoplastic thumbs, coloboma of choroid, cataracts, developmental delay, and sensorineural hearing loss

Ward et al. (1) described two sibs with hypoplasia of thumbs, developmental delay, hypoplastic anthelices, bilateral choroid coloboma, cataract, and severe sensorineural hearing loss. Inheritance is probably autosomal recessive.

Reference

1. Ward JR et al: Upper limb defect associated with developmental delay, unilaterally poorly developed anthelix, hearing deficit, and bilateral choroid coloboma: a new syndrome. *J Med Genet* 29:589–591, 1992.

Duane anomaly, upper limb malformation, and sensorineural hearing loss (Okihiro syndrome)

In 1977, Okihiro et al. (10) described a family of five members of three generations with Duane syndrome (bilateral absence of adduction with widening on attempted abduction) (Fig. 8–42A). Four members also had congenital hypoplasia of the thenar eminences (Fig. 8–42B), one had Hirschsprung disease, and another had congenital severe sensorineural hearing loss. Another member did not manifest Duane syndrome but exhibited more extensive anomalies of the upper extremities, hypoplasia of ulna, radius, and thumbs, and unilateral sensorineural hearing loss. The association of upper limb malformation associated with Duane syndrome was probably first observed by Crisp (4). Further reports have identified a significant range of upper limb malformations (Fig. 8–42C–E) as well as variable associated findings including ASD, VSD, anal stenosis, choanal stenosis, renal malformation, and external ear malformations (3,6,8,11). Hearing loss (50 dB) was found in only 1 of 11 affected individuals in one kindred (6). McGowan and Pagon (9) noted unilateral hearing loss. Review of other case reports has not suggested that hearing loss is a frequent finding (2). Inheritance is clearly autosomal dominant (3,5–8,10,11).

Pathogenic mutations have been identified in the human *SALL4* gene at 20q13 in affected individuals (1,7). Reporting nonsense and frameshift mutations in five of eight families studied, Kohlhase et al. drew attention to the clinical overlap with Holt-Oram syndrome, acro-renal-ocular syndrome and cases mistakenly diagnosed as representing thalidomide embryopathy (7). Further mutation at *SALL4* has been recorded by Al-Baradie et al., including patients with hearing loss (1).

Duane anomaly may also be seen as an isolated finding or an autosomal dominant trait. It is also found in Wildervanck syndrome and has been reported in association with chromosome 8q deletion involving the region of the *EYA1* locus, which causes branchio-oto-renal syndrome (12).

Kohlhase et al. (7) have drawn attention to the slit-like configuration of the external ear canal in an affected father and daughter (Fig. 8–42F,G).

References

1. Al-Baradie R et al: Duane radial ray syndrome (Okihiro syndrome) maps to 20q13 and results from mutations in *SALL4*, a new member of the SAL family. *Am J Hum Genet* 71: online publication Oct 22, 2002.
2. Becker K et al: Okihiro syndrome and acro-renal-ocular syndrome: clinical overlap, expansion of the phenotype, and absence of *PAX2* mutations in two new families. *J Med Genet* 39:68–71, 2002.
3. Collins A et al: Okihiro syndrome: thenar hypoplasia and Duane anomaly in 3 generations. *Clin Dysmorphol* 2:237–240. 1993.

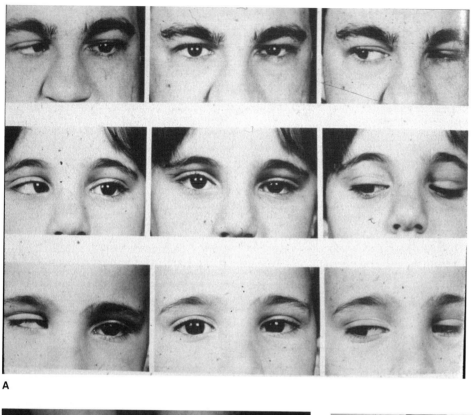

A

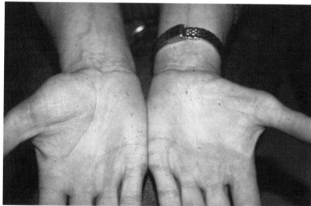

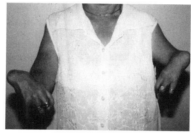

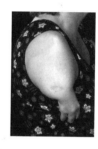

B

C

D

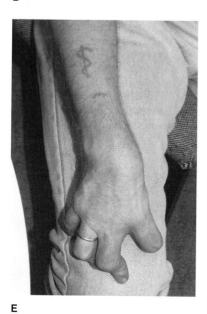

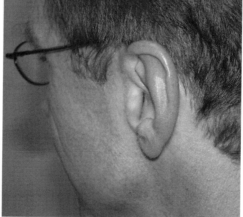

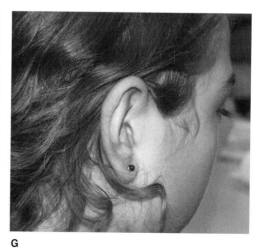

E

F

G

Figure 8–42. *Okihiro syndrome*. (A) Duane anomaly, (B) thenar hypoplasia, (C-E) variability of limb defects, (F,G) slit-like configuration of external ear canal. [From W. Reardon, Dublin, Ireland, and J Kohlhase, Göttingen, Germany.]

4. Crisp WH. Congenital paralysis of the external rectus muscle. *Am J Ophthalmol* 1:172–176, 1918.
5. Halal F et al: Acro-renal-ocular syndrome: autosomal dominant thumb hypoplasia, renal ectopia, and eye defect. *Am J Med Genet* 27:753–762, 1984.
6. Hayes A et al: The Okihiro syndrome of Duane anomaly, radial ray abnormalities, and deafness. *Am J Med Genet* 22:273–280, 1985.
7. Kohlhase J et al: Mutations at the SALL4 locus on chromosome 20 result in a range of clinically overlapping phenotypes, including Okihiro syndrome, Holt-Oram syndrome, acro-renal-ocular syndrome, and patients previously reported to represent thalidomide embryopathy. *J Med Genet* 40:473–478, 2003.
8. MacDermot KD, Winter RM: Radial ray defect and Duane anomaly: report of a family with autosomal dominant transmission. *Am J Med Genet* 27:313–319, 1987.
9. McGowan KF, Pagon RA: Okihiro syndrome. *Am J Med Genet* 51:89, 1994.
10. Okihiro MM et al: Duane syndrome and congenital upper-limb anomalies. *Arch Neurol* 34:174–177, 1977.
11. Temtamy SA, McKusick VA: The genetics of hand malformations. *Birth Defects* 14:133–135, 1978.
12. Vincent C et al: A proposed new contiguous gene syndrome on 8q consists of branchio-oto-renal syndrome, Duane syndrome, a dominant form of hydrocephalus and trapeze aplasia: implications for the mapping of the BOR gene. *Hum Mol Genet* 3:1859–1866, 1994.

Triphalangeal thumbs, Glanzmann thrombasthenia, and sensorineural hearing loss

Wiedemann et al. (2), in 1985, and Schlegelburger et al. (1), in 1986, described a 22-year-old woman with triphalangeal thumbs, Glanzmann thrombasthenia, and sensorineural hearing loss. She reported severe epistaxis several times a year, menorrhagia, spontaneous hematomas, and purpura since the first year of life. The bleeding disorder became evident in infancy when oozing was observed. There was severe reduction in concentrations of glycoprotein IIb–IIIa.

In addition to hemorrhagic diathesis, there was a somewhat unusual face characterized by a mild hypertelorism, broad nasal root, mild prognathism, and alopecia areata (Fig. 8–43A).

Musculoskeletal system. Finger-like thumbs were noted bilaterally. One thumb was hypoplastic and had flexion contracture. The thenar eminences were hypoplastic (Fig. 8–43B,C). The carpal bones were abnormal (Fig. 8–43D).

Auditory system. Hearing loss was sensorineural but otherwise was not described.

Heredity. The disorder was thought to be autosomal recessive because the parents had reduced concentrations of glycoprotein IIb-IIIa.

Diagnosis. To be excluded are IVIC syndrome, Fanconi pancytopenia syndrome, and Holt-Oram syndrome.

References

1. Schlegelburger B et al: Probable autosomal recessive syndrome with triphalangia of thumbs, thrombasthenia (Glanzmann) and deafness of internal ear. *Klin Pädiatr* 198:337–339, 1986.
2. Wiedemann H-R et al: Syndrome of triphalangism of the first ray of the hands, thrombocytopathy, and inner ear hearing impairment. In: *An Atlas of Characteristic Syndromes: A Visual Aid to Diagnosis,* Wolfe Medical Publications, London, 1985, pp 434–435.

Wildervanck syndrome (cervico-oculo-acoustic syndrome, Klippel-Feil anomaly plus)

The major clinical features of Wildervanck syndrome are fused cervical vertebrae, abducens palsy with retracted globe (Duane syndrome),

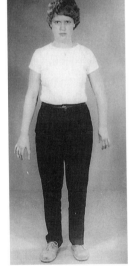
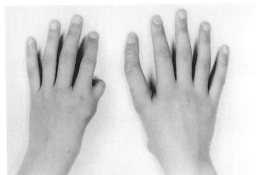
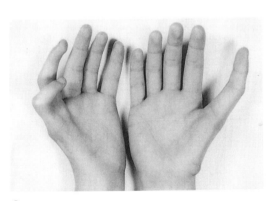

A   B   C

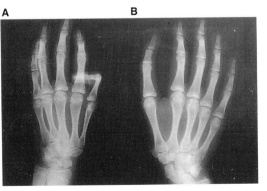

D

Figure 8–43. *Triphalangeal thumbs, Glanzmann thrombasthenia, and sensorineural hearing loss.* (A) Twenty-two-year-old female with triphalangeal thumbs, Glanzmann thrombasthenia, and sensorineural hearing loss. (B,C) Bilateral triphalangeal thumbs. Right thumb lies in same plane as other digits. Left thumb is hypoplastic with flexion contracture. (D) Radiograph showing different anomalies in the two hands. Note hypoplasia of the left first metacarpal and unusual carpal bone changes as well as triphalangeal thumbs. [From B Schlegelburger et al., *Klin Pädiatr* 19:337, 1986.]

and sensorineural and/or conductive hearing loss (60,62). Different phenotypic definitions are evident (29,30,38,59,62). We will consider Klippel-Feil anomaly and Duane syndrome as part of a broader spectrum.

Facial and ocular findings. Facial asymmetry (15–17) and nonprogressive hemifacial weakness, present since birth, have been described (Fig. 8–44A–F). Unilateral or bilateral Duane syndrome is a major feature (6,14,17,28,31,37–39,43,56,60). Duane syndrome consists of abducens paralysis that prevents external rotation of the affected eye. On adduction, the lid fissure of the affected eye narrows, and the globe retracts (Fig. 8–43E,F). Abducens paralysis without retraction has also been reported (12). Pseudopapilledema (28), unilateral epibulbar dermoid (15,28), and bilateral temporal subluxation of the lens (56) have been observed. Cleft palate may be present (17,31) and an anterior glottic web has been noted. Some patients have abnormal bony masses in the mandibular ramus region that has occasionally been reported as duplication phenomena (2,11,33).

Musculoskeletal system. Klippel-Feil anomaly, consisting of fusion of one or more cervical and sometimes thoracic vertebrae, is characteristic (7,12,15,19,21,28,31,60). The neck is short, thick, and webbed, and the head appears to sit directly on the trunk (14, 16,17,28,56). Flexion, extension, and lateral mobility of the neck are severely restricted (12,14,16,17,28,31) and there may be torticollis (15,16,37). Spina bifida occulta (12,15–17,37), Sprengel deformity (28), kyphosis (13,37), scoliosis (14,15,37), and basilar impression (12,14–16) have been described.

Central nervous system. A few reports have noted mild (6) or severe (17) mental retardation. Facial paralysis (30) and mirror movements (12) have been described, as has brain stem hypoplasia (5).

Auditory system. Among patients having just Duane's anomaly (49), hearing loss, both sensorineural and conductive, has been found in about 15%. However, in Wildervanck syndrome, hearing loss is noted in at least 30%. It may be sensorineural (15–18,28,31,39,41,56), conductive (9,12,25,49,50,53–55,57), or mixed (7,15,41). Although age of onset is usually in the first decade (7,52,60,61) and may be profound (28,31), the severity and age of onset have not been well documented. The loss may be unilateral (14,59). In addition, preauricular tags (15,28,41), cheek skin tags, malformation of the pinna (28), atresia or absence of the external auditory canal (12), stenotic or short internal auditory meatus (14), abnormal and absent ossicles (35), stapes fixation (7), stapes gusher (8), abnormal semicircular canals (14,35,63), and underdevelopment of the bony labyrinth (Mondini defect) (3,14, 26,41,45,48,51,58,59,63,64) have been described.

Vestibular findings. Caloric areflexia is usually found (3,14,24,61).

Heredity. All cases with this triad of abnormalities are sporadic. The overwhelming majority of affected individuals reported are females, although a few males with the condition have been described (15,16). Several modes of inheritance have been proposed (10,27,31,32,62,63) and nongenetic causes cannot be excluded (6).

Diagnosis. Differential diagnosis is complicated because many patients with Klippel-Feil anomaly have been incompletely described; some may have Wildervanck syndrome. Klippel-Feil anomaly and associated abnormalities have been particularly well reviewed by Helmi and Pruzansky (23). There is overlap with oculo-auriculo-vertebral spectrum (15,28). A number of unusual cases with some Wildervanck syndrome features are difficult to classify (4,6,13,31,36,56). Okihiro syndrome consists of autosomal dominant inheritance of Duane anomaly with congenital hypoplasia of the thenar eminence and sensorineural hearing loss (22,44). The hand anomalies resemble those seen in Stewart-Bergstrom syndrome. MURCS association (Rokitansky-Küster-Hauser syndrome) consists of müllerian duct aplasia, renal aplasia, and cervicothoracic somite dysplasia. Vertebral defects occur from C_5 to T_1. Other clinical manifestations include Klippel-Feil anomaly, absent

uterus and vagina, renal agenesis, and conductive hearing loss (1, 13,20,34,40,42,46,47) (Fig. 8–43G–I).

Summary. Characteristics include (*1*) doubtful genetic etiology; (*2*) fused cervical vertebrae; (*3*) abducens palsy with retracted globe; and (*4*) sensorineural, conductive, or mixed hearing loss.

References

1. Baird PA, Lowry RB: Absent vagina and the Klippel-Feil anomaly. *Am J Obstet Gynecol* 118:290–291, 1974.
2. Ball IA: Klippel-Feil syndrome associated with accessory jaws. *Br Dent J* 161:20–23, 1986.
3. Baumeister S, Terrahe K: Innenohrmissbildungen beim Klippel-Feil-Syndrom. *Laryngol Rhinol* 53:120–130, 1974.
4. Brik M, Athayde A: Bilateral Duane's syndrome, paroxysmal lacrimation and Klippel-Feil anomaly. *Ophthalmologica* 167:1–8, 1973.
5. Brodsky MC et al: Brainstem hypoplasia in the Wildervanck (cervico-oculo-acoustic) syndrome. *Arch Ophthalmol* 116:383–385, 1998.
6. Corsello G et al: Cervico-oculo-acusticus (Wildervanck's) syndrome: a clinical variant of Klippel-Feil sequence? *Klin Pädiatr* 202:176–179, 1990.
7. Cremers CWRJ et al: Hearing loss in the cervico-oculo-acoustic (Wildervanck) syndrome. *Arch Otolaryngol* 110:54–57, 1984.
8. Daniilidis J et al: Stapes gusher and Klippel-Feil syndrome. *Laryngoscope* 88:1178–1181, 1978.
9. Daniilidis J et al: Otological findings in cervico-oculo-auditory dysplasia. *J Laryngol Otol* 94:533–544, 1980.
10. Da Silva EO et al: Autosomal recessive Klippel-Feil syndrome. *J Med Genet* 19:130–134, 1982.
11. Douglas PS et al: Abnormal bone masses in Klippel-Feil syndrome. *Br J Oral Maxillofac Surg* 30:382–386, 1992.
12. Eisemann ML, Sharma GK: The Wildervanck syndrome: cervico-oculo-acoustic dysplasia. *Otolaryngol Head Neck Surg* 87:892–897, 1979.
13. Everberg G: Congenital absence of the oval window. *Acta Otolaryngol (Stockh)* 66:320–332, 1968.
14. Everberg G et al: Wildervanck's syndrome: Klippel-Feil's syndrome associated with deafness and retraction of the eyeball. *Br J Radiol* 36:562–567, 1963.
15. Franceschetti A, Klein D: Dysmorphie cervico-oculo-faciale avec surdité familiale. (Klippel-Feil, retractio bulbi, asymétrie cránio-faciale autres anomalies congénitales). *J Génét Hum* 3:176–213, 1954.
16. Franceschetti A et al: An extensive form of cervico-oculo-facial dysmorphia (Wildervanck-Franceschetti-Klein). *Acta Fac Med Univ Brun* 25:53–61, 1965.
17. Fraser WI, MacGilivray RC: Cervico-oculo-acoustic dysplasia ("the syndrome of Wildervanck"). *J Ment Defic Res* 12:322–329, 1968.
18. Giroud M et al: Le syndrome cervico-oculo-acoustique. *Pédiatrie* 36:479–482, 1981.
19. Giroud M et al: Les anomalies radiologiques dans le syndrome de Wildervanck. *J Radiol* 64:131–132, 1983.
20. Griffin JE et al: Congenital absence of the vagina. Mayer-Rokitansky-Küster-Hauser syndrome. *Ann Intern Med* 85:224–236, 1976.
21. Gupte G et al: Wildervanck syndrome (cervico-acoustic syndrome). *J Postgrad Med* 38:180–184, 1992.
22. Hayes A et al: The Okihiro syndrome of Duane anomaly, radial ray abnormalities, and deafness. *Am J Med Genet* 22:273–280, 1985.
23. Helmi C, Pruzansky S: Craniofacial and extracranial malformations in the Klippel-Feil syndrome. *Cleft Palate J* 17:65–88, 1980.
24. Hughes PJ et al: Wildervanck or cervico-oculo-acoustic syndrome and MRI findings. *J Neurol Neurosurg Psychiatry* 54:503–504, 1991.
25. Jarvis JF, Sellars SL: Klippel-Feil deformity associated with congenital conductive deafness. *J Laryngol Otol* 88:285–289, 1974.
26. Jensen J, Rovsing H: Dysplasia of the cochlea in a case of Wildervanck syndrome. *Adv Oto-Rhino-Laryngol* 21:32–39, 1974.
27. Juberg RC, Gershanik JJ: Cervical vertebral fusion (Klippel-Feil) syndrome with consanguineous parents. *J Med Genet* 13:246–248, 1976.
28. Kirkham TH: Cervico-oculo-acousticus syndrome with pseudopapilloedema. *Arch Dis Child* 44:504–508, 1969.
29. Kirkham TH: Duane's syndrome and familial perceptive deafness. *Br J Ophthalmol* 53:335–339, 1969.
30. Kirkham TH: Inheritance of Duane's syndrome. *Br J Ophthalmol* 54:323–329, 1969.
31. Kirkham TH: Duane's retraction syndrome and cleft palate. *Am J Ophthalmol* 70:209–212, 1970.
32. Konigsmark BW, Gorlin RJ: *Genetic and Metabolic Deafness.* W.B. Saunders, Philadelphia, 1976, pp 188–191.

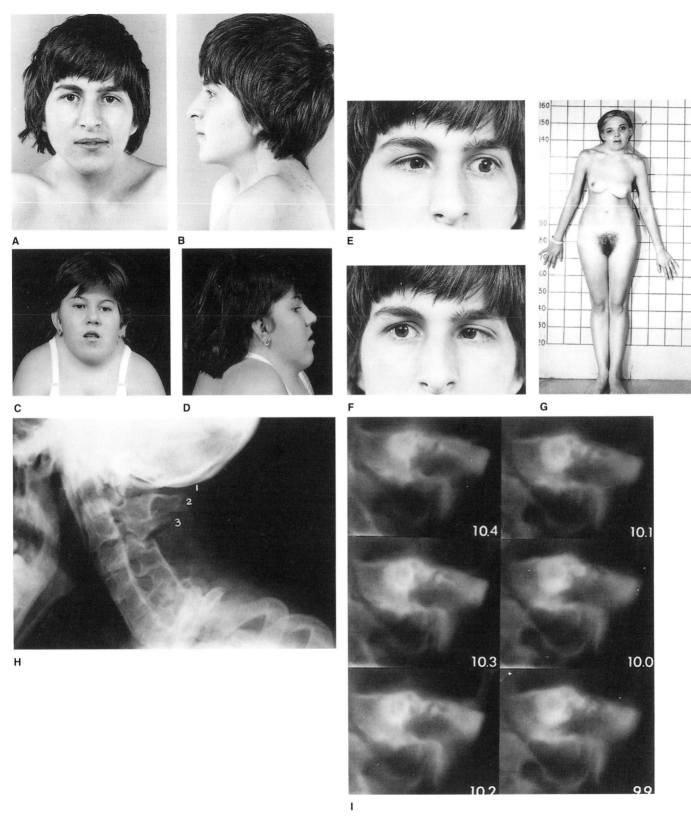

Figure 8–44. *Wildervanck syndrome.* (A,B) Short neck and Sprengel's deformity. (C,D) More severe examples of Wildervanck syndrome. (E,F) Congenital bilateral abducens palsy evident when patient looks to right and to left. (G) *MURCS variant.* Patient has absent vagina but has normal secondary sexual characteristics. (H) Multiple fusions of cervical spine. (I) Polyto-mogram of petrous pyramid. Note indentation of middle cranial fossa, downslanting external auditory canal, and ossicular malformations including fusion of malformed malleus. [(A,B,E,F) from CWRJ Cremers et al., *Arch Otolaryngol* 110:54, 1984; (C,D) from RT Miyamoto et al., *Am J Otol* 5:113, 1983; (G–I) from IJ Park and HW Jones Jr, *Birth Defects* 7(6):311, 1971.]

33. Lawrence TM et al: Congenital duplication of mandibular rami in Klippel-Feil syndrome. *J Oral Med* 40:120–122, 1985.

34. Leduc B et al: Congenital absence of the vagina. Observations on 25 cases. *Am J Obstet Gynecol* 100:512–520, 1968.

35. Lindsay JR: Inner ear histopathology in genetically determined congenital deafness. *Birth Defects* 7:21–32, 1971.

36. Livingstone G, Delahunty JE: Malformation of the ear associated with congenital ophthalmic and other conditions. *J Laryngol Otol* 82:495–504, 1968.

37. Magnus JA: Congenital paralysis of both external recti treated by transplantation of eye muscles. *Br J Ophthalmol* 28:241–245, 1949.

38. Mayer B et al: Zervikal ausgelöste neurootologische Symptome des Klippel-Feil-Syndroms. *Laryngol Rhinol Otol* 63:364–370, 1984.

39. McLay K, Maran AGD: Deafness and the Klippel-Feil syndrome. *J Laryngol* 83:175–184, 1969.

40. Mecklenburg RS, Krueger PM: Extensive genitourinary anomalies associated with Klippel-Feil syndrome. *Am J Dis Child* 125:92–93, 1974.

41. Miyamoto RT et al: Klippel-Feil syndrome and associated ear deformities. *Am J Otol* 5:113–119, 1983.

42. Moore WB et al: Genitourinary anomalies associated with Klippel-Feil syndrome. *J Bone Joint Surg Am* 57:355–357, 1975.

43. Nagib MG et al: Klippel-Feil syndrome in children: clinical features and management. *Childs Nerv Syst* 1:255–263, 1985.

44. Okihiro MM et al: Duane syndrome and congenital upper-limb anomalies. *Arch Neurol* 34:174–177, 1979.

45. Palant DI, Carter BL: Klippel-Feil syndrome and deafness. *Am J Dis Child* 123:218–221, 1972.

46. Park IJ, Jones HW Jr: A new syndrome in two unrelated females: Klippel-Feil deformity, conductive deafness and absent vagina. *Birth Defects* 7(6):311–317, 1971.

47. Ramsay J, Bliznak J: Klippel-Feil syndrome with renal agenesis and other anomalies. *AJR Am J Roentgenol* 113:460–463, 1971.

48. Regenbogen L, Godel V: Cervico-oculo-acoustic syndrome. *Ophthalmol Paediatr Genet* 6:183–187, 1985.

49. Ro A et al: Auditory function in Duane's retraction syndrome. *Am J Ophthalmol* 109:75–78, 1990.

50. Sakai M et al: Klippel-Feil syndrome with conductive deafness and histological findings of removed stapes. *Ann Otol Rhinol Laryngol* 92:113–117, 1983.

51. Schild JA et al: Wildervanck syndrome—the external appearance and radiographic findings. *Int J Pediatr Otorhinolaryngol* 7:305–310, 1984.

52. Sherk HH, Nicholson JT: Cervico-oculo-acusticus syndrome. *J Bone Joint Surg Am* 54:1776–1778, 1972.

53. Singh SP et al: Klippel-Feil syndrome with unexplained apparent conductive hearing loss. *Laryngoscope* 79:113–117, 1969.

54. Stark EW, Borton TE: Klippel-Feil syndrome and associated hearing loss. *Arch Otolaryngol* 97:415–419, 1973.

55. Stewart EJ, O'Reilly BF: Klippel-Feil syndrome and conductive deafness. *J Laryngol Otol* 103:947–949, 1989.

56. Strisciuglio P et al: Wildervanck's syndrome with bilateral subluxation of lens and facial paralysis. *J Med Genet* 20:72–73, 1983.

57. Van Rijn PM, Cremers CWRJ: Surgery for congenital conductive deafness in Klippel-Feil syndrome. *Ann Otol Rhinol Laryngol* 97:347–352, 1988.

58. Veldman JE, Franken PL: Binnenooranomalieen. Een patient met het syndroom van Wildervanck. *Ned Tidj Geneesk* 120:1730–1733, 1976.

59. West PDB et al: Wildervanck's syndrome—unilateral Mondini dysplasia identified by computed tomography. *J Laryngol Otol* 103:408–411,1989.

60. Wildervanck LS: Een geval aandoening van Klippel-Feil gecombineerd met abducensparalyse, retractio bulbi en doofst omheid. *Ned Tijdschr Geneeskd* 96:2752–2756, 1952.

61. Wildervanck LS: Een cervico-oculo-acusticussyndroom. *Ned Tijdschr Geneeskd* 104:2600–2605, 1960.

62. Wildervanck LS: The cervico-oculo-acusticus syndrome. In: *Handbook of Clinical Neurology*, Vol. 32, Vinken PJ, Bruyn GW, Myrianthopoulos NC (eds), North-Holland Publishing, Amsterdam, 1978, pp 123–130.

63. Wildervanck LS et al: Radiological examination of the inner ear of deaf-mutes presenting the cervico-oculo-acusticus syndrome. With a summary of roentgenologic and pathologico-anatomical findings in other endogenous forms of deafness. *Acta Otolaryngol (Stockh)* 61:445–453, 1966.

64. Windle-Taylor PC et al: Ear deformities associated with the Klippel-Feil syndrome. *Ann Otol Rhinol Laryngol* 90:210–216, 1981.

Miscellaneous Musculoskeletal Disorders

In this section, two types of disorders are described: (*1*) rare conditions with hearing loss and (*2*) well-known conditions with occasional or rarely occurring hearing loss.

Rare Conditions with Hearing Loss

Tibial agenesis and congenital hearing loss (Carraro syndrome)

In 1931, Carraro (1) described a syndrome characterized by absence of one or both tibiae and severe congenital hearing loss in four of six sibs. Wandler and Schwarz (6) described an isolated patient.

The affected sibs reported by Carraro (1) were normal except for abbreviation of one or both lower legs. Two sibs had marked shortening of the right leg and mild shortening of the left, whereas another sib had marked shortening of the left leg and moderate shortening of the right lower leg (Fig. 8–45A–C).

Radiographs of the lower legs in one boy showed a striking shortening and mild thickening of both tibiae. The fibulae were of normal length and appeared to project above the knee joint (Fig. 8–45D,E). Radiographs of the remaining three sibs showed somewhat similar findings with a variable degree of bowing of the fibula.

Auditory system. Each of the four sibs described by Carraro (1) was congenitally deaf. No further audiometric testing was mentioned. The patient of Wandler and Schwarz (6) had profound hearing loss but no further details were given.

Heredity. Autosomal recessive inheritance is likely (1).

Diagnosis. A syndrome of multiple bony anomalies (aplasia of tibiae, heptadactyly of toes and/or fingers), prognathism, and hypodontia was described by Pashayan et al. (2). Pfeiffer and Roeskau (3) indicated that this was genetically heterogeneous and delineated four different syndromes, none of which had associated hearing loss. All showed autosomal dominant inheritance. Excellent reviews are those of Richieri-Costa and coworkers (4,5), Wiedemann and Opitz (7), and Yujnovsky et al. (8).

Summary. Characteristics include (*1*) probable autosomal recessive inheritance; (*2*) significant shortening of the tibiae; and (*3*) congenital profound hearing loss, not otherwise designated.

References

1. Carraro A: Assenza congenita della tibia e sordomutismo nel quattro fratelli. *Chir Organi Mov* 16:429–438, 1931.

2. Pashayan H et al: Bilateral aplasia of the tibia, polydactyly and absent thumbs in a father and daughter. *J Bone Joint Surg Br* 53:495–499, 1971.

3. Pfeiffer RA, Roeskau M: Agenesie der Tibia, Fibulaverdoppelung und spiegelbildliche Polydaktylie (Diplopodie) bei Mutter und Kind. *Z Kinderheilk* 111:38–50, 1971.

4. Richieri-Costa A: Tibial hemimelia–cleft lip/palate in a Brazilian child born to consanguineous parents. *Am J Med Genet* 28:325–329, 1987.

5. Richieri-Costa A et al: Autosomal dominant tibial hemimelia-poly-syndactyly-triphalangeal thumbs syndrome: report of a Brazilian family. *Am J Med Genet* 36:1–6, 1990.

6. Wandler H, Schwarz R: Carraro-Syndrom. *Roefo* 133:43–46, 1980.

7. Wiedemann H-R, Opitz JM: Unilateral partial tibia defect with preaxial polydactyly, general micromelia, and trigonocephaly with a note on "developmental resistance." *Am J Med Genet* 14:467–471, 1974.

8. Yujnovsky O et al: A syndrome of polydactyly-syndactyly and triphalangeal thumbs in three generations. *Clin Genet* 6:51–59, 1974.

Broad terminal phalanges, abnormal face, and sensorineural hearing loss (Keipert syndrome, nasodigitoacoustic syndrome)

Keipert et al. (3) described two brothers with severe sensorineural hearing loss, unusual face, and broad terminal phalanges. Balci and Dagli (1) reported two brothers and Cappon and Khalifa (2) and Reardon and Hall (5) each reported a single boy with similar findings.

Craniofacial findings. Facial appearance was marked by prominent frontal bone, hypertelorism, large nose with high bridge, hypoplastic

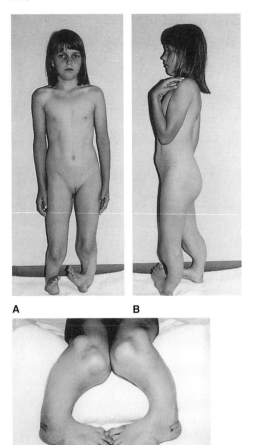

A   B

C

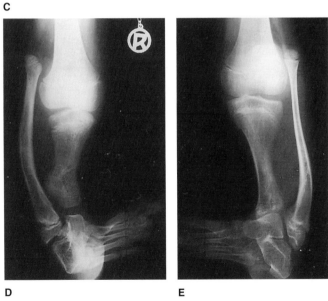

D   E

Figure 8–45. *Tibial agenesis and congenital hearing loss (Carraro syndrome).* (A,B) Nine-year-old female with congenital shortening of both lower extremities. Patient had congenital profound hearing loss. (C) Talipes equinovarus and marked shortening of tibiae. (D,E) Radiographs showing markedly abbreviated tibiae and severe talipes. [From H Wandler and R Schwarz, *Roefo* 133:43, 1980.]

maxilla, large rounded columella, and prominent nasal alae. The upper lip protruded, had a cupid's bow configuration, and laterally overlapped the rather straight lower lip. Head circumference was large (Fig. 8–46A,B).

Extremities. The distal phalanges of the thumbs, first, second, and third fingers, and all toes were markedly broad. The fifth fingers were short and clinodactylous. The toes were rotated medially (Fig. 8–46C,D). A third fontanelle was present during infancy. Radiographically, one sib had bifid terminal phalanges in both index fingers. In the halluces of both brothers, the proximal phalanges were short, and the terminal phalanges were markedly abbreviated with large, rounded epiphyses.

Other findings. One sib noted by Keipert et al. (3) had severe mental deficiency. The child reported by Cappon and Khalifa (2) had developmental delay and abnormal behavior. Dermatoglyphic findings included an increased number of digital whorls. Pulmonic stenosis and hoarseness were found (1).

Auditory system. One brother reported by Keipert et al. had severe sensorineural hearing loss in one ear but normal hearing in the other ear. The other sib exhibited moderately severe bilateral high-tone sensorineural hearing loss (3). Both brothers noted by Balci and Dagli (1) had mild sensorineural loss. The boy reported by Cappon and Khalifa (2) had severe bilateral sensorineural loss.

Heredity. Autosomal recessive inheritance is likely; however, all reported patients have been male, thus X-linked recessive inheritance cannot be ruled out.

Diagnosis. Keipert syndrome is distinctive in its overall pattern. Broad thumbs and halluces are found in Rubinstein-Taybi syndrome (6), Pfeiffer syndrome, and Palant syndrome (4).

Figure 8–46. *Broad terminal phalanges, abnormal facies, and sensorineural hearing loss (Keipert syndrome).* (A,B) Sibs exhibiting cupid's bow mouth and unusual nasal form. Younger sib also had ptosis of left lid and mild hydrocephalus. (C) Right hand of older boy showing broad terminal phalanx of thumb and first three fingers as well as clinodactyly of fifth finger. (D) Right foot of same child showing broad terminal phalanges and medial rotation of toes. [From JA Keipert et al., *Aust Paediatr J* 9:10, 1973.]

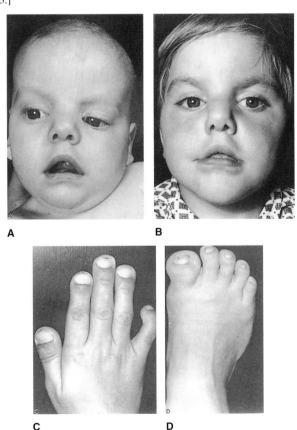

A   B

C   D

Summary. Characteristics include (*1*) autosomal inheritance; (*2*) unusual facial phenotype; (*3*) broad terminal phalanges; and (*4*) sensorineural hearing loss.

References

1. Balci S, Dagli S: Two brothers with Keipert syndrome from Turkey. *Clin Genet* 50:223–228, 1996.
2. Cappon SM, Khalifa MM: Additional case of Keipert syndrome and review of the literature. *Med Sci Monit* 6:776–778, 2000.
3. Keipert JA et al: A new syndrome of broad terminal phalanges and facial abnormalities. *Aust Paediatr J* 9:10–13, 1973.
4. Palant DI et al: Unusual facies, cleft palate, mental retardation and limb abnormalities in siblings—a new syndrome. *J Pediatr* 78:686–689, 1971.
5. Reardon W, Hall CM: Broad thumbs and halluces with deafness: a patient with Kiepert syndrome. *Am J Med Genet* 118A:86–89, 2003.
6. Rubinstein JH: The broad thumbs syndrome. *Birth Defects* 5(2):25–41, 1969.

Joint fusions, mitral insufficiency, and conductive hearing loss

A mother and two daughters with conductive hearing loss, fusion in the carpus, tarsus, and cervical vertebrae, and mitral insufficiency were described by Forney et al. (1).

All had short stature, with both children being below the third centile in height. Large numbers of freckles were noted on the face, particularly on the cheeks and shoulders (Fig. 8–47A).

Cardiovascular system. Cardiac murmurs consistent with mitral insufficiency were heard in all affected individuals. An electrocardiogram showed incomplete bundle branch block in each patient. Cardiac catheterization in two cases revealed moderate mitral insufficiency.

Musculoskeletal system. From two to five vertebrae were fused in each patient (Fig. 8–47B). In one, the capitate and hamate as well as the lunate and navicular were fused bilaterally. In another patient, the lunate and triquetrum were fused. The phalanges were shortened (Fig. 8–47C). The navicular, first cuneiform, and cuboidal bones were fused in both feet in one patient. In another patient, the tarsal bones were normal.

Auditory system. Moderate hearing loss was present in childhood and may have been congenital. Pure-tone audiograms on each patient showed a 30–70 dB conductive hearing loss. Surgical exploration of one ear in each of the two children showed fixation of the footplate of the stapes.

Heredity. Autosomal dominant inheritance is likely.

Diagnosis. LEOPARD syndrome is similar but readily distinguishable.

Reference

1. Forney WR et al: Congenital heart disease, deafness, and skeletal malformations: a new syndrome? *J Pediatr* 68:14–26, 1966.

Acrofacial dysostosis, type Kelly

In 1977, Kelly et al. (1) described three males, two of whom were sibs, with short stature, mild mental retardation (IQ 50–60), downslanting palpebral fissures, maxillary and mandibular hypoplasia, hypospadias, cryptorchidism, symphalangism of thumbs and distal interphalangeal joints of index fingers, and radioulnar synostosis. All had bilateral, high-frequency hearing loss. In two families, the parents were cousins. Autosomal recessive inheritance is likely.

Reference

1. Kelly TE et al: Acrofacial dysostosis with growth and mental retardation, one with simultaneous Hermansky-Pudlak syndrome. *Birth Defects* 13(3B):45–52, 1977.

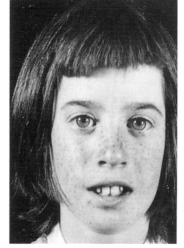
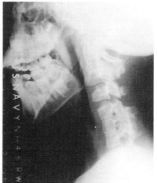
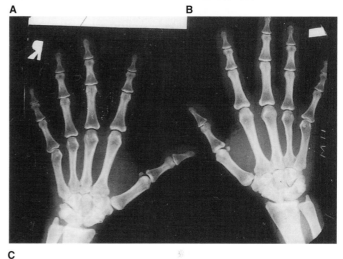

C

Figure 8–47. *Joint fusions, mitral insufficiency, and conductive hearing loss.* (A) Numerous freckles on face and shoulders were present in all affected members. (B) Fusion of cervical vertebrae. (C) Fusion of carpal bones. Tarsal bones similarly affected. [From WR Forney et al., *J Pediatr* 68:14, 1966.]

Acrofacial dysostosis, type Reynolds

Reynolds et al. (1) described a family manifesting autosomal dominant inheritance of a previously undescribed acrofacial dysostosis syndrome. The craniofacial manifestations were those of mild mandibulofacial dysostosis and included prominent forehead, ptosis, downslanting palpebral fissures, malar hypoplasia, highly arched palate with dental malocclusion, and micrognathia. The pinnae were normal. However, mild congenital mixed hearing loss was a feature.

The variable acral abnormalities affected predominantly the radial ray, manifesting as mild hypoplasia of the first metacarpal and first proximal phalanx. This was more evident on metacarpal–phalangeal pattern profile than on clinical examination in some affected individuals.

There is some resemblance of the face to that of maxillofacial dysostosis.

Reference

1. Reynolds JF et al: A new autosomal dominant acrofacial dysostosis syndrome. *Am J Med Genet* (Suppl)2:143–150, 1986.

Acrofacial dysostosis, type Rodriguez

In 1990, Rodriguez et al. (4) reported three male sibs with a lethal acrofacial dysostosis. Death occurred in the neonatal period from respiratory problems secondary to severe mandibular underdevelopment. Other examples have been described (1,3). A 100-year-old example has been noted (2).

In addition to severe micrognathia, there are malar hypoplasia, malformed pinnae with atretic canals, prominent nasal bridge and, in most cases, cleft palate.

Skeletal alterations are variable but include short or absent humerus, absent forearm, preaxial (predominantly) and/or postaxial digital anomalies, lower limb defects, including digital deficiencies, shoulder and pelvic girdle hypoplasia, and rib defects.

Cardiac malformations, CNS malformations, and absent lung lobation can also be seen.

To be excluded are Genée-Wiedemann syndrome and Nager syndrome.

References

1. Fryns J-P, Kleckowska A: New lethal acrofacial dysostosis syndrome. *Am J Med Genet* 39:223–224, 1991.
2. Oostra RJ et al: Severe acrofacial dysostosis with orofacial clefting and tetraphocomelia in the plaster cast of a 100-year-old anatomical specimen. *Am J Med Genet* 78:195–197, 1998.
3. Petit P et al: Acrofacial dysostosis type Rodriguez: a new lethal MCA syndrome. *Am J Med Genet* 42:343–345, 1992.
4. Rodriguez JI et al: New acrofacial dysostosis syndrome in 3 sibs. *Am J Med Genet* 35:484–489, 1990.

Brachydactyly A1, dwarfism, ptosis, microcephaly, mental retardation, and mixed hearing loss

In 1989, Tsukahara et al. (1) described a single case of a child with type A1 brachydactyly, disproportionate dwarfism, ptosis, microcephaly, mental retardation, and moderate mixed hearing loss. The child also had persistent iridopupillary membranes and myopia. The parents were second cousins. Inheritance is possibly autosomal recessive.

A gene for A1 brachydactyly has been mapped to 2q35–q36 (2).

References

1. Tsukahara M et al: Type A1 brachydactyly, dwarfism, ptosis, mixed hearing loss, microcephaly, and mental retardation. *Am J Med Genet* 33:7–9, 1989.
2. Yang X et al: A locus for brachydactyly type A-1 maps to chromosome 2q35–q36. *Am J Hum Genet* 66:892–903, 2000.

Brachyphalangy, polydactyly, absent tibiae, dysmorphic pinnae, and hearing loss

Baraitser et al. (1) reported lower limb preaxial polydactyly and severe finger brachydactyly. Similar cases were reported by Pierson et al. (4), Faravelli et al. (2), and Olney et al. (3).

Malformed pinnae with tags and/or pits in some individuals, small nose, thin eyebrows, short philtrum, low posterior hairline, short neck, micrognathia, short syndactylous fingers with absence of nails on some fingers, preaxial polydactyly of toes, tibial absence, and micropenis were found.

Radiographically, metacarpals, metatarsals, and short middle phalanges of fingers and toes, dislocated hips, absent tibiae, preaxial polydactyly of toes, hypoplastic ischiae, and dysplastic acetabulae and pubic rami were documented.

Sensorineural hearing loss was noted (1,4).

References

1. Baraitser M et al: A syndrome of brachyphalangy, polydactyly and absent tibiae. *Clin Dysmorphol* 6:111–121, 1997.
2. Faravelli F et al: Brachyphalangy, feet polydactyly, absent hypoplastic tibiae: a further case and review of main diagnostic findings. *Clin Dysmorphol* 10:101–103, 2001.
3. Olney RS et al: Limb/pelvis hypoplasia/aplasia with skull defect (Schinzel phocomelia): distinctive features and prenatal detection. *Am J Med Genet* 103:295–301, 2001.

4. Pierson DM et al: Total anomalous pulmonary venous connection and a constellation of craniofacial, skeletal, and urogenital anomalies in a newborn and similar features in his 36-year-old father. *Clin Dysmorphol* 10:95–100, 2001.

Temtamy preaxial brachydactyly syndrome

Temtamy et al. (2) described a boy with short stature, sensorineural hearing loss, moderate mental retardation, minor facial anomalies (round face, large-appearing eyes, midface hypoplasia, and small mouth and jaw), dental anomalies, and digital anomalies. The dental anomalies included microdontia, diastema between mandibular incisors, and talon cusp formation of the maxillary central incisors. Digital anomalies included low insertion of the thumbs and great toes, radial clinodactyly of fingers 2–5, and tibial deviation of toes 2–5. There was partial soft tissue syndactyly of fingers and toes. An older brother, who died at age 1.5 years, was thought to be similarly affected. Parents were second cousins, thus inheritance was thought to be autosomal recessive. There are similarities to the condition described by Camera and Costa (1), but distinguished by lack of cardiac defect and presence of dental anomalies in this condition.

References

1. Camera G, Costa M: Unusual type of brachydactyly associated with intraventricular septal defect and deafness: a new condition? *Clin Dysmorphol* 6:31–33, 1997.
2. Temtamy SA et al: A new multiple congenital anomaly, mental retardation syndrome with preaxial brachydactyly, hyperphalangism, deafness and orodental anomalies. *Clin Dysmorphol* 7:249–255, 1998.

Brachydactyly, type Char, and congenital profound sensorineural hearing loss

In 1977, Char (1) briefly described a female child with a unique form of brachydactyly and sensorineural hearing loss. The child was one of eight sibs and the parents were not consanguineous. Inheritance is unknown. Char (personal communication, November, 1992) indicated that the patient was about 20 years old, still living at home, and unmarried.

The nasal bridge was broad (Fig. 8–48A). The teeth were noted to have darkened enamel.

The fingers and toes were markedly shortened, with two phalanges in each digit. Nails were absent in both fingers and toes (Fig. 8–48B–E). Dermatoglyphics showed vestigial digital pattern.

Char (personal communication, November, 1992), reported that the hearing loss was congenital and profound.

Reference

1. Char F: An unusual form of brachydactyly associated with deafness. *Birth Defects* 13(3C):228, 1977.

Brachydactyly B, macular colobomas, and severe mixed hearing loss (Sorsby syndrome)

In 1935, Sorsby (1) reported a mother and five children with bilateral colobomas of the macula and brachydactyly B (bifid thumb and halluces, no nails or second digits) (Fig. 8–49). When reexamined in 1988, the kindred spanned four generations and included nine individuals (2). Two had severe bilateral mixed hearing loss, worse in higher frequencies. It is possible that this is an incidental finding and not part of the syndrome.

Radiographic examination showed duplication of distal phalanges of thumbs and halluces, hypoplastic distal phalanges of hands and feet, and two phalanges in fifth digits of hands.

References

1. Sorsby A: Congenital coloboma of the macula together with an account of the familial occurrence of bilateral macular colobomas in association with apical dystrophy of the hands and feet. *Br J Ophthalmol* 19:65–90, 1935.
2. Thompson EM, Baraitser M: Sorsby syndrome. A report on further genetics of the original family. *J Med Genet* 25:313–321, 1988.

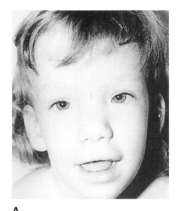

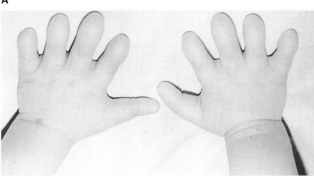

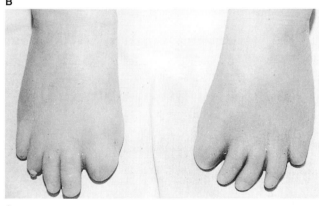

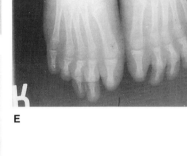

Figure 8–48. *Brachydactyly, type Char, and congenital profound sensorineural hearing loss.* (A) Two-and-one-half-year-old child. Nose is straight due to broad nasal bridge. (B) Hands are brachydactylic, there being only two phalanges in all fingers. Note absent nails. (C) Nails are also absent in toes, except for a rudimentary one in right fourth toe. (D,E) Radiographs of hands and feet show absence of middle phalanges in all fingers. Distal phalanges are rudimentary in left second and fourth toes and absent in right fourth toe. There is only a single phalanx in both fifth toes. [From F Char, *Birth Defects* 13(3C):228, 1977.]

Van der Woude syndrome with hearing loss and minor limb anomalies

Kantaputra et al. (1) described a four-generation family in which several members had manifestations of van der Woude syndrome (cleft lip/palate and lip pits) but in addition had, in variable combinations, sensorineural hearing loss, large facial sinuses, dental pulp stones, long tooth roots, ankyloglossia, and minor limb anomalies. The limb anomalies included brachydactyly, 2/3 syndactyly of the toes, short distal phalanges of toes 2 and 3, and short middle phalanges of toe 4. The hearing loss was detected before age 10 in those affected. Van der Woude syndrome is heterogeneous, with loci at 1q32–41 and 1p34 identified (2,3). It is unknown if this condition is a variant form of either of these entities.

References

1. Kantaputra PN et al: Van der Woude syndrome with sensorineural hearing loss, large craniofacial sinuses, dental pulp stones, and minor limb anomalies: report of a four-generation Thai family. *Am J Med Genet* 108:275–280, 2002.
2. Koillinen H et al: Mapping of the second locus for the van der Woude syndrome to chromosome 1p34. *Eur J Hum Genet* 9:747–752, 2001.
3. Kondo S et al: Mutations in *IRF6* cause Van der Woude and popliteal pterygium syndromes [letter]. *Nat Genet* 32:285–287, 2002.

Brachydactyly, broad first digits, hyperopia, and congenital conductive hearing loss

In 1990, Teunissen and Cremers (4) described a syndrome of hyperopia, broad first digits of hands and feet, short distal phalanges, syndactyly of toes 2–3, and conductive hearing loss in five members of a family in three generations. Other kindreds were added by Hilhorst-Hofstee et al. (2) and Milunsky et al. (3).

Ocular findings. All had hyperopia of 5-11 diopters.

Musculoskeletal system. Broad thumbs and halluces, short distal phalanges, and syndactyly of toes 2–3 were found in five patients. Two exhibited fused C_6–C_7 vertebrae (Fig. 8–50).

Auditory findings. Conductive hearing loss of 50–60 dB was noted. On tympanotomy, in addition to ankylosis of the stapes, a short process of the incus was fixed in the fossa incudis.

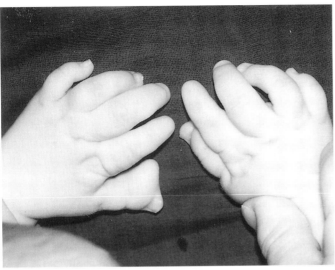

A

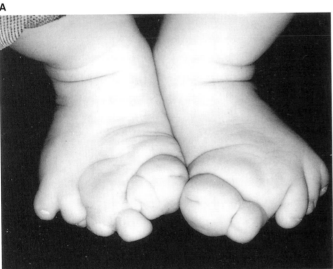

B

Figure 8–49. *Brachydactyly B, macular colobomas, and severe mixed hearing loss (Sorsby syndrome).* (A,B) Note bifid thumbs and halluces, agenesis of nails. [Courtesy of M Baraitser and E Thompson, London, England.]

Heredity. Autosomal dominant inheritance is evident. Recently Brown et al. (1) identified mutations in noggin (*NOG*) in two affected families, thus this condition is allelic to proximal symphalangism with conductive hearing loss.

References

1. Brown DJ et al: Autosomal dominant stapes ankylosis with broad thumbs and toes, hyperopia, and skeletal anomalies is caused by heterozygous nonsense and frameshift mutations in *NOG*, the gene encoding noggin. *Am J Hum Genet* 71:618–624, 2002.
2. Hilhorst-Hofstee Y et al: The autosomal dominant syndrome with congenital stapes ankylosis, broad thumbs, and hyperopia. *Clin Dysmorphol* 6:195–203, 1997.
3. Milunsky J et al: Congenital stapes ankylosis, broad thumbs and hyperopia: report of a family and refinement of a syndrome. *Am J Med Genet* 82:404–408, 1999.
4. Teunissen B, Cremers CWRJ: An autosomal dominant inherited syndrome with congenital stapes fixation. *Laryngoscope* 100:380–384, 1990.

Dysplasia of capital femoral epiphyses, severe myopia, and sensorineural hearing loss

In 1973, Pfeiffer et al. (4) described a syndrome consisting of severe myopia, epiphyseal dysplasia of femoral heads, and sensorineural hearing loss in three brothers.

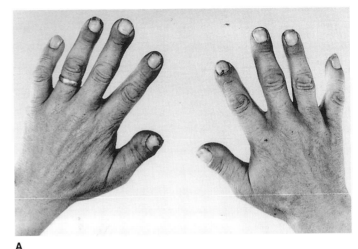

A

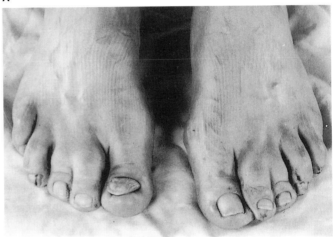

B

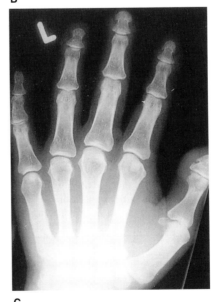

C

Figure 8–50. *Brachydactyly, broad first digits, hyperopia, and congenital conductive hearing loss.* (A) Note broad thumb. (B) Note broad hallux and soft tissue syndactyly involving digits 2–3. (C) Short terminal phalanges of digits 1, 2, 3, and 4. No symphalangism or carpal fusions were evident. [From B Teunissen and CWRJ Cremers, *Laryngoscope* 100:380, 1990.]

Musculoskeletal findings. Height was normal. Mild pectus excavatum and hypermobility of joints, manifested by genua valga and recurvata, were noted in all three brothers. One brother had inguinal hernias.

Radiographic study of each boy showed flattened, irregularly shaped femoral heads with fragmentation (Fig. 8–51). The distal metaphyses of the radius and ulna were irregular. There were two accessory centers of ossification in the carpus. Identical twin brothers showed atypical ossification of the talus.

Ocular findings. Myopia of about 10 diopters became evident at 5 years of age in each brother. Fundus examination showed supertraction of the retina on the nasal side of the disc, atrophy of the pigmentary epithelium, diminution of the choroid nasally, and scattered diffuse peripheral pigmentation.

Auditory system. Symmetrical, sensorineural hearing loss with abrupt high-tone loss above 3000 to 4000 Hz was noted in all brothers. Speech reception threshold was at 30–35 dB. Speech discrimination showed a 20% loss.

Heredity. The parents were consanguineous. Inheritance is likely autosomal recessive.

Diagnosis. This combination of symptoms is unique but most closely resembles spondyloepiphyseal dysplasia, myopia, and sensorineural hearing loss described by MacDermot et al (3). However, inheritance in that family was autosomal dominant. Severe myopia and sensorineural hearing loss occur in a number of syndromes including Stickler syndrome and spondyloepiphyseal dysplasia congenita. A similar but distinctly different disorder was reported by Chitty et al. (1). Aseptic necrosis of the femoral heads (Perthes disease) must be excluded. A dominantly inherited Perthes-like dysplasia associated with brachydactyly was described by Robinson et al. (5). Multiple epiphyseal dysplasia (2) must also be excluded.

References

1. Chitty L et al: Two brothers with deafness, femoral epiphyseal dysplasia, short stature and developmental defect. *Clin Dysmorphol* 5:17–25, 1996.
2. Hunt DD et al: Multiple epiphyseal dysplasia in two siblings. *J Bone Joint Surg Am* 49:1611–1627, 1967.
3. MacDermot KD et al: Epiphyseal dysplasia of femoral head, mild vertebral abnormality, myopia and sensorineural deafness: report of a pedigree with autosomal dominant inheritance. *J Med Genet* 24:602–608, 1987.
4. Pfeiffer RA et al: Epiphyseal dysplasia of the femoral head, severe myopia, and perceptive hearing loss in three brothers. *Clin Genet* 4:141–144, 1973.
5. Robinson GC et al: Hereditary brachydactyly and hip disease. *J Pediatr* 72:539–543, 1968.

Spondyloepiphyseal dysplasia, myopia, and sensorineural hearing loss

In 1987, MacDermot et al. (1) reported a four-generation family in which females exhibited short stature, epiphyseal dysplasia limited to the femoral heads, very mild vertebral alterations, and sensorineural hearing loss. Some affected members of the family had myopia and retinal detachment.

There is some overlap with spondyloepiphyseal dysplasia congenita and with Stickler syndrome. It most closely resembles dysplasia of capital femoral epiphyses, severe myopia, and sensorineural hearing loss, a syndrome having autosomal recessive inheritance.

Reference

1. MacDermot KD et al: Epiphyseal dysplasia of the femoral head, mild vertebral abnormality, myopia, and sensorineural deafness: report of a pedigree with autosomal dominant inheritance. *J Med Genet* 24:602–608, 1987.

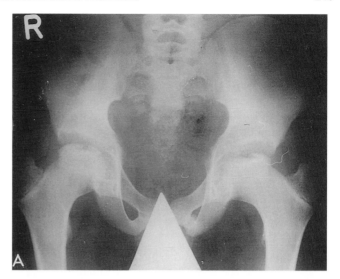

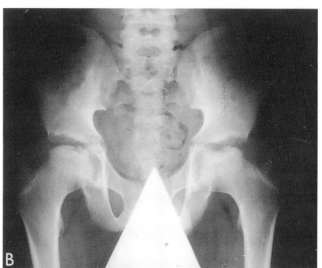

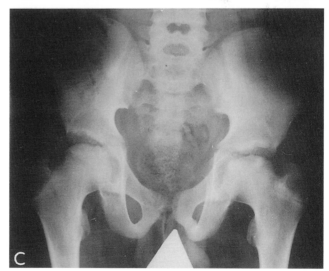

Figure 8–51. *Dysplasia of capital femoral epiphyses, severe myopia, and sensorineural hearing loss.* (A–C) Radiographs of male patient taken at 10, 11, and 12 years of age and showing regression of epiphyseal deformity. [From RA Pfeiffer et al., *Clin Genet* 4:141, 1973.]

Multiple epiphyseal dysplasia, myopia, and conductive hearing loss

Beighton et al. (2) described an Afrikaner mother and three children with reduced stature due to multiple epiphyseal dysplasia, myopia, and conductive hearing loss.

The face was round and the nose small, somewhat resembling that of Marshall syndrome. Bone changes resembled multiple epiphyseal dysplasia. The fingers appeared shortened. The femoral necks were widened and coxa valga was present. Progressive myopia, retinal thinning, asteroid hyalosis, and crenated cataract were noted. Visual defects dated from the third year of life.

Conductive hearing loss was noted in early childhood and was probably congenital and profound.

MacDermot et al. (3) described spondyloepiphyseal dysplasia, myopia, and sensorineural hearing loss. This also has autosomal dominant inheritance. There was epiphyseal dysplasia of the femoral head, mild vertebral abnormality, myopia, and sensorineural hearing loss. In addition to severe capital femoral epiphyseal dysplasia, there was mild flattening of vertebral bodies. Some resemblance to spondylo-epiphyseal dysplasia congenita was noted. No member of the kindred had ophthalmologic changes seen in the kindred described by Beighton et al. (2) and the face was not remarkable. The changes most resembled those of dysplasia of capital femoral epiphyses, severe myopia, and sensorineural hearing loss, but that disorder had autosomal recessive inheritance (4).

Ballo et al. (1) noted a dominant negative mutation in the *COL2A1* gene.

References

1. Ballo R et al: Stickler-like syndrome due to a dominant negative mutation in the *COL2A1* gene. *Am J Med Genet* 80:6–11, 1998.
2. Beighton P et al: Dominant inheritance of multiple epiphyseal dysplasia, myopia and deafness. *Clin Genet* 14:173–177, 1978.
3. MacDermot KD et al: Epiphyseal dysplasia of femoral head, mild vertebral abnormality, myopia and sensorineural deafness: report of a pedigree with autosomal dominant inheritance. *J Med Genet* 24:602–608, 1987.
4. Pfeiffer RA et al: Epiphyseal dysplasia of the femoral head, severe myopia, and perceptive hearing loss in three brothers. *Clin Genet* 4:141–144, 1973.

Synostosis (metacarpals/metatarsals 4–5), hypospadias, and profound sensorineural hearing loss

In 1988, Pfeiffer and Kapferer (3) described a male with synostosis of metacarpals and metatarsals 4–5, truncal obesity, first degree hypospadias, and sensorineural hearing loss. The fifth fingers were short and malplaced. Radiographs showed fusion of metacarpals 4–5 with a distally articulating fifth finger on one side and proximal synostosis on the other. The fifth toe was short with proximal fusion of metatarsals 4–5.

Hearing loss, noted at 3 years, was probably congenital and profound. It was conceivably not recognized, since psychomotor development was quite delayed. Evoked potentials were not recorded, even at 100 dB.

Somewhat similar examples were reported by Ruvalcaba et al. (4) and Küster (1), but no mention was made of hearing loss. Milewski (2) described five males, including two brothers, with hypospadias and profound congenital sensorineural hearing loss, who were otherwise normal.

References

1. Küster W: Die Synostosen des Metarcarpe 4 und 5. Inauguration Dissertation, University of Münster, 1980.
2. Milewski C: Beidseitige konnatale Resthörigkeit und Hypospadie—ein neues Syndrom? *Laryngo-Rhino-Otologie* 69:145–149, 1990.
3. Pfeiffer RA, Kapferer L: Sensorineural deafness, hypospadias, and synostosis of metacarpals and metatarsals 4 and 5: a previously apparently undescribed MCA/MR syndrome. *Am J Med Genet* 31:5–10, 1988.
4. Ruvalcaba RHA et al: Smith-Lemli-Opitz syndrome. *Arch Dis Child* 43:620–623, 1968.

Carpal and tarsal abnormalities, cleft palate, oligodontia, and conductive hearing loss

Gorlin et al. (1) reported a syndrome of cleft palate, oligodontia, carpal and, especially, tarsal anomalies, and stapes fixation in two sisters.

Facial and oral findings. The two sisters, 19 and 21 years old, each exhibited mild primary telecanthus. Both had cleft soft palate. Neither ever had more than three or four primary teeth and no permanent teeth.

Musculoskeletal system. The halluces were short and dorsiflexed with wide separation between the hallux and the rest of the toes (Fig. 8–52A).

Auditory system. Reduced hearing was noted prior to puberty. Audiometric testing demonstrated bilateral conductive hearing loss in both patients, being more marked in the right ear of one. Exploratory surgery revealed that each had bilateral congenital fixation of the footplate of the stapes.

Vestibular system. Vestibular studies were not carried out.

Radiographic findings. Radiographic findings showed that the third toe was the longest. There was shortening of the first metatarsal, which was fused with the navicular. The second and third cuneiforms, the talus and navicular, and the talus and calcaneus were fused. The talus was malformed and showed a hump on the superior and medial surfaces. There was underdevelopment of the joint surface of the tibia with only the posterior two-thirds being in articulation (Fig. 8–52B). In the hands, there was underdevelopment of the navicular bones bilater-

Figure 8–52. Carpal and tarsal abnormalities, cleft palate, oligodontia, and conductive hearing loss. (A) Shortening of dorsiflexed halluces with wide space between halluces and rest of toes. (B) Radiograph showing shortening of first metatarsal, talonavicular, and talocalcaneal fusions. Malformed talus with hump on superior surface. (C) Radiograph show-

ing bilateral underdevleopment of navicular bones with small sesamoid bones at distal facet. (D) Cephalogram showing absence of alveolar processes. This demonstrates lack of original teeth, since the alveolar process develops after the teeth are present. [From RJ Gorlin et al., *Birth Defects* 7(7):87, 1971.]

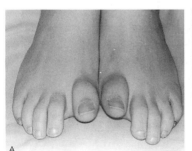
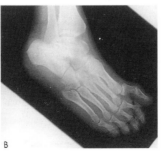
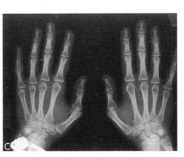
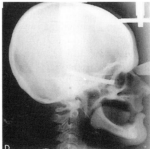

ally with small sesamoid bones associated with the distal facet of the navicular (Fig. 8–52C). The skull was normocephalic. No alveolar ridges were evident (Fig. 8–52D).

Heredity. The parents were second cousins. Two younger sibs were normal. Inheritance appears to be autosomal recessive.

Diagnosis. The combination of abnormalities in this syndrome is unique. In oligodontia and congenital sensorineural hearing loss, there were no carpal or tarsal abnormalities. In spondylocarpotarsal coalition syndrome with or without unilateral unsegmented bar, there is some overlap. For example, both share autosomal recessive inheritance, carpal and tarsal abnormalities, and cleft palate. However, the spinal anomalies make the syndrome distinctive. Further, there is no oligodontia.

Summary. Characteristics of the syndrome include (*1*) autosomal recessive inheritance; (*2*) dorsiflexion of halluces, talonavicular and talocalcaneal fusion, second and third cuneiform bone fusion, malformed talus, abnormal talotibial articulation, hypoplasia of carponavicular bones; (*3*) oligodontia; (*4*) cleft palate; and (*5*) conductive hearing loss due to stapes fixation.

Reference

1. Gorlin RJ et al: Cleft palate, stapes fixation, and oligodontia: A new autosomal recessively inherited syndrome. *Birth Defects* 7(7):87–88, 1971.

Spondylocarpotarsal coalition syndrome with or without unilateral unsegmented bar

Langer and Moe (6) first described congenital scoliosis with carpal fusions in Iranian male and female sibs. The same sibs were again reported by Akbarnia and Moe (1). About 20 other patients have subsequently been reported with the same condition (2–5,7–10). Gorlin et al. (3) suggested that it be called "spondylocarpotarsal coalition syndrome, with or without unilateral unsegmented bar."

Musculoskeletal findings. Height is reduced below the third centile, the trunk being especially shortened. Thoracic scoliosis, which becomes evident within the first few years of life, is progressive and due to unilateral tethering of the vertebral bodies and posterior elements, i.e., formation of a unilateral unsegmented bar involving several vertebrae (Fig. 8–53A,B). Block vertebrae are found in the neck.

In the wrists, capitate–hamate and lunate–triquetrum coalitions are noted. The navicular bones are small and deformed (Fig. 8–53C). In the feet, there is calcaneonavicular, talocalcaneal, and talonavicular coalitions. The calves may be small and the feet are flat.

Craniofacial findings. The face tends to be round and the neck short. Cleft palate and/or bifid uvula have been noted in several cases (2,3).

Auditory findings. Hearing loss has been noted in childhood. Both sensorineural and conductive loss have been documented (2,3).

Heredity. Inheritance is clearly autosomal recessive (1–3,6,9,10).

Diagnosis. To be differentiated is the syndrome of carpal and tarsal abnormalities, cleft palate, oligodontia, and conductive hearing loss.

Summary. Characteristics include (*1*) autosomal recessive inheritance; (*2*) scoliosis with or without unilateral unsegmented bar; (*3*) cervical vertebral fusion; (*4*) carpal and tarsal coalition; (*5*) flat feet; (*6*) variable cleft palate; and (*7*) sensorineural or mixed hearing loss.

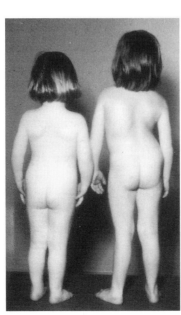
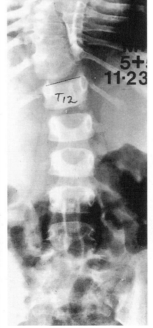
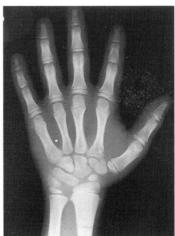

Figure 8–53. *Spondylocarpotarsal coalition syndrome with or without unilateral unsegmented bar.* (A) Sibs showing scoliosis more marked in older child. Also note flat feet. (B) Scoliosis with unilateral unsegmented bar. (C) Note carpal bone fusion. [Courtesy of RJ Gorlin.]

A B C

References

1. Akbarnia BA, Moe JH: Familial congenital scoliosis with unilateral unsegmented bar. Case report of two siblings. *J Bone Joint Surg Am* 60:259–261.
2. Coelho KEFA et al: Three new cases of spondylocarpotarsal synostosis syndrome. Clinical and radiological studies. *Am J Med Genet* 77:12–15, 1998.
3. Gorlin RJ et al: Spondylocarpotarsal synostosis syndrome (with or without unilateral unsegmented bar). Presented at the European Society of Pediatric Genetics, Samos, Greece, 1993.
4. Hunter A et al: A man with abnormal vertebral segmentation and carpal bone fusions. Unpublished, 1993.
5. Jones KL et al: Case report 8. *Syndrome Ident* I(2):10–11, 1973.
6. Langer LO Jr, Moe JH: A recessive form of congenital scoliosis different from spondylothoracic dysplasia. *Birth Defects* 11(6):83–86, 1975.
7. Seaver LH, Boyd E: Spondylocarpotarsal synostosis and cervical instability. *Am J Med Genet* 91:340–344, 2000.
8. Steiner CL et al: Spondylocarpotarsal synostosis with ocular findings. *Am J Med Genet* 91:131–134, 2000.
9. Ventruto V, Catani L: New syndrome: progressive scoliosis by unilateral unsegmented fusion bar, foot deformity, joint laxity, congenital inguinal herniae, peculiar face. *Am J Med Genet* 25:429–432, 1986.
10. Wiles CR et al: Congenital synspondylism. *Am J Med Genet* 42:288–295, 1992.

Coarse facial appearance, skeletal dysplasia, and mixed hearing loss

In 1991, Reardon et al. (1) reported male and female sibs with somewhat coarsened facial appearance, skeletal dysplasia, and mixed hearing loss.

Height (25%), weight (10%), and head circumference (3%) were all significantly reduced in the male but normal in the female.

The face was coarsened with mild frontal bossing, hypertelorism, and somewhat prominent supraorbital ridges. The nose was broad with mandibular prognathism (Fig. 8–54A,B).

Intelligence was estimated at less than 50 IQ in the male and 70 in the female.

Bilateral mixed hearing loss was evident in the male sib prior to 2 years of age. Hearing deteriorated but some speech developed. His sister showed hearing loss at 4 years.

Radiologic examination in both sibs showed sclerosis of the vault and cranial base with thickening of the supraorbital region and obliteration of the frontal sinuses (Fig. 8–54C). The metaphyses of long bones were widened, poorly modeled, and sclerotic (Fig. 8–54D). The lumbar ver-

Figure 8–54. *Coarse facial appearance, skeletal dysplasia, and mixed hearing loss.* (A,B) Mild frontal bossing, hypertelorism, and somewhat prominent supraorbital ridges together with broad nasal bridge and mandibular prognathism make for coarsened facies. (C) Sclerosis of vault and cranial base with thickening of supraorbital region and obliteration of frontal sinuses. (D) Metaphyses are widened, poorly modeled, and sclerotic. (E) Ribs are widened. [From W Reardon et al., *J Med Genet* 28:622, 1991.]

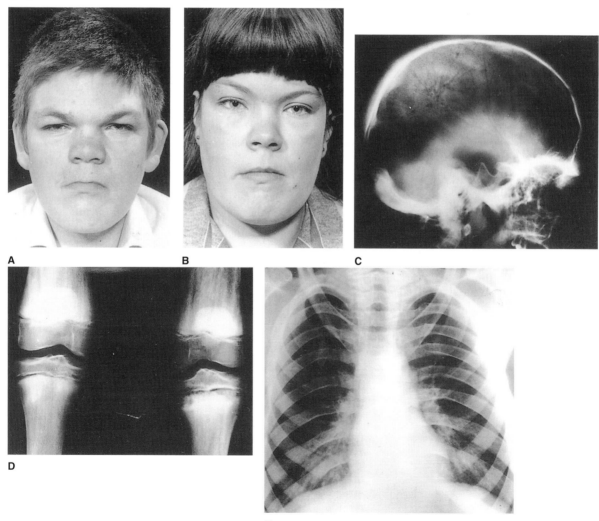

A   B   C

D

E

tebrae showed biconcave flattening. The vertebral endplates were irregular with narrowing of disc spaces. The ribs were mildly widened (Fig. 8–54E).

The parents were normal and nonconsanguineous but autosomal recessive inheritance seems likely.

Biochemical studies were stated to be normal.

Reference

1. Reardon W et al: Sibs with mental retardation, supraorbital sclerosis, and metaphyseal dysplasia: frontometaphyseal dysplasia, craniometaphyseal dysplasia, or a new syndrome? *J Med Genet* 28:622–626, 1991.

Lenz-Majewski syndrome

The syndrome characterized by large head, characteristic facial phenotype, loose skin, mental retardation, and skeletal findings was first reported by Braham (1) in 1969. This report went largely ignored until the entity was rediscovered by Lenz and Majewski (7) in 1974. Macpherson et al. (8) reported an example in the same year. Eleven published examples were reviewed in 1983 by Gorlin and Whitley (4). Additional examples are those of Elefant et al. (3), Chrzanowska et al. (2), and Saraiva et al. (11).

Craniofacial findings. The head appears disproportionately great with large fontanels and widely separated sutures that close late (Fig. 8–55A). The size of the head contrasts sharply with the reduced trunk and limbs. Prominent veins, especially in the scalp, are evident. The ears are very large and floppy. Choanal atresia or stenosis and nasolacrimal duct obstruction are common. Hypertelorism is evident.

Musculoskeletal findings. The fingers are extremely short (Fig. 8–55B). Inguinal hernia is common. The digits are hyperflexible and there may be generalized hypotonia (5). Radiographic features include progressive sclerosis of the skull (especially at the base), facial bones, and vertebrae (Fig. 8–55C,D). The clavicles and ribs are broad (Fig. 8–55E). The middle phalanges are short or absent (Fig. 8–55F). The long bones exhibit diaphyseal undermodeling and midshaft cortical thickening. However, there is marked hypostosis of the metaphyses and epiphyses (8) (Fig. 8–55G). In general, skeletal maturation is retarded.

Genitourinary system. Cryptorchidism has been a uniform finding in affected males. Hypospadias and/or chordee have been noted (6,10). The anus may be anteriorly displaced.

Central nervous system. All children with the disorder have been mentally retarded, their IQs ranging from 20 to 40. Agenesis of the corpus callosum has been documented (11).

Integumentary system. The skin is thin, loose, wrinkled, and atrophic. Veins, especially in the scalp, are prominent and cutis marmorata is evident (5). Proximal interdigital webbing of the fingers is frequent (4).

Auditory findings. Sensorineural hearing loss is frequent, but not well documented.

Laboratory aids. While alkaline phosphatase levels have been elevated in some cases (4,10), the significance is not known.

Heredity. All patients have been isolated examples. Paternal age appears to be advanced (4). Chromosome studies have been normal. Inheritance may be autosomal dominant, with each case representing a new mutation. Nishimura et al. (9) reported a child with similar findings but the child lacked diaphyseal hyperostosis and had, in addition, proximal symphalangism.

Diagnosis. Radiographically, the disorders most often mistaken for Lenz-Majewski syndrome are craniometaphyseal dysplasia and craniodiaphyseal dysplasia. One child was thought to have Camurati-Engelmann syndrome (1).

Summary. Characteristics include (1) unknown inheritance; (2) macrocephaly; (3) loose skin and prominent veins; (4) progressive sclerosis of skull; (5) mental retardation; and (6) hearing loss, possibly sensorineural.

References

1. Braham RL: Multiple congenital abnormalities with diaphyseal dysplasia (Camurati-Engelmann's syndrome). *Oral Surg* 27:20–26, 1969.
2. Chrzanowska KH et al: Skeletal dysplasia syndrome with progeroid appearance, characteristic facial and limb anomalies, multiple synostoses, and distinct skeletal changes: a variant example of the Lenz-Majewski syndrome. *Am J Med Genet* 32:470–474, 1989.
3. Elefant E et al: Acrogeria: A case report. *Ann Paediatr* 204:273–280, 1965.
4. Gorlin RJ, Whitley CB: Lenz-Majewski syndrome. *Radiology* 149:129–131, 1983.
5. Hood OJ et al: Cutis laxa with craniofacial, limb, genital and brain defects. *J Clin Dysmorphol* 2(4):23–26, 1984.
6. Kaye CI et al: Cutis laxa, skeletal anomalies, and ambiguous genitalia. *Am J Dis Child* 127:115–117, 1974.
7. Lenz WD, Majewski F: A generalized disorder of the connective tissues with progeria, choanal atresia, symphalangism, hypoplasia of dentine and craniodiaphyseal hypostosis. *Birth Defects* 10(12):133–136, 1974.
8. Macpherson RI: Craniodiaphyseal dysplasia, a disease or group of diseases. *J Can Assoc Radiol* 25:22–23, 1974 (case 3).
9. Nishimura G et al: Craniotubular dysplasia with severe postnatal growth retardation, mental retardation, ectodermal dysplasia, and loose skin: Lenz-Majewski-like syndrome. *Am J Med Genet* 71:87–92, 1997.
10. Robinow M et al: The Lenz-Majewski hyperostotic dwarfism: a syndrome of multiple congenital anomalies, mental retardation, and progressive skeletal sclerosis. *J Pediatr* 91:417–421, 1977.
11. Saraiva JM: Dysgenesis of corpus callosum in Lenz-Majewski hyperostotic dwarfism. *Am J Med Genet* 91:198–200, 2000.

Cranial hyperostosis and mixed hearing loss

Moesker and Tange (3) reported a mother and daughter from Curaçao with cranial hyperostosis and conductive hearing loss. Probably the same disorder was described by Manni et al. (1,2).

Clinical findings. Head circumference was enlarged (63 cm). The nasal bridge was broad and the chin somewhat prominent. Other than hearing loss, there was no other cranial nerve involvement in one family (3). In the other (1,2), however, cranial nerves I, II, VII, and VIII exhibited variable involvement from late childhood onward. Facial palsy appeared first. The palsy abated and recurred in most cases.

Radiographic findings. The calvaria was greatly thickened but the rest of the skeleton was almost normal (Fig. 8–56A,B). There was progressive hyperostosis and osteosclerosis. The internal auditory canals were severely narrowed (Fig. 8–56C).

Auditory system. Symmetric mixed hearing loss was found from late childhood. The ossicles were thickened and the malleus and incus were fixed in the epitympanum (Fig. 8–56C,D). In one kindred, there was diminished caloric response. Sequential vestibular tests and brain stem auditory evoked potentials indicated nerve entrapment (2).

Laboratory findings. Alkaline phosphatase was somewhat elevated.

Heredity. Inheritance is clearly autosomal dominant (1–3).

References

1. Manni JJ et al: Hyperostosis cranialis interna. A new hereditary syndrome with cranial nerve entrapment. *N Engl J Med* 332:450–454, 1990.

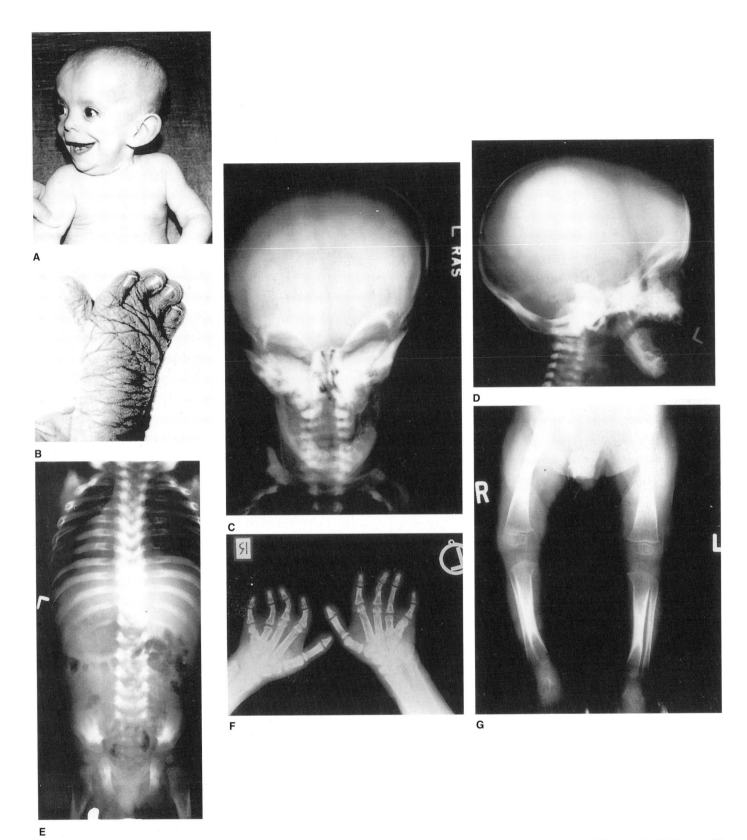

A

B

C

D

E

F

G

Figure 8–55. *Lenz-Majewski syndrome.* (A) Head disproprtionately large. Note thin atrophic skin with prominent superficial veins. (B) Loose, wrinkled atropic skin with short digits and partial syndactyly of fingers. (C,D) Thickening of calvaria, increased density of skull base, orbital rims, maxilla and mandible, and widely patent anterior fontanel. (E) Wide and sclerosed ribs and radiolucent medial ends, patchy sclerosis of vertebral bodies, and sclerosis of central portions of iliac and ischial bones. (F) Abbreviated digits, absent middle phalanges, fused metacarpals 4–5, and clinodactyly. (G) Long bones show marked osteoporotic epiphyses with radiolucent metaphyses that are flared and elongated. The diaphyses are short and exhibit sclerosis and thickening of cortex with diminution of medullary canal.

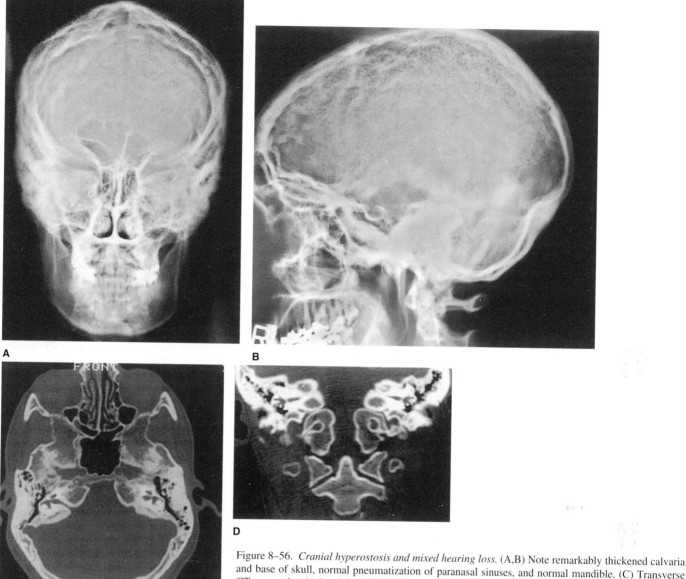

A   **B**

C   **D**

Figure 8–56. *Cranial hyperostosis and mixed hearing loss.* (A,B) Note remarkably thickened calvaria and base of skull, normal pneumatization of paranasal sinuses, and normal mandible. (C) Transverse CT scan at level of ossicles of middle ear. Note massive overgrowth of bone at base of skull, narrow right internal auditory canal, and normal tympanic cavities and ossicles. (D) Cranial CT scan showing massive overgrowth of bone at base of skull and narrow internal auditory canals. [(A–C) fom *JJ Manni et al., N Engl J Med* 322:450, 1990; (D) from *JJ Manni et al., Acta Otolaryngol (Stockh)* 112:75,1992.]

2. Manni JJ et al: Eighth cranial nerve dysfunction in hyperostosis cranialis interna. *Acta Otolaryngol (Stockh)* 112:75–82, 1992.
3. Moesker WH, Tange RA: Cranial hyperostosis and hearing loss (A new syndrome?). *J Laryngol Otol* 100:1187–1193, 1986.

Grebe-like chondrodysplasia and mixed hearing loss

In 1986, Teebi et al. (3) described two unrelated patients with a severe, nonlethal short limb bone dysplasia. One patient had been briefly described earlier by Romeo et al. (1,2).

The disorder was characterized by round face, prominent forehead, hypertelorism, depressed nasal bridge, bulbous nasal tip, and downslanting palpebral fissures. One patient had submucous cleft palate (Fig. 8–57A).

Skeletal changes included short humeri, short deformed forearms and lower legs, and unequal shortness and distortion of fingers and toes. Radiographically, the ribs were irregular, the vertebral bodies somewhat irregular, the humeri short and distorted, tubular bones of the hands and feet anarchic in development, and tibiae and fibulae short and dysplastic (Fig. 8–57B–F).

Hearing loss was mixed and moderate to severe in both patients.

There is superficial resemblance to otopalatodigital syndrome, type II.

References

1. Romeo G et al: Grebe chondrodysplasia and similar forms of severe short-limbed dwarfism. *Birth Defects* 13(3C):105–115, 1977 (case 3).
2. Romeo G et al: Heterogeneity of nonlethal severe short-limbed dwarfism. *J Pediatr* 91:918–923, 1977.
3. Teebi AS et al: Severe short-limb dwarfism resembling Grebe chondrodysplasia. *Hum Genet* 74:386–390, 1986.

Radial hypoplasia, psychomotor retardation, and sensorineural hearing loss

In 1985, Wiedemann et al. (1) described a boy with mild bilateral radial hypoplasia and hypoplasia of thenar musculature and thumbs.

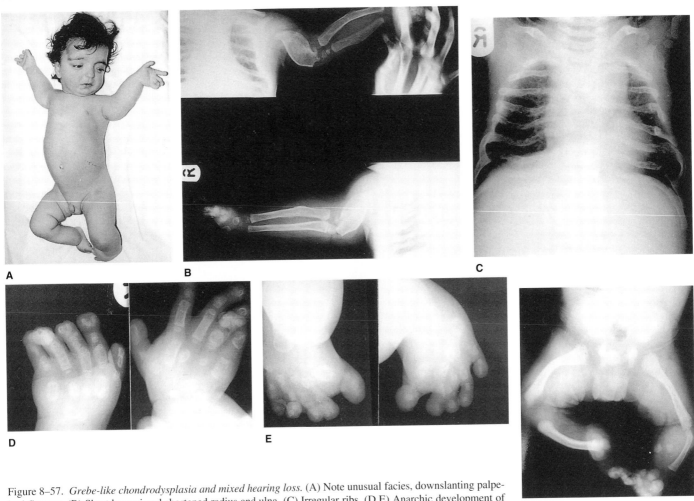

Figure 8–57. *Grebe-like chondrodysplasia and mixed hearing loss.* (A) Note unusual facies, downslanting palpebral fissures. (B) Short humeri and shortened radius and ulna. (C) Irregular ribs. (D,E) Anarchic development of tubular bones of hands and feet. (F) Dysplastic tibiae and fibulae. [From AS Teebi, *Hum Genet* 74:386, 1986.]

Marked mental retardation and poor motor coordination were evident.

Other than a high broad forehead, the face was unremarkable. The pinnae were small and cup-shaped with diminished helices.

Hearing loss was bilateral and congenital but was not otherwise defined.

The reader should also refer to IVIC syndrome.

Reference

1. Wiedemann H-R et al: Syndrome of deafness, radial hypoplasia, and psychomotor retardation. In: *An Atlas of Characteristic Syndromes,* Wolfe Medical Publishers, London, 1985, pp 284–285.

Nasal bone hypoplasia, hand contractures, and sensorineural hearing loss

In 1977, Bogard and Lieber (2) very briefly described three males in three generations with hypoplastic nasal bones, contractures of fingers 2, 3, and 4, and congenital bilateral sensorineural hearing loss (Fig. 8–58). Sommer et al. (3) reported a similarly affected mother and daughter. The family reported by Sommer et al. was subsequently found to have a *PAX3* mutation identical to that reported in an individual with Waardenburg syndrome, type 3 (1). It is highly likely the family reported by Bogard and Lieber (2) also has involvement of *PAX3*.

Figure 8–58. *Nasal bone hypoplasia, hand contractures, and sensorineural hearing loss.* (A,B) Child with hypoplastic nasal bones, lack of nasal alar flare, contractures of digits 2, 3, and 4, and congenital bilateral sensorineural hearing loss. [Courtesy of E Lieber, New Hyde Park, New York.]

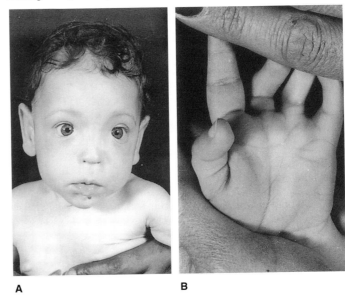

References

1. Asher JH Jr et al: Missense mutation in the paired domain of PAX3 causes craniofacial-deafness-hand syndrome. *Hum Mutat* 7:30–35, 1996.
2. Bogard B, Lieber E: Males with deafness, nasal bone abnormalities and hand contractures in three generations. *Birth Defects* 13(3C):226, 1977.
3. Sommer A et al: Previously undescribed syndrome of craniofacial, hand anomalies, and sensorineural deafness. *Am J Med Genet* 15:71–77, 1983.

Brachycephaly, cataracts, mental retardation, and sensorineural hearing loss (Fine-Lubinsky syndrome)

In 1993, Suthers et al. (6) reported a distinctive syndrome of brachycephaly, cataracts, mental retardation, and sensorineural hearing loss in a male.

The face was characterized by brachycephaly, prominent frontal bones, flat face, shallow orbits, mild ocular hypertelorism, long eyelashes, and small nose. Brain stem auditory evoked response confirmed severe bilateral sensorineural hearing loss.

Radiographic findings included craniosynostosis, hydrocephalus, hydronephrosis secondary to pelvo-ureteric obstruction, but normal renal function. Mild central nuclear cataracts were found. Other findings included short neck, pectus, camptodactyly of the fifth fingers, and shawl scrotum.

In discussing differential diagnosis, Suthers et al. (6) noted that Fine and Lubinsky (2) reported a boy with cloverleaf skull, mental retardation, hydrocephalus, cataracts, small mouth, and hearing loss. There was also severe growth failure. Preus et al. (5) described a child with somewhat similar manifestations, including flat facial profile, small mouth, submucous cleft palate, sensorineural hearing loss, and clinodactyly. Ayme and Philip (1) described a child with a phenotype resembling that of the patient described by Preus et al. (5) and suggested that all four children had the same condition, despite some differences in phenotype. All had in common abnormal skull shape that worsened over time, microstomia, deafness, abnormal central nervous system development, hypotonia, and genital abnormalities. Nakane et al. (4) described a boy without craniosynostosis whom they also believed had Fine-Lubinsky syndrome. Gripp et al. may also have reported cases (3). All cases have been sporadic, and a submicroscopic deletion was postulated as the cause (1).

References

1. Ayme S, Philip N: Fine-Lubinsky syndrome: a fourth patient with brachycephaly, deafness, cataract, microstomia and mental retardation. *Clin Dysmorphol* 5:55–60, 1996.
2. Fine BA, Lubinsky M: Craniofacial and CNS anomalies with body asymmetry, severe retardation, and other malformations. *J Clin Dysmorphol* 1(4):6–9, 1983.
3. Gripp KW et al: Apparently new syndrome of congenital cataracts, sensorineural deafness, Down syndrome–like facial appearance, short stature, and mental retardation. *Am J Med Genet* 61:382–386, 1996.
4. Nakane T et al: A variant of Fine-Lubinsky syndrome: a Japanese boy with profound deafness, cataracts, mental retardation, and brachycephaly without craniosynostosis. *Clin Dysmorphol* 11:195–198, 2002.
5. Preus M et al: Case report 117: Sensorineural hearing loss, small facial features, submucous cleft palate, and myoclonic seizures. *J Clin Dysmorphol* 2:30–31, 1984.
6. Suthers GK et al: A distinctive syndrome of brachycephaly, deafness, cataracts, and mental retardation. *Clin Dysmorphol* 2:342–345, 1993.

Facial, skeletal, and genital anomalies and sensorineural hearing loss

In 1976, Rippberger and Aase (1) described a 26-year-old male with normal intelligence and height. The nose was somewhat small and broad with anteverted nostrils and midfacial hypoplasia. There was clefting of the distal phalanges of both thumbs, inguinal and umbilical hernias, hypospadias, and urethral stricture.

The pinnae were of essentially normal form but appeared to be somewhat low-set. There were preauricular pits and large ear canals. The hearing test, not otherwise defined, revealed 30–60 dB sensorineural loss at high frequencies.

References

1. Rippberger CW, Aase JM: Case report 42: facial, skeletal and genital abnormalities. *Synd Ident* 4(1):16–19, 1976.

Cleft lip and palate, short stature, and sensorineural hearing loss

D. Flannery (personal communication, 1992) reported twin boys with cleft lip and palate, short stature, brachycephaly, inguinal hernia, hyperreflexia, and sensorineural hearing loss. In addition, both boys had narrow shoulders with winged scapulae and pectus as well as mild hyperextensibility of fingers, short fifth fingers, broad hallluces, hallux valgus, and a wide space between first and second toes. The boys seemed to have some spasticity with a somewhat crouched stance. One boy had glaucoma in the right eye and a maternal cousin was reported to have a cleft.

Lymphedema–lymphangiectasia–mental retardation (Hennekam) syndrome

In 1989, Hennekam et al. (5) described an inbred family with the combination of lymphedema, intestinal lymphangiectasia, minor facial anomalies, and mental retardation. Several other patients have since been described (1–4,6–12), and Van Balkom et al. (11) present a recent review of all cases. The lymphedema is congenital and can affect the face and/or limbs. Lymphangiectasia almost always affects the intestinal tract, but can affect other organs (e.g., pleura and pericardium) as well. The underlying cause is thought to be maldevelopment of the lymphatic system (11). The face was described as being flat, with flat and broad nasal bridge and hypertelorism being nearly constant findings (Fig 8–59). Other facial findings include dental anomalies, small mouth, ear anomalies (including duplicated ear in one patient (11)), and craniosynostosis (2). Variable skeletal anomalies also occurred, with some patients having pectus excavatum, narrow thorax, equinovarus feet, and hypoplasia of distal phalanges. Cutaneous syndactyly involving digits 2, 3, and 4 has been described. Seizures affect approximately 33%. Cognitive achievement ranges from normal to severely mentally impaired. Hearing loss has not been well described, but in the comprehensive review of Van Balkom et al. (11), 4 of the 24 patients had hearing loss of some kind. Inheritance is autosomal recessive.

References

1. Angle B, Hersh JH: Expansion of the phenotype in Hennekam syndrome: a case with new manifestations. *Am J Med Genet* 71:211–214, 1997.
2. Cormier-Daire V et al: Craniosynostosis and kidney malformations in a case of Hennekam syndrome. *Am J Med Genet* 57:66–68, 1995.
3. Erkan et al: Syndrome de Hennekam. *Arch Pediatr* 5:1344–1346, 1998.
4. Gabrielli O et al: Intestinal lymphangiectasia, lymphedema, mental retardation, and typical face: confirmation of the Hennekam syndrome. *Am J Med Genet* 40:244–247, 1991.
5. Hennekam RCM et al: Autosomal recessive intestinal lymphangiectasia and lymphedema, with facial anomalies and mental retardation. *Am J Med Genet* 34:593–600, 1989.
6. Huppke P et al: Two brothers with Hennekam syndrome and cerebral abnormalities. *Clin Dysmorphol* 9:21–24, 2000.
7. Rockson SG et al: Lymphoscintigraphic manifestations of Hennekam syndrome—a case report. *Angiology* 50:1017–1020, 1999.
8. Rosser E et al: Hennekam syndrome (autosomal recessive intestinal lymphangiectasia and lymphedema with facial anomalies and mental retardation) in a preterm infant. Presented at the 9th Manchester Birth Defects Conference November 7–10, Manchester, UK, 2000.
9. Scarcella A et al: Hennekam syndrome: two fatal cases in sisters. *Am J Med Genet* 93:181–183, 2000.
10. Sombolos KI et al: End-stage renal disease and hemodialysis in a patient with congenital lymphangiectsia and lymphedema. *Pediatr Nephrol* 16:151–153, 2001.

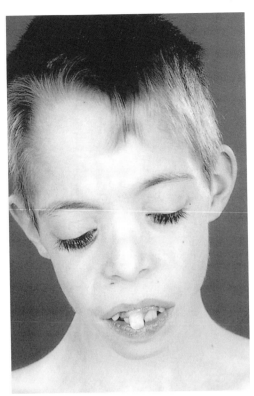

Figure 8–59. *Hennekam syndrome.* Note flat face, flat nasal bridge, smooth philtrum, and dental anomalies. [From IDC VanBalkom, Am J Med Genet 112:415, 2002, reprinted by permission of Wiley-Liss, Inc., a subsidiary of John Wiley & Sons, Inc.]

11. Van Balkom IDC et al: Lymphedema–lymphangiectasia–mental retardation (Hennekam) syndrome: a review. *Am J Med Genet* 112:412–421, 2002.
12. Yasunaga M et al: Protein-losing gastroenteropathy with facial anomaly and growth retardation: a mild case of Hennekam syndrome. *Am J Med Genet* 45:477–480, 1993.

Lymphedema of the lower limbs, hematologic abnormalities, and sensorineural hearing loss

In 1979, Emberger et al. (1) described a syndrome of lymphedema of the lower extremities, hematologic abnormalities, and congenital profound sensorineural hearing loss in three sibs and in the child of one of them.

Acute myeloblastic leukemia at 11 years was found in one sib, anemia and granulocytopenia in another at 21 years, and transient granulocytopenia at 3 years in a third member of the kindred.

Firm lymphedema involving the feet and lower legs appeared around the age of 4 years in one sib, at age 13 years in another, and at 3 years in the son of one of the affected sibs.

Repeated episodes of lymphangitis were experienced. These findings in no way differed from Meige late-onset lymphedema (Fig. 8–60).

All affected exhibited congenital profound sensorineural hearing loss.

Although inheritance may be autosomal dominant, one cannot exclude autosomal recessive inheritance.

Reference

1. Emberger JM et al: Sordi-mutité, lymphoedeme des membres inferieurs et anomalies hematologiques (leukose aigue, cytopenies) a transmission autosomique dominante. *J Génét Hum* 27:237–245, 1979.

Skeletal malformations, ptosis, and conductive hearing loss

In 1978, Jackson and Barr (1) reported two female sibs with unusual facial appearance, ptosis, skeletal abnormalities, and conductive hearing loss. There was marked eyelid ptosis and thin pinched nose.

Craniofacial findings. The face was unusual with severe ptosis of upper eyelids, narrow palpebral fissures, moderate epicanthus, and thin pinched nose with hypoplastic alae (Fig. 8–61A).

Musculoskeletal system. Both sibs exhibited internal rotation of the hips with a toe-in walk. There was limitation of pronation–supination of the forearms and clinodactyly of fifth fingers (Fig. 8–61B). Radiographic studies showed subluxation of the radial heads.

Auditory system. The pinnae were of unusual form (Fig. 8–61C). The external auditory canals were narrow. Epithelial ingrowth into the middle ear with subsequent infection destroyed the ossicles. Hearing loss was marked. Exploration revealed destruction of ossicles.

Heredity. Affected female sibs with normal parents suggest autosomal recessive inheritance.

Reference

1. Jackson LG, Barr MA: Conductive deafness with ptosis and skeletal malformations in sibs: a probably autosomal recessive disorder. *Birth Defects* 14(6B):199–204, 1978.

Mental and somatic retardation, short clubbed digits, EEG abnormalities, and mixed hearing loss

Pfeiffer (1) reported mental and somatic retardation, short clubbed digits, EEG abnormalities, and mixed hearing loss in female monozygotic twins.

Clinical findings. Stature was proportionate. Narrow forehead, short broad nose, and long eyelashes characterized the facial appearance. The digits were mildly clubbed with watchglass nail form, with the thumbs, fifth fingers, and toes being especially short.

Neurologic findings. A dysrhythmic EEG was demonstrated at 6 years in both girls although neither exhibited seizures. The IQs were in the 60–70 range.

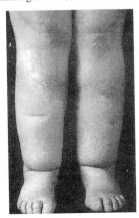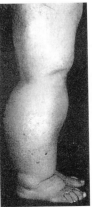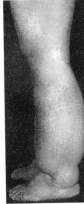

Figure 8–60. *Lymphedema of the lower limbs, hematologic abnormalities, and sensorineural hearing loss.* Note swollen lower extremities. [From JM Emberger et al., *J Génét Hum* 27:237, 1979.]

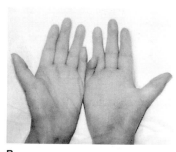

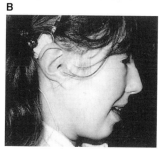

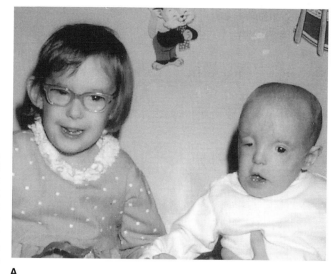

Figure 8–61. *Skeletal malformations, ptosis, and conductive hearing loss.* (A) Affected ribs showing ptosis of upper eyelids, narrow palpebral fissures, thin pinched nose with hypoplastic alae. (B) Clinodactyly of fifth fingers. (C) Postsurgical enlargement of extreme auditory opening. Note unusual form of pinna. [Courtesy of L Jackson, Philadelphia, Pennsylvania.]

A   **C**

Auditory system. The mixed hearing loss was probably congenital. In one girl, there was retention of hearing up to 500 Hz. The other child was considered deaf, with retention of hearing at 90 dB and within speech limits until 4000 Hz.

Diagnosis. Although some overlap was posited with Keipert syndrome (broad terminal phalanges, and sensorineural hearing loss) and Winkelmann syndrome (hypopituitary dwarfism and sensorineural hearing loss), we believe them to be very distinct.

Reference

1. Pfeiffer RA: Mixed hearing loss, mental deficiency, growth retardation, short clubbed digits and EEG abnormalities in monozygous female twins. *Am J Med Genet* 27:639–644, 1987.

Horizontal gaze palsy, scoliosis, and sensorineural hearing loss

In 1974, Dretakis and Kondoyannis (1) described five children (from two families) affected by horizontal gaze palsy and scoliosis. Several other families were reported (2–4).

Ocular findings. Difficulty with lateral eye movements was generally noted soon after birth but, in some cases, experienced in childhood (2).

Musculoskeletal findings. The neck was short. Scoliosis was noted at about the age of 4–5 years. The trunk was shortened secondary to the scoliosis.

Auditory findings. Sensorineural hearing loss was noted only by Riley and Swift (3). It may have been adventitious.

Heredity. Parental consanguinity and multiple sib involvement were present in all cases (1–4). Autosomal recessive inheritance is clearly demonstrated.

References

1. Dretakis EK, Kondoyannis PN: Congenital scoliosis associated with encephalopathy in five children of two families. *J Bone Joint Surg Am* 56:1747–1750, 1974.
2. Granat M et al: Familial infantile scoliosis associated with bilateral paralysis of conjugate gaze. *J Med Genet* 16:448–452, 1979.
3. Riley E, Swift M: Congenital horizontal gaze palsy and kyphoscoliosis in two brothers. *J Med Genet* 16:314–316, 1979.

4. Sharpe JA et al: Familial paralysis of horizontal gaze. *Neurology* 25:1035–1040, 1975.

Humero-radio-ulnar synostosis and congenital sensorineural hearing loss

Shih et al. (1) described two sisters with elbows flexed at approximately 90 degrees (Fig. 8–62A). Radiographs demonstrated bilateral humero-radio-ulnar synostosis (Fig. 8–62B). Other skeletal anomalies included

Figure 8–62. *Humero-radio-ulnar synostosis and congenital sensorineural hearing loss.* (A) One of two sisters showing fixation at elbows. (B) Radiograph showing humero-radio-ulnar synostosis. (C) Note hypoplastic scapulae, disunited acromion ossification centers, and short, drooping clavicles. [From LY Shih et al., March of Dimes Birth Defects Conference, 1979.]

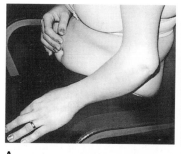

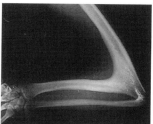

A   **B**

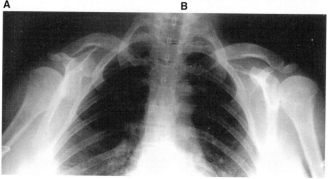

C

hypoplastic scapulae, disunited acromion ossification centers, and short, drooping clavicles (Fig. 8–62C). Congenital sensorineural hearing loss of marked degree was present in both sisters. Although there was no parental consanguinity, autosomal recessive inheritance is likely.

Reference

1. Shih LY et al: Deafness associated with humero-radio-ulnar synostosis. A new syndrome? March of Dimes Birth Defects Conference, June 24–27, Chicago, 1979, p 211.

Osteoma of the middle ear

Osteoma of the middle ear is rare. In a review of 53 extracanalicular osteomas of the temporal bone, not one occurred in the middle ear (3). Only three reports are known that describe osteomas located in the middle ear (2,4,5). Sporadic cases were reported by Ombredanne (4) and by Cremers (2). Both patients had hearing loss. Thomas (5) described two examples in a 10-year-old boy and in his 6-year-old sister. Their parents and two older sibs were normal. Exploration of the boy's middle ears showed a smooth, broad-based osteoma arising in the region of the pyramid. The tumor extended forward to become adherent to the incudostapedial joint. The tympanic membranes were normal, and hearing was normal according to audiometric tests. A unilateral, but smaller, osteoma was found in the sister. Her reduced hearing returned to normal postoperatively. Exudative otitis, present in both sibs, was suggested as a possible cause of new bone formation in the middle ear.

Several patients with Proteus syndrome have had osteomas of the external ear canal (1).

References

1. Cohen MM Jr: Proteus syndrome: clinical evidence for somatic mosaicism and selective review. *Am J Med Genet* 47:645–652, 1993.
2. Cremers CWRJ: Osteoma of the middle ear. *J Laryngol Otol* 99:383–386, 1985.
3. Denia A et al: Extracanalicular osteomas of the temporal bone. *Arch Otolaryngol* 105:706–709, 1979.
4. Ombredanne M: Ostéome exceptionnel de l'orielle moyenne. *Ann Otolaryngol (Paris)* 83:433–436, 1966.
5. Thomas TR: Familial osteoma of the middle ear. *J Laryngol* 78:805–807, 1964.

Dyschondrosteosis (Madelung's deformity, Leri-Weil disease)

Dyschondrosteosis is characterized by deformity of the distal radius and ulna and proximal carpal bones and by mesomelic dwarfism (2,4) (Fig.

8–63). Nassif and Harboyan (7) described brothers with 40–50 dB bilateral conductive hearing loss. DeLeenheer et al. (3) reported a single case with a 20–35 dB loss. The external auditory canals were narrow. The malleus was absent, and the incus was vestigial with no connection with the deformed stapes. In one ear, the chorda tympani could not be identified. Three sisters had the skeletal deformity but normal hearing.

The condition is inherited in a dominant pattern (5). The causative gene is *SHOX*, which maps to the pseudoautosomal region of the sex chromosomes (1,8). Langer-type mesomelic dysplasia appears to result from homozygosity of the gene (6).

References

1. Belin V et al: *SHOX* mutations in dychondrosteosis (Leri-Weill sydrome). *Nat Genet* 19:67–69, 1998.
2. Dawe C et al: Clinical variation in dyschondrosteosis: a report on 13 individuals in 8 families. *J Bone Joint Surg Br* 64:377–381, 1982.
3. DeLeenheer EM et al: Congenital conductive hearing loss in dyschondrosteosis. *Ann Otol Rhinol Laryngol* 112:153–158, 2003.
4. Herdman RC et al: Dyschondrosteosis. *J Pediatr* 68:432–441, 1966.
5. Jackson LG: Dyschondrosteosis: clinical study of a sixth generation family. *Proc Greenwood Genet Ctr* 4:147–148, 1985.
6. Kunze J, Klemm T: Mesomelia dysplasia, type Langer—a homozygous state for dyschondrosteosis. *Eur J Pediatr* 134:269–272, 1980.
7. Nassif R, Harboyan G: Madelung's deformity with conductive hearing loss. *Arch Otolaryngol* 91:175–178, 1970.
8. Shears DJ et al: Mutation and deletion of the pseudoautosomal gene *SHOX* causes Levi-Weill dyschondrosteosis. *Nat Genet* 19:70–73, 1998.

Cleft lip-palate, mental and somatic retardation, postaxial polydactyly, and sensorineural hearing loss

Gorlin and Cervenka (1) saw a family with autosomal dominant inheritance of cleft lip–palate, micrognathia, sensorineural hearing loss, mental and somatic retardation, and postaxial polydactyly.

Reference

1. Gorlin RJ et al: *Syndromes of the Head and Neck*, 4th ed. Oxford University Press, New York, 2001.

Cleft lip and palate, sacral lipomas, misplaced supernumerary digits, and sensorineural hearing loss

In 1991, Lowry and Yong (1) described two Chinese brothers with cleft lip–palate, sacral lipomas, and profound sensorineural hearing loss. In-

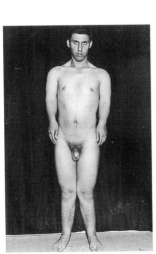

A

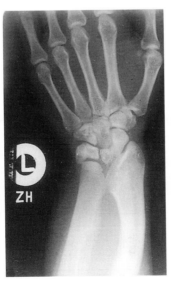

B

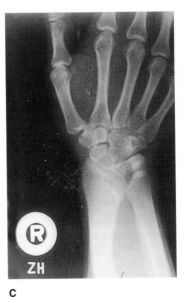

C

Figure 8–63. *Dyschondrosteosis (Madelung's deformity, Leri-Weil disease).* (A) Note shortened forearms and subluxation of the ulna and elbows with limited wrist motion. (B,C) Radiographs show increased distance between radius and ulna, which are curved and short. Note altered alignment of carpal bones. [From R Nassif and G Harboyan, *Arch Otolaryngol* 91:175, 1970.]

telligence and growth were normal. RJ Gorlin saw a similarly affected boy in Iowa City, Iowa, in 1993.

Both boys exhibited lower limb asymmetry and functional constipation. One sib had focal cutis aplasia of the scalp, an extra digit on the right foot attached at the heel (Fig. 8–64), and another digit attached to the right thigh. The other sib had a dislocated hip, an anterior sacral meningocoele, and a rotation defect of the penis.

The profound sensorineural hearing loss was not otherwise defined.

Inheritance could be autosomal recessive or X-linked recessive. Perhaps there is some relationship to the mouse mutant "disorganization" described by Winter and Donnai (3), and reviewed by Robin et al. (2).

References

1. Lowry RB, Yong SL: Cleft lip and palate, sensorineural deafness, and sacral lipoma in two brothers: a possible example of the disorganization mutant. *J Med Genet* 28:135–137, 1991.
2. Robin NH et al: Disorganisation in mice and humans and its relation to sporadic birth defects. *Am J Med Genet* 73:425–436, 1998.
3. Winter RM, Donnai D: A possible human homologue for the mouse mutant disorganization. *J Med Genet* 26:417–420, 1989.

Metaphyseal dysplasia, retinal pigmentary changes, and sensorineural hearing loss

LeMerrer and Maroteaux (1) described two sibs with metaphyseal dysplasia, retinal pigmentary changes, and hearing loss. The height of the two children was normal for chronologic age. Both had blue sclerae, and one had a large depigmented patch on the trunk and shoulder. Fingernails and toenails were hypoplastic. In spite of pigmented retinal lesions, there was no visual defect. Radiographically, distal metaphyseal changes without flaring were noted in the wrists and ankles. In the knees and hands, the changes in the metaphyses were more moderate.

Both children had profound congenital sensorineural hearing loss.

Reference

1. LeMerrer M, Maroteaux P: Unknown syndrome. Presented at the First Meeting—Bone Dysplasia Society, June, 1993, Chicago, Illinois.

Mental and somatic retardation, generalized muscular hypertrophy, joint limitation, unusual facial appearance, and mixed hearing loss (Myhre syndrome, GOMBO syndrome)

In 1981, Myhre et al. (4) described a syndrome of growth and mental deficiency, unusual facial phenotype, generalized muscular hypertrophy, joint limitation, skeletal deformities, and mixed hearing loss in two unrelated males. Other examples were reported by Soljak et al. (5), Garcia-Cruz et al. (3), Farrell (2), Whiteford et al. (8), and Verloes et al. (1,6,7). Verloes et al. (1,6) suggested that Myhre syndrome is the same as GOMBO syndrome, an acronym that indicates combination of *g*rowth retardation, *o*cular abnormalities, *m*icrocephaly, *b*rachydactyly, and *o*ligophrenia.

Figure 8–64. *Cleft lip and palate, sacral lipomas, misplaced supernumerary digits, and sensorineural hearing loss.* Note finger-like appendage attached to heel. [Courtesy of RB Lowry, Calgary, Alberta.]

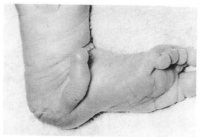

There was both prenatal and postnatal growth deficiency. The muscles were enlarged and there was decreased joint mobility. The midface was hypoplastic with relative mandibular prognathism (Fig. 8–65A,B). Blepharophimosis and short philtrum were evident. One patient had cleft lip–palate (3). Hypospadias and cryptorchidism were noted.

Radiographically, the calvaria was thickened (Fig. 8–65C). The iliac wings were hypoplastic (champagne-glass configuration), the ribs broad. The long and short tubular bones were somewhat abbreviated (Fig. 8–65D) and the vertebrae were large and somewhat flattened with large pedicles (Fig. 8–65E).

Mixed hearing loss ranged from moderate to severe (4,5). In the patient reported by Soljak et al. (5), no mention was made of hearing loss. Six of seven patients were isolated male patients, but Verloes et al. (7) demonstrated a cryptic translocation involving the short arm of chromosome 3 and the long arm of chromosome 2. Verloes and coworkers combined Myhre and GOMBO syndromes (1,6,7).

References

1. Bottani A, Verloes A: Myhre-GOMBO syndrome: possible lumping of two "old" new syndromes? *Am J Med Genet* 59:523–524, 1995.
2. Farrell SA: Microcephaly, markedly short stature, hearing loss, and developmental delay: extension of the phenotype of GOMBO syndrome? *Am J Med Genet* 72:18–23, 1997.
3. Garcia-Cruz D et al: The Myhre syndrome. Report of two cases. *Clin Genet* 44:203–207, 1993.
4. Myhre SA et al: A new growth deficiency syndrome. *Clin Genet* 20:1–5, 1981.
5. Soljak MA et al: A new syndrome of short stature, joint limitation and muscle hypertrophy. *Clin Genet* 23:441–446, 1983.
6. Verloes A et al: GOMBO syndrome of growth retardation, ocular abnormalities, microcephaly, brachydactyly, and oligophrenia: a possible "new" recessively inherited MCA/MR syndrome. *Am J Med Genet* 32:15–18, 1989.
7. Verloes A et al: GOMBO syndrome: another "pseudorecessive" disorder due to a cryptic translocation. *Am J Med Genet* 95:185–186, 2000.
8. Whiteford ML et al: A new case of Myhre syndrome. *Clin Dysmorphol* 10:135–140, 2001.

Spondyloperipheral dysplasia

In 1977, Kelly et al. (1) described a new skeletal disorder that they named "spondyloperipheral dysplasia." Additional examples were added by Sybert et al. (3), Vanek (4), and Sorge et al. (2).

Craniofacial findings. Nasal septum deviation and a "pugilistic" face have been observed. There may be associated nasal respiratory obstruction.

Musculoskeletal findings. Short stature and short hands are evident. The terminal phalanges are somewhat bulbous. The feet are similarly affected. The chest is barrel-shaped.

Radiographic changes include generalized platyspondyly and thoracic kyphosis. Thoracic and lumbar vertebrae manifest large superior and inferior indentations of the posterior portions of the endplates without loss of height of the intervertebral disc spaces. The hands show brachydactyly with shortening of the metacarpals 3–5 and distal phalanges. Bone age is delayed.

Auditory findings. Sensorineural hearing loss of mild degree is noted in early childhood. The hearing loss is progressive, becoming mixed in adulthood in one patient (2).

Heredity. Inheritance is autosomal dominant with variable expression.

References

1. Kelly TE et al: An unusual familial spondyloepiphyseal dysplasia: spondyloperipheral dysplasia. *Birth Defects* 13(3B):149–165, 1977.

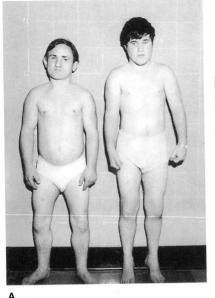

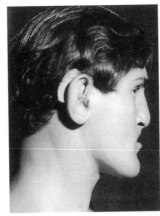

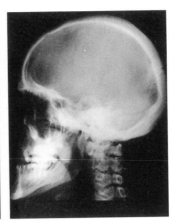

A   B   C

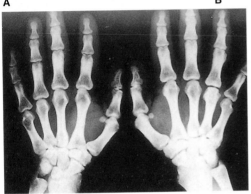

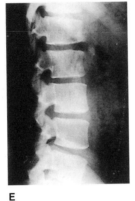

D   E

Figure 8–65. *Myhre syndrome.* (A) Two unrelated males with short stature, decreased joint mobility, and blepharophimosis. Note cleft lip in patient on the left. (B) Note midface hypoplasia, cleft lip, and relative mandibular prognathism. Patient wears hearing aid. (C) Note thickened calvaria, midface hypoplasia, and relative mandibular prognathism. (D) Short tubular bones are somewhat abbreviated. (E) Vertebrae, large, somewhat flattened with large, short pedicles. [From SA Myhre et al., *Clin Genet* 20:1, 1981.]

2. Sorge G et al: Spondyloperipheral dysplasia. *Am J Med Genet* 59:139–142, 1995.
3. Sybert VP et al: Variable expression in a dominantly inherited skeletal dysplasia with similarities to brachydactyly E and spondyloepiphyseal-spondyloperipheral dysplasia. *Clin Genet* 15:160–166, 1979.
4. Vanek J: Spondyloperipheral dysplasia. *J Med Genet* 20;117–121, 1983.

Bowed tibiae, dislocated elbows, scoliosis, microcephaly, cataract, and sensorineural hearing loss

Mégarbané et al. (1) noted four male and female sibs with dislocated elbows, bowed tibiae, and scoliosis. All had microcephaly and mental retardation. Some exhibited ptosis of eyelids. Two had cataracts. Mental retardation was relatively mild.

Hearing loss was sensorineural with a 40–55 dB deficit. The loss was not otherwise characterized.

Inheritance is autosomal recessive.

Reference

1. Mégarbané A et al: Four sibs with dislocated elbows, bowed tibiae, scoliosis, deafness, cataract, microcephaly, and mental retardation. *J Med Genet* 35:755–758, 1998.

Rigid mask-like face, ear anomalies, preaxial polydactyly, toe malformations, and mixed hearing loss

Franceschini et al. (1) reported a 15-year-old boy with rigid mask-like face, profound mixed hearing loss, thick lower lip, microtia, preaxial

polydactyly with triphalangeal thumbs, synectrodactyly of toes, and hypospadias. The child is an isolated example.

Reference

1. Franceschini P et al: Rigid mask-like face, ear anomalies, deafness, preaxial polydactyly, and toe malformations in a patient with normal intelligence: a new entity? *Clin Dysmorphol* 3:234–237, 1994.

Müllerian dysgenesis, bilateral forearm deformity, spinal stenosis and scoliosis, flat face, and conductive hearing loss

In 1977, Kumar and Masel (1) described a 23-year-old woman with unusual facial phenotype, various skeletal anomalies, and conductive hearing loss.

The face was characterized by prominent supraorbital ridges, flat facial profile, downslanting palpebral fissures, high prominent nasal bridge, hypoplastic ear lobes, and bifid nasal tip (Fig. 8–66A). The external ear canals were narrow and obliquely set.

In addition to the flat facial bones, there were hypoplastic clavicles, bowed forearm bones, kyphoscoliosis, spinal stenosis, hypoplastic ilia, and brachydactyly (Fig. 8–66B,C).

Urogenital sinus, vestigial uterus, and very small vagina were noted.

Reference

1. Kumar D, Masel JP: A new multiple malformation syndrome of müllerian dysgenesis and conductive hearing loss with facial hypoplasia, bilateral forearm deformity, brachydactyly, spinal stenosis and scoliosis. *Clin Genet* 52:30–36, 1997.

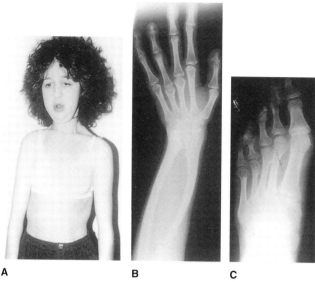

A   **B**   **C**

Figure 8–66. *Müllerian dysgenesis, bilateral forearm deformity, skeletal abnormalities, flat face, and conductive hearing loss.* (A) Young female with long, flat profile, high prominent nasal bridge, and micrognathia. (B,C) Short metapodial bones of hands and feet. [Courtesy of D Kumar, Sheffield, England.]

Histiocytosis, joint contractures, and sensorineural hearing loss

Moynihan et al. (1) described a highly inbred Pakistani kindred in which there were seven individuals affected by histiocytosis, joint contractures, and sensorineural hearing loss.

Histiocytosis. The patient presented at 3 years with rubbery swellings of the eyelids. Recurrent swellings occurred with failure to thrive and generalized lymphadenopathy.

Joint contractures. Progressive joint contractures were observed after puberty.

Auditory findings. From the age of 5–10 years, there was progressive sensorineural hearing loss to profound deafness.

Other findings. Ovarian failure was noted.

Heredity. Inheritance is clearly recessive. The gene was mapped to 11q25 (1).

Laboratory findings. Biopsies showed histiocytes with plasma cells and some eosinophils. Elevated sedimentation rates and hypergammaglobulinemia were found.

Reference

1. Moynihan LM et al: Autozygosity mapping, to chromosome 11q25, of a rare autosomal recessive syndrome causing histiocytosis, joint contractures, and sensorineural deafness. *Am J Hum Genet* 62:1123–1128, 1998.

Caudal appendage, short terminal phalanges, sensorineural hearing loss, cryptorchidism, and mental retardation

Lynch et al. (1) noted two male sibs (the third of triplets being a female). The boys were monozygotic. Both males had short stature, short

terminal phalanges, caudal appendage (Fig. 8–67C), mental retardation, and mixed hearing loss. Upslanting palpebral fissures and wide mouth were evident (Fig. 8–67A,B).

The IQ estimates are in the 50–60 range.

Reference

1. Lynch SA et al: Caudal appendage, short terminal phalanges, deafness, cryptorchidism, and mental retardation: a new syndrome? Clin Dysmorphol 3:340–346, 1994.

Figure 8–67. *Caudal appendage and other anomalies.* (A,B) Triangular face, long, upslanting palpebral fissures, wide mouth, and prominent ears. (C) Caudal appendage. [From S Lynch, *Clin Dysmorphol* 3:341, 1994.]

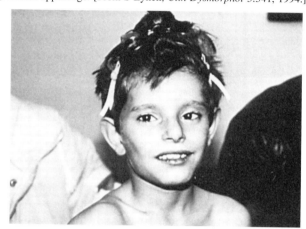

A

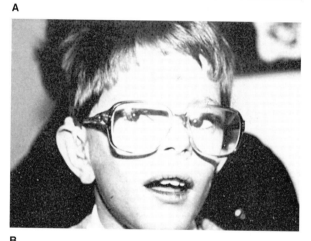

B

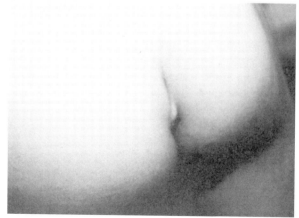

C

Unusual face, microcephaly, joint laxity, and conductive hearing loss

In 1977, Bartsocas et al. (1) described two mildly retarded male and female sibs, the offspring of a consanguineous marriage. Both had microcephaly, long nose, and micrognathia (Fig. 8–68). The boy had cleft palate as well as meningocele, hypoplastic penis with chordee, and scrotal hypospadias. Both had joint laxity and genua valga. Thumbs were broad. Audiograms of both sibs revealed bilateral conductive hearing defect of unspecified degree. Autosomal recessive inheritance appears likely.

Reference

1. Bartsocas CS et al: A new syndrome of multiple congenital anomalies, partial deafness, and mental subnormality. Presented at the 5th International Conference on Birth Defects, Montreal, June 21–27, 1977.

Macrocephaly, hypertelorism, short limbs, developmental delay, and conductive hearing loss

Bagatelle and Cassidy (1) reported a boy with macrocephaly, hypertelorism, short stature, relatively short limbs, and delayed milestones. The hearing loss was conductive but was otherwise not defined.

Reference

1. Bagatelle R, Cassidy SB: New syndrome of macrocephaly, hypertelorism, short limbs, hearing loss, and developmental delay. *Am J Med Genet* 55:367–371, 1995.

Common Syndromes with Occasional Hearing Loss

Cleidocranial dysplasia

Cleidocranial dysplasia is a syndrome of absence or hypoplasia of the clavicles and various other skeletal anomalies (wormian bones, delayed

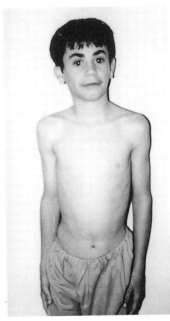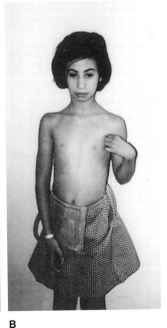

Figure 8–68. *Unusual facies, microcephaly, joint laxity, and conductive hearing loss.* (A,B) Mildly retarded male and female sibs with somewhat long nose, full eyebrows. Both had joint laxity, genua valga, and conductive hearing loss. (From *CS Bartsocas et al.,* 5th Int Conf Birth Defects, Montreal, 21–27 June 1977.)

A   B

closure of cranial sutures and fontanelles and pubic symphysis, delayed development of chondral portion of supraoccipital bone, hypoplastic paranasal sinuses, anteverted foramen magnum, upward distortion of clivus, absent nasal bones, unerupted and supernumerary teeth, etc.) (11,20) (Fig. 8–69). The syndrome has been discussed exhaustively elsewhere (9). The development of the skull and teeth has been presented in elegant papers (12–15).

Auditory system. Conductive or mixed hearing impairment has been described in some cases with concentric narrowing of the external auditory canals (2,3,5–7,10,18,19). Tomography has demonstrated deformed ear ossicles (5). The mastoid air cells are absent.

Vestibular findings. A vestibular study (6) showed somewhat reduced response to caloric stimulation, but patients of Føns (5) were normal.

Heredity. Autosomal dominant inheritance has been clearly demonstrated (1). About 30% represent new mutations. The gene for cleidocranial dysplasia is at 6p21 (4,8,16). The gene, *CFBA1*, controls differentiation of precursor cells into osteoblasts (8,17). Genotype–phenotype correlation has been discussed (21).

Diagnosis. The face and body habitus in cleidocranial dysplasia are characteristic. Brachycephaly, frontal and parietal bossing, unerupted teeth, and supernumerary teeth may be found in a variety of disorders. For differential diagnosis, see Gorlin et al. (9).

References

1. Chitayat D et al: Intrafamilial variability in cleidocranial dysplasia: a three-generation family. *Am J Med Genet* 42:298–302, 1992.
2. Das BC, Majumdar NK: An unusual case of congenital deafness associated with malformation of clavicle. *Calcutta Med J* 66:204–206, 1969.
3. Davis PL: Deafness and cleidocranial dysostosis. *Arch Otolaryngol* 59:602–603, 1954.
4. Feldman GJ et al: A gene for cleidocranial dysplasia maps to the short arm of chromosome 6. *Am J Hum Genet* 56:938–943, 1995.
5. Føns M: Ear malformations in cleidocranial dysostosis. *Acta Otolaryngol (Stockh)* 67:483–489, 1969.
6. Forland M: Cleidocranial dysostosis. *Am J Med* 33:792–799, 1962.
7. Gay I: A case of dysostosis cleidocranialis with mixed deafness. *J Laryngol* 72:915–919, 1958.
8. Gelb BD et al: Genetic mapping of the cleidocranial dysplasia (CCD) locus on chromosome band 6p21 to include a microdeletion. *Am J Med Genet* 58:200–205, 1995.
9. Gorlin RJ et al: *Syndromes of the Head and Neck,* 4th ed. Oxford University Press, New York, 2001.
10. Hawkins HB et al: The association of cleidocranial dysostosis with hearing loss. *AJR Am J Roentgenol* 125:944–947, 1975.
11. Järvinen S: Cephalometric findings in three cases of cleidocranial dysostosis. *Am J Orthod* 79:184–191, 1981.
12. Jarvis JL, Keats TE: Cleidocranial dysostosis, a review of 40 new cases. *AJR Am J Roentgenol* 121:5–16, 1974.
13. Jensen BL, Kreiborg S: Development of the dentition in cleidocranial dysplasia. *J Oral Pathol Med* 19:89–93, 1990.
14. Jensen BL, Kreiborg S: Development of the skull in infants with cleidocranial dysplasia. *J Craniofac Genet Dev Biol* 13:89–97, 1993.
15. Jensen BL, Kreiborg S: Craniofacial abnormalities in 52 school-age and adult patients with cleidocranial dysplasia. *J Craniofac Genet Dev Biol* 13:98–108, 1993.
16. Mundlos S et al: Genetic mapping of cleidocranial dysplasia and incidence of a microdeletion in the family. *Hum Mol Genet* 4:71–75, 1995.
17. Mundlos S et al: Mutations involving the transcription factor CBFA1 cause cleidocranial dysplasia. *Cell* 89:773–779, 1997.
18. Nager FR, DeReynier JP: Das Gehörorgan bei den angeborenen Kopfmissbildungen. *Pract Otorhinolaryngol (Basel)* 10(Suppl 2):43–59, 1948.
19. Pou JW: Congenital anomalies of the middle ear. *Laryngoscope* 81:831–839, 1971.
20. Tan KL, Tan LKA: Cleidocranial dysplasia in infancy. *Pediatr Radiol* 11:14–116, 1981.
21. Zhou G et al: *CBFA1* mutation analysis and functional correlation with phenotypic variability in cleidocranial dysplasia. *Hum Mol Genet* 8:2311–2316, 1999.

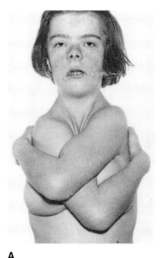
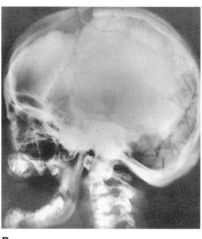
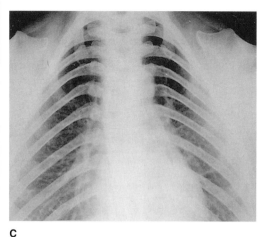

A   **B**   **C**

Figure 8–69. *Cleidocranial dysplasia.* (A) Frontal and parietal bossing, glabellar groove in 13-year-old girl attempting to approximate shoulders. (B) Numerous wormian bones found in lambdoid sutures, delayed cranial bone formation. Wide open anterior fontanelle. (C) Radiograph demonstrating aplasia of clavicles. [(A) from M Føns, *Acta Otolaryngol (Stockh)* 67:483, 1969; (B) from M Forland, *Am J Med* 33:792, 1962.]

Frontonasal malformation

Frontonasal malformation consists of hypertelorism, broad nasal root, lack of nasal tip, widow's peak, and anterior cranium bifidum occultum (Fig. 8–70). There are many associated defects, both cephalic and extracephalic. Frontonasal malformation is both etiologically and pathogenetically heterogeneous. Several conditions associated with frontonasal malformation and various etiologic factors are discussed by Gorlin et al. (2). Various limb defects have been reported including preaxial polydactyly, tibial hypoplasia, brachydactyly, and clinodactyly (2). Only rarely is hearing loss an associated feature. Conductive hearing loss has been reported (1,4). Roizenblatt et al. (3) noted a case with severe sensorineural hearing loss. Preauricular tags have been described in some cases of frontonasal malformation (2).

References

1. Gaard RA: Ocular hypertelorism of Greig: a congenital craniofacial deformity. *Am J Orthod* 47:205, 1961 (case 2).
2. Gorlin RJ et al: *Syndromes of the Head and Neck*, 4th ed. Oxford University Press, New York, 2001.

Figure 8–70. *Frontonasal malformation.* (A,B) Marked variability in expression from severe to mild. Note ocular hypertelorism, frontal bossing, and mild pseudocleft of upper lip and separated nostrils in child on left and lesser degree of all of the aforementioned in the child on right.

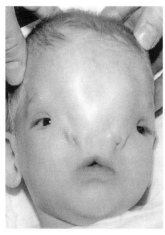
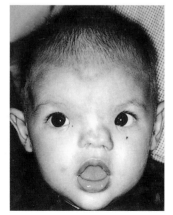

A   **B**

3. Roizenblatt J et al: Median cleft face syndrome or frontonasal dysplasia: a case report with associated kidney malformation. *J Pediatr Ophthalmol* 16:16–20, 1979.
4. Sedano HO, Gorlin RJ: Frontonasal malformation as a field defect and in syndromal associations. *Oral Surg* 65:704–710, 1988.

Larsen syndrome

Larsen syndrome is characterized by flat facial profile, multiple congenital joint dislocations, clubfoot deformities, and, frequently, cleft palate (Fig. 8–71). The syndrome is discussed exhaustively by Gorlin et al. (2).

Auditory system. Hearing loss is noted in 20% of cases and has been conductive (3,4,7), mixed (9), or sensorineural (8). An incudostapedial joint anomaly and fixed stapes footplate were found (7). Deformity or dislocation of the malleus, incus, and stapes footplate was noted (4,5). Renault et al. (8) described a family with hearing loss and retinal dysplasia. Hearing loss may have been independently inherited in a family described by Ventruto et al. (10). It is surprising that hearing loss has not been more frequently reported, as at least 25% of patients have cleft palate.

Heredity. Autosomal dominant transmission has been reported in many families. At least 150 cases have been reported. The gene for the dominant form has been mapped to 3p21.1–p14.1 (11). However, affected sibs have also been noted. Some recessive cases may occur because of reduced penetrance or gonadal mosaicism. A true recessive form has been found in the island of La Réunion in the Indian Ocean (1,6).

References

1. Bonaventure J et al: Linkage studies of four fibrillar collagen genes in three pedigrees with Larsen-like syndrome. *J Med Genet* 29:465–470, 1992.
2. Gorlin RJ et al: *Syndromes of the Head and Neck*, 4th ed. Oxford University Press, New York, 2001.
3. Herrmann J et al: The association of a hearing deficit with Larsen's syndrome. *J Otolaryngol* 10:45–48, 1981.
4. Horn KL et al: Stapedectomy in Larsen's syndrome. *Am J Otol* 11:205–206, 1990.
5. Kaga K et al: Temporal bone pathology of two infants with Larsen's syndrome. *Int J Pediatr Otorhinolaryngol* 22:257–268, 1991.
6. Laville JM et al: Larsen's syndrome: review of the literature and analysis of thirty-eight cases. *J Pediatr Orthop* 14:63–73, 1994.
7. Maack RW, Muntz HR: Ossicular abnormality in Larsen's syndrome. *Am J Otolaryngol* 12:51–53, 1991.

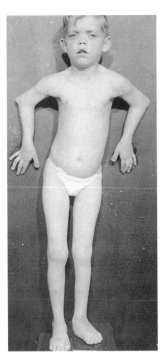
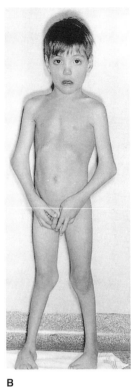
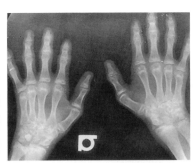
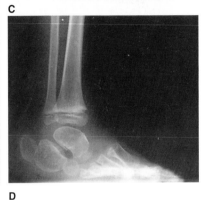

Figure 8–71. *Larsen syndrome.* (A,B) Compare children in A and B. Both have broad nasal bridge, flattened midface, and dislocated elbows. Both have dislocated knees and talipes. (C) Carpal bones, late to appear, are supernumerary. (D) Juxta-calcaneal bone will fuse with calcaneus just prior to puberty.

A   B   D

8. Renault F et al: Le syndrome de Larsen: Aspects cliniques et génétiques. *Arch Fr Pédiatr* 39:35–38, 1982.
9. Stanley CS et al: Mixed hearing loss in Larsen syndrome. *Clin Genet* 33:395–398, 1988.
10. Ventruto V et al: Larsen syndrome in two generations of an Italian family. *J Med Genet* 13:538–539, 1976.
11. Vujic M et al: Localization of a gene for autosomal dominant Larsen syndrome to chromosome region 3p21.1–14.1 in the proximity of, but distant from, the *COL7A1* locus. *Am J Med Genet* 57:1104–1113, 1995.

Fanconi pancytopenia syndrome

Fanconi anemia syndrome consists of pancytopenia, small stature, patchy melanotic hyperpigmentation of the skin, and various malformations (microcephaly, strabismus, dysplastic kidneys, hypoplastic or aplastic thumbs or radii, or thumb duplication). The bone marrow is hypocellular. Although occasionally congenital, the pancytopenia initially presents in young children and by young adulthood is often fatal because of hemorrhage or infection. There is also an increased incidence of malignancy (leukemia, squamous cell carcinoma, hepatocellular carcinoma). Giampietro et al. (3) provide a good review of the clinical manifestations. Cultured fibroblasts show a high prevalence of chromosomal instability (breaks, rings, endoreduplication). There are increased levels of fetal hemoglobin.

Hearing loss has been documented in 5%–15% of patients (1,2,6,7,10). The auricles are malformed in about 5% (6–8,11). The external auditory meatus may be atretic (4,6,10,11) and the ossicles have been fused or malformed (9). In still other cases there is hearing loss without demonstrable abnormality (6). An excellent survey of auricular and auditory changes is that of Harada et al. (6). Inner ear changes have also been described. Inheritance is autosomal recessive. To date, eight different causative genes have been identified (5). Individuals who are severely affected with numerous malformations may be misdiagnosed as having VACTERL association.

References

1. Dawson JP: Congenital pancytopenia associated with multiple congenital anomalies (Fanconi type). *Pediatrics* 15:325–333, 1955.
2. Esparza A, Thompson WR: Familial hyperplastic anemia with multiple congenital anomalies (Fanconi's syndrome). *Rhode Island Med J* 49:103–110, 1966.
3. Giampietro PF et al: The need for more accurate and timely diagnosis in Fanconi anemia: a report from the International Fanconi Anemia Registry. *Pediatrics* 91:1116–1120, 1993.
4. Goldstein LR: Hypoplastic anemia with multiple congenital anomalies (Fanconi syndrome). *Am J Dis Child* 89:618–622, 1955.
5. Grompe M and D'Andrea A: Fanconi anemia and DNA repair. *Hum Mol Genet* 10:2253–2259, 2001.
6. Harada T et al: Temporal bone histopathologic features in Fanconi's anemia syndrome. *Arch Otolaryngol* 106:275–279, 1980.
7. Jeune M et al: Pancytopenia constitutionelle avec malformations (anemie de Fanconi). *Pédiatrie* 13:543–570, 1958.
8. Jones R: Fanconi anemia: simultaneous onset of symptons in two siblings. *J Pediatr* 88:152, 1976.
9. McDonough ER: Fanconi anemia syndrome. *Arch Otolaryngol* 92:284–285, 1970.
10. Nilsson LR: Chronic pancytopenia with multiple congenital anomalies (Fanconi's anemia). *Acta Paediatr* 49:518–529, 1960.
11. Prindull G: Fanconi's anemia. *Z Kinderheilkd* 120:37–49, 1975.

Trichorhinophalangeal syndromes

The trichorhinophalangeal syndromes are characterized by clinodactyly, cone-shaped epiphyses, sparse fine hair, bulbous nose with lack of alar flare, protruding ears, and variable growth retardation (Fig. 8–72). Type I has been reported in kindreds, consistent with autosomal dominant transmission. Type II (Langer-Giedion syndrome) has, in addition, multiple cartilaginous exostoses that present from 3 to 5 years of age, frequent mental retardation, mild microcephaly, loose redundant skin in infancy, and lax joints. Type I is due to a deletion of 8q24.12. The more severe type II appears to result from larger deletions of material within the same chromosomal region (3). Hearing deficit has been reported in some cases of type II, although the frequency, age of onset, and degree of severity are not well documented (1,2). Oorthuys and Beemer (4) found a 60–80 dB sensorineural loss. Vantrappen et al. (5) reported mild to moderate conductive hearing loss. In a personally examined exam-

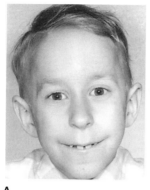
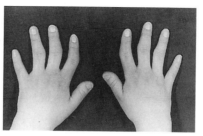
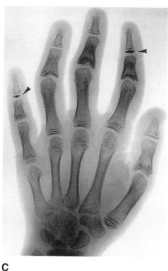

Figure 8–72. *Trichorhinophalangeal syndrome.* (A) Typical facies characterized by high forehead, thin hair, lack of nasal alar flare. (B) Note deviation of fingers. (C) Note numerous cone-shaped epiphyses, short fifth metacarpal. Arrows point to eburnated epiphyses. [(C) courtesy of A Giedion, Zürich, Switzerland.] **A** **B** **C**

ple of type II, RJ Gorlin (unpublished, 1992) found a progressive bilateral mixed hearing loss of moderate to severe degree.

References

1. Gorlin RJ et al: *Syndromes of the Head and Neck*, 4th ed. Oxford University Press, New York, 2001.
2. Hall BD et al: Langer-Giedion syndrome. *Birth Defects* 10(12):147–164, 1974.
3. Lüdecke H-J et al: Molecular definition of the shortest region of deletion overlap in the Langer-Giedion syndrome. *Am J Hum Genet* 49:1197–1206, 1991.
4. Oorthuys JWE, Beemer FA: The Langer-Giedion syndrome (tricho-rhino-phalangeal syndrome, type II). *Eur J Pediatr* 132:55–59, 1979.
5. Vantrappen G et al: Conductive hearing loss in the tricho-rhino-phalangeal syndrome (TRPII) or in the Langer-Giedion syndrome. *Am J Med Genet* 72:372–373, 1997.

Coffin-Lowry syndrome

Coffin et al. (2), in 1966, and Lowry et al. (17), in 1971, independently reported patients with mental and somatic retardation, characteristic facial appearance, large soft hands with distally tapering fingers, and various skeletal anomalies. Well over 100 cases have been described (4,7). Hanauer and Young (8) provide an excellent review.

Craniofacial findings. Characteristic facial changes become more marked with age but are apparent by the second year of life. Scalp hair is straight and coarse in males. The forehead is prominent and broad. There are prominent supraorbital ridges, hypertelorism, downslanting narrow palpebral fissures, heavy arched eyebrows, ptotic upper eyelids, and somewhat hypoplastic midfacial development with relative mandibular prognathism. The nose is large with a broad base, flared alae, and anteverted nostrils. The lips are thick and pouting and the mouth is usually held open (Fig. 8–73A). There is progressive coarsening with age, and the glabellar prominence and lip protrusion become more pronounced (8). The facial features in females are variable, ranging from no phenotypic manifestations to a facial phenotype similar to that of an affected male (8).

Musculoskeletal system. Although usually normal at birth, height and weight become reduced below the third centile in hemizygotes and in 50% of heterozygotes. Delayed ambulation and a clumsy, broad-based gait are seen. At birth, hypotonia and/or loose ligaments with pes planus and inguinal hernia may be noted. The hands are broad and soft with distally tapering fingers in both sexes (Fig. 8–73B). This is the most striking feature at birth (25,26). The finger joints are hyperextensible. Because of increased subcutaneous fat, the forearms are described as being full (12). Radiographically, the calvaria, especially the frontal

tables, is thickened in 60% of patients. The anterior fontanel is large and suture closure is markedly delayed (24). Pectus carinatum or excavatum, found in 80% of hemizygotes and in 30% of heterozygotes, is associated with thoracolumbar kyphosis/scoliosis. Pseudoepiphyses at the base of each metacarpal may be seen in males during childhood. The distal phalanges are short or tufted. The middle phalanges are poorly modeled. Female heterozygotes tend to be obese.

Central nervous system. Intelligence quotients in males have ranged from 5 to 50 and speech is severely retarded. In female carriers, intelligence varies, with 20% having normal IQ, another 20% with severe mental retardation, and the remainder in between (27). Psychiatric illness appears more frequently in heterozygotes, with onset around the age of 20 years (8). Internal communicating hydrocephaly or ventricular dilatation has been noted in hemizygotes, and over 40% exhibit severe generalized seizures (5). Males do not appear to be prone to psychosis, and in general are described as cheerful, easygoing, and friendly (7).

Older individuals experience loss of ambulation and quadriplegia (15).

Oral manifestations. The lips are large, thick, and pouting. The tongue may have a deep midline furrow (15). The palate is high, arched,

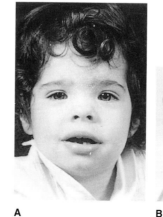
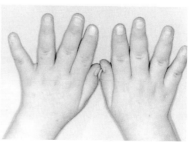

Figure 8–73. *Coffin-Lowry syndrome.* (A) Broad forehead, prominent supraorbital ridges, mild ptosis, depressed nasal bridge with flared alae and anteverted nostrils, relative mandibular prognathism. Lips are thick and pouting, and mouth is usually held open. (B) Digits are thick at base and tapered distally.

A **B**

and narrow. The lower permanent incisors may be absent, or, more often, have reduced crown form in 80% of affected males and in 20% of females (11,15,17,21). Malocclusion with overjet and/or overbite appears to be a nearly constant feature. Early tooth loss has been noted (16,19).

Auditory findings. The prevalence of sensorineural hearing loss in Coffin-Lowry syndrome is not known. It has been reported in few families (3,10,13,15,26). Hearing loss has ranged from moderate to severe and is not correlated with the degree of mental retardation, which suggests that they are independent traits (2,17,20).

Heredity. The disorder has X-linked inheritance, with most cases being sporadic (i.e., due to fresh mutation) (8). The gene locus is on the short arm of the X chromosome at Xp22.2 (1,9,20) and has been identified as the *RSK2* gene (4,23). There is also some evidence of heterogeneity, in that an individual with a Coffin-Lowry phenotype was found to have an interstitial deletion of chromosome 10q (18).

Diagnosis. During infancy, several children have presented with a diagnosis of possible hypothyroidism. With age, diagnosis becomes easier but coarseness of features may suggest a mucopolysaccharidosis or oligosaccharidosis. Alpha-thalassemia-mental retardation syndrome has also been confused with Coffin-Lowry syndrome (6).

Laboratory aids. Dermatoglyphic changes include a characteristic horizontal hypothenar crease in both sexes (22). Mutation analysis of the *RSK2* gene may be helpful, but not all individuals with the Coffin-Lowry phenotype will be found to have a causative mutation (8,23).

Summary. Characteristics include (*1*) X-linked inheritance with milder expression in female heterozygotes; (*2*) characteristic face; (*3*) short stature; (*4*) large soft hands; (*5*) pectus and scoliosis; (*6*) variable mental retardation; and (*7*) sensorineural hearing loss.

References

1. Biancalana V et al: Confirmation and refinement of the genetic localization of the Coffin-Lowry syndrome locus in Xp22.1–p22.2. *Am J Hum Genet* 50:981–987, 1992.
2. Coffin GS et al: Mental retardation with osteocartilaginous anomalies. *Am J Dis Child* 112:205–213, 1966.
3. Collacott RA et al: Coffin-Lowry syndrome and schizophrenia: a family report. *J Ment Defic Res* 31:199–207, 1987.
4. Delauney JP et al: Mutations in the X-linked *RSK2* gene (RPS6KA3) in patients with Coffin-Lowry syndrome. *Hum Mutat* 17:103–116, 2001.
5. Fryns JP et al: The Coffin syndrome. *Hum Genet* 36:271–276, 1977.
6. Gibbons RJ, Higgs DR: Molecular-clinical spectrum of the ATR-X syndrome. *Am J Med Genet* 97:204–212, 2000.
7. Gilgenkrantz S et al: Coffin-Lowry syndrome: a multicenter study. *Clin Genet* 34:230–245, 1988.
8. Hanauer A, Young ID: Coffin-Lowry syndrome: clinical and molecular features. *J Med Genet* 39:705–713, 2002.
9. Hanauer A et al: Probable localization of the Coffin-Lowry locus in Xp22–p22.1 by multipoint linkage analysis. *Am J Med Genet* 30:523–530, 1988.
10. Hartsfield JK Jr et al: Pleiotropy in Coffin-Lowry syndrome: sensorineural hearing deficit and premature tooth loss as early manifestations. *Am J Med Genet* 45:552–557, 1993.
11. Haspeslagh M et al: The Coffin-Lowry syndrome. *Eur J Pediatr* 143:82–86, 1984.
12. Hersh JH et al: Forearm fullness in Coffin-Lowry syndrome: a misleading yet possible early diagnostic clue. *Am J Med Genet* 18:185–189, 1984.
13. Higashi K, Matsuki C: Coffin-Lowry syndrome with sensorineural deafness and labyrinthine anomaly. *J Laryngol Otol* 108:147–148, 1994.
14. Hunter AG. Coffin-Lowry syndrome: a 20-year follow-up and review of long-term outcomes. *Am J Med Genet* 111:1:345–355, 2002.
15. Hunter AGW et al: The Coffin-Lowry syndrome: experience from four centres. *Clin Genet* 21:321–335, 1982.
16. Kousseff BG: Coffin-Lowry syndrome in an Afro-American family. *Am J Med Genet* 11:373–375, 1982.
17. Lowry B et al: A new dominant gene mental retardation syndrome. *Am J Dis Child* 121:491–500, 1971.
18. McCandless SE et al: Adult with an interstitial deletion of chromosome 10 [(del(10)(q25.125.3)]: overlap with Coffin-Lowry syndrome. *Am J Med Genet* 95:93–98, 2000.
19. Padley S et al: The radiology of Coffin-Lowry syndrome. *Br J Radiol* 63:72–75, 1990.
20. Partington MW et al: A family with the Coffin-Lowry syndrome revisited: localization of CLS to Xp21–pter. *Am J Med Genet* 30:509–521, 1988.
21. Sylvester PE et al: The syndrome of Coffin, Siris and Wegienka: report of a case. *J Ment Def Res* 20:35–54, 1976.
22. Temtamy SA et al: The Coffin-Lowry syndrome: an inherited faciodigital mental retardation syndrome. *J Pediatr* 86:724–731, 1975.
23. Touraine RL et al: A syndromic form of X-linked mental retardation: the Coffin-Lowry syndrome. *Eur J Pediatr* 161:179–187, 2002.
24. Trivier E et al: Mutations in the kinase Rsk-2 associated with Coffin-Lowry syndrome. *Nature* 384:567–570, 1996.
25. Vles JSH et al: Early clinical signs in Coffin-Lowry syndrome. *Clin Genet* 26:448–452, 1984.
26. Wilson WG, Kelly T: Early recognition of the Coffin-Lowry syndrome. *Am J Med Genet* 8:215–220, 1981.
27. Young ID: The Coffin-Lowry syndrome. *J Med Genet* 25:344–348, 1988.

FG (Opitz-Kaveggia) syndrome (unusual face, mental retardation, congenital hypotonia, and imperforate anus)

In 1974, Opitz and Kaveggia (12) described a syndrome that included short stature, unusual face, congenital hypotonia, hyperextensible joints, relative macrocephaly, mental retardation, and anal stenosis (or imperforate or anteriorly placed anus) leading to severe constipation (1). Approximately 30% of patients die during the neonatal period. Over 50 patients have been reported (1–19).

The face is characterized by relative macrocephaly and a broad high forehead with upswept frontal hairline (13). The scalp hair tends to be soft, silky, and sparse. Anterior fontanel closure is delayed. The lower lip is prominent. Strabismus, hypertelorism, and enlarged corneae are frequent. The philtrum is long (Fig. 8–74A). Cranial imaging often demonstrates agenesis of the corpus callosum (17).

Fetal finger and toe pads are maintained through childhood (Fig. 8–74B).

Ears are generally simple. The canals are stenotic in 25%. Sensorineural hearing loss is found in 35% of the patients (5,10) but otherwise has not been defined.

Inheritance is clearly X-linked with about 30% of heterozygotes manifesting stigmata (17,18). The gene locus was identified as Xq12–21 (2,8); however, following the identification of a family in which a para-

Figure 8–74. *FG (Opitz-Kaveggia) syndrome.* (A) Tall forehead, upswept frontal hair, wide nasal bridge, long philtrum, open mouth. (B) Persistence of fetal toe pads. [From EM Thompson et al., *Clin Genet* 27:582, 1985.]

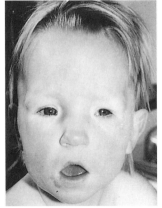
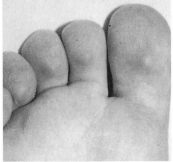

A   B

centric inversion of the X occurred, a second locus for FG syndrome was postulated (3,4). In addition, DeVries et al. (7) described a boy with an FG phenotype who was found to have a submicroscopic deletion of 22q. Therefore it is likely that there may be several distinct conditions which all superficially resemble FG syndrome.

References

1. Bianchi DW: FG syndrome in a premature male. *Am J Med Genet* 19:383–386, 1984.
2. Briault S et al: A gene for FG syndrome maps in the Xq12–q21.31 region. *Am J Med Genet* 73:87–90, 1997.
3. Briault S et al: Paracentric inversion of the X chromosome [inv(X)(q12q28)] in familial FG syndrome. *Am J Med Genet* 86:112–114, 1999.
4. Briault S et al: Mapping of the X chromosome inversion breakpoints [inv(X)(q11q28)] associated with FG syndrome: a second FG locus [FGS2]? *Am J Med Genet* 95:178–181, 2000.
5. Burn J, Martin N: Two retarded male cousins with odd facies, hypotonia, and severe constipation: possible examples of the X-linked FG syndrome. *J Med Genet* 20:97–99, 1983.
6. Cohen MM Jr: The FG syndrome. *J Pediatr* 89:687, 1976.
7. DeVries BBA et al: A boy with a submicroscopic 22qter deletion, general overgrowth and features suggestive of FG syndrome. *Clin Genet* 58:483–487, 2000.
8. Graham JM Jr et al: FG syndrome: report of three new families with linkage to Xq12–q22.1. *Am J Med Genet* 89:145–156, 1998.
9. Keller MA et al: A new syndrome of mental deficiency with craniofacial limb and anal anomalies. *J Pediatr* 88:589–591, 1976.
10. Neri G et al: Sensorineural deafness in the FG syndrome: report on four new cases. *Am J Med Genet* 19:369–378, 1984.
11. Opitz JM: The FG syndrome. *J Pediatr* 89:687, 1976.
12. Opitz JM, Kaveggia EG: The FG syndrome: an X-linked recessive syndrome of multiple congenital anomalies and mental retardation. *Z Kinderheilkd* 117:1–18, 1974.
13. Opitz JM et al: The FG syndrome. Further studies on three affected individuals from the FG family. *Am J Med Genet* 12:147–154, 1982.
14. Opitz JM et al: FG syndrome update 1988. Note of 5 new patients and bibliography. *Am J Med Genet* 30:309–328, 1988.
15. Riccardi VM et al: The FG syndrome—further characterization: report of a third family and of a sporadic case. *Am J Med Genet* 1:47–58, 1977.
16. Richiera-Costa A: FG syndrome in a Brazilian child with additional, previously unreported signs. *Am J Med Genet* (Suppl) 2:247–254, 1986.
17. Thompson E, Baraitser M: FG syndrome. *J Med Genet* 24:139–143, 1987.
18. Thompson EM et al: The FG syndrome: 7 new cases. *Clin Genet* 27:582–594, 1985.
19. Thompson EM et al: Necropsy findings in a child with FG syndrome. *J Med Genet* 23:372–373, 1986.

de Lange syndrome

de Lange syndrome, characterized by severe mental retardation, low birth weight, microbrachycephaly, synophrys, small nose with anteverted nostrils, thin lips with downturned angles, micromelia, proximal thumb implantation, clinodactyly of fifth fingers, limitation of elbow flexion, hirsutism, and cutis marmorata, is usually easily recognized (Fig. 8–75). It has been estimated to occur in about 1/10,000 live births with no sexual predilection (5). A mild form clearly exists (2,11). Children with duplication of the distal long arm of chromosome 3 can have a de Lange phenotype (8,9)

Hearing loss has been recognized as a component (1–16). Yet, although over 500 cases of the de Lange (Cornelia de Lange) syndrome have been published, only a few audiologic studies (brain stem-evoked response, pure-tone audiometry) have been carried out (4,10,14). Marres et al. (10), studying seven patients, found one patient with moderate sensorineural hearing loss and two with slight impairment. Egelund (4) also found mild to moderate loss. In a systematic analysis of 45 children with de Lange syndrome attending a national meeting, Sataloff et al. (14), found that 9 had mild, 9 had moderate, and 20 had profound sensorineural hearing loss.

References

1. Aberfeld DC, Pourfar M: de Lange's Amsterdam dwarfs syndrome. *Dev Med Child Neurol* 7:35–41, 1965.

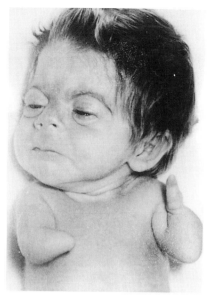

Figure 8–75. *de Lange syndrome.* Characteristic phenotype showing hirsutism, synophrys, small nose with anteverted nostrils, thin lips with downturned angles, and marked limb reduction.

2. Allanson J et al: De Lange syndrome: subjective and objective comparison of the classical and mild phenotypes. *J Med Genet* 34:645–650, 1997.
3. Cherington M et al: Cornelia de Lange syndrome in an adult male. *Neurology* 19:879–883, 1969.
4. Egelund EP: Congenital hearing loss in patients with Cornelia de Lange syndrome. *J Laryngol Otol* 101:1276–1279, 1987.
5. Gorlin RJ et al: *Syndromes of the Head and Neck*, 4th ed. Oxford University Press, New York, 2001, pp. 372–377.
6. Hacek LJ et al: The Cornelia de Lange syndrome. *J Pediatr* 63:1000–1020, 1963.
7. Hawley PP et al: Sixty-four patients with Brachmann-de Lange syndrome: a survey. *Am J Med Genet* 20:453–459, 1985.
8. Holder SE et al: Partial trisomy 3q causing mild Cornelia de Lange phenotype. *J Med Genet* 31:150–152, 1994.
9. Ireland M et al: Partial trisomy 3q and the mild Cornelia de Lange syndrome phenotype [letter]. *J Med Genet* 32:837–838, 1995.
10. Marres HAM et al: Hearing levels in the Cornelia de Lange syndrome. A report of seven cases. *Int J Pediatr Otorhinolaryngol* 18:31–37, 1989.
11. Moeschler JB, Graham JM Jr: Mild Brachmann–de Lange syndrome. Phenotypic and developmental characteristics of mildly affected individuals. *Am J Med Genet* 47:969–976, 1993.
12. Moore MV: Speech, hearing and language in de Lange syndrome. *J Speech Hear Disord* 35:66–69, 1970.
13. Robinson LK et al: Brachmann–de Lange syndrome: evidence for autosomal dominant inheritance. *Am J Med Genet* 22:109–115, 1985.
14. Sataloff RT et al: Cornelia de Lange syndrome. Otolaryngologic manifestations. *Arch Otolaryngol Head Neck Surg* 116:1044–1046, 1990.
15. Silver HK: The de Lange syndrome. *Am J Dis Child* 108:523–529, 1964.
16. Watson A: Cornelia de Lange syndrome: occurrence in twins. *Australas J Dermatol* 20:7–9, 1979.

SHORT syndrome

SHORT syndrome is an acronym given by Gorlin et al. (4) for *s*hort stature, *h*yperextensibility of joints, *o*cular depression, *R*ieger anomaly, and delayed *t*eething. Other consistent findings are intrauterine growth retardation, slow weight gain, distinctive facial abnormalities, and partial lipodystrophy. In four cases, sensorineural hearing loss was noted (3,5,7,11). Inheritance was thought to be autosomal recessive (3,9). Families with apparent autosomal dominant inheritance have also been described (2,6,8). It may be that at least some of these represent confusion with the clinically overlapping condition of Rieger anomaly with partial lipodystrophy (1,10).

References

1. Aarskog D et al: Autosomal dominant partial lipodystrophy associated with Rieger anomaly, short stature, and insulinopenic diabetes. *Am J Med Genet* 15:29–38, 1983.
2. Bankier A et al: Absent iris stroma, narrow body build and small facial bones: a new association or variant of SHORT syndrome? *Clin Dysmorphol* 4:304–312, 1995.
3. Brodsky MC et al: Rieger anomaly and congenital glaucoma in the SHORT syndrome. *Arch Ophthal* 114:1146–1147, 1996.
4. Gorlin RJ et al: Rieger anomaly and growth retardation (the S-H-O-R-T syndrome). *Birth Defects* 11(2):46–48, 1975.
5. Joo SH et al: Case report on SHORT syndrome. *Clin Dysmorphol* 8:219–221, 1999.
6. Koenig R et al: SHORT syndrome. *Clin Dysmorphol* 12:45–49, 2003.
7. Schwingshandl J et al: SHORT syndrome and insulin resistance. *Am J Med Genet* 47:907–909, 1993.
8. Sorge G et al: SHORT syndrome: a new case with probably autosomal dominant inheritance. *Am J Med Genet* 61:178–181, 1996.
9. Stratton RF et al: Sibs with growth deficiency, delayed bone age, congenital hip dislocation, and iridocorneal abnormalities with glaucoma. *Am J Med Genet* 32:330–332, 1989.
10. Temple IK. Personal communication at 10th Manchester Birth Defects Conference, 2002.
11. Toriello HV et al: Report of a case and further delineation of the SHORT syndrome. *Am J Med Genet* 22:311–314, 1985.

Appendix

Other conditions with musculoskeletal findings

Entity	Musculoskeletal Finding	Chapter in this Book
Nager syndrome	Radial ray anomalies	6 (external ear)
Miller syndrome	Postaxial limb anomalies	6 (external ear)
Townes-Brocks syndrome	Radial ray anomalies	6 (external ear)
LADD syndrome	Radial ray anomalies	6 (external ear)
Coxoauricular syndrome	Hip dislocation	6 (external ear)
IVIC syndrome	Radial ray anomalies	7 (eye)
BRESHECK	Postaxial polydactyly, contractures	9 (renal)
Weaver-Williams syndrome	Thin limbs, bone hypoplasia, other skeletal	10 (neurologic)
Stewart-Bergstrom syndrome	Arthrogrypotic hands	10 (neurologic)
Davenport syndrome	Joint contractures	14 (integumentary)
Goodman-Moghadam syndrome	Triphalangeal thumbs	14 (integumentary)
Dominant onychodystrophy, type B brachydactyly, ectrodactyly	Ectrodactyly, brachydactyly	14 (integumentary)
Radial dysplasia, hyperkeratosis, enterocolitis	Radial ray anomalies	14 (integumentary)

Chapter 9
Genetic Hearing Loss Associated with Renal Disorders

MARIA BITNER-GLINDZICZ, KAREN E. HEATH, and ANGEL CAMPOS-BARROS

In this chapter, we have attempted to place the conditions considered here into groups such as specific nephritides, nephroses, and renal acidoses. Molecular genetic studies are rapidly clarifying the molecular basis of various syndromes, confirming genetic heterogeneity in some while identifying allelic disorders in others.

Alport syndrome (nephritis and sensorineural hearing loss)

The syndrome of hereditary progressive glomerulonephritis with intermittent or gross hematuria and sensorineural hearing loss was first described by Alport (1) in 1927. Earlier reports of the same family were published by Guthrie (45) and Kendall and Hurst (67). Classic Alport syndrome represents a defect in type IV collagen. What has been called Alport syndrome is now known to represent a genetically heterogeneous group of at least six different disorders (Table 9–1) that exhibit unique ultrastructural and antigenic abnormalities in basement membranes due to defective type IV collagen (7,59,60,62,64,106). The gene frequency is about 1/5000 (30,33). The syndrome is seen in at least 1% of those with congenital hearing loss and in 0.6% of those seeking renal replacement (30).

Three of the following four criteria must be fulfilled for individuals to be considered to have one of the Alport syndromes: (1) positive family history of hematuria with or without renal failure, (2) electron microscopic evidence on renal biopsy, (3) characteristic ophthalmologic signs, and (4) high-tone sensorineural hearing loss which is usually progressive during childhood.

Renal system. All types show similar renal symptomatology. X-linked Alport syndrome can be divided into those with early-onset end-stage renal disease with death before 31 years (juvenile form) and those with onset after 31 years (adult form) (27,40,41,49,102). This variability likely correlates with the nature of the gene mutation (54). Hematuria is the cardinal clinical finding and is twice as common in males (67% vs. 36%). Often the initial sign appears early as "red diapers." By the age of 5 years, affected males have persistent microhematuria and may have episodes of macrohematuria during intercurrent infections. In females heterozygous for the X-linked form, microhematuria is present by the age of 20 years. It is a more reliable sign than proteinuria and pyuria, which are usually minimal and asymptomatic in children (42,89). Albuminuria tends to increase with age. Nephrotic syndrome eventuates in at least 45% (40–43). Hypertension appears during the teenage years with renal failure and death by 20–40 years in about 50%–75% of males and 10%–35% of females (33,49). Children with the autosomal recessive form develop chronic renal failure between the ages of 5–15 years (30).

During pregnancy, affected women with mild renal disease have no problems while those with advanced disease may have exacerbation of high blood pressure and renal dysfunction. It should be emphasized that at least 12% of females with the X-linked form show no signs of renal disease, even hematuria (107). Life span of these females is usually normal.

Individuals with the autosomal recessive form generally develop renal failure in adulthood. Most heterozygotes show hematuria (24,108).

Ocular system. Bilateral anterior lenticonus may be found with or without macular and perimacular flecks and gradual development of axial myopia (4,6,16,36,38,43,46,86,91) in 35%–70% of those with juvenile onset of the disease and is more common in males (6,8,32). The "oil droplet" appearance of the red reflex aids in diagnosis. Anterior lenticonus often progresses to anterior capsule cataract and this sometimes has been followed by spontaneous rupture of the capsule. Prior suggestions that spherophakia was found probably represent misdiagnosis of lenticonus. Visual acuity is usually compatible with the degree of lens opacity present. Govan (38) concluded that Alport syndrome can be diagnosed if one of three characteristic features is seen: anterior lenticonus, macular flecks, or peripheral coalescing flecks, but their absence does not preclude the diagnosis, especially in females. Colville et al. (22) examined the eyes of a family with autosomal recessive Alport syndrome and concluded that the ocular manifestations of autosomal recessive Alport syndrome are identical to those for the X-linked form. In 1997, Rhys et al. (97) observed three brothers with Alport syndrome and a history of spontaneous attacks of recurrent corneal erosion. To assess the prevalence of recurrent corneal erosion in Alport syndrome, Rhys et al. (97) surveyed 41 patients with Alport syndrome and renal failure and 67 control patients who received transplants for another form of nephropathy. A history of recurrent corneal erosion, first manifested between the ages of 12 and 21 years, was found at a statistically significant level in Alport syndrome patients.

Ultrastructural changes include thinning of the basement membrane of the lens capsule (38,105).

Esophageal, tracheal, and vulval leiomyomatosis. Leiomyomatosis of the esophagus and/or trachea, bronchi, and vulva has been found in more than 40 cases (2,11,12,20,21,29,35,45,52, 56,68,74–76,95,99,101,111) (Fig. 9–1A–C). Lerone et al. (78) noted rectal leiomyomatosis. These examples involve contiguous gene deletion (see Heredity).

Clinically, bronchitis, stridor and/or apnea, dysphagia, and epigastric pain are not rare in these cases. There is no sex predilection. In all cases, hearing loss has been demonstrated in affected males before 15 years of age, and posterior cataracts have been evident in 40%. Age of onset of manifestations is earlier in affected males (7 years) than in carrier females (13 years). In one family, however, renal failure had late onset (82), and may have been related to the nature of the deletion.

Auditory system. Bilateral sensorineural hearing loss is progressive and variable in degree (37,39). Cassady et al. (14) and Chiricosta et al. (18) found that 55% of males and 40% of females had hearing loss. Somewhat lower figures were noted by others (6,28,50). In females the hearing loss tends to occur later than in males. It may be relatively mild or even subclinical; rarely it may be the first component to be clinically evident (88). Children below 10 years of age usually have normal hearing (104). Beginning in the second decade, a sensorineural hearing loss of about 50 dB, most marked in the higher (2000–4000 Hz) frequencies, is found (40,42,43,98). Speech discrimination is usually normal. Recruitment is frequently present. The SISI test has been positive in about 50% while tone-decay test has rarely been positive (81,103). Most patients retain some hearing capacity (53). Abnormal brain stem auditory-evoked response (BAER) findings have been reported (25).

Table 9–1. Alport syndrome—various forms, phenotypes, and genes involved

Hereditary	End-Stage Renal Disease	Hearing Loss	Other Anomalies	Gene Chromosomal Location	Mutations in Gene
XL	Juvenile	Yes	Ocular	Xq22.3	COL4A5
XL	Adult	Yes/no	None	Xq22.3	COL4A5
XL	Adult	Yes	Ocular, leiomyomatosis	Xq22.3	Contiguous gene deletion of COL4A5 and COL4A6
XL		Yes	Ocular, mental retardation, midface hypoplasia, and elliptocytosis	Xq22.3	Contiguous gene deletion of COL4A5, FACL4, and AMMECR1
AR	Juvenile	Yes	Ocular	2q36-q37	COL4A3 or COL4A4
AD	Juvenile	Yes	Ocular		
AD[1]	Juvenile/adult	Yes	Macrothrombocytopenia, ocular	22q11–13	MYH9

[1]This form of Alport-like syndrome is classified now as MYHIIA syndrome and Fechtner or Epstein syndrome (50).

Figure 9–1. *Alport syndrome (nephritis and sensorineural hearing loss).* (A) Massive enlargement and thickening of lower esophagus due to leiomyomatosis. (B) CT scan showing marked enlargement. (C) Leiomyomatosis of vulva. (D–F) Reactivity of Alport patient serum with epidermal basement membranes (EBM) of urea-denatured skin from three members of a kindred. (a) Normal person. Note brilliant fluorescence of EBM (arrows). (b) Affected female. Note discontinuity or gap in fluorescence of EBM. Nonreactive EBM is designated by bracket. (c) Affected male. Note absence of EBM fluorescence (arrows). Arrows, EBM; E, epidermis; D, dermis. (G) Electron pho-tomicrograph of a glomerular capillary loop from male illustrating pathognomonic lesion of glomerular basement membrane (GBM). The GBM is markedly thickened, with irregular epithelial aspect, and appears to consist of many interweaving strands or layers of electron-dense material. Round, electron-dense bodies of varying size are scattered throughout the GBM. BS, Bowman's space; CL, capillary lumen; En, endothelial cell cytoplasm; Ep, visceral epithelial cell cytoplasm. [(A–C) courtesy of Prof J Le Borgne and Prof Y Heloury, Nantes, France; (D–F) from C Kashtan et al., *J Clin Invest* 78:1035, 1986; (G) courtesy of C Kashtan, Minneapolis, Minnesota.]

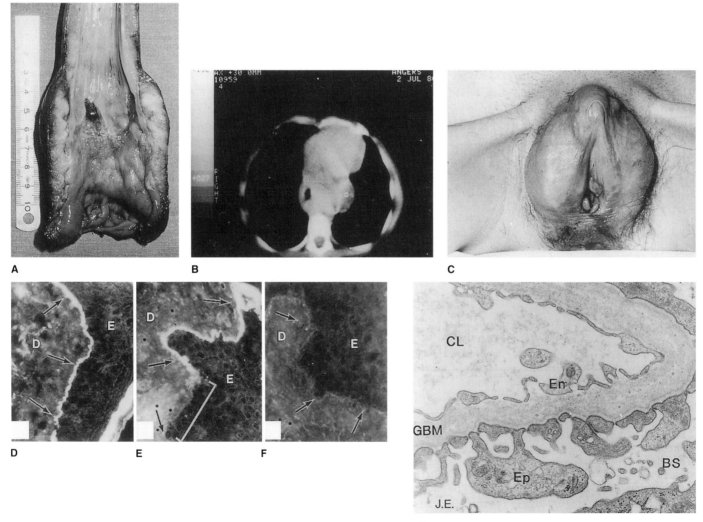

The cochlea and kidney share antigens and are injured by the same drugs (5,55,95). Experimentally induced glomerulonephritis in animals has produced associated strial changes in the cochlea (5). The Alport antigen, a 26 dKa noncollagenous peptide of a type IV collagen chain, has been localized to the basement membrane of the spiral limbus inner sulcus, and the spiral prominence in the cochlea. It is also found in the vascular basement membranes in these same structures (70).

Recently, a canine model of X-linked Alport syndrome was studied to determine the expression of type IV collagen α-chains in the inner ear (47). By 1 month in normal adult dogs, the $\alpha3$, $\alpha4$, and $\alpha5$ chains were co-expressed in a thin internal and external sulci, with the strongest expression along the lateral aspect of the spiral ligament in the basal turn of the cochlea. Affected dogs showed complete absence of the $\alpha3/\alpha4/\alpha5$ network.

Ultrastructural changes in the cochlea of affected patients show multi-layering of the vas spirale consistent with changes found in the glomerular basement membrane and lens capsule (112).

Temporal bone pathology studies have been inconsistent and non-specific. Variable hair cell loss and/or primary loss of cochlear neurons have been reported by a number of authors (8,23,39,55,73,81,84,112–114). Other investigators (10,34,84,109,113,114) were unable to find hair cell degeneration. Hearing loss has been reported to both improve (79) and deteriorate (58) following renal transplantation. It is not convincing that the auditory defect in Alport syndrome is specifically affected by renal function. The loss of neurons may have resulted from uremia, the alterations in the organ of Corti from ototoxic drugs, and the vascular changes from repeated dialysis.

Vestibular system. Caloric stimulation has shown mild to insignificantly decreased response (15,37,81).

Heredity. There is clearly genetic heterogeneity (7), summarized in Table 9–1. The types are separated on the basis of (1) mode of inheritance, (2) juvenile or middle-age onset of end-stage renal disease, (3) hearing loss, and (4) other anomalies. To further compound the confusion, there are kindreds in which extrarenal anomalies are not evident (49,89,114). Females are, as a rule, less severely affected. For many years, because of less severe expression in females and because father-to-son transmission has been noted in only a few families, earlier investigators suggested autosomal dominant inheritance with reduced penetrance in the sons of affected males (93). Linkage and mutation studies have established several genetic loci and associated inheritance patterns.

The most common and classic form is X-linked with expression in the female heterozygote (32). This form was first extensively reported by Perkoff et al. (90) and studied in depth by O'Neill et al. (89) and Hasstedt and Atkin (48). The midregion of the long arm of the X chromosome (Xq21.3–q22) is the site for the locus of this X-linked dominant form (7,13,31–33,49,61,63,83–85,106). The X-linked dominant form of Alport syndrome is attributable to mutations in the gene *COL4A5*, which encodes for the type IV collagen $\alpha5$ chain (9). Many different mutations and deletions have been demonstrated in up to 50% of patients (3,72,96), with some correlation between genotype and phenotype (54). Males with missense or splice site mutations are less likely to develop end-stage renal failure by age 30 than are males with large deletions, nonsense mutations, or mutations which change the reading frame. The risk of developing hearing loss before age 30 is less in males with missense mutations than in males with other types of mutations.

In 1992, Antignac et al. (2) presented evidence that the syndrome of diffuse esophageal leiomyomatosis and Alport syndrome represents a contiguous gene deletion syndrome. They found patients with deletions in the 5′ part of the *COL4A5* gene, extending 700 bp upstream. Zhou et al. (116) then demonstrated that this leiomyomatosis–nephropathy syndrome represents a contiguous gene syndrome due to deletions that disrupt the *COL4A5* and the *COL4A6* genes. Those cases with leiomyomatosis of the esophagus, vulva, and rectum have a contiguous gene deletion (2,116) with mutations extending upstream from the 5′ end of the *COL4A5* into the *COL4A6* genes (116).

Jonsson et al. (57) described a family with features of X-linked Alport syndrome, but the affected males had mental retardation, dysmorphic face with midface hypoplasia, and elliptocytosis. Molecular characterization suggested a submicroscopic deletion of the X chromosome including the *COL4A5* gene. Jonsson et al. (57) proposed that the additional features in the affected males might be due to disruption of the genes adjacent to the *COL4A5*, which could correspond to a new contiguous gene deletion syndrome, the AMME (Alport syndrome, mental retardation, midface hypoplasia, and elliptocytosis) complex, at Xq22.3. Piccini et al. (92) presented evidence that the AMME complex was indeed a contiguous gene deletion syndrome involving *COL4A5* and another gene, *FACL4*, which encodes a long-chain acyl-CoA synthetase. Viteli et al. (110) also identified another gene from the deleted region, which they designated *AMMECR1* (AMME chromosomal region gene-1).

Autosomal recessive forms were thought to exist because in some kindreds parental consanguinity occurs; the severity of the disorder in males and females is identical and the parents exhibit no renal impairment (44,77). Autosomal recessive inheritance was established by the demonstration of mutations in the *COL4A3* and *COL4A4* genes, which are located on chromosome 2 (44,77). Gubler et al. (44) stated that up to 15% of Alport syndrome cases represent the autosomal recessive form.

Autosomal dominant inheritance with male-to-male transmission seems to exist in other kindreds (14,17,18,23,26,71,93). A caveat should be issued, however, that some of these actually stand for the classic X-linked form in which the mother is a heterozygote, or they are in fact misdiagnosed Fechtner or Epstein syndrome affected kindreds with the additional hematological abnormalities (see MYHIIA syndrome).

Laboratory findings. In patients with more severe renal disease, intravenous pyelography demonstrates atrophied, somewhat lobulated kidneys.

Immunohistochemical methods may be used to identify the X-linked dominant form of Alport syndrome. A human antibody probe demonstrates a defect in type IV collagen in basement membranes (10,49,53,54,56,58,59) (Fig. 9–1D–F). The Goodpasture antigen has been identied with type IV collagen. The antigen is absent in hemizygous males but present in deficient amounts in female heterozygotes, thus following the X-linked pattern of inheritiance. Amyloid P component is missing in the basement membranes of males with X-linked Alport syndrome (80).

Microscopic hematuria is common, even in females. Proteinuria and pyuria are uncommon in children but increase with age. Cellular casts containing red blood cells may be found. The level of blood urea nitrogen (BUN) increases with the severity of the disease. By age 25, nearly all affected males but only about 3% of carrier females have elevated serum creatinine (33).

Pathology. Renal changes in Alport syndrome exhibit combined features of nonspecific chronic glomerulonephritis, pyelonephritis, and interstitial nephritis but lack some characteristics of each one and are nonspecific. In children up to the age of 10 years, the kidneys appear normal by light microscopy.

The earliest microscopic lesion is marked by thinning of the glomerular basement membrane. Lipid-laden foam cells, derived from tubular epithelial cells, present in most cases, may form macroscopic yellow streaks, particularly in the lower cortex. The glomeruli may appear fetal-like. There are progressive glomerular changes and late development of interstitial nephritis. Ultrastructurally there is irregular but marked thickening and splitting of the glomerular basement membrane into many thin strands with electron-lucent areas that may contain dense granulations of various sizes between the layers (20,41,46,87,100,103,115) (Fig. 9–1G). Dagher et al. (24) described differences between carriers of X-linked and autosomal recessive Alport syndrome.

Immunofluorescence studies using polyclonal and monoclonal Goodpasture-like anti-glomerular basement membrane (GBM) antibodies have shown absence of the typical linear staining of glomerular basement membranes seen when these probes are applied to normal kidney (60,88).

Pathogenesis. The pathogenesis appears to be the result of mutations of structural components of the basement membranes, i.e., the α subunits of collagen IV. Quick et al. (94) and Weidauer and Arnold (112) noted similarity of the cochlea and kidney in several modalities (fluid and electrolyte balance, common ototoxic and nephrotoxic drugs) and demonstrated by immunochemistry and immunohistochemistry evidence for a shared antigen between kidney and cochlea.

Diagnosis. Diagnosis depends on kidney pathology, family history, and ophthalmologic examination (anterior lenticonus, macular flecks, peripheral coalescing flecks). Diagnosis of the X-linked form may be confirmed by appropriate ultrastructural and immunohistochemical studies of kidney biopsy specimens or skin biopsy for absence of Alport antigen. The heterozygote may exhibit abnormal epidermal basement membrane by immunohistology (60,65,69).

Alport syndrome must be separated from all other causes of hematuria and proteinuria in childhood since the autosomal dominant disorders, Epstein syndrome, Fechtner syndrome, and Alport-like syndrome with macrothrombocytopenia (now collectively known as MYHIIA syndrome) (51) are clinically similar to Alport syndrome, but have macrothrombocytopenia and characteristic leukocyte inclusions (Döhle-like bodies).

Kawakami et al. (66) reported a 5-year-old male with ultrastructural changes of the kidney similar to those of Alport syndrome. Goodpasture antigen and amyloid P component were found in GBM. In addition, growth and developmental retardation, hyperkinesis, and cleft palate were noted. There was congenital sensorineural hearing loss as demonstrated by BAER testing. The authors considered this condition to be distinct from Alport syndrome.

Prognosis. Prognosis is variable. See Jais et al. (54) for a discussion of genotype–phenotype correlation. In some patients the disease may be mild and show practically no effect, whereas renal failure occurs in other patients at a relatively early age. For patients who develop terminal chronic renal failure, renal transplant can be carried out, but the patient may occasionally develop anti-GBM–mediated disease. A small percentage of patients with the X-linked form of the disease who lack an antigen in the collagen IV component of the glomerular basement membrane develop an anti-GBM nephritis following renal transplantation (60). In 1994, Lemmink et al. (77) went on to investigate 46 patients with transplants (45 with the juvenile form), among whom were 41 with a *COL4A5* mutation, 4 with a *COL4A3* mutation, and 1 with a *COL4A4* mutation. In nine patients with transplants (20% of the total number of transplants), a specific anti-GBM nephritis was detected. Comparison of mutations and anti-GBM nephritis suggested that Alport syndrome patients with a type IV collagen mutation resulting in the absence of the noncollagenous domain have an increased risk of developing anti-GBM nephritis after renal transplantation.

Summary. Characteristics of this syndrome include (*1*) genetic heterogeneity with X-linked dominant inheritance being most common; but autosomal dominant or recessive inheritance in some kindreds; (*2*) progressive nephritis with uremia; (*3*) lens abnormalities, including lenticonus or cataracts in those with early-onset end-stage renal disease; (*4*) leiomyomatosis of the esophagus and vulva occasionally; and (*5*) progressive sensorineural hearing loss beginning during the first or second decades and showing variable expressivity.

References

1. Alport AC: Hereditary familial congenital hemorrhagic nephritis. *BMJ* 1:504–506, 1927.
2. Antignac C et al: Alport syndrome associated with diffuse oesophageal leiomyomatosis. Deletions at the 5' end and upstream region of the *COL4A5* collagen gene. *Kidney Int* 42:1178–1183, 1992.
3. Antignac C et al: Deletions in the *COL4A5* collagen gene in X-linked Alport syndrome: characterization of the pathological transcripts in nonrenal cells and correlation with disease expression. *J Clin Invest* 93:1195–1207, 1994.
4. Arenberg IK et al: Alport's syndrome: reevaluation of the associated ocular abnormalities and report of a family study. *J Pediatr Ophthalmol* 4:21–32, 1967.
5. Arnold W et al: Experimental demonstration of an identical antigenicity of the inner ear and kidney [author's transl]. *Arch Otorhinolaryngol* 212:699–717, 1976.
6. Arnott EJ et al: Anterior lenticonus and Alport's syndrome. *Br J Ophthalmol* 50:390–403, 1966.
7. Atkin CL et al: Mapping of Alport syndrome to the long arm of the X chromosome. *Am J Hum Genet* 42:249–255, 1988.
8. Babai F, Bettez P: Auditory lesions in Alport's syndrome (hereditary hematuric nephritis). *Ann Anat Pathol (Paris)* 13:289–302, 1968.
9. Barker DF et al: Identification of mutations in the *COL4A5* collagen gene in Alport syndrome. *Science* 248:1224–1226, 1990.
10. Bergstrom L et al: Hearing loss in renal disease: clinical and pathological studies. *Ann Otol Rhinol Laryngol* 82:555–576, 1973.
11. Blank E, Michael TD: Muscular hypertrophy of the esophagus: report of a case with involvement of the entire esophagus. *Pediatrics* 32:595–598, 1963.
12. Bourque M et al: Esophageal leiomyoma in children: two case reports and review of the literature. *J Pediatr Surg* 24:1103–1107, 1989.
13. Brunner H et al: Localization of the gene for X-linked Alport's syndrome. *Kidney Int* 34:507–510, 1988.
14. Cassady G et al: Hereditary renal dysfunction and deafness. *Pediatrics* 35:967–979, 1965.
15. Celes-Blaubach A et al: Vestibular disorders in Alport's syndrome. *J Laryngol Otol* 88:663–674, 1974.
16. Chavis RMR, Groshong T: Corneal arcus in Alport's syndrome. *Am J Ophthalmol* 75:793–794, 1973.
17. Chazan JA et al: Hereditary nephritis. Clinical spectrum and mode of inheritance in five new kindreds. *Am J Med* 50:764–771, 1971.
18. Chiricosta A et al: Nephropathy with hematuria (Alport's syndrome). *Can Med Assoc J* 102:396–401, 1970.
19. Churg J, Sherman RL: Pathologic characteristics of hereditary nephritis. *Arch Pathol* 95:374–379, 1973.
20. Cochat P et al: Diffuse leiomyomatosis in Alport syndrome. *J Pediatr* 113:339–344, 1988.
21. Cochat P et al: Alport syndrome and diffuse leiomyomatosis. *Am J Dis Child* 147:791–792, 1993.
22. Colville D et al; Ocular manifestations of autosomal recessive Alport syndrome. *Ophthalmol Genet* 18:119–128,1997.
23. Crawfurd M d'A, Toghill PJ: Alport's syndrome of hereditary nephritis and deafness. *Q J Med* 37:563–576, 1968.
24. Dagher H et al: A comparison of the clinical, histopathologic, and ultrastructural phenotypes in carriers of X-linked and autosomal recessive Alport's syndrome. *Am J Kidney Dis* 38:1217–1228, 2001.
25. DiPaola B et al: Significance of brain stem auditory evoked responses in Alport's syndrome. *Contrib Nephrol* 80:88–94, 1990.
26. Evans SH et al: Apparently changing patterns of inheritance of Alport's hereditary nephritis: genetic heterogeneity versus altered diagnostic criteria. *Clin Genet* 17:285–292, 1980.
27. Feingold J et al: Genetic heterogeneity of Alport syndrome. *Kidney Int* 27:672–677, 1985.
28. Ferguson RJ, Rance CP: Hereditary nephropathy with nerve deafness (Alport's syndrome). *Am J Dis Child* 124:84–88, 1972.
29. Fernandes JP et al: Diffuse leiomyomatosis of the esophagus. A case report and review of the literature. *Digest Dis Rel Res* 20:684–690, 1975.
30. Flinter A. Alport's syndrome. *J Med Genet* 34:326–330, 1997.
31. Flinter FA, Bobrow M: The molecular genetics of Alport syndrome: report of the workshops. *J Med Genet* 29:352–353, 1992.
32. Flinter FA et al: Alport's syndrome. A clinical and genetic study. *Contrib Nephrol* 80:9–16, 1990.
33. Flinter FA et al: Molecular genetics of Alport's syndrome. *Q J Med* 86:289–292, 1993.
34. Fujita S, Hayden RC Jr: Alport's syndrome. *Arch Otolaryngol* 90:453–466, 1969.
35. Garcia Torres R, Guarner V: Leiomyomatosis of the esophagus, tracheobronchi and genitals associated with Alport type hereditary nephropathy: a new syndrome. *Rev Gastroenterol Mex* 48:163–170, 1983.
36. Gelisken O et al: Retinal abnormalities in Alport's syndrome. *Acta Ophthalmol* 66:713–717, 1988.
37. Gleeson MJ: Alport's syndrome. Audiological manifestations and implications. *J Laryngol Otol* 98:449–465, 1984.
38. Govan JAA: Ocular manifestations of Alport's syndrome: a hereditary disorder of basement membranes? *Br J Ophthalmol* 57:493–503, 1983.
39. Gregg JB, Becker SF: Concomitant progressive deafness, chronic nephritis, and ocular lens disease. *Arch Ophthalmol* 69:293–299, 1963.

40. Grunfeld JP: The clinical spectrum of hereditary nephritis. *Kidney Int* 27:83–92, 1985.

41. Grunfeld JP et al: Progressive and non-progressive hereditary chronic nephritis. *Kidney Int* 4:216–228, 1973.

42. Gubler MC et al: Alport's syndrome: natural history and ultrastructural lesions of glomerular and tubular basement membranes. *Contrib Nephrol* 2:163–169, 1976.

43. Gubler M et al: Alport's syndrome: a report of 58 cases and a review of the literature. *Am J Med* 70:493–505, 1981.

44. Gubler MC et al: Autosomal recessive Alport syndrome: immunohistochemical study of type IV collagen chain distribution. *Kidney Int* 47:1142–1147, 1995.

45. Guthrie KJ: Idiopathic muscular hypertrophy of oesophagus, pylorus, duodenum and jejunum in a young girl. *Arch Dis Child* 20:176–178, 1945.

46. Habib R et al: Alport's syndrome: experience at Hospital Necker. *Kidney Int* 21 (Suppl 11):20–28, 1982.

47. Harvey SJ et al: The inner ear of dogs with X-linked nephritis provides clues to the pathogenesis of hearing loss in X-linked Alport syndrome. *Am J Pathol* 159:1097–1104, 2001.

48. Hasstedt SJ, Atkin CL: X-linked inheritance of Alport syndrome: family P revisited. *Am J Hum Genet* 35:1241–1251, 1983.

49. Hasstedt SJ et al: Genetic heterogeneity among kindreds with Alport syndrome. *Am J Hum Genet* 38:940–953, 1986.

50. Hauser J: Chronic hereditary nephropathy with deafness and ocular lesions. Chronic hereditary nephropathy with deafness and eye involvment. *Schweiz Med Wochenschr* 104:724–728, 762–772, 1974.

51. Heath KE et al: Nonmuscle myosin heavy chain IIA (MYHIIA) mutations define a spectrum of autosomal dominant macrothrombocytopenias: May-Hegglin anomaly, Fechtner, Sebastian, Epstein and Alport-like syndromes. *Am J Hum Genet* 69:1033–1045, 2001.

52. Heloury Y et al: Diffuse esophageal leiomyomatosis. Apropos of 3 cases. *Chir Paediatr* 31:1–4, 1990.

53. Iverson UM: Hereditary nephropathy with hearing loss—'Alport's syndrome.' *Acta Paediatr Scand Suppl* 245:1–25, 1974.

54. Jais JP et al: X-linked Alport syndrome: natural history in 195 families and genotype–phenotype correlations in males. *Am Soc Nephrol* 11:649–657, 2000.

55. Johnsson L-G, Arenberg IK: Cochlear abnormalities in Alport's syndrome. *Arch Otolaryngol* 107:340–349, 1981.

56. Johnston JB et al: Smooth-muscle tumours of the oesophagus. *Thorax* 8:251–265, 1953 (case 3).

57. Jonsson JJ et al: Alport syndrome, mental retardation, midface hypoplasia, and elliptocytosis: a new X-linked contiguous gene deletion syndrome? *J Med Genet* 35:273–278, 1998.

58. Jordan B et al: Renal transplantation and hearing loss in Alport's syndrome. *Transplantation* 38:308–309, 1984.

59. Kashtan C, Michael AF: Hereditary nephritis. *Semin Nephrol* 9:135–146, 1989.

60. Kashtan C et al: Nephritogenic antigen determinants in epidermal and renal basement membranes of kindreds with Alport-type familial nephritis. *J Clin Invest* 78:1035–1044, 1986.

61. Kashtan CE et al: The Alport locus associated with a defect in type IV collagen NC1 domain maps to region Xp21.3–q22. *Kidney Int* 35:205, 1989.

62. Kashtan CE et al: Identification of variant Alport phenotypes using an Alport-specific antibody probe. *Kidney Int* 36:669–674, 1989.

63. Kashtan CE et al: Gene mapping in Alport families with different antigenic phenotypes. *Kidney Int* 38:925–930, 1990.

64. Kashtan CE et al: Alport syndrome, basement membranes and collagen. *Pediatr Nephrol* 4:523–532, 1990.

65. Kashtan CE et al: Post-transplant anti-glomerular basement membrane nephritis in related males with Alport syndrome. *J Lab Clin Med* 116:508–515, 1990.

66. Kawakami H et al: Chronic nephritis, sensorineural deafness, growth and developmental retardation, hyperkinesis, and cleft soft palate in a 5-year-old boy. *Nephron* 56:214–217, 1990.

67. Kendall G, Hurst AF: Hereditary familial congenital haemorrhagic nephritis. *Guys Hosp Rep* 66:137–141, 1912.

68. Kenney LJ: Giant intramural leiomyomas of oesophagus: a case report. *J Thorac Surg* 26:93–100, 1953.

69. Kleppel MM et al: Distribution of familial nephritis antigen in normal tissue and renal basement membranes of patients with homozygous and heterozygous Alport familial nephritis. *Lab Invest* 61:278–289, 1989.

70. Kleppel MM et al: Immunochemical studies of the Alport antigen. *Kidney Int* 41:1629–1637, 1992.

71. Kluka V, Tischler V: The genetics of Alport's syndrome. *Cesk Pediatr* 41:574–581, 1986.

72. Knebelmann B et al: Spectrum of mutations in the *COL4A5* collagen gene in X-linked Alport syndrome. *Am J Hum Genet* 59:1221–1232, 1996.

73. Lachhein L et al: Hereditary nephritis with inner ear deafness (Alport syndrome). *Dtsch Med Wochenschr* 93:1891–1898, 1968.

74. Leborgne J et al: Diffuse esophageal leiomyomatosis. Apropos of 5 cases with 2 familial cases. *Chirurgie* 115:277–286, 1989 (same cases as in ref. 51).

75. Legius E et al: Muscular hypertrophy of the oesophagus and 'Alport-like' glomerular lesions in a boy. *Eur J Pediatr* 149:623–627, 1990.

76. Leichter H et al: Alport's syndrome and achalasia. *Pediatr Nephrol* 2:312–314, 1988.

77. Lemmink HH: Mutations in the type IV collagen alpha-3 (COL4A3) gene in autosomal recessive Alport syndrome. *Hum Mol Genet* 3:1269–1273, 1994.

78. Lerone M et al: Leiomyomatosis of oesophagus, congenital cataracts and hematuria. Report of a case with rectal involvement. *Pediatr Radiol* 21:578–579, 1991.

79. McDonald TJ et al: Reversal of deafness after renal transplantation in Alport's syndrome. *Laryngoscope* 88:38–42, 1978.

80. Melvin T et al: Amyloid P component is not present in the glomerular basement membrane in Alport-type hereditary nephritis. *Am J Pathol* 125:460–464, 1986.

81. Miller GW et al: Alport's syndrome. *Arch Otolaryngol* 92:418–432, 1970.

82. Mothes H et al: Alport syndrome associated with diffuse leiomyomatosis, Col4A5–Col4A6 deletion associated with mild form of Alport nephropathy. *Nephrol Dial Transplant* 17:70–74, 2002.

83. M'Rad R et al: Alport syndrome: a genetic study of 31 families. *Hum Genet* 90:420–426, 1992.

84. Myers GJ, Tyler HR: The etiology of deafness in Alport's syndrome. *Arch Otolaryngol* 96:333–340, 1972.

85. Myers HC et al: Molecular cloning of alpha 5(IV) collagen and assignment of the gene to the region of the X chromosome containing the Alport syndrome locus. *Am J Hum Genet* 46:1024–1033, 1990.

86. Nielsen CE: Lenticonus anterior and Alport's syndrome. *Acta Ophthalmol (Kbh)* 56:518–530, 1978.

87. Noel LH et al: Inherited defects of renal basement membranes. *Adv Nephrol* 18:77–94, 1989.

88. Olson DL et al: Diagnosis of hereditary nephritis by failure of glomeruli to bind antiglomerular basement membrane antibodies. *J Pediatr* 96:697–699, 1980.

89. O'Neill WM Jr et al: Hereditary nephritis: a re-examination of its clinical and genetic features. *Ann Intern Med* 88:176–182, 1978.

90. Perkoff GT et al: A clinical study of hereditary interstitial pyelonephritis. *Arch Intern Med* 88:191–200, 1951.

91. Perrin D et al: Perimacular changes in Alport's syndrome. *Clin Nephrol* 13:163–167, 1980.

92. Piccini M et al: *FACL4*, a new gene encoding long-chain acyl-coA synthetase 4, is deleted in a family with Alport syndrome, elliptocytosis, and mental retardation. *Genomics* 47:350–358, 1998.

93. Preus M, Fraser FC: Genetics of hereditary nephropathy with deafness (Alport's disease). *Clin Genet* 2:331–337, 1971.

94. Quick CA et al: The relationship between cochlea and kidney. *Laryngoscope* 83:1469–1482, 1973.

95. Rabushka LS et al: Diffuse esophageal leiomyomatosis in a patient with Alport syndrome: CT demonstration. *Radiology* 179:176–178, 1991.

96. Renieri A et al: X-linked Alport syndrome: an SSCP-based mutation survey over all 51 exons of the *COL4A5* gene. *Am J Hum Genet* 58:1192–1204, 1996.

97. Rhys C et al: Recurrent corneal erosion associated with Alport's syndrome. *Kidney Int* 52:208–211, 1997.

98. Rintelmann WF: Auditory manifestations of Alport's disease syndrome. *Trans Am Acad Ophthalmol Otolaryngol* 82:375–387, 1976.

99. Roussel B et al: Familial esophageal leiomyomatosis associated with Alport's syndrome in a 9-year-old boy. *Helv Paediatr Acta* 41:359–368, 1986.

100. Rumpelt H-J: Hereditary nephropathy (Alport syndrome): correlation of clinical data with glomerular basement membrane alterations. *Clin Nephrol* 13:203–207, 1980.

101. Schapiro RL, Sandrock AR: Esophagogastric and vulvar leiomyomatosis: a new radiologic syndrome. *J Can Assoc Radiol* 24:184–187, 1973.

102. Schneider RG: Congenital hereditary nephritis with nerve deafness. *NY State J Med* 15:2644–2648, 1963.

103. Spear GS, Slusser RJ: Alport's syndrome: emphasizing electron microscopic studies of the glomerulus. *Am J Pathol* 69:213–223, 1972.

104. Spear GS et al: Hereditary nephritis with nerve deafness. *Am J Med* 49:52–63, 1970.

105. Streeten BW et al: Lens capsule abnormalities in Alport's syndrome. *Arch Ophthalmol* 105:1693–1697, 1987.

106. Szpiro-Tapia S et al: Linkage study in X-linked Alport's syndrome. *Hum Genet* 81:85–87, 1988.

107. Tishler PV: Healthy female carriers of a gene for the Alport syndrome: importance for genetic counseling. *Clin Genet* 19:291–294, 1979.

108. Torra R et al: Autosomal recessive Alport syndrome: linkage analysis and clinical features in two families. *Nephrol Dial Transplant* 14:627–630, 1999.

109. Turner JS Jr: Hereditary hearing loss with nephropathy (Alport's syndrome). *Acta Otolaryngol Suppl* 271:1–26, 1970.

110. Vitelli F et al: Identification and characterization of a highly conserved protein absent in the Alport syndrome (A), mental retardation (M), midface hypoplasia (M), and elliptocytosis (E) contiguous gene deletion syndrome (AMME). *Genomics* 55:335–340, 1999.

111. Wahlaen T, Anstedt B: Familial occurrence of coexisting leiomyoma of the vulva and oesophagus. *Acta Obstet Gynecol Scand* 44:197–203, 1965.

112. Weidauer H, Arnold W: Morphological changes in the inner ear of Alport's syndrome [author's transl]. *Laryngol Rhinol Otol* 55:6–16, 1976.

113. Westergaard O et al: Alport's syndrome. Histopathology of human temporal bones. *Otol Rhinol Laryngol* 34:263–273, 1972.

114. Winter LE et al: Hearing loss in hereditary renal disease. *Arch Otolaryngol* 88:238–241, 1968.

115. Yoshikawa N et al: Familial hematuria: clinico-pathologic correlations. *Clin Nephrol* 17:172–182, 1982.

116. Zhou J et al: Deletion of the paired alpha-5(IV) and alpha-6(IV) collagen genes in inherited smooth muscle tumors. *Science* 261:1167–1169, 1993.

Nonmuscle myosin heavy chain IIA (MYHIIA) syndrome [macrothrombocytopenia, nephritis, sensorineural deafness, and cataracts (Epstein and Fechtner syndromes and Alport syndrome with macrothrombocytopenia, included)]

In 1972, Epstein et al. (7) reported a syndrome consisting of giant platelets associated with thrombocytopenia, nephritis, and sensorineural hearing loss in two unrelated kindreds. The syndrome was named "Epstein syndrome" (EPS). Since that report, several multigenerational kindreds as well as a few sporadic cases have been reported (2,4,6).

Fechtner syndrome (FTNS) refers to the report of a four-generation family with macrothrombocytopenia, characteristic leukocyte inclusions, known as Döhle-like bodies, nephritis, and high-tone sensorineural hearing loss in varying degrees within the family (18). Many cases have since then been reported (3,8–10).

After the study of 32 families with Alport syndrome, M'Rad et al. (19) in 1992 reported one family presenting a particularly severe form of the disease with deafness and end-stage renal disease by the age of 14, but without the ocular signs of Alport syndrome. In both mother and son, macrothrombocytopenia with Döhle-like bodies was observed. They suggested that this was an X-linked heterogeneous form of Alport syndrome with macrothrombocytopenia (APSM), but it is now known that the phenotype is consistent with FTNS, which is an autosomal dominant disorder (11).

Although the three syndromes are clinically very similar, they have commonly been reported as separate entities. Recently, molecular genetic studies identified that the same gene, nonmuscle myosin heavy chain 9 (*MYH9*), is involved in all three of these and two other syndromes (1,12,17,22).

Renal system. Renal involvement usually presents in the second decade, with occasional exceptions (18). Males and females are equally affected. Proteinuria is usual. Hematuria, though noted, is more variable than in Alport syndrome. The normal course is of progressive renal compromise, often requiring transplantation (18).

Hematopoietic system. With the exception of a single case (7), affected individuals have all presented early, even neonatally, with variable combinations of bleeding, epistaxis, and anemia. Macrothrombocytopenia with large platelets and platelet counts ranging from 25,000 to 96,000 have also occurred (Fig. 9–2A).

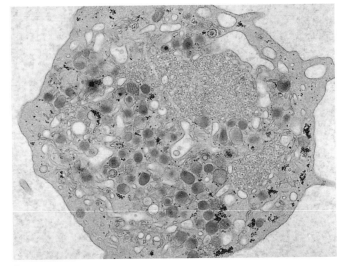

A

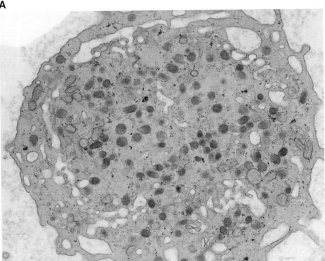

B

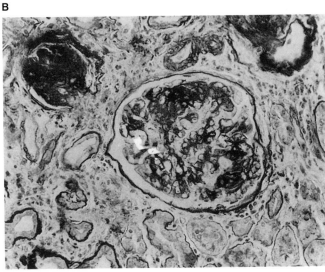

C

Figure 9–2. *Macrothrombocytopathia, nephritis, and sensorineural hearing loss (Epstein syndrome).* (A,B) Thin sections of giant platelets similar in size to lymphocytes. Note random distribution of organelles and channels of the surface-connected system. (C) Kidney showing interstitial fibrosis, focal glomerular proliferation, and sclerotic glomerulus. [(A,B) courtesy of JG White, Minneapolis, Minnesota; (C) from CJ Epstein et al., *Am J Med Genet* 52:299, 1972.]

Ocular system. Congenital cataract and juvenile glaucoma are described in FTNS (8) but not in EPS. Anterior lenticonus and dot-and-fleck retinopathy described in Alport syndrome are not seen (5).

Auditory system. Audiograms have revealed bilateral moderate to severe sensorineural hearing loss, more marked in higher frequencies. It usually presents between the ages of 5 and 10 years, i.e., slightly earlier than in males with classic Alport syndrome. In at least two individuals, however, hearing loss appeared prior to 5 years of age (7). The initially moderate auditory deficits progress gradually to severe loss, unrelated to severity of the renal disease or hemorrhagic episodes. The only temporal bone study showed partial loss of the stria vascularis (4).

Vestibular system. Vestibular function tests have not been reported in this syndrome.

Laboratory findings. Thrombocytopenia is a consistent finding. Platelet counts average about 40,000 but may be as low as 25,000. The platelets are large and spherical with diameters sometimes as large as lymphocytes. Abnormalities of platelet aggregation in response to ADP, collagen, and epinephrine are variable within the syndrome. The patients reported by Eckstein et al. (6) and Peterson et al. (21) had normal platelet aggregation and function, but in other patients platelet aggregation was decreased (2,4,7).

In FTNS patients, the neutrophils contain one to several small (1–2 μm) irregularly shaped inclusions, or Döhle-like bodies, that appear pale blue with May-Grünwald Giemsa stain (Fig. 9–2B). These leukocyte inclusions have not been observed in EPS patients, but Döhle-like bodies are generally only visible if a blood smear is stained in a time-dependent manner (9,10). Thus, the diagnosis may be missed or incorrectly interpreted depending on the availability or appropriate testing facilities. Among the published cases, differences in the morphology and appearance of the inclusions in patients with FTNS, May-Hegglin anomaly (MHA), and Sebastian syndrome (SBS) have also been described. The Döhle-like bodies or paracrystalline inclusions appear as highly parallel bodies in MHA but seem smaller and less organized in SBS and FTNS, although this does not always seem to hold true (KE Heath, personal observation). Moreover, these ultrastructural features are only detectable by electron microscopy (EM) and this preparation is also time-sensitive.

Microscopic hematuria and proteinuria are variable findings in individuals with the renal disorder. Hematuria has been a variable and intermittent finding. Azotemia occurred in the few patients who had chronic renal insufficiency.

Pathology. Renal findings have included extensive hyalinization of glomeruli, scarring, and some crescent formation. The arterial walls have been thickened and hyalinized (Fig. 9–2C). The findings are nonspecific and are compatible with a chronic nephritic process. However, EM studies performed in one patient (4) showed lamellation of the thickened glomerular basement membrane and round, dense granules consistent with the ultrastructural findings of classic Alport syndrome. However, the finding was not constant (20).

Renal biopsy has shown hyalinized glomeruli. There was patchy tubular atrophy, with the remaining tubules appearing dilated. The blood vessels demonstrated moderate medial thickening and a diffuse interstitial cellular infiltrate. The findings were felt to be suggestive of "hereditary nephritis." Electron microscopy of glomerular basement membranes showed that they were thickened with focal areas of attenuation. However, the basement membrane was not described as having the characteristic "basket weave" pattern of classic Alport syndrome.

Neutrophils and eosinophils show small, irregularly shaped cytoplasmic inclusions, or Döhle-like bodies. The inclusions are small and spindle-shaped and thought to consist of clusters of ribosomes and small segments of rough endoplasmic reticulum without an enclosing membrane. Kunishima et al. (14) have shown that the inclusions in leukocytes are aggregates of MYHIIA.

Pathogenesis. Although the pathogenesis of the macrothrombocytopenia, nephritis, and sensorineural hearing loss in EPS and FTNS is still unknown, MYHIIA, the protein encoded by the affected gene, *MYH9*, has been shown to be expressed in all affected organs and tissues, thus supporting a role for the mutated protein in the molecular pathogenesis of these syndromes (1,15,23,24). Hu et al. (12) showed impaired enzymatic function in those with MYH9 mutations.

Heredity. Epstein, Fechtner, and Alport-with-macrothrombocytopenia syndromes are allelic disorders and inherited in an autosomal dominant mode. They and two other purely hematological disorders, MHA and SBS, are caused by mutation in the *MYH9* gene on chromosome 22q11–13 (4,11,13,16,17,25). *MYH9* encodes the nonmuscle myosin heavy chain IIA (MYHIIA), which is expressed ubiquitously but is the only myosin expressed in the platelets.

Genotype–phenotype correlation studies (11) found a common mutation, R702C, in FTNS, EPS, and APSM. A different mutation at the same codon, R702H, was identified in a further individual diagnosed with APSM. Therefore, substitutions at codon 702 appear consistently associated with the manifestation of nephritis and high-tone neurosensorial deafness in addition to macrothrombocytopenia, indicating that the preservation of this region is critical for the maintenance of MYHIIA function in the affected organs. In this regard, it has also been shown that a specific missense mutation in *MYH9*, R705H, located just three amino acid residues away from codon 702, results in a form of nonsyndromic deafness, DFNA17, an autosomal dominant high-tone sensorineural deafness without platelet abnormalities [(15) and personal communication].

Altogether, the molecular and clinical data indicate that these six disorders with a broad phenotypic spectrum represent variants of a single syndrome, to which the name *MYHIIA syndrome* has been applied (11).

Diagnosis. The combination of sensorineural hearing loss and nephritis resembles classic Alport syndrome. Ultrastructural findings of the glomerular basement membrane in EPS and FTNS are similar to those for the classic Alport syndrome. However, onset of hearing loss is generally earlier in the EPS and FTNS, and males and females are equally affected. In addition, the presence of macrothrombocytopenia easily distinguishes this syndrome from classic Alport syndrome.

Prognosis. Because of the chronic and progressive nature of the renal insufficiency, prognosis is poor. As in classic Alport syndrome, transplantation and hemodialysis are options and provide opportunities for a better outcome.

The natural history of renal impairment is more variable in FTNS than in EPS or classic Alport syndrome. In each of the families reported, a few individuals progressed to chronic renal insufficiency in middle age (2,7), whereas other individuals appear to have had no significant renal disease. Most individuals do well with the bleeding problem, which rarely causes life-threatening bleeding episodes.

Summary. The MYHIIA syndrome is characterized by (*1*) autosomal dominant inheritance; (*2*) mutations in the nonmuscle myosin heavy chain 9 gene (*MYH9*); (*3*) nephropathy that is more variable than in classic Alport syndrome, with males and females being equally affected; (*4*) giant platelets with thrombocytopenia; (*5*) leukocyte inclusions, which are characteristic of this syndrome but may not always be detectable; and (*6*) high-tone sensorineural hearing loss.

References

1. Arrondel C et al: Expression of the nonmuscle myosin heavy chain IIA in the human kidney and screening for *MYH9* mutations in Epstein and Fechtner syndromes. *J Am Soc Nephrol* 13:65–74, 2001.
2. Bernheim J et al: Thrombocytopenia, macrothrombocytopathia, nephritis and deafness. *Am J Med* 61:145–150, 1976.
3. Brivet RG et al: Hereditary nephritis associated with May-Hegglin anomaly. *Nephron* 29:59–62, 1981.
4. Clare NM et al: Alport's syndrome associated with macrothrombopathic thrombocytopenia. *Am J Clin Pathol* 72:111–117, 1974.

5. Colville D et al: Absence of ocular manifestations in autosomal dominant Alport syndrome associated with haematological abnormalities. *Opthalmic Genet* 21:217–25, 2000.
6. Eckstein JD et al: Hereditary thrombocytopenia, deafness, and renal disease. *Ann Intern Med* 82:639–645, 1977.
7. Epstein CJ et al: Hereditary macrothrombocytopathia, nephritis and deafness. *Am J Med Genet* 52:299–310, 1972.
8. Gershoni-Baruch R et al: Fechtner syndrome: clinical and genetic aspects. *Am J Med Genet* 31:357–367, 1988.
9. Greinacher A, Mueller-Eckhardt C: Hereditary types of thrombocytopenia with giant platelets and inclusion bodies in the leukocytes. *Blut* 60:53–60, 1990.
10. Greinacher A et al: May-Hegglin anomaly: a rare cause of thrombocytopenia. *Eur J Pediatr* 151:668–671, 1992.
11. Heath KE et al: Nonmuscle myosin heavy chain IIA (MYHIIA) mutations define a spectrum of autosomal dominant macrothrombocytopenias: May-Hegglin anomaly, Fechtner, Sebastian, Epstein and Alport-like syndromes. *Am J Hum Genet* 69:1033–1045, 2001.
12. Hu A et al: Mutations in human nonmuscle myosin IIA found in patients with May-Hegglin anomaly and Fechtner syndrome result in impaired enzymatic function. *J Biol Chem* 277:46512–46517, 2002.
13. Kelley MJ et al: Mutations of MYH9, encoding non-muscle myosin heavy chain A, in May-Hegglin anomaly. *Nat Genet* 26:108–109, 2000.
14. Kunishima S et al: Mutations in the NMMHC-A gene cause autosomal dominant macrothrombocytopenia with leukocyte inclusions (May-Hegglin anomaly/Sebastian syndrome). *Blood* 97:1147–1149, 2001.
15. Lalwani AK et al: Human nonsyndromic hereditary deafness DFNA17 is due to a mutation in nonmuscle myosin MYH9. *Am J Hum Genet* 67:1121–8, 2000.
16. Martignetti JA et al: The May-Hegglin anomaly (MHA) gene localizes to a <1Mb region on chromosome 22q12.3–13.1. *Am J Hum Genet* 66:1449–1454, 2000.
17. May Hegglin/Fechtner Syndrome Consortium: Mutations in *MYH9* result in May-Hegglin anomaly, Fechtner and Sebastian syndrome. *Nat Genet* 26:103–105, 2000.
18. Moxey-Mims MM, et al: End-stage renal disease in two pediatric patients with Fechtner syndrome. *Pediatr Nephrol* 13:782–786, 1999.
19. M'Rad R et al: Alport syndrome: a genetic study of 31 families. *Hum Genet* 90:420–426, 1992.
20. Parsa KP et al: Hereditary nephritis, deafness and abnormal thrombopoiesis: study of a new kindred. *Am J Med* 60:665–672, 1976.
21. Peterson LC et al: Fechtner syndrome—a variant of Alport syndrome with leukocyte inclusions and macrothrombocytopenia. *Blood* 65:397–406, 1985.
22. Seri M et al: *MYH9*-related disease. May-Heggelin anomaly, Sebastian syndrome, Fechtner syndrome, and Epstein syndrome are not distinct entities but represent a variable expression of a single illness. *Medicine* 82:203–215, 2003.
23. Simons M et al: Human nonmuscle myosin heavy chains are encoded by two genes located on two different chromosomes. *Circ Res* 69:530–539, 1991.
24. Toothhaker LE et al: Cellular myosin heavy chain in human leukocytes: isolation of 5' cDNA clones, characterization of the protein, chromosomal localization and up regulation during myeloid differentiation. *Blood* 78:1826–1833, 1991.
25. Toren A et al: Autosomal dominant giant platelet syndromes: a hint of the same genetic defects as in Fechtner syndrome owing to a similar linkage to chromosome 22q11–13. *Blood* 96:3447–3451, 2000.

Nephritis, motor and sensory neuropathy (Charcot-Marie-Tooth disease), and sensorineural hearing loss (Lemieux-Neemeh syndrome)

In 1967, Lemieux and Neemeh (8) described a syndrome in two families, characterized by childhood onset of progressive distal muscle atrophy, nephropathy with proteinuria and hematuria, and progressive sensorineural hearing loss. A sporadic case was reported by Hanson et al. (4) in 1970. Gherardi et al. (3) reported the variable presence of nephropathy and peroneal muscular atrophy in a four-generation kindred. The fact that two of the well-studied cases did not have hearing loss suggests heterogeneity or variable expression in this disorder.

Renal system. The nephritis is characterized by proteinuria and microscopic hematuria. The proteinuria progresses to nephrotic syndrome

and in the index case in the family described by Gherardi et al. (3), renal failure and hypertension occurred, requiring hemodialysis at age 16. Lennert et al. (9), in an abstract cited by Gherardi et al. (3), collected follow-up information on all cases published prior to 1978. Five of six cases progressed to renal failure with hypertension. In a review of the literature, Fillod et al. (2) noted that 9 of 13 reported patients with Charcot-Marie-Tooth disease (CMT) and nephritis progressed to end-stage renal failure after 6 months to 17 years of follow-up (2). Sensorineural deafness, uncommon in CMT, was present in 7 out of the 13 cases with CMT and nephritis.

Peripheral nervous system. Weakness and atrophy of the distal legs and feet began in childhood and were slowly progressive. Later the weakness resulted in difficulty in walking and holding objects. Inturning of the toes and steppage gait were noted at 1 year by Hanson et al. (4). Involvement of the hands developed by 13–15 years and slowly evolved to claw hand deformity. Neurologic examination showed marked atrophy and weakness of the distal musculature of the legs and the intrinsic musculature of the hands with normal strength in proximal muscles (Fig. 9–3A). Affected individuals had an awkward gait with bilateral foot drop, but no true ataxia. In the older individuals, deep tendon reflexes were normal to absent in the arms and absent at the knees and ankles. Sensory examination was usually normal.

Motor nerve conduction velocities in the ulnar and median nerves were markedly decreased in the four patients in whom this study has been done (3,4,8). Electromyography revealed a diffuse denervation process. The findings are consistent with a motor neuropathy, similar to hereditary sensory motor neuropathy (Charcot-Marie-Tooth syndrome).

Auditory system. Hearing loss began in childhood and was slowly progressive. Two of the three patients reported by Lemieux and Neemeh (8) as well as the patient described by Hanson et al. (4) had progressive sensorineural hearing loss. In the latter patient, there was moderate hearing loss, more marked in higher frequencies and first noted at 7 years of age. Hearing loss was present in the case of Lennert et al. (8) by 8 years of age. A 50 dB hearing loss was documented in the cases of Lemieux and Neemeh (8). Kousseff et al. (6), studying CMT and deafness, found that sensorineural hearing loss became apparent in the second decade, and was severe to profound in most affected persons after the third decade.

Pathology. In one report biopsy of the sural nerve showed no abnormalities (4). However, in the study of Gherardi et al. (3), sections of the peroneal nerve showed a severe myelinated fiber loss and an excessive number of Schwann cell nuclei, increased endoneural collagen, and onion bulb formations. This latter finding is consistent with hereditary sensory motor neuropathy, type I. Muscle biopsy showed marked atrophy with small foci of hypertrophic muscle fibers (4,9). This was consistent with denervation (3).

Gherardi et al. (3) described the histopathologic findings of the kidney in all six cases as being consistent with focal glomerulosclerosis (Fig. 9–3B). Electron microscopic findings showed no splitting, lamellation, or thinning of the basal laminae; vacuolated podocytes were frequently observed as well as numerous clear nuclear inclusion bodies. These findings are not consistent with the ultrastructural findings of Alport syndrome (4).

Heredity. It is not clear whether the combination of neuropathy, nephritis, and variable deafness is a discrete entity, a heterogeneous collection of disorders, or even coincidental occurrences within the families.

In the family described by Lemieux and Neemeh (6), 4 of 11 siblings were affected. One had neuropathy, one had nephropathy, and two had both disorders. The two index cases with both disorders also had hearing loss. The remainder of the family was not available for evaluation but was not known to have components of the disorder. In the second family in that report, the 21-year-old proband had distal muscle wasting and nephropathy but no hearing loss. A 12-year-old

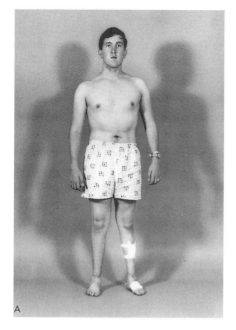

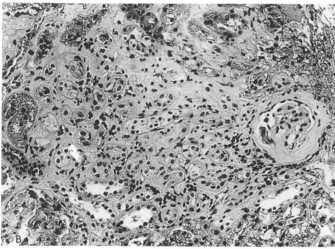

Figure 9–3. *Nephritis, motor and sensory neuropathy (Charcot-Marie-Tooth disease), and sensorineural hearing loss (Lemieux-Neemeh syndrome).* (A) Sixteen-year-old patient showing tapering extremities and claw hands. (B) Renal biopsy showing zone of tubular atrophy and hyalinization of glomerular tuft. [(A) from PA Hanson et al., *Neurology* 20:426, 1970; (B) from G Lemieux and JA Neemeh, *Can Med Assoc J* 97:1193, 1967.]

thy, suggests that this is a discrete entity rather than a set of coincidences.

Diagnosis. While the nephropathy has some similarities to Alport syndrome, the ultrastructural findings are different. The combination of motor and sensory neuropathy and sensorineural hearing loss has been described in autosomal dominant, autosomal recessive, as well as the X-linked form (10). Profound hearing impairment has been noted in one of two individuals homozygous for the CMT gene (5), which is the ganglioside-induced differentiation-associated protein (*GDAP1*) gene (1), and deafness and CMT have been shown in the family reported by Kousseff et al. (6) to be due to point mutation in the *PMP22* gene (7).

Prognosis. Gherardi et al. (3) cited an abstract by Lennert et al. (9) which indicated that in follow-up of five of the reported six cases, there was a rapid renal failure with hypertension. Thus, the renal failure is more severe than originally thought from the two earlier reports. The CMT syndrome seemed quite classic in its behavior.

Summary. The syndrome is characterized by (*1*) an autosomal dominant inheritance with variable expression and incomplete penetrance; (*2*) nephropathy consisting of nephrotic syndrome and some progression to renal insufficiency; (*3*) progressive neuropathy similar to hereditary motor and sensory neuropathy, type I (Charcot-Marie-Tooth syndrome); and (*4*) variable presence of sensorineural hearing loss beginning in childhood.

References

1. Baxter RV et al: Ganglioside-induced differentiation-associated protein-1 is mutant in Charcot-Marie-Tooth disease type 4A/8q21. *Nat Genet* 30:21–22, 2001
2. Fillod I et al: Nephropathy and Charcot-Marie-Tooth disease. A case report. *Pediatrie* 45:319–322 ,1990.
3. Gherardi R et al: Focal glomerulosclerosis associated with Charcot-Marie-Tooth disease. *Nephron* 40:357–361, 1985.
4. Hanson PA et al: Distal muscle wasting, nephritis and deafness. *Neurology* 20:426–434, 1970.
5. Killian JM, Klopfer HW: Homozygous expression of a dominant gene for Charcot-Marie-Tooth neuropathy. *Ann Neurol* 5:515–522, 1979.
6. Kousseff BG et al: Charcot-Marie-Tooth disease with sensorineural hearing loss—an autosomal dominant trait. *Birth Defects* 18:223–228, 1982.
7. Kovach MJ et al: A unique point mutation in the *PMP22* gene is associated with Charcot-Marie-Tooth disease and deafness. *Am J Hum Genet* 64:1580–1593, 1999.
8. Lemieux G, Neemeh JA: Charcot-Marie-Tooth disease and nephritis. *Can Med Assoc J* 97:1193–1198, 1967.
9. Lennert T et al: Charcot-Marie-Tooth disease and chronic nephropathy. Presented at the European Society of Pediatric Nephrology, 10th meeting, Barcelona, Spain, 1976.
10. Young P et al: Mutation analysis in Chariot-Marie Tooth disease type 1: point mutations in the *MPZ* gene and the *GJB1* gene cause comparable phenotypic heterogeneity. *J Neurol* 248:410–415, 2001.

sister, a 13-year-old brother, and their 46-year-old mother had distal muscle wasting. Urinalysis done on seven members of the family, including the mother and 12-year-old sister with distal muscle wasting, showed proteinuria. The family reported by Gherardi et al. (3) showed variable findings within three generations of the kindred. Although the proband had nephropathy and peroneal muscular atrophy, neither parent nor siblings were affected. The mother had two brothers with pes cavus, one of whom had a daughter with minor foot deformities. The other had a son with the same neurologic and renal disorder as the propositus. The proband's maternal great-aunt also appeared to have the complete syndrome of nephropathy and muscular atrophy. No one in this family had clear-cut hearing loss, although the proband had minor bilateral loss of 30 dB at high frequency. The pattern of disorders in this family would suggest the existence of an autosomal dominant trait of variable expression of nephropathy and neuropathy and incomplete penetrance. The set of conditions in the family reported by Lemieux and Neemeh (8) is also impressive and, together with the association of nerve deafness in cases of CMT and nephropa-

Nephritis, urticaria, amyloidosis, and sensorineural hearing loss (Muckle-Wells syndrome) (MWS)

This autosomal dominant syndrome was first described by Muckle and Wells (13) in nine members of a Derbyshire family in 1962 and is characterized by recurrent episodes of fever, abdominal pain, arthritis, and urticaria. Later on it is complicated by progressive sensorineural hearing loss, multiorgan amyloidosis of the amyloid A (AA) type, and end-stage renal failure. The disease usually begins in adolescence with attacks of transient urticaria-like rash accompanied by chills, mild fever, ill-defined malaise, episcleritis, abdominal pain, and aching limbs. The flu-like bouts, noted in 85% of affected individuals, last 12–36 hours and occur with variable intensity every few weeks. Concurrently, progressive sensorineural hearing loss is noticed. In middle age, some patients develop a nephrotic syndrome secondary to amyloidosis and die of uremia. Disease course and clinical expression among families varies considerably (1,5). It is now known to be allelic with the phenotypically similar familial cold autoinflammatory syndrome (FCAS), also called familial cold urticaria (FCU).

Renal system. During the third and fourth decades, about 35% of patients develop a nephrotic syndrome with proteinuria, uremia, anemia, and edema. Renal amyloidosis, of the AA type (derived from serum amyloid-associated protein) has been found on kidney biopsy in over one-half of this group (7), but this complication may be delayed in the course of the disease and it can even be clinically latent (11).

Integumentary system. An urticaria-like rash extends over most of the body but is most pronounced over the extremities. The rash consists of slightly erythematous papules, 1–7 cm in diameter, which are painful but infrequently pruritic.

Central nervous system. Distal limb pains usually begin in the second decade of life. Arthralgias, fever, and urticarial-like rash accompany these bouts. Pes cavus has occurred occasionally.

Auditory system. Bilateral sensorineural hearing loss is noted in 85% of cases and usually appears in childhood or adolescence. It progresses slowly to severe loss in the third or fourth decade of life (Fig. 9–4A).

Laboratory findings. When acute clinical episodes occur, there is an elevated erythrocyte sedimentation rate, high leukocyte blood counts, and hypergammaglobulinemia. With kidney failure the hemoglobin is decreased to 7–8 g/dl, serum urea nitrogen may be elevated, and albuminuria is common.

Pathology. The kidneys are small with multiple surface adhesions. Histologic sectioning shows amyloid throughout the parenchyma, in most glomeruli, in many tubules, and in vessel walls (Fig. 9–4B). In the spleen, amyloid is noted throughout the parenchyma, follicles, and vessel walls. The testes are small with atrophic seminiferous tubules infiltrated by amyloid, both in tubules and vessel walls. In liver and adrenal cortices, amyloid involves the vessels. Amyloid has also been noted in the sciatic nerve and the dorsal root ganglia (14) (Fig. 9–4C,D). The amyloid has been characterized as being of the AA type (6).

Histopathologic examination of the inner ear has shown absence of the organ of Corti and vestibular sensory epithelium, atrophy of the cochlear nerve, and ossification of the basilar membrane. Amyloid was not present (12) (Fig. 9–4E).

Heredity. The syndrome shows an autosomal dominant inheritance with variable expressivity. It is not known whether sporadic cases represent incomplete penetrance in families or new mutations.

Linkage to chromosome 1q (1) followed by mutation studies (3) identified the *CIAS1* gene, so named for *Cold-Induced Autoinflammatory Syndrome*, as the cause of the syndrome. At the same time three *CIAS1* mutations were also identified in FCAS, thus demonstrating that these two disorders are allelic. The *CIAS1* gene encodes a pyrin-like protein, cryopyrin, which is expressed predominantly in peripheral blood leukocytes. Cryopyrin has significant amino acid homology to other proteins involved in inflammation, particularly that causing familial Mediterranean fever (FMF) in a domain that has since been called the "pyrin" domain, pyrin being the protein encoded by the gene mutated in FMF. Pyrin domains have now been found in a number of recently identified proteins involved in apoptosis and inflammation. There is growing evidence that the dysregulation of leukocyte apoptosis may be a common molecular pathway leading to inflammatory disease (4).

Diagnosis. There is clinical overlap with the phenotypically similar but distinct familial cold autoinflammatory syndrome (or familial cold urticaria). This syndrome is distinguished from MWS by the presence of cold sensitivity (absent in MWS) and a higher incidence of conjunctivitis, which is present in 84% of cases (3). In FCAS, deafness is not a feature and amyloidosis is rare, affecting only 2% (3). There is also considerable similarity with other hereditary periodic inflammatory

diseases including familial Mediterranean fever, hyperimmunoglobulinemia D and periodic fever (HIDS), and familial Hibernian fever. Renal amyloidosis may complicate about 25% of cases of the autosomal recessive condition familial Mediterranean fever, and uremia can result. Hearing loss does not occur in this condition. Several reports of possible variants of MWS have been published. Throssell et al. reported a family with periodic urticaria, arthralgia, and a nephropathy (manifest as hematuria) but without amyloidosis or sensorineural deafness (15). Asymptomatic hematuria was present in individuals in two other generations and renal biopsies in this family were either normal or showed mild, nondiagnostic glomerular abnormalities, but in no case was there any evidence of amyloidosis. Given the phenotypic overlap between this condition and MWS, and between MWS and FCAS that are now known to be allelic, this may well be a variant of MWS, as postulated by the authors. Similarly, the syndrome reported by McDermott et al. (8) consisted of arthralgia, skin rashes, and early-onset AA amyloidosis, in the absence of deafness and without cold as a precipitating factor, and is likely to be another variant. They described a third-generation family from the Indian subcontinent in which three affected males died between 26 and 35 years of age from amyloidosis. Male-to-male transmission was demonstrated, but females appeared to be less severely affected. A number of individuals also complained of intermittent periorbital edema and the disorder mapped to the same chromosomal region as the *CAIS1* gene. Gerbig et al. (2) suggested that some of the sporadic cases of MWS in particular had probably been confounded with other disorders, particularly chronic infantile neurologic, cutaneous, and auricular (CINCA) syndrome (14).

Systemic amyloidosis may be dominantly inherited either alone or in several syndromes: neuropathy with vitreous opacities, neuropathy with carpal tunnel syndrome, neuropathy with cutis laxa, cardiac form, visceral form, etc. (9,10). Patients with these conditions do not suffer from urticaria or hearing loss. However, Van Allen et al. (16) reported a family with what McKusick (9) calls amyloidosis IV, Iowa type. In addition to early neuropathy and late nephropathy, cataracts and severe peptic ulcer disease were common and sensorineural hearing loss was frequent. Inheritance was autosomal dominant. It appears to be a disorder different from MWS. Amyloidosis may also occur with hypersensitivity as a dominantly inherited syndrome (9). However, amyloidosis is not required for the diagnosis of MWS since it may be late in onset, may be occult, and may not occur in some families (1,11).

Prognosis. Prognosis is poor. The hearing loss is slowly progressive, resulting in severe deafness in all patients. Affected individuals usually die of uremia in the third to fifth decades of life.

Summary. Characteristics of this syndrome include (*1*) autosomal dominant transmission with variable expressivity; (*2*) mutations in the *CIAS1* gene; (*3*) adolescent onset of recurrent episodes of urticaria, fever, and limb and joint pain; (*4*) variable amyloidosis resulting in nephropathy and uremia; and (*5*) childhood onset of progressive sensorineural hearing loss.

References

1. Cuisset L et al: Genetic linkage of the Muckle-Wells syndrome to chromosome 1q44. *Am J Med Genet* 65:1054–1059, 1999.
2. Gerbig AW et al: Circadian elevation of IL-6 levels in Muckle-Wells syndrome: a disorder of the neuro-immuno axis? *Q J Med* 91:489–492, 1998.
3. Hoffman HM et al: Mutation of a new gene encoding a putative pyrin-like protein causes familial cold autoinflammatory syndrome and Muckle-Wells syndrome. *Nat Genet* 29:301–305, 2001.
4. Kastner DL, O'Shea JJ: A fever gene comes in from the cold. *Nat Genet* 29:241–242, 2001.
5. Lagrue G et al: Syndrome de Muckle et Wells. Cinquième observation familiale. *Nouv Presse Méd* 1:2223–2226, 1972.
6. Linke RP et al: Identification of amyloid A protein in a sporadic Muckle-Wells syndrome. *Lab Invest* 48:698–704, 1983.
7. Mamou H et al: Maladie periodique et syndrome de Muckle et Wells. *Nouv Presse Med* 3:1363–1364, 1974.
8. McDermott MF et al: An autosomal dominant periodic fever associated with AA amyloidosis in a North Indain family maps to distal chromosome 1q. *Arthritis Rheum* 43:2034–2040, 2000.

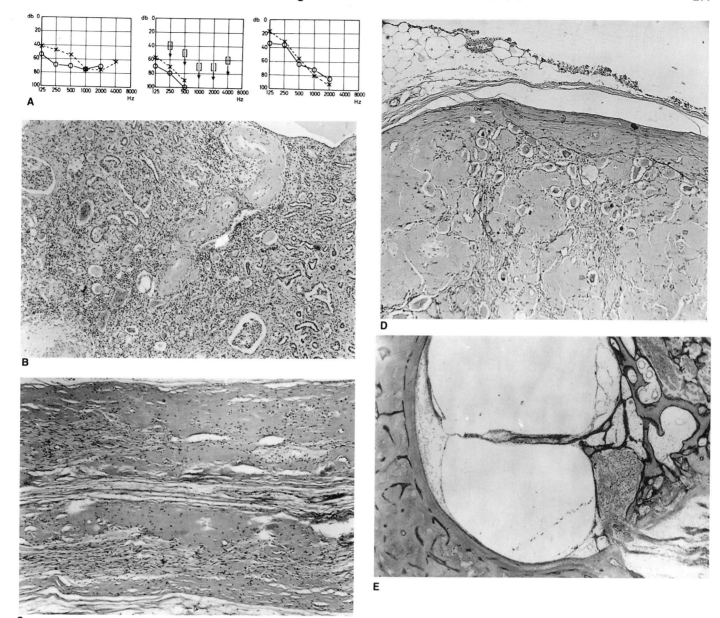

Figure 9–4. *Nephritis, urticaria, amyloidosis, and sensorineural hearing loss (Muckle-Wells syndrome).* (A) Left: audiogram of patient at 7 years of age; center: audiogram of same patient at 30 years of age; right: audiogram of patient's brother at 10 years of age. (B) Section of kidney showing amyloid deposits primarily affecting large blood vessels. Renal parenchyma is scarred and atrophic. (C) Sciatic nerve showing amyloid deposits effacing nerve trunk architecture. (D) Dorsal root ganglion with dispersion of ganglion cells by amyloid masses. (E) Section of inner ear showing absence of organ of Corti and a line of ossification in the basilar membrane. [(A) from V Andersen et al., *Am J Med* 42:449, 1967; (B–D) from MW Van Allen et al., *Neurology (Minneap)* 19:10, 1968; (E) from TJ Muckle and M Wells, *Q J Med* 31:235, 1962.]

9. McKusick VA: *Mendelian Inheritance in Man*, 9th ed. Johns Hopkins University Press, Baltimore, 1990.
10. Mertoja J: Genetic aspects of familial amyloidosis with corneal lattice dystrophy and cranial neuropathy. *Clin Genet* 4:175–185, 1973.
11. Messier G et al: Overt or occult renal amyloidosis in the Muckle-Wells syndrome. *Kidney Int* 34:566, 1988.
12. Muckle TJ: The 'Muckle-Wells' syndrome. *Br J Dermatol* 100:87–92, 1979.
13. Muckle TJ, Wells M: Urticaria, deafness, and amyloidosis: a new heredofamilial syndrome. *Q J Med* 31:235–248, 1962.
14. Prieur AM et al: A chronic, infantile, neurological, cutaneous and articular (CINCA) syndrome: a specific entity analysed in 30 patients. *Scand J Rheum Suppl* 66:57–68, 1987.
15. Throssell D et al: Urticaria, arthralgia, and nephropathy without amyloidosis: another variant of the Muckle-Wells syndrome? *Clin Genet* 49:130–133, 1996.
16. Van Allen MW et al: Inherited predisposition to generalized amyloidosis. Clinical and pathological studies of a family with neuropathy, nephropathy, and peptic ulcer. *Neurology (Minneap)* 19:10–25, 1968.

Nephritis, myopathy, corneal crystals, and conductive hearing loss

In 1987, Arnold et al. (1) reported an adolescent female with renal abnormalities, myopathy, ocular problems, and conductive hearing loss.

Renal system. Chronic urinary infections, vesicoureteral reflex, and pyelonephritis became evident at age 10 years. Hypertension appeared at 13 years.

Neuromuscular system. Progressive dysphonia and dysphagia began at about 10 years of age. The facies became myopathic, the palate akinetic, and the tongue atrophic (Fig. 9–5A). Atrophy of the hypothenar and thenar eminences was manifested at age 13 (Fig. 9–5B). Gag reflex was absent and speech was dysarthric. Intelligence was normal.

Optical system. At age 8, deep corneal crystals were observed (Fig. 9–5C). Retinal epithelial mottling was found at 13 years (Fig. 9–5D). Lateral nystagmus was also noted.

Auditory system. Conductive hearing loss was first noted at the age of 5.

Laboratory findings. Albuminuria was marked.

Heredity. Family history was unremarkable.

Reference

1. Arnold RW et al: Corneal crystals, myopathy and nephropathy: a new syndrome. *J Pediatr Ophthalmol Strabismus* 24:151–155, 1987.

Nephritis, anorectal malformations, and sensorineural hearing loss

In 1983, Lowe et al. (1) reported five males in three generations with nephritis, anorectal malformations, and sensorineural hearing loss.

Renal system. Hereditary nephritis was documented in three of the males in two generations.

Anorectal findings. Low imperforate anus with anoperineal fistula or anal stenosis was found in four of the affected individuals.

Auditory system. Sensorineural hearing loss was found in the patients affected by kidney failure. Two children had preauricular tags and large pinnae.

Heredity. Autosomal dominant inheritance with variable expression best fits the family.

Diagnosis. There is great overlap with Townes-Brocks syndrome. However, no radial defects were evident in any of this kindred.

Reference

1. Lowe J et al: Dominant ano-rectal malformation, nephritis and nerve deafness: a possible new entity? *Clin Genet* 24:191–193, 1983.

Membranous glomerulonephritis and sensorineural hearing loss

In 1990, Meroni et al. (1) reported two brothers with membranous glomerulonephritis (MGN) with sensorineural hearing loss.

Membranous glomerulonephritis has been considered to be an immune complex–mediated disorder on the basis of electron microscopic and immunofluorescent findings. Yet, there is an association with HLA-DRw3 in 65%–75% of whites with MGN (20%–25% controls) and a strong association with HLA-DR2 in Japanese with MGN.

Renal system. Nephrotic syndrome (hypertension, pretibial edema, hematuria, proteinuria) was found. Light microscopy using Jones's silver staining showed diffuse thickening of the glomerular capillary walls with characteristic membranous spikes. Immunofluorescence revealed fine granular deposition of IgG and C3 along glomerular capillary walls. Ultrastructural changes included thickening of glomerular basement membrane with subepithelial electron-dense deposits (Fig. 9–6).

Auditory system. Both sibs, aged 33 and 36 years, showed moderate sensorineural hearing loss in the higher ranges. Both parents showed a similar hearing loss but did not have kidney disease. No further information was available, however.

Heredity. Hearing loss in parents and sons, with kidney disease in the sons and in a son of one of the sons, may represent independent inheritance of two disorders. In the absence of further information concerning the nature of the hearing loss in the parents, we cannot comment further.

Summary. Characteristics of this syndrome include (*1*) unclear inheritance; (*2*) moderate sensorineural hearing loss; and (*3*) membranous glomerulonephritis in some individuals.

Reference

1. Meroni M et al: Two brothers with idiopathic membranous nephropathy and familial sensorineural deafness. *Am J Kidney Dis* 15:269–272, 1990.

Figure 9–5. *Nephritis, myopathy, corneal crystals, and conductive hearing loss.* (A) Note myopathic facies. Patient had marked hypophonia, could not purse lips. (B) Marked atrophy of thenar and hypothenar muscles. (C) Deep corneal crystals. (D) Retinal epithelial mottling. [(A) courtesy of G Stickler, Lake City, Minnesota; (B–D) from RW Arnold et al, *J Pediatr Ophthalmol Strabismus* 24:151, 1987.]

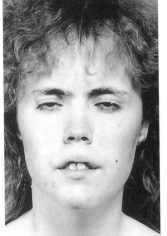

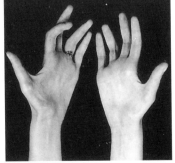

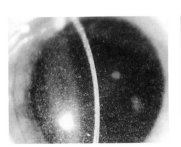

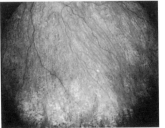

A　　　　　　　　　**B**　　　　　　　　　**C**　　　　　　　　　**D**

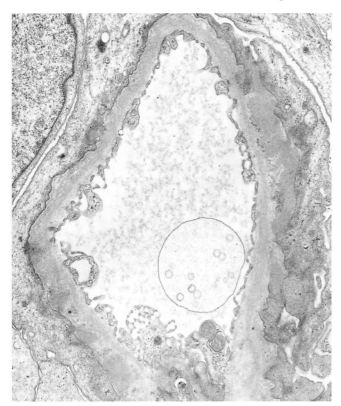

Figure 9–6. *Membranous glomerulonephritis and sensorineural hearing loss.* Almost total fusion of epithelial foot processes and scattered subepithelial deposits in epimembranous portion. [From M Meroni et al., *Am J Kidney Dis* 15:269, 1990.]

Mesangial IgA nephropathy, spastic paraplegia, mental retardation, and sensorineural hearing loss (Fitzsimmons syndrome)

In 1988, Fitzsimmons et al. (3) described a syndrome of progressive nephropathy, spastic paraplegia, mental retardation, and sensorineural hearing loss in a woman and three children by two separate fathers. In a family reported by Bizzarri et al. (1) in 1990, an affected mother, her son, and two daughters had all of the above findings except for that of spastic paraplegia.

Birth weight was normal in two of the three children, but low in the other (3). Subsequent weight and height followed the 3rd to 10th centile, while occipitofrontal circumference (OFC) followed the 50th centile.

Renal system. In the first family (3), initial evidence of renal disease was proteinuria, followed by hypertension. The course was progressive with manifestations of nephrotic syndrome. In the mother, renal failure occurred at 34 years and was treated with transplantation. In the second family, all manifested hematuria (1).

Central nervous system. In the family reported by Fitzsimmons et al. (3), motor development was delayed in the children. There were increased falling and gait abnormality at 4–8 years. These progressed to spastic paraplegia with spasticity, hyperreflexia, and extensor plantar responses in the legs. Increased reflexes were present in the arms. Mild spastic paraplegia was noted in the mother at age 28 years, although it probably began earlier.

In both families, IQs of 40–50 were recorded.

Auditory system. In the first family (3), the males showed hearing loss before the fifth year of life, eventually requiring hearing aids.

Speech development was delayed. Audiometry showed sensorineural hearing loss at 60–90 dB. Females were more moderately affected.

In the second family, sensorineural hearing loss was found in the son and one daughter. It was first diagnosed in the son in his 20s and involved high frequencies. It was not otherwise documented.

Laboratory findings. Proteinuria was found in all individuals. Other abnormalities included reduced serum albumin and glomerular filtration rate, and other evidence of nephrotic syndrome. Tests for mitochondrial disease were not described.

Pathology. In both families, kidney biopsies exhibited areas of glomerular sclerosis and tubular atrophy (Fig. 9–7A,B) combined with focal and segmental mesangial proliferative lesions with positive immunofluorescence for IgA and C3, and electron-dense mesangial deposits on electron microscopy (Fig. 9–7C). The basement membrane did not show the changes characteristic of Alport syndrome.

Heredity. In both families, the mothers transmitted the disorder to their children. Inheritance is probably autosomal dominant, but X-linked or mitochondrial inheritance cannot be excluded (Fig. 9–7D).

Diagnosis. The most common familial nephropathy with hearing loss is Alport syndrome, but the pathological changes in these families differed. Autosomal dominant inheritance of spastic paraplegia has been reported but was not previously associated with hearing loss or nephropathy. Spastic paraplegia is also seen with the Gemignani syndrome (ataxia, amyotrophy of hands, spastic paraplegia, hypogonadism, short stature, and sensorineural hearing loss). It is also found in binary combination with X-linked sensorineural hearing loss (Wells syndrome) (5). Spastic paraplegia (2) and mesangial IgA nephropathy (4) have each had myriad associations, but hearing loss has not been reported.

Prognosis. Neurologic and kidney problems can lead to early death.

Summary. This disorder is characterized by (*1*) probable autosomal dominant inheritance; (*2*) early developmental delay; (*3*) mental retardation; (*4*) progressive spastic paraplegia; (*5*) progressive nephropathy; and (*6*) progressive sensorineural hearing loss.

References

1. Bizzarri D et al: Familial IgA nephropathy and sensorineural hearing deafness. *Contrib Nephrol* 80:113–117, 1990.
2. Chevenix-Trench G et al: Spastic paresis, glaucoma and mental retardation—a probable autosomal recessive syndrome. *Clin Genet* 30:416–421, 1986.
3. Fitzsimmons JS et al: Familial spastic paraplegia, bilateral sensorineural deafness, and intellectual retardation associated with a progressive nephropathy. *J Med Genet* 25:168–172, 1988.
4. Kinkaid-Smith P, Nicholls K: Mesangial IgA nephropathy. *Am J Kidney Dis* 3:90–102, 1983.
5. Wells CR, Jankovic J: Familial spastic paraparesis and deafness. A new neurodegenerative disorder. *Arch Neurol* 43:943–946, 1986.

Renal disease, urinary tract and digital anomalies, and conductive hearing loss

A syndrome characterized by renal anomalies, nephrosis, digital anomalies, cleft uvula, and conductive hearing loss was described in 1962 by Braun and Bayer (1) in five male sibs.

Renal findings. Several types of renal disease were noted. Two boys had nephrosis with severe proteinuria beginning in infancy. Intravenous pyelograms done on all five affected sibs showed no abnormalities in two. In one patient, the pelvis and ureters were not visualized; in another, congenital ureterovesical obstruction and malfunction of one kidney were noted; in a third, unilateral duplication of the renal pelvis and upper ureter was evident. The occurrence of duplication of the ureter in the normal population is 1 in 100.

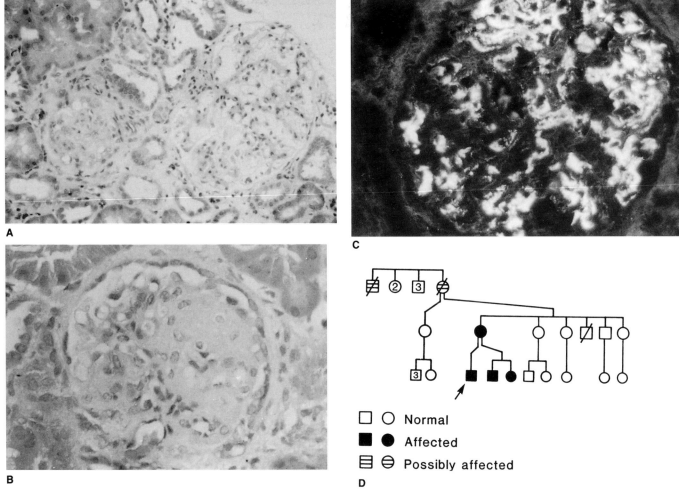

A

B

C

D

☐ ○ Normal

■ ● Affected

⊟ ⊝ Possibly affected

Figure 9–7. *Mesangial IgA nephropathy, spastic paraplegia, mental retardation, and sensorineural hearing loss (Fitzsimmons syndrome).* (A) Renal biopsy showing patchy tubular atrophy, interstitial fibrosis, hyalinization of one glomerulus, and mild mesangial proliferation in another. (B) Glomerulus exhibiting sclerosis of a segment proliferation lesion. (C) Fluorescent immunochemistry showing IgA deposits in mesangium.(D) Pedigree showing probable autosomal dominant pattern, although X-linked dominant or maternal inheritance cannot be excluded. [(A,B,D) from JS Fitzsimmons et al., *J Med Genet* 25:168, 1968; (C) courtesy of T Mauch, Minneapolis, Minnesota.]

Musculoskeletal system. The thumbs and great toes in three sibs had a short, broad, bulbous appearance.

Oral findings. The uvula was bifurcated in two sibs. This may be significant since the frequency of cleft uvula in whites is about 1 in 85.

Auditory system. Two males had a 30–40 dB conductive hearing loss. One boy had a 60–80 dB mixed hearing loss; conductive loss was 20–40 dB bilaterally. Other audiometric tests were not reported.

Laboratory findings. Radiographs of the abnormal digits of three of the boys showed short and rudimentary distal phalanges, each exhibiting bifurcation of the distal ends.

Proteinuria was found in two sibs. Intravenous pyelograms were abnormal in three of the five sibs.

Heredity. Five brothers among a sibship of 12 had the same general features. None of five sisters was affected. The parents were normal and not related (Fig. 9–8). It appears that the syndrome has X-linked or, less likely, autosomal recessive inheritance.

Diagnosis. Alport syndrome is associated with a progressive sensorineural hearing loss in contrast to the rather stable conductive hearing loss found in the syndrome described here.

Prognosis. Prognosis is rather poor because of the renal disease. The sibs with nephrosis had no other renal abnormalities. One died from renal failure, whereas another sib at 5 years of age was in moderately good health.

Figure 9–8. *Renal disease, digital anomalies, and conductive hearing loss.* Pedigree showing affected persons in kindred. [From FC Braun Jr and JF Bayer, *J Pediatr* 60:33, 1962.]

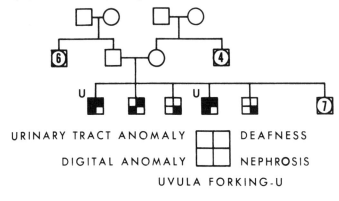

URINARY TRACT ANOMALY ☐ DEAFNESS

DIGITAL ANOMALY ☐ NEPHROSIS

UVULA FORKING-U

Summary. Characteristics of this syndrome include (*1*) X-linked or, less likely, autosomal recessive inheritance; (*2*) shortened bulbous thumbs and halluces with bifurcation of the distal end of the terminal phalanx; (*3*) renal anomalies, including ureteral constriction and duplication of the renal pelvis; (*4*) bifurcation of the uvula; and (*5*) congenital moderate to severe conductive hearing loss.

Reference

1. Braun FC Jr, Bayer JF: Familial nephrosis associated with deafness and congenital urinary tract anomalies in siblings. *J Pediatr* 60:33–41, 1962.

Renal disease, hyperprolinuria, ichthyosis, and sensorineural hearing loss

In 1968, Goyer et al. (2) found renal disease, hearing loss, hyperprolinuria, and ichthyosis in various combinations in 23 members of a kindred.

Physical findings. The proband was admitted to the hospital when she was 12 years old because of progressive fatigue and failure to gain weight.

Renal findings. Nephropathy of variable degree was present in eight individuals (2). The proband developed albuminuria and hematuria at 13 years of age. Blood urea nitrogen gradually increased. A 9-year-old brother had mild proteinuria, and another sib developed gross hematuria at 14 years. An intravenous pyelogram revealed a large cyst in one kidney and a small calculus in a cortical cyst in the other. The mother experienced gross hematuria at 22 years of age. Later, renal calculus was found.

Integumentary system. Dry skin was present in many members of the kindred (2), and a brownish scaling ichthyosis was found in 6 of 23 individuals (Fig. 9–9A).

Figure 9–9. *Renal disease, hyperprolinuria, ichthyosis, and sensorineural hearing loss.* (A) Ichthyosis on ventral surface of legs of proband. (B) Photomicrograph showing sclerosis of renal parenchyma. (C) Note mild infiltration of lymphocytes and foam cells into scarred areas of the kidney. (D) Electron microscopic view showing mesangial deposits. [From RA Goyer et al., *Am J Med Sci* 256:166, 1968.]

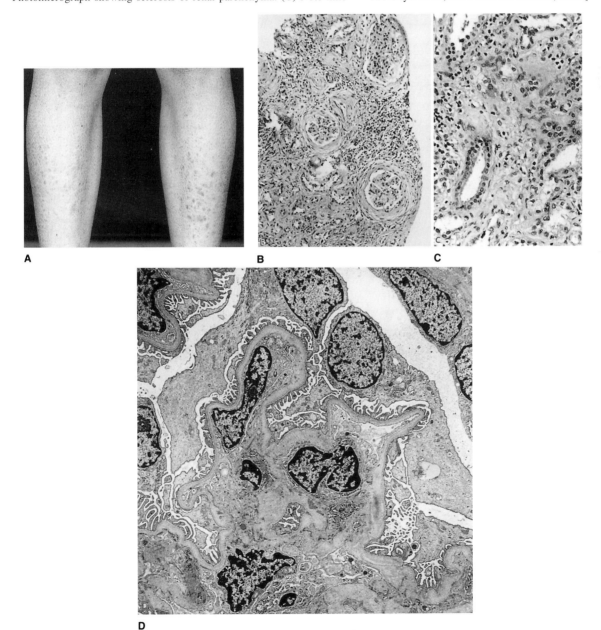

A   B   C

D

Laboratory findings. The only radiographic abnormalities found in the kindred were the bilateral renal cysts noted in the proband's 15-year-old brother and the calculi noted above.

Plasma proline levels were elevated to approximately three times the normal level in the proband. Urinary proline and hydroxyproline levels were also elevated. A sib had normal plasma levels but developed elevated urinary levels of proline, which suggests decreased renal tubular reabsorption. Two other members of the kindred had elevated plasma proline levels.

Pathology. Renal biopsy on the proband showed glomerular sclerosis. The interstitial tissue was infiltrated largely by lymphocytes. Arteries showed variable degrees of medial hypertrophy and subendothelial sclerosis (Fig. 9–9B,C). Electron micrographs revealed thickened mesangial basement membranes with dense deposits in the matrix (Fig. 9–9D).

Heredity. There were 23 persons in five generations affected by different components of this syndrome (2). The evidence suggests that this disease is an autosomal dominant trait with variable expressivity (Fig. 9–9E).

Diagnosis. The combination of hyperprolinemia and microscopic hematuria has been described as an autosomal dominant disorder in an Amerindian family, but no hearing loss was demonstrable (3).

Ichthyosis, convergent strabismus, and sensorineural hearing loss were noted in a girl who was the offspring of a consanguineous union (1). Among the 10 sibs in this kindred, 7 had a combination of two or more traits. No kidney anomalies or hyperprolinuria were found (1).

Prognosis. This syndrome, in spite of the uremia, did not appear to decrease life span. The hearing loss is probably slowly progressive, resulting in rather severe impairment in the later decades of life.

Summary. Characteristics of this syndrome include: (*1*) autosomal dominant inheritance with variable expressivity; (*2*) nephropathy of variable degree; (*3*) hyperprolinuria; (*4*) ichthyosis; and (*5*) slowly progressive sensorineural hearing loss.

References

1. Fishman JE, Crystal N: Sensorineural hearing loss: familial incidence and additional defects—study of a school for deaf children. *Am J Med Sci* 266:111–117, 1973.
2. Goyer RA et al: Hereditary renal disease with neurosensory hearing loss, prolinuria, and ichthyosis. *Am J Med Sci* 256:166–179, 1968.
3. Perry TL et al: Hyperprolinemia in two successive generations of a North American Indian family. *Ann Hum Genet* 31:401–408, 1968.

Renal failure, severe hypertension, abnormal steroidogenesis, hypogenitalism, and sensorineural hearing loss

In 1973, Hamet et al. (2) reported three sibs with severe hypertension, hypogenitalism, renal failure, and sensorineural hearing loss.

Renal system. All three sibs exhibited progressive renal failure, with death occurring in two sibs before age 40. On autopsy, the male sib had malignant nephrosclerosis and his sister had focal nephritis.

Cardiovascular system. Marked hypertension was noted in all three sibs during late adolescence.

Endocrine system. Cryptorchidism and small testes with reduced spermatogenesis were found in the male sib. Both female sibs exhibited primary amenorrhea. The ovaries were fibrotic streaks, and the uterus was infantile. Breast development was deficient, and axillary, pubic, and body hair was absent in the female sibs.

Auditory system. Progressive hearing loss was first noted in the male sib at age 5 with total loss of hearing resulting within the next few years. A female sib had bilateral moderate sensorineural hearing loss. No audiometric information was available on the second female sib.

Laboratory findings. Bone age was delayed in the two female sibs. An adrenal biosynthetic defect compatible with incomplete 17-hydroxylation and 11-hydroxylation abnormalities was demonstrated.

Heredity. The three affected sibs, of French-Canadian origin, had two normal sibs and healthy, nonconsanguineous parents. Inheritance is apparently autosomal recessive.

Diagnosis. Alport syndrome may be excluded on the basis of hypogenitalism, recessive inheritance, and hypertension, which occurs late in the course of this disorder. A disorder that is clinically similar but does not present with renal failure is ovarian dysgenesis (Perrault syndrome), which is also inherited in an autosomal recessive manner (1,3,4).

Prognosis. Prognosis is poor. The male sib and one female sib died of cerebral hemorrhage at the age of 30 and 35 years, respectively.

Summary. Characteristics of this syndrome include: (*1*) autosomal recessive inheritance; (*2*) progressive renal failure; (*3*) severe hypertension appearing during adolescence; (*4*) hypogenitalism manifested by cryptorchidism or primary amenorrhea; and (*5*) progressive sensorineural hearing loss appearing in childhood.

References

1. Christakos AC et al: Gonadal dysgenesis as an autosomal recessive condition. *Am J Obstet Gynecol* 104:1027–1030, 1969.
2. Hamet P et al: Hypertension with adrenal, genital, renal defects, and deafness. *Arch Intern Med* 131:563–569, 1973.
3. Josso N et al: Le syndrome de Turner familiale. *Ann Pediatr* 10:163–167, 1963.
4. Linssen WHJP et al: Deafness, sensory neuropathy, and ovarian dysgenesis: a new syndrome or a broader spectrum of Perrault syndrome? *Am J Med Genet* 51: 81–82, 1994.

Renal tubular acidosis with progressive sensorineural hearing loss

Primary distal renal tubular acidosis (dRTA) is inherited as either an autosomal dominant or autosomal recessive trait. Patients with recessive dRTA are severely affected and hearing loss is confined to a subset of patients. In 1973, Cohen et al. (6) reported a syndrome of congenital sensorineural hearing loss and infantile renal tubular acidosis. Many cases have been reported since, but the largest study to date has been by Karet et al., (12) who demonstrated mutations in the B1 subunit of H^+-ATPase, although there is clearly genetic heterogeneity. The study included four outbred kindreds with 2 or more affected sibs and 27 kindreds with parental consanguinity, of which 7 had more than one affected individual. They presented either with acute dehydration and vomiting or with failure to thrive and/or growth impairment.

Physical findings. One of the two presenting factors was failure to thrive and/or growth impairment. There is marked growth retardation, often being below the third centile. Growth has been reported to respond to treatment with alkali supplementation (14). In five of the kindreds studied, rickets was also noted (12).

Renal system. At birth or soon thereafter, the infants presented with vomiting, dehydration, polydipsia, polyuria, and hyposthenuria (inability to concentrate urine) or with failure to thrive and/or growth failure. They were diagnosed as having renal tubular acidosis, a disorder in which there is inability to maximally acidify the urine despite severe metabolic acidosis. The acidosis is out of proportion to any reduction in glomerular filtration rate. Other features include low potassium, due to renal potassium wasting and elevated urinary calcium. If untreated the acidosis may result in dissolution of bone, giving rise to osteomalacia and rickets. Renal stones are common as is nephrocalcinosis. The female sib described by Konigsmark BW, unpublished data, and Walker et al. (20) had bilateral renal calculi removed at 12 years of age. She had recurrent bouts of renal colic and passed numerous small stones. Renal tubular acidosis, ascertained on laboratory study, was mild (20). Despite the nephrocalcinosis described in all the kindreds studied by Karet et al. (12), the renal function was normal in every case and remained so in all but one female, who developed end-stage renal disease at the age of 18 years.

Other findings. Wilms tumor and aniridia/glaucoma have been reported in one sibship. One child developed insulin-dependent diabetes mellitus (8).

Auditory system. Mild to profound sensorineural hearing loss, more pronounced at higher frequencies, has been demonstrated in childhood (Fig. 9–10A). However, in one patient, only moderate hearing loss was found at 17 years, although this case was atypical because of the associated features. (8). Mutations in the *ATP6B1* gene may cause dRTA without deafness but 87% of families with mutations in *ATP6B1* were shown to have hearing loss, which tended to be severe to profound, and this bred true in families (12). In several cases the hearing loss has been reported to be progressive (3,4). High-resolution magnetic resonance imaging (MRI) performed in three consecutive cases with dRTA and progressive sensorineural hearing loss showed enlarged vestibular aqueducts (bilateral in two and unilateral in two) (2). Hearing loss does not respond to alkali treatment. Because of the possibility of enlarged vestibular aqueducts (see Vestibular system) it is likely that hearing may deteriorate following head trauma and sudden atmospheric pressure variation.

Vestibular system. No studies have been published. It is known, however, that vestibular symptoms are present in one-third of those who have enlarged vestibular aqueducts associated with other conditions.

Laboratory findings. The urine is alkaline. Hyperchloremic acidosis is confirmed by blood pH and serum electrolytes. Acid loading studies reveal impairment of urinary acidification. Radiographic studies showed nephrocalcinosis and signs of renal rickets (7). Ultrasonography may also be employed as an accurate monitor for nephrocalcinosis.

Heredity. The inheritance pattern of dRTA with sensorineural hearing loss is autosomal recessive, as proven by mutation analysis of *ATP6B1*, normal parents, affected sibs, and parental consanguinity (12).

This gene encodes B1α subunit of the H⁺ATPase, the apical proton pump mediating distal nephron acid secretion. Consistent with the associated hearing loss, Karet et al. (12) demonstrated expression of ATP6B1 in the cochlea and endolymphatic sac. The expression pattern and the known requirement for active proton secretion to maintain proper endolymph pH implicated ATP6B1 in endolymph pH homeostasis and in normal auditory function.

Diagnosis. In the families studied by Karet et al. (12), the diagnosis was based on inappropriately alkaline urine (pH >5.5) and the presence of systemic metabolic acidosis with normal anion gap, evidence of renal potassium wasting, and no evidence of secondary causes of dRTA. Dominant dRTA is usually milder and involves no hearing loss (1).
Carbonic anhydrase II deficiency may be seen in the syndrome of osteopetrosis, renal tubular acidosis, and sensorineural hearing loss (3,16,17). Mutations in the carbonic anhydrase 2 (*CA2*) gene were first identified by Moore et al. (13), in 1971. Sensorineural hearing loss can be found with the congenital magnesium-losing kidney syndrome (9).

There are other renal acidoses that are clinically similar except that in all syndromes sensorineural deafness is absent. In these syndromes, mutations have been identified in different genes (reviewed in 1,15). These include mutations in the *ATP6N1B* encoding the B-subunit of the apical pump (ATP6B1) in autosomal recessive distal RTA with preserved hearing (18), in the *SLC4A4* gene encoding Na⁺HCO₃-cotransporter in proximal RTA with ocular abnormalities (10), and in the gene *SLC4A1*, encoding Cl⁻-HCO₃-exchanger (AE1) in autosomal dominant distal RTA (1,5,11).

Prognosis. Prognosis is reasonably good. Life expectancy does not seem to be reduced if the disorder is recognized and treated early. The RTA is mild, and although renal calcinosis is associated, it may be treated effectively. Growth retardation, however, is persistent.

Summary. This syndrome is characterized by: (*1*) autosomal recessive inheritance; (*2*) mutations in the *ATP6B1* gene; (*3*) renal tubular acidosis with onset in infancy, adolescence, or early adulthood; (*4*) growth retardation; and; (*5*) mild to profound progressive sensorineural hearing loss.

References

1. Battle D et al: Hereditary distal renal tubular acidosis: new understandings. *Annu Rev Med* 52:471–484, 2001.
2. Berettini SB et al: Large vestibular aqueduct in distal renal tubular acidosis. High resolution MR in three cases. *Acta Radiol* 42:320–322, 2001.
3. Bourke E et al: Renal tubular acidosis and osteopetrosis in siblings. *Nephrosis* 28:268–272, 1981.

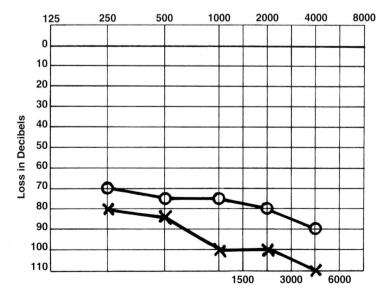

Figure 9–10. *Infantile renal tubular acidosis and progressive sensorineural hearing loss.* Audiogram of patient at 6 years of age. [From T Cohen et al., *Clin Genet* 4:275, 1973.]

4. Brown MT et al: Progressive sensorineural hearing loss in association with distal renal tubular acidosis. *Arch Otolaryngol Head Neck Surg* 119:458–460, 1993.

5. Bruce LJ et al: Familial distal renal tubular acidosis is associated with mutations in the red cell anion exchanger (band 3, AE1) gene. *J Clin Invest* 100:1693–1707, 1997.

6. Cohen T et al: Familial infantile renal tubular acidosis and congenital nerve deafness: an autosomal recessive syndrome. *Clin Genet* 4:275–278, 1973.

7. Cremers CWRJ et al: Renal tubular acidosis and sensorineural deafness. *Arch Otolaryngol* 106:287–289, 1980.

8. De Chadarévian JP et al: Aniridia/glaucoma and Wilms tumor in a sibship with renal tubular acidosis and sensorineural nerve deafness. *Am J Med Genet* (Suppl 3):323–328, 1987.

9. Evans RA et al: The congenital 'magnesium-losing kidney'. *Q J Med* 50:39–52, 1981.

10. Igarashi T et al: Mutations in *SLC4A4* cause permanent isolated proximal RTA with ocular abnormalities. *Nat Genet* 23:264–265, 1999.

11. Karet FE et al: Mutations in the chloride-bicarbonate exchanger gene *AE1* cause autosomal dominant but not autosomal recessive distal renal tubular acidosis. *Proc Natl Acad Sci USA* 95:6337–6342, 1997.

12. Karet FE et al: Mutations in the gene encoding B1 subunit of H(+)-ATPase cause renal tubular acidosis with sensorineural deafness. *Nat Genet* 21:84–90, 1999.

13. Moore MJ et al: A new carbonic anhydrase type isozyme in erythrocytes of American Negros. *Biochem Genet* 5:497–504, 1997.

14. Peces R et al: Long-term follow-up in distal renal tubular acidosis with sensorineural deafness. *Pediatr Nephrol* 15:63–65, 2000.

15. Rodriguez-Soriano J: New insights into the pathogenesis of renal tubular acidosis—from functional to molecular studies. *Pediatr Nephrol* 14:1121–1136, 2000.

16. Shapira E et al: Enzymatically inactive red cell carbonic anhydrase B in a family with renal tubular acidosis. *J Clin Invest* 53:59–63, 1974.

17. Sly WS et al: Carbonic anhydrase II deficiency in 12 families with autosomal recessive syndrome of osteopetrosis with renal tubular acidosis and cerebral calcifications. *N Engl J Med* 313:139–145, 1985.

18. Smith AN et al: Mutations in *ATP6N1B*, encoding a new kidney vacuolar proton pump 116-kD subunit, cause recessive distal renal tubular acidosis with preserved hearing. *Nat Genet* 26:71–75, 2000.

19. Walker WG: Renal tubular acidosis and deafness. *Birth Defects* 7(4):126, 1971.

20. Walker WG et al: Syndrome of perceptive deafness and renal tubular acidosis. *Birth Defects* 10(4):163, 1974.

Bartter syndrome with sensorineural deafness

Landau et al. first described the combination of infantile variant of Bartter syndrome and sensorineural deafness in a consanguineous Bedouin kindred (10). There were five living affected children born in different branches of the same extended family, a history of stillbirth with polyhydramnios, and two other stillbirths. The presentation of this condition is that of maternal polyhydramnios, premature birth, postnatal profound renal salt and water wasting, failure to thrive, sensorineural deafness, and motor retardation. The children described by Landau had similar characteristic features of triangular face, wide prominent forehead, prominent eyes, large ears, and small mouth unlike that of the unaffected siblings.

Renal system. The antenatal presentation with polyhydramnios is due to fetal polyuria, resulting in premature birth between 28 and 34 weeks. After birth, polyuria may result in dramatic weight loss and failure to thrive, with increased excretion of sodium, potassium chloride, and calcium in the urine. There is hyperreninemic hyperaldosteronism and hypokalemic hypochloremic metabolic alkalosis (10). Nephrocalcinosis was apparent on renal ultrasound scan in one of Landau's cases by the age of 7 months. In one of the cases described by Jeck et al. (9), ultrasound showed hyperechoic parenchyma with loss of corticomedullary differentiation. Histology has shown tubulointerstitial fibrosis and tubular atrophy with focal calcifications as well as global glomerular sclerosis.

Central nervous system. There is severe muscular hypotonia and deep tendon reflexes are reported to be normal or slightly decreased.

Motor milestones are markedly delayed, with a mean age of head control and sitting of 12 months and 26 months, respectively. Mean age of independent walking was between 3 and 5 years of age (9). Fine motor development and social skills appear to be less affected than gross motor skills. Convulsions have been reported but these are likely to be secondary to electrolytic disturbances (10). Two of Landau's cases are said to have had persisting developmental delay whereas two others are reported to have had normal psychomotor development (9). Jeck et al. (9) noted that "marked" mental retardation was not regularly observed, which together with Landau's findings suggest that any persistent developmental delay may be secondary to hypovolaemia and acute renal failure.

Auditory findings. Complete sensorineural hearing loss, probably of congenital (or prenatal) nature, is a consistent feature. In the family reported by Landau et al., absent brain stem auditory evoked responses (BAER) were documented in the proband at 7 months and in a cousin at the age of 3 weeks. In all of the cases described by Jeck et al. (9) hearing loss was diagnosed between the ages of 3 months and 2 years. Several children have undergone cochlear implant with positive results on speech development (9,10).

Vestibular system. No data have been published. Although there is muscular hypotonia in this condition, the Barttin protein is known to be expressed in the crista ampullaris of the vestibular organ and so there is likely to be a vestibular component to this motor delay (2).

Pathogenesis. Bartter syndrome with deafness is caused by mutation in the *BSND* gene, encoding the protein Barttin (2), which is thought to be an accessory subunit for a chloride ion channel. Chloride ions need to be transported across the surface of the luminal cells of the thick ascending loop of Henle by ClC-K family channels. Barttin is expressed with ClC-K channels in the stria vascularis and the kidney, and is needed for chloride efflux to occur [reviewed in Hunter (7)]. In the absence of barttin, no measurable Cl^- currents are recorded from ClC-K channels in vitro (4,7).

Laboratory findings. Hypochloremic hypokalemic metabolic alkalosis with marked increase in excretion of sodium, potassium, and calcium in the urine is found. Increased plasma renin and aldosterone with normal blood pressure and increased urinary prostaglandin E2 levels are observed.

Heredity. Inheritance is undoubtedly autosomal recessive in the cases reported to date. Nearly all the affected individuals have been the offspring of consanguineous marriages, and recessive inheritance is confirmed by mutation analysis of the *BSND* gene (2,3,10,16). The condition is now known to be caused by mutation in the *BSND* gene, encoding the protein Barttin, which is thought to be an accessory subunit for a chloride ion channel (2,4).

Diagnosis. The major differentiation is between other types of Bartter syndrome (familial hypokalemic hypochloremic metabolic alkalosis), which do not include deafness—i.e., infantile Bartter syndrome without deafness, Gitelman syndrome, and "classic" Bartter syndrome (1,5,6,8). In classic Bartter syndrome presentation is within the first few years of life and laboratory findings show moderate to severe hypokalemia with metabolic alkalosis, high urinary K and prostaglandin E2 excretion, and normal to increased urinary calcium. It may be caused by defects in the *KCNJ1* gene (*ROMK*) or by mutations in *CLCNKB* (14,15). Gitelman syndrome has an onset in childhood or adolescence, tends to be milder, and is caused by mutations in the thiazide sensitive sodium-chloride (Na-Cl) cotransporter, encoded by the *SLC12A3* gene (12). There is normal urinary prostaglandin excretion, hypocalciuria, and usually marked hypomagnesemia. In infantile, or antenatal, Bartter syndrome, presentation is that of intrauterine polyhydramnios and premature delivery but there is no deafness (6), and this is caused by mutation in *ROMK* (8) or Na-K-2Cl (encoded by the *SLC12A1* gene) (13).

Prognosis. There is suggestive evidence that affected individuals may die in utero or suffer the effects of prematurity as a result of polyhydramnios (10). After birth, supportive treatment and indomethacin may help electrolyte imbalance, but this therapy does not always appear to have a significant effect on subsequent growth (9). Response to indomethacin therefore appears to be less successful than in other forms of Bartter syndrome. Some individuals have required parenteral nutrition or gastrostomy feeding to maintain their weight. All patients reported by Jeck et al. developed chronic renal failure (9). Miyamura et al. (11) recently described a mildly affected young adult who had a *barttin* mutation, indicating clinical heterogeneity likely exists.

Summary. This syndrome is characterized by (*1*) autosomal recessive inheritance; (*2*) maternal polyhydramnios and premature birth; (*3*) postnatal polyuria and hypokalemic hypochloremic metabolic alkalosis; (*4*) profound congenital sensorineural deafness; and (*5*) mutation in the BSND gene.

References

1. Bettinelli A et al: Phenotypic variability in Bartter syndrome type 1. *Pediatr Nephrol* 14:10–11, 2000.
2. Birkenhäger R et al: Mutation of *BSND* causes Bartter syndrome with sensorineural deafness and kidney failure. *Nat Genet* 29:310–314, 2001.
3. Brennan T et al: Linkage of infantile Bartter syndrome with sensorineural deafness to chromosome 1p. *Am J Hum Genet* 62:355–361, 1998.
4. Estevez R et al: Barttin is a Cl⁻ channel β-subunit crucial for renal Cl⁻ reabsorption and inner ear K⁺ secretion. *Nature* 414:558–561, 2001.
5. Feldman D et al: Large deletion of the 5′ and of *ROMK1* gene causes antenatal Bartter syndrome. *J Am Soc Nephrol* 9:2357–2359, 1998.
6. Guay-Woodford L: Bartter syndrome: unravelling the pathophysiologic enigma. *Am J Med* 105:151–161, 1998.
7. Hunter M: Accessory to kidney disease. *Nature* 414:502–503, 2001.
8. International Collaborative study group for Bartter-like syndromes: Mutations in the gene encoding the inwardly rectifying real potassium channel, *ROMK*, cause the antenatal variant of Bartter syndrome: evidence for genetic heterogeneity. *Hum Mol Genet* 6:17–26, 1997.
9. Jeck N et al: Hypokalemic salt-losing tubulopathy with chronic renal failure and sensorineural deafness. *Pediatrics* 108:E5, 2001.
10. Landau D et al: Infantile variant of Bartter syndrome and sensorineural deafness: a new autosomal recessive disorder. *Am J Med Genet* 59:454–459, 1995.
11. Miyamura N et al: Atypical Barrter syndrome with sensorineural deafness with G47R mutation of the beta-subunit for CK-Ka and CK-Kb chloride channels, *barrtin. J Clin Endo Metab* 88:781–786, 2003.
12. Simon DB et al: Gitelman's variant of Bartter syndrome, inherited hypokalemic alkalosis, is causd by mutations in the thiazide sensitive Na-Cl cotransporter. *Nat Genet* 12:24–30, 1996.
13. Simon DB et al: Bartter's syndrome, hypokalemic alkalosis with hypercalciuria is caused by mutations in the Na-K-2Cl cotransporter NKCC2. *Nat Genet* 13:183–188, 1996.
14. Simon DB et al: Genetic heterogeneity of Bartter's syndrome revealed by mutations in the K⁺ channel, ROMK. *Nat Genet* 14:152–156, 1996.
15. Simon DB et al: Mutations in the chloride channel gene *CLCNKB* cause Bartter syndrome type III. *Nat Genet* 17:171–178, 1998.
16. Vollmer M et al: Antenatal Bartter syndrome with sensorineural deafness: refinement of the locus on chromosome 1p31. *Nephrol Dial Transplant* 15:970–974, 2000.

Renal rickets, retinitis pigmentosa, and progressive sensorineural hearing loss

In 1993, Beighton et al. (1) identified 14 affected individuals in nine Afrikaner families in South Africa. Onset occurred in early infancy, and patients presented with renal dysfunction of the Fanconi type leading to ricket-like skeletal changes and renal failure, sensorineural hearing loss, and relentless progression of visual handicap due to retinitis pigmentosa. Most of the children died of renal failure before reaching adulthood.

Renal system. Renal dysfunction usually presented with albuminuria during the first 5 years, leading to rickets-like skeletal changes,

stunted stature, and malalignment of the weight-bearing bones, resulting in renal failure.

Auditory and optical system. Onset of auditory and visual dysfunction was usually before the age of 5 and invariably before the age of 10.

Diagnosis. The condition is to be separated from the HDR/Barakat syndrome and Yumita syndrome. In neither of these syndromes is there mention of retinitis pigmentosa. In the family described, retinitis pigmentosa or Usher syndrome had initially been diagnosed in every child.

Prognosis. Eight of the 11 children died between the ages of 3 and 20 years; in most patients, the cause of death was reported to be renal failure.

Heredity. None of the parents were affected, thus autosomal recessive inheritance is suggested. Although minor changes were found in the eyes of the father of two affected sibs, none of the parents were known to be consanguineous. However, the Afrikaner population is derived from a comparatively small number of founders.

Summary. This syndrome is characterized by (*1*) autosomal recessive inheritance; (*2*) to date, sole identification in Afrikaners; (*3*) renal rickets leading to renal failure; (*4*) retinitis pigmentosa and progressive sensorineural hearing loss before the age of 10; and (*5*) poor prognosis.

Reference

1. Beighton P et al: Rod-cone dystrophy, sensorineural deafness, and renal dysfunction: an autosomal recessive syndrome. *Am J Med Genet* 47:832–836, 1993

Renal-coloboma syndrome (renal hypoplasia, ocular coloboma, and high-frequency hearing loss)

Karcher (11) reported a father and son with a glomerulonephritis resulting in renal failure. They both had optic nerve abnormalities, myopia, and reduced visual acuity. Later, Bron et al. (2) reported a father and two sons with coloboma of the optic nerve (one with a type of morning glory syndrome—Handmann's optic nerve anomaly). The other son was reported to have had microphthalmos, but he died in childhood.

Weaver et al. (21) reported two brothers with optic nerve colobomata, renal immune complex disease, interstitial fibrosis, and tubular atrophy. The parents were clinically normal. Sanyanusin et al. (17) reported that this condition was caused by mutation of the paired box transcription factor PAX2 in a father and three sons with optic nerve colobomas, renal anomalies, vesicoureteric reflux, and variable sensorineural hearing loss inherited in an autosomal dominant manner, and proved the same in the family originally reported by Weaver (16). This was based on the known expression pattern of the gene and the phenotype of the *krd* mouse, caused by transgenic insertion and deletion of a region of mouse chromosome 19, which included *Pax2* (12).

The hallmarks of this condition are renal hypoplasia and ocular coloboma, but affected individuals may also have high-frequency sensorineural hearing loss, vesico-ureteric reflux, central nervous system anomalies, and, occasionally, joint hyperextensibility and genital anomalies. The disorder is highly variable in all of its manifestations.

Renal system. The phenotype ranges from lethal prenatal hypoplasia, asymptomatic proteinuria leading in some cases to childhood renal failure, and vesicoureteric reflux, to normal renal development and function (10,14–17). Bilateral renal hypoplasia appears to be the most common renal manifestation. Ford et al. (10) described a multigeneration family with variable manifestations in whom the propositus was detected with severe renal hypoplasia and oligohydramnios on routine ultrasound scan at 18 weeks. Other members of the same family suffered from renal dysplasia with vesico-ureteric reflux, renal hypoplasia, or asymptomatic renal failure, whereas others enjoyed normal function. Several individuals with renal-coloboma syndrome (RCS) have required renal transplantation. Intrafamilial variability is also demonstrated in the large Brazilian family described by Porteous et al. (15), in which phenotypes ranged from normal renal appearance and function, to small cystic kidneys, cortical hyperechogenicity, and nephro- and urolithiasis. Amiel et al. described cases of unilateral renal cystic hypoplasia and also of a single pelvic kidney (1). In the single affected patient reported by Cunliffe et al. (4) the patient had no recognizable right kidney, which was replaced by a cystic structure, with no functional renal tissue.

At present there is no evidence that mutation of *PAX2* in humans causes isolated vesicoureteric reflux (3,9), although it has been reported in a family with isolated renal hypoplasia (14). Dressler and Woolf (6) provide a nice overview of *Pax2* in renal development.

Studies in mice [particularly the heterozygous $Pax2^{1Neu}$ mouse, caused by a 1 bp insertion in *Pax2* identical to a mutation also described in humans (8,16)], have shown that renal hypoplasia is common (60%). Unilateral renal agenesis and cystic abnormalities do occur but are much rarer (1% each of heterozygous mutant mice). Developing murine kidneys contain fewer nephrons and glomeruli than wild-type animals although early morphology appears to be normal, and this has been shown to be due to enhanced apoptosis (15).

Ocular system. The classic abnormality, as the name of the condition suggests, is optic disc coloboma, occasionally with the appearance of "morning glory," in which vision is severely impaired. Retinal and iris colobomata have also been reported (1), as has microphthalmia. Milder changes may include unusual patterns of retinal vessels or mild optic disc dysplasia or optic pit (5,7) which may be asymptomatic, being discovered upon routine examination, although in others vision is severely impaired and individuals present with myopia or visual inattention. Lens opacities have been reported (18).

However, *Pax2* mutations do not seem to be responsible for the occurrence of ocular colobomata, microphthalmos, or retinal anomalies, either in isolation or in association with urogenital conditions, in a significant number of patients (4).

Auditory system. Hearing loss is not a universal feature of RCS, but it is a recurrent finding (15,17,18); it is likely that in many reports it has not been specifically excluded by audiometry. When present it tends to be a high-frequency sensorineural hearing loss. *Pax2* is expressed in the developing otic vesicle, in the ventral part from which the cochlea, utricle, and saccule develop (19). *Pax2* null mice show agenesis or truncation of the cochlea and spiral ganglion (20) but the vestibular system develops normally.

Central nervous system. Porteus et al. (15) reported a child with febrile seizures and cognitive impairment in a large Brazilian kindred. Microcephaly and mental retardation (18) and abnormal EEG have also been reported in single cases and within families. In the $Pax2^{1neu}$ mutant, 26% of homozygous mutants have a deletion of the mid-hindbrain region (8) and 5% have exencephaly. However, heterozygous $Pax2^{+/-}$ animals may also have exencephaly, although penetrance is low and depends on the genetic background of the mouse (20).

Muscuolskeletal system. Hyperextensibility of the joints has been reported (10,18), as has soft skin (16,18).

Pathology. A minority of patients with RCS have had renal biopsy. Autopsy of the fetus reported by Ford et al. (10) revealed small nephritic buds associated with miniscule ureters. There was no evidence of glomeruli or other renal tissue on histology and the bladder was noted to be hypoplastic. Renal biopsy of another member of the same family who was 14 years of age was reported to show "oligonephric hypoplasia." Several members of the family reported by Devriendt et al. (5) have documented biopsy findings: a cortical biopsy of a 16-year-old family member showed six glomeruli, one of which was said to be ob-

solete. Glomeruli had an increased diameter and an increased number of capillaries. One glomerulus showed focal and segmental hyalinization. In another family member the cortex was thin and few glomeruli were found. The papillae contained few collecting ducts, and the cortex and medulla contained cysts.

Pathogenesis. Studies of mouse mutants have shed light on pathogenetic mechanisms in RCS. In the $Pax2^{1neu}$ heterozygotes, mutants show reduced fetal kidney size in comparison to wild-type littermates (60% of wild-type) and on histology there is reduced branching of the ureteric bud with increased apoptosis in fetal collecting ducts (15). The $krd/^+$ mouse has thinner renal cortex on day 4 of life, with fewer glomeruli, less well-developed proximal convoluted tubules, and a reduced number of mature neprons (12). Nephrons that are formed appear to be morphologically normal.

Heredity. There is autosomal dominant inheritance caused by haploinsufficiency for *PAX2* (13). Germline mosaicism has been reported (1).

Summary. Characteristics of this syndrome include (*1*) renal hypoplasia; (*2*) optic nerve coloboma, although minor asymptomatic anomalies such as optic disc dysplasia and pits may be found; (*3*) varaiable sensorineural hearing loss; and (*4*) haploinsufficiency for the *PAX2* gene.

References

1. Amiel J et al: *PAX2* mutations in renal-coloboma syndrome: mutational hotspot and germline mosaicism. *Eur J Hum Genet* 8:820–826, 2000.
2. Bron AJ et al: Papillo-renal syndrome: an inherited association of optic disc dysplasia and renal disease. Report and review of the literature. *Ophthalmol Paediatr Genet* 10:185–198, 1989.
3. Cho K-L et al: Absence of *PAX2* gene mutations in patients with primary vesicoureteric reflux. *J Med Genet* 35:338, 1998.
4. Cunliffe HE et al: The prevalence of *PAX2* mutations in patients with isolated colobomas or colobomas associated with urogenital anomalies. *J Med Genet* 35:800–812, 1998.
5. Devriendt K et al: Missense mutation and hexanucleotide duplication in the *PAX2* gene in two unrelated families with renal-coloboma syndrome. *J Med Genet* 103:149–153, 1998.
6. Dressler GR, Woolf AS: PAX2 in development and renal disease. *Int J Dev Biol* 43:463–468, 1999.
7. Dureau P et al: Renal coloboma syndrome. *Ophthalmology* 108:1912, 2001.
8. Favor J et al: The mouse $Pax2^{1Neu}$ mutation is identical to a human *PAX2* mutation in a family with renal-coloboma syndrome and results in developmental defects of the brain, ear, eye and kidney. *Proc Natl Acad Sci USA* 93:13870, 1996.
9. Feather S et al: Exclusion of key nephrogenesis genes as candidates for familial vesicoureteric reflux. *J Am Soc Nephrol* 8:388A, 1997.
10. Ford B et al: Renal-coloboma syndrome: prenatal detection and clinical spectrum in a large family. *Am J Med Genet* 99:137–141, 2001.
11. Karcher H. Zum morning glory Syndrom. *Klin Monatsbl Augenheilkd* 175:835–840, 1979.
12. Keller KA et al: Kidney and retinal defects (*Krd*), a transgene-induced mutation with a deletion of mouse chromosome 19 that includes the *pax2* locus. *Genomics* 23:309, 1994.
13. Narahara K et al: Localisation of a 10q breakpoint within the *PAX2* gene in a patient with a de novo t(10;13) translocation and optic nerve coloboma-renal disease. *J Med Genet* 34:213–216, 1997.
14. Nishimoto K et al: *PAX2* gene mutation in a family with isolated renal hypoplasia. *J Am Soc Nephrol* 12:1769, 2001.
15. Porteous S et al: Primary renal hypoplasia in humans and mice with *PAX2* mutations: evidence of increased apoptosis in fetal kidneys of $PAX2^{1\ Neu}$ +/− mutant mice. *Hum Med Genet* 9:1–11, 2000.
16. Sanyanusin P et al: Mutation of *PAX2* in two siblings with renal-coloboma syndrome. *Hum Mol Genet* 1995;4:2183–2184.
17. Sanyanusin P et al: mutation of the *PAX2* gene in a family with optic nerve colobomas, renal anomalies and vesicoureteric reflux. *Nat Genet* 9:358, 1995.
18. Schimmenti LA et al: Further delineation of renal-coloboma syndrome in patients with extreme variability of phenotype and identical *PAX2* mutations. *Am J Hum Genet* 60:869–878, 1997.
19. Tellier A-J et al: Expression of the *PAX2* gene in human embryos and exclusion in the CHARGE syndrome. *Am J Med Genet* 93:85–88, 2000.

20. Torres M et al: Pax2 contributes to inner ear patterning and optic nerve trajectory. *Development* 122:3381, 1996.
21. Weaver RG et al: Optic nerve coloboma associated with renal disease. *Am J Med Genet* 1988;29:597–605.

Hirschsprung disease, polydactyly, unilateral renal agenesis, hypertelorism, and congenital sensorineural hearing loss

In 1988, Santos et al. (2) described a brother and sister with a unique disorder. The boy had aganglionic megacolon, polydactyly of toes, unilateral renal agenesis, hypertelorism, and congenital sensorineural hearing loss of about 60 dB (Fig. 9–11). The sister died at 2 weeks of age. She had aganglionic megacolon and polydactyly of hands and feet. No additional information was available. Santos et al. (2) thought that this family did not have the same disorder found in another family described by Laurence et al. (1), where two male infants presented with Hirschsprung disease, ulnar polydactyly, and ventricular septal defect, as there was no mention of hearing loss.

Heredity. Unaffected but consanguineous parents and affected sibs suggest autosomal recessive inheritance.

Diagnosis. Although Hirschsprung disease (aganglionic megacolon) is usually an isolated finding (1/5000 births) with a 4M:1F sex predilection and multifactorial inheritance, there are several syndrome associations. One of the most common is with all types of Waardenburg syndrome.

Summary. Characteristics of this syndrome include (*1*) autosomal recessive inheritance; (*2*) Hirschsprung disease, polydactyly, and hypertelorism; (*3*) unilateral renal agenesis; and (*4*) congenital sensorineural hearing loss.

References

1. Laurence KM et al: Hirschsprung's disease associated with congenital heart malformation, broad big toes, and ulnar polydactyly in sibs: a case for fetoscopy. *J Med Genet* 12:334–338, 1975.
2. Santos H et al: Hirschsprung disease associated with polydactyly, unilateral renal agenesis, hypertelorism, and congenital deafness: a new autosomal recessive syndrome. *J Med Genet* 25:204–205, 1988.

Prune belly syndrome with pulmonic stenosis, mental retardation, and sensorineural hearing loss

In 1979, Lockhart et al. (1) described three male siblings with absence of abdominal muscles, undescended testes, megaureters, pulmonary

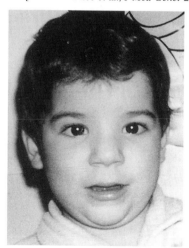

Figure 9–11. *Hirschsprung disease, polydactyly, unilateral renal agenesis, hypertelorism, and congenital sensorineural hearing loss.* Note hypertelorism and broad nasal root. [From H Santos et al., *J Med Genet* 25:204, 1988.]

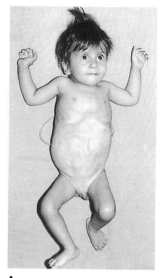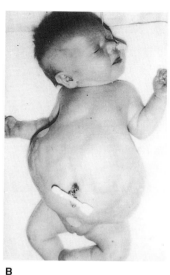

A   **B**

Figure 9–12. *Prune belly syndrome with pulmonic stenosis, mental retardation, and sensorineural hearing loss.* (A,B) Prune belly due to hypoplastic abdominal musculature. Note scar-like appearance of midabdomen due to loose skin. [(A) courtesy of J Spranger, Mainz, Germany; (B) courtesy of D Donnai, Manchester, England.]

stenosis, mental retardation, and sensorineural hearing loss. A sister was less severely affected. One male sib died soon after birth. In 1975, Welling et al. (2), reported two isolated males with prune belly and sensorineural hearing loss.

Physical findings. Short stature and genua valga due to renal osteodystrophy were noted in the eldest male reported by Lockhart et al. (1). All males had protuberant abdomen with markedly underdeveloped abdominal musculature. The female sib had hypotonic abdominal muscles (1) (Fig. 9–12).

Central nervous system. Intelligence quotients in all three sibs reported by Lockhart et al. (1) ranged from 59 to 75. The patients of Welling et al. (2) were stated to be mentally retarded.

Genitourinary system. Urinary tract infection, vesicoureteral reflux with megaureters, megacystis, and hydronephrosis with renal failure occurred in all sibs. One male sib died at 3 years of kidney failure. All three males had cryptorchidism (1).

Cardiovascular system. At least two male sibs had pulmonary stenosis. The female sib had a murmur consistent with that diagnosis (1).

Musculoskeletal system. One boy reported by Welling et al. (2) had bilateral hip joint dislocation and kyphoscoliosis.

Auditory system. Two male and female sibs described by Lockhart et al. (1) had bilateral sensorineural hearing loss. In one, hearing impairment was detected between 3 and 6 years of age. The degree of severity was not mentioned. The children reported by Welling et al (2) had severe congenital hearing loss.

Heredity. Because the involvement in the female was less marked than in the males, the possibility of X-linked inheritance was suggested.

Diagnosis. At least 500 cases of prune belly have been well documented in the literature. Talipes (20%) and hip joint dysplasia are frequently associated findings. With few exceptions, prune belly has been limited to males, familial occurrence is rare, and identical twins have always been discordant.

Summary. Characteristics include (*1*) probable X-linked inheritance; (*2*) lack of abdominal muscles; (*3*) renal anomalies; (*4*) pulmonary stenosis; (*5*) mild mental retardation; and (*6*) sensorineural hearing loss.

References

1. Lockhart JL et al: Siblings with prune belly syndrome and associated pulmonic stenosis, mental retardation, and deafness. *Urology* 14:140–142, 1979.
2. Welling P et al: Observations on the prune-belly syndrome. *Z Kinderheilkd* 118:315–335, 1975 (cases 4, 5).

Renal, genital, and middle ear anomalies (Winter syndrome)

A syndrome characterized by renal hypoplasia, internal genital malformations, and malformations of the middle ear appearing in four female sibs was described by Winter et al. (8) in 1968. Sibs with possibly the same syndrome were reported briefly by Turner (6). King et al. (3) also described affected female sibs. A patient who also had Mayer-Rokitansky-Küster syndrome was briefly reported (7).

Renal system. All four patients described by Winter et al. (8) had renal anomalies. Both sibs that died in infancy had bilateral renal agenesis, absent or hypoplastic ureters, and hypoplastic bladder (5). In both living sibs, intravenous pyelograms revealed a normal kidney on one side and absence or hypoplasia of the kidney and ureter on the other side. Turner's patient had unilateral kidney agenesis and ipsilateral hemiaplasia of the bladder (6). King et al. (3) also described unilateral renal agenesis in both sisters.

Genitourinary system. The female infants that died in infancy had variable genital anomalies, including normal ovaries but thin, coiled fallopian tubes in one and markedly hypoplastic ovaries and uterus, and vaginal atresia in the other. In the two living sibs, the urethral opening was shifted posteriorly in one, and the vaginal opening was absent in both (8). One girl reported by Turner (6) had an anteriorly placed stenotic rectum and vaginal atresia. King et al. (3) also observed vaginal atresia in both sibs.

Auditory system. The two living sibs described by Winter et al. (8) had narrowed external auditory canals; the younger sib had low-set ears. Hearing loss was suspected in the latter when she was 1 year old. Audiometric tests at 3 years showed a 50 dB bilateral conductive hearing loss. Surgery revealed a malformed incus with fixation of the malleus and incus in the attic. Hearing loss was suspected in the older girl in early childhood. Otologic examination at 20 years showed severe conductive loss in one ear and a moderate high-tone conductive loss in the other. Tympanotomy revealed an absent incus (5). The patient reported by Turner (6) had very narrow external auditory canals and mild hearing loss. King et al. (3) found mild conductive hearing impairment and stenotic external auditory canals.

Laboratory findings. Intravenous pyelograms revealed renal anomalies in two sibs (3). Autopsies performed on two children showed the renal and genital anomalies as noted above. In one child, atrial septal defect and patent ductus arteriosus were also noted (3).

Heredity. Affected sibs (3,6,8) and parental consanguinity (3) suggest autosomal recessive inheritance (Fig. 9–13).

Diagnosis. Patients with renal disease, digital anomalies, and conductive hearing loss (1) have bulbous distal phalanges and cleft uvula, which are not described in the syndrome discussed above. However, until more cases are reported, the possibility of the disorders being identical cannot be excluded. Franek (2) described a small female with mild cryptotia, clitoral enlargement, hypoplasia of the labia minora, aplasia of the kidney, and sensorineural hearing loss. Litterie and Vauss described an association between Müllerian tract abnormalities (mainly bicornuate uterus), renal anomalies (unilateral renal agenesis and bifid ureter), and high-frequency sensorineural deafness (4).

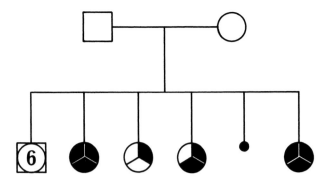

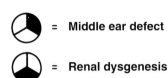
= **Middle ear defect**

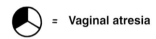
= **Renal dysgenesis**

= **Vaginal atresia**

Figure 9–13. *Renal, genital, and middle ear anomalies (Winter syndrome).* Pedigree showing 4 affected persons among 10 sibs. [From JSD Winter et al., *J Pediatr* 72:88, 1968.]

Prognosis. There is moderate variation in the degree of severity of the lesions in affected persons. If a single kidney is involved, a patient can live an essentially normal life.

Summary. This syndrome is characterized by (*1*) autosomal recessive transmission; (*2*) unilateral or bilateral renal hypoplasia or agenesis; (*3*) variable involvement of the genital system with occasional hypoplastic ovaries, tubes, or vagina; and (*4*) moderate to severe conductive hearing loss with malformation of the ossicles.

References

1. Braun FC Jr, Bayer JF: Familial nephrosis associated with deafness and congenital urinary tract anomalies in siblings. *J Pediatr* 60:33–41, 1962.
2. Franek A: An oto-uro-genital syndrome with microsomia. *Monatschr Kinderheilkd* 130:731–733, 1982.
3. King LA et al: Syndrome of genital, renal and middle ear anomalies: a third family and report of a pregnancy. *Obstet Gynecol* 69:491–493, 1987.
4. Litterie GS, Vauss N: Müllerian tract abnormalities and associated auditory defects. *J Reprod Med* 36:765–768, 1991.
5. Schmidt ECH et al: Renal aplasia in sisters. *Arch Pathol* 54:403–406, 1952.
6. Turner G: A second family with renal, vaginal, and middle ear anomalies. *J Pediatr* 76:641, 1970.
7. Willemsen WNP: Renal-skeletal-ear and facial anomalies in combination with the Mayer-Rokitansky-Küster (MRK) syndrome. *Eur J Obstet Gynecol Reprod* 14:121–130, 1982.
8. Winter JSD et al: A familial syndrome of renal, genital, and middle ear anomalies. *J Pediatr* 72:88–93, 1968.

Renal failure, cataracts, recurrent infections, and conductive hearing loss

In 1992, Siegler et al. (1) described a syndrome in sibs involving visual, auditory, respiratory, gastrointestinal, and renal systems.

Ocular system. Both sibs had cataracts, first identified at around 3 or 4 years of age.

Gastrointestinal system. Both sibs first manifested failure to thrive at age 5 or 6. This was accompanied by steatorrhea and metabolic acidosis, followed in both by chronic diarrhea.

Renal system. Initially, both sibs presented with hyposthenuria. This was followed by proteinuria, progressive azotemia, and anemia.

Respiratory system. Both suffered from bronchitis, sinusitis, and recurrent pneumonia. Death ensued just prior to puberty.

Auditory findings. Conductive hearing loss was present in both children, possibly the result of otitis media.

Heredity. Inheritance is possibly autosomal recessive. There was distant parental consanguinity.

Summary. Characteristics include (*1*) possible autosomal recessive inheritance; (*2*) cataracts in childhood; (*3*) early renal failure; (*4*) steatorrhea and chronic diarrhea; (*5*) recurrent respiratory problems; and (*6*) conductive hearing loss.

Reference

1. Siegler RL et al: New syndrome involving visual, auditory, respiratory, gastrointestinal, and renal systems. *Am J Med Genet* 44:461–464, 1992.

BRESHECK syndrome (*B*rain anomalies, *R*etardation of mentality and growth, *E*ctodermal dysplasia, *S*keletal malformations, *H*irschsprung disease, *E*ar deformity and deafness, eye hypoplasia, *C*left palate, cryptorchidism, and *K*idney dysplasia/hypoplasia)

Reish et al. (1) described two maternal half brothers both with microhydrocephaly, growth delay, mental retardation, ectodermal dysplasia, hemivertebrae/scoliosis, abnormal ears and conductive hearing loss, eye anomalies, cryptorchidism, and renal dysplasia/hypoplasia (1). Submucous cleft palate, Hirschsprung disease, and unilateral testicular agenesis were additional features present in only one of the two siblings. Only one brother survived the neonatal period; the other showed profound developmental delay.

Physical findings. Marked growth delay was noted in the surviving twin.

Central nervous system. The first half-sibling was found to have enlarged lateral cerebral ventricles with dilatation of the spinal canal at postmortem, absent septum pellucidum, and fusion of the thalami. The surviving half-sib developed complex partial neonatal seizures and had a thin corpus callosum with enlarged ventricles on MRI scanning. There was marked plagiocephaly but no craniosynostosis. Development of the

survivor was markedly delayed with a developmental age of 9 months at chronological age of 7 years.

Integumentary system. The authors described lamellar desquamation and diffuse scaling most prominent on the scalp but also on the trunk. There was also generalized alopecia of the scalp, eyebrows, and eyelashes. On microscopy there was marked epidermal hyperkeratosis with hyperkeratinized hair follicles. On some sections there was a reduction in hair follicle number but eccrine glands were normal. The findings were said to be consistent with an ectodermal dysplasia. Sweating and teeth were normal in the surviving child.

Skeletal system. Postaxial polydactyly was noted in the first child, together with bilateral talipes and multiple flexion contractures and dislocation of one hip. In the second surviving child there were hemivertebrae and abnormal segmentation of the ribs.

Ocular system. One half-sibling had microphthalmia and the other had small, oval-shaped optic nerves.

Renal. One half-sibling had dysplastic muticystic kidneys with a hypoplastic bladder and absent ureters. This led to Potter sequence and his early death. The other had a unilateral hypoplasia/aplasia, a small bladder, and severe ureteric reflux.

Auditory findings. External ears were described as large, low-set, and posteriorly angulated. Brain stem evoked responses in the surviving child showed bilateral mixed hearing loss affecting mainly the high frequencies.

Heredity. Inheritance would be consistent with X-linkage but also compatible with gonadal mosaicism for an autosomal dominant gene or contiguous gene deletion.

Summary. The syndrome characteristics are (*1*) X-linked or autosomal dominant inheritance; and (*2*) multiple congenital anomalies consisting of brain anomalies, retardation of growth and development, ectodermal dysplasia, skeletal deformities, Hirschsprung disease, ear/eye anomalies, cleft palate, cryptorchidism, and kidney dysplasia/hypoplasia and reflux.

Reference

1. Reish O et al: Brain anomalies, retardation of mentality and growth, ectodermal dysplasia, skeletal malformations, Hirschsprung disease, ear deformity and deafness, eye hypoplasia, cleft palate, cryptorchidism and kidney dysplasia/hypoplasia (BRESEK/BRESHECK): new X-linked syndrome? *Am J Med Genet* 68:386–390, 1997.

Appendix

Other conditions with renal anomalies

Entity	Renal Finding	Chapter in this Book
Branchio-oto-renal syndrome	Renal agenesis, polycystic kidneys	6 (external ear)
Beighton syndrome	Fanconi type nephropathy	7 (eye)
Fraser cryptophthalmos syndrome	Renal agenesis	7 (eye)
Renal tubulopathy, diabetes mellitus, cerebellar ataxia	Renal tubulopathy	10 (neurologic)
Cutler syndrome	Nephropathy	10 (neurologic)
Feigenbaum syndrome	Nephropathy	10 (neurologic)
Hypoparathyroidism, deafness, and renal disease	Renal dysplasia	12 (endocrine)
Hyperparathyroidism, nephropathy, and sensorineural hearing loss	Renal failure	12 (endocrine)

Chapter 10
Genetic Hearing Loss Associated with Neurologic and Neuromuscular Disorders

HELGA V. TORIELLO

Many progressive neurodegenerative diseases are associated with sensorineural hearing loss, but the classification of these disorders remains controversial. This chapter combines reports of families with similar disorders and different ages of onset, but separates similar families if the pattern of inheritance was different. It is apparent that some neurological manifestations of these diseases tend to cluster. For example, ataxia is frequently associated with spastic paraplegia ("spinocerebellar ataxia") and with motor and sensory neuropathy. Pigmentary retinopathies (which include retinitis pigmentosa) are often associated with optic atrophy. Some are considered in this chapter, but others were assigned to Chapter 7. In many older reports, modern neurodiagnostic tests often were not available, making clinical distinctions more difficult. Because of the clinical similarity, it is possible that some disorders described in this section represent unrecognized mitochondrial encephalomyopathies.

Neurofibromatosis, type 2 (vestibular schwannomas and sensorineural hearing loss)

In 1920, Feiling and Ward (9) described a large family affected with acoustic neuromas (vestibular schwannomas) and neural hearing loss. As early as a century before, others (3,50) noted isolated examples. Follow-up of a family first reported in 1930 (10,11) showed that almost 100 individuals were involved (52). Many additional kindreds have been described (6,14,23,31,36,49). Diagnostic prevalence has been estimated at one per million in one study (16), and 1/200,000 in another (5). Birth prevalence is approximately 1/40,500 (5) in one study, and 1/87,410 in another (1). About 4% of individuals with acoustic neuromas have type 2 neurofibromatosis (NF-2) (8). It has been estimated that NF-2 accounts for 5%–10% of all neurofibromatosis cases. The reader is referred to many excellent reviews of the subject (2,5,6,15,19,21,25,26,29,34).

Diagnostic criteria for NF-2 were recently established by a National Institutes of Health (NIH) Consensus Development Conference (35). Accepted criteria include bilateral eighth nerve masses, a first-degree relative with NF-2 and unilateral eighth nerve mass, or a first-degree relative with NF-2 and any two of the following: glioma, meningioma, neurofibroma, schwannoma, or juvenile posterior subcapsular lenticular opacity. More recently it has been suggested that there should be additional criteria for evaluation of NF-2, including having a family history of NF-2; for persons younger than 30 presence of unilateral vestibular schwannoma or meningioma; and presence of multiple spinal tumors (12).

Central nervous system. Tumors of the central or peripheral nervous system are hallmarks of NF-2 and may result in virtually any type of focal neurological deficit. Besides hearing loss, other common symptoms include headaches, facial weakness, sensory or visual changes, or unsteadiness. In most patients, symptoms begin in the teens or 20's, but it is not uncommon to remain asymptomatic past age 30. Rarely, the tumors will present as early as the first or as late as the seventh decade of life. The most common type of tumor is schwannoma, which often involves the vestibular nerve (acoustic neuromas). They may be unilat-

eral or bilateral and often are not synchronous. Schwann cell tumors may also occur on any of the cranial nerves or spinal roots, especially on sensory nerves or roots. Using magnetic resonance imaging (MRI), one group found the frequency of spinal tumors to be 63% (38). Wertelecki et al. (49) found 9 of 11 patients had nontumoral intracranial calcifications. However, these are not considered a diagnostic feature (13). Other tumor types include gliomas that are usually low grade, ependymomas, meningiomas, and neurofibromas. While less frequent than acoustic neuromas, gliomas and meningiomas often become symptomatic at an earlier age (14,23,40,52). The cumulative neurological effects may be devastating and often lead to severe morbidity and death.

Bilateral vestibular schwannomas (acoustic neuromas) occur in 95% of those affected (Fig. 10–1A). Clinical data on 100 patients indicated that the average age of onset was 20 years (range 15–30 years) (5,52). The clinical course was variable and, in some cases, relatively benign. Rarely did signs become manifest in infancy (42) and only about 5% did not have symptoms until age 35 years or older. Physical examination of affected persons showed no evidence of type 1 neurofibromatosis (NF-1). Wertelecki et al. (49), by contrast found that nearly one-half of their patients were asymptomatic for the first 30 years of life. Kanter et al. (21) and Evans et al. (5,6) suggested that there is earlier onset if the affected child is born to an affected mother. In a large study of 334 individuals with NF-2, 18% presented before 15 years of age. Not all patients presented with vestibular schwannomas; many had meningioma, spinal tumor, or cutaneous tumor as the presenting sign (7).

Three types of nervous system signs develop: those caused by encroachment on adjacent cranial nerves by the vestibular schwannomas, those caused by increased intracranial pressure, and those caused occasionally by other nervous system tumors. In some affected persons, palsies of the fifth, sixth, seventh, ninth, and tenth cranial nerves as well as cerebellar ataxia develop. Impaired intelligence is not part of the syndrome.

Peripheral nervous system. Schwannomas or neurofibromas may develop from deeper nerves and result in a subtle subcutaneous mass or localized sensory disturbance or weakness.

Ocular system. Progressive visual loss is common. Slightly over 50% of those who died with known disease were blind, and 8% had markedly decreased vision due to increased intracranial pressure with papilledema (52). More recent estimates suggest that as many as 75% have visual impairment (24). Subcapsular cataracts develop early (<16 years) in about 50% (6,20,24,36,39) and may be seen in as many as 80% (37). Retinal hamartomas and epiretinal membranes occur in 9%–22% of those with NF-2, and these are likely to be present from a young age (13). Over 10% of patients have juvenile amblyopia/strabismus (24). Lisch nodules, common in NF-1, are not found in NF-2, nor are optic gliomas (4). Because the lens opacities develop prior to the tumors, they may allow identification of those at risk.

Integumentary system. From 20% to 65% have a few small (<2 cm) cutaneous neurofibromas, especially in the scalp. In half of patients, skin tumors are the first clinical sign of NF-2 (22). They are of three types. The most common type is discrete, somewhat raised, roughened,

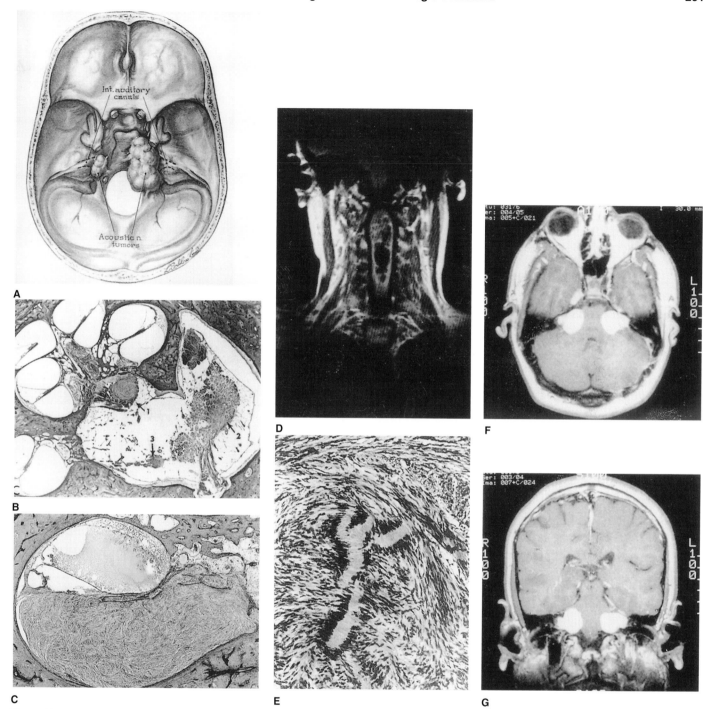

Figure 10–1. *Neurofibromatosis, type 2.* (A) Bilateral acoustic neuromas (schwannomas) in a 20-year-old woman. (B) Midmodiolar section through cochlea showing three neurinomas in auditory canal. (C) Total destruction of hair cells in organ of Corti. Severe degeneration of stria vascularis and spiral ligament. Tumor mass invades entire space of scala tympani. Note total destruction of ganglion cells. (D) A T$_1$-weighted image of the cervical spine in the coronal plane after administration of gadolinium shows a large, loculated, irregular cyst involving most of the cervical spinal cord. Note enhancement of cyst wall and of mass projecting into upper portion of cyst. At surgery, this tumor proved to be an ependymoma. (E) Marked palisading of cell nuclei in an area of fibrillary architecture. (F,G) Axial and coronal MRI with gadolinium enhancement showing 18-year-old male with synchronous, bilateral, moderate-sized acoustic neuromas. [(A,B,E) from GT Nager, *Arch Otolaryngol* 89:252, 1969; (C) from JT Benitez et al., *Int Audiol* 6:181, 1967; (D) courtesy of W Wertelecki, Mobile, Alabama; (F,G) courtesy of JB Nadol Jr, Boston, Massachusetts.]

usually pigmented skin, accompanied by excessive hair. The next most common type consists of well-circumscribed, mobile, often spherical tumors, associated with peripheral nerves. The least common are similar to the intradermal violaceous lesion of NF-1. Histologically most tumors of all three types are found to contain Schwann cells (27). About 40% have a few (less than six) small café-au-lait spots (5,6,9,16,21,52). Intertriginous freckling does not occur (2,5).

Auditory system. About 45% of patients present with hearing loss that is unilateral in over 75% of cases. The loss is often noted when using a telephone. In some cases of unilateral involvement, as many as 10 years elapse before the other ear becomes affected (4,49). In general, the risk of patients with a sporadic unilateral vestibular schwannoma developing a contralateral tumor in the absence of positive family history or other features of NF-2 is low, but those who have a positive family history and/or other typical tumors have a much higher risk of developing contralateral tumors (8). Hearing loss, usually first noted in the second or third decade, is progressive, resulting in total deafness within 5–10 years. Hearing loss due to unilateral or bilateral vestibular schwannomas is the first symptom in 50% of cases, with tinnitus or roaring sound in 10%–30%, imbalance in 10%, and facial twitching in 5% being the presenting sign. Audiograms generally show no or slow pure-tone change, progressive loss of discrimination, and more marked loss at higher frequencies (14,30,40).

Vestibular system. Vestibular abnormalities may occur before audiometric change (4,52). Several persons in the family described by Young et al. (52) nearly drowned because they had lost direction under water; three other members, not known to be affected, did drown. It is possible that they were in the early stage of the disorder and had only vestibular involvement.

Radiographic studies. These studies may show enlarged internal auditory meatuses due to the vestibular schwannomas. Computed tomography (CT) scan and MRI studies are employed to visualize the tumors.

Pathology. Multiple schwannomas arise from cranial nerves, especially from the vestibular branch of the eighth nerve, dorsal and ventral roots, and deep peripheral nerves (Fig. 10–1A–C). Gliomas and ependymomas are usually low grade, but may be located anywhere in the neuroaxis, including the brain stem and spinal cord (Fig. 10–1D). Meningiomas are usually multiple. Bilateral vestibular schwannomas often measure from 1 to 6 cm in diameter and encroach upon the basis pontis and adjacent cranial nerves (10,11,32,45). Histologic sections show characteristic interlacing bundles of elongated cells forming palisades (31,40) (Fig. 10–1E).

Heredity. NF-2 has autosomal dominant inheritance with high penetrance. About 50% of carriers become symptomatic by 25 years of age. NF-2 is caused by a mutation in the responsible gene, *merlin* (12,33,43,44,48,49), a tumor-suppressor gene that maps to 22q12 (51). There is preliminary evidence that there may be genotype–phenotype correlations (12,46) with the type of mutation, but studies have not produced consistent results. About 50% of cases are new mutations (5). Evans et al. (5) suggested maternal imprinting with a greater transmission by females (almost 2:1). They further suggested heterogeneity, with one type having earlier onset, a rapid course, bilateral vestibular schwannomas, and other tumors (Wishart type); the other type having late onset, a more benign course, and usually just bilateral vestibular schwannomas (Gardner type). This latter discrepancy may be due to genotype–phenotype correlations (12,46), however. Recently, Zhao et al. (54) have demonstrated that there is strong intrafamilial correlation of clinical manifestations, particularly for age at onset of hearing loss and number of meningiomas.

Diagnosis. Audiological and vestibular assessment [pure-tone, speech impedance audiography, brain stem auditory evoked response (BAER), internal auditory tomograms, electronystagmography] are indicated, with auditory evoked response being the most sensitive technique (19). Imaging for vestibular schwannomas can be performed using CT scans or MRI with gadolinium-DPTA contrast enhancement (37,53) (Fig. 10–1F,G). Air cisternography has been especially effective (18).

NF-2 should be distinguished from NF-1 because clinical manifestations, gene localization, and management are distinct. About 5% of patients with NF-1 have meningiomas or astrocytomas and 2%–4% have vestibular schwannomas but only rarely are they bilateral (16,21). NF-1 also has autosomal dominant transmission and characteristically (95%) is associated with café-au-lait spots and cutaneous neurofibromatosis, which are present in NF-2 with considerably less frequency (2,16). Lisch nodules of the iris are not found with increased frequency in NF-2. Incidentally, a few small café-au-lait spots may be seen in 5%–10% of the normal population. Bilateral vestibular schwannomas differ in sev-

eral ways from unilateral ones. The former are hereditary, develop earlier in life, and are harder to manage. Bilateral vestibular schwannomas can reach remarkable size, effecting severe distortion of the brain stem, enlarging and eroding the bony walls of the internal meatus, and finally extending extradurally into the middle cranial fossa. The tumors tend to invade the marrow spaces and mastoid air cells (16). Nontumoral intracranial calcifications are found in both NF-1 and NF-2.

A condition called *neurilemmomatosis*, which consists of multiple peripheral and/or spinal schwannomas but without acoustic tumors or other signs of NF-1 or NF-2, has been described (47). It has recently been found, however, that the gene locus for neurilemmomatosis lies within the NF-2 region, thus this condition may be allelic with NF-2 (17).

Prognosis. After puberty, growth of vestibular schwannomas is unpredictable. In some patients, there may be only minimal growth for many years; in others, there is inexorable progress with resultant hearing loss, chronic headache, visual loss, and severe gait disturbance (41). Death may eventuate from pressure on and displacement of the brain stem. Mayfrank et al. (28) suggested that sporadic cases of NF-2 are more often associated with multiple meningiomas and spinal tumors. Unlike in NF-1, there is no apparent malignant transformation of the tumors.

Patients live an average of about 20 years (range 2–44 years) after onset of symptoms, which occurs, at about 35 years.

Summary. Characteristics of NF-2 include (*1*) autosomal dominant inheritance; (*2*) bilateral vestibular schwannomas (acoustic neuromas); (*3*) schwannomas involving other nerves; (*4*) brain tumors, especially meningiomas and gliomas; (*5*) juvenile posterior subcapsular cataracts; (*6*) sometimes café-au-lait spots and subcutaneous neurofibromas (but fewer than in NF-1); and (*7*) neural hearing loss and altered vestibular function.

References

1. Antinheimo J et al: Population-based analysis of sporadic and type 2 neurofibromatosis–associated meningiomas and schwannomas. *Neurology* 54:71–76, 2000.
2. Baldwin RL, Le Master K: Neurofibromatosis-2 and bilateral acoustic neuromas. Distinction from neurofibromatosis-1 (von Recklinghausen's disease). *Am J Otol* 10:439–442, 1989.
3. Cushing H: *Tumors of the Nervus Acusticus*, W.B. Saunders, Philadelphia, 1917.
4. Eldridge R: Central neurofibromatosis with bilateral acoustic neuroma. *Adv Neurol* 29:57–65, 1981.
5. Evans DGR et al: A genetic study of type 2 neurofibromatosis in the United Kingdom. *J Med Genet* 29:841–846,847–852, 1992.
6. Evans DGR et al: A clinical study of type 2 neurofibromatosis. *Q J Med* 84:603–618, 1992.
7. Evans DGR et al: Paediatric presentation of type 2 neurofibromatosis. *Arch Dis Child* 81:496–499, 1999.
8. Evans DGR et al: Probability of bilateral disease in people presenting with a unilateral vestibular schwannoma. *J Neurol Neruosurg Psychiatry* 66:764–767, 1999.
9. Feiling A, Ward E: A familial form of acoustic tumour. *BMJ* 1:496–497, 1920.
10. Gardner WJ, Frazier CH: Bilateral acoustic neurofibromas: a clinical study and field survey of a family of five generations with bilateral deafness in thirty-eight members. *Arch Neurol Psychiatry* 23:266–300, 1930.
11. Gardner WJ, Turner O: Bilateral acoustic neurofibromas. Further clinical and pathologic data onhereditary deafness and von Recklinghausen's disease. *Arch Neurol Psychiatry* 44:76–99, 1940.
12. Gutmann DH: Review: molecular insights into neurofibromatosis 2. *Neurobiol Dis* 3:247–261, 1997.
13. Gutmann DH et al: The diagnostic evaluation and multidisciplinary management of neurofibromatosis 1 and neurofibromatosis 2. *JAMA* 278:51–57, 1997.
14. Hitselberger WE, Hughes RL: Bilateral acoustic tumors and neurofibromatosis. *Arch Otolaryngol* 88:700–711, 1968.
15. Hughes GB et al: Management of bilateral acoustic tumors. *Laryngoscope* 92:1351–1359, 1982.
16. Huson SM, Thrush DC: Central neurofibromatosis. *Q J Med* 55:213–224, 1985.

17. Iyengar V et al: Neurilemmomatosis, NF2, and juveniile xanthogranuloma. *J Am Acad Dermatol* 39:831–834, 1998.

18. Johnson DW: Air cisternography of the cerebellopontine angle using high resolution computed tomography. *Radiology* 151:401–403, 1984.

19. Jones RM et al: Familial central neurofibromatosis. *Otolaryngol Head Neck Surg* 91:527–531, 1983.

20. Kaiser-Kupfer MI et al: The association of posterior lens opacities with bilateral acoustic neuromas in patients with neurofibromatosis type 2. *Arch Ophthalmol* 107:541–544, 1989.

21. Kanter WR et al: Central neurofibromatosis with bilateral acoustic neuroma: genetic, clinical and biochemical distinctions from peripheral neurofibromatosis. *Neurology* 30:851–859, 1980.

22. Kluwe I et al: Mutations and allelic loss of the NF2 gene in neurofibromatosis 2-associated skin tumors. *J Invest Dermatol* 114:1017–1021, 2000.

23. Lee DK, Abbott ML: Familial central nervous system neoplasia. *Arch Neurol* 20:154–160, 1969.

24. MacCollin M, Mautner V-F: The diagnosis and management of neurofibromatosis 2 in childhood. *Semin Pediatr Neurol* 5:243–252, 1998.

25. Martuza RL, Eldridge R: Neurofibromatosis 2 (bilateral acoustic neurofibromatosis). *N Engl J Med* 318:684–688, 1988.

26. Martuza RL, Ojemann RG: Bilateral acoustic neuromas: clinical aspects, pathogenesis, and treatment. *Neurosurgery* 10:1–12, 1982.

27. Mautner VF et al: Skin abnormalities in neurofibromatosis 2. *Arch Dermatol* 133:1539–1543, 1997.

28. Mayfrank L et al: Neurofibromatosis 2: a clinically and genetically heterogeneous disease? Report on 10 sporadic cases. *Clin Genet* 38:362–370, 1990.

29. McKennan KX, Bard A: Neurofibromatosis type 2: report of a family and review of current evaluation and treatment. *Laryngoscope* 101:109–113, 1991.

30. Miyamoto RT et al: Preservation of hearing in neurofibromatosis. 2. *Otolaryngol Head Neck Surg* 103:619–624, 1990.

31. Moyes PD: Familial bilateral acoustic neuromas affecting 14 members from four generations. *J Neurosurg* 29:78–82, 1968.

32. Nager GT: Acoustic neurinomas. Pathology and differential diagnosis. *Arch Otolaryngol* 89:252–279, 1969.

33. Narod SA et al: Neurofibromatosis type 2 appears to be a genetically homogenous disease. *Am J Hum Genet* 51:486–496, 1992.

34. Neary WJ et al: A clinical, genetic and audiological study of patients and families with bilateral acoustic neurofibromas. *J Laryngol Otol* 107:6–11, 1993.

35. NIH Consensus Development Conference: Neurofibromatosis. *Arch Neurol* 45:575–578, 1988.

36. Parry DM et al: Neurofibromatosis 2 (bilateral acoustic or central neurofibromatosis), a treatable cause of deafness. *Ann NY Acad Sci* 630:305–307, 1991.

37. Pastores GM et al: Early childhood diagnosis of acoustic neuromas in presymptomatic individuals at risk for neurofibromatosis 2. *Am J Med Genet* 41:325–329, 1991.

38. Patronas NJ et al: Intramedullary and spinal canal tumors in patients with neurofibromatosis 2: MR imaging findings and correlation with genotype. *Radio* 218:434–442, 2001.

39. Pearson-Webb MA et al: Eye findings in bilateral acoustic (central) neurofibromatosis: association with presenile lens opacities and cataracts but absence of Lisch nodules. *N Engl J Med* 315:1553–1554, 1986.

40. Perez De Moura LF et al: Bilateral neurinoma and neurofibromatosis. *Arch Otolaryngol* 90:28–34, 1969.

41. Piffko P, Pasztor E: Operated bilateral acoustic neurinoma with preservation of hearing and facial nerve function. *ORL Otorhinolaryngol Relat Spec* 43:255–261, 1981.

42. Rosenberg D et al: Le neurinome bilat;aeral de l'acoustique chez l'enfant. *Ann Pédiatr (Paris)* 21:257–263, 1974.

43. Rouleau GA et al: Genetic linkage of bilateral acoustic neurofibromatosis to a DNA marker on chromosome 22. *Nature* 329:246–248, 1987.

44. Rouleau GA et al: Flanking markers bracket the neurofibromatosis type 2 (NF2) gene on chromosome 22. *Am J Hum Genet* 46:323–328, 1990.

45. Rubenstein LJ: The malformative central nervous system lesions in the central and peripheral forms of neurofibromatosis. *Ann NY Acad Sci* 486:14–29, 1986.

46. Sainio M et al: Mild familial neurofibromatosis 2 associates with expression of merlin with altered COOH-terminus. *Neurology* 54:1132–1138, 2000.

47. Shishiba T: Follow-up study of a patient with neurilemmomatosis. *J Am Acad Dermatol* 37(5 pt 1):797–799, 1997.

48. Trofatter JA et al: A novel moesin-, ezrin-, radixin-like gene is a candidate for the neurofibromatosis 2 tumor suppressor. *Cell* 72:1–20, 1993.

49. Wertelecki W et al: Neurofibromatosis 2: clinical and DNA linkage studies of a large kindred. *N Engl J Med* 319:278–283, 1988.

50. Wishart JH: Case of tumours in the skull, dura mater and brain. *Edinb Med Surg J* 393–397, 1822.

51. Wolff RK et al: Analysis of chromosome 22 deletions in neurofibromatosis type 2–related tumors. *Am J Hum Genet* 51:478–485, 1992.

52. Young DF et al: Bilateral acoustic neuroma in a large kindred. *JAMA* 214:347–353, 1970.

53. Young IR et al: The role of NMR imaging in the diagnosis and management of acoustic neuroma. *AJNR Am J Neuroradiol* 4:223–224, 1983.

54. Zhao Y et al: Intrafamilial correlation of clinical manifestations in neurofibromatosis 2 (NF2). *Genet Epidemiol* 23:245–259, 2002.

Cockayne syndrome

In 1936, Cockayne (5) first described a syndrome of progressive growth failure, neurologic deterioration superimposed on mental retardation, visual and hearing loss, facial and skeletal changes, photodermatitis, and other abnormalities. Subsequently, over 150 patients with Cockayne syndrome (CS) were reported (26,31). Four forms exist: the classic form is designated type 1, the congenital form is type 2, a later-onset form with normal development is type 3, and the fourth form, which shows overlap between Cockayne syndrome and xeroderma pigmentosum, is CS-XP (15,20,25,26). These divisions are based on clinical features. Cockayne syndrome has also been divided into groups A and B, based on protein complementation, which generally correspond to the two genes identified so far, *ERCC8* and *ERCC6*.

For clinical diagnosis of type 1 CS there must be severe and progressive postnatal growth failure with relatively normal birth weight, mental retardation, later neurological dysfunction consistent with prominent white matter involvement, and at least three of the following: skin photosensitivity, pigmentary retinopathy, cataracts, optic atrophy, sensorineural hearing loss, marked dental caries, and characteristic appearance of cachectic dwarfism (26).

Children with type 2 CS have the same manifestations, but with earlier onset and more severe symptoms. The latter consist of low birth weight, little postnatal growth, minimal or no developmental progress, early onset of characteristic cachectic appearance, and congenital or early childhood cataracts (13,20,25,26,30). Some children who have been diagnosed as having cerebrooculofacioskeletal (COFS) syndrome have been found to have CS type 2, on the basis of molecular studies (22).

Physical findings. Growth failure is profound and begins within the first year of life, although birth weight and other growth indices are usually normal in CS type 1. Weight is more affected than length, which has led to use of the term "cachectic dwarfism" in describing CS patients. Height or weight measurement over the fifth centile in a child over 2 years is incompatible with the diagnosis of CS type 1. Although head circumference may be normal during the first 6 months of life in type 1 CS, almost all patients over 2 years have microcephaly (26). Children with CS type 2 have low birth weight, low head circumference, and extremely poor postnatal growth. Weight never exceeds 8 kg and occipitofrontal circumference (OFC) is never more than 38 cm (20,25,26).

Appearance is relatively normal during the first year in CS type 1. Subsequently, a recognizable appearance emerges that consists of generalized decrease in subcutaneous fat involving the face, microcephaly, sunken eyes, beaked nose, large ears, small jaw, and relatively large hands and feet, all of which impart a senile appearance (26,31) (Fig. 10–2). In CS type 2, the same appearance is evident at birth or during the first year. Marked dental caries was described in 86% of CS patients (3,35).

Central nervous system. The earliest sign of neurologic dysfunction is developmental delay, which usually becomes apparent at about 1 year, when walking and speech should develop. About 10% of cases come to medical attention earlier because of weak cry or poor feeding, but diagnosis is rarely made unless a sib is affected. All patients with CS type 1 have mental retardation, most frequently in the mild or moderate range. Over 20% never progress beyond use of single words. Still,

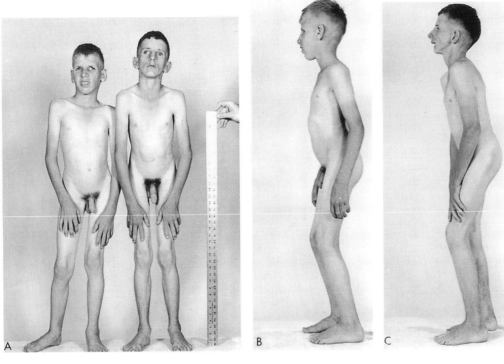

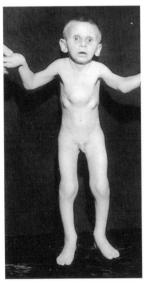

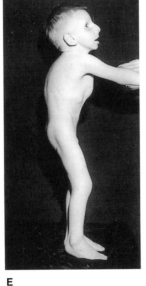

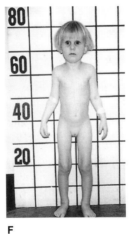

Figure 10–2. *Cockayne syndrome, type 1.* (A–C) Fourteen-and sixteen-year-old sibs with marked mental and somatic retardation, eye difficulties, and sensorineural hearing loss. Note wizened appearance, photodermatitis of sun-exposed areas, horse-riding stance, and large hands and feet. (D,E) Wizened appearance of 6-year-old boy with kyphosis and flexion deformities of the joints. (F) Note similar phenotype including horse-riding stance and sunken eyes. [(A–C) from RM Paddison et al., *Dermatol Trop* 2:196, 1963; (D,E) from A Moosa and V Dubowitz, *Arch Dis Child* 45:674, 1970.]

they are often characterized as happy and socially interactive. Early signs of generalized spasticity are apparent by 5–10 years and remain stable for several years. Patients with CS type 2 have profound mental retardation and earlier onset of spasticity.

Among higher-functioning patients, behavioral and intellectual deterioration often occur, usually in teen years. Motor signs progress to spastic quadriplegia with hyperactive tendon reflexes and extensor plantar responses, flexion contractures, and scoliosis. These signs are usually accompanied by dysarthria, coarse tremor, ataxia, and sometimes choreoathetosis. Gait disorder, striking and progressive, results from a combination of leg spasticity, ataxia, and contractures of the hips, knees, and ankles. Later there may be further wasting and decreased tendon reflexes due to peripheral neuropathy. Seizures are reported in 5%–10%, but rarely present initially. Progression becomes more rapid during the last few years before death, leading to a cachectic, bedridden state (26,31). Cranial CT and MRI scans in older patients show diffuse white matter hypomyelination or demyelination, bilateral basal ganglia and subcortical calcifications, and cerebellar atrophy (1,2,19,41).

Peripheral nervous system. Neuropathic changes, such as further weakness and wasting, and decreased or absent tendon reflexes often occur during teen years. Nerve conduction studies are slow (20–38 m/sec), consistent with demyelinating motor and sensory neuropathy. Some patients have diminished lacrimation or sweating, miotic pupils, and cool limbs. These symptoms may be due to autonomic dysfunction, but no autonomic testing has been reported (8).

Ocular system. Sunken eyes are a virtually constant feature. Progressive visual loss due to retinal pigmentary degeneration, usually of the "salt-and-pepper" type, has been reported in a majority but certainly not in all patients. The true incidence may be very high, as reports of normal fundus in early childhood do not exclude it. In most patients, visual loss is noticed at about 2 years and progresses to blindness after about 10 years. Optic atrophy and cataracts have been reported in about 35% of patients (13). Cataracts, present at birth or within the first 3 years of life, are a predictor of CS type 2 and poor prognosis (13). Congenital malformations of the eye, such as iris hypoplasia and microphthalmos, have been reported in a few patients with CS type 2. Less common eye abnormalities include nystagmus, photophobia, and corneal scarring (4,26).

Musculoskeletal system. Common skeletal changes include kyphoscoliosis, pectus carinatum, small clavicles, disproportionately long limbs with large hands and feet, joint contractures, pes valgus, and short second toes. Skeletal X-rays show thickened calvaria and skull base, small facial bones, early appearance of epiphyseal centers in long bones, sclerotic "ivory" epiphyses most prominent in the fingers, vertebral body abnormalities such as anterior notching, wedging, and flattening, long thin ribs, pelvic abnormalities including small, "squared-off" pelvis, and hypoplastic iliac wings, coxa valga, and osteoporosis (1,30,40).

Integumentary system. A scaly rash occurs in over–sun-exposed areas by age 2 or before in at least 75% of cases, and is often one of the earliest signs of the disease. Decrease in subcutaneous tissue, scarring, pigmentary changes, and thin dry hair are seen in older patients.

Genitourinary system. Renal complications occur in about 10% of CS patients. Most have elevated renal function tests such as blood urea nitrogen (BUN), creatinine, or decreased creatinine clearance, which do not require treatment. Some have hypertension and a few have died of renal failure (26). About a third of affected males have cryptorchidism and small testes (26).

Auditory system. Sensorineural hearing loss occurs in most patients with CS, with onset during childhood or teen years. The frequency and severity have not been well documented, perhaps because of the underlying neurological disorder, which makes testing difficult. Audiograms show bilateral sensorineural loss that varies from mild to severe (23,26,41).

Vestibular system. No study has been reported.

Laboratory findings. Cells from patients with CS are usually sensitive to killing by ultraviolet light and chemicals that produce DNA damage (38,43,45). Also, the normal recovery of DNA and RNA synthesis after exposure does not occur. Cell fusion studies, using ultraviolet sensitivity, showed at least two complementation groups (16), designated A and B.

Pathology. At autopsy, the brain is small, with strikingly reduced white matter, and shows severe atrophy of the brain stem and cerebellum. Microscopic changes include patchy demyelination and gliosis of white matter, widespread mineralization primarily in vessel walls of the basal ganglia, subcortex, and cerebellum, atrophy of corticospinal and other tracts, and poor myelinization of optic nerves. Sural nerve biopsy shows segmental demyelination and remyelination with onion bulb formation that is consistent with a demyelinating neuropathy (12,13,18,23,27,40–42,47).

The retina of one child showed lipofuscin deposition in the retinal pigment epithelium, large pigment-laden cells in a perivascular distribution, cell loss in the ganglion cell and outer nuclear layers, disintegration of the outer segments of the photoreceptors, and some loss of inner segments. The optic nerve had marked thinning of nerve fiber bundles with axonal loss and partial demyelination of the remaining fibers. The cornea showed some accumulation of pigment-laden macrophages (18). A keratotomy specimen from another child showed marked corneal dystrophy (4).

The cochlea exhibits marked atrophy of the spiral ganglion and cochlear division of the eighth nerve, with transsynaptic degeneration in the ventral cochlear nucleus, medial dorsal olivary nucleus, and inferior colliculus (4,10,39).

Renal abnormalities consist of thickening of the basement membranes of the glomeruli, mesangium, and tubules, interstitial fibrosis, tubular atrophy, hyalinization of glomeruli, and thickening or atrophy of capillary loops. Immune complex deposits in glomerular basement membrane were found in two patients (34).

Heredity. Inheritance is autosomal recessive, as there have been repeated observations of families with several affected sibs with normal parents and increased frequency of parental consanguinity (1,13,29–31). Two genes have been identified and are designated *ERCC6* and *ERCC8* (which generally correspond to CSB and CSA, respectively). The clinical phenotype does not correlate with the genotype, however; for example, mutations in *CSB* can cause both Cockayne type 1 and type 2 phenotypes (6,7,21). Fryns et al. (9) suggested that the gene for late-onset CS may be located at 10q21.1. Some of the children with XP-CS have mutations in some of the xeroderma pigmentosum complementation group genes, including XPB, XPD, and XPG (14,28,33,44).

Diagnosis. Cockayne syndrome must be differentiated from progeria, as both have early-onset growth deficiency, decreased subcutaneous tissue, and premature senility. Patients with progeria do not have visual or hearing loss, mental retardation, or photosensitivity. The facial appearance of CS has some similarity to that of Seckel syndrome, but other manifestations differ. The brain and neurologic changes in CS are similar to those in infantile familial encephalopathy with cerebral calcifications and leukodystrophy except that onset of symptoms is consistently earlier in the latter syndrome. It also lacks manifestations in other systems (32). Somewhat similar phenotypes are seen in a syndrome of nephrogenic diabetes mellitus, somatic and mental retardation, and intracerebral calcifications (36). Prenatal diagnosis is possible using an assay on colony-forming ability or RNA synthesis following UV irradiation (17).

A defect in the nucleotide excision-repair pathway has been demonstrated in both CS and in XP. Some mutations in at least three of seven genes known to be involved in XP can result in partial or complete CS (11,24,37,46).

Prognosis. Many patients with CS type 1 have died in their 20's or 30's, of a variety of causes. Children with CS type 2 usually succumb before age 10 (15).

Summary. This disorder is characterized by (*1*) autosomal recessive inheritance; (*2*) severe growth failure; (*3*) mental retardation; (*4*) dementia; (*5*) spastic quadriplegia; (*6*) ataxia; (*7*) motor and sensory neuropathy; (*8*) pigmentary retinopathy; (*9*) optic atrophy; (*10*) cataracts; (*11*) photodermatitis; (*12*) decreased subcutaneous tissue; (*13*) abnormal facial appearance; (*14*) defective DNA repair; and (*15*) sensorineural hearing loss.

References

1. Bensman A et al: The spectrum of X-ray manifestations in Cockayne's syndrome. *Skeletal Radiol* 7:173–177, 1981.
2. Boltshauser E et al: MRI in Cockayne syndrome type I. *Neuroradiology* 31:276–277, 1989.
3. Borazo RA: Cockayne's syndrome: literature review and case report. *Pediatr Dent* 13:227–230, 1991.
4. Brodrick JD, Dark AJ: Corneal dystrophy in Cockayne's syndrome. *Br J Ophthalmol* 57:391–399, 1973.
5. Cockayne EA: Dwarfism with retinal atrophy and deafness. *Arch Dis Child* 11:1–8, 1936.
6. Colella S et al: Alterations in the CSB gene in three Italian patients with the severe form of Cockayne syndrome (CS) but without clinical photosensitivity. *Hum Mol Genet* 8:935–942, 1999.
7. Colella S et al: Identical mutations in the CSB gene associated with either Cockayne syndrome or the DeSanctis-Cacchione variant of xeroderma pigmentosum. *Hum Mol Genet* 9:1171–1175, 2000.
8. Dabbagh O, Swaiman KF: Cockayne syndrome: MRI correlates of hypomyelination. *Pediatr Neurol* 4:113–117, 1988.
9. Fryns JP et al: Apparent late-onset Cockayne syndrome and interstitial deletion of the long arm of chromosome 10(del(10)(q11.23q21.2)). *Am J Med Genet* 40:343–344, 1991.
10. Gandolfi A et al: Deafness in Cockayne's syndrome: morphological, morphometric, and quantitative study of the auditory pathway. *Ann Neurol* 15:134–143, 1984.

11. Greenhaw GA et al: Xeroderma pigmentosum and Cockayne: overlapping clinical and biochemical phenotypes. *Am J Hum Genet* 50:677–689, 1992.

12. Grunnet ML et al: Ultrastructure and electrodiagnosis of peripheral neuropathy in Cockayne's syndrome. *Neurology* 33:1606–1609, 1983.

13. Houston CS et al: Identical male twins and brother with Cockayne syndrome. *Am J Med Genet* 13:211–213, 1982.

14. Jaeken J et al: Clinical and biochemical studies in three patients with severe early infantile Cockayne syndrome. *Hum Genet* 83:339–346, 1989.

15. Kennedy RM et al: Cockayne syndrome: an atypical case. *Neurology* 30:1268–1272, 1980.

16. Lehmann AR: Three complementation groups in Cockayne syndrome. *Mutat Res* 106:347–356, 1982.

17. Lehmann AR et al: Prenatal diagnosis of Cockayne's syndrome. *Lancet* 1:486–488, 1985.

18. Levin PS et al: Histopathology of the eye in Cockayne's syndrome. *Arch Ophthalmol* 101:1093–1097, 1983.

19. Levinson ED et al: Cockayne syndrome. *J Comput Assist Tomogr* 6:1172–1174, 1982.

20. Lowry RB: Early onset Cockayne syndrome. *Am J Med Genet* 13:209–210, 1982.

21. Mallery DL et al: Molecular analysis of mutations in the CSB (*ERCC6*) gene in patients with Cockayne syndrome. *Am J Hum Genet* 62:77–85, 1999.

22. Meira LB et al: Manitoba Aboriginal kindred with original cerebro-oculo-facio-skeletal syndrome has a mutation in the Cockayne syndrome group B (CSB) gene. *Am J Hum Genet* 66:1221–1228, 2000.

23. Moossy J: The neuropathology of Cockayne's syndrome. *J Neuropathol Exp Neurol* 10:644–660, 1967.

24. Mounkes LC et al: A *Drosophilia* model for xeroderma pigmentosum haywire encodes the fly homolog of *ERCC3*, a human excision repair gene. *Cell* 71:925–937, 1992.

25. Moyer DB et al: Brief clinical report: Cockayne syndrome with early onset of manifestations. *Am J Med Genet* 13:225–230, 1932.

26. Nance MA, Berry SA: Cockayne syndrome: review of 140 cases. *Am J Med Genet* 42:68–84, 1992.

27. Ohnishi A et al: Primary segmental demyelination in the sural nerve in Cockayne's syndrome. *Muscle Nerve* 10:163–167, 1987.

28. Okinaka RT et al: Heritable genetic alterations in a xeroderma pigmentosum group G/Cockayne syndrome pedigree. *Mutat Res* 385:107–114, 1997.

29. Otsuka F, Robbins JH: The Cockayne syndrome—an inherited multisystem disorder with cutaneous photosensitivity and defective repair of DNA. *Am J Dermatopathol* 7:387–392, 1985.

30. Patton MA et al: Early onset Cockayne's syndrome: case reports with neuropathological and fibroblast studies. *J Med Genet* 26:154–159,1989.

31. Proops R et al: A clinical study of a family with Cockayne's syndrome. *J Med Genet* 18:288–293, 1981.

32. Razavi-Encha F et al: Infantile familial encephalopathy with cerebral calcifications and leukodystrophy. *Neuropediatrics* 19:72–79, 1988.

33. Riou L et al: The relative expression of mutated *XPB* genes results in xeroderma pigmentosum/Cockayne's syndrome or trichothiodystrophy cellular phenotypes. *Hum Mol Genet* 8:1125–1133, 1999.

34. Sato H et al: Renal lesions in Cockayne's syndrome. *Clin Nephrol* 29:206–209, 1988.

35. Schneider PE: Dental findings in a child with Cockayne's syndrome. *J Dent Child* 30:58–64, 1983.

36. Schofer O et al: Mental retardation syndrome with renal concentration deficiency and intracerebral calcification. *Eur J Pediatr* 149:470–474, 1990.

37. Scott RJ et al: Xeroderma pigmentosum-Cockayne syndrome complex in two patients: absence of skin tumors despite severe deficiency of DNA excision. *J Am Acad Dermatol* 29:883–889, 1993.

38. Seguin LR et al: Ultraviolet light–induced chromosomal aberrations in cultured cells from Cockayne syndrome and complementation group C xeroderma pigmentosum patients: lack of correlation with cancer susceptibility. *Am J Hum Genet* 42:468–475, 1988.

39. Shemen LJ et al: Cockayne's syndrome—an audiologic and temporal bone analysis. *Am J Otol* 5:300–307, 1984.

40. Silengo MC et al: Distinctive skeletal dysplasia in Cockayne syndrome. *Pediatr Radiol* 16:264–266, 1986.

41. Smits MG et al: Peripheral and central myelinopathy in Cockayne's syndrome: report of 3 siblings. *Neuropediatrics* 13:161–167, 1982.

42. Smits MG et al: Calcium phosphate metabolism in autosomal recessive idiopathic strio-pallido-dentate calcinosis and Cockayne's syndrome. *Clin Neurol Neurosurg* 85:145–153, 1983.

43. Sugita K et al: Cockayne syndrome with delayed recovery of RNA synthesis after ultraviolet irradiation but normal ultraviolet survival. *Pediatr Res* 21:34–37, 1987.

44. Van Hoffen A et al: Cells from XP-D and XP-D-CS patients exhibit equally inefficient repair of UV-induced damage in transcribed genes but different capacity to recover UV-inhibited transcription. *Nucleic Acids Res* 27:2898–2904, 1999.

45. Venema J et al: The genetic defect in Cockayne syndrome is associated with a defect in repair of UV-induced DNA damage in transcriptionally active DNA. *Proc Natl Acad Sci USA* 87:4707–4711, 1990.

46. Vermeulen W et al: Xeroderma pigmentosum complementation group G associated with Cockayne syndrome. *Am J Hum Genet* 53:185–192,1993.

47. Vos A et al: The neuropathology of Cockayne syndrome. *Acta Neuropathol* 61:153–156, 1983.

Friedreich ataxia and Friedreich-like ataxia syndromes

Friedreich ataxia is the most common of the spinocerebellar ataxias. The diagnosis has often been used indiscriminately. Diagnostic criteria proposed by Harding (10) include onset of symptoms before 25 years, progressive and unremitting ataxia of limbs and gait, and absent knee and ankle tendon reflexes. Secondary criteria observed in later stages include dysarthria, extensor plantar responses, and diminished vibration sense and proprioception. Patients with similar or later onset and slower progression are classified as having Acadian ataxia, but both map to the same region of chromosome 9 and are probably allelic. While audiograms are often abnormal, less than 10% of patients have clinical hearing loss. A good review of Friedreich ataxia has recently been published (7). Friedreich-like ataxia syndrome with vitamin E deficiency, which maps to 8q13.1–13.3, is briefly discussed under Diagnosis.

Central nervous system. This disorder presents with gait ataxia in most patients, with mean age of onset at 10.5 years (range 1.5–27 years). Examination during early stages shows gait and limb ataxia and absent tendon reflexes, especially at the knees and ankles. Biceps jerks are occasionally preserved. As the disease progresses, additional abnormalities occur, especially nystagmus, broken-up pursuit eye movements, ataxic dysarthria, distal or generalized wasting, pyramidal weakness, extensor plantar responses, and diminished vibration sense and proprioception. The mean age at which ambulation is lost is 25 years (range 11–58 years), and mean time from onset to loss of ambulation is 15.5 years (range 3–44 years). Dementia does not occur (2,10,26).

Peripheral nervous system. Several of the foregoing signs or symptoms may be attributed, all or in part, to peripheral nerve dysfunction, especially reflex loss, wasting, and large fiber sensory loss. Sensory nerve conduction studies are absent (>90%) or diminished in all patients early in the course of the disease. Motor nerve conduction studies show borderline slowing and normal distal latency. These changes are consistent with a chronic, slowly progressive dying-back neuropathy producing axonal degeneration of large myelinated fibers (22).

Musculoskeletal system. Scoliosis (80%), pes cavus (55%), and contractures are sequelae of the neurological degeneration.

Ocular system. Optic atrophy occurs in up to 30% of patients during the course of the disease, although visual evoked potential studies suggest subclinical involvement in many more. Only 5% have severe visual loss. Significant clustering occurs between optic atrophy and hearing loss (10).

Cardiovascular system. Cardiac symptoms are noted in about 40% of most series, with mean age of onset at 25 years (range 13–39 years), which corresponds to about 17 years (range 9–22 years) after onset of neurological disease. It is likely that almost all patients eventually have cardiac symptoms. Common signs and symptoms include palpitations, dyspnea, orthopnea, easy fatigability, irregular rhythm, apical holosystolic murmur, and eventually congestive heart failure or arrest.

Electrocardiograms show repolarization abnormalities and later, atrial dysrhythmias. Echocardiograms show asymmetric septal thickening, concentric left ventricular thickening, or dilated cardiomyopathy, all of which are progressive. Left ventricular mass is increased. There is no correlation between the extent of cardiac and neurological involvement except that patients with dilated cardiomyopathy more often have severe neurological disability (1).

Endocrine system. Diabetes occurs in about 10% of patients. Mean onset is 25 years, which corresponds to about 15 years after onset of neurological manifestations (10).

Auditory system. Mild or moderate hearing loss has been found in about 8% of patients. Severe loss is rare (10). Audiograms show slightly decreased acuity without significant tone decay. Brain stem auditory evoked responses are normal in early stages of the disease but later show dysfunction in the pontomesencephalic region (waves III–V) and, less often, the auditory nerves (waves I–II). In advanced stages, all waves are absent (8,14).

Vestibular system. Nystagmus occurs in about 20% of cases (10). Vestibular testing shows reduced duration of responses to rotational stimuli, variability in amplitude and irregular insertion of the fast phase of nystagmus, and reduced slow-phase velocities. Thresholds to angular acceleration have been elevated (8).

Pathology. Pathological changes involve multiple systems within the neuraxis (14). Sensory cranial nerves (sensory V, VIII, IX, X), peripheral nerves, and posterior roots show moderate to marked loss of myelinated fibers, which is often more marked among large myelinated fibers. Mild myelin pallor is sometimes seen in the optic nerves. The spinal cord has marked loss of myelinated fibers in the posterior columns and less severe loss in the spinocerebellar and corticospinal tracts. There is moderate atrophy and loss of neurons in Clarke's column. The anterior and intermediolateral horns are normal. The brain stem has moderate degeneration of corticospinal tracts up to the medulla and pons, but appears more normal in the cerebral peduncles. Mild or moderate degeneration occurs in the superior cerebellar peduncle, tractus solitarius, restiform body, and medial lemniscus. Moderate loss of neurons is seen in the gracile, cuneate, and vestibular nuclei, and in the inferior colliculus with astrocytic proliferation. The cerebellum shows mild or moderate loss of Purkinje cells, with some bizarre shapes and fusiform swellings of axons and dentate neurons, and loss of myelinated fibers in white matter. The cerebrum has moderate loss of neurons with proliferation of astrocytes in the thalamus and, less often, in the pallidum (16).

Temporal bone studies show loss of cochlear nerve fibers and ganglion cells (13).

Histologic changes in the heart include diffuse interstitial fibrosis, myocellular hypertrophy, and necrosis (1).

Heredity. Many studies have confirmed autosomal recessive inheritance (7,9). One gene for Friedreich ataxia has been mapped to the pericentromeric region of chromosome 9 at 9q13–q21.1 (4,17,24) and is called the *FRDA* gene (7). In 98% of affected individuals, an intronic expansion of a GAA repeat is present in both alleles. In 2% of individuals, there is heterozygosity for an expanded region in one allele and point mutation in the other (17), both which cause decreased expression of the gene. The similar but milder Acadian ataxia maps to the same region (5). A second locus for Friedreich ataxia, which is clinically indistinguishable, maps to 9p23–p11 (15).

Diagnosis. As the clinical manifestations are so well known, disorders with any atypical features should be excluded, such as those with autosomal dominant inheritance, retinal degeneration, or onset with symptoms other than gait ataxia, scoliosis, or cardiac disease. Harding (11) described a condition with early-onset cerebellar ataxia (EOCA) with retained reflexes. Sensorineural hearing loss was noted in 2 of 20 patients by Harding (11) and, by employing BAEP, in 1 of 4 patients by Vanasse et al. (27) and in 15 of 20 patients by Filla et al. (9). Mielke et al. (19) also described patients with this condition. Initially considered a distinct condition, Friedreich ataxia with retained tendon reflexes (FARR) has been mapped to 9q, and recent studies have identified mu-

tations in the *FRDA* gene in individuals diagnosed with FARR (6,21). Another Friedreich-like ataxia is an entity with vitamin E deficiency. This syndrome of progressive gait ataxia, areflexia, and selective vitamin E deficiency was first described by Harding et al. (12) in 1985. Others (3,25,28) have reported similarly affected patients. It is distinguished from Friedreich ataxia by the improvement of neurologic signs following administration of high doses of α-tocopherol (23). In addition, hearing loss has not been described in this condition. The gene was mapped to the proximal 8q area in 1993 (18), and has been identified as the α-tocopherol transfer protein (TTPA) (20). Sylvester syndrome should be excluded.

Prognosis. All signs and symptoms are slowly but relentlessly progressive and result in severe disability and eventually death. Mean age of death is about 37 years (range 21–69 years) (2,16).

Summary. This disorder is characterized by (*1*) autosomal recessive inheritance; (*2*) onset before 25 years; (*3*) progressive ataxia; (*4*) absent tendon reflexes in legs; and (*5*) mild motor and sensory neuropathy. Later manifestations include (*6*) mild spastic diplegia; (*7*) scoliosis and pes cavus; (*8*) infrequent optic atrophy; and (*9*) infrequent sensorineural hearing loss.

References

1. Alboliras ET et al: Spectrum of cardiac involvement in Friedreich's ataxia: clinical, electrocardiographic and echocardiographic observations. *Am J Cardiol* 58:518–524, 1986.
2. Barbeau A: Friedreich's ataxia 1976—an overview. *Can J Neurol Sci* 3:389–397, 1976.
3. Ben Hamida C et al: Localization of Friedreich ataxia phenotype with selective vitamin E deficiency to chromosome 8q by homozygosity mapping. *Nat Genet* 5:195–200, 1993.
4. Chamberlain S et al: Mapping of mutation causing Friedreich's ataxia to human chromosome 9. *Nature* 334:248–250, 1988.
5. Chamberlain S et al: Genetic homogeneity at the Friedreich ataxia locus on chromosome 9. *Am J Hum Genet* 44:518–521, 1989.
6. Coppola G et al: Why do some Friedreich's ataxia patients retain tendon reflexes? A clinical, neurophysiological and molecular study. *J Neurol* 246:353–357, 1999.
7. Delatycki MB et al: Friedreich ataxia: an overview. *J Med Genet* 37:1–8, 2000.
8. Ell J et al: Neuro-otological abnormalities in Friedreich's ataxia. *J Neurol Neurosurg Psychiatry* 47:26–32, 1984.
9. Filla A et al: Clinical and genetic heterogeneity in early onset cerebellar ataxia with retained tendon reflexes. *J Neurol Neurosurg Psychiatry* 53:667–670, 1990.
10. Harding AE: Friedreich's ataxia: a clinical and genetic study of 90 families with an analysis of early diagnostic criteria and intrafamilial clustering of clinical features. *Brain* 104:589–620, 1981.
11. Harding AE: Early-onset cerebellar ataxia with retained tendon reflexes: a clinical and genetic study of a disorder distinct from Friedreich's ataxia. *J Neurol Neurosurg Psychiatry* 44:503–508, 1981.
12. Harding AE et al: Spinocerebellar degeneration associated with a selective defect of vitamin E absorption. *N Engl J Med* 313:32–35, 1985.
13. Igarashi M et al: Temporal bone findings in Friedreich's ataxia. *ORL* 44:145–155, 1982.
14. Jabbari B et al: Early abnormalities of brainstem auditory evoked potentials in Friedreich's ataxia: evidence of primary brainstem dysfunction. *Neurology* 33:1071–1074, 1983.
15. Kostrzewa M et al: Locus heterogeneity in Friedreich ataxia. *Neurogenetics* 3:127–132, 2001.
16. Lamarche JB et al: The neuropathology of "typical" Friedreich's ataxia in Quebec. *Can J Neurol Sci* 11:592–600, 1984.
17. Massimo P: Molecular pathogenesis of Friedreich ataxia. *Arch Neurol* 56:1201–1208, 1999.
18. Mendel JL, Koenig M: Localization of Friedreich ataxia phenotype with selective vitamin E deficiency to chromosome 8q by homozygosity mapping. *Nat Genet* 5:195–200, 1993.
19. Mielke R et al: Early onset cerebellar ataxia (EOCA) with retained reflexes: reduced cerebellar benzodiazepine-receptor binding, progressive metabolic and cognitive impairment. *Mov Disord* 13:739–745, 1998.
20. Ouahchi K et al: Ataxia with isolated vitamin E deficiency is caused by mutations in the alpha-tocopherol transfer protein. *Nat Genet* 9:141–145, 1995.

21. Palau F et al: Early-onset ataxia with cardiomyopathy and retained tendon reflexes maps to the Friedreich's ataxia locus on chromosome 9q. *Ann Neurol* 37:359–362, 1995.
22. Peyronnard JM et al: Nerve conduction studies and electromyography in Friedreich's ataxia. *Can J Neurol Sci* 3:313–317, 1976.
23. Schuelke M et al: Treatment of ataxia in isolated vitamin E deficiency caused by alpha-tocopherol transfer protein deficiency. *J Pediatr* 134:240–244, 1999.
24. Shaw J et al: Regional localization of the Friedreich ataxia locus to human chromosome 9q13–q21.1. *Cytogenet Cell Genet* 53:221–224, 1990.
25. Sokol RJ et al: Isolated vitamin E deficiency in the absence of fat malabsorption—familial and sporadic cases: characterization and investigation of causes. *J Lab Clin Med* 111:548–559, 1988.
26. Ülkü A et al: Friedreich's ataxia: a clinical review of 20 childhood cases. *Acta Neurol Scand* 77:493–497, 1988.
27. Vanasse M et al: Evoked potential studies in Friedreich's ataxia and progressive early onset cerebellar ataxia. *Can J Neurol Sci* 15:292–298,1988.
28. Yokota T et al: Adult onset spinocerebellar syndrome with idiopathic vitamin E deficiency. *Ann Neurol* 22:84–87, 1987.

Ataxia and sensorineural hearing loss (autosomal recessive) (Lichtenstein-Knorr syndrome)

In 1930, Lichtenstein and Knorr (6) first described a syndrome of severe progressive hearing loss and ataxia. This syndrome appears to be distinct from Friedreich ataxia. Several other familes have been described subsequently (1,6–10).

Central nervous system. Mild intention tremor and gait ataxia usually begin between 10 and 20 years of age and progress slowly to involve all four limbs and speech. Most patients are unable to walk by 30 years. In others, onset is later and progression slower. One mildly affected individual had weakness and wasting without ataxia at 32 years (7), and another was still able to walk at 47 years (9). Examination usually showed dysarthric and sometimes explosive speech, and signs of both upper and lower motor neuron disease including muscle wasting, weakness, diminished deep tendon reflexes in the legs, hyperactive deep tendon reflexes in the arms that later decrease, and extensor plantar responses. Electromyography (EMG) often showed decreased amplitudes and slowing on nerve conduction studies and neurogenic changes on needle exam. A CT scan in one patient showed cerebellar atrophy. In another, an MRI scan revealed normal cerebellum, but diminished cerebral white matter and mild atrophy.

Musculoskeletal system. Associated neuromuscular problems included lordosis, scoliosis, and pes cavus. Foot deformity was particularly common.

Ocular system. One patient had unilateral and another had bilateral cataracts (6).

Cardiovascular system. One patient died of heart failure at 20 years, but most had no cardiac symptoms.

Auditory system. Sensorineural hearing loss most often began in early childhood and progressed rapidly to profound loss. In others, including sibs of some patients with congenital onset, hearing loss began between 10 and 20 years of age and progressed more slowly. In one family, both hearing loss and ataxia consistently began at a later age (9).

Vestibular system. Vestibular function was normal.

Heredity. The syndrome has autosomal recessive inheritance, based on reports of four families with several affected children. The parents were healthy and, in one family (6), consanguineous.

Diagnosis. Patients with the autosomal dominant ataxia and sensorineural hearing loss have had mild hearing deficiency (4,5). Patients with Friedreich ataxia have preadolescent onset, cardiac dysfunction in 40%, and diabetes mellitus in 10%. Hearing loss is mild and occurs in only about 10% (2). Hearing impairment has also been reported in a

few patients with "early-onset ataxia with retained tendon reflexes" (3). As noted earlier, this selective disorder of vitamin E deficiency has been mapped to chromosome 8q. Several syndromes can be distinguished from this syndrome because of retinal involvement. In ataxia, hypogonadism, mental retardation, and sensorineural hearing loss (Richards-Rundle syndrome), mental deficiency, and hypogonadism are present.

Prognosis. The ataxia, associated amyotrophy, and hearing loss are all progressive and disabling.

Summary. This syndrome is characterized by (*1*) autosomal recessive inheritance; (*2*) ataxia; (*3*) associated musculoskeletal problems such as scoliosis and pes cavus; and (*4*) sensorineural hearing loss.

References

1. Barbieri F et al: Clinical and CT-scan study of a case of cerebellar ataxia and progressive hearing loss: Lichtenstein-Knorr disease? *Acta Neurol (Napoli)* 8:159–163, 1986.
2. Harding AE: Friedreich's ataxia: a clinical and genetic study of 90 families with an analysis of early diagnostic criteria and intrafamilial clustering of clinical features. *Brain* 104:589–620, 1981.
3. Harding AE: Early onset cerebellar ataxia with retained tendon reflexes: a clinical and genetic study of a disorder distinct from Friedreich's ataxia. *J Neurol Neurosurg Psychiatry* 44:503–508, 1981.
4. Heras Pérez JA et al: Ataxia y sorderahereditarias (enfermedad de Lichtenstein-Knorr): estudio de una familia a lo largo de cinco generaciones. *Med Clin (Barcelona)* 87:508–509, 1986.
5. Klippel M, Durante G: Affections nerveuses familiales et héréditaires. *Rev Méd (Paris)* 12:745–785, 1892.
6. Lichtenstein H, Knorr A: Über einige Fälle von fortschreitender Schwerhörigkeit beihereditärer Ataxie. *Dtsch Z Nervenheilkd* 114:1–28, 1930.
7. Matthews WB: Familial ataxia, deaf-mutism, and muscular wasting. *J Neurol Neurosurg Psychiatry* 13:307–311, 1950.
8. Pires W, de Carvalho AH: Doença de Friedreich com surdez em dois irmãos. *Rev Neuropsiquatr (Sao Paulo)* 1:435–441, 1935.
9. Schimke RN: Adult-onset hereditary cerebellar ataxia and neurosensory deafness. *Clin Genet* 6:416–421, 1974.
10. Striano S et al: Hearing loss associated with progressive ataxia (Lichtenstein-Knorr disease?). Report of a sporadic case with peculiar neuroradiological findings. *Acta Neurol (Napoli)* 11:351–359, 1989.

Spinocerebellar ataxia with blindness and deafness (SCABD)

Bomont et al. (1) described an uncle and niece with a Freidreich ataxia–like condition that mapped to 6p23–p21 and was distinct from Freidreich ataxia. This may be the same condition described by van Bogaert and Martin (4) and Spoendlin (3) as Friedreich ataxia with optic and cochleovestibular degeneration.

Peripheral nervous system. Onset of gait ataxia is in early childhood, with loss of ambulation by early adulthood.

Ocular system. Individuals begin to lose vision in the early teens, with optic atrophy, nystagmus, and visual decline common manifestations. One studied individual had abnormal electroretinograms at age 14.

Musculoskeletal system. Hand contractures were described in one individual.

Auditory system. Hearing loss also has onset in late childhood and, in the cases described by Van Bogaert and Martin (4) and Spoendlin (3), cochlear degeneration occurred.

Pathology. Muscle biopsy in the niece (1) showed mild fiber disproportion. Evaluation of the cochlea done by Spoendlin (3) demonstrated loss of nerve fibers and spiral ganglion cells.

Heredity. This condition is autosomal recessive in inheritance. The gene has not yet been identified, but has been mapped to 6p23–p21. For comparison basis, Friedreich ataxia has been mapped to 9q13–21 (2).

References

1. Bomont P et al: Homozygosity mapping of spinocerebellar ataxia with cerebellar atrophy and peripheral neuropathy to 9q33–34, and with hearing impairment and optic atrophy to 6p21–23. *Eur J Hum Genet* 8:986–990, 2000.
2. Delatycki M et al: Friedreich ataxia: an overview. *J Med Genet* 37:1–8, 2000.
3. Spoendlin H: Optic and cochleo-vestibular degenrations in hereditary ataxias. II. Temporal bone pathology in two cases of Friedreich's ataxia with
vestibulo-cochlear disorders. *Brain* 97:41–48, 1974.
4. van Bogaert L, Martin L: Optic and cochleo-vestibular degenerations in the hereditary ataxias. I. Clinicopathological and genetic aspects. *Brain* 97:15–40, 1974.

Ataxia and sensorineural hearing loss (autosomal dominant) (Klippel-Durante syndrome)

Klippel-Durante syndrome is not well documented but appears to resemble autosomal recessive ataxia and sensorineural hearing loss. Hearing loss may be less severe (1,2).

Central nervous system. Onset of ataxia varied from childhood to
later adulthood.

Auditory system. The hearing loss began later and was less severe
than in the recessive form of the disease.

Heredity. Autosomal dominant inheritance is most likely because affected individuals came from two generations in each family (Fig. 10–3).

Prognosis. The symptoms were all progressive, but probably were
milder than in the autosomal recessive form.

Diagnosis. There is marked resemblance to ataxia and sensorineural
hearing loss (autosomal recessive) (Lichtenstein-Knorr syndrome).

Summary. This disorder is characterized by (*1*) autosomal dominant
inheritance, possibly with decreased penetrance; (*2*) ataxia; and (*3*) sensorineural hearing loss.

References

1. Heras Pérez JA et al: Ataxia y sorderahereditarias (enfermedad de Lichtenstein-Knorr): Estudio de una familia a lo largo de cinco generaciones. *Med
Clin (Barcelona)* 87:508–509, 1986.
2. Klippel M, Durante G: Affectiones nerveuses familiales et héréditaires. *Rev
Méd (Paris)* 12:745–785, 1892.

Ataxia, amyotrophy of hands, spastic paraplegia, hypogonadism, short stature, and sensorineural hearing loss (Gemignani syndrome)

Gemignani (1) described two brothers with ataxia, amyotrophy of hands,
spastic paraplegia, hypogonadism, short stature, and sensorineural hearing loss.

Central nervous system. Gait ataxia probably began in the 20's.
It was definitely present by the 40's and progressed slowly thereafter.
Ataxia was much less prominent in the arms. Unusual atrophy, weakness, and diminished reflexes (amyotrophy) of hands and distal arms
began at the same time and were also slowly progressive. Spastic paraparesis was evident when examined at 60–70 years. Speech and intelligence were normal in one brother, while communication was poor in
the other who was considered mentally retarded. Cranial CT scans
showed generalized cerebellar atrophy. A myelogram indicated a small
cervical spinal cord in one but was normal in the other.

Peripheral nervous system. Examination showed absent vibration, diminished position sense, and slightly decreased light touch in the
legs. Nerve conduction studies were normal although one brother had
mild slowing in the right peroneal nerve.

Endocrine system. Small, atrophic testes, small genitalia, and short
stature were present in both brothers. Onset of hypogonadism was probably in childhood or young adulthood. Neither was able to have sexual
intercourse. Height was 152 and 148 cm, respectively (more than 2 SD
below the mean).

Integumentary system. Vitiligo restricted to the right hand was
noted in one brother.

Auditory system. Hearing loss likely began in the 20's, and progressed to profound loss by 50–70 years. Brain stem auditory evoked
potentials were done when hearing loss was profound and showed absent responses.

Laboratory findings. Endocrine testing revealed increased levels
of luteinizing hormone (LH), follicle-stimulating hormone (FSH), and
estradiol.

Pathology. Muscle biopsy showed moderate denervation changes.
Nerve biopsy showed demyelination, more marked in the older brother.

Heredity. Inheritance could be either autosomal or X-linked recessive.

Diagnosis. The onset of symptoms in ataxia, hypogonadotrophic
hypogonadism, mental retardation, and sensorineural hearing loss
(Richards-Rundle syndrome) and ataxia, mental retardation, motor and
sensory neuropathy, spastic diplegia, and sensorineural hearing loss
(Berman syndrome) occurs earlier than in this syndrome. In addition,
mental retardation may not occur.

Prognosis. Both brothers were living at 60–70 years of age. One
had normal intelligence and the other was probably retarded. Thus, it
is not known whether retardation is related to the disease.

Summary. The syndrome is manifested by (*1*) autosomal or X-
linked recessive inheritance; (*2*) ataxia; (*3*) localized amyotrophy of

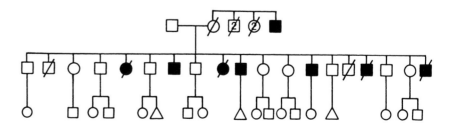

Figure 10–3. *Ataxia and sensorineural hearing loss (autosomal dominant) (Klippel-Durante syndrome).* Pedigree
of family showing probable autosomal dominant inheritance. [From JA Heras Pérez et al., *Med Clin (Barcelona)*
87:508, 1986.]

□ ○ △   Normal
■ ●   Affected

hands; (4) spastic paraparesis; (5) hypogonadism; (6) short stature; and (7) sensorineural hearing loss.

Reference

1. Gemignani F: Spinocerebellar ataxia associated with localized amyotrophy of the hands, sensorineural deafness and spastic paraparesis in two brothers. *J Neurogenet* 3:125–133, 1986.

Ataxia, cataracts, dementia, and sensorineural hearing loss (Strömgren syndrome)

In 1970, Strömgren et al. (2) reported a syndrome of ataxia, cataracts, psychosis and dementia, and sensorineural hearing loss in 11 individuals from four generations of a large Danish family (1,2).

Ocular system. Posterior polar cataracts were a constant feature, usually appearing between 20 and 30 years of age and slowly maturing over several decades. Intrabulbar hemorrhage and nystagmus were also common. In some individuals, the pupils did not react to light.

Central nervous system. Ataxia without spinal cord involvement appeared after the age of 40. Other abnormalities included staggering gait, intention tremor involving the trunk and all limbs, slurred speech, central nystagmus, and hypotonia. None had pyramidal signs. Paranoid psychosis developed after age 50 in several individuals and was followed by organic dementia.

Other findings. Ichthyosis and gastric achylia were variable findings. Several had intractable diarrhea during their terminal illness.

Auditory system. Impaired hearing began some years after the ocular symptoms and progressed to severe loss by 45 years.

Vestibular system. Vestibular reflexes were diminished or lost.

Pathology. In one patient, autopsy showed diffuse atrophy of the brain. The cranial nerves were very thin and nearly completely demyelinated. The main pathological change was accumulation of cholesterol and related compounds freely in the tissues and within glial cells and vessel walls. Subsequent evaluations have found severe cerebral amyloid angiopathy, hippocampal plaques, and neurofibrillary tangles (3).

Heredity. Inheritance is autosomal dominant. A mutation in the *ITM2B* (integral membrane protein 2B) gene was identified by Vidal et al. (3). This is the same gene that causes familial British dementia.

Diagnosis. The disorder resembles Refsum syndrome, but the pattern of inheritance is different. It also resembles ataxia, motor and sensory neuropathy, mental retardation, cataracts, and sensorineural hearing loss (Begeer syndrome).

Prognosis. Affected individuals become demented and bedridden by about age 50 and usually die by age 60 from complications such as pneumonia, intractable diarrhea, and strokes.

Summary. This disorder is characterized by (1) autosomal dominant inheritance; (2) posterior polar cataracts appearing during the third decade; (3) intrabulbar hemorrhage; (4) late-onset ataxia; (5) later onset of paranoid psychosis and dementia; (6) late-onset severe sensorineural hearing loss; and (7) loss of vestibular function.

References

1. Strömgren E: Heredopathia ophthalmo-oto-encephalica. In: *Handbook of Clinical Neurology, Vol. 42. Neurogenetics Directory*, Vinken PJ et al. (eds), North Holland Publishing Co., Amsterdam, 1981, pp 150–152.
2. Strömgren E et al: Cataract, deafness, cerebellar ataxia, psychosis and dementia—a new syndrome. *Acta Neurol Scand* 43(Suppl):261–262, 1970.

3. Vidal R et al: A decamer duplication in the 3′ region of the BRI gene originates an amyloid peptide that is associated with dementia in a Danish kindred. *Proc Natl Acad Sci USA* 97:4920–4925, 2000.

Ataxia, motor and sensory neuropathy, mental retardation, cataracts, and sensorineural hearing loss (Begeer syndrome)

In 1991, Begeer et al. (1) briefly described two sisters with ataxia, polyneuropathy, mental retardation, cataracts, and progressive hearing loss.

Physical findings. Both affected sisters had short stature.

Central nervous system. No information regarding early development was available, but both sisters were mentally retarded. Ataxia was first observed in their 20's. Exam in their 50's showed mild mental retardation, mild spasticity, absent tendon reflexes, normal plantar responses, and ataxia that was more prominent in the trunk than in the limbs. Cranial CT scan was normal.

Peripheral nervous system. The ataxia was attributed primarily to diminished proprioception. In their 50's both sisters showed absent tendon reflexes and probably decreased sensation for light touch, pain, and temperature. Sensory nerve conduction study (NCS) showed no response to stimulation in the arms. Motor NCS exhibited decreased velocity in the legs and normal velocity in the arms; specific results were not given.

Ocular system. Both sisters had congenital cataracts that required surgery. Their exam showed postsurgical changes after cataract removal, impaired visual acuity (in at least one of the two), normal fundi, and nystagmus.

Auditory system. Progressive sensorineural hearing loss was first noticed in their 20's. One had a hearing loss of 60 dB below and 100 dB loss above 1000 Hz.

Laboratory findings. Routine laboratory studies were normal, as were blood and cerebrospinal fluid (CSF) lactate, blood phytanic acid and ceruloplasmin, and blood and urine amino and organic acid levels.

Pathology. Sural nerve biopsy in the proband showed severe axonal atrophy.

Heredity. Two females among six sibs were affected and their parents were not related. Thus, autosomal recessive inheritance is likely.

Diagnosis. Patients with ataxia, cataracts, dementia, and sensorineural hearing loss (Strömgren syndrome) are not retarded but later develop dementia. Patients with ataxia, motor and sensory neuropathy, cataracts, myopia, pigmentary retinopathy, skeletal abnormalities, and sensorineural hearing loss (Flynn-Aird syndrome) have several other abnormalities such as pigmentary retinopathy. Both syndromes have autosomal dominant inheritance. Patients with ataxia, mental retardation, motor and sensory neuropathy, spastic diplegia, and sensorineural hearing loss (Berman syndrome) lack cataracts. Tuck and McLeod (3) described a patient with similar abnormalities who also had pigmentary retinopathy. Schaap et al. (2) described three brothers who had some similar manifestations, but in whom hearing loss occurred at an earlier age. Although the oldest patient was 13 at the time of the report, no neurologic symptoms had developed.

Prognosis. Both sisters were disabled but alive and healthy in their 50's.

Summary. This disorder is characterized by (1) autosomal recessive inheritance; (2) cataracts; (3) mental retardation; (4) ataxia; (5) motor and sensory neuropathy; and (6) sensorineural hearing loss.

References

1. Begeer JH et al: Two sisters with mental retardation, cataract, ataxia, progressive hearing loss, and polyneuropathy. *J Med Genet* 28:884–885, 1991.
2. Schaap C et al: Three mildly retarded siblings with congenital cataracts, sensorineural deafness, hypogonadism, hypertrichosis, and short stature: a new syndrome? *Clin Dysmorphol* 4:283–288, 1995.
3. Tuck RR, McLeod JG: Retinitis pigmentosa, ataxia, and peripheral neuropathy. *J Neurol Neurosurg Psychiatry* 46:206–213, 1983.

Ataxia, motor and sensory neuropathy, cataracts, myopia, pigmentary retinopathy, skeletal abnormalities, and sensorineural hearing loss (Flynn-Aird syndrome)

In 1965, Flynn and Aird (1) described this syndrome in 15 members of a single family. No similar families have been described.

Ocular system. Myopia appeared in childhood and became severe enough to interfere with schoolwork after 10 years (Fig. 10–4A). Con-striction of peripheral visual fields and night blindness were noticed in the 20's and 30's. Later abnormalities included severe myopia (90%), bilateral cataracts (50%), and atypical retinitis pigmentosa (20%), all of which may have contributed to severe blindness (Fig. 10–4B).

Peripheral nervous system. Poor muscular development was apparent from early in life (Fig. 10–4C). Symptoms of a combined motor and sensory neuropathy began during the teens or 20's. This at first consisted of ataxia, muscle atrophy, and intense neuropathic pain (Fig. 10–4D). The ataxia was presumably sensory in origin. Distal weakness, diminished deep tendon reflexes, and sensory loss for light touch, pain, and vibration and joint position were noticed later. An EMG needle exam in one patient showed neuropathic changes.

Central nervous system. Academic achievement was poor despite normal intelligence. Many affected individuals had unusual spells consisting of expressive aphasia with normal comprehension, patches of blurred vision that varied from spell to spell, and paresthesias of the face and limbs. Several had epileptiform discharges on electroencephalogram (EEG) and one had convulsive movements. The spells

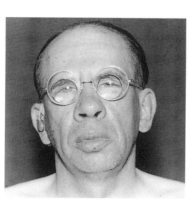

A

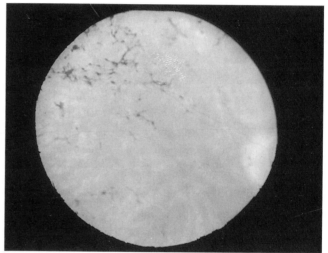

B

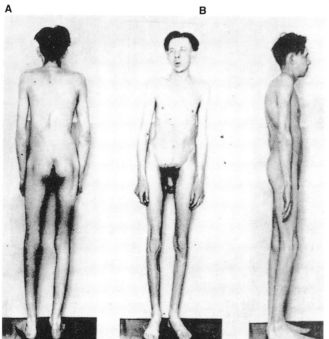

C

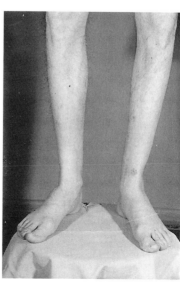

D

Figure 10–4. *Ataxia, motor and sensory neuropathy, cataracts, myopia, pigmentary retinopathy, skeletal abnormalities, and sensorineural hearing loss (Flynn-Aird syndrome).* (A) Facial photograph showing coarse features and myopia. (B) Fundus photograph shows atypical retinitis pigmentosa. (C) Full body views. (D) Leg photo showing atrophy of the skin and muscles. [From P Flynn and RB Aird, *J Neurol Sci* 2:161, 1965.]

were interpreted as atypical seizures, but other explanations such as transient ischemic attacks or vasospasm are possible.

Musculoskeletal system. Kyphoscoliosis appeared only after the neuropathy was established and progressed slowly. Later skeletal changes consisted of osteoporosis and bone cysts measuring up to 3 cm in diameter, mostly in the pelvis.

Integumentary system. Atrophy of skin and subcutaneous tissue was seen in most patients and predisposed to chronic ulcers, especially over the feet and ankles. Severe dental caries was common. Baldness occurred as a late manifestation.

Endocrine system. Insulin-resistant diabetes mellitus occurred in one patient.

Auditory system. Bilateral sensorineural hearing loss began in childhood, usually as the first sign of the disease, and progressed at a variable rate to severe impairment by the second to sixth decade. No further hearing tests were described.

Laboratory findings. Routine blood and urine tests were normal. Several patients had elevated spinal fluid protein.

Pathology. Generalized atrophy of the brain and unspecified microscopic changes "typical of ischemia" were described. Nerve biopsy in one patient was "characteristic of peripheral neuritis." Skin biopsies showed atrophy, hyperkeratosis with absence of rete ridges, and sparse sweat glands and hair follicles. Basophilic hyperplasia of the pituitary, associated with bilateral adrenal hyperplasia, and adrenal atrophy were rare manifestations.

Heredity. The pedigree was consistent with autosomal dominant inheritance with variable expressivity.

Diagnosis. Werner syndrome shares the skin ulceration, osteoporosis, cataracts, and other signs of early aging but lacks neurologic abnormalites, hearing loss, etc. Usher syndrome shares retinitis pigmentosa and hearing loss but lacks other manifestations. Refsum syndrome is similar but lacks the skin changes and may be diagnosed by elevated phytanic acid levels. Although another patient was stated to have Flynn-Aird syndrome, we are skeptical regarding this diagnosis (2).

Prognosis. The hearing and visual deficits combined to cause severe disability. The neuropathy was slowly progressive and probably predisposed patients to pneumonia and other complications.

Summary. This disorder is characterized by (*1*) autosomal dominant inheritance; (*2*) ataxia; (*3*) cataracts; (*4*) motor and sensory neuropathy that results in neuropathic pain; (*5*) myopia; (*6*) pigmentary retinopathy; (*7*) skeletal abnormalities such as kyphoscoliosis; (*8*) skin atrophy; (*9*) unusual spells; and (*10*) sensorineural hearing loss.

References

1. Flynn P, Aird RB: A neuroectodermal syndrome of dominant inheritance. *J Neurol Sci* 2:161–182, 1965.
2. Kalb R: Über einen Patientin mit Flynn-Aird-Symptomatik. *Lebensversicherungsmedizin* 36:59–62, 1984.

Ataxia, dementia, myocardial fibrosis, and sensorineural hearing loss (Jeune-Tommasi syndrome)

In 1963, Jeune et al. (1) described male and female Gypsy sibs who developed ataxia, myocardial fibrosis, mental deficiency, and progressive sensorineural hearing loss. Through personal communication (Jeune, 1974), we learned of a third affected sib, a male, and of other relatives with the same disorder.

Central nervous system. At about 6 years of age, the sibs developed mild ataxia with intention tremor, adiadochokinesia, and hypotonia. The older sib had marked mental deterioration and increased severity of the other abnormalities by age 12. She also had nystagmus, depressed deep tendon reflexes, and extensor plantar responses.

Ocular system. The affected female had mild pigmentary retinopathy and nystagmus at 12 years.

Cardiovascular system. In all affected sibs, the heart was moderately enlarged, and electrocardiogram (ECG) showed left ventricular hypertrophy. Terminally, the children developed atrioventricular conduction block.

Integumentary system. Many freckles or lentigines were present over the face, arms, and legs.

Auditory system. Hearing loss was first noticed at about 6 years and was progressive. Audiometry showed bilateral sensorineural loss.

Vestibular system. No vestibular tests were described.

Laboratory findings. A chest radiograph of the oldest child showed cardiomegaly.

Pathology. Autopsy was performed on the 12-year-old girl. Gross examination of the brain including the cerebellum was normal, but there was mild myelin pallor of the white matter. The spinal cord showed moderate degeneration of spinocerebellar tracts and fasciculis gracilis. The heart exhibited diffuse myocardial fibrosis.

Heredity. Inheritance is autosomal recessive as three of five sibs were affected, and the parents were first cousins and unaffected.

Diagnosis. Ataxia, pigmentary retinopathy, and sensorineural hearing loss (Hallgren syndrome), ataxia-telangiectasia, Friedreich ataxia, Refsum syndrome, and Usher syndrome must be considered in differential diagnosis. It is not known whether pigmentary retinopathy is a consistent manifestation. Lentigines also occur in LEOPARD syndrome.

Prognosis. By age 12 years, disability is severe and one child had died, presumably due to the neurologic and cardiac abnormalities.

Summary. This disorder is characterized by (*1*) autosomal recessive inheritance; (*2*) progressive ataxia; (*3*) childhood-onset dementia; (*4*) myocardial fibrosis associated with cardiac conduction abnormalities; (*5*) skin pigmentary changes; (*6*) possible retinitis pigmentosa; and (*7*) sensorineural hearing loss.

Reference

1. Jeune M et al: Syndrome familial associant ataxie, surdité et oligo-phrénie. Sclérose myocardique d'evolution fatale chez l'un des enfants. *Pédiatrie* 18:984–987, 1963.

Ataxia, optic atrophy, esotropia, dysphagia, and sensorineural hearing loss with episodic worsening (Schmidley syndrome)

In 1987, Schmidley et al. (1) reported a single family with ataxia, optic atrophy, dysphagia, esotropia, and sensorineural hearing loss with episodic worsening of neurological symptoms.

Central nervous system. The earliest abnormalities consisted of hypotonia, and episodes of choking or vomiting between 1 and 5 months of age. Early developmental milestones were delayed, and later milestones such as walking and speech were never achieved. Ataxia, dysphagia, and more chronic problems with choking and vomiting began between age 10 months and 2 years. Seizures appeared at 3–4 years. All individuals had hypotonia and ataxia. Spasticity, diminished deep tendon reflexes, and upgoing plantar responses were reported in older boys. The disorder was progressive and associated with episodes of weakness, lethargy, hypoventilation, and worsening of the ataxia and dysphagia.

The mother of an affected boy had two episodes of transient ataxia. Cranial MRI scan showed cerebellar atrophy and enlarged fourth ventricle.

Peripheral nervous system. Diminished or absent deep tendon reflexes were described in the older boys but NCS and EMG were not performed. These tests were normal in the youngest child.

Ocular system. Esotropia (occurring as early as 3 months) and optic atrophy were noted on initial clinical exam between 10 months and 2 years in all three boys. Paralysis of vertical and left conjugate gaze was present at 6 years in the oldest child.

Auditory system. Sensorineural hearing loss was noticed as early as 10 months and was progressive. Audiograms revealed 70 dB loss in one child at 16 months and 85 dB loss in another at 2 years.

Laboratory findings. Pertinent negative tests included serum ammonia, lactate, pyruvate and amino acids, and urine amino acids.

Pathology. Skin biopsy, electron microscopic examination, and bone marrow biopsy were normal. The brains of three boys were examined pathologically. Consistent lesions were limited to the brain stem, cerebellum, and optic system. In the brain stem, neuronal loss and gliosis were observed in the dorsal motor nucleus of the vagus, inferior colliculus, medial and lateral vestibular nuclei, cochlear nucleus, superior and inferior olives, and red nucleus. The cerebellum showed neuronal loss and gliosis of the dentate nucleus and loss of myelinated fibers with gliosis in adjacent white matter. There was moderate loss of fibers of both optic nerves with atrophy of neurons and gliosis in the lateral geniculate nuclei. Variability in severity between affected boys was marked and not always related to age. For example, the cochlear and vestibular nuclei, colliculi, and geniculates were normal in the boy who died at age 7 years.

Heredity. Inheritance is X-linked recessive. Carrier females may have mild manifestations (Fig. 10–5A).

Diagnosis. Ataxia, optic atrophy, and hearing loss occur together in several other syndromes, none of which is X-linked. Both types of ataxia, optic atrophy, and sensorineural hearing loss (autosomal domi-

nant and recessive) and optico-cochleo-dentate degeneration (Muller-Zeman syndrome) lack episodic worsening and ophthalmoplegia. Cockayne syndrome includes many other abnormalities such as pigmentary retinopathy. Kearns-Sayre syndrome differs because of later onset, absence of optic atrophy, and milder clinical course. X-linked ataxia of somewhat later onset has been described (2).

Prognosis. One boy died during such an episode at 10 months. The others died of pneumonia at 3.5 and 7 years. Cranial CT scan in the former showed possible cerebellar atrophy (Fig. 10–5B).

Summary. This syndrome is characterized by (1) X-linked recessive inheritance; (2) onset in infancy with subsequent progression; (3) discrete episodes of neurologic deterioration; (4) ataxia; (5) dysphagia and choking; (6) early hypotonia and later spasticity and areflexia; (7) mental retardation; (8) seizures; (9) esotropia that evolves to ophthalmoplegia; (10) optic atrophy; and (11) sensorineural hearing loss.

References

1. Schmidley JW et al: Infantile X-linked ataxia and deafness: a new clinicopathologic entity? *Neurology* 37:1344–1349, 1987.
2. Spira PJ et al: A spinocerebellar degeneration with X-linked inheritance. *Brain* 102:27–41, 1987.

Fatal X-linked ataxia with deafness and loss of vision (Arts syndrome)

Arts et al. (1) described 12 boys in three generations who were affected by a combination of optic atrophy, deafness, susceptibility to infection, and neurologic degeneration.

Nervous system. The condition is characterized by onset of neurologic signs in infancy. Achievement of motor milestones was delayed, and once attained was lost soon thereafter. For example, one child could stand and walk with support at age 2 years, but lost that skill within 6 months. Truncal and extremity ataxia accompanied by loss of deep tendon reflexes was characteristic. Hypotonia was also fairly common. Arts et al. (1) suggested that there was involvement of the posterior columns, peripheral motor and sensory neurons, and second and eighth cranial nerves.

Ocular abnormalties. Optic atrophy developed during the first 1–2 years of life, with nystagmus developing soon thereafter. Other ocular signs included ptosis and paralytic squint.

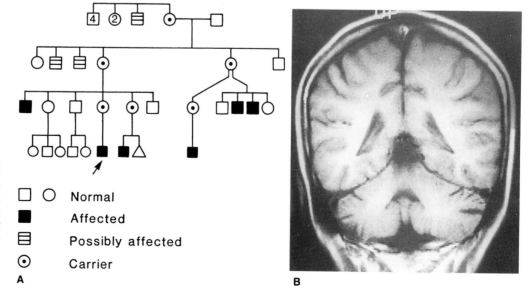

Figure 10–5. *Ataxia, optic atrophy, dysphagia, esotropia, and sensorineural hearing loss with episodic worsening (Schmidley syndrome).* (A) Pedigree showing X-linked recessive inheritance. (B) Coronal MRI scan of patient showing prominent cerebellar folia and enlarged fourth ventricle. [(B) from JW Schmidley et al., *Neurology* 37:1344, 1987.]

□ ○ Normal
■ Affected
▤ Possibly affected
⊙ Carrier

A   B

Immune system. This condition is characterized by an apparent increased susceptibility to infection, particularly involving the respiratory system. No disturbance of the immune system was identified, however.

Auditory system. Hearing loss is thought to be congenital and severe. Female carriers generally developed hearing loss during adulthood, which was severe enough to necessitate the use of hearing aids.

Imaging studies. Computed tomography and MRI results were normal.

Laboratory findings. Metabolic screening, lactate and pyruvate testing, chromosome analysis for increased breakage and fragile X, creatine kinase testing, and screening for congenital infections were all negative.

Pathology. Muscle biopsy showed in all but one individual signs of denervation and strong type I fiber grouping. Skin biopsy did not demonstrate abnormal storage products. Autopsy on one individual demonstrated absence of myelination in the dorsal columns, but not in the other tracts. The brain was entirely normal as well.

Heredity. This is an X-linked condition, which maps to Xq21.33–q24 (2).

Diagnosis. This condition most resembles the entity described above by Schmidley et al. (3), except in that condition brain abnormalities are found.

Prognosis. Death occurred by age 5 years in all but one boy; that boy was alive at age 12.

References

1. Arts WFM et al: X-linked ataxia, weakness, deafness, and loss of vision in early childhood with a fatal course. *Ann Neurol* 33:535–539, 1993.
2. Kremer H et al: Localization of the gene (or genes) for a syndrome with X-linked mental retardation, ataxia, weakness, hearing impairment, loss of vision and a fatal course in early childhood. *Hum Genet* 98:513–517, 1996.
3. Schmidley JW et al: Infantile X-linked ataxia and deafness: a new clinicopathologic entity? *Neurology* 37:1344–1349, 1987.

Ataxia, hypogonadotrophic hypogonadism, mental retardation, and sensorineural hearing loss (Richards-Rundle syndrome)

Richards and Rundle (6) described a syndrome consisting of slowly progressive ataxia, mental retardation, and sensorineural hearing loss in five sibs. Several other families were subsequently reported (1–3).

Central nervous system. Delay or lack of walking and language development were noticed in early childhood, and mental retardation was evident later. Several patients had IQs in the 65–70 range, while others appeared more severely retarded (perhaps magnified by the hearing loss). Progressive intellectual decline was not reported. At least one had seizures including status epilepticus.

In the family reported by Richards and Rundle (6), gait ataxia began before age 5 years and resulted in loss of walking within a few years. In other affected individuals, gait and limb ataxia appeared later and progressed more slowly. Male sibs seen by W.B. Dobyns were able to walk in their 20's. Deep tendon reflexes were present in early childhood, but were later lost in most patients. Hyperactive reflexes were reported in two sisters with late onset. Other abnormalities consisted of nystagmus, weakness, and distal wasting.

Peripheral nervous system. Nerve conduction studies showed slow conduction in the brothers examined by W.B. Dobyns. In other patients, the motor signs suggest peripheral nerve involvement.

Musculoskeletal system. All affected individuals had muscle wasting, particularly of the distal extremities. Skeletal abnormalities usually developed during the second decade, especially pes cavus, pes varus or equinovarus, flexion contractures of the fingers, and scoliosis (Fig. 10–6A).

Ocular system. Most patients had nystagmus.

Endocrine system. All patients had primary hypogonadism and failed to develop secondary sexual characteristics (Fig. 10–6B). Males had scanty axillary and pubic hair, higher-pitched (prepubertal) voice, normal penis, and descended testes. Females had scanty axillary and pubic hair, minimal breast tissue, prepubertal areolas, small labia, and infrequent or absent menses. Some patients also had diabetes mellitus, which was insulin-dependent in some cases.

Integumentary system. There was general disappearance of subcutaneous fat.

Auditory system. Sensorineural hearing loss began in the first few years of life (in the sibs who also had early onset of ataxia) and progressed rapidly to severe loss or began in adolescence and progressed more slowly. The brothers examined by W.B. Dobyns had mild loss with no need for hearing aids in their 20's.

Laboratory findings. Richards and Rundle (6) described marked reduction of urinary estrogen, pregnanediol, and total neutral 17-ketosteroid levels. Franceschi et al. (2) reported two adult females in whom plasma FSH levels were consistently higher than LH, growth hormone levels did not rise with provocative testing, and prolactin levels showed low peaks, all consistent with hypogonadotrophic hypogonadism. Thyroid and adrenal cortex functions were normal. Glucose tolerance tests were abnormal.

Pathology. Two sibs reported by Richards and Rundle (6) later died and were studied at autopsy (7). Principal neuropathologic changes consisted of nerve cell loss, myelin loss, and gliosis that affected selective areas of the brain stem, cerebellum, and spinal cord. Cell loss was most prominent within the dentate and other deep cerebellar nuclei, inferior olives, nuclei of gracilis and cuneatus, and Clarke's column. Large nerve fibers were severely depleted in the medial lemnisci and pyramids. Myelin loss involved the olivocerebellar tracts, spinocerebellar tracts, dorsal columns, and lateral corticospinal tracts. Gliosis involved these and many other areas within the brain stem and cerebellum. Peripheral nerves were small and had concentric thickening of fibrous tissue, hyaline degeneration, and reduced axons with normal myelination of those remaining. Changes typical of hypertrophic neuropathy with onion bulbs were not seen.

In the inner ear, lesions consisted of severe depletion of nerve tissue, atrophy of neuroepithelium, degenerate hair cells, abnormal attachment of Reissner's membrane, and prominent vessels with hemorrhage in the basal coils.

Ovaries were very small and consisted of ovarian fibrous stroma with no follicle formation. Testes were descended and showed nearly complete spermatogenic arrest at the spermatocyte stage. Leydig cells showed no evidence of function. The adrenals had good histologic differentiation, but lipid content was decreased.

Heredity. Inheritance is autosomal recessive, given observations of multiple affected sibs in four families, normal parents, and recognized consanguinity in one of the families (Fig. 10–6C).

Diagnosis. Several other syndromes have manifestations that overlap with this disorder. In Friedreich ataxia, hearing loss is less frequent, and hypogonadism and mental retardation do not occur. The syndrome of ataxia, mental retardation, motor and sensory neuropathy, spastic diplegia, and sensorineural hearing loss (Berman syndrome) also lacks hypogonadism. Hypogonadism also occurs in ataxia, amyotrophy of

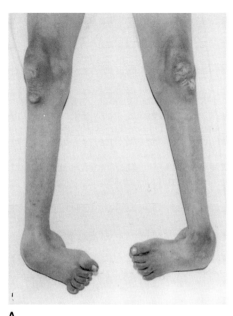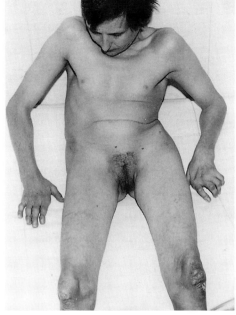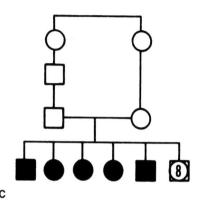

A   B   C

Figure 10–6. *Ataxia, hypogonadotrophic, hypogonadism, mental retardation, and sensorineural hearing loss (Richards-Rundle syndrome).* (A) Muscle atrophy and flexion deformities. (B) The patient, a deaf-mute, exhibits claw hands and wasting of peroneal muscles. The breasts are prepubescent and the pubic hair is scanty. (C) Pedigree showing 5 affected persons among 13 sibs from a consanguineous mating. [From BW Richards and AT Rundle, *J Ment Defic Res* 3:33, 1959.]

hands, spastic paraplegia, hypogonadism, short stature, and sensorineural hearing loss (Gemignani syndrome) and in spastic paraplegia, hypogonadism, and sensorineural hearing loss (Wells-Jankovic syndrome), although other manifestations differ. Ataxia and hypogonadism without hearing loss have been reported in several families (4,5).

Prognosis. All symptoms except possibly mental retardation are slowly progressive and lead to severe disability. At least three affected persons have died in early adulthood from pneumonia or status epilepticus.

Summary. This syndrome is characterized by (*1*) autosomal recessive inheritance; (*2*) ataxia; (*3*) distal amyotrophy; (*4*) mental retardation; (*5*) diabetes mellitus; (*6*) absent development of secondary sex characteristics; and (*7*) sensorineural hearing loss.

References

1. Fehlow P, Walther F: Richards-Rundle-Syndrom. *Klin Pädiatr* 203:184–186, 1991.
2. Franceschi M et al: Richards-Rundle syndrome, cochleovestibular dysfunction and neurofibromatosis in a family. *J Neurol* 231:11–13, 1984.
3. Koennecke W: Friedreichsche Ataxie und Taubstummheit. *Z Gesamte Neurol Pathol* 53:161–165, 1920.
4. Matthews WB, Rundle AT: Familial cerebellar ataxia and hypogonadism. *Brain* 87:463–468, 1964.
5. Neuhauser G, Opitz JM: Autosomal recessive syndrome of cerebellar ataxia and hypogonadotropic hypogonadism. *Clin Genet* 7:426–434, 1975.
6. Richards BW, Rundle AT: A familial hormonal disorder associated with mental deficiency, deaf mutism, and ataxia. *J Ment Defic Res* 3:33–55,1959.
7. Sylvester PE: Spino-cerebellar degeneration, hormonal disorder, hypogonadism, deaf mutism and mental deficiency. *J Ment Defic Res* 16:203–214, 1972.

Cerebellar ataxia and hypergonadotropic hypogonadism (Amor syndrome)

Amor et al. (1) described two sisters with the combination of ataxia, hypergonadotropic hypogonadism, and sensorineural hearing loss.

Nervous system. Onset of ataxia was during adulthood. Tendon reflexes were decreased in both.

Ocular system. Mild nystagmus was present.

Endocrine system. Both individuals (1) had menses for at least a few years before undergoing amenorrhea, one at age 16 and the other at age 32.

Auditory system. Hearing loss was sensorineural and mild to moderate in severity.

Vestibular function. Vestibular function was mildly impaired.

Imaging studies. Magnetic resonance imaging showed marked cerebellar atrophy.

Laboratory findings. Gonadotropins were in the postmenopausal range,

Heredity. This condition is most likely inherited as an autosomal recessive trait.

Diagnosis. This condition resembles, but is distinct from, other conditions that include the combination of ataxia, hypogonadism, and deafness (2). Perrault syndrome (3,4) has an earlier age of onset and is characterized by total lack of menstruation. However, see also discussion of Perrault syndrome in Chapter 12.

Prognosis. This condition is slowly progressive, but the sisters in the report were able to function quite well in their 40's.

References

1. Amor DJ et al: New variant of familial cerebellar ataxia with hypergonadotropic hypogonadism and sensorineural deafness. *Am J Med Genet* 99:29–33, 2001.

2. De Michele G et al: Heterogeneous findings in four cases of cerebellar ataxia associated with hypogonadism (Holmes' type ataxia). *Clin Neurol Neurosurg* 95:23–28, 1993.
3. Linssen WH et al: Deafness, sensory neuropathy, and ovarian dysgenesis: a new syndrome or a broader spectrum of Perrault syndrome? *Am J Med Genet* 51:81–82, 1994.
4. Nishi Y et al: The Perrault syndrome: clinical report and review. *Am J Med Genet* 31:623–629, 1988.

Ataxia, mental retardation, motor and sensory neuropathy, spastic diplegia, and sensorineural hearing loss (Berman syndrome)

A syndrome of slowly progressive ataxia, mental retardation, and sensorineural hearing loss was described in six children from two unrelated families by Berman et al. (1) in 1973 and Koletzko et al. (3) in 1987. Hanft and Haddad (2) reported a child with earlier onset of the ataxia and a more rapid progression. It is unknown if this is the same condition.

Central nervous system. Early motor development and speech were delayed. Walking was attained between 16 months and 4 years and was considered clumsy. Truncal ataxia began between 5 and 10 years and was followed by severe generalized ataxia and signs of both spasticity and peripheral neuropathy. The latter symptoms were all progressive. One child stopped walking at 15 years. All were mentally retarded with IQ scores between 35 and 60 (Fig. 10–7).

Myopathic-like facial appearance, horizontal nystagmus, marked truncal and extremity ataxia, spastic diplegia (weakness, spasticity, hyperreflexia, and extensor plantar responses), and sometimes neuropathic

Figure 10–7. *Ataxia, mental retardation, motor and sensory neuropathy, spastic diplegia, and sensorineural hearing loss (Berman syndrome). Two affected sibs and their normal brother (in the middle). Note myopathic facies, broad-based stance, and wasting of the legs.* [From W Berman et al., *Arch Neurol* 29:258, 1973.]

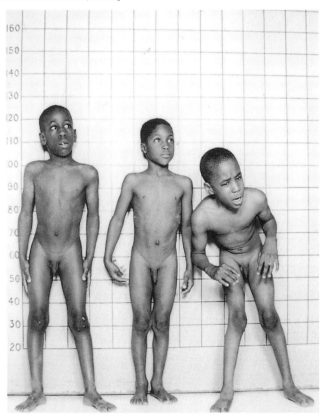

changes as described below were evident on examination. Cranial CT scans showed slight enlargement of lateral ventricles and atrophy of the cerebellar cortex and vermis.

Peripheral nervous system. Most affected individuals had subtle signs of clinical neuropathy superimposed on other neurological abnormalities, such as distal amyotrophy, reduced deep tendon reflexes, pes cavus, and hammer toes. Motor and sensory nerve conduction studies were normal in younger patients but became abnormal in older individuals with slowing of motor velocity and absent sensory responses. An EMG needle examination demonstrated a neurogenic pattern with fibrillation and denervation potentials in distal leg muscles.

Auditory system. Progressive sensorineural hearing loss began as early as 15 months in one child and was always present by age 8 years. Audiograms revealed bilateral sensorineural hearing loss of 40–90 dB. The hearing loss may have contributed to the observed speech delay.

Vestibular system. Caloric vestibular tests were normal.

Pathology. Muscle biopsy showed changes consistent with mild denervation. Sural nerve biopsy showed nonspecific changes with loss of large myelinated fibers and many hypomyelinated fibers, without onion bulb formation.

Heredity. Three affected boys in the first family and three affected girls in the second with healthy parents suggest autosomal recessive inheritance. However, onset of ataxia was at age 8–10 years in one family and in infancy in another, so there may be genetic heterogeneity.

Diagnosis. Patients having ataxia, hypogonadotrophic hypogonadism, mental retardation, and sensorineural hearing loss (Richards-Rundle syndrome) have hypogonadism in addition to ataxia. Patients with ataxia, dementia, myocardial fibrosis, and sensorineural hearing loss (Jeune-Tommasi syndrome) have ataxia but also myocardial fibrosis. Several different syndromes have ataxia with optic atrophy or congenital cataracts, which this syndrome lacks.

Summary. This syndrome is characterized by (*1*) autosomal recessive inheritance; (*2*) ataxia; (*3*) mental retardation; (*4*) spastic diplegia; (*5*) motor and sensory neuropathy; and (*6*) sensorineural hearing loss.

References

1. Berman W et al: A new familial syndrome with ataxia, hearing loss, and mental retardation: report of three brothers. *Arch Neurol* 29:258–261, 1973.
2. Hanft KL, Haddad J: Progressive sensorineural hearing loss (SNHL) and peripheral neuropathy: a case report. *Int J Pediatr Otorhinolaryngol* 28:229–234, 1994.
3. Koletzko S et al: Ataxia-deafness-retardation syndrome in three sisters. *Neuropediatrics* 18:18–21, 1987.

Olivopontocerebellar atrophy and deafness (Pratap-Chand syndrome)

Pratap-Chand et al. (2) described 11 Omani children who had the combination of progressive ataxia and hearing loss with onset in infancy. Eight were sporadic and three had an affected sib.

Central nervous system. Onset of neurologic symptoms occurred in the first year of life. Presentation was as progressive imbalance in sitting, standing, and walking. Spasticity and increased deep tendon reflexes occurred in some. Speech delay was also present (but may have been secondary to hearing loss). Seizures also occurred in two children.

Ocular system. Convergent squint and nystagmus occurred in less than half of the children. One child also had retinal coloboma and optic atrophy.

Growth. Height, weight, and head circumference were below the third centile in 8 of 11 individuals.

Auditory system. Hearing loss was fairly severe and may have been congenital; it was clearly present in infancy.

Imaging findings. Computed tomography demonstrated variable degrees of olivopontocerebellar atrophy. Enlargement of the fourth ventricle, cisterna magna, and foramen of Magendie was also noted in most children.

Heredity. This is almost certainly an autosomal recessive entity.

Diagnosis. This condition is similar to X-linked ataxia with deafness (3) but differs in mode in inheritance. It can also be distinguished from Berman syndrome (1) by age of onset and lack of peripheral neuropathy.

References

1. Berman W et al: A new familial syndrome with ataxia, hearing loss, and mental retardation: report of three brothers. *Arch Neurol* 29:258–261, 1973.
2. Pratap-Chand R et al: A syndrome of olivopontocerebellar atrophy and deafness with onset in infancy. *Acta Neurol Scand* 91:133–136, 1995.
3. Schmidley JW et al: Infantile X-linked ataxia and deafness. A new clinicopathologic entity. *Neurology* 37:1344–1349, 1987.

Ataxia, optic atrophy, and sensorineural hearing loss (autosomal recessive) (Dobyns syndrome)

A syndrome consisting of early-onset optic atrophy, ataxia, and sensorineural hearing loss was observed in two brothers by W. Dobyns (unpublished, 1994). The optic atrophy began earlier and was more severe than in Friedreich ataxia.

Ocular system. The proband began sitting closer to the television at 3.5 years. Visual impairment progressed rapidly during the following months. At 4 years, there were severe, bilateral optic atrophy and normal retinas with visual acuity of 4/30, but no nystagmus. By age 6 years, he had lost all but light perception and had prominent nystagmus. Electroretinogram at 4 years showed moderate depression to dark adapted blue and red flash stimuli and minimal depression to scotopic white flash stimulus. His younger brother had mild optic atrophy at 4 years of age.

Central nervous system. The proband had mild gait and truncal ataxia at 4 years. By age 6 years, he had mild hypotonia, moderate dysmetria of the hands, more obvious gait and truncal ataxia, and positive Romberg test. Intelligence was normal. Cranial MRI scan was unremarkable. His brother was asymptomatic at age 2 years but had mild ataxia at 4 years of age.

Peripheral nervous system. Deep tendon reflexes were absent in the older boy. They were normal in his brother at 2 years but diminished by age 4 years. Motor nerve conduction studies (NCS) were normal, while sensory NCS were absent on repeated exams in both the proband and his brother. The younger brother was 2 years old and asymptomatic at the time of the study.

Auditory system. The proband began turning up the television volume at 3.5 years of age. Audiometry revealed mild to moderate sensorineural loss at age 4 years, which was progressive (Fig. 10–8). A hearing aid was recommended at 5 years. His brother's last audiogram at age 3 years was normal.

Laboratory findings. Chromosome analysis in the older brother revealed mosaic Klinefelter syndrome in 20% of his cells (46,XY/ 47,XXY). This is probably unrelated to his progressive neurological disease. Extensive metabolic investigations, including amino and organic

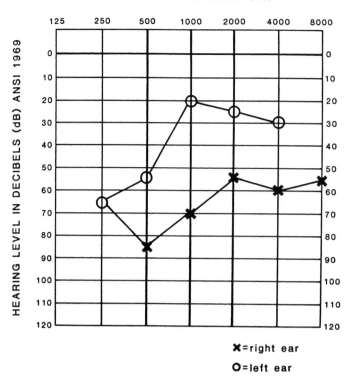

FREQUENCY IN HERTZ (Hz)

✗=right ear

O=left ear

Figure 10–8. *Ataxia, optic atrophy, and sensorineural hearing loss (autosomal recessive) (Dobyns syndrome).* Audiogram at 6 years shows decreased hearing for low frequencies on the right, and decreased hearing at all frequencies on the left.

acid analysis, serum lactate and pyruvate, and tests for lysosomal and peroxisomal diseases, were negative.

Pathology. Muscle and nerve biopsies in the proband showed only nonspecific changes.

Heredity. Inheritance is either autosomal or X-linked recessive, as two brothers were affected and both parents were normal.

Diagnosis. The late onset form of optico-cochleo-dentate degeneration (Muller-Zeman syndrome) presents at a similar age with mixed spastic and ataxic gait and hyperactive deep tendon reflexes. However, optic atrophy occurs much later if at all, and sensory nerve conduction abnormalities have not been described. In Friedreich ataxia, both optic atrophy and hearing loss occur later and remain mild. Behr syndrome consists of ataxia and optic atrophy with later onset. Hearing loss has not been described. The combination of ataxia, optic atrophy, and sensorineural hearing loss (autosomal dominant) (Sylvester syndrome) was described in a single, unusual family.

Prognosis. Follow-up has been insufficient to determine prognosis.

Summary. This disorder is characterized by (1) autosomal or X-linked recessive inheritance; (2) ataxia; (3) optic atrophy; (4) motor and sensory neuropathy; and (5) sensorineural hearing loss.

Ataxia, optic atrophy, and sensorineural hearing loss (autosomal dominant) (Sylvester syndrome)

In 1958, Sylvester (1) described a family in which six of nine children had ataxia, optic atrophy, and sensorineural hearing loss. Their father had optic atrophy and hearing loss but no ataxia.

Ocular system. Visual loss began before age 10 years and was slowly progressive. The optic discs appeared normal at first but became pale as the disorder progressed. The retina otherwise appeared normal. Visual fields showed peripheral constriction without central scotoma. Nystagmus was described after onset of ataxia.

Central nervous system. Development was apparently normal in early childhood although the children were described as dull. Neurologic changes beginning with unsteady gait were present by age 10 years and progressed thereafter. Associated abnormalities included nystagmus, limb ataxia, spasticity, increased or decreased deep tendon reflexes, extensor plantar responses, and muscle wasting, which was most prominent in the shoulders and hands. Some children had dysesthesias and diminished vibratory sensation. The father had none of these abnormalities, but was said to have had poliomyelitis as a child. The EMG was reported to be normal in one child.

Musculoskeletal system. Musculoskeletal complications of the neurologic disorder include kyphosis, scoliosis, pes cavus, and clawhand.

Auditory system. Hearing loss also started before age 10 years, but progression was uncertain. The hearing impairment was mild in three affected sibs and moderate or severe in the father and other sibs. No audiometric testing was reported.

Laboratory findings. Most routine and CSF fluid tests were normal.

Pathology. Histologic changes in the brain and spinal cord consisted of loss of myelinated fibers in the dorsal and ventral spinocerebellar tracts and posterior columns, and demyelination of the corticospinal tracts and optic nerves. Cell loss was prominent in the ventral and dorsal horns of the spinal cord, Clarke's column, cuneate nucleus, trigeminal nucleus, and substantia nigra (Fig. 10–9). The eighth nerve and auditory pathways were not described. Some of the material was lost prior to the report and was not available for review. Muscle biopsy was normal.

Heredity. Inheritance was probably autosomal dominant. Because the father lacked ataxia, the nosological place of this disorder is uncertain.

Diagnosis. The syndrome of ataxia, optic atrophy, and sensorineural hearing loss (autosomal recessive) (Dobyns syndrome) differs primarily because of the different pattern of inheritance. Optico-cochleodentate degeneration (Muller-Zeman syndrome) usually follows a more severe course. The combination of ataxia, optic atrophy, esotropia, dysphagia, and sensorineural hearing loss (Schmidley syndrome) is more severe and is X-linked. Clinical differentiation between these disorders and Friedreich's ataxia may be difficult.

Prognosis. The father had only visual and hearing deficits in middle age while three of his affected children died between 2 and 19

months after onset. Such extreme variation is unusual and adds to the questions regarding this syndrome.

Summary. This disorder is characterized by (*1*) probable autosomal dominant inheritance; (*2*) ataxia; (*3*) variable spasticity and amyotrophy; (*4*) optic atrophy; and (*5*) sensorineural hearing loss.

References

1. Sylvester PE: Some unusual findings in a family with Friedreich's ataxia. *Arch Dis Child* 33:217–221, 1958.

Cerebellar ataxia, areflexia, pes cavus, optic atrophy, and sensorineural hearing loss (CAPOS)

Nicolaides et al. (1) described a mother and her two children with early-onset ataxia, progressive optic atrophy, and sensorineural hearing loss.

Peripheral nervous system. Febrile illness during infancy seemed to trigger episodes of cerebellar ataxia, which then showed a pattern of relapse and remission. The ataxia seemed to become permanent during mid- to late childhood. Affected individuals also had absent deep tendon reflexes and pes cavus, which developed over time.

Ocular. Horizontal nystagmus was one of the earliest ocular manifestations, followed by progressive optic atrophy.

Auditory system. Sensorineural hearing loss was of postnatal onset but progressive, so that by adulthood hearing loss was profound in the mother. One child only had low-frequency loss at 9 months.

Heredity. This condition is inherited as either an autosomal dominant or mitochondrial trait.

Diagnosis. There are similarities to SCABD (spinocerebellar ataxia with blindness and deafness), but inheritance of that condition is autosomal recessive. There is also no indication that febrile episodes trigger ataxic episodes in that condition.

Reference

1. Nicolaides P et al: Cerebellar ataxia, areflexia, pes cavus, optic atrophy, and sensorineural hearing loss (CAPOS): a new syndrome. *J Med Genet* 33:419–421, 1996.

Cerebellar ataxia, deafness, and narcolepsy

Melberg et al. (2) described a four-generation family of five affected individuals in which all had ataxia and deafness and four had narcolepsy.

Central nervous system. Age of onset of neurologic symptoms was generally in the fourth and fifth decade, although some individuals showed signs of incoordination before the age of 20. Narcolepsy generally occurred before age 20, but in one individual it did not occur until the late 30's. Psychosis (paranoia, hallucinations) developed in the 40's in two individuals whereas seizures occurred in one at age 48.

Ocular system. Optic atrophy developed after the age of 38. Nystagmus was common, as was defective color vision in these individuals.

Endocrine system. Diabetes mellitus developed in the late 40's in two individuals.

Other findings. Excessive sweating was noted in two individuals.

Auditory system. Adult-onset sensorineural hearing loss progressed to total hearing loss in three of four adults. High tones were affected first, but then hearing loss progressed to include lower tones as

Figure 10–9. *Ataxia, optic atrophy, and sensorineural hearing loss (autosomal dominant) (Sylvester syndrome).* Sections of spinal cord from cervical, thoracic, and sacral levels show loss of myelinated fibers and demyelination of dorsal and ventral spinocerebellar tracts and dorsal columns. There is less marked demyelination of corticospinal tracts. [From PE Sylvester, *Arch Dis Child* 33:217, 1958.]

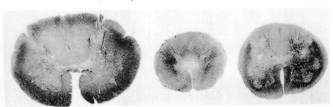

well. One individual, however, had a unilateral hearing loss affecting high tones at age 4 years.

Imaging studies. Computed tomography done 5 or more years after the onset of ataxia demonstrated rapidly progressing cerebellar and cerebral atrophy. Magnetic resonance imaging also showed brain stem atrophy. The MRIs done when individuals were in their 40's showed poor cerebral cortex–white matter differentiation and periventricular white matter changes (1).

Pathology. Muscle biopsy results in one individual were suggestive of mitochonrial dysfunction with decreased ATP production for certain substrates. However, analysis of the electron transport chain enzymes did not reveal any abnormalities.

Heredity. Autosomal dominant inheritance seems most likely. Although Melberg et al. (2) speculated that a mitochondrial disorder seemed likely, the presence of male-to-male transmission rules out mitochondrial inheritance.

Diagnosis. This disorder is distinguished from other adult-onset cerebellar ataxias by the presence of narcolepsy.

References

1. Melberg A et al: Neuroimaging study in autosomal dominant cerebellar ataxia, deafness, and narcolepsy. *Neurology* 53:2190–2192, 1999.
2. Melberg A et al: Autosomal dominant cerebellar ataxia deafness and narcolepsy. *J Neurol Sci* 134:119–129, 1995.

Optico-cochleo-dentate degeneration (Muller-Zeman syndrome)

This rare disorder of progressive spastic quadriplegia and visual and sensorineural hearing loss was first described by Muller and Zeman (3) in 1965. It has been reported in at least 13 individuals from six sibships. While age of onset and rate of progression have varied greatly, clinical signs and symptoms and pathological changes have been consistent (1–5).

Central nervous system. The earliest sign of the disease in most children (77%) is abnormal motor development during infancy. Most sibs have been concordant in this regard, although two sibs had discordant onset at birth and 5 years, respectively (4). Characteristic abnormalities include diminished spontaneous movements, poor head control, inability to sit, stand, or walk, hypotonia, and severe mental retardation. In one patient, cranial CT scan at 4 months showed mild cerebral atrophy, which progressed to severe cerebral and cerebellar atrophy by 11 months (1). In most patients with early onset, the disease progressed rapidly to immobility with flexor contractures, opisthotonos, extensor spasms of the legs, kyphoscoliosis, and, eventually, death. In children with later onset, the earliest motor sign was usually mixed spastic and ataxic gait. This progressed to more generalized spasticity and ataxia and hyperactive tendon reflexes. Later, reflexes became hypoactive or absent. Associated abnormalities vary and may include intention tremor, "cerebellar" myoclonus, foot deformity (pes cavus and equinovarus), scoliosis, and choreoathetosis. These disturbances may progress (albeit slowly) to complete immobility (Fig. 10–10). Mental abilities may be preserved for years, with rapid dementia occurring only terminally. Thus, this disorder follows a pattern in which early clinical onset is followed by a shorter and more severe clinical course.

Ocular system. In children with early onset, visual loss began during the first several years of life and was among the earliest well-defined signs. In those with later onset and slower course, visual signs occurred later or not at all (2). Once begun, visual loss progressed rapidly to blindness, usually over several years. The fundus appeared normal at first, but optic atrophy was observed later.

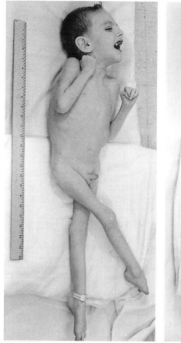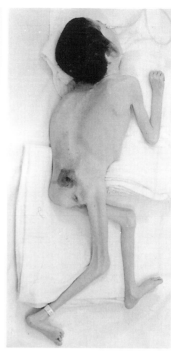

A   **B**

Figure 10–10. *Optico-cochleo-dentate degeneration (Muller-Zeman syndrome).* (A) Photograph of patient at 4 years showing multiple contractures, extensor spasm of legs, and cachexia. (B) Photograph of his brother at 10 years showing more severe cachexia, kyphoscoliosis, and severe contractures. [From J Muller and W Zeman, *Acta Neuropathol* 5:26, 1965.]

Auditory system. Hearing loss began several years after visual loss and progressed to severe loss over the following months to several years. Few hearing tests were carried out, but sensorineural hearing loss seems certain, given the pathological changes.

Laboratory findings. Cerebrospinal fluid lactate and pyruvate were normal in one child (1).

Pathology. The pathologic changes comprise a multisystem atrophy predominantly involving the optic, cochlear, dentatofugal, and medial lemniscal pathways. The optic nerves, chiasm, and tracts appeared diffusely demyelinated with degeneration of the lateral geniculate nuclei. The cochlear, superior olivary, inferior colliculi, and medial geniculate nuclei were atrophied and gliosed with demyelination and atrophy of the eighth nerve and lateral lemnisci. The dentate and inferior olivary nuclei were also severely atrophied and gliosed, with demyelination of the dentate hilus and superior cerebellar peduncles. Similar, severe changes were seen in the gracilis and cuneate nuclei in most patients, with degeneration of the medial lemnisci and posterior columns. Other less severe changes were widespread, affecting especially the cerebral and cerebellar cortices (1-5).

Heredity. Inheritance is autosomal recessive, given the observation of five sibships with two or more affected children, equal sex ratio, and no other affected relatives.

Prognosis. This disease results in cachexia, bedridden state, and shortened life span, especially for early-onset cases.

Diagnosis. The combination of ataxia, optic atrophy, and sensorineural hearing loss occurs in several disorders that may be difficult to differentiate. Ataxia, optic atrophy, and sensorineural hearing loss (Dobyns syndrome) might represent the same disorder without pathological confirmation, except that optic atrophy is prominent appearing well before any other symptoms begin, and a sensory neuropathy occurs, which probably causes the ataxia. The combination of ataxia, optic atrophy, esotropia, dysphagia, and sensorineural hearing loss (Schmidley syndrome) differs because of the episodic worsening, ophthalmoplegia, and X-linked pattern of inheritance.

Summary. This disorder is characterized by (1) autosomal recessive inheritance; (2) early developmental delay; (3) early hypotonia that evolves to (4) spastic quadriplegia; (5) ataxia; (6) dementia; (7) optic atrophy; and (8) sensorineural hearing loss associated with striking degeneration of optic, cochlear, dentate, and medial lemniscal pathways.

References

1. Ferrer I: Dégénérescence systématisée optico-cochléo-dentelée. *J Neurol* 234:416–420, 1987.
2. Hasaerts R: Sur une dégénérescence optico-cochléo-dentelée avec extension strio-thalamique des abiotrophies. *Encéphale* 46:81–107, 1957.
3. Muller J, Zeman W: Dégénérescence systématisée optico-cochléo-dentelée. *Acta Neuropathol* 5:26–39, 1965.
4. Nyssen R, van Bogaert L: La dégénérescence systématisée optico-cochléo-dentelée. (Etude anatomiclinique d'un type familial). *Rev Neurol* 2:321–345, 1934.
5. Zeman W: Dégénérescence systématisée optico-cochléo-dentelée. In: *Handbook of Clinical Neurology, Vol. 21. System Disorders and Atrophies, Part I,* Vinken PJ et al. (eds), North Holland Publishing Co., Amsterdam, 1975, pp 535–551.

Ataxia, pigmentary retinopathy, and sensorineural hearing loss (Hallgren syndrome)

Although most patients with ataxia, pigmentary retinopathy, and sensorineural hearing loss, including the large Swedish family reported by Hallgren (2) in 1959, have Usher syndrome, several patients have had later onset of symptoms and generalized, rather than gait, ataxia. It is likely that these patients (1,3,4) have a separate disorder described in this section. Even among these patients, heterogeneity is likely. None was evaluated for a mitochondrial disorder.

Central nervous system. Ataxia was noted by age 6 in one patient, but not until the 30's or 40's in the others, and was always slowly progressive. Examination showed generalized ataxia involving the arms and trunk as well as the legs and gait, normal or diminished tendon reflexes, and sometimes extensor plantar responses and diminished sensation in the distal legs. Mental retardation and schizophrenia were each observed in one patient. Cranial CT scan showed cerebellar atrophy in all patients studied (2,3). One patient also had cerebral atrophy, abnormal low density lesions around the frontal horns, and calcifications in the globus pallidus (2).

Peripheral nervous system. Some (but not all) patients had wasting of the hands and pes cavus. Sensory abnormalities varied, but some patients had decreased perception of light touch, pain, and joint position. Nerve conduction studies showed normal or slightly decreased motor conduction velocities and diminished sensory action potentials (3).

Ocular system. The first symptoms of visual loss were constriction of visual fields and night blindness. These were first noticed between 10 and 30 years of age and were slowly progressive. Examination showed nystagmus, pigmentary retinopathy, and, sometimes, optic atrophy and cataracts.

Other systems. The patient with mental retardation also had short stature and elevated CSF protein, which suggest the possibility of a mitochondrial disorder. Another had small testes.

Auditory system. Sensorineural hearing loss began between ages 15 and 40 years as high-frequency loss. It usually progressed to severe loss over many years.

Laboratory findings. Two patients had elevated serum triglycerides and pre-β lipoproteins, and one had elevated CSF protein. Tests for mitochondrial disorders were not described.

Pathology. Sural nerve biopsies showed reduced densities of myelinated fibers. Large-diameter fibers were predominantly affected in some patients, and smaller fibers in others (3).

Heredity. None of the patients had affected relatives. Thus, the inheritance pattern is unknown but is most likely autosomal recessive.

Diagnosis. Patients with severe Usher syndrome have congenital hearing loss and sometimes ataxia of gait with normal hand and trunk coordination. The same group of symptoms occurs in some patients with various mitochondrial disorders.

Prognosis. Several were still able to walk in later adult life.

Summary. This disorder is characterized by (1) possible autosomal recessive inheritance; (2) ataxia; (3) mild motor and sensory neuropathy; (4) pigmentary retinopathy; and (5) sensorineural hearing loss.

References

1. Bitoun P et al: A hereditary syndrome with retinopathy and ataxia or deafness in two consanguineous brothers. *Ophthalmol Paediatr Genet* 12:149–152, 1991.
2. Hallgren B: Retinitis pigmentosa combined with congenital deafness; with vestibulo-cerebellar ataxia and mental abnormality in a proportion of cases. A clinical and genetico-statistical study. *Acta Psychiatr Neurol Scand* 34(Suppl 138):1–101, 1959.
3. Koizumi J et al: CNS changes in Usher's syndrome with mental disorder: CT, MRI and PET findings. *J Neurol Neurosurg Psychiatry* 51:987–990, 1988.
4. Tuck RR, McLeod JG: Retinitis pigmentosa, ataxia, and peripheral neuropathy. *J Neurol Neurosurg Psychiatry* 46:206–213, 1983.

Ataxia, mental retardation, and sensorineural hearing loss (Reardon syndrome)

In 1993, Reardon et al. (3) described two brothers with ataxia, global developmental delay, and sensorineural hearing loss.

Central nervous system. Initial development was slightly delayed. One sib sat at age 10 months, walked independently at 18 months, and had several single words by the age of 2 years. Thereafter, progress was extremely slow. There was no history of seizures. At age 4, there were clear signs of cerebellar incoordination in upper limbs and gait was broad-based. Tone, power, and sensation were normal. His brother sat at 9 months, crawled at 9–10 months, and walked at 18 months. Gait was unsteady from the beginning. By age 3, he used simple sentences but no further progress was made. Unlike his brother, he had six generalized seizures, all associated with febrile episodes. His gait was ataxic, and there was finger–nose incoordination. Tone was reduced but power and reflexes were normal.

Auditory system. Both brothers had severe bilateral sensorineural hearing loss with normal middle ear function as confirmed by tympanometry.

Vestibular system. Vestibular tests were not performed.

Heredity. Inheritance is either autosomal or X-linked recessive. A maternal first cousin was said to be similarly affected but was not assessed.

Diagnosis. The syndrome of ataxia, mental retardation, motor and sensory neuropathy, spastic diplegia, and sensorineural hearing loss (Berman syndrome) is characterized by progressive ataxia, mental retardation, and sensorineural hearing loss (initially noted at age 2–3 years) (1). However, the patients had myopathic faces and marked muscle wasting of the lower limbs present by age 6. Hyperreflexia of lower limbs was observed with extensor plantar responses, and heel contractures developed. The EMG and sural nerve biopsy suggested mild peripheral neuropathy, and hearing loss was progressive, resulting in severe sensorineural loss.

Koletzko et al. (2) described three sisters with myopathic faces, extensor plantar responses, peripheral neuropathy, and ataxia at age 8–10 years. In contrast, the sibs reported by Berman et al. (1) had ataxia present from infancy.

Summary. Characteristics include (*1*) autosomal or X-linked recessive inheritance; (*2*) ataxia with onset in infancy; (*3*) global delay; and (*4*) sensorineural hearing loss with onset at 2–3 years.

References

1. Berman W et al: A new familial syndrome with ataxia, hearing loss and mental retardation. *Arch Neurol* 29:258–261, 1973.
2. Koletzko S et al: Ataxia-deafness-retardation syndrome in three sisters. *Neuropediatrics* 18:18–21, 1987.
3. Reardon W et al: A new form of familial ataxia, deafness, and mental retardation. *J Med Genet* 30:694–695, 1993.

IOSCA: Infantile-onset spinocerebellar ataxia (formerly OHAHA and SCA8)

Eleven individuals from Finland were first reported with this disorder (2). These families were then the subject of a series of clinical and gene localization and identification studies (6–8). The term *OHAHA syndrome* (MIM 258120) was originally suggested as an acronym for *o*phthalmoplegia, *h*ypotonia, *a*taxia, *h*ypoacusis, and *a*thetosis (3), but the preferred term is now IOSCA, an acronym for *i*nfantile-*o*nset *s*pino*c*erebellar *a*taxia.

Central nervous system. Ataxia and hypotonia appeared between ages 10 and 18 months (4,5). Motor function then improved somewhat and remained static until age 10–13 when it progressively diminished. The inability to speak was almost complete. Athetotic dyskinesia of the face and upper limbs varied considerably among patients. Intelligence was normal but strabismus and open mouth caused the patients to appear retarded. Epilepsy was a late manifestation (3).

Ocular system. Ophthalmoplegia was noted at 3–12 years. It too progressed, being almost complete with only convergence persisting, producing marked strabismus. No retinal pigmentary anomalies were evident.

Auditory system. Sudden hearing loss occurred between 1 and 4 years of age with steady progression to 90 dB or more in a few years. The eighth cranial nerve and nucleus were atrophic (5); however, otoacoustic emissions were absent, suggesting that a cochlear auditory pathology was also present. No auditory brain stem response (ABR) results have been published.

Vestibular system. Total loss of caloric responses was demonstrated in all patients tested (1).

Other findings. Primary hypogonadism was observed in female patients (3).

Heredity. The incidence of several affected sib pairs with normal parents indicates autosomal recessive inheritance. Consanguinity was noted in one family (2). The gene has been mapped to chromosome 10q24 (6).

Laboratory findings. No biochemical abnormalities were found. No ragged-red fibers or abnormal mitochondria were noted on muscle biopsy.

Diagnosis. Ophthalmoplegia is found in a host of disorders. In association with hearing loss, one must exclude Kearns-Sayre syndrome and other mitochondropathies such as MELAS and MERRF syndromes. Separation from IVIC syndrome should be evident.

Summary. The chief characteristics include (*1*) autosomal recessive inheritance; (*2*) ataxia, hypoacusis, athetosis, and ophthalmoplegia; (*3*) hypotonia; (*4*) sudden and rapid progressive sensorineural hearing loss; and (*5*) marked vestibular dysfunction.

References

1. Johnsson LG et al: Labyrinthine pathology in deaf patients with infantile onset of spinocerebellar ataxia (IOSCA). In: *Progress in Human Auditory and Vestibular Histopathology*, Iurato S, Veldman JE (eds), Amsterdam, Kugler, 1997, pp. 103–108.
2. Kallio AK, Jauhiainen T: A new syndrome of ophthalmoplegia, hypoacusis, ataxia, hypotonia and athetosis (OHAHA). *Adv Audiol* 3:84–90, 1985.
3. Koskinen T et al: Primary hypogonadism in females with infantile onset spinocerebellar ataxia. *Neuropediatrics* 26:263–266, 1995.
4. Koskinen T et al: Infantile onset spinocerebellar ataxia with sensory neuropathy: a new inherited disease. *J Neurol Sci* 121:50–56, 1994.
5. Lönnqvist T et al: Infantile onset spinocerebellar ataxia with sensory neuropathy (IOSCA): neuropathological features. *J Neurol Sci* 161:57–65, 1998.
6. Nikali K et al: Toward cloning of a novel ataxia gene: refined assignment and physical map of the IOSCA locus (SCA8) on 10q24. *Genomics* 39:185–191, 1997.
7. Nikali K et al: Random search for shared chromosomal regions in four affected individuals: the assignment of a new hereditary ataxia locus. *Am J Hum Genet* 56:1088–1095, 1995.
8. Varilo T et al: Tracing an ancestral mutation: genealogical and haplotype analysis of the infantile onset spinocerebellar ataxia locus. *Genome Res* 6:870–875, 1996.

Spastic paraplegia, hypogonadism, and sensorineural hearing loss (Wells-Jankovic syndrome)

In 1986, Wells and Jankovic (3) reported six males from two generations of a family with spastic paraplegia, hypogonadism, and sensorineural hearing loss.

Central nervous system. Weakness, falling, and other signs of spastic paraplegia began at age 10–15 years and progressed slowly. Essential (postural) and intention tremors of the head and arms often began at about the same time and resulted in deteriorating handwriting. One person had side-to-side head tremor and oscillopsia beginning at age 2. Examination at 10–30 years showed mild to moderate spastic paraplegia with moderate involvement of legs, minimal involvement of arms, and diminished joint position and vibration in the feet.

The EEG and EMG were normal when performed. Cranial CT scan showed cerebral atrophy in the proband at 28 years. Somatosensory and brain stem auditory evoked responses were prolonged.

Musculoskeletal system. Diminished growth velocity, especially after 10 years, and short stature were common. The proband began to walk with flexed knees at age 10. Radiographs later showed dysplastic hips and other changes of spondyloepiphyseal dysplasia. No other family members had any similar bony changes, so these findings might be unrelated.

Ocular system. Small lens opacities resembled suture lines. Fine granularity or pigment stippling of the macula was seen after 10 years. The lens changes progressed to white opacities involving the subcapsular region and lens cortex. Despite these changes, visual acuity was normal or only slightly decreased.

Endocrine system. Small, soft testes and other signs of hypogonadism were found in the proband at 28 years. Endocrine laboratory studies included increased corticotropin, FSH, LH and prolactin, and azospermia. Serum testosterone, morning and evening cortisol levels, adrenal response to corticotropin, growth hormone, and urine 17-keto-steroids and 17-hydroxysteroids were normal.

Auditory system. Sensorineural hearing loss began in childhood and progressed slowly. The proband had mild loss below 2000 Hz and moderate loss above 2000 Hz by age 15 years, while his brother had moderate to severe loss at 13 years.

Laboratory findings and pathology. Cerebrospinal fluid findings, except for elevated protein, were normal. Conjunctival biopsy in the proband showed a single abnormal inclusion similar to but larger than those seen in adrenoleukodystrophy. However, serum very long-chain fatty acids were normal.

Heredity. Inheritance is X-linked recessive as there are six affected males from two generations, all related through females (Fig. 10–11). Linkage studies excluded this disorder from the Xq28 region but did not establish the location (1). At least two genes for X-linked spastic paraplegia without deafness have been identified, one linked to probes from Xq28 and the other to probes from the Xq13–q22 region (2). Thus, the disease in this family might result from variable expressivity of the Xq13–q22 gene.

Diagnosis. At least two forms of X-linked spastic paraplegia exist, based on the linkage data. Clinical heterogeneity is also apparent as some families have pure spastic paraplegia (Strumpell form), while others have complex disorders that may include mental retardation or mild ataxia. The late-onset variant of X-linked adrenoleukodystrophy, known as adrenomyeloneuropathy, presents with spastic paraplegia without hearing loss, but may be excluded by measurement of very long-chain fatty acids. Autosomal dominant and recessive forms of familial spastic paraplegia are more common than X-linked forms. Spastic paraplegia, syndactyly, and sensorineural hearing loss (Opjordsmoen-Nyberg-Hansen syndrome) may be differentiated by autosomal dominant inheritance and usually by syndactyly. Many forms of spinocerebellar ataxia have a component of spastic paraplegia. Ataxia, amyotrophy of hands, spastic paraplegia, hypogonadism, short stature, and sensorineural hearing loss (Gemignani syndrome) may be related.

Prognosis. Disability was moderate to severe by mid-adulthood, but neither of the older affected individuals had died. Intellectual function was apparently normal.

Summary. This disorder is characterized by (*1*) X-linked recessive inheritance; (*2*) spastic paraplegia; (*3*) cataracts; (*4*) mild pigmentary retinopathy; (*5*) hypogonadism; and (*6*) sensorineural hearing loss.

Figure 10–11. *Spastic paraplegia, hypogonadism, and sensorineural hearing loss (Wells-Jankovic syndrome).* Pedigree of family showing X-linked recessive inheritance. [From CR Wells and J Jankovic, *Arch Neurol* 43:943, 1986.]

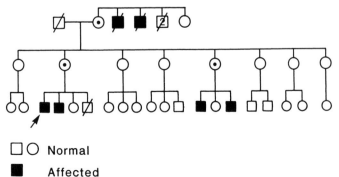

□○ Normal

■ Affected

⊙ Carrier

References

1. Fishbeck K-H et al: Linkage studies of X-linked spastic paraplegia. *Am J Hum Genet* 41:A165, 1987.
2. Goldblatt J et al: X-linked spastic paraplegia: evidence for homogeneity with a variable phenotype. *Clin Genet* 35:116–120, 1989.
3. Wells CR, Jankovic J: Familial spastic paraparesis and deafness: a new X-linked neurodegenerative disorder. *Arch Neurol* 43:943–946, 1986.

Spastic paraplegia, syndactyly, and sensorineural hearing loss (Opjordsmoen-Nyberg-Hansen syndrome)

In 1980, Opjordsmoen and Nyberg-Hansen (1) described spastic paraplegia, syndactyly, and sensorineural hearing loss in nine individuals from three generations of a Norwegian family.

Central nervous system. Bladder disturbances began before age 10 and consisted of urgency, frequency, and incontinence, especially at night. Gait disturbance began later (range 10–40 years) while the arms remained relatively uninvolved. All symptoms progressed slowly. Examination of the proband at age 46 showed weakness, spasticity, hyperreflexia and extensor plantar responses in the legs, and hyperreflexia only in the arms.

Musculoskeletal system. Syndactyly of fingers 4 and 5 served as a marker for the neurological symptoms. This anomaly was present in eight of nine affected individuals.

Auditory system. Mild bilateral sensorineural hearing loss probably began in adulthood, since it was described in only three of nine persons, all 40 years of age or older.

Laboratory findings. Visual evoked potentials were abnormal, suggesting subclinical involvement of the optic pathways.

Heredity. Inheritance is autosomal dominant with nine affected individuals from three generations and several instances of male-to-male transmission. Both spastic paraplegia and syndactyly have been reported as autosomal dominant traits, so this disorder could represent a contiguous gene deletion syndrome.

Diagnosis. Familial spastic paraplegia is genetically heterogeneous, as autosomal dominant, autosomal recessive, and X-linked recessive forms have been described. In some cases, a "pure" spastic paraplegia occurs, while others have more complex disorders, such as spastic quadriparesis, dementia/mental retardation, optic atrophy, pigmentary retinopathy, and sensorineural hearing loss (Gordon syndrome). A single family with X-linked spastic paraplegia and sensorineural hearing loss has been described.

Prognosis. While the gait and bladder disturbances are disabling, life span and intelligence are normal.

Summary. This disorder is characterized by (*1*) autosomal dominant inheritance; (*2*) spastic paraplegia; (*3*) syndactyly; and (*4*) sensorineural hearing loss.

Reference

1. Opjordsmoen S, Nyberg-Hansen R: Hereditary spastic paraplegia with neurogenic bladder disturbances and syndactylia. *Acta Neurol Scand* 61:35–41, 1980.

Spastic quadriparesis, dementia/mental retardation, optic atrophy, pigmentary retinopathy, and sensorineural hearing loss (Gordon syndrome)

This disorder was described in two brothers originating from a small genetic isolate in Maryland by Gordon et al. (1) in 1976.

Physical findings. Height, weight, and head circumference all followed the third centile. Both sibs had low-set, malformed ears and dull expression.

Central nervous system. The first signs were apparent as newborns: weak cry and suck, "quietness," and probably hypotonia. Motor development was delayed because of spasticity and weakness, which first affected the legs and later the arms. The brothers learned to walk with braces and to use a few words by 2–4 years of age. Examination showed expressionless face, drooling, mild spastic diplegia, and IQ of about 30–40 (Fig. 10–12A,B). The disorder progressed to include exotropia, nystagmus, severe spastic quadriplegia with dysphagia and loss of walking, progressive wasting, tremors, and myoclonic jerks by age 9 years. Speech was also lost.

Musculoskeletal system. Skeletal anomalies consisted of brachydactyly, especially of the third digit, clinodactyly, and congenital hip dislocation.

Ocular system. Vision was normal at first, but visual loss began in early childhood and progressed to severe loss with response only to bright lights. Fundus exam showed a pigmentary retinopathy with coarse, granular pigment throughout the retina, optic atrophy with small discs, and arteriolar narrowing. Electroretinograms were abnormal because of elevated electrical thresholds, subnormal cone response, and decreased light and dark adapted responses.

Auditory system. One child had profound sensorineural hearing loss (90 dB) by 2–4 years of age, while the other had subclinical or mild loss that became significant by 4–5 years. In later childhood, both responded only to loud noises. Neither child developed speech.

Vestibular system. Caloric vestibular tests were normal at 2–4 years.

Laboratory findings. Most routine studies were normal, but extensive metabolic testing for potentially similar disorders (i.e., mitochondrial or peroxisomal disorders) was not possible at the time.

Pathology. Bone marrow and rectal and sural nerve biopsies were normal.

Heredity. The parents were remotely related and came from a small genetic isolate in Maryland. Inheritance was probably autosomal recessive, although X-linked recessive inheritance could not be excluded (Fig. 10–12C).

Diagnosis. The combination of sensorineural hearing loss and retinitis pigmentosa occurs in several other diseases. Usher syndrome lacks neurologic manifestations except possibly for variable ataxia. The combination of ataxia, pigmentary retinopathy, and sensorineural hearing loss (Hallgren syndrome) is characterized by a slower clinical course with ataxia rather than spastic quadriplegia. Alström syndrome, Cockayne syndrome, and Refsum syndrome include many associated abnormalities that differ from this syndrome. Optico-cochleo-dentate degeneration (Muller-Zeman syndrome) lacks retinitis pigmentosa.

Prognosis. Both brothers were bedridden and completely disabled by 9 years. Prolonged survival seemed unlikely.

Summary. This disorder is characterized by (*1*) autosomal recessive or X-linked inheritance; (*2*) spastic quadriparesis; (*3*) both mental retardation and dementia; (*4*) optic atrophy; (*5*) pigmentary retinopathy; and (*6*) sensorineural hearing loss.

Reference

1. Gordon AM et al: Progressive quadriparesis, mental retardation, retinitis pigmentosa, and hearing loss: report of two sibs. *Johns Hopkins Med* J 138:142–145, 1976.

Chorea and sensorineural hearing loss

In 1977, Damasio et al. (2) described chorea and sensorineural hearing loss in two sibs, but the same movement disorder without hearing loss has been reported in several other families (1).

Central nervous system. Involuntary movements began insidiously before age 10 and progressed over several years to severe chorea involving the head and all limbs. It eventually reached a plateau, after which further progression did not occur. The chorea did not prevent walking. Examination showed hypotonia and involuntary movements. Dementia, mental retardation, seizures, and other neurologic abnormalities were not present.

Figure 10–12. *Spastic quadriparesis, dementia/mental retardation, optic atrophy, pigmentary retinopathy, and sensorineural hearing loss (Gordon syndrome).* (A,B) Two sibs showing short stature, lack of facial expression, and low-set, malformed ears. (C) Pedigree of family supports autosomal recessive inheritance. [From AM Gordon et al., *Johns Hopkins Med* J 138:142, 1976.]

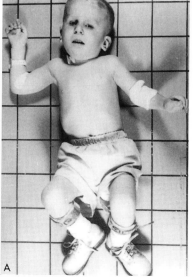
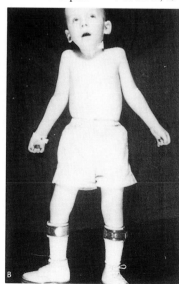
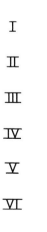
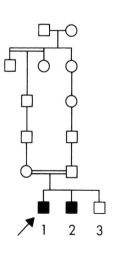

Auditory system. Congenital hearing loss was evident. Audiometry suggested localization of the defect in the cochlea, in the eighth nerve, or in both the cochlea and eighth nerve.

Heredity. Inheritance is probably autosomal recessive, based on multiple affected sibs of each sex and normal parents.

Diagnosis. Familial chorea occurs in several other diseases such as Huntington disease, autosomal dominant late-onset chorea, chorea with acanthocytosis, paroxysmal dystonic choreoathetosis, and paroxysmal kinesiogenic choreoathetosis, none of which includes hearing loss.

Prognosis. While the chorea is disabling, it does not progress indefinitely, and other neurologic manifestations do not occur.

Summary. This disorder is characterized by (*1*) autosomal recessive inheritance; (*2*) childhood onset, nonprogressive chorea; (*3*) mild hypotonia; and (*4*) sensorineural hearing loss.

References

1. Chun RWM et al: Benign familial chorea with onset in childhood. *JAMA* 225:1603–1607, 1973.
2. Damasio H et al: Familial nonprogressive involuntary movements of childhood. *Ann Neurol* 1:602–603, 1977.

Choreoathetosis, mental retardation, microcephaly, spastic quadriplegia, strabismus, and sensorineural hearing loss (Schimke-Horton syndrome)

In 1984, Schimke et al. (2) first described a striking syndrome of severe basal ganglia disorder, mental retardation, strabismus, postnatal microcephaly, short stature, and sensorineural hearing loss in four boys from two unrelated families.

Physical findings. Length and weight were normal at birth, but postnatal growth was slow, leading to growth deficiency and microcephaly. All affected individuals had a similar appearance characterized by microcephaly, sunken eyes, internal strabismus, and narrow nasal bridge. This gave the appearance of a "pinched" face in older individuals.

Central nervous system. Hypotonia and poor feeding were evident in the newborn period and gradually evolved to mixed hypotonia and spastic quadriplegia. Examination showed (postnatal) microcephaly, profound mental retardation, axial hypotonia, spasticity of limbs, hyperreflexia, and extensor plantar responses. Random, dyskinetic movements began in infancy and progressed to frank choreoathetosis. These movements became less prominent as spasticity progressed and contractures developed. Cranial CT scan at 1 year showed only atrophy, although basal ganglia calcifications would be expected in older patients on the basis of autopsy observations.

Ocular system. None of the patients appeared to be able to see, although it was not determined whether this was due to brain or eye abnormalities. All had internal strabismus, which the authors referred to as "apparent external ophthalmoplegia."

Renal system. Bilateral ureteral reflux and hydronephrosis were found in one child.

Auditory system. Severe hearing loss was present, probably from birth. Brain stem auditory evoked responses were decreased or absent, while impedance studies were normal, suggesting sensorineural hearing loss.

Laboratory findings. Blood lactate and pyruvate levels were normal.

Pathology. Autopsy studies in one patient showed moderate atrophy, especially of the cerebellum and cystic basal ganglia. Microscopic examination showed extensive calcification of the thalamus and globus pallidus, spongy degeneration in the same area, extensive gliosis in the thalamus, periaqueductal tissues and cerebellum, and loss of cerebellar Purkinje cells.

Heredity. Three males in the first family were affected, including the proband, his maternal uncle, and maternal first cousin (Fig. 10–13). His mother and maternal aunt (mother of the affected cousin) had mild congenital hearing loss. In the second family, only the male proband was affected. X-linked recessive inheritance appears likely.

Diagnosis. Similar neurological abnormalities occur with kernicterus and in Lowe oculocerebrorenal syndrome, but without hearing loss. Other X-linked mental retardation–hearing loss syndromes to be excluded are X-linked mental and somatic retardation, genital hypoplasia, and sensorineural hearing loss (Juberg-Marsidi syndrome) and optic atrophy, mental retardation, seizures, spasticity, restricted joint mobility, and sensorineural hearing loss (Gustavson syndrome); see Table 10–1. Golabi et al. (1) described an X-linked syndrome of somatic and mental retardation, microcephaly, seizures, spasticity, obesity, and sensorineural hearing loss.

Prognosis. This disease results in severe disability and shortened life span.

Summary. This disorder is characterized by (*1*) X-linked recessive inheritance; (*2*) congenital hypotonia; (*3*) choreoathetosis; (*4*) later spastic quadriplegia with contractures; (*5*) mental retardation; (*6*) typical facial appearance with "pinched" nasal bridge; (*7*) postnatal microcephaly; (*8*) postnatal growth deficiency; (*9*) apparent blindness; and (*10*) sensorineural hearing loss.

References

1. Golabi M et al: A new X-linked multiple congenital anomalies/mental retardation syndrome. *Am J Med Genet* 17:367–374, 1984.
2. Schimke RN et al: A new X-linked syndrome comprising progressive basal ganglion dysfunction, mental and growth retardation, external ophthalmoplegia, postnatal microcephaly and deafness. *Am J Med Genet* 17:323–332, 1984.

Dystonia and sensorineural hearing loss (Scribanu-Kennedy syndrome)

In 1976, Scribanu and Kennedy (6) described a French family with X-linked dystonia and hearing loss. Because X-linked dystonia without

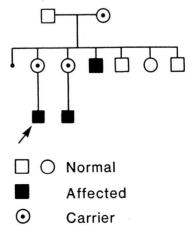

Figure 10–13. *Choreoathetosis, mental retardation, microcephaly, spastic quadriplegia, strabismus, and sensorineural hearing loss (Schimke-Horton syndrome).* Pedigree of the family shows X-linked recessive inheritance. [From RN Schimke et al., *Am J Med Genet* 17:323, 1984.]

☐ ○ Normal
■ Affected
⊙ Carrier

Table 10–1. X-linked mental retardation syndromes and hearing loss

Manifestation	Juberg-Marsidi Syndrome	Golabi-Ito-Hall Syndrome	Schimke-Horton Syndrome	Gustavson Syndrome	Martin Syndrome
Early death	+	–	–	+	–
Growth retardation	+	+	+	+	+
Mental retardation	+	+	+	+	+
Microcephaly	+	+	+	+	+
Optic atrophy	+	–	–	+	
Ophthalmoplegia	+	–	+	–	
Hearing loss	+	+	+	+	+
Spasticity	+	+		+	
Epileptic seizures	+	+	+	+	
Renal abnormalities			+	–	+
Hypogonadism	+	–		–	+
Endocrine disorders	+	+		–	+
Restricted joint mobility		–	+	+	

Adapted from K-H Gustavson et al., *Am J Med Genet* 45:654, 1993.

hearing loss has been reported in an isolated Filipino population (3,4), this disorder might represent a rare contiguous gene deletion syndrome.

Central nervous system. Motor and probably speech development were normal in early childhood, although speech became worse following the onset of hearing loss. Dystonic movements began at 5–7 years and were progressive. By age 9 years, the proband was unable to walk. A trial on L-dopa resulted in dramatic, albeit shortlived, improvement. After several months, he began to regress. Both he and his uncle became bedridden and died. During the therapeutic respite, psychometric testing showed an IQ of 74 in the proband; it is uncertain whether this represents mental retardation or dementia. The nephew was mentally retarded, but no dystonia was noted by age 6 years. In the Filipino population (without hearing loss), the mean age of onset was 38 years with a range of 12 to 52 years, and the dystonia became generalized within 10 years after onset (3).

Auditory system. Hearing loss began in early childhood (2–6 years) and progressed to severe or profound impairment. The nephew of the proband, who had been born prematurely, had sensorineural hearing loss.

Pathology. Major pathological changes in the brain consisted of neuronal loss and gliosis of the caudate, putamen, and globus pallidus bilaterally. The brain stem and spinal cord were normal. Changes in the vestibular nerve and inner ear were not described.

Heredity. The three affected males came from three generations of a family and were related through females, a pattern consistent with X-linked recessive inheritance (Fig. 10–14). Both X-linked dystonia without hearing loss (2) and X-linked sensorineural hearing loss have been described, so it is possible that this disorder is caused by deletion of contiguous genes on the X chromosome. Mapping studies in several large Filipino families (without hearing loss) showed linkage to probes at Xq21 (1). There is a significant similarity to the condition first described by Mohr and Mageroy (5) (now called the Mohr-Tranebjaerg syndrome), which includes optic atrophy as an additional manifestation. This condition has been mapped to Xq22 and is caused by mutations in the *DDP* gene (1,7). The best evidence for Scribanu-Kennedy syndrome being the same condition is that Jin et al. (1) found *DDP* mutations in individuals who had dystonia and deafness, but no ocular manifestations.

Diagnosis. Several genetic diseases associated with dystonia have been described, especially dystonia musculorum deformans (familial torsion dystonia), which has been mapped to chromosome 9q32–q34. X-linked dystonia has been described in a large Filipino family originating on Panay Island (4). The only similar disorder associated with hearing loss is chorea and sensorineural hearing loss.

Prognosis. The proband and his uncle both became bedridden and mute; they died during their teens or 20's.

Summary. This disorder is characterized by (*1*) X-linked recessive inheritance; (*2*) dystonia; (*3*) probable dementia; and (*4*) sensorineural hearing loss.

References

1. Jin H et al: A novel X-linked gene, *DDP*, shows mutations in families with deafness (DFN-1), dystonia, mental deficiency, and blindness. *Nat Gent* 14:177–180, 1996.
2. Kupke KG et al: Assignment of the X-linked torsion dystonia gene to Xq21 by linkage analysis. *Neurology* 40:1438–1442, 1990.
3. Kupke KG et al: X-linked recessive torsion dystonia in the Philippines. *Am J Med Genet* 36:237–242, 1990.
4. Lee L et al: Torsion dystonia in Panay, Philippines. *Adv Neurol* 14:137–151, 1976.
5. Mohr J, Mageroy K: Sex-linked deafness of a possibly new type. *Acta Genet Statist Med* 10:54–62, 1960.
6. Scribanu N, Kennedy C: Familial syndrome with dystonia, neural deafness, and possible intellectual impairment: clinical course and pathological findings. *Adv Neurol* 14:235–243, 1976.
7. Tranebjaerg L et al: A de novo missense mutation in a critical domain of the X-linked *DDP* gene causes the typical deafness-dystonia-optic atrophy syndrome. *Eur J Hum Genet* 8:464–467, 2000.

Figure 10–14. *Dystonia and sensorineural hearing loss (Scribanu-Kennedy syndrome). Pedigree shows X-linked recessive inheritance.* (From N Scribanu and C Kennedy, *Adv Neurol* 14:235, 1976.]

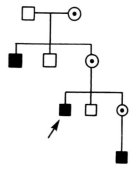

□ Normal
■ Affected
⊙ Carrier

Progressive myoclonus epilepsy, ataxia, and sensorineural hearing loss (May-White syndrome)

In 1968, May and White (3) first described a syndrome of progressive myoclonus epilepsy, ataxia, and sensorineural hearing loss. Several other families have subsequently been described (1,2,5).

Central nervous system. Progressive ataxia was first observed during the teens and 20's in six of eight patients, while the other two had later onset. Gait ataxia usually preceded limb and speech ataxia, and several patients became unable to walk. Myoclonic jerks were reported in five of eight patients and were often frequent. Onset of the jerks and the ataxia occurred at about the same age as the ataxia. Photic stimulation during EEG precipitated electrical and sometimes clinical myoclonic seizures in several patients, including two with no history of myoclonic jerks (Fig. 10–15A). In one patient, a seizure was precipitated during pattern shift visual evoked potential testing. Some patients also had generalized tonic clonic seizures, but these were never frequent. Intelligence was normal and no patient had weakness or atrophy. One patient became demented at 70 years of age.

Peripheral nervous system. Mild peripheral neuropathy was documented in two patients who were asymptomatic, but tendon reflexes were absent in the legs (1,4). Nerve conduction studies in one patient showed slowing in the peroneal nerve and reduced amplitude of sensory nerve action potentials (1).

Ocular system. One patient developed cataracts in his late 50's.

Auditory system. Progressive sensorineural hearing loss was first noted as early as age 4 years and as late as 70 years (1–4). In most patients, it preceded onset of neurological symptoms by several years. Audiometry in two patients showed moderately severe hearing loss (30–50 dB) and full recruitment without tone decay. Stapedius reflex thresholds were normal. The abnormalities were considered cochlear in origin (1).

Vestibular system. Vestibular testing in the same two patients was abnormal. In one of these patients, caloric responses were absent; in the other the caloric responses showed a marked directional preponderance to the right with superimposed canal paresis. Optokinetic nystagmus was abnormal in both. There was no positional nystagmus. The abnormalities were considered consistent with semicircular canal involvement (1).

Laboratory findings. No laboratory tests were reported. However, both myoclonus epilepsy and ataxia are known to occur in several disorders of mitochondrial metabolism. Thus, similar patients should be evaluated for abnormalities of mitochondrial metabolism.

Pathology. Autopsy was performed in one patient who died at age 74 (1). Gross examination of the brain showed mild atrophy of the dentate nuclei of the cerebellum and small areas of old softening in the left basis pontis. Histologic examination of the cerebrum showed foci of laminar necrosis in the right pericallosal gyrus and loss of pyramidal neurons from Ammon's horn. The brain stem had an area of cavitation in the left basis pontis and some gliosis of the inferior olive. The cochlear nuclei were normal. The cerebellum showed atrophy of the vermis and hemispheres, decreased density of Purkinje cells, and reduced volume of white matter. The spinal cord showed pallor of the gracile tracts.

Heredity. The pedigrees in the four families were most consistent with autosomal dominant inheritance (Fig. 10–15B). However, maternal inheritance remains a possibility.

Diagnosis. Both myoclonus epilepsy and ataxia occur in some disorders of mitochondrial metabolism. The clinical manifestations of several mitochondrial encephalomyopathies overlap with this syndrome, but muscle biopsy usually shows ragged-red fibers, and biochemical studies such as serum lactate may be helpful. For example, mitochondrial encephalomyopathy plus myoclonus epilepsy with ragged-red fibers (MERRF) is very similar (5). Mitochondrial encephalomyopathy with progressive myoclonus epilepsy, ataxia, dementia, diabetes mellitus, nephropathy, and sensorineural hearing loss (Herrmann syndrome) differs because of renal disease and diabetes and may also have maternal inheritance, indicating that it may be a mitochondrial disorder. The combination of progressive myoclonus epilepsy, dementia, and hearing loss (Latham-Munro) usually has earlier onset, follows a more severe course, lacks ataxia, and is autosomal recessive.

Prognosis. This disorder is very disabling because of the ataxia, myoclonus epilepsy, and hearing loss. In the late-onset family (1), two patients died at 60 and 74 years of age from problems related, at least in part, to the disease. Follow-up on the families with earlier onset is not available, but prognosis is presumably worse.

Summary. This syndrome is characterized by (*1*) autosomal dominant inheritance; (*2*) ataxia; (*3*) myoclonic and other seizures; and (*4*) sensorineural hearing loss.

References

1. Baraitser M et al: Autosomal dominant late-onset cerebellar ataxia with myoclonus, peripheral neuropathy and sensorineural deafness: a clinicopathological report. *J Neurol Neurosurg Psychiatry* 47:21–25, 1984.

Figure 10–15. *Progressive myoclonus epilepsy, ataxia, and sensorineural hearing loss (May-White syndrome).* (A) EEG shows spike discharges and myoclonic jerks in response to photic stimulation. (B) Pedigree showing six affected individuals in four generations. [From DL May and HH White, *Arch Neurol* 19:331, 1968.]

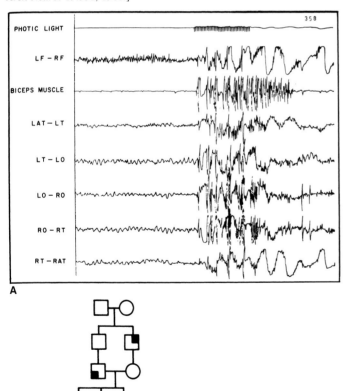

2. Chayasirisobhon S, Walters B: Familial syndrome of deafness, myoclonus, and cerebellar ataxia. *Neurology* 34:78–79, 1984.
3. May DL, White HH: Familial myoclonus, cerebellar ataxia, and deafness. *Arch Neurol* 19:331–338, 1968.
4. Melo TP, Ferro JM: Autosomal dominant cerebellar ataxia with deafness, myoclonus and amyotrophy. *J Neurol Neurosurg Psychiatry* 52:1448–1449, 1989.
5. Vaamonde J et al: Abnormal muscle and skin mitochondria in family with myoclonus, ataxia, and deafness (May-White syndrome). *J Neurosurg Psychiatry* 55:128–132, 1992.

Progressive myoclonus epilepsy, dementia, and sensorineural hearing loss (Latham-Munro syndrome)

In 1937, Latham and Munro (1) reported progressive myoclonus epilepsy, dementia, and sensorineural hearing loss in five sibs born to normal parents.

Central nervous system. Frequent episodes of generalized myoclonus began at about 10–12 years and gradually progressed in frequency and severity. They were soon followed by generalized tonic clonic seizures, often during the night after a prolonged episode of myoclonus. Early development and intelligence were considered normal. As the disease progressed, more frequent myoclonic and other seizures, abnormal behavior, and dementia were observed. In some patients, more rapid deterioration occurred in their 20's, while this was delayed until the 40's or 50's in others. All patients eventually became bedridden and several had died at the time of the report.

Cardiovascular system. One patient succumbed suddenly from dilated cardiomyopathy at 24 years.

Auditory system. All affected individuals had profound congenital hearing loss and none learned to speak. Results of hearing tests were not described, but sensorineural loss was presumed.

Laboratory findings. No laboratory tests were reported. However, myoclonus epilepsy is known to occur in several disorders of mitochondrial metabolism. The report of cardiomyopathy in one patient suggests that this disorder might also involve mitochondrial metabolism. Similar patients should be evaluated for abnormalities of mitochondria.

Pathology. No pathologic findings were described.

Heredity. Inheritance is autosomal recessive on the basis of parental consanguinity (second cousins) and multiple affected children of both sexes. Neither parent had any evidence of disease.

Diagnosis. Mitochondrial encephalomyopathy, myoclonus epilepsy with ragged-red fibers (MERRF), and sensorineural hearing loss and other mitochondrial disorders may be difficult to differentiate clinically; but muscle biopsy usually shows ragged-red fibers, and biochemical studies may be helpful. Mitochondrial encephalomyopathy with progressive myoclonus epilepsy, ataxia, dementia, diabetes mellitus, nephropathy, and sensorineural hearing loss (Herrmann syndrome) differs because of renal disease, diabetes, and probable maternal inheritance. The syndrome of progressive myoclonus epilepsy, ataxia, and sensorineural hearing loss (May-White syndrome) differs because of ataxia and autosomal dominant inheritance.

Prognosis. The neurological disorder led to death in early or middle adult life.

Summary. This disorder is characterized by (*1*) autosomal recessive inheritance; (*2*) progressive myoclonus epilepsy; (*3*) dementia; and (*4*) profound congenital sensorineural hearing loss.

Reference

1. Latham AD, Munro TA: Familial myoclonus epilepsy associated with deaf-mutism in a family showing other psychobiological abnormalities. *Ann Eugen* 8:166–175, 1937.

Myoclonic epilepsy, congenital hearing loss, macular dystrophy, and psychiatric disorders (Megarbane syndrome)

Megarbane et al. (2) described two sibs, one male, one female, with the title combination. Additional manifestations included incomplete bundle branch block. Hearing loss was congenital, but the onset of neurologic signs did not develop until adulthood.

Nervous system. The neurologic manifestations could best be described as episodes. These episodes did not develop until after the age of 30 years. The episode began with a fever of unknown origin accompanied by vomiting and seizures. Coma lasting 3 days then usually occurred, followed by psychiatric manifestations such as hallucinations, delirium, and depression. Episodes occurred once or twice a year, with seizures becoming myoclonic with successive episodes.

Ocular findings. Ophthalmologic investigation demonstrated deposits of yellow pigment in the macula; vision did not appear to be affected.

Cardiac findings. Both had incomplete right bundle branch block as demonstrated by ECG.

Auditory system. Both sibs had fairly severe congenital bilateral sensorineural hearing loss.

Imaging studies. The woman had mild brain atrophy noted on MRI at age 40.

Laboratory studies. Mitochondrial mutations were not found, and skin and muscle biopsy did not demonstrate any evidence of a respiratory chain disorder.

Heredity. This condition is most likely autosomal recessive, particularly since the parents are second cousins.

Diagnosis. This condition most resembles the entity described by Latham and Munro (1), but can be distinguished by the much earlier age of onset and rapid deterioration and death by early adulthood.

Prognosis. This condition seems to be slowly progressive, but life span is unknown.

References

1. Latham AD, Munro TA: Familial myoclonus epilepsy associated with deaf-mutism in a family showing other psychobiological abnormalities. *Ann Eugen* 8:166–175, 1937.
2. Megarbane A et al: Two sibs with myoclonic epilepsy, congenital deafness, macular dystrophy, and psychiatric disorders. *Am J Med Genet* 87:289–293, 1999.

Dystonia, pigmentary retinopathy, and sensorineural hearing loss (Coppeto-Lessell syndrome)

In 1990, Coppeto and Lessell (1) described dystonia (with blepharospasm) and pigmentary retinopathy in male and female sibs, one of whom had congenital sensorineural hearing loss.

Physical findings. Both sibs had high-arched palate, and the proband had marked lumbar lordosis.

Central nervous system. The proband developed excessive blinking (blepharospasm), dysarthria, and poor coordination of the arms at age 17 years. Initial examination showed normal cognitive skills, marked blepharospasm, dysarthria, poor arm coordination, and stiff and stooped gait. Over the next several years, her gait became more clumsy, stiff, and narrow-based, and she fell frequently. At 30 years, she had inappropriate affect and poor judgment but intellectual function was otherwise normal. Her exam showed mask-like face, slight restriction of upgaze, severe blepharospasm, facial grimacing, unintelligible speech, writhing neck movements, poor coordination, chorea (primarily in the arms), cogwheel rigidity, hyperactive tendon reflexes with bilateral ankle clonus, loss of superficial abdominal reflexes, normal plantar responses, and slow gait with retropulsion. She did not have ataxia. Her brother had poor coordination by age 3 years. By 23 years, he had abnormalities similar to but less severe than those of his sister. He was also considered intellectually slow and had impaired memory. A CT scan of the proband showed bilateral calcification of basal ganglia.

Ocular system. When examined at 17 years, the proband had a mild decrease in visual acuity to 20/40 in both eyes, mild constriction of visual fields, slightly pale optic discs, and mild, macular pigmentary retinopathy. Over the next few years, she had gradual visual loss. By age 30 years she had night blindness, visual acuity of 20/400, severe constriction of visual fields to 15 degrees, and advanced pigmentary retinopathy with marked pigment clumping around the macula and bone corpuscles in the periphery.

Auditory system. The brother's severe, bilateral sensorineural hearing loss, discovered in infancy, progressed to complete loss over several years. The sister had normal hearing and audiogram at 30 years.

Laboratory findings. Normal studies included thyroid and parathyroid function tests, complete blood count, red cell morphology, blood lactate and pyruvate, serum very long-chain fatty acids, phytanic acid, copper and ceruloplasmin, and urine amino acids.

Pathology. Muscle biopsies showed increased variation of fiber size and slightly increased central nuclei. Muscle mitochondria appeared normal. Nerve biopsy showed mild loss of myelinated fibers with occasional thinly myelinated fibers.

Heredity. Two sibs of different sex were affected. While not known to be consanguineous, the parents came from the same small village in Italy. Thus, inheritance is probably autosomal recessive.

Diagnosis. Patients with Usher syndrome have pigmentary retinopathy and hearing loss. Patients with ataxia, pigmentary retinopathy, and sensorineural hearing loss (Hallgren syndrome) may have diverse neurologic symptoms, but not dystonia. Patients with dystonia and sensorineural hearing loss (Scribanu-Kennedy syndrome) lack the visual abnormalities, and inheritance is X-linked.

Prognosis. The disorder was slowly progressive and resulted in severe disability before 30 years of age.

Summary. This disorder is characterized by (1) autosomal recessive inheritance; (2) dystonia including blepharospasm; (3) pigmentary retinopathy; (4) possible dementia; and sometimes (5) sensorineural hearing loss.

References

1. Coppeto JR, Lessell S: A familial syndrome of dystonia, blepharospasm, and pigmentary retinopathy. *Neurology* 40:1359–1363, 1990.

Late infantile neuroaxonal dystrophy (Seitelberger disease)

In 1952, Seitelberger (3,4) first described a disorder of rapidly progressive dementia, hypotonia, spastic quadriplegia, and optic atrophy. Hearing loss occurs in the later stages of the disease. It has been reported in more than 50 patients, making it one of the more common and better known neurodegenerative diseases of childhood (1).

Central nervous system. Early developmental milestones are normal. Between 1 and 2 years of age (occasionally as early as 6 months), the rate of motor and mental development slows and then stops. Within a few months, regression of previously acquired skills, including loss of speech, walking, standing, and sitting, begins. By age 2 years, examination shows hypotonia with poor head control, weakness, hyperactive tendon reflexes, extensor plantar responses, and sometimes subtle evidence of spasticity in the legs. With progression, both upper motor neuron (spasticity) and lower motor neuron (amyotrophy, diminished tendon reflexes) signs become more prominent. By 3 years, examination usually shows severe axial hypotonia, spastic quadriplegia with extensor plantar responses, decreased or absent tendon reflexes in the legs (usually brisk or normal in the arms), generalized muscle wasting (amyotrophy), and decreased responses to painful and other stimuli.

With further progression of the disease, reemergence of primitive reflexes, opisthotonos, decerebrate posture, and other complex motor reactions to external stimuli are observed. Seizures may occur late, although some reported seizures might be only episodes of opisthotonos, etc. Extrapyramidal signs may be seen but are rare. Terminally, brain stem signs such as difficulty swallowing, apnea, other respiratory abnormalities, and sphincter disturbances are common. All affected children are helpless and bedridden, and most die within 10 years of onset.

Ocular system. Visual loss and strabismus are first noticed between age 1 and 2 years, at the same time as the first neurological symptoms. The visual loss progresses rapidly to blindness by 3 or 4 years. Examination shows strabismus, optic atrophy (in 40% by 3 years and 70% by 3.5 years), pendular nystagmus, and uncoordinated eye movements (1).

Other systems. Bradycardia and sinus tachycardia, presumed to be due to "central" mechanisms, were reported in one patient.

Auditory system. Loss of response to auditory stimuli is observed later in the course of this disease in some children. This symptom is probably underreported because of the severe dementia. Given the pathological changes, hearing loss is probably sensorineural.

Laboratory findings. Cerebrospinal fluid studies are normal. Electroencephalograms during the early stages of the disease are normal or show only nonspecific changes such as slowing or spikes. Between age 2 and 3 years, a characteristic EEG pattern emerges that consists of high-amplitude, nonreactive fast rhythms at 16–22 Hz. Visual evoked responses are normal at first, but later show decreased amplitude and may be absent in the later stages of the disease. Electroretinograms are normal (1).

Pathology. Neuropathological changes include generalized atrophy, diffuse loss of neurons and spongy changes in cortex, iron deposits in basal ganglia, especially the globus pallidus, and sometimes the frontal cortex, and mild demyelination and gliosis of white matter. The most striking abnormalities are numerous axonal spheroids that appear as round, homogeneous, or granular eosinophilic structures. These are numerous in cellular zones such as cortex, basal ganglia, brain stem, and central spinal cord, but may be seen in white matter as well (2).

Axonal spheroids may also be seen in peripheral nerves, although they are less numerous. Thus, the disease may be confirmed by biopsy of nerve, skin, conjunctiva, or rectal mucosa (1,2).

Heredity. Inheritance is autosomal recessive.

Diagnosis. This disorder must be differentiated from other neurodegenerative disorders with early onset. Several lysosomal storage diseases may begin early and have similar symptoms, especially Krabbe disease and the infantile variant of metachromatic leukodystrophy. Optico-cochleo-dentate degeneration begins at about the same age and has similar visual and hearing deficits, as well as hypotonia and ataxia. Seitelberger disease lacks ataxia, and pathological changes are also different.

Prognosis. Progression is rapid during the first year of the illness but slower thereafter. Most affected children die within 10 years of onset (1).

Summary. This disease is characterized by (1) autosomal recessive inheritance; (2) early regression and dementia; (3) hypotonia; (4) spastic quadriplegia; (5) optic atrophy; (6) nystagmus; and often (7) sensorineural hearing loss.

References

1. Aicardi J, Castelmein P: Infantile neuroaxonal dystrophy. *Brain* 102:727–748, 1979.
2. Hinton GG et al: A neurodegenerative disorder in a 10-year-old boy. *Can J Neurol Sci* 14:319–324, 1987.
3. Seitelberger F: Eine unbekannte Form von infantiler Lipoidspeicher-Krankheit des Gehirns. In: *Proceedings of the First Congress on Neuropathology, Vol. 3,* Rosenberg and Sellier, Turin, 1952, pp 323–333.
4. Seitelberger F: Infantile neuroaxonal dystrophy. In: *Handbook of Clinical Neurology, Vol. 42. Neurogenetics Directory, Part I,* Bruyn GW, Myrianthopoulos NC (eds), North Holland Publishing Co., Amsterdam, 1981, pp 229–230.

Congenital neuroaxonal dystrophy with peripheral gangrene

In 1985–1987, Hunter et al. (1,2) described two male sibs with dysmorphic appearance, congenital hypotonia, severe developmental delay and mental retardation, blindness, hearing loss, and unusual distal gangrene of the ears and digits. Pathological examination showed changes typical of neuroaxonal dystrophy.

Craniofacial findings. Both affected sibs had intrauterine growth deficiency, congenital microcephaly, sloping forehead, broad nasal bridge (possible hypertelorism), short and blunt nose, large ears with deficient cartilage, small jaw, and high palate. One had upslanting palpebral fissures and the other unilateral cleft lip and palate.

Musculoskeletal system. Both sibs had congenital equinovarus foot deformities, mild to moderate contractures in many joints, ulnar deviation of fingers, thumb contractures in adduction, bilateral transverse palmar creases, and short neck. The second sib had dimples over the elbows.

Central nervous system. Prenatal onset of this disorder is likely based on observations of polyhydramnios in one affected sib and congenital hypotonia in both. Examination during the newborn period showed severe hypotonia and absent primitive reflexes. Neither sib made any developmental progress, and tube feedings were required. The second sib had myoclonic jerks by 2 months and generalized seizures afterwards.

Ocular system. No response to any visual stimuli was observed. Eye examination showed hypoplastic optic nerves and a few small hemorrhages around the disc.

Cardiovascular system. At about 2 months, the tips of all digits and the ears, especially the superior helices, became discolored. This process then progressed through dry gangrene to autoamputation of most distal digits and the tips of the ears, with normal healing.

Integumentary system. Both sibs had dry and scaly (ichthyotic) skin, chronic conjunctivitis, papery nails, and sparse hair.

Genitourinary system. Both sibs had undescended testes, small scrotum, and small penis.

Auditory system. Neither sib had any response to sounds. Brain stem auditory evoked response in the younger sib showed no response beyond wave 2.

Laboratory findings. Both had chronic relative neutropenia, monocytosis, and lymphocytosis. Brain CT scan in one showed indistinct white–gray matter differentiation and atrophy. Chest X-ray showed only 11 ribs in the older sib.

Pathology. Neuropathological abnormalities included marked cerebral and mild vermis atrophy, but the major changes were similar to those observed in late infantile form of neuroaxonal dystrophy. Numerous axonal spheroids, axonal thickening, and varicosities were seen throughout the brain and spinal cord, although the distribution was variable. Many of the spheroids were undergoing or had undergone regressive changes, especially in the upper layers of the cerebral cortex. They appeared to be replaced by scattered microglial nodules. Also, all cortical layers had variable gliosis, and neuronal loss was marked in the second, third, and sixth layers. Demyelination and reactive gliosis were prominent in the central white matter, brain stem, and spinal cord. The brain stem, especially the medulla, had focal intraneuronal vacuoles and spheroid-like inclusions. The granular layer of the cerebellum and the dentate nuclei were rich in spheroids, while Purkinje cells were virtually absent. The optic nerves were atrophied (2). The sural nerve had marked demyelination, dystrophic axons, and various stages of onion bulb formation. Electron microscopy showed typical lamellar fragments. The myenteric plexus of the bowel showed thickened axons, but spheroids were rare. The skeletal muscles had mild to moderate denervation changes (2).

Heredity. Two brothers were affected and both parents were healthy. While X-linked inheritance cannot be excluded, autosomal recessive inheritance is more likely because all previously described forms of neuroaxonal dystrophy have had autosomal recessive inheritance. This includes rare cases of prenatal onset type.

Diagnosis. While several disorders have overlapping symptoms, the severe course and distal gangrene seem to be unique. Optico-cochleodentate degeneration may begin early in life but not before birth. Also, the pathological changes are different. It is not known whether the connatal form of neuroaxonal dystrophy without gangrene is the same or a different disorder. The pathological changes are very similar to late infantile neuroaxonal dystrophy (Seitelberger disease), but the onset of the latter is much later, progression is slower, and distal gangrene has not been described.

Prognosis. Both affected children died early, one at 9 months and the other at 14 months.

Summary. This disorder is characterized by (1) probable autosomal recessive inheritance; (2) dysmorphic appearance; (3) congenital hypotonia; (4) severe developmental delay and mental retardation; (5) blindness; (6) distal gangrene; (7) ichthyosis; (8) pathological changes of neuroaxonal dystrophy; and (9) sensorineural hearing loss.

References

1. Hunter AGW et al: Microcephaly with cerebral gliosis, unusual facies and postnatal distal gangrene. *J Clin Dysmorphol* 3:26–31, 1985.
2. Hunter AGW et al: Neuroaxonal dystrophy presenting with neonatal dysmorphic features, early onset of peripheral gangrene, and a rapidly lethal course. *Am J Med Genet* 28:171–180, 1987.

Meningitic migraine, rash, arthropathy, chorioretinitis, and sensorineural hearing loss (Campbell-Clifton syndrome)

This striking disorder was first reported in 1950 by Campbell and Clifton (2) as an example of familial toxoplasmosis affecting several indivials from three generations of an English/Australian family. In retrospect, it probably represents a rare genetic disease (4).

Central nervous system. Episodes of meningitic migraine began in childhood (5–14 years) and continued, apparently for the lifetime. The headaches were severe and often incapacitating, occurred frequently, and were sometimes associated with fever. Cerebrospinal fluid examination usually showed pleocytosis (20–200 white cells) with lymphocytic predominance and slight eosinophilia. Examination in older individuals showed mild spastic diplegia with leg spasticity and extensor plantar responses.

Peripheral nervous system. According to McKusick (4), peripheral neuropathy was found subsequent to the report.

Integumentary system. A striking maculopapular rash was first noticed in early childhood, possibly from birth. The extent of the rash varied greatly from day to day. Suffusion of the conjunctiva also occurred with similar variation. This was the only abnormality noted in a 3-year-old girl.

Musculoskeletal system. Recurrent joint pains and swelling were described, beginning in late childhood.

Ocular system. Visual loss was reported in older individuals, but the age of onset was uncertain. Examination showed chorioretinitis involving the periphery and sometimes the macula, optic atrophy, and diminished pupillary reactions to light and accommodation.

Cardiovascular system. According to McKusick (4), one person developed gangrene after a small dose of ergotamine. This suggests some type of peripheral arterial disease, which might help explain many of the other manifestations.

Auditory system. Sensorineural hearing loss began at about age 10 and progressed slowly to severe loss.

Laboratory findings. Peripheral eosinophilia and elevated CSF protein were reported, but no information regarding pathology was available.

Heredity. The pedigree is most consistent with autosomal dominant inheritance with four affected individuals from three generations.

Diagnosis. Meningitic migraine with cerebral edema and ataxia was reported in another Australian family. Inheritance was also autosomal dominant, but hearing loss, rash, arthropathy, and visual changes were not described (3). Meningitic migraine also occurs as an episodic disorder without affected relatives (1).

Prognosis. Many of the symptoms are disabling, but all affected persons were still living at the time of the report.

Summary. This disorder is characterized by (1) autosomal dominant inheritance; (2) meningitic migraine; (3) arthropathy; (4) chorioretinitis; (5) rash; and (6) sensorineural hearing loss, all possibly related to peripheral arterial disease.

References

1. Bartelson JD et al: A migrainous syndrome with cerebrospinal fluid pleocytosis. *Neurology* 31:1257–1262, 1981.
2. Campbell AMG, Clifton F: Adult toxoplasmosis in one family. *Brain* 73:281–290, 1950
3. Fitzsimmons RB, Wolfenden WH: Migraine coma: meningitic migraine with cerebral oedema associated with a new form of autosomal dominant cerebellar ataxia. *Brain* 108:555–577, 1985.
4. Online Mendelian Inheritance in Man, OMIM™. Johns Hopkins University, Baltimore, MD. 124950, 1994. World Wide Web URL: http//www.ncbi.nlm.nih/gov/omim/.

Navajo brain stem syndrome

Friedman et al. (2) described seven children of Athabaskan descent who had the combination of congenital horizontal gaze palsy, hearing loss, and central hypoventilation. The Athabaskans are the ancestors of several Native American groups, including the Navajo and Apache. They were thought to have crossed the Bering Strait approximately 4000 years ago (1).

Nervous system. All children had global developmental delay and central hypoventilation; three also had seizures.

Ocular system. All children had horizontal gaze palsy secondary to lack of conjugate horizontal gaze.

Cardiac defects. Three children had cardiac defects, which were outflow tract anomalies in two.

Other findings. Vocal cord weakness was present in 20%.

Auditory system. Hearing loss was congenital and severe. Brain stem auditory evoked response testing evoked no response.

Vestibular system. Cold caloric testing indicated no response.

Heredity. This is an autosomal recessive condition, which to date has not been described in other ethnic groups.

Diagnosis. There are some similarities to Moebius syndrome, but in Moebius syndrome the gaze palsy is secondary to sixth nerve palsy. Hearing loss and cardiac defects do not occur in Moebius syndrome.

Prognosis. Life span is unknown, but one child reportedly died of sudden infant death syndrome, which may have been caused by central hypoventilation.

References

1. Erickson RP: Southwestern Athabaskan (Navajo and Apache) genetic diseases. *Genet Med* 1:151–157, 1999.
2. Friedman BD et al: Congenital horizontal gaze palsy, deafness, central hypoventilation, and developmental impairment: a brain stem syndrome prevalent in the Navajo population. *Proc Greenwood Genet Ctr* 16:160–161, 1997.

N syndrome (mental retardation, multiple congenital anomalies, growth deficiency, spastic quadriplegia, blindness, risk for neoplasia, increased chromosomal breakage, and sensorineural hearing loss) (Hess-Opitz syndrome)

Hess et al. (2) first reported this striking disorder in two brothers in 1974. The occurrence of neoplasia in both boys and their normal mother and chromosome breakage abnormalities were described in later reports (1,3).

Physical findings. Birth weight and length were normal in both boys, but severe postnatal growth deficiency occurred with parameters below the fifth centile. Craniofacial changes included dolichocephaly, high forehead, flat supraorbital ridges, shallow orbits, long and narrow face, mild hypotelorism, small jaw, and malformed ears (Fig. 10–16A,B). Wide-spaced nipples, pectus excavatum, and diastasis recti were also noted.

Central nervous system. Both boys had global developmental delay that was apparent within the first year of life. Examination during childhood showed profound mental retardation and spastic quadriplegia. Seizures also occurred.

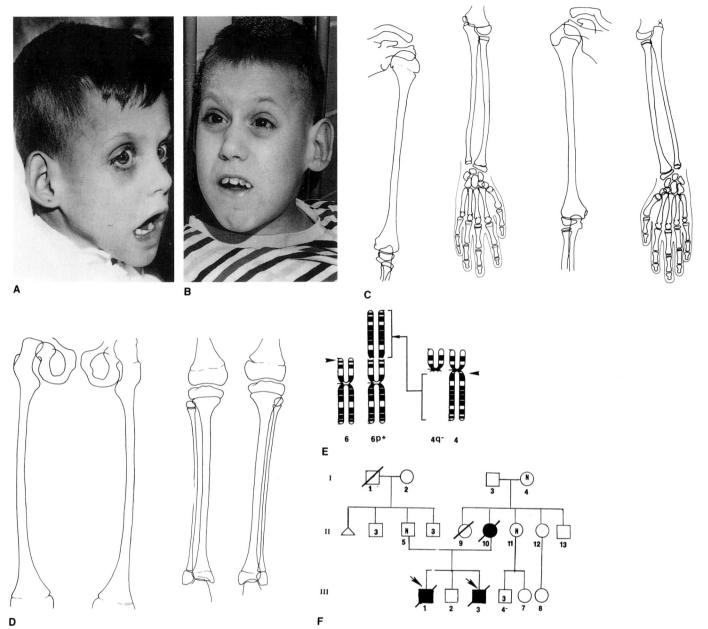

Figure 10–16. *N syndrome (mental retardation, multiple congenital anomalies, growth deficiency, spastic quadriplegia, blindness, risk for neoplasia, increased chromosomal breakage, and sensorineural hearing loss) (Hess-Opitz syndrome).* (A,B) Two brothers with severe mental and growth retardation, visual impairment, and hearing loss. Note laterally overlapping upper eyelid, large corneas, and abnormal pinae. (C,D) Overtubulation and relative shortness of distal long bones. (E) Translo-

cation (4;6)(q12;p25) found in about one-half the cells in fibroblast culture. (F) Pedigree of N family with propositi designated by arrows. Persons with chromosome instability are shown by darkened squares or circles; relatives whose chromosomes were studied and found to be normal are designated by the letter N. [(A–D) from RO Hess et al., *Clin Genet* 6:237, 1974; (E,F) from RO Hess et al., *Am J Med Genet* (Suppl) 3:383, 1987.]

Ocular system. Severe visual impairment and congenital nystagmus were apparent early in life. Examinations showed large corneas, eccentric pupils, prominent upper tarsal plates, and downslanting palpebral fissures. The appearance of the fundus was not described.

Musculoskeletal system. Skeletal changes included narrow thorax, kyphoscoliosis, proximally placed thumbs, hypoplastic thenar eminences, camptodactyly, metatarsus varus, pes cavus, and abnormal dermatoglyphics with high ridge count. Skeletal X-rays showed wide cervical spinal canal, straight cervical spine, wedging of dorsal vertebral bodies, bilateral cervical ribs, overtubulation of long bones with

flaring of metaphyses, shortening of long bones (distal greater than proximal), and delayed bone age (Fig. 10–16C,D).

Genitourinary system. Both boys had hypospadias and cryptorchidism.

Neoplasia. Both brothers died of acute malignancies resembling T-cell leukemia at 5 and 19 years, respectively. Their mother succumbed to acute leukemia at 37 years.

Auditory system. Although hearing tests were not reported, neither boy responded to sounds and hearing loss was suspected.

Laboratory findings. Chromosome analysis showed increased chromosome breakage and rearrangement in one boy and the normal mother (Fig. 10–16E). Chromosome breakage studies were done using bleomycin with or without added aphidicolin (which inhibits repair by DNA polymerase alpha). In contrast to controls, N syndrome fibroblasts showed no increased breakage when aphidicolin was added. On the basis of these results, the authors suggested that the N syndrome was caused by a mutation affecting the gene for DNA polymerase alpha, which is located at Xp21.3–p22.1 (1,4).

Pathology. Partial review of brain sections showed several abnormalities often seen with systemic diseases such as malignancies, combined with primary structural changes of congenital origin. The latter included patchy distribution of neurons in the temporal lobe and vertical columns of neurons in the occipital lobe.

Heredity. In this family, two boys expressed the complete phenotype, while their mother appeared normal but also had increased chromosomal breakage and died of leukemia. The latter might be explained by expression of an X-linked trait in cells in which the normal X is inactivated. Chromosome breakage studies suggested a defect in DNA polymerase alpha, which is located on the X chromosome. Thus, X-linked inheritance of N syndrome is very likely (Fig. 10–16F).

Diagnosis. The most striking aspect of this syndrome is the combination of birth defects and mental retardation with susceptibility to neoplasia, especially hematologic. Ataxia telangiectasia consists of ataxia, dementia, and risk for malignancies, especially hematologic, but lacks congenital anomalies. Fanconi syndrome comprises multiple congenital anomalies, occasional mental retardation, and risk for aplastic anemia. Both syndromes are also associated with increased chromosomal breakage.

Prognosis. This disorder causes severe disability and shortened life span in hemizygous males and may result in fatal malignancies in heterozygous females as well.

Summary. This disorder is characterized by (1) X-linked recessive inheritance of the complete phenotype with partial expression in carrier females; (2) mental retardation; (3) multiple congenital anomalies; (4) growth deficiency; (5) spastic quadriplegia; (6) visual loss; (7) susceptibility to neoplasia, especially hematologic; (8) increased chromosomal breakage; and (9) hearing loss.

References

1. Floy KM et al: DNA polymerase alpha defect in the N syndrome. *Am J Med Genet* 35:301–305, 1990.
2. Hess RO et al: Studies of malformation syndromes in man XXVII: The N syndrome, a "new" multiple congenital anomaly—mental retardation syndrome. *Clin Genet* 6:237–246, 1974.
3. Hess RO et al: Updating the N syndrome: occurrence of lymphoid malignancy and possible association with an increased rate of chromosome breakage. *Am J Med Genet* (Suppl) 3:383–388, 1987.
4. Wang TS et al: Assignment of the gene for human DNA polymerase alpha to the X chromosome. *Proc Natl Acad Sci USA* 82:5270–5274, 1985.

Holoprosencephaly, myelomeningocoele, abducens paralysis, and sensorineural hearing loss

Burck et al. (2) described a boy with a probable forme fruste of holoprosencephaly (hypotelorism, developmental delay, and mild spasticity), abducens paralysis and hearing loss, whose sib had severe holoprosencephaly with cyclopia. Another sib had thoracolumbar myelomeningocoele.

Physical findings. The proband had mild facial asymmetry and hypotelorism, with inner canthal distance of 1.2 cm (less than third centile). A younger sib had fetal demise at about 15–16 weeks gestation. Examination after delivery showed cyclopia with a proboscis above the

eye, and a posterior neck mass that might have been a cephalocele or cystic hygroma.

Central nervous system. The proband had congenital hypotonia and global developmental delay (he sat at 1 year and walked at 19 months), but subsequent mental development was normal. Examination at 6 years showed apparently normal olfactory function, mild spastic quadriplegia, poor fine motor coordination, and broad-based gait. Cranial CT scan revealed mild asymmetry of the lateral ventricles.

Although autopsy was not performed, the younger sib must have had a severe form of holoprosencephaly, given the observed cyclopia. An older sib had thoracolumbar myelomeningocoele and died in the newborn period. Further description was not available.

Ocular system. The proband had a right abducens (sixth nerve) palsy.

Auditory system. Severe hearing loss was noticed at 3 months in the proband. Hearing tests at 6 years showed severe hearing loss with responses only at 80–100 dB.

Laboratory findings. Chromosome analysis was normal in the proband and in his sib with cyclopia. Thyroid function tests, corticoids, testosterone, and growth hormone assays were normal in the proband.

Heredity. Varying degrees of defects in neural tube closure suggest common etiology. The parents were unrelated and had no subtle dysmorphic signs such as hypotelorism, single central upper incisor, mild mental retardation, or spina bifida. Autosomal recessive inheritance appears likely, but a small deletion is possible.

Diagnosis. Relatives of patients with holoprosencephaly are known to have an increased incidence of mental retardation, spina bifida, myelomeningocoele, endocrine disorders, and sensorineural hearing loss. Holoprosencephaly has also occurred in the autosomal recessive form, and there is an autosomal dominant type associated with mild hypotelorism, midfacial hypoplasia, hyposmia, mild mental retardation, and single upper central incisor (1). Holoprosencephaly can also be associated with various other syndromes (3,4).

Prognosis. The prognosis is related to the severity of the brain abnormality. The sib with cyclopia had fetal demise and the sib with myelomeningocoele died in the newborn period.

Summary. This syndrome consists of (1) autosomal recessive inheritance; (2) holoprosencephaly or a mild form of holoprosencephaly; (3) possibly other brain malformations; (4) abducens paralysis; and (5) hearing loss.

References

1. Berry S et al: Single central incisor in familial holoprosencephaly. *J Pediatr* 104:877–880, 1984.
2. Burck U et al: Occurrence of cyclopia, myelomeningocele, deafness, and abducens paralysis in siblings. *Am J Med Genet* 11:443–448, 1982.
3. Cohen MM Jr: Perspectives on holoprosencephaly: Part I. Epidemiology, genetics, and syndromology. *Teratology* 40:211–235, 1989.
4. Gorlin RJ et al: *Syndromes of the Head and Neck*, 4th ed. Oxford University Press, New York, 2001, pp. 714–715.

Chudley-McCullough syndrome

Chudley et al. (1) described sibs with the combination of multiple brain abnormalities and hearing loss. Lemire and Stoeber (3), Hendriks et al. (2), and Welch et al. (4), also reported cases.

Nervous system. All children had brain malformations, with hydrocephalus being the most consistent finding. Other anomalies found in some included corpus callosum dysgenesis or partial agenesis, arachnoid cysts, cortical dysplasia, and cerebellar dysgenesis.

Auditory system. Profound bilateral sensorineural hearing loss is a constant finding.

Heredity. This is likely an autosomal recessive condition, as demonstrated by the occurrence of the condition in children of both sexes and those born to consanguineous parents.

Prognosis. Development in two female children was described as normal (2); both girls had partial agenesis of the corpus callosum and arachnoid cysts in addition to hydrocephalus.

References

1. Chudley AE et al: Bilateral sensorineural deafness and hydrocephalus due to foramen of Monro obstruction in sibs: a newly described autosomal recessive disorder. *Am J Med Genet* 68:350–356, 1997.
2. Hendriks YMC et al: Bilateral sensorineuraal deafness, partial agenesis of the corpus callosum, and arachnoid cysts in two sisters. *Am J Med Genet* 86:183–186, 1999.
3. Lemire EG, Stoeber GP: Chudley-McCullough syndrome: bilateral sensorineural deafness, hydrocephalus, and other structural brain abnormalities. *Am J Med Genet* 90:127–130, 2000.
4. Welch KO et al: Chudley-McCullough syndrome: expanded phenotype and review of the literature. *Am J Med Genet* 119A:71–76, 2003.

Microcephaly, dysmorphic facial phenotype, mental retardation, cleft palate, weight deficiency, skeletal abnormalities, and hearing loss (Weaver-Williams syndrome)

In 1977, Weaver and Williams (1) described an unusual multiple congenital anomalies/mental retardation syndrome in a brother and sister.

Physical findings. Birth weight and length were normal. Subsequent growth was poor despite adequate caloric intake. Height was mildly reduced, while weight was well below the third centile (>4 SD) for height age (Fig. 10–17A). Facial appearance was unusual because of severe microcephaly (>5 SD), small facial structures, sparse scalp and facial hair, deep-set eyes, midface hypoplasia, hypoplastic ears, broad nasal tip, small mouth with downturned corners, small jaw, and small, malformed, or missing teeth (Fig. 10–17B,C). The brother had orbital hypertelorism by skull X-ray, cupped ears, unilateral preauricular pit, and complete cleft palate, while his sister had cleft soft palate only. Her facial appearance was very similar to that of her brother when young, but by her 20's she had developed coarser facial features including eyes that were less deeply set and prognathism (Fig. 10–17D).

Central nervous system. Both sibs had global developmental delay and severe mental retardation. However, the brother was able to sit at 2.5 years, walk at 8 years, and use limited speech at 8–10 years. His sister was profoundly retarded and unable to sit, stand, walk, or speak. She was difficult to feed and had onset of myoclonic seizures and left hemiparesis at age 12. Examination showed diminished muscle bulk and strength, mild spastic diplegia with brisk knee reflexes and clonus at the ankles, and poor balance. The sister had severe flexion contractures and limited movement.

Musculoskeletal system. Both sibs had strikingly thin limbs, due to diminished subcutaneous and muscle mass, and delayed bone age during childhood. The proband held his neck in an extended position. His sister had kyphoscoliosis, barrel-shaped chest, and short neck. Skeletal X-rays showed generalized bone hypoplasia, delayed skeletal maturation, tall but narrow vertebral bodies, unusual downsloping ribs, narrow pelvis with shallow acetabula, coxa valga, increased tubulation of long bones, and short ulnas and fibulas.

Ocular system. Strabismus was noted in the sister.

Auditory system. Hearing examination of the proband at age 31 showed speech reception threshold of 60 dB in the right and 25 dB in the left. Hearing status of the sister was uncertain.

Heredity. Two sibs of different sex were affected. The parents were unrelated and healthy and had three healthy children. The mother also

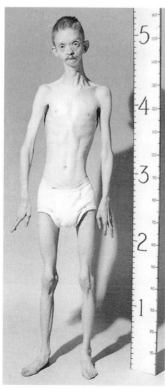
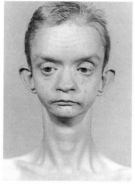
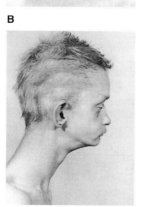
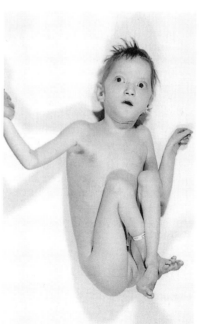

Figure 10–17. *Microcephaly, dysmorphic facies, mental retardation, cleft palate, weight deficiency, skeletal abnormalities, and hearing loss (Weaver-Williams syndrome).* (A–C) Proband at 24 and 32 years shows microcephaly, cupped ears, broad nose, small mouth and jaw, long neck, thin limbs, relatively normal height, and normal leg and trunk proportions. (D) His sister also is affected. [From DD Weaver and CPS Williams, *Birth Defects* 13(3B):69, 1977.]

A   B   C   D

had six unexplained miscarriages. Inheritance is probably autosomal recessive, although a cryptic chromosome translocation is possible.

Diagnosis. This syndrome appears to be unique.

Prognosis. Both sibs had severe or profound mental retardation, but their health was good.

Summary. This syndrome is characterized by (*1*) autosomal recessive inheritance; (*2*) microcephaly; (*3*) weight deficiency; (*4*) mental retardation; (*5*) dysmorphic facial appearance; (*6*) cleft palate; (*7*) skeletal abnormalities; and (*8*) hearing loss.

Reference

1. Weaver DD, Williams CPS: A syndrome of microcephaly, mental retardation, unusual facies, cleft palate and weight deficiency. *Birth Defects* 13(3B):69–84, 1977.

Microcephaly, mental retardation, epilepsy, spastic paraplegia, and sensorineural hearing loss (Renier syndrome)

Renier et al. (2) described a syndrome of mental retardation, microcephaly, epilepsy, spastic diplegia, and hearing loss in a Dutch family.

Physical findings. Birth parameters and postnatal somatic growth were normal, but head growth decelerated, resulting in microcephaly by 1 year. No characteristic facial changes were described.

Central nervous system. All affected males had congenital hypotonia and global developmental delay in infancy. Examination at 1–2 years showed microcephaly, spasticity, and severe mental retardation. None learned to speak, although some were able to walk. Epilepsy, usually consisting of generalized tonic clonic seizures, began in early childhood. Pneumoencephalogram in one child showed moderate dilatation of lateral ventricles. Each mother of an affected male and several of their sisters had "subnormal" intelligence without other abnormalities.

Auditory system. All affected males had severe sensorineural hearing loss, but audiograms were not described.

Pathology. Brain biopsy from the right second frontal gyrus was performed on the proband at 17 months. It showed poor differentiation of cortical layers 3 and 4 consisting of immature neurons with round cell shape and increased nucleus-to-cytoplasm ratio. All other layers were normal.

Heredity. The proband, two maternal uncles, and two maternal first cousins were affected. Many females in the family, including each obligatory carrier, had borderline or mild mental retardation. The pedigree is consistent with X-linked recessive inheritance with partial expression in females (Fig. 10–18).

Diagnosis. Many X-linked mental retardation syndromes are known, but few are associated with hearing loss. X-linked mental and somatic retardation, genital hypoplasia, and sensorineural hearing loss (Juberg-Marsidi syndrome) may be differentiated, based on the genital abnormalities and lack of spasticity. It should be noted that Gustavson et al. (1) have suggested that this is the same as Juberg-Marsidi syndrome.

Prognosis. Several affected males died during childhood.

Summary. This disorder is characterized by (*1*) X-linked inheritance with partial expression in females; (*2*) mental retardation; (*3*) microcephaly; (*4*) epilepsy; (*5*) spastic paraplegia; and (*6*) sensorineural hearing loss.

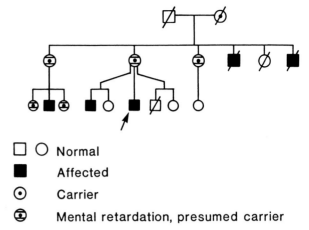

□ ○ Normal

■ Affected

⊙ Carrier

🛈 Mental retardation, presumed carrier

Figure 10–18. *Microcephaly, mental retardation, epilepsy, spastic paraplegia, and sensorineural hearing loss (Renier syndrome).* Pedigree of family shows X-linked recessive inheritance with partial expression in females.

References

1. Gustavson K-H et al: New X-linked syndrome with severe mental retardation, severely impaired vision, severe hearing defect, epileptic seizures, spasticity, restricted joint mobility, and early death. *Am J Med Genet* 45:654–658, 1993.
2. Renier WO et al: An X-linked syndrome with microcephaly, severe mental retardation, spasticity, epilepsy and deafness. *J Ment Defic Res* 26:27–40, 1982.

Microcephaly, mental retardation, spastic diplegia or quadriplegia, persistent hyperplastic primary vitreous, microphthalmia, cleft palate, asthma, and conductive hearing loss (oculo-palato-cerebral dwarfism)

In 1985, Frydman et al. (1) described three sibs with an unusual multiple congenital anomaly/mental retardation syndrome that included persistent hyperplastic primary vitreous (PHPV). Pellegrino et al. (2) described another case.

Physical findings. All affected individuals had low birth weight, subsequent short stature, microcephaly, deep-set eyes, and bulbous nose. One child had midline cleft palate, two had cleft soft palate, and one had highly arched palate.

Central nervous system. The three affected sibs had congenital hypotonia and spasticity; all four had microcephaly and mental retardation or developmental delay. Developmental delay was variable, with the case reported by Pellegrino et al. (2) having mild delays, and the girl reported by Frydman et al. (1) at 15 years having mild microcephaly, borderline retardation (IQ 76), and mild spastic diplegia. Her two affected brothers had severe microcephaly (>5 SD), profound mental retardation, and severe spastic quadriplegia. Cranial CT scan in one of the brothers showed focal atrophy of the left temporal lobe and moderate ventricular dilatation; MRI of the head in the single case showed cerebral atrophy in the frontal region and thinning of the corpus callosum.

Ocular system. The most unusual manifestation of this syndrome was PHPV, which was unilateral or bilateral. The affected eyes were small with mild microcornea and shallow anterior chambers. The sister also had secondary glaucoma, which progressed to cataracts, glaucoma of the right eye, and bulbar atrophy of the left. An ultrasound on the younger brother showed a retrolental mass but no retinal detachment.

Musculoskeletal system. All patients had subjectively soft skin, visible veins, and joint hypermobility. Pectus excavatum, limited elbow extension, kyphoscoliosis, 13 ribs on one side, and umbilical hernia were each observed occasionally.

Genitourinary system. Undescended testes occurred in two of the boys.

Pulmonary system. All three of the sibs had severe asthma, often complicated by pneumonia and requiring frequent hospitalization. No other relatives had asthma or other forms of atopy. Thus, the authors considered it a component of the syndrome. The child described by Pellegrino et al. (2) did not have asthma, so it is not clear if asthma really is a component manifestation.

Auditory system. All three sibs had frequent episodes of otitis. The sister had thickened and scarred tympanic membranes and mild hearing loss that was presumably conductive. The brothers were suspected of having hearing loss.

Heredity. Three sibs, both male and female, were affected. Their parents were first cousins, once removed, of Moroccan Jewish origin and unaffected. Thus, autosomal recessive inheritance is probable.

Diagnosis. The most unusual aspect of this syndrome is familial PHPV. Norrie disease can be associated with PHPV, as well as microcephaly, growth retardation, cryptorchidism, sensorineural hearing loss, and mental retardation. Norrie disease is inherited as an X-linked recessive trait, however. Several of the reported cases may represent examples of trisomy 13. PHPV may also be observed in Walker-Warburg syndrome, which consists of type II lissencephaly, cerebellar malformation, retinal abnormality, congenital muscular dystrophy, and often hydrocephalus. Rarely, familial PHPV has been described in individuals without other abnormalities (3). Because the inheritance of asthma is probably multifactorial, it is uncertain whether asthma is a true component of this syndrome.

Prognosis. The degree of mental retardation ranged from borderline to profound.

Summary. This syndrome is characterized by (*1*) autosomal recessive inheritance; (*2*) microcephaly; (*3*) mental retardation; (*4*) spastic diplegia or quadriplegia; (*5*) persistent hyperplastic primary vitreous; (*6*) microphthalmia; (*7*) cleft or highly arched palate; and (*8*) conductive hearing loss.

References

1. Frydman M et al: Oculo-palato-cerebral syndrome: a new syndrome. *Clin Genet* 27:414–419, 1985.
2. Pellegrino JE et al: Oculo-palatal-cerebral syndrome: a second case. *Am J Med Genet* 99:200–203, 2001.
3. Wang MK, Phillips CI: Persistent hyperplastic primary vitreous in nonidentical twins. *Acta Ophthalmol* 51:434–437, 1973.

X-linked mental retardation, microcephaly, unusual face, and sensorineural hearing loss (Golabi-Ito-Hall syndrome)

In 1984, Golabi et al. (1) reported a new X-linked syndrome in three affected males in one kindred. The main features included congenital microcephaly, postnatal growth retardation, dry brittle hair, narrow triangular face with ridged metopic suture, upslanting palpebral fissures, laterally displaced inner canthi, macrodontia, and prominent ears. Two affected individuals had atrial septal defect.

Mild sensorineural hearing loss was noted.

For diagnosis, see Table 10–1.

Reference

1. Golabi M et al: A new X-linked multiple congenital anomalies/mental retardation syndrome. *Am J Med Genet* 17:367–374, 1984.

X-linked mental and somatic retardation, genital hypoplasia, and sensorineural hearing loss (Juberg-Marsidi syndrome)

In 1980, Juberg and Marsidi (2) reported a male child and two maternal uncles with mental and somatic retardation, unusual face, microgenitalism, and sensorineural hearing loss. Mattei et al. (3) described an additional large kindred with seven males, and Tsukahara et al. (6) described a single possible case.

Clinical findings. Birth weight was low and growth did not exceed the third centile. Head circumference was reduced.

Craniofacial findings. All affected individuals had high forehead, upslanting palpebral fissures, prominent epicanthal folds, and flat nasal bridge (Fig. 10–19A). The pinnae were hyperfolded with a large helix.

Ocular system. Small palpebral fissures were found in most of the affected individuals. Light retinal pigmentation was noted in some of the patients (2).

Central nervous system. Severe global delay was evident in all affected individuals. Hypotonia was evident in infancy. Most patients learned to walk. Some had seizures.

Musculoskeletal system. Camptodactyly of the second or third finger, clinodactyly of the index finger, asymmetrically sized halluces, and retarded bone age were found.

Genitourinary system. All affected individuals had rudimentary scrotum, undescended testes, and micropenis (2,3) (Fig. 10–19B). Some had vesicoureteric reflex and small kidneys.

Auditory findings. Bilateral sensorineural hearing loss dating from infancy ranged from moderate to severe but was not otherwise characterized because of severe mental retardation. In one child, hearing deficit involved higher tones below 60 dB.

Laboratory findings. Delayed bone age was a constant finding.

Heredity. Inheritance in the two kindreds is clearly X-linked. The gene has been mapped to Xq12-q21 (5) and has been identified as the

Figure 10–19. *X-linked mental and somatic retardation, genital hypoplasia, and sensorineural hearing loss (Juberg-Marsidi syndrome).* (A) Face of patient showing high forehead, upslanting palpebral fissures, flat nasal bridge. (B) Genital hypoplasia in the same patient. [From JF Mattei et al., *Clin Genet* 23:70, 1983.]

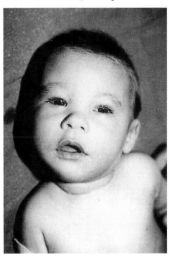
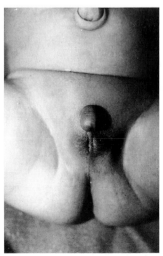

A   B

X-linked helicase-2 (*XH2*) gene (7). This is the same gene that is mutant in X-linked α-thalassemia/mental retardation syndrome.

Diagnosis. Renier et al. (4) reported three male sibs and two maternal uncles with microcephaly, mental retardation, epilepsy, spastic paraplegia, and sensorineural hearing loss with X-linked inheritance. In Gustavson syndrome, an affected kindred similar to that of Juberg and Marsidi was described (1), but the genitalia were normal. See Table 10–1.

Prognosis. The two uncles reported by Juberg and Marsidi (2) died at 9 years and 20 months, respectively. One child described by Mattei et al. (3) died at 10 months.

Summary. This syndrome is characterized by (*1*) X-linked recessive inheritance; (*2*) mental and somatic retardation; (*3*) genital hypoplasia; and (*4*) sensorineural hearing loss.

References

1. Gustavson K-H et al: New X-linked syndrome with severe mental retardation, severely impaired vision, severe hearing defect, epileptic seizures, spasticity, restricted joint mobility, and early death. *Am J Med Genet* 45:654–657, 1993.
2. Juberg RC, Marsidi I: A new form of X-linked mental retardation with growth retardation, deafness and microgenitalism. *Am J Hum Genet* 32:714–722, 1980.
3. Mattei JF et al: X-linked mental retardation, growth retardation, deafness and microgenitalism: a second familial report. *Clin Genet* 23:70–74, 1983.
4. Renier WO et al: An X-linked syndrome with microcephaly, severe mental retardation, spasticity, epilepsy and deafness. *J Ment Def Res* 26:27–40, 1982.
5. Saugier-Veber P et al: The Juberg-Marsidi syndrome maps to the proximal long arm of the X chromosome (Xq12–121). *Am J Hum Genet* 52:1040–1045, 1993.
6. Tsukahara M et al: Juberg-Marsidi syndrome: report of an additional case. *Am J Med Genet* 58:353–355.
7. Villard L et al: XNP mutation in a large family with Juberg-Marsidi syndrome. *Nat Genet* 12:359–360, 1996.

Optic atrophy, mental retardation, seizures, spasticity, restricted joint mobility, and sensorineural hearing loss (Gustavson syndrome)

In 1993, Gustavson et al. (2) reported a syndrome involving microcephaly, severe mental retardation, optic atrophy with severely impaired vision or blindness, spasticity, seizures, restricted movement of large joints, and severe sensorineural hearing loss.

Central nervous system. Microcephaly, severe mental retardation, spasticity, apneic spells, and seizures were evident.

Ocular system. Optic atrophy with apparent total blindness was found in all affected individuals.

Auditory system. There seemed to be no response to auditory stimuli.

Heredity. X-linked inheritance was clearly evident. Among seven affected persons, six were males. Two generations were involved. Maternal inheritance appeared to be excluded on the basis of normal appearance of mitochondria in cultured fibroblasts. Preliminary evidence seemed to suggest linkage at Xq26 (3,4).

Prognosis. Death occurred in infancy or early childhood.

Diagnosis. To be excluded are other X-linked mental retardation syndromes with hearing loss such as X-linked mental and somatic retardation, genital hypoplasia, and sensorineural hearing loss (Juberg-Marsidi syndrome); Golabi-Ito-Hall syndrome; and choreoathetosis, mental retardation, microcephaly, spastic quadriplegia, strabismus, and sensorineural hearing loss (Schimke-Horton syndrome); see Table 10–1. In addition, Barth et al. (1) reported a syndrome with a similar phenotype, but inheritance was autosomal recessive and no hearing loss was evident.

References

1. Barth PG et al: Inherited syndrome of microcephaly, dyskinesia and pontocerebellar hypoplasia: a systemic atrophy with early onset. *J Neurol Sci* 97:25–42, 1990.
2. Gustavson KH et al: New X-linked syndrome with severe mental retardation, severely impaired vision, severe hearing defect, epileptic seizures, spasticity, restricted joint mobility, and early death. *Am J Med Genet* 45:654–658, 1993.
3. Malmgren H et al: Linkage analysis of a new type of X-linked mental retardation. Abstract from the 3rd Chromosome Workshop, Amalfi, Italy, 3–4 April, 1992.
4. Malmgren H et al: Linkage mapping of a severe X-linked mental retardation syndrome. *Am J Hum Genet* 52:1046–1052, 1993.

Mental retardation, behavior disturbance, and sensorineural hearing loss

In 1988, Saul and Stevenson (1) described three sibs with mental retardation, behavior disturbance characterized by emotional lability, and sensorineural hearing loss. Spells of hypotonia occurred as early as 3 weeks of age and were noted intermittently through the first several years of life. Development was delayed. Emotional lability, with severe outbursts, was noted in childhood. Speech was severely limited, and both fine and gross motor incoordination were evident. Intelligence tests indicated IQs of 26–42. All three sibs had severe sensorineural hearing loss not otherwise described.

Reference

Saul RA, Stevenson RE: Deafness, mental retardation, and behavior disturbance in three siblings. *Proc Greenwood Genet Ctr* 7:7–8, 1988.

X-linked mental retardation with characteristic facial features and hearing loss (Martin syndrome)

Martin et al. (1) described a three-generation kindred with the combination of unusual facial appearance and sensorineural hearing loss. Ages of the affected individuals ranged from 12 to 54 years at the time of the report. Facial features included telecanthus, epicanthal folds, narrow palpebral fissures, malar hypoplasia, full lower lip, and micrognathia (Fig. 10–20). The article describes the ears as being low-set, but they do not appear to be so in the pictures provided. Congenital sensorineural hearing loss affected all individuals and was characterized as severe to profound. Cognitive development was borderline normal to mildly impaired in the younger two males; in the oldest male, cognitive function was described as moderately to severely retarded. Additional manifestations included renal anomalies (unilateral dysplasia in one, bilaterally small kidneys in another), telangiectasias, and pancytopenia. Mapping studies placed the gene within a 48 cM region on Xq1–21, although no specific gene mutation was identified.

Reference

1. Martin DM et al: Characterisation and genetic mapping of a new X-linked deafness syndrome. *J Med Genet* 37:836–841, 2000.

Neuromuscular Disorders with Hearing Loss

Neuromuscular diseases form a large group of disorders that are frequently genetic and involve dysfunction of the lower motor unit and associated structures such as the anterior horn cell, spinal roots, peripheral nerves, neuromuscular junction, and muscle. Classification is based on the primary site of involvement. Motor neuron diseases affect anterior horn cells and are divided into bulbospinal disorders that are very rare, spinal muscular atrophies that are relatively common and often severe, and hereditary motor neuropathies (HMN) that represent the spinal form of motor neuropathy. Electromyography (EMG) shows normal motor and sensory nerve conduction studies (NCS) and denervation by needle exam.

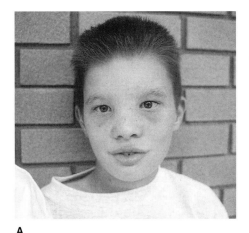
A

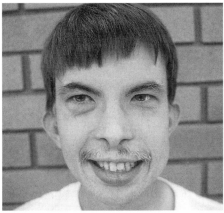
B

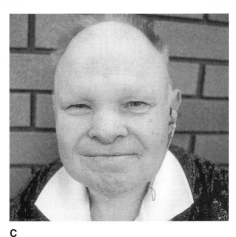
C

Figure 10–20. *X-linked mental retardation with characteristic facial features and hearing loss (Martin syndrome).* Note telecanthus or hypertelorism, epicanthal folds, wide nasal bridge, and broad mouth. [From DM Martin et al., *J Med Genet* 37:836–841, 2000. Reprinted with permission of the BMJ Publishing Group.]

Hereditary neuropathies have been subclassified into three major groups based on results of clinical examination and electrophysiologic tests. Patients in the first two groups usually present with weakness in the legs and feet. In HMN, sensory symptoms are absent, NCS are normal, and EMG shows denervation. In hereditary motor and sensory neuropathies (HMSN), sensory symptoms may be mild or absent, while sensory NCS are slow or absent. Motor NCS may be very slow (type I) or borderline normal (type II). Electromyography shows denervation. Patients with hereditary sensory and autonomic neuropathy (HSAN) have severe loss of sensation and usually come to medical attention because of repeated injuries and medical complications, especially wound infections. Sensory NCS are absent, while motor NCS may be normal or borderline slow. Autonomic symptoms such as poor control of body temperature are most frequent with HSAN, but may occur with HMSN as well (2).

Diseases of muscle are divided into the muscular dystrophies and other, usually congenital, myopathies. The former are uniformly progressive and have evidence of fibrosis and scarring (dystrophic changes) on muscle biopsy. The latter may be static or progressive, and muscle biopsy results are variable.

Mitochondrial encephalomyopathies. Suspected or proven abnormalities in mitochondrial metabolism, especially those involving the respiratory chain, usually affect either muscle alone (pure myopathies) or multiple systems, especially muscle and brain (encephalomyopathies). Sensorineural hearing loss occurs frequently in the latter group. Patients with the multisystem form show striking clinical heterogeneity. Some present with an overwhelming metabolic disorder, which is fatal within the first few months of life. Others begin later with a wide spectrum of symptoms that may include any of those listed in Table 10–2. Several relatively discrete clinical disorders have been described. Even among these, however, substantial clinical overlap and biochemical heterogeneity exist (1,3).

Because so many combinations of symptoms have been described, it is not possible to review them all. Several of the best known mitochondrial encephalomyopathies associated with sensorineural hearing loss, as well as rarer disorders in which hearing loss is prominent, will be summarized in the following sections. However, a mitochondrial disorder should be suspected and appropriate investigations obtained whenever any combination of two or more of these manifestations occurs. Keep in mind that it is possible that several of the multisystem disorders described elsewhere in this chapter represent mitochondrial diseases in patients evaluated before adequate laboratory studies were available.

References

1. DiMauro S et al: Mitochondrial myopathies. *Ann Neurol* 17:521–538, 1985.
2. Vance MJ: Hereditary motor and sensory neuropathies. *Am J Med Genet* 18:1–5, 1991.
3. Zeviani M et al: Mitochondrial diseases. *Neurol Clin* 7:123–156, 1989.

Table 10–2. Manifestations of mitochondrial encephalomyopathies

Auditory System

Sensorineural hearing loss

Cardiovscular System

Cardiac conduction defects (heart block)
Cardiomyopathy (e.g., histiocytoid cardiomyopathy of infancy)

Central Nervous System

Ataxia
Brain stem dysfunction
Dementia, mental retardation
Hypotonia
Pyramidal signs
Seizures, especially myoclonic seizures
Stroke-like episodes

Peripheral Nervous System

Motor, sensory, and autonomic neuropathy
Myopathy, exercise intolerance, weakness

Ocular System

Ophthalmoplegia, ptosis
Optic atrophy
Pigmentary retinopathy

Other Systems

Endocrine dysfunction (i.e., diabetes mellitus)
Gastrointestinal dysfunction (e.g., cyclic vomiting, pseudo-obstruction)
Hepatic dysfunction
Renal dysfunction

Laboratory Findings and Pathology

Enzyme deficiencies (complexes I–V)
Lactic and pyruvic acidosis
Myopathy with ragged-red fibers

Anterior Horn Cell and Miscellaneous Neuromuscular Disorders

Pontobulbar palsy and sensorineural hearing loss (Brown–Vialetto–Van Laere syndrome)

Progressive pontobulbar palsy and sensorineural hearing loss, first described by Brown (7) in 1894, has now been reported in over 30 patients (1–14,17–28).

Central nervous system. Hearing loss is rarely preceded by ptosis. More often, it is accompanied or followed within a few years by lower cranial nerve palsies. Typical symptoms include facial weakness, dysarthria due to vocal cord paralysis, swallowing difficulties, and weakness, wasting, and fasciculations of the tongue (Fig. 10–21A). Many patients have lower motor neuron signs involving the body that may present as weakness and wasting of the arms, hypoactive reflexes, diaphragmatic weakness causing hypoventilation, respiratory failure, daytime sleepiness, and exaggerated lumbar lordosis (Fig. 10–21B). Fewer patients have upper cranial nerve palsies, or upper motor neuron signs in the legs including spasticity, hyperreflexia, and extensor plantar responses. Progression of any manifestations may be gradual or episodic with sudden development or worsening of symptoms. Some patients have had only mild manifestations. Electromyography shows abnormalities consistent with mild or severe chronic denervation. Age of onset of neurologic symptoms has been variable, with usual onset in the second decade. However, cases with onset as early as 2 years have been reported (18). Apparently rate of progression of the condition does not correlate well with age of onset.

Auditory system. The first clinical symptom in most patients is sensorineural hearing loss, which usually begins in mid-childhood with a range of 1 to 20 years (4). The onset is variable, and progression may be either rapid or slow. Brain stem auditory evoked potentials show normal waves 1–3, with absent waves 4 and 5 in one patient and absence of all responses in another.

Figure 10–21. *Progressive pontobulbar palsy and sensorineural hearing loss (Brown–Vialetto–Van Laere syndrome).* (A) Wasting of tongue in anterior horn cell disease. (B) Generalized muscle wasting. [(A) from SA Hawkins et al., *J Med Genet* 27:176, 1990.]

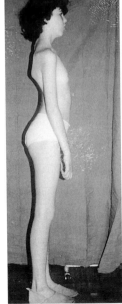

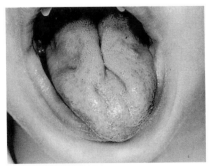

A   B

Vestibular system. Caloric abnormalities have been observed by several investigators (4,6,26,27).

Pathology. The few patients studied showed cell loss and gliosis in the lower cranial nerve nuclei, ventral cochlear nuclei, and anterior horns of the spinal cord, gross loss of axons in the lower cranial nerves, and degeneration of the eighth or cochleovestibular nerves. Other abnormalities were variable (2,8,13,17).

Heredity. In five families, one or more sibs were affected with no recognized symptoms in parents or other relatives (6,13,17,18,26,28). Consanguinity was described in one family (18). Most authors proposed autosomal recessive inheritance. In one family, hearing loss was present on both sides of the family (27). In another family, both the proband and her paternal aunt had hearing loss, facial weakness, and respiratory insufficiency. The father, paternal uncle, and paternal first cousin (son of an affected aunt) had sensorineural hearing loss without other symptoms (14). Given transmission through the father and a preponderance of females among reported patients, maternal (mitochondrial) inheritance is excluded and X-linked inheritance is unlikely. Thus, autosomal recessive inheritance seems most likely, although autosomal dominant with variable penetrance and perhaps sex-related expression cannot be excluded. It may also be possible that there is causal heterogeneity with both autosomal dominant and recessive forms of the condition.

Laboratory studies. A few individuals have been tested for mutations in the *SMN* and *NAIP* genes, but no mutations were found.

Diagnosis. The Madras form of motor neuron disease is very similar and could be the same disorder (16,22). It has also been suggested that the Madras form could be an environmentally caused entity, with viral or autoimmune causes possible (18). Motor neuropathy, vocal cord paralysis, and sensorineural hearing loss (Boltshauser syndrome) are similar, but brain stem signs were restricted to vocal cord paralysis, and age of onset and severity of hearing loss were more variable. Juvenile motor neuron disease (Fazio-Londe disease) lacks hearing loss but is otherwise identical (16). Khaldi et al. (15) described a patient who also had optic atrophy.

Prognosis. This disease results in severe disability and shortened life span, especially in those with more rapid progression.

Summary. This disorder is characterized by (*1*) probable autosomal dominant inheritance; (*2*) pontobulbar paralysis; (*3*) motor neuron disease, predominantly affecting the cervical cord; and (*4*) sensorineural hearing loss.

References

1. Abarbanel JM et al: Bulbo-pontine paralysis with deafness: the Vialetto-Van Laere syndrome. *Can J Neurol Sci* 18:349–351, 1991.
2. Alberca R et al: Progressive bulbar paralysis associated with neural deafness: a nosological entity. *Arch Neurol* 37:214–221, 1980.
3. Arnould G et al: Paralysie bulbo-pontine chronique progressive avec surdite—a propos d'une observation de syndrome de Fazio-Londe. *Rev Otoneuroophtal* 40:158–161, 1968.
4. Athertino Tavares CC et al: Données cochléo-vestibulaires dans la sclérose latérale amyotrophique (forme de Van Laere). *Rev Laryngol (Paris)* 106:375–378, 1985.
5. Ben Hamida M, Hentati F: Maladie de Charcot et sclérose latérale amyotrophique juvénile. *Rev Neurol* 140:202–206, 1984
6. Boudin G et al: Cas familial de paralysie bulbo-pontine chronique progressive avec surdité. *Rev Neurol* 124:90–92, 1971.
7. Brown CH: Infantile amyotrophic lateral sclerosis of the family type. *J Nerv Ment Dis* 21:707–716, 1894.
8. Brucher JM et al: Progressive pontobulbar palsy with deafness. Clinical and pathological study of 2 cases. *Arch Neurol* 38:186–190, 1981.
9. Davenport RJ, Mumford CJ: The Brown-Vialetto-Van Laere syndrome: a case report and literature review. *Eur J Neurol* 1:51–54, 1994.
10. De Mattos et al: Esclerose lateral amiotrofica com surdez: relato de um caso e revisao da literatura. *Arq Neuropsiquiatr* 40:201–207, 1982.

11. De Oliveira JT et al: Brown-Vialetto-Van Laere syndrome: report of 2 cases. *Arq Neuropsiquiatr* 53:789–791, 1995.
12. Francis DA et al: Brown-Vialetto-Van Laere syndrome: *Neuropathol Appl Neurobiol* 19:91–94, 1993.
13. Gallai V et al: Ponto-bulbar palsy with deafness (Brown-Vialetto-Van Laere syndrome). *J Neurol Sci* 50:259–275, 1981.
14. Hawkins SA et al: Pontobulbar palsy and neurosensory deafness (Brown–Vialetto–Van Laere syndrome) with possible autosomal dominant inheritance. *J Med Genet* 27:176–179, 1990.
15. Khaldi F et al: Un nouveau cas de paralysie bulbo-pontine progressive avec surdité et atrophie optique. *Ann Pédiatr* 34:731–733, 1987.
16. Jagganathan K: Juvenile motor neuron disease. In: *Tropical Neurology*, Spillane JD (ed), Oxford University Press, London, 1973, pp 127–130.
17. Lombaert A et al: Progressive ponto-bulbar palsy with deafness: A clinico-pathological study. *Acta Neurol Belg* 76:309–314, 1976.
18. Megarbane A et al: Brown–Vialetto–Van Laere syndrome in a large inbred Lebanese family: confirmation of autosomal recessive inheritance? *Am J Med Genet* 92:117–121, 2000.
19. Orrel RW et al: The relationship of spinal muscular atrophy to motor neuron disease: investigation of *SMN* and *NAIP* gene deletions in sporadic and familial ALS. *J Neurol Sci* 145:55–61, 1997.
20. Piccolo G et al: Recovery from respiratory muscle failure in a sporadic case of Brown–Vialetto–Van Laere syndrome with unusually late onset. *J Neurol* 239:355–356, 1992.
21. Serratrice G, Gastaut JL: Amyotrophies degeneratives et lesions du neurone moteur (a propos de 32 observations). *Marseille Med* 109:821–840, 1972.
22. Summers BA et al: Juvenile-onset bulbospinal muscular atrophy with deafness: Vialetto–Van Laere syndrome or Madras-type motor neuron disease. *J Neurol* 234:440–442, 1987.
23. Szatjzel R et al: Syndrome de Brown–Vialetto–Van Laere. Un cas avec anticorps anti-ganglioside GM1 et revue de la litterature. *Rev Neurol (Paris)* 154:51–54, 1998.
24. Tridon P et al: Syndrome pseudo-bulbaire cortical congénitale et surdité verbale associée. *Rev Otoneuroophtalmol* 46:83–88, 1974.
25. Trillet M et al: La paralysie bulbo-pontine chronique progressive familiale avec surdité. *Lyon Med* 223:145–153, 1960.
26. Van Laere J: Paralysie bulbo-pontine chronique progressive familiale avec surdité. Un cas de syndrome de Klippel-Trenaunay dans la meme fratrie. Problèmes diagnostiques et génétiques. *Rev Neurol* 115:289–295, 1966.
27. Van Laere J: Over een nieuw geval van chronische bulbopontiene paralysis met doofheid. *Verh Vlaam Akad Beneesk Belg* 30:288–308, 1967.
28. Vialetto E: Contributo alla forma ereditaria della paralisi bulbare progressiva. *Riv Sper Freniat* 40:1–24, 1936.

Spinal muscular atrophy, cardiac conduction disorder, cataracts, hypogonadism, and sensorineural hearing loss (Nathalie syndrome)

In 1975, Cremers et al. (1) reported four sibs with spinal muscular atrophy, cardiac conduction disorder, cataracts, hypogonadism, and sensorineural hearing loss in a family of Dutch and Ukrainian descent. They named the condition "Nathalie syndrome," after the oldest affected child.

Physical findings. The patients appeared younger than their chronologic age. Weight was below the third centile in all. Adult height was below 165 cm in three of the four sibs.

Central nervous system. Mild weakness and wasting began insidiously at 10–20 years and progressed very slowly. Muscle wasting, most prominent in the shoulders, thighs, and legs, and diminished deep tendon reflexes were evident. Nerve conduction studies were normal. Electromyographic needle exams were interpreted as most consistent with spinal muscular atrophy, but the description did not allow clear distinction between neurogenic and myopathic changes. Intelligence was normal.

Ocular system. Bilateral, visually significant cataracts were discovered in mid-childhood with a range of 4–10 years. When left untreated, the cataracts became denser and the anterior chamber more shallow.

Musculoskeletal system. Osteochondrosis might be part of this disorder as two of the sibs had Perthes disease and one had Scheuermann disease.

Endocrine system. Hypogonadism became apparent in adolescence. The two oldest girls had irregular menses, immature breasts, and sparse axillary and pubic hair. Laboratory studies were not reported.

Cardiovascular system. The oldest child had frequent palpitations, episodic perspiration, and murmur. Electrocardiogram showed ventricular extra systoles with aberrant intraventricular conduction and wandering pacemaker. The others had less severe repolarization abnormalities.

Auditory system. Sensorineural hearing loss began before 5 years and progressed slowly, especially for higher frequencies.

Vestibular system. Vestibular tests were normal.

Heredity. Four children including both sexes were affected, and their parents were healthy and nonconsanguineous. Thus, autosomal recessive inheritance is probable.

Diagnosis. Muscular weakness, cataracts, and cardiac conduction abnormalities occur in myotonic dystrophy. Walker (4) reported juvenile cataract and Perthes disease in three sisters, and van den Heuvel (3) reported cataract, arthropathy, and sensorineural hearing loss in two sisters. Pfeiffer et al. (2) noted dysplasia of the capital femoral epiphyses, severe myopia, and sensorineural hearing loss in three brothers.

Prognosis. This disease results in significant disability but no patients had died at the time of the report. The long-term prognosis is unknown.

Summary. This disorder is characterized by (*1*) autosomal recessive inheritance; (*2*) spinal muscular atrophy; (*3*) cardiac conduction abnormalities; (*4*) cataracts; (*5*) hypogonadism; (*6*) osteochondrosis; and (*7*) sensorineural hearing loss.

References

1. Cremers CWRJ et al: The Nathalie syndrome. A new hereditary syndrome. *Clin Genet* 8:330–340, 1975.
2. Pfeiffer RA et al: Epiphyseal dysplasia of the femoral head, severe myopia, and perceptive hearing loss in three brothers. *Clin Genet* 4:141–145, 1973.
3. van den Heuvel JEA: Cataracta brunescens, deafness, and arthropathy. *Ophthalmologica* 160:100–102, 1970.
4. Walker BA: Juvenile cataract and multiple epiphyseal dysplasia in three sisters. *Birth Defects* 5(2):315–318, 1969.

Arthrogrypotic hand abnormality and sensorineural hearing loss (Stewart-Bergstrom syndrome)

In 1971, Stewart and Bergstrom (3) first reported the combination of congenital arthrogrypotic hand anomaly and nonprogressive sensorineural hearing loss. Akbarnia et al. (1) described a second family. In the two families, a total of 22 individuals were affected. An isolated patient was reported by Martinón et al. (2).

Neuromuscular system. The hand anomaly is present at birth and resembles arthrogryposis. It consists of nonopposing, digitalized thumbs and spindle-shaped fingers with absent flexion creases at both proximal and distal joints. Muscle mass of the thenar, hypothenar, and interosseous muscles is decreased (Fig. 10–22). Ulnar deviation of the fingers and sometimes of the hand occurs, and wrist dorsiflexion is decreased. Some individuals had decreased elbow extension, and forearm pronation and supination. One possibly affected child had normal appearance of the hands with poor modeling of the metacarpals on X-ray. Most had normal feet except for decreased toe flexion. Unilateral clubfoot was

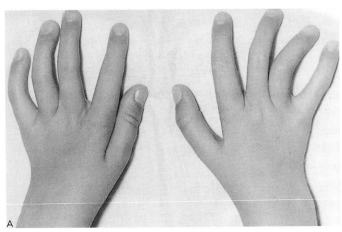

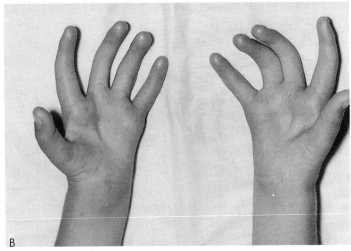

Figure 10–22. *Arthrogrypotic hand abnormality and sensorineural hearing loss (Stewart-Bergstrom syndrome).* (A,B) Dorsal and palmar views of hands showing absence of flexion creases and diminished muscle mass. [From JM Stewart and L Bergstrom, *J Pediatr* 78:102, 1971.]

observed in one person and coxa vara in another. No progression of the anomalies was reported. The basis of these abnormalities has not been adequately investigated.

Auditory system. Sensorineural hearing loss was documented by audiogram in 8 of 11 persons tested. It was bilateral and severe (up to 90 dB loss) in some, but unilateral or mild in others. The hearing loss was probably congenital and nonprogressive (1–3).

Heredity. Vertical transmission over several generations and two instances of male-to-male transmission are consistent with autosomal dominant inheritance.

Diagnosis. The lack of progression and other findings are apparently unique. Okihiro syndrome is characterized by dominant inheritance of Duane anomaly with congenital hypoplasia of the thenar eminences and sensorineural hearing loss.

Prognosis. Motor disability was usually moderate and nonprogressive, but hearing loss was sometimes severe.

Summary. This disorder is characterized by (*1*) autosomal dominant inheritance; (*2*) congenital hand deformity that resembles arthrogryposis; and (*3*) congenital sensorineural hearing loss.

References

1. Akbarnia BA et al: Familial arthrogryposis-like hand abnormality and sensorineural deafness. *Am J Dis Child* 133:403–405, 1979.
2. Martinón F et al: Sindrome de Stewart y Bergstrom. Aportacion de una nueva observacion. *An Esp Pediatr* 12:549–552, 1979.
3. Stewart JM, Bergstrom L: Familial hand abnormality and sensorineural deafness: a new syndrome. *J Pediatr* 78:102–110, 1971.

Motor and Sensory Neuropathies with Hearing Loss

Motor neuropathy, vocal cord paralysis, and sensorineural hearing loss (Boltshauser syndrome)

In 1989, Boltshauser et al. (1) reported three individuals with distal spinal muscular atrophy (hereditary motor neuropathy), vocal cord paralysis, and sensorineural hearing loss in three generations of a single family. Young and Harper (4) and Pridmore et al. (3) described kindreds with similar abnormalities but with normal hearing. These two families were later found to be related to each other (2).

Central nervous system. In the proband, stridor was noticed from about 6 months. Abduction palsy of the right vocal cord was diagnosed, and arytenoidectomy of the left vocal cord was performed at 10 years. Her mother had no voice changes, while her maternal grandfather had a hoarse voice from about 40 years of age. Both of the latter had abduction palsies of the left cord.

Weakness and wasting of the hands developed during childhood in all three. Leg weakness was noted by 13 years in the proband, but not until the 50's in her grandfather. Examination showed distal muscular atrophy, most marked in the hands, weakness that was most severe in distal muscle groups but also involving proximal muscles in later stages, absent tendon reflexes, intact sensation, and normal intelligence. The proband had an abnormal gait and scapular winging. Motor and sensory nerve conduction velocities were normal, but some sensory nerve amplitude was diminished. Electromyographic needle exams showed denervation changes including reduced recruitment pattern and large polyphasic units of long duration in small hand muscles.

Auditory system. In the proband, mild hearing loss was detected on testing at 13 years, while the mother's hearing loss was not noticed until her 30's. Hearing loss was slowly progressive, and the grandfather required hearing aids in his 50's. Audiograms showed that hearing loss started in the middle frequencies in early childhood and progressed to involve higher frequencies. Tympanometry and BAER indicated primarily cochlear location of the hearing loss, although a slight neural component could not be excluded.

Laboratory findings. Serum creatine kinase values were minimally elevated in all three affected individuals.

Pathology. Muscle biopsy in the mother showed moderate changes in the quadriceps and severe abnormalities in the gastrocnemius. The latter consisted of long-standing denervation atrophy with fiber atrophy involving whole fascicles, areas of hypertrophic fibers, and slightly increased endomysial connective tissue. Sural nerve biopsy showed normal architecture, although myelinated fiber density was significantly decreased.

Heredity. The three affected individuals came from three generations of a single family. There were no instances of male-to-male transmission. Thus, autosomal dominant inheritance is most likely, although X-linked dominant inheritance cannot be excluded. In the families with motor neuropathy and vocal cord paralysis with normal hearing, inheritance was also autosomal dominant (2). The gene that causes that condition has been mapped to 2q14 (2).

Diagnosis. The neuromuscular abnormalities observed in this disorder are most similar to hereditary motor neuropathy (the spinal form that the authors described as "distal spinal muscular atrophy"). The slightly raised serum creatine kinase values are compatible with this diagnosis. However, the mild abnormalities observed on sensory nerve conduction studies suggest additional sensory involvement, possibly from loss of cells in the dorsal root ganglia. Thus, classification as a form of HMSN might be more accurate. This disorder must be differentiated from motor neuropathy and vocal cord paralysis without deafness (4), and from pontobulbar palsy and sensorineural hearing loss (Brown-Vialetto-Van Laere syndrome), which includes many additional signs of brain stem involvement other than vocal cord paralysis. Motor and sensory neuropathy and sensorineural hearing loss (several types) may be separated on the basis of EMG results.

Prognosis. Clinical expression of this disorder varied greatly, but always caused significant disability.

Summary. This syndrome is characterized by (*1*) autosomal dominant inheritance; (*2*) mild motor neuropathy; (*3*) vocal cord paralysis; and (*4*) sensorineural hearing loss.

References

1. Boltshauser E et al: Hereditary distal muscular atrophy with vocal cord paralysis and sensorineural hearing loss: a dominant form of spinal muscular atrophy? *J Med Genet* 26:105–108, 1989.
2. McEntagart M et al: Localization of the gene for distal hereditary motor neuronopathy VII (dHMN-VII) to chromosome 2q14. *Am J Hum Genet* 68:1270–1276, 2001.
3. Pridmore C et al: Distal spinal muscular atrophy with vocal cord paralysis. *J Med Genet* 29:197–199, 1992.
4. Young ID, Harper PS: Hereditary distal spinal muscular atrophy with vocal cord paralysis. *J Neurol Neurosurg Psychiatry* 43:413–418, 1980.

Charcot-Marie-Tooth hereditary neuropathies [hereditary motor and sensory neuropathies (HMSN)]

The Charcot-Marie Tooth (CMT) or hereditary motor and sensory neuropathies are a group of conditions characterized by chronic motor and sensory neuropathy. On the basis of electrophysiology, CMT has been subdivided into type 1, which is characterized by reduced motor nerve conduction velocities, and type 2, which is characterized by normal or slightly reduced motor nerve conduction velocities and reduced amplitudes (2). The neuropathology of CMT type 1 has prominent demyelination, whereas that of CMT type 2 has prominent axonal loss.

Charcot-Marie-Tooth syndrome can be inherited as autosomal dominant, autosomal recessive, or X-linked traits, and several attempts have been made to incorporate genetics into the earlier clinical classification scheme. Currently the autosomal dominant forms are designated CMT1; the axonal neuropathies, which include autosomal dominant and recessive forms, are designated CMT2; and the recessive demyelinating forms are termed CMT4. In addition, there are at least three X-linked forms (CMTX), some of which have not been well characterized. Within each group, there is further subdivision with the addition of a letter, with each group presumably having a different molecular cause. The genes for CMT1A and CMT1B, respectively, are *PMP22* and *MPZ*. CMT1C encompasses the remaining autosomal dominant causes of CMT1 including *EGR2* (8) and a gene mapped to 16p13.1–p12.3 (1). This latter gene has recently been identified to be a protein degradation gene, *LITAF/SIMPLE* (7). Among the autosomal dominant CMT2 entities, genes have been identified for CMT2A (*KIF1B*) and CMT2E (*NEFL*); CMT2B and CMT2D have been mapped to 3q12–q22 and 7p14, respectively. The cause or gene locus for CMT2C is unknown. One autosomal recessive form, CMT2B1, is caused by homozygous mutations in lamin A/C (*LMNA*); the gene responsible for CMT2B2 is unknown, but maps to 19q13.3 (3). CMT4 encompasses seven forms, with not all of the responsible genes identified as of end of 2002 (1). However, the genes that have not been identified have been mapped. The most common form of CMTX is that caused by *GJB1* mutations, although heterogeneity within this group is also present. For reviews of the molecular genetics of CMT see references 4–6. In addition, there is a database in which what is known about the molecular genetics of the inherited peripheral neuropathies is frequently updated (http://molgen-www.uia.ac.be/CMTMutations/).

Hearing loss has been described in only a very few families with CMT, so only those will be described in more detail. In addition, there are several reports of conditions that resemble CMT but have not been designated as specific forms of CMT that include hearing loss. Those will also be reviewed.

References

1. Berger P et al: Molecular cell biology of Charcot-Marie-Tooth disease. *Neurogenetics* 4:1–18, 2002.
2. Harding AE, Thomas PK: The clinical features of hereditary motor and sensory neuropathy types I and II. *Brain* 103:259–280, 1980.
3. Leal A et al: A second locus for axonal form of autosomal recessive Charcot-Marie-Tooth disease maps to chromosome 19q13.3. *Am J Hum Genet* 68:269–277, 2001.
4. Nelis E et al: Mutations in the peripheral myelin genes and associated genes in inherited peripheral neuropathies. *Hum Mutat* 13:11–28, 1999.
5. Pareyson D: Charcot-Marie-Tooth disease and related neuropathies: molecular basis for distinction and diagnosis. *Muscle Nerve* 22:1498–1509, 1999.
6. Shy ME et al: A molecular basis for hereditary motor and sensory neuropathy disorders. *Curr Neurol Neurosci Rep* 1:77–88. 2001.
7. Street VA et al: Mutation of a putative protein degradation gene *LITAF/SIMPLE* in Charcot-Marie-Tooth disease 1C. *Neurology* 14:22–26, 2003.
8. Venken K et al: Search for mutations in the EGR2 corepressor proteins, NAB1 and NAB2, in human peripheral neuropathies. *Neurogenetics* 4:37–41, 2002.

Autosomal dominant Charcot-Marie-Tooth (AD HMSN) with hearing loss

Since many of these conditions were described prior to molecular characterization, it is unknown in which CMT group they may belong. When known, however, that information is provided.

In 1974, De Weerdt and Heerspink (4) described a single large family with autosomal dominant inheritance of neuropathy, most similar to HMSN type I, and hearing loss. Clinical manifestations were similar to those of the autosomal recessive form (2,3). Kousseff et al. (7) reported a large kindred, as did Gummerson et al. (5). An isolated example with hearing loss has been described (9). Hamiel et al. (6) also reported another kindred, but in that family hearing loss was noted in infancy or early childhood. In this family linkage studies excluded CMT1A and CMT1B. Boerkoel et al. (1) identified hearing loss in 2 of 82 individuals with CMT1A; one had a 17p12 duplication, and the other a *PMP22* mutation.

Peripheral nervous system. Weakness and wasting were noticed at about the same age and progressed slowly. Examination showed severe atrophy and weakness involving feet, calves, and hands, foot drop, diminished reflexes in the legs, and wide-based, steppage gait. Electromyogram evaluation showed severe slowing of nerve conduction and variable denervation on needle exam, which are consistent with demyelination and similar to findings in HMSN type I.

Auditory system. De Weerdt and Heerspink (4) noted that hearing loss began in the 30's or 40's and was slowly progressive. Kousseff et al. (7) reported hearing loss beginning in childhood and progressing to severe loss in 61 of 72 affected members. Perez et al. (11) noted hearing loss in almost 30% of patients with CMT. Musiek et al. (10) briefly described hearing loss in a woman with dominantly inherited CMT, not otherwise specified. Onset of hearing loss was in her late 40's. Satya-Murti et al. (13) reported abnormal auditory evoked potentials in two brothers who were thought to have HSMN type II. No other family members had hearing loss. Raglan et al. (12) also described abnormal auditory evoked potentials. Hamiel et al. (6) described childhood onset with variable degrees of sensorineural hearing loss. In this family hearing loss sometimes preceded onset of neurologic signs.

Laboratory findings. In the kindred described by De Weerdt and Heerspink (4), several individuals had elevated serum alkaline phosphatase levels, but its significance is not known.

Heredity. These entities are inherited as autosomal dominant traits. The family reported by Kousseff et al. (7) was found to have a mutation in the *PMP22* gene at 17p11.2 (8) and thus has CMT1A with associated hearing loss. In the family reported by Hamiel et al. (6) linkage to *PMP22* was excluded, thus indicating clearly that CMT1A is not the only autosomal dominant CMT associated with hearing loss.

Diagnosis. Diagnostic considerations are the same as those for the recessive form.

Prognosis. Both the hearing loss and neuropathy are progressive, but no other systems are involved.

Summary. This disorder is characterized by (*1*) autosomal dominant inheritance; (*2*) hereditary motor and sensory neuropathy; and (*3*) sensorineural hearing loss.

References

1. Boerkoel CF et al: Charcot-Marie-Tooth disease and related neuropathies: mutation distribution and genotype–phenotype correlation. *Ann Neurol* 51:190–201, 2002.
2. Bouldin TW et al: Clinical and pathological features of an autosomal recessive neuropathy. *J Neurol Sci* 46:315–323, 1980.
3. Cornell J et al: Autosomal recessive inheritance of Charcot-Marie-Tooth disease associated with sensorineural deafness. *Clin Genet* 25:163–165, 1984.
4. De Weerdt CJ, Heerspink W: Family with Charcot-Marie-Tooth disease showing unusual biochemical, clinical and genetic features. *Eur Neurol* 12:253–260, 1974.
5. Gummerson E, personal communication: MIM Number: 118300: 6/14/99. In: *Online Mendelian Inheritance in Man, OMIM* (TM), Johns Hopkins University, Baltimore, MD.
6. Hamiel OP et al: Hereditary motor-sensory neuropathy (Charcot-Marie-Tooth disease) with nerve deafness: A new variant. *J Pediatr* 123:431–434, 1993.
7. Kousseff BG et al: Charcot-Marie-Tooth disease with sensorineural hearing loss—an autosomal dominant trait. *Birth Defects* 18(3B):223–228, 1982.
8. Kovach MJ et al: A unique point mutation in the *PMP22* gene is associated with Charcot-Marie-Tooth disease and deafness. *Am J Hum Genet* 64:1580–1593, 1999.
9. Laubert A: Schwerhörigkeit als Symptom der neuralen Muskelatrophie (Charcot-Marie-Tooth Krankheit). *HNO* 34:434–437, 1986.
10. Musiek FE et al: Auditory findings in Charcot-Marie-Tooth disease. *Arch Otolaryngol* 108:595–599, 1982.
11. Perez H et al: Audiologic evaluation in Charcot-Marie-Tooth disease. *Scand Audiol Suppl* 30:211–213, 1988.
12. Raglan E et al: Auditory function in hereditary motor and sensory neuropathy (Charcot-Marie-Tooth disease). *Acta Otolaryngol (Stockh)* 103:50–55, 1987.
13. Satya-Murti S et al: Abnormal auditory evoked potentials in hereditary motor-sensory neuropathy. *Ann Neurol* 5:445–448, 1979.

Neuropathy and sensorineural hearing loss, autosomal dominant

Lopez-Bigas et al. (1) described a unique family in which the combination of peripheral neuropathy and sensorineural hearing loss occurred secondary to mutations in the connexin 31 (*GJB3*) gene.

Peripheral nervous system. Affected individuals presented with variable degrees of peripheral nerve involvement, with some showing minor abnormalities on electrophysiologic studies, whereas others showed severe symmetrical motor and sensory demyelinating neuropathy. In the more severely affected persons, distal chronic trophic ulcerations and osteomyelitic changes were common, leading to amputations of the feet in some.

Auditory findings. Degree and distribution of hearing loss was also variable within the family, with some individuals having unilateral loss that was quite severe, and others having bilateral involvement that was fairly mild.

Heredity. The inheritance of this condition is autosomal dominant, and caused by mutations in connexin 31 (*GJB3*) at 1p35.1. This gene also causes nonsyndromic hearing loss and erythrokeratodermia variabilis. The phenotype in this family was thought to be caused by the nature of the mutation, which was a deletion of codon 66. It is noteworthy that deletions of codon 66 in *GJB1* (connexin 32) causes X-linked Charcot-Marie-Tooth disease, and deletion of codon 66 in *GJB2* (connexin 26) causes Vohwinkel syndrome.

Reference

1. Lopez-Bigas N et al: Connexin 31 (GJB3) is expressed in the peripheral and auditory nerves and causes neuropathy and hearing impairment. *Hum Mol Genet* 10:947–952, 2001.

Hereditary motor and sensory neuropathy Lom (CMT4D)

Kalaydjieva et al. (3,4) described a provisionally unique neuropathy that was originally described in Bulgarian Gypsies living in the community of Lom. Colomer et al. (1) described a Spanish family of Gypsy descent.

Nervous system. Disturbance of gait was the presenting symptom in all affected individuals, occurring between the ages of 5 and 10 years. Lower limb weakness was progressive, and muscle wasting was common. Some patients were no longer walking, the earliest age at which this occurred being 26 years. Upper limbs were also affected, but occurrence of weakness and wasting was later and involvement was less severe.

Sensation was impaired in both upper and lower limbs, but more so in lower limbs. Pes cavus and clawing of toes and fingers were common but not consistent.

Auditory system. Onset of hearing loss was between the ages of 13 and 26 years, and affected approximately two-thirds of the patients. All had sensorineural loss, affecting high tones more than low tones. Some also had a conductive component to the hearing loss, as demonstrated by the loss of the stapedial reflex. Brain stem auditory evoked potentials were abnormal, suggesting a defect in the central auditory pathways.

Laboratory findings. Nerve conduction studies showed severely reduced velocities.

Pathology. Sural nerve biopsy specimens were obtained from a number of individuals, and showerd hypertrophic changes with multiple "onion bulbs" in the younger individuals, whereas in the older individuals the onion bulbs had regressed.

Heredity. This is an autosomal recessive condition that has been mapped to 8q24.3 (4). The gene has subsequently been identified as N-myc downstream regulated gene 1 (*NDRG1*) (5).

Diagnosis. This condition closely resembles an autosomal recessive neuropathy with deafness described in a South African family (2), but hearing loss was present in infancy. The Rosenberg-Chutorian syndrome is also similar, but that condition also includes optic atrophy in the phenotype (6).

References

1. Colomer J et al: Hereditary motor and sensory neuropathy-Lom (HMSNL) in a Spanish family: clinical, electrophysiological, pathological and genetic studies. *Neuromuscl Disord* 10:578–583, 2000.
2. Cornell J et al: Autosomal recessive inheritance of Charcot-Marie-Tooth disease associated with sensorineural deafness. *Clin Genet* 25:163–165, 1983.
3. Kalaydjieva L et al: Gene mapping in gypsies identifies a novel demyelinating neuropathy on chromosome 8q24. *Nat Genet* 14:214–217, 1996.

4. Kalaydjieva L et al: Hereditary motor and sensory neuropathy–Lom, a novel demyelinating neuropathy associated with deafness in gypsies. *Brain* 121:399–408, 1998.
5. Kalaydjieva L et al: N-myc downstream-regulated gene 1 is mutated in hereditary motor and sensory neuropathy–Lom. *Am J Hum Genet* 67:47–58, 2000.
6. Rosenberg RN, Chutorian A: Familial opticoacoustic nerve degeneration and polyneuropathy. *Neurology* 17:827–832, 1967.

Motor and sensory neuropathy with sensorineural hearing loss, Bouldin type

In 1980, Bouldin et al. (1) described a brother and sister with onset of motor and sensory neuropathy, most similar to HMSN type I, and hearing loss in their 30's.

Peripheral nervous system. Weakness began in the 30's (range 15–50 years) and progressed slowly. Scoliosis occurred in childhood (2). Examination was typical for sensorimotor neuropathy with severe atrophy and weakness involving the feet, calves, and hands, foot drop, diminished or absent reflexes (especially in the legs), and wide-based, steppage gait. Sensory loss in a stocking-glove distribution occurred in some families, being severe enough in one family to result in foot ulcers. None had pseudohypertrophy of involved nerves. Electromyographic evaluation demonstrated severe slowing of nerve conduction and variable denervation on needle exam. These results are typical of demyelination and similar to HMSN type I without hearing loss.

Musculoskeletal system. Both sibs from one family (2) had progressive scoliosis during childhood.

Auditory system. Hearing loss began in the 30's or 40's and progressed slowly. Audiograms showed mild or moderate sensorineural loss.

Pathology. Sural nerve biopsy in a 45-year-old affected man showed marked loss of myelinated fibers, occasional demyelinated axons, increased endoneurial fibrous tissue, and only rare clusters of regenerating myelinated fibers. All sizes of myelinated fibers were affected. Axonal degeneration and onion bulb formation were not seen. The lack of nerve enlargement, onion bulb formation, and demyelinated axons differs significantly from the usual forms of hereditary sensorimotor neuropathy.

Heredity. Autosomal recessive inheritance is likely given observation of multiple affected sibs of both sexes and apparently unaffected parents.

Diagnosis. In sporadic patients, it may not be possible to separate the recessive and dominant forms. Hereditary motor and sensory neuropathy with deafness, mental retardation, and absence of sensory large myelinated fibers differs by age of onset and other clinical manifestations (2). Motor and sensory neuropathy, trigeminal neuralgia, and sensorineural hearing loss (Cruse syndrome) may be a variant presentation of this disorder. Motor and sensory neuropathy and sensorineural hearing loss (X-linked) (Cowchock syndrome) may be separated by both EMG studies and pattern of inheritance. Motor and sensory neuropathy, optic atrophy, and sensorineural hearing loss with autosomal dominant, autosomal recessive, or X-linked inheritance all include optic atrophy. The syndrome of motor and sensory neuropathy, nephritis, and sensorineural hearing loss (Lemieux-Neemeh syndrome) differs by virtue of the renal disease.

Prognosis. Both the hearing loss and neuropathy are progressive, but no other systems are involved.

Summary. This disorder is characterized by (1) autosomal recessive inheritance; (2) hereditary motor and sensory neuropathy (most similar to HMSN type I); and (3) sensorineural hearing loss.

References
1. Bouldin TW et al: Clinical and pathological features of an autosomal recessive neuropathy. *J Neurol Sci* 46:315–323, 1980.
2. Sabatelli M et al: Hereditary motor and sensory neuropathy with deafness, mental retardation, and absence of sensory large myelinated fibers: confirmation of a new entity. *Am J Med Genet* 75:309–313, 1998.

Hereditary motor and sensory neuropathy with deafness, mental retardation, and absence of large myelinated fibers

In 1984, Cornell et al. (1) reported three brothers with onset of neuropathy and deafness that occurred in the first year of life. Sabatelli et al. (3) and Mancardi et al. (2) described similar cases, and it is likely these individuals have the same condition.

Central nervous system. Degree of mental retardation, when stated, is mild.

Peripheral nervous system. Results of nerve conduction studies resemble those found for CMT1. Electrophysiologic studies in two boys (3) demonstrated slowed motor nerve conduction velocity and absent sensory action potentials.

Auditory system. Severe to profound bilateral sensorineural hearing loss occurred before age 1 year.

Pathology. Sural nerve biopsy in two patients, who were sibs, demonstrated absence of large myelinated fibers. Density of small myelinated fibers and unmyelinated fibers was found (3).

Heredity. The presence of this condition in affected sibs with unaffected parents, who were confirmed to be consanguineous in two cases and suspected to be consanguineous in the third case, suggests autosomal recessive inheritance. It is noteworthy that all affected individuals are male. The precise gene defect is unknown.

Diagnosis. This condition can be distinguished from other recessively inherited motor and sensory neuropathies by the constellation of manifestations.

Prognosis. Life span appears to be unaffected. Degree of mental retardation is suspected to be mild, although speech may never develop (1).

Summary. This condition is characterized by (1) autosomal recessive inheritance; (2) motor and sensory neuropathy resembling HMSN type 1; and (3) early-onset sensorineural hearing loss with mild mental retardation.

References
1. Cornell J et al: Autosomal recessive inheritance of Charcot-Marie-Tooth disease associated with sensorineural deafness. *Clin Genet* 25:163–165, 1984.
2. Mancardi GL et al: Hereditary motor and sensory neuropathy with deafness, mental retardation and absence of large myelinated fibers. *J Neurol Sci* 110:121–130, 1992.
3. Sabatelli M et al: Hereditary motor and sensory neuropathy with deafness, mental retardation, and absence of sensory large myelinated fibers: confirmation of a new entity. *Am J Med Genet* 75:309–313, 1998.

X-linked Charcot-Marie-Tooth disease

Charcot-Marie-Tooth disease, X-linked form, is caused by mutations in at least three genes. The most common is attributable to mutations in connexin 32, although most cases are not associated with hearing loss. However, Stojkovic et al. (2) described one family in which several individuals had hearing loss, and Lee et al. (1), in their description of six families with *GJB1* mutations, noted that in three of these families some individuals had hearing loss that was likely associated with the disease process.

References

1. Lee MJ et al: Six novel connexin32 (*GJB1*) mutations in X-linked Charcot-Marie-Tooth disease. *J Neurol Neurosurg Psychiatry* 73:304–306, 2002.
2. Stojkovic T et al: Sensorineural deafness in X-linked Charcot-Marie-Tooth disease with connexin 32 mutation (*R142Q*). *Neurology* 52:1010–1014, 1999.

Motor and sensory neuropathy and sensorineural hearing loss (X-linked) (Cowchock syndrome, X-L recessive Charcot-Marie-Tooth syndrome)

In 1985, Cowchock et al. (2) reported a family in which seven males from two generations were affected with hereditary motor and sensory neuropathy, most similar to HMSN type II, and sensorineural hearing loss.

Peripheral nervous system. Weakness and wasting were probably present from birth. The proband was evaluated at 8 weeks because his mother noted weakness of the dorsiflexors of the great toes, a characteristic of other boys affected in infancy. Examination in infancy showed profound, generalized weakness and areflexia, often mistaken for infantile spinal muscular atrophy. Motor development was delayed.

Older affected individuals had generalized weakness, which was most severe in distal muscle groups. The peroneal muscles were always affected, and older males had pes cavus and hammer toes. Sensory examination was limited by young age, poor commuication, or previous ankle surgery. The clinical course was slowly progressive although older affected males were able to walk. The oldest affected male had decreasing hand strength and could walk only a few steps without assistance at 25 years. Motor nerve conduction studies were moderately delayed to normal (33–55 m/sec) in three affected males and were normal in two carrier females. Sensory nerve conduction was abnormal (usually absent) in the affected males, while one of two carriers had mild prolongation of sural nerve latency. These results are most similar to those of HMSN type II.

Central nervous system. One of the older affected males was considered mentally retarded and deaf by his family and was institutionalized. He died at 14 years from gastric hemorrhage due to ingested foreign objects. Delay in motor milestones could be attributed to the neuromuscular disease. However, two younger affected boys apparently had evidence of delay in social development as well. Because of the presence of weakness and hearing loss and absence of psychometric data, it is not possible to conclude whether mental retardation is a component of this disorder.

Auditory system. Sensorineural hearing loss, usually diagnosed by 5 years, was present in all but one affected male. Audiograms confirmed the abnormality in four boys. Brain stem auditory evoked potentials were normal in an affected boy with apparently normal hearing, and further tests were not done. One woman (at 50% risk for being a carrier) had unilateral, mild sensorineural hearing loss.

Pathology. Sural nerve biopsy in one affected male showed decreased myelinated fibers, mostly of fine to moderate size. Connective tissue was greatly increased. Electron microscopy showed a paucity of myelinated axons and stacking of Schwann cell cytoplasm, suggesting involvement of small nonmyelinated nerves. There was no onion bulb formation or evidence of an active process.

Heredity. This disorder was diagnosed in seven males from two generations, all related through females (Fig. 10–23). Minor abnormalities in sensory nerve conduction and hearing were identified in female relatives but were not consistent enough to be useful in identification of gene carriers. One female had mild hearing loss and was presumed to be a carrier. These observations are consistent with X-linked recessive

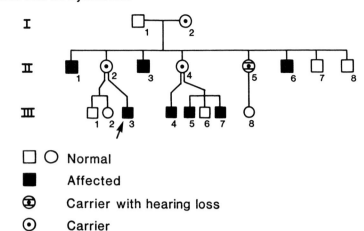

Figure 10–23. *Motor and sensory neuropathy and sensorineural hearing loss (X-linked) (Cowchock syndrome, X-L Charcot-Marie-Tooth syndrome).* Pedigree of family showing X-linked recessive inheritance.

inheritance with mild signs in some carriers. This disorder was originally thought to be a contiguous gene syndrome that mapped to the Xq13 area, the site of the X-linked dominant CMT gene (1,3,4). However, recent studies have mapped this gene to Xq24–q26, indicating that it is a distinct condition (6).

Diagnosis. The clinical presentation in this disorder is distinguished by the very early, probably congenital, onset of weakness, which is unusual for hereditary neuropathies, and by X-linked inheritance. It is important to note that in some families with X-linked dominant CMT sensorineural hearing loss occurs in some members (5,7). The syndrome of motor and sensory neuropathy, type I, optic atrophy, and sensorineural hearing loss (Rosenberg-Chutorian syndrome) is characterized by slightly later onset and visual abnormalities.

Prognosis. All affected males were very weak but still able to walk as adults.

Summary. This syndrome is characterized by (*1*) X-linked recessive inheritance; (*2*) congenital onset of hereditary motor and sensory neuropathy (most similar to HMSN type II); (*3*) possible mental retardation in some individuals; and (*4*) early-onset sensorineural hearing loss.

References

1. Bergoffen J et al: Connexin mutations in X-linked Charcot-Marie-Tooth disease. *Science* 262:2039–2042, 1993.
2. Cowchock FS et al: X-linked motor-sensory neuropathy type-II with deafness and mental retardation: a new disorder. *Am J Med Genet* 20:307–315, 1985.
3. Fischbeck KH et al: Linkage studies of X-linked neuropathy and spinal muscular atrophy. *Cytogenet Cell Genet* 46:614, 1987.
4. Ionanescu VV et al: Heterogeneity in X-linked recessive Charcot-Marie-Tooth neuropathy. *Am J Hum Genet* 48:1075–1083, 1991.
5. Lee MJ et al: Six novel connexin32 (*GJB1*) mutations in X-linked Charcot-Marie-Tooth disease. *J Neurol Neurosurg Psychiatry* 73:304–306, 2002.
6. Priest JM et al: A locus for axonal motor-sensory neuropathy with deafness and mental retardation maps to Xq24–q26. *Genomics* 20:409–412, 1995.
7. Stojkovic T et al: Sensorineural deafness in X-linked Charcot-Marie-Tooth disease with connexin 32 mutation (R142Q). *Neurology* 52:1010–1014, 1999.

Motor and sensory neuropathy, optic atrophy, and sensorineural hearing loss (autosomal dominant) (Hagemoser syndrome)

In 1989, Hagemoser et al. (1) described this disorder with at least eight families manifesting the combination of motor and sensory neuropathy, optic atrophy, and hearing loss with apparent genetic heterogeneity.

When organized by which symptom was first to appear, three separate syndromes with different patterns of inheritance may be distinguished. In the autosomal dominant form, optic atrophy is the first symptom and the neuropathy is most similar to HMSN type II (1). Autosomal recessive and X-linked forms are reviewed in the following sections.

Ocular system. Decreased visual acuity associated with optic atrophy was usually noticed during early school years but could be recognized even earlier on eye examination. The visual deficit progressed gradually over many years to the point where only finger counting was possible. Visual fields first showed mild constriction, which progressed to central and paracentral scotomas. Later testing showed normal electroretinograms, but absent visual evoked responses.

Peripheral nervous system. Neuropathic symptoms were mild but sometimes unrecognized for many years. Neurologic testing was normal in childhood, but mild weakness, diminished deep tendon reflexes, and decreased position and vibration sense began in early adulthood. One affected person was unable to walk at age 62. Nerve conduction studies showed mild slowing and prolonged distal latencies consistent with axonal motor and sensory neuropathy, probably most similar to HMSN type II.

Auditory system. Bilateral sensorineural hearing loss was most often recognized soon after the visual loss but could be detected earlier with hearing tests. Hearing loss, never as severe as visual loss, progressed slowly. Audiometry showed mild to moderately severe hearing loss and absent acoustic reflexes.

Vestibular system. Vertigo was an occasional complaint.

Heredity. Vertical transmission through several generations, and several instances of male (including male-to-male) transmission occurred in the two families reported. These observations establish autosomal dominant (and exclude maternal) inheritance of this disorder.

Diagnosis. The three disorders presenting with this triad can be distinguished by family history and, possibly, by clinical presentation. Sporadic cases should be counseled for different possible patterns of inheritance. Given the subtlety of the neuropathy, it is possible that some reports describing hearing loss with optic atrophy have missed this component.

Prognosis. Visual loss is eventually severe, but other disabilities are moderate. Life span is probably normal.

Summary. This disorder consists of (1) autosomal dominant inheritance; (2) motor and sensory neuropathy (most similar to HMSN type II); (3) optic atrophy; and (4) sensorineural hearing loss.

Reference

1. Hagemoser K et al: Optic atrophy, hearing loss, and peripheral neuropathy. *Am J Med Genet* 33:61–65, 1989.

Motor and sensory neuropathy, pigmentary retinopathy, and sensorineural hearing loss (Pauli syndrome)

In 1984, Pauli (1) described 99 individuals from three generations of a family (family B) with variable neuropathy, pigmentary retinopathy, and sensorineural hearing loss.

Ocular system. Night blindness and decreased visual fields were observed in two of nine affected individuals. Examination showed a pigmentary retinal degeneration.

Peripheral nervous system. Although the ages of onset of symptoms were not described, motor and sensory neuropathy was confirmed by nerve conduction studies in two of nine affected individuals.

Auditory system. Sensorineural hearing loss began in early childhood, and progressed to moderate or severe loss. This was the only manifestation in six of the nine affected individuals.

Heredity. In this family, vertical transmission through three generations and observed male-to-male transmission suggest autosomal dominant inheritance (Fig. 10–24). However, neuropathy and pigmentary retinopathy occurred in only three of nine affected individuals from one branch of the family. Thus, this might represent cosegregation of two different genetic disorders.

Diagnosis. An unrecognized mitochondrial encephalomyopathy, but with autosomal dominant inheritance, is possible because each of the clinical manifestations is known to occur in this group of disorders. For example, Kearns-Sayre syndrome (ophthalmoplegia plus) differs clinically because of ophthalmoplegia and ptosis as early signs and by ragged-red fibers on muscle biopsy. Usher syndrome lacks the peripheral neuropathy. The syndrome of ataxia, retinitis pigmentosa, and sensorineural hearing loss (Hallgren syndrome) differs because of ataxia and mental retardation, although some peripheral nerve involvement may be present.

Prognosis. Clinical severity varied greatly among affected individuals.

Summary. This disorder is characterized by (1) autosomal dominant inheritance; (2) motor and sensory neuropathy; (3) pigmentary retinopathy; and (4) sensorineural hearing loss.

Reference

1. Pauli RM: Sensorineural deafness and peripheral neuropathy. *Clin Genet* 26:383–384, 1984 (family B).

Motor and sensory neuropathy, trigeminal neuralgia, and sensorineural hearing loss (Cruse syndrome)

In 1977, Cruse et al. (1) reported hypertrophic peripheral neuropathy, most similar to HMSN type I, hearing loss, and trigeminal neuralgia (tic douloureux) in four generations of a family originating in Haywood County, North Carolina.

Peripheral nervous system. Pes cavus was frequently noted in infancy and always during childhood. Gait abnormalities occurred in all 14 affected individuals and were slowly progressive. Examination showed changes typical of sensorimotor neuropathy including pes

Figure 10–24. *Motor and sensory neuropathy, pigmentary retinopathy, and sensorineural hearing loss (Pauli syndrome). Pedigree of family showing probable autosomal dominant inheritance.*

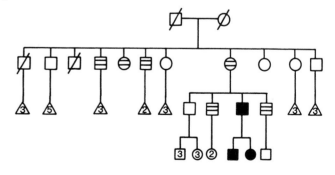

□ ○ Normal

■ ● Affected

⊟ ⊖ Hearing loss only

cavus, distal atrophy and weakness, loss of deep tendon reflexes, and distal sensory loss. Peripheral nerves were not enlarged to palpation. Electromyography showed slow or absent sensory evoked responses, slow motor nerve conduction studies, and chronic denervation on needle examination, similar to HMSN type I.

Central nervous system. Unilateral trigeminal neuralgia affected 6 of 10 family members over age 30, with onset between 30 and 51 years. This differs from idiopathic trigeminal neuralgia, which is usually a disease of older age.

Other systems. None of the affected individuals had optic atrophy or known renal disease.

Auditory system. Sensorineural hearing loss was documented in 4 of 10 family members over age 30 years, with onset usually in the 30's. One 6-year-old boy had conductive loss but no evidence of sensorineural hearing impairment.

Laboratory findings. Cerebrospinal fluid protein was elevated to 116 mg/dl in the 60-year-old proband.

Pathology. Sural nerve biopsy showed severe myelin loss with relative axonal preservation. Electron microscopy confirmed Schwann cell hyperplasia, severe demyelination, and abortive remyelination. Muscle biopsy showed chronic denervation.

Heredity. This disorder occurred in 11 of 31 at-risk individuals from four generations of a single family. There were no instances of male-to-male inheritance. Thus, autosomal dominant inheritance with variable penetrance is probable, although X-linked dominant inheritance cannot be excluded (Fig. 10–25).

Diagnosis. A similar family was reported by Kalyanaraman et al. (2), but affected individuals had an earlier age of onset of both neuropathy and trigeminal neuralgia. Hearing loss was not reported in these individuals. Patients with motor and sensory neuropathy and sensorineural hearing loss (autosomal dominant, autosomal recessive, and X-linked forms) lack trigeminal neuralgia, although this appears to be a variable manifestation. Thus, it could be the same as the autosomal dominant form. Patients with motor and sensory neuropathy, optic atrophy, and sensorineural hearing loss (autosomal dominant, autosomal recessive, and X-linked) all have optic atrophy, and all but those with the X-linked form have more normal nerve conduction studies.

Figure 10–25. *Motor and sensory neuropathy, trigeminal neuralgia, and sensorineural hearing loss (Cruse syndrome).* Pedigree showing autosomal dominant inheritance with incomplete penetrance.

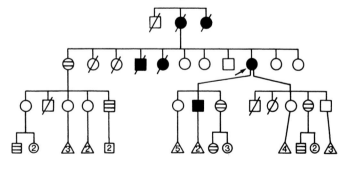

Prognosis. Both the neuropathy and hearing loss are progressive. One person died of complications of intracranial surgery to relieve her facial pain.

Summary. This syndrome consists of (*1*) autosomal dominant inheritance; (*2*) motor and sensory neuropathy (most similar to HMSN type I) with onset in childhood; (*3*) trigeminal neuralgia; and (*4*) sensorineural hearing loss.

References

1. Cruse RP et al: Hereditary hypertrophic neuropathy combining features of tic douloureux, Charcot-Marie-Tooth disease, and deafness. *Cleve Clin Q* 44:107–111, 1977.
2. Kalyanaraman K et al: Hereditary hypertrophic neuropathy with facial and trigeminal involvement: report of a case and comments on its possible identity with Hellsing syndrome 1. *Arch Neurol* 31:15–17, 1974.

Peripheral neuropathy, intestinal pseudo-obstruction, and deafness

Pingault et al. (2) described a single patient with hypomyelination of peripheral nerves, chronic intestinal pseudo-obstruction, and congenital hearing loss. Early development was characterized by hypotonia and weak spontaneous movements, but eventually the child achieved walking and other motor skills. Intestinal pseudo-obstruction was diagnosed after birth and treated with a colostomy that was closed after 1 year. Nerve biopsy demonstrated hypomyelination. Sequencing of the *SOX10* gene demonstrated a truncated mutation. *SOX10* mutations usually cause Waardenburg syndrome 4 (1), but this girl had no pigmentary disturbances.

References

1. Pingault V et al: *Sox10* mutations in patients with Waardenburg-Hirschsprung disease. *Nat Genet* 18:171–173, 1998.
2. Pingault V et al: Peripheral neuropathy with hypomyelination, chronic intestinal pseudo-obstruction and deafness: a developmental "neural crest syndrome" related to *Sox10* mutation. *Ann Neurol* 48:671–676, 2000.

Motor and sensory neuropathy, optic atrophy, and sensorineural hearing loss (autosomal recessive) (Iwashita syndrome)

In 1970, Iwashita et al. (1) reported recessively inherited motor and sensory neuropathy, optic atrophy, and sensorineural hearing loss. Additional cases were described (2–4).

Peripheral nervous system. Early development, including walking, was normal. Unusual hand postures consisting of ulnar deviation and flexion of the fingers were noted in late childhood (about 8 years). This was followed within several years by progressive weakness and wasting of the hands (10–11 years) and later the legs (13 years), associated with difficulty in walking. Examination showed distal atrophy that was worse in the arms, absent tendon reflexes, and wide-based gait. Diminished sensation, especially position sense and vibration, and scoliosis occurred in some older individuals. Electromyography showed denervation, but motor nerve conduction studies were normal, which is most similar to HMSN type II.

Ocular system. Visual problems were evident by age 13–15 years. Exam showed bilateral optic atrophy, more severe in the temporal than nasal half, and poor visual acuity. Visual fields were normal. No patients had evidence of pigmentary retinopathy.

Auditory system. Hearing loss began at 11–13 years, soon after the neuropathic symptoms. Audiometry showed severe, bilateral sensorineural loss.

Pathology. Muscle biopsies showed severe neurogenic atrophy. Sural nerve biopsy in a 25-year-old man showed a nonspecific hypertrophic neuropathy with onion bulb formation (3).

□ ○ Normal

■ ● Affected

⊟ ⊖ Affected but without trigemial neuralgia

Heredity. This disorder occurred in two of five sibs born to healthy and unrelated Korean parents. The older was male and the younger female. The parents in the other families were also unaffected. Thus, autosomal recessive inheritance is probable.

Diagnosis. This disorder differs from motor and sensory neuropathy, optic atrophy, and sensorineural hearing loss (autosomal dominant and X-linked forms) because of later onset of most symptoms, normal nerve conduction studies, and different inheritance pattern.

Prognosis. This disorder eventually causes severe disability, but there have been no reported deaths.

Summary. This disorder is characterized by (*1*) autosomal recessive inheritance; (*2*) hereditary motor and sensory neuropathy, type II; (*3*) optic atrophy; and (*4*) sensorineural hearing loss.

References

1. Iwashita H et al: Optic atrophy, neural deafness, and distal neurogenic amyotrophy. *Arch Neurol* 22:357–364, 1970.
2. Kim I et al: Three cases of Charcot-Marie-Tooth disease with nerve deafness. The classification and sural nerve pathology. *Rinsho Shinkeigaku* 20:264–270, 1980 (case 2).
3. Ohta M: Electron microscopic observations of sural nerve in familia opticoacoustic nerve degeneration with polyneuropathy. *Acta Neuropathol* 15:114–127, 1970.
4. Taylor J: Peroneal atrophy. *Proc R Soc Med* 6(2):50–51, 1912.

Hearing loss, optic atrophy, and ataxia (Jequier-Deonna syndrome)

Jequier and Deonna (1) described two sisters who developed hearing loss, vision loss, and ataxia, in that order, during late childhood/early adolescence.

Nervous system. Sensory ataxia became manifest after the age of 15 years and was accompanied by loss of deep tendon reflexes. There was no muscle weakness, muscle atrophy, or pyramidal or cerebellar signs. The ataxia was progressive, however.

Ocular system. Optic atrophy developed after the age of 11 years, with progressive loss of vision.

Auditory system. The first manifestation of this condition was bilateral hearing loss, which was rapidly progressive and led to significant hearing loss.

Vestibular system. Progressive vestibular areflexia was noted.

Laboratory findings. Nerve conduction studies were normal, as was a basic metabolic screen.

Heredity. This condition is likely autosomal recessive.

Diagnosis. Rosenberg-Chutorian syndrome (2) is similar, but the mode of inheritance of that condition is X-linked recessive.

Prognosis. The condition is rapidly progressive for the first 8–10 years, then more slowly progressive in adulthood.

References

1. Jequier M, Deonna T: A propos des degenerescences neuro-sensorielles Surdite, atrophie optique et ataxie sensitive progressives chez deux soeurs. *Arch Suisses Neurol Neurochir Psychiatrie* 112:219–227, 1973.
2. Rosenberg RN, Chutorian A: Familial opticoacoustic nerve degeneration and polyneuropathy. *Neurology* 17:827–832, 1967.

Motor and sensory neuropathy, adrenocortical deficiency, hepatosplenomegaly, optic atrophy, pigmentary retinopathy, and sensorineural hearing loss (Dyck syndrome)

In 1981, Dyck et al. (1) described a multisystem disorder in two brothers. Lipid studies showed reduced tissue arachidonic and related fatty acids.

Central nervous system. Early development was delayed in one of the boys. Psychometric testing suggested borderline retardation (mental age of 5.5 years at age 7 years) in the older child and milder delay in the younger. The EEG studies showed nonspecific slowing. Cranial CT scans were normal.

Peripheral nervous system. Clumsy gait was noticed at about 4 years of age and progressed to obvious distal amyotrophy. Examination at 5–7 years showed mild distal weakness in the arms, severe weakness and wasting in the legs, especially involving foot dorsiflexors, absent deep tendon reflexes, down-going plantar responses, and grossly normal sensation. Mild slowing and other abnormalities of motor and sensory nerve conduction studies were observed in the older boy, most similar to HMSN type II. Electromyographic needle exam showed neurogenic changes including increased duration of motor unit potentials and frequent polyphasic potentials. The EMG on the younger boy was normal.

Ocular system. Visual loss was also noticed in infancy as the children responded only to large objects. By 4–7 years, visual acuity was poor and visual fields were severely constricted. Examination showed bilateral optic atrophy and pigmentary retinopathy that consisted of depigmented areas and pigment clumps in the retinal periphery. Follow-up was not sufficient to determine if any of the visual changes were progressive.

Gastrointestinal and other systems. Gastrointestinal symptoms such as poor feeding, frequent vomiting and diarrhea, and poor weight gain occurred in the older boy, but resolved by 1 year. Darkening of the skin occurred by about 4 years of age in both boys. The lower edge of the liver and the spleen tip were palpable on exam.

Auditory system. Hearing loss was apparent in infancy, as neither boy turned his head to sounds. Follow-up was insufficient to determine if this was progressive. In the older boy, hearing loss ranged from 65 dB at 250 Hz to 90 dB at 2000 Hz, consistent with moderate to severe sensorineural loss.

Laboratory findings. Endocrine studies showed normal thyroid function tests, low serum estrogen, low normal fasting cortisol, and striking elevation of basal corticotropin level. Routine studies were normal except for mild elevation of serum glutamic–oxaloacetic transaminase (SGOT).

Complex abnormalities of serum and tissue lipids were discovered in both boys. Levels of arachidonic and related polyunsaturated fatty acids were decreased, and certain precursors increased in serum, red cells, and liver. The authors suggested a defect of synthesis of long-chain highly unsaturated fatty acids.

Pathology. The sural nerves including teased fiber preparations appeared normal by light microscopy. Electron microscopy showed an increased density of profiles, which appeared to be degenerative mitochondria, abnormal myelin figures with different configurations, and rare focal accumulation of glycogen in axons especially adjacent to Schmidt-Lantermann incisures. Liver biopsies revealed portal cirrhosis.

Heredity. In this family, two brothers were affected. Their parents were healthy, unrelated, and of German descent. Thus, inheritance could be either autosomal or X-linked recessive.

Diagnosis. This disorder resembles both the X-linked and neonatal forms of adrenoleukodystrophy as well as Refsum syndrome, but the specific lipid abnormalities differ. Several mitochondrial disorders such as MNGIE syndrome are similar except for hepatosplenomegaly, but the biochemical abnormalities again differ. The syndrome of motor and sensory neuropathy, optic atrophy, and sensorineural hearing loss (all types) lacks pigmentary retinopathy, adrenal dysfunction, and hepatosplenomegaly. Motor and sensory neuropathy, pigmentary retinopathy, and sensorineural hearing loss is autosomal dominant.

Prognosis. The clinical status was stable at last report when the brothers were 4 and 7 years old.

Summary. This disorder is characterized by (*1*) autosomal or X-linked recessive inheritance; (*2*) motor and sensory neuropathy; (*3*) adrenocortical insufficiency; (*4*) hepatosplenomegaly; (*5*) opticatrophy; (*6*) pigmentary retinopathy; and (*7*) sensorineural hearing loss.

References

1. Dyck PJ et al: Multisystem neuronal degeneration, hepatosplenomegaly, and adrenocortical deficiency associated with reduced tissue arachidonic acid. *Neurology* 31:925–934, 1981.

Motor and sensory neuropathy (polyneuropathy), ophthalmoplegia, leukoencephalopathy, intestinal pseudo-obstruction, and sensorineural hearing loss (POLIP syndrome)

A syndrome consisting of neuropathy most similar to HMSN type I, ophthalmoplegia, intestinal pseudo-obstruction, and sensorineural hearing loss has been described in at least 10 individuals from five unrelated families. The consistent and early involvement of the gastrointestinal (GI) tract sets this disorder apart from most other known inherited disorders of the peripheral nervous system (2,3). It was named POLIP syndrome as an acronymic mnemonic (2).

Gastrointestinal system. The earliest and most severe symptoms involve the GI tract and begin between 3 and 30 years of age. Typical symptoms include poor appetite, intolerance of large meals, and episodic nausea, vomiting, abdominal distension, cramps, and diarrhea. These invariably progress and may result in growth deficiency, malnutrition, and death. Radiologic studies fail to show any obstruction but do show signs of severe dysmotility. The stomach and duodenum, dilated and fluid-filled, empty slowly.

Peripheral nervous system. Weakness and numbness of hands and feet begin at about the same time or soon after the GI symptoms commence. Examination shows atrophy, weakness, hyporeflexia, and diminished sensation, most prominent in the distal extremities. Although severity varies, the neuropathy is progressive and often results in loss of ambulation. Other signs of visceral neuropathy, such as orthostatic drop in blood pressure, are sometimes found. Cranial neuropathies may occur, resulting in facial diplegia and dysphagia in addition to hearing and oculomotor deficits.

Nerve conduction studies show reduced motor conduction velocities without conduction block, and diminished amplitude or absence of motor and sensory action potentials. Electromyographic needle exam shows typical neuropathic changes. These abnormalities are most similar to HMSN type I.

Central nervous system. There are few if any symptoms of brain disease. However, MRI scans show diffuse abnormally high signal in white matter on T_2-weighted images, which extends to the gray–white border and arcuate fibers, and relatively spares the corpus callosum and internal capsule.

Ocular system. Neuropathies of the oculomotor nerves typically begin after the peripheral and autonomic neuropathy and result in severe ptosis and ophthalmoplegia.

Auditory system. Sensorineural hearing loss begins well after the other problems and remains mild. It was, however, the presenting symptom in one woman who had bilateral hearing loss at age 10 years, which progressed to profound loss by age 30 years.

Laboratory findings. Elevated levels of CSF protein were found in two of four patients.

Pathology. Pathologic studies of the stomach and intestines showed a visceral neuropathy consisting of fibrosis of autonomic ganglia and plexuses, decreased terminal nerve branches to smooth muscle, loss of nerve fibers in the muscularis, which varied between segments, and vacuolation of neurons in Auerbach plexus.

Cranial and peripheral nerve abnormalities consisted of increased endoneurial collagen, thinning or loss of myelin sheaths, distal axonal loss with relative preservation proximally, and little or no onion bulb formation. The cells of origin in the brain stem, spinal cord, and dorsal root ganglia remained intact. These changes are consistent with either primary demyelinating neuropathy or "dying-back" neuropathy with remodeling of myelin sheaths due to axonal atrophy.

Brain abnormalities consisted of a nonspecific leukoencephalopathy that was more severe with myelin than axonal stains and closely matches the MRI scan changes. Grossly, there was pallor of the white matter with prominent involvement of the centrum semiovale, patchy involvement of the internal capsule and cerebellar white matter, and sparing of the corpus callosum. These changes, resulting from both attenuation of myelin sheaths and reduced numbers of myelinated fibers, were not accompanied by glial reaction. Pallor and attenuation of central fascicles of the optic nerves were seen.

Heredity. Several families were reported with multiple affected sibs and apparently normal parents (Fig. 10–26). Two reported families were of Iranian Jewish ancestry, and the others were of Mexican ancestry. None were known to be consanguineous. Inheritance is probably autosomal recessive.

Diagnosis. Chronic intestinal pseudo-obstruction may result from either neuropathic or myopathic disorders of the gut, which may be associated with neurologic abnormalities similar to those of this disorder but with different pathological changes and usually lacking hearing loss (1). The MNGIE syndrome is a rare mitochondrial encephalomyopathy with a very similar clinical course, but showing ragged-red fibers on muscle biopsy.

Figure 10–26. *Motor and sensory neuropathy (polyneuropathy), ophthalmoplegia, leukoencephalopathy, intestinal pseudo-obstruction, and sensorineural hearing loss (POLIP) syndrome. Pedigrees of three families reported by Simon et al. (2) showing autosomal recessive inheritance.*

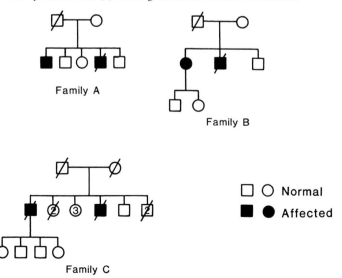

Prognosis. This disorder is progressive and eventually results in significant morbidity. Most patients have become bedridden, and death from malnutrition has been common.

Summary. This disorder is characterized by (*1*) autosomal recessive inheritance; (*2*) chronic intestinal pseudo-obstruction; (*3*) motor and sensory neuropathy (most similar to HMSN type I) with associated cranial neuropathy; (*4*) ophthalmoplegia and ptosis; (*5*) asymptomatic leukoencephalopathy; and (*6*) sensorineural hearing loss.

References

1. Ionasescu V et al: Inherited ophthalmoplegia with intestinal pseudo-obstruction. *J Neurol Sci* 59:215–228, 1983.
2. Simon LT et al: Polyneuropathy, ophthalmoplegia, leukoencephalopathy, and intestinal pseudo-obstruction: POLIP syndrome. *Ann Neurol* 28:349–360, 1990.
3. Steiner I et al: Familial progressive neuronal disease and chronic idiopathic intestinal pseudo-obstruction. *Neurology* 37:1046–1050, 1987.

Motor and sensory neuropathy, optic atrophy, and sensorineural hearing loss (X-linked) (Rosenberg-Chutorian syndrome)

In three families reported by Rosenberg and Chutorian (3) in 1967 and by Pauli (2) in 1984 (family A in that report), hearing loss was usually the first symptom, and the pedigrees were most consistent with X-linked recessive inheritance. This was supported by observation of manifesting carriers in some families. Case 1 of Kim et al. (1) may be another example.

Peripheral nervous system. Walking was delayed until age 2 years. Weakness and atrophy of the lower legs were evident by 5 years. There was deterioration of gait between 5 and 10 years of age, and later the distal arms and hands became involved (Fig. 10–27A,B). Most patients required canes and braces by age 15 years. Examination showed severe weakness and wasting involving the distal upper and lower extremities, pes cavus, absent tendon reflexes, normal plantar responses,

and broad steppage gait. Motor exam was normal in a 3-year-old boy except for absent deep tendon reflexes. Sensory exam showed decreased sensation for all modalities below the knees and elbows in the adults, but was found to be normal in the boy. Motor nerve conduction studies were decreased, a result most similar to HMSN type I.

Ocular system. Visual impairment was first noted at about 20 years and progressed slowly. The earliest symptom was impaired night vision, followed by impaired visual acuity. Exam showed bilateral optic atrophy more severe in the temporal than the nasal side, and concentric constriction of visual fields. Corrected visual acuity in one man was 20/100 in both eyes; in his brother it was 20/400. Only gross hand movements were perceived. No patients had retinitis pigmentosa. Eye exam in the 3-year-old boy was normal.

Auditory system. Hearing loss was evident in infancy and became severe by age 5 years. Speech was slow in onset and remained rudimentary. Audiograms showed severe sensorineural loss of 60–90 dB or more at 500–2000 Hz. Mild sensorineural loss was discovered in some carrier females in both families.

Vestibular system. No vestibular tests were described.

Laboratory findings. Electroretinograms, serum creatine kinase, CSF analysis, and many other routine studies were normal.

Pathology. Muscle biopsies showed severe neurogenic atrophy. Sural nerve biopsy revealed demyelination with preservation of axons.

Heredity. In the family reported by Rosenberg and Chutorian (3), two brothers and their nephew (son of their sister) were affected. In the family described by Pauli (2), two brothers and their nephew (son of their maternal half-sister) were affected. Mild hearing loss was noted in several definite and possible carrier females. There was no male-to-male transmission. Thus, inheritance appears to be X-linked recessive with partial expression in carriers (Fig. 10–27C).

Figure 10–27. *Motor and sensory neuropathy, optic atrophy, and sensorineural hearing loss (X-linked) (Rosenberg-Chutorian syndrome).* (A,B) Photographs showing distal muscle atrophy with sparing of face and trunk.

(C) Pedigrees reported by Rosenberg and Chutorian (3) (family A on left), and Pauli (2) (family B on right) showing X-linked recessive inheritance. [(A,B) from RM Pauli, *Clin Genet* 26:383, 1984.]

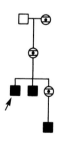

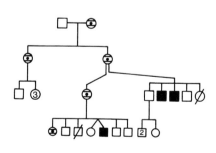

□ ○ Normal

■ Affected

⊕ Carrier with hearing loss

C

Diagnosis. The syndrome of motor and sensory neuropathy, optic atrophy, and sensorineural hearing loss (autosomal dominant) differs primarily by earlier onset of visual loss. The syndrome of motor and sensory neuropathy, optic atrophy, and sensorineural hearing loss (autosomal recessive) has later onset. Several other disorders with neuropathy and hearing loss lack optic atrophy.

Prognosis. This disorder results in significant disability, due primarily to early hearing loss, with additional disability from the visual and motor disorders.

Summary. This disorder is characterized by (1) X-linked recessive inheritance with partial expression in carrier females; (2) motor and sensory neuropathy (most similar to HMSN type I); (3) optic atrophy; and (4) sensorineural hearing loss.

References

1. Kim I et al: Three cases of Charcot-Marie-Tooth disease with nerve deafness. The classification and sural nerve pathology. *Rinsho Shinkeigaku* 20:264–270, 1980 (case 1).
2. Pauli RM: Sensorineural deafness and peripheral neuropathy. *Clin Genet* 26:383–384, 1984.
3. Rosenberg RN, Chutorian A: Familial opticoacoustic nerve degeneration and polyneuropathy. *Neurology* 17:827–8321, 1967.

Sensory and Autonomic Neuropathies with Hearing Loss

Hereditary sensory and autonomic neuropathy (HSAN), dementia, and sensorineural hearing loss (Hicks syndrome)

Hicks (8), in 1922, and Denny-Brown (3), in 1951, reported progressive sensory loss, perforating ulcers of the feet, shooting radicular pains, and progressive sensorineural hearing loss in four generations of an English family. At least eight additional families have been described (5–7,9,10,13–16), including some in which dementia also occurred (9,10,16, Robert B Layzer, personal communication, 1989).

Peripheral nervous system. The first symptom of this disorder is usually sensory loss affecting the distal legs and later the arms, which usually begins in childhood (Fig. 10–28A). However, most patients do not become aware of the disorder until later when calluses and ulcers of the feet appear. This usually occurs in young adulthood with a range of 15 to 36 years. The classic description was given by Hicks (8), who described a painless callus of the great toe that gave way to an ulcer with indurated edges and purulent discharge. The ulcer extended to the bone with extrusion of small pieces of bare bone (Fig. 10–28B). With treatment, the ulcers healed but broke down again, and the process of ulceration and healing then went on for the rest of the patient's life. The process affected other areas of the foot and finally resulted in severe deformity. Several years after onset of the ulcers, brief but often severe radicular shooting pains affected first the legs and then other areas. However, ulcers, considered not a primary part of disorder, are less common in the arms than in the feet. Dyck (4) stated that avoidance of trauma to the foot and more careful hygiene will prevent most foot ulcers.

Examination shows severe sensory loss involving the distal legs and feet and, to a lesser extent, the arms. In most patients, loss of sensation of temperature is greater than loss of pain, and loss of pain greater than loss of touch. Vibratory sensation is decreased in some patients, while position sense is usually preserved. Strength is normal, but reflexes are diminished or absent. Mild sensory ataxia was observed in two families (14). When tested, sensory nerve conduction is severely diminished or absent, while motor nerve conduction velocities are normal. These results and early adult age of onset are similar to those of HSAN type I (4).

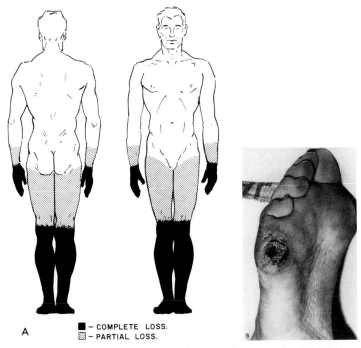

A   ■ – COMPLETE LOSS.
             ▦ – PARTIAL LOSS.

Figure 10–28. *Hereditary sensory and autonomic neuropathy (HSAN), dementia, and sensorineural hearing loss (Hicks disease).* (A) Areas of involvement. (B) Perforating ulcer of foot.

Central nervous system. Yee et al. (16) reported two families with mental symptoms beginning between 20 and 40 years of age, several years before hearing loss was recognized. At first, these consisted of personality change, difficulty in concentration, memory loss, and, less frequently, psychosis and seizures. Slowly progressive intellectual decline followed and resulted in severe dementia with early death between 40 and 60 years of age. Horoupian (10) described low intellect and possible dementia in another patient. Although Hicks (8) and Denny-Brown (3) did not describe mental changes, most affected family members died at relatively early ages from causes unrelated to the ulcers.

Other systems. Recurrent, unexplained diarrhea occurred in several older individuals in one family (3,8). A few patients had diabetes. One had primary hyperparathyroidism (16).

Auditory system. Bilateral sensorineural hearing loss began at about the same time as the shooting pains and progressed slowly to severe impairment over the next 10–20 years. Audiometry suggested cochlear lesions in one patient (5).

Vestibular system. While mild vestibular symptoms were reported only occasionally, vestibular testing in one patient showed no response to bithermal or cold water caloric stimulation and no response on the torsion swing test (5).

Radiographic findings. Hojo et al. (9) performed neuroimaging via positron emission tomography (PET) scan on their patients and found frontal hypometabolism or hypoperfusion. Magnetic resonance imaging demonstrated frontal atrophy in one patient.

Laboratory findings. Cerebrospinal fluid analysis showed 11 white cells/cmm and 200 mg/dl protein in one patient (16).

Pathology. At autopsy, brain weight was decreased in the two patients in whom this was reported. Neuronal and severe dendritic loss and gliosis were described in the auditory and sensory cortex in one patient (10). Mild but more widespread changes were seen with associated dementia in another patient who also had neuronal loss and gliosis of the cerebellum, inferior olive, medial vestibular nuclei, and dorsal cochlear nuclei (16). Degenerative changes in the inner ear consisted of neuronal loss and fibrosis involving the spiral ganglion, cochlear nerve, Scarpa's ganglion, and vestibular nerve, and severe atrophy of the organ of Corti and sensory epithelium. Only mild atrophy was noted in the ventral cochlear nucleus (6,10).

Abnormalities in the spinal cord consisted of atrophy of the posterior columns, loss of myelinated fibers and gliosis of the gracile tracts, and slight neuronal dropout in Clarke's column. The dorsal root ganglia were atrophic with great neuronal loss and increased connective tissue, and there was severe fiber loss of the dorsal nerve roots. This was most severe in the L_4–S_2 ganglia, with less severe changes in the C_8–T_1 ganglia. The ventral roots were normal. The peripheral nerves were atrophic with fiber loss most severe distally (3,10).

Heredity. This disorder is inherited as an autosomal dominant trait with variable severity but apparently high penetrance. The gene for HSAN type I was mapped to 9q22.1–23.1 by Nicholson et al. (12). Eventually, Dawkins et al. (2) and Bejaoui et al. (1) independently found mutations in the *SPTLC1* gene. It is unknown whether HSAN with deafness is caused by mutations in this gene or not.

Diagnosis. This disorder must be differentiated from HSAN types I (similar onset and inheritance) and II (childhood onset, more severe and autosomal recessive inheritance), neither of which is associated with hearing loss. Munro (11) and Ogden et al. (13) reported a child with nonprogressive sensory neuropathy, congenital sensorineural hearing loss, and abnormal vestibular function. Patients with sensory and autonomic neuropathy, ataxia, scoliosis, and sensorineural hearing loss (Robinson syndrome) have milder sensory symptoms and absence of ulcers. Patients with sensory and autonomic neuropathy, gastrointestinal motility disorder, small bowel diverticulitis, and sensorineural hearing loss (Groll-Hirschowitz syndrome) have less severe sensory symptoms and gastrointestinal complications. Syringomyelia and leprosy may present with similar sensory loss but are not genetic.

Prognosis. The sensory neuropathy and hearing loss are slowly progressive and eventually result in severe disability. Most affected individuals have died at relatively young ages of causes apparently unrelated to the ulcers. This may reflect the associated dementia, which is probably more common than previously realized.

Summary. This disorder is characterized by (*1*) autosomal dominant inheritance; (*2*) sensory and autonomic neuropathy (most similar to HSAN type I); (*3*) dementia; and (*4*) sensorineural hearing loss.

References

1. Bejaoui K et al: *SPTLC1* is mutated in hereditary sensory neuropathy, type 1. *Nat Genet* 27:261–262, 2001.
2. Dawkins JL et al: Mutations in *SPTCL1*, encoding serine palmitoyltransferase, long chain base subunit-1, causes hereditary sensory neuropathy type 1. *Nat Genet* 27:309–312, 2001.
3. Denny-Brown D: Hereditary sensory radicular neuropathy. *J Neurol Neurosurg Psychiatry* 14:237–252, 1951.
4. Dyck PJ: Neuronal atrophy and degeneration predominantly affecting peripheral sensory and autonomic neurons. In: *Peripheral Neuropathy*, Dyck PJ et al. (eds), W.B. Saunders, Philadelphia, 1984, pp 1557–1599.
5. Fitzpatrick DB et al: Hereditary deafness and sensory radicular neuropathy. *Arch Otolaryngol* 102:552–557, 1976.
6. Hallpike CS: Observations on the structural basis of two rare varieties of hereditary deafness. In: *CIBA Foundation Symposium: Myotatic, Kinesthetic, and Vestibular Mechanisms*, DeReuch AVS, Knight J (eds), Little, Brown, Boston, 1967, pp 285–294.
7. Hamanishi H et al: Familial case of hereditary sensory radicular neuropathy. *Seikeigeka* 39:371–375, 1988.
8. Hicks EP: Hereditary perforating ulcer of the foot. *Lancet* 202:319–321, 1922.
9. Hojo K et al: Hereditary sensory neuropathy with deafness and dementia: a clinical and neuroimaging study. *Eur J Neurol* 6:357–361, 1999.
10. Horoupian DS: Hereditary sensory neuropathy with deafness: a familial multisystem atrophy. *Neurology* 39:244–248, 1989.
11. Munro M: Sensory radicular neuropathy in a deaf child. *BMJ* 1:541–544, 1956.
12. Nicholson GA et al: The gene for hereditary sensory neuropathy type 1 (HSN-1) maps to chromosome 9q22.1–q22.3. *Nat Genet* 13:101–104, 1996.
13. Ogden TE et al: Some sensory syndromes in children: indifference to pain and sensory neuropathy. *J Neurol Neurosurg Psychiatry* 22:267–276, 1959.
14. Stanley RJ et al: Sensory radicular neuropathy. *Arch Dermatol* 111:760–762, 1975.
15. Van Bogaert L: Familial ulcers, mutilating lesions of the extremities, and also acro-osteolysis. *BMJ* 2:367–371, 1957.
16. Yee MHC et al: Hereditary sensory neuropathy with deafness and dementia: a new syndrome. *Neurology* 36(Suppl):115–116, 1986.

Sensory and autonomic neuropathy, ataxia, scoliosis, and sensorineural hearing loss (Robinson syndrome)

In 1977, Robinson et al. (1) reported a single large family of West Coast Indians with sensory loss, ataxia, scoliosis, and sensorineural hearing loss.

Peripheral nervous system. Mild sensory neuropathy, probably present from childhood, was usually not recognized until careful clinical examination after onset of other symptoms. Slowly progressive (sensory) ataxia with an unsteady gait was most often recognized in later childhood, although in some it began in infancy, in others as late as age 60 years. Affected individuals did not have mutilating acropathy or signs of autonomic dysfunction. Examination showed minimally slurred speech in some, absent reflexes, ataxia without intention tremor, and abnormal Romberg test. Loss of touch and pressure sensation was mild and generalized, more severe distally. Pain and temperature sensation was less impaired.

Musculoskeletal system. All affected individuals had slowly progressive thoracolumbar scoliosis beginning at about the same time as the ataxia.

Auditory system. Bilateral sensorineural hearing loss occurred in most affected individuals, but details were not given.

Laboratory findings. Sensory action potentials were impaired or absent, while motor nerve conduction velocities were normal. Spine X-rays confirmed scoliosis without evidence of structural anomalies.

Pathology. Sural nerve biopsy showed severe loss of myelinated fibers and some loss of smaller unmyelinated axons (Fig. 10–29A). Inflammatory cells and evidence of myelin breakdown were not seen.

Heredity. The disorder probably has autosomal dominant inheritance with variable severity and age of onset (Fig. 10–29B).

Diagnosis. Patients with sensory and autonomic neuropathy, dementia, and sensorineural hearing loss (Hicks disease) have more severe loss of sensation that results in ulcers, etc., and mental changes that progress to dementia. The syndrome of sensory and autonomic neuropathy, gastrointestinal motility disorder, small bowel diverticulitis, and sensorineural hearing loss (Groll-Hirschowitz syndrome) differs because of the severe gastrointestinal symptoms and autosomal recessive inheritance.

Prognosis. Life span was not limited by this disorder, and affected individuals were able to hold jobs satisfactorily.

Summary. This disorder is characterized by (*1*) autosomal dominant inheritance; (*2*) mild sensory neuropathy with sensory ataxia; (*3*) thoracolumbar scoliosis; and (*4*) sensorineural hearing loss.

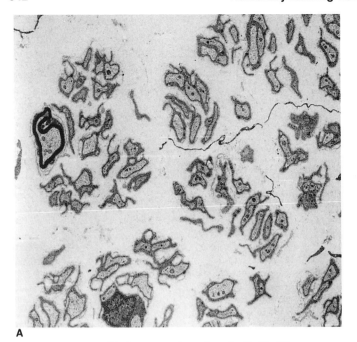

A

B

□ male   ●■ affected   † dead
○ female   ↗ propositus   ⊙□ infantile
                                       polymyoclonus

Reference

1. Robinson GC et al: A new variety of hereditary sensory neuropathy. *Hum Genet* 35:153–161, 1977.

Sensory and autonomic neuropathy, gastrointestinal motility disorder, small bowel diverticulitis, and sensorineural hearing loss (Groll-Hirschowitz syndrome)

Groll and Hirschowitz (1), in 1966, and Hirschowitz et al. (2), in 1972, reported a syndrome of progressive sensory neuropathy with trophic changes, progressive loss of gastrointestinal motility, multiple small inflamed intestinal diverticula, and profound sensorineural hearing loss in three sisters. Potasman et al. (4) reported two sisters from another family.

Gastrointestinal system. The first symptoms were episodes of abdominal cramping, vomiting, diarrhea, and weight loss. These usually began between 5 and 15 years of age and progressed to chronic abdominal pain, distension, vomiting, steatorrhea, and emaciation. X-rays and other tests showed progressive loss of gastric and intestinal motility consistent with intestinal pseudo-obstruction. The motility disorder was attributed to functional impairment of the gastric motor vagus. Episodes of intestinal obstruction led to surgery in several patients, during which ulcerated diverticulitis, fibrotic mesentery, and massive lymph node enlargement were found. The oldest of the sisters reported by Hirschowitz et al. (2) died at age 18 years from massive gastrointestinal hemorrhage, while the sibs described by Potasman et al. (4) died at 13 and 24 years, respectively.

Peripheral nervous system. The first signs of the neuropathy were diminished tendon reflexes in the legs and pes cavus, usually noted between ages 14 and 16 years when sensation was still normal. Sensory loss began soon after and progressed slowly. Later examinations showed absent knee and ankle reflexes, absent corneal and abdominal reflexes, and distal loss of touch and pain sensation. Loss of touch was more severe than loss of pain, and both were much more severe than loss of vibration. Both motor and sensory nerve conduction velocities were decreased in all affected individuals, with sensory conduction unobtainable in one. Sensory and motor nerve conduction studies in the father of the sisters reported by Hirschowitz et al. (2) showed mild slowing.

Cardiovascular system. Sinus tachycardia was discovered soon after the onset of gastrointestinal symptoms. Normal pulse eventually returned, but the carotid sinus reflex remained absent and pulse did not increase after exercise, indicating functional impairment of the cardiac vagus. Impairment of autonomic function was confirmed by reduced wheal and flare reaction to intradermal histamine at the ankle.

Integumentary system. Acanthosis nigricans developed in most of the affected individuals (Fig. 10–30A).

Other findings. Teeth were lost prematurely in at least two individuals (3).

Auditory system. Bilateral sensorineural hearing loss was discovered between 3 and 9 years of age, and progressed to total loss within a period of 2 to 8 years after onset. In the family reported by Hirschowitz et al. (2), the father and several other paternal relatives had late-onset, mild hearing loss most consistent with otosclerosis.

Figure 10–29. *Sensory and autonomic neuropathy, ataxia, scoliosis, and sensorineural hearing loss (Robinson syndrome).* (A) Electron microscopic section of nerve showing marked reduction of myelinated axons. (B) Pedigree showing autosomal dominant inheritance. [From GC Robinson et al., *Hum Genet* 35:153, 1977.]

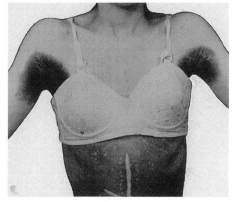

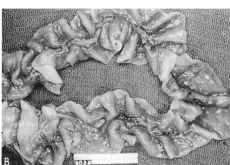

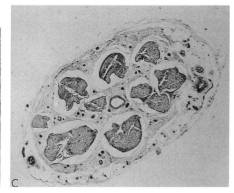

A

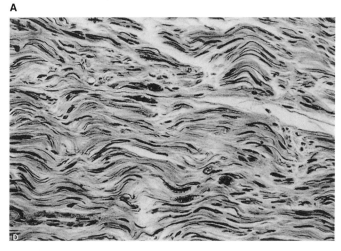

Figure 10–30. *Sensory and autonomic neuropathy, gastrointestinal motility disorder, small bowel diverticulitis, and sensorineural hearing loss (Groll-Hirschowitz syndrome).* (A) Acanthosis nigricans in both axillae and over the abdomen. (B) Specimen of small bowel shows thickened ileum, fibrosed mesentery, which made full extension of bowel impossible, and a long serpiginous ulcer at the mesenteric implantation through length of specimen. (C) Sural nerve is thin and fibrosed with nerve bundles separated by connective tissue. (D) High-power view of nerve shows reduced axons with swollen and vacuolated myelin sheaths. [From BI Hirschowitz et al., *Birth Defects* 8(2):27, 1972.]

Vestibular system. Vestibular function was found to be normal in the three sisters (3,4).

Laboratory findings. Multiple laboratory abnormalities resulted from malnutrition. These included low serum albumin, found in three of five patients, and low serum carotene, which occurred in all patients (4). Serum zinc levels were also depressed (B. Hirschowitz, personal communication, 1974).

Pathology. At autopsy in one patient, the small intestine was shortened by severe thickening and fibrosis of the mesenteric root. Large lymph nodes filled the retroperitoneum. Multiple small polyps, scattered diverticula, and occasional ulcers were seen in the intestines. The stomach was dilated and thickened (Fig. 10–30B). Grossly, the brain appeared normal, but histologic exam showed loss of fibers in the roots of the vagus nerve, especially at the level of the fasciculus solitarius. Examination of the temporal bones showed collapsed Reissner's membrane and destruction of the organ of Corti (3).

In her younger sister, sural nerve biopsy showed marked atrophy of nerve bundles, which were encased in a thick layer of fibrous tissue (Fig. 10–30C). Demyelination was severe with only occasional myelin coats, vacuolized and fragmented, preserved. Axons were better preserved but varied greatly in thickness (Fig. 10–30D). Macrophages filled with fatty debris were prominent.

Heredity. In these two families, there were multiple affected sibs, and the parents were healthy. In one of the two families, the parents were consanguineous. Thus, autosomal recessive inheritance is probable (2,4).

Diagnosis. The relatively mild sensory loss and severe autonomic disturbances differ significantly from sensory and autonomic neuropathy, dementia, and sensorineural hearing loss (Hicks syndrome) in which severe sensory loss is accompanied by recurrent ulcers, radicular shooting pains, and often dementia. While the sensory changes are similar, the lack

of ataxia and scoliosis separated this disorder from sensory and autonomic neuropathy, ataxia, scoliosis, and sensorineural hearing loss (Robinson syndrome). Intestinal pseudo-obstruction is also seen in POLIP syndrome, but there one finds ophthalmoplegia and leukoencephalopathy.

Prognosis. Prognosis is poor because of the severity and progressive nature of the disorder. One sib died and others were bedridden. Hearing loss was profound in all.

Summary. This syndrome is characterized by (*1*) autosomal recessive inheritance; (*2*) sensory and autonomic neuropathy; (*3*) cardiac rhythm disturbances due to loss of autonomic regulation; (*4*) intestinal pseudo-obstruction; (*5*) small bowel diverticulitis; and (*6*) sensorineural hearing loss.

References

1. Groll A, Hirschowitz BI: Steatorrhea and familial deafness in two siblings. *Clin Res* 14:47, 1966.
2. Hirschowitz BI et al: Hereditary nerve deafness in three sisters with absent gastric motility, small bowel diverticulitis and ulceration and progressive sensory neuropathy. *Birth Defects* 8(2):27–41, 1972.
3. Igarashi M et al: Cochleo-saccular degeneration in one of three sisters with hereditary deafness, absent gastric motility, small bowel diverticulitis and progressive sensory neuropathy. *ORL* 43:4–16, 1981.
4. Potasman I et al: The Groll-Hirschowitz syndrome. *Clin Genet* 28:76–79, 1985.

Muscular Dystrophies

Facioscapulohumeral muscular dystrophy and sensorineural hearing loss

Facioscapulohumeral muscular dystrophy (FSHD) is characterized by considerable variability in clinical course. It is rarer than Duchenne and myotonic dysotrophies. Involvement of other systems has rarely been reported. Some patients have sensorineural hearing loss, especially those with early-onset muscular weakness (2,12,15,20). The combination of FSHD, exudative telangiectasia of the retina (Coats disease), and sensorineural hearing impairment was first reported in 1968 by Small (23). The combination subsequently was described in at least 22 individuals from 13 unrelated families (1–8,11,14,19,23,24,26,28,31). Molecular genetic studies have suggested genetic homogeneity regardless of time of onset (4,17,29). However, Gilbert et al. (9) noted heterogeneity. Prevalence is about 5/100,000 (17).

Neuromuscular system. In adult-onset FSHD, facial and shoulder girdle weakness and wasting (especially lower trapezius, upper deltoid, pectoral, biceps, and triceps with relative preservation of lower deltoid and prominence of upper trapezius due to elevation of the scapulae on arm abduction) generally appear late in the first decade or during the second decade (range 7–30 years) (Fig. 10–31A–E). The weakness spreads to involve other muscle groups, especially the upper arms, abdomen, pelvic girdle, and foot extensors. In general, progression occurs slowly over many decades, interspersed with periods of relatively rapid deterioration. Facial mask-like weakness is characterized by difficulty in eye closure, whistling, drinking through straws, playing wind instruments, etc. Other difficulties are experienced in combing hair and hanging laundry out to dry.

In contrast to later-onset FSHD, infantile-onset FSHD is usually noticed within the first 2 years of life because the child never smiles and the eyes remain open during sleep (4). Weakness in other muscle groups,

especially in the shoulder girdle, is severe. Many patients use wheelchairs by 10 years of age.

Although onset of weakness occurs within the first years of life in most patients with both FSHD and hearing loss (14,23), an affected parent had much later onset of weakness than the proband in four families.

Central nervous system. Among eight families, 5 of 18 children had mental retardation (19,23).

Ocular system. Bilateral severe tortuosity of retinal vessels, microaneurysms, vessel occlusions, or exudative telangiectasia of the retina (Coats disease) in the macular area and peripheral retina with visual loss have been described in FSHD and hearing loss (1–8,12,17,19,23,24,26,28,31) (Fig. 10–31F). Diagnosis requires indirect ophthalmoscopy or fluorescein angiography. There is no correlation between the retinal abnormality and the severity of muscle involvement (7). However, there is correlation with childhood onset. Padberg et al. (21) noted that 16 sibs from 11 families (50%) exhibited retinal changes.

Auditory system. While hearing loss is rare in adult-onset FSHD, it occurs often in those with infantile onset of weakness (1–5,7,8,11,19,28). The loss is bilateral sensorineural and has ranged from 20 to 100 dB with especially marked high-tone loss (3,20). Stapedial reflexes are reduced. The loss first becomes manifest at 3–4 years of age. Audiomet-

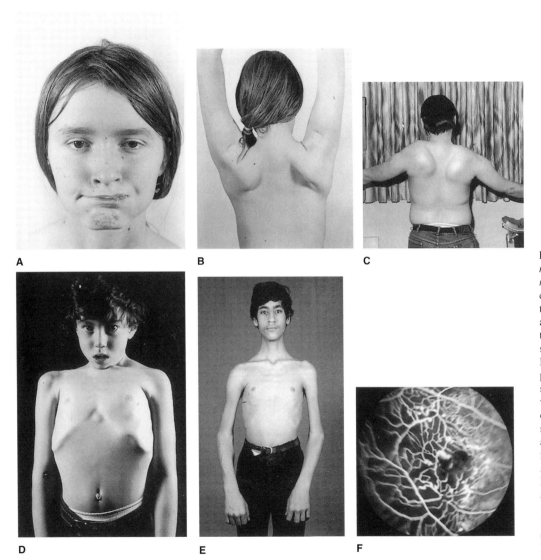

Figure 10–31. *Facioscapulohumeral muscular dystrophy and sensorineural hearing loss.* (A) Marked facial weakness leads to smooth, relatively inanimate face. Patient is attempting to inflate cheeks. (B) Extreme wasting of muscles is responsible for scapular stabilization. (C) Difficulty raising arms because of proximal weakness that accentuates scapular winging. (D,E) Bifacial weakness and atrophy around shoulder girdle. (F) Fluorescein angiogram showing dilatation of capillary bed and microaneurysms in peripheral fundus. [(A,B) from KF Swaiman, *Pediatric Neurology,* C.V. Mosby, St. Louis, 1989; (C) from UR Desai and FN Sabates, *Am J Ophthalmol* 110:568, 1990; (D,E) courtesy of BR Korf, Boston, Massachusetts; (F) courtesy of R Fitzsimons and AC Bird, London, England.]

A   B   C

D   E   F

ric studies have indicated a cochlear origin with intact pathways from the cochlea to the temporal lobe (8,28). Brouwer et al. (3) found there was no correlation between hearing loss and severity of muscle weakness. Most patients had normal hearing but a few had severe loss. Padberg et al. (21) found 20 sibs from 14 families (62%) with various degrees of high-tone deficit.

Laboratory findings. Serum creatine kinase is moderately elevated in 50%–80% of patients with FSHD, except in older patients in whom it is much more likely to be normal. Thus, there is limited usefulness in presymptomatic testing, as elevated levels are found in only 80% of affected males and 50% of affected females under 40 years of age (17). Few patients have elevation of lactate dehydrogenase (LDH), aldolase, SGOT, and serum glutamic–pyruvic transaminase (SGPT) (9).

Pathology. Although changes are variable, most muscles show advanced histological changes including replacement by fat and connective tissue, variation in fiber diameter, central nuclei, occasional fiber necrosis and regeneration, and a few scattered inflammatory cells. In a small proportion of patients, the inflammatory infiltrates are extensive and indistinguishable from polymyositis.

Heredity. From among 22 probands with FSHD and hearing loss, the disorder was isolated in several cases (7,14,19,24,26). In others, a parent was mildly affected (2,14,20), and several authors described the syndrome in several generations (6,8,10,11,15). In two families, however, multiple affected sibs were noted (23,31). Nevertheless, we believe that this represents autosomal dominant inheritance with variable expressivity.

Molecular genetic studies indicate that the gene is located at 4q35 (3,4,9,18,22,27,29,30). Heterogeneity has not been indicated (17). However, Gilbert et al. (9) found that two kindred did not map to 4q35. Penetrance is 70% at 15 years and 95% after 20 years (17). Anticipation has been noted (25) and is related to deletion size.

Diagnosis. Coats' disease has been reported with retinitis pigmentosa as an autosomal recessive syndrome (16). OJ Hood (Greenville, North Carolina, personal communication, 1992) has seen an isolated patient with Coats disease, sensorineural hearing loss, short stature, and significant brachydactyly of digits 2–3–4–5 of hands and feet. Patients with juvenile spinal muscular atrophy may have similar clinical presentation, but examination and EMG should lead to correct diagnosis. Several mitochondrial encephalomyopathies may present with muscle weakness and hearing loss, but have other findings. Polymyositis may simulate the disorder (13).

Prognosis. Severity varies greatly among the affected individuals.

Summary. This disorder is characterized by (*1*) autosomal dominant inheritance with high penetrance and marked variability in expression; (*2*) weakness in face and shoulder girdle with spread to other groups; (*3*) retinal telangiectasia with progression to Coats disease; (*4*) occasional mental retardation; and (*5*) sensorineural hearing loss.

References

1. Akiyama C: Facioscapulohumeral muscular dystrophy with infantile spasms, sensorineural deafness and retinal vessel abnormalities. *No To Hattatsu* 23:395–399, 1991.
2. Brooke MH: *A Clinician's View of Neuromuscular Diseases,* 2nd ed. Williams & Wilkins, Baltimore, 1986.
3. Brouwer OF et al: Hearing loss in facioscapulohumeral muscular dystrophy. *Neurology* 41:1878–1881, 1991.
4. Brouwer OF et al: Facioscapulohumeral muscular dystrophy: the impact of genetic research. *Clin Neurol Neurosurg* 95:9–21, 1993.
5. Desai UR, Sabates FN: Long-term follow-up of facioscapulohumeral dystrophy and Coats' disease. *Am J Ophthalmol* 110:568–569, 1990.
6. Fitzsimons RB et al: Retinal vascular abnormalities in facioscapulohumeral muscular dystrophy. *Brain* 110:631–648, 1987.
7. Fujimara H et al: A case of facioscapulohumeral muscular dystrophy with sensorineural hearing loss and retinal angioma. *Clin Neurol* 29:1387–1391, 1989.
8. Gieron MA et al: Facioscapulohumeral dystrophy with cochlear hearing loss and tortuosity of retinal vessels. *Am J Med Genet* 22:143–147, 1985.
9. Gilbert JR et al: Evidence for heterogeneity in facioscapulohumeral muscular dystrophy (FSHD). *Am J Hum Genet* 53:401–408, 1993.
10. Griggs RC et al: Genetics of facioscapulohumeral muscular dystrohy: new mutation in sporadic cases. *Neurology* 43:2369–2372, 1993.
11. Gurwin EB et al: Retinal telangiectasis in facioscapulohumeral muscular dystrophy with deafness. *Arch Ophthalmol* 103:1695–1700, 1985.
12. Kamata T et al: Facioscapulohumeral syndrome with sensorineural hearing loss and abnormality of retinal vessels. *Intern Med* 32:678–680, 1993.
13. Kaner J et al: The facioscapulohumeral syndrome: a report of two cases. *Henry Ford Hosp Med J* 30:30–36, 1982.
14. Korf BR et al: Facioscapulohumeral dystrophy presenting in infancy with facial diplegia and sensorineural deafness. *Ann Neurol* 17:513–516, 1985.
15. Kousseff B et al: Facioscapulohumeral dystrophy and hearing loss. Presented at the March of Dimes Birth Defects Conference, Seattle, June 20, 1983.
16. Lanier JD et al: Autosomal recessive retinitis pigmentosa and Coats disease. *Arch Ophthalmol* 94:1737–1742, 1976.
17. Lunt PW, Harper PS: Genetic counseling in facioscapulohumeral muscular dystrophy. *J Med Genet* 28:655–664, 1991.
18. Mathews KD et al: Linkage localization of facioscapulohumeral dystrophy (FSHD) in 4q35. *Am J Hum Genet* 51:428–431, 1992.
19. Matsuzaka T et al: Facioscapulohumeral dystrophy associated with mental retardation, hearing loss and tortuosity of retinal arterioles. *J Child Neurol* 1:218–223, 1986.
20. Meyerson MD et al: Facioscapulohumeral muscular dystrophy and accompanying hearing loss. *Arch Otolaryngol* 110:261–266, 1984.
21. Padberg GW et al: Retinal vascular disease and sensorineural deafness are part of facioscapulohumeral muscular dystrophy. Abstract #405. American Society of Human Genetics meeting, 1992. *Am J Hum Genet* 51:A104, 1992.
22. Sarfarazi M et al: Regional mapping of facioscapulohumeral muscular dystrophy gene on 4q35: combined analysis of an international consortium. *Am J Hum Genet* 51:396–439, 1992.
23. Small RG: Coats' disease and muscular dystrophy. *Trans Am Acad Ophthalmol Otolaryngol* 72:225–231, 1968.
24. Suehara M et al: Facioscapulohumeral type myopathy with hearing loss and retinal vessel abnormality. *Shinkeinaika* 25:268–272, 1986.
25. Tawil R et al: Evidence for anticipation and association of deletion size with severity in facioscapulohumeral muscular dystrophy. *Ann Neurol* 39:744–748, 1996.
26. Taylor DA et al: Facioscapulohumeral dystrophy associated with hearing loss and Coats disease. *Ann Neurol* 12:395–398, 1982.
27. Upadhyaya M et al: The mapping of chromosome 4q markers in relation to facioscapulohumeral muscular dystrophy. *Am J Hum Genet* 51:404–410, 1992.
28. Voit T et al: Hearing loss in facioscapulohumeral dystrophy. *Eur J Pediatr* 145:280–285, 1986.
29. Wijmenga C et al: Mapping of facioscapulohumeral muscular dystrophy gene to chromosome 4q35–qter by multipoint linkage analysis and in situ hybridization. *Genomics* 9:570–575, 1991.
30. Wijmenga C et al: Chromosome 4q DNA rearrangements associated with facioscapulohumeral muscular dystrophy. *Nat Genet* 2:26–30, 1992.
31. Yasukohchi S: Facioscapulohumeral dystrophy associated with sensorineural hearing loss, tortuosity of retinal arterioles, and an early onset and rapid progression of respiratory failure. *Brain Dev* 10:319–324, 1988.

Myotonic dystrophy

Myotonic dystrophy affects multiple organs, although neuromuscular symptoms are the most prominent (2,6,11,19).

Physical findings. The facial appearance is striking and recognizable because of the combination of wasting of facial muscles that results in temporal hollowing, sunken eyes and sagging jaw, and premature baldness (Fig. 10–32A). Children with congenital myotonic dystrophy also have a highly arched palate and narrow facial structure.

Neuromuscular system. The age of onset is difficult to determine because of the long asymptomatic period. Median age of onset is 20–25 years, and at least 80% of patients are affected by age 50. A striking and severe clinical variant, known as congenital myotonic dystrophy, occurs in about 20% of those born to affected mothers.

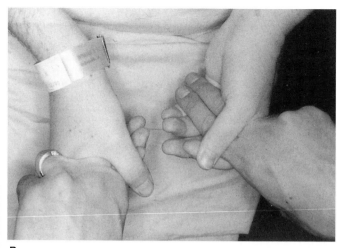

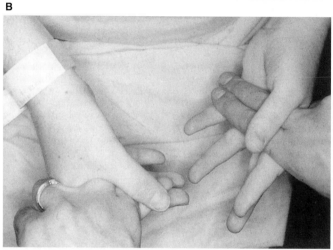

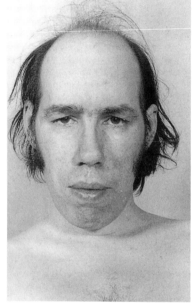

Figure 10–32. *Myotonic dystrophy.* (A) Affected man shows facial weakness, temporal wasting, and frontal balding. (B) Patient gripping fingers of examiner. (C) Note myotonia, i.e., inability to relax muscles of the hand, when asked to release examiner's fingers. [Courtesy of WB Dobyns, Chicago, Illinois.]

In most patients, the earliest neuromuscular symptoms are weakness and wasting of facial and jaw muscles, including ptosis, which are often present for years before diagnosis. Jaw weakness often results in sagging jaw and temporomandibular joint dislocation. Sternocleidomastoid weakness and wasting are prominent, while posterior neck and shoulder girdle muscles are less affected. Limb involvement early in the course is usually mild and first noticed in the small muscles of the hands and feet, wrist extensors, and foot dorsiflexors. Proximal limb weakness occurs much later, allowing most patients to remain ambulatory throughout their lives. It is relatively unusual for patients to be confined to a wheelchair, even when otherwise severely affected.

The other striking neuromuscular abnormality observed is myotonia, which consists of a delay in relaxation of normal muscle contractions (Fig. 10–32B,C). It is best elicited in the hand or with percussion of the tongue, as generalized myotonia is rare. Many patients seem unaware of the myotonia, even if it is obvious on exam. Those who are aware of it usually describe it as "stiffness" that is often aggravated by cold.

In congenital myotonic dystrophy, the disease begins before birth and results in much more severe manifestations. This severe form is always inherited from the affected mother. During the pregnancy, diminished fetal movements and polyhydramnios are common. At birth, respiratory distress is frequent and is the major cause of mortality. Facial and jaw muscle weakness and wasting are severe, result in a "tented" upper lip, and contribute to severe feeding problems. Generalized hypotonia is present and usually severe. Other abnormalities may include talipes, congenital hip dislocation, undescended testes, and hernias. The weakness and hypotonia slowly improve during infancy, and virtually all surviving children learn to walk. Speech and swallowing difficulties usually improve, but residual problems persist (15).

The EMG changes are striking and consist of excessive insertional activity, other signs of electrical irritability, and myotonic potentials. The latter are repetitive potentials that wax and wane in frequency and amplitude, resulting in the so-called dive-bomber sound.

Central nervous system. Mental symptoms such as apathy, inertia, reluctance to seek medical advice, and social decline are common, and efforts to help may not be welcomed. Hypersomnia is very common and has been observed even after correction of alveolar hypoventilation, suggesting a central cause. Most, if not all, patients with the congenital form and some with childhood (but not congenital) onset have mild to moderate mental retardation. Thus, mental retardation correlates with onset of neuromuscular symptoms and maternal inheritance, but not with severity of weakness or the sex of the patient. The MRI scans in mentally retarded individuals may show generalized or focal cerebral atrophy, focal white matter abnormalities especially in the anterior temporal lobe, and increased skull thickness (7).

Ocular system. Many patients have cataracts, most often consisting of multihued specks in the anterior and posterior subcapsular zones. Involvement of the retina may result in either peripheral or macular pigmentary degeneration. Changes in the electroretinograms are often prominent and may be useful in screening relatives of affected individuals (16). Other ocular abnormalities include ptosis, strabismus, low intraocular pressure, blepharitis, corneal lesions, and extraocular muscle weakness.

Cardiovascular system. Cardiac involvement is common and not confined to severely disabled patients. Most patients have cardiac conduction defects, and sudden death has been reported frequently (9). The most common abnormality is first-degree heart block, but other arrhythmias such as atrial flutter may occur. Hypotension is common. Few patients have signs of cardiac failure, despite histopathological changes of cardiomyopathy.

Respiratory system. Involvement of the diaphragm, shown by elevation on X-rays and functional studies, results from both weakness and myotonia. Alveolar hypoventilation, frequent in patients with either mild or severe disease, may have a central component.

Gastrointestinal system. The muscles of the gastrointestinal tract are involved, resulting in abnormal swallowing, frequent aspiration, reduced esophageal motility, occasional malabsorption, megacolon, and fecal impaction.

Endocrine system. While laboratory studies have shown many abnormalities of endocrine function, only a few are significant. Overt diabetes mellitus is rare although most patients have hyperinsulinism. Testicular atrophy occurs in 60%–80% of males and results from primary tubular degeneration. There is a high rate of fetal loss and major complications of pregnancy.

Auditory system. Hearing loss has not been widely recognized but appears to be common (8). Wright et al. (22) reported moderate to severe, usually sensorineural, hearing loss in 17 of 25 patients. It is more frequent in older individuals (21). On the other hand, Stephens et al. (17) did not find a higher incidence of middle ear or cochlear dysfunction, or tinnitus in a cohort of 42 patients with myotonic dystrophy. This issue awaits further resolution.

Vestibular system. Vestibular dysfunction is seen to some degree in patients with long-standing disease (21).

Laboratory findings. Serum creatine kinase and other muscle enzymes are often abnormal but are of little help in establishing the diagnosis.

Pathology. There is no single abnormality that is diagnostic, but the overall pattern is distinctive. The most characteristic changes on muscle biopsy include increased central nuclei, nuclear chains, ringed fibers, sarcoplasmic masses, type 1 fiber atrophy, increased fiber splitting in muscle spindles, and increased arborization of nerve endings. Less prominent changes include small angular fibers, moth-eaten fibers, type 2 fiber hypertrophy, and increased fibrosis.

Heredity. Inheritance is autosomal dominant. Molecular genetic studies mapped the gene to 19q13.2–q13.3, and a large number of flanking markers have been found (4,18). A second locus has been identified at 3q13.3-924 (12). A trinucleotide (CTG) repeat undergoes expansion in patients with myotonic dystrophy (3,5,10,20). Unaffected individuals have between 5 and 30 copies. Patients with mild symptoms have at least 50–80 repeats, while more severely affected patients have expansion of up to 2000 or more copies. The number of repeats often increases with transmission from affected parent to child, thus explaining the phenomenon of anticipation (14). Infants with the neonatal form are almost always born to mothers with the disease. The CTG repeat segment is transcribed and is located in the 3′ untranslated region of a polypeptide that is a member of the protein kinase family (1). The severe form of the disease is due to hypermethylation (17). Both prenatal and presymptomatic diagnosis is possible using flanking markers or the CTG repeat (13).

Diagnosis. Patients with facioscapulohumeral muscular dystrophy have similar weakness and wasting of the face and sternocleidomastoids, but the posterior neck and shoulder girdle muscles are more severely affected. Distribution of the weakness is proximal rather than distal. They also have retinal vascular abnormalities that differ from the retinal dystrophy and cataracts observed in myotonic dystrophy and lack involvement of other systems.

Prognosis. Affected individuals may have a normal life span but are at increased risk for death from cardiac conduction defects (sudden death) and aspiration. These risks are higher for children with congenital myotonic dystrophy. Disability is variable but may be severe.

Summary. Myotonic dystrophy is characterized by (1) autosomal dominant inheritance; (2) weakness and wasting of the face and distal muscles, with later weakness of proximal muscles; (3) myotonia; (4) cataracts; (5) cardiac conduction defects; (6) mental symptoms, especially apathy; and sometimes (7) mental retardation; (8) retinal degeneration; and (9) sensorineural hearing loss.

References

1. Brook JD et al: Molecular basis of myotonic dystrophy: expansion of a trinucleotide (CTG) repeat at the 3′ end of a transcript encoding a protein kinase family member. *Cell* 68:799–808, 1992.
2. Brooke MH: *A Clinician's View of Neuromuscular Diseases,* 2nd ed. William & Wilkins, Baltimore, 1986.
3. Gennarelli M et al: Prediction of myotonic dystrophy clinical severity based on the number of intragenic [CTG]n trinucleotide repeats. *Am J Med Genet* 65:342–347, 1996.
4. Harley HG et al: Localization of the myotonic dystrophy locus to 19q13.2–19q13.3 and its relationship to twelve polymorphic loci on 19q. *Hum Genet* 87:73–80, 1991.
5. Harley HG et al: Size of the unstable CTG repeat sequence in relation to phenotype and parental transmission in myotonic dystrophy. *Am J Hum Genet* 52:1164–1174, 1993.
6. Harper PS: Myotonic disorders. In: *Myology,* Engel AG, Banker BQ (eds), McGraw-Hill, New York, 1986, pp 1267–1296.
7. Huber SJ et al: Magnetic resonance imaging and clinical correlates of intellectual impairment in myotonic dystrophy. *Arch Neurol* 46:536–540, 1989.
8. Huygen PLM et al: Auditory abnormalities including "precocious presbycusis" in myotonic dystrophy. *Audiology* 33:73–84, 1994.
9. Josefowitz RF, Griggs RC: Myotonic dystrophy. *Neurol Clin* 6:455–472, 1988.
10. Martorell L et al: Comparison of CTG repeat length expansion and clinical progression of myotonic dystrophy over a five-year period. *J Med Genet* 32:593–596, 1995.
11. Morgenlander JC, Massey JM: Myotonic dystrophy. *Semin Neurol* 11:236–243, 1991.
12. Ranum L LPW et al: Genetic mapping of a second myotonic dystrophy locus. *Nat Genet* 19:196–198, 1998.
13. Reardon W et al: Five years experience of predictive testing for myotonic dystrophy using linked DNA markers. *Am J Med Genet* 43:1006–1011, 1992.
14. Roig M et al: Presentation, clinical course, and outcome of the congenital form of myotonic dystrophy. *Pediatr Neurol* 11:208–213, 1994.
15. Salomonson J et al: Velopharyngeal incompetence as the presenting symptom of myotonic dystrophy. *Cleft Palate J* 25:296–300, 1988.
16. Sandrini G et al: Electroretinographic and visual evoked potential abnormalities in myotonic dystrophy. *Electroenceph Clin Neurophysiol* 64:215–217, 1986.
17. Steinbach P et al: The *DMPK* gene of severely affected myotonic dystrophy patients is hypermethylated proximal to the largely expanded CTG repeat. *Am J Hum Genet* 62:278–285, 1998.
18. Stephens SDG et al: Neuro-otological function in patients with myotonic dystrophy. *J Audiol Med* 3:8–22, 1994.
19. Tapscott SJ: Deconstructing myotonic dystrophy. *Science* 289:1701–1702, 2000.
20. Tsilfidis C et al: Correlation between CTG trinucleotide repeat length and frequency of severe congenital myotonic dystrophy. *Nat Genet* 1:192–195, 1992.
21. Verhagen WIM et al: Oculomotor, auditory, and vestibular responses in myotonic dystrophy. *Arch Neurol* 49:954–960, 1992.
22. Wright RB et al: Hearing loss in myotonic dystrophy. *Ann Neurol* 23:202–203, 1988.

Oculopharyngeal muscular dystrophy

Oculopharyngeal muscular dystrophy has its onset late, usually in midlife. Facial musculature is weakened to the point of flaccid paralysis. Involvement of the masticatory muscles is reflected in hollowing of the temporal areas and sagging of the mandible. Blepharoptosis is striking. The brow is usually furrowed. There is increasing difficulty encountered in eating and drinking (5).

Heredity. The autosomal dominant form maps to 14q11.3–q13, a gene encoding poly(A)-binding protein-2 (*PABP2*) (2,3). Many cases are of French-Canadian origin. The recessive form maps to the same site.

Auditory system. Slowly progressive sensorineural hearing loss has been reported in a kindred by Graf (1). Conversely, Roberts and Bamforth (6) noted no hearing loss among 26 patients. In contrast, Kuhn and Ey (4) reported that 8 of 23 patients with myotonic dystrophy exhibited hearing loss; of these, 4 were the result of chronic middle ear infections.

References

1. Graf K: Myopathia oculo-pharyngealis tarda hereditaria. *Pract Otorhinolaryngol (Basel)* 33:203–208, 1971.
2. Brais B et al: The oculopharyngeal muscular dystrophy locus maps to the region of the cardiac alpha and beta myosin heavy-chain genes on chromosome 14q11.2–q13. *Hum Mol Genet* 4:429–434, 1995.
3. Brais B et al: Short GCG expansions in the *PABP2* gene cause oculopharyngeal muscular dystrophy. *Nat Genet* 18:164–167, 1998.
4. Kuhn E, Ey W: Innenohrschwerhörigkeit bei Dystrophia myotonica und Dystrophia muscularis progressiva. *Dtsch Med Wochenschr* 91:947–951, 1966.
5. Lewis I: Late-onset muscle dystrophy: oculopharyngeal variety. *Can Med Assoc J* 95:146–150, 1966.
6. Roberts AH, Bamforth J: The pharynx and esophagus in ocular muscular dystrophy. *Neurology (Minneap)* 18:645–652, 1968.

Scapuloperoneal syndrome

Scapuloperoneal syndrome is a progressive muscle disorder with predominant weakness in the shoulder girdle and peroneal muscles. Facial involvement is late and mild. Both neuropathic and myopathic forms have been described.

Auditory system. Ansher et al. (1) reported an affected family with severe sensorineural hearing loss.

Heredity. Inheritance is autosomal dominant, the gene mapping to 12q13.3–q15 (2).

Diagnosis. In facioscapulohumeral muscular dystrophy, facial involvement is early and prominent.

References

1. Ansher M et al: Autosomal dominant scapuloperoneal syndrome with sensorineural hearing loss. *Otolaryngol Head Neck Surg* 100:242–244, 1989.
2. Isozumi K et al: Linkage of scapuloperoneal spinal muscular atrophy to chromosome 12q24.1–q24.31. *Hum Mol Genet* 5:1377–1382, 1996.

Established Mitochondrial Syndromes with Hearing Loss

Mitochondrial syndromes constitute a vast array of disorders associated with impaired energy production (1,10). These syndromes occur as a result of the inability of mitochondria to meet the metabolic demands of tissues. Originally thought of as neuromuscular disorders (6), it has become clear that mitochondrial dysfunction can present with varied phenotypes. This section will be limited to discussion of those disorders with hearing loss. Several good reviews of the subject have been published as well (2,5,7).

Thousands of mitochondria are present in cells and retain the ability to direct the production of many of the enzymes necessary for oxidative phosphorylation by the presence of their own genome. This genome (mtDNA), which is present in 2 to 10 copies per mitochondrion, works in concert with the nuclear genome to produce all of the enzymes needed for energy production (1). Human mtDNA encodes 13 polypeptides of

the respiratory chain subunits, 28 ribosomal RNAs, and 22 transfer RNAs. However, these mitochondrial gene products are insufficient to support the full function of the mitochondrion, and thus a significant proportion of mitochondrial proteins are coded for by nuclear genes.

Since dual genomes direct enzyme production in the mitochondrion, inheritance patterns can be maternal (8) or autosomal recessive (9). Cases of mitochondrial disorders can also be sporadic. These generally result from deletions in the mitochondrial genome (3,4).

Diagnosis of mitochondrial disorders is difficult. Patients that present with a wide variety of dysfunctions in varied organ systems should raise suspicion of a mitochondrial syndrome (Table 10–2). Investigation for these disorders should include assay of serum lactate/pyruvate, CSF lactate, and muscle biopsy for the presence of abnormal collections of mitochondria, the so-called ragged-red fibers, and fatty infiltration. Muscle levels of mitochondrial enzymes should be assayed (1,6). Molecular techniques can be used to confirm the diagnosis and give clues to the inheritance pattern of the specific disorder.

References

1. DiMauro S et al: Mitochondrial encephalomyopathies. *Neurol Clin North Am* 8:483–506, 1990.
2. Fischel-Ghodsian N: Mitochondrial deafness mutations reviewed. *Hum Mutat* 13:261–270, 1999.
3. Harding AE, Hammans SR: Deletions of the mitochondrial genome. *J Inherit Metab Dis* 15:480–486, 1992.
4. Holt IJ et al: Deletions of muscle mitochondrial DNA in patients with mitochondrial myopathies. *Nature* 331:717–719, 1988.
5. Hutchin TP, Cortopassi GA: Mitochondrial defects and hearing loss. *CMLS Cell Mol Life Sci* 57:1927–1937, 2000.
6. Munnich A et al: Clinical aspects of mitochondrial disorders. *J Inherit Metab Dis* 15:448–455, 1992.
7. Van Camp G, Smith RJH: Maternally inherited hearing impairment. *Clin Genet* 57:409–414, 2000.
8. Wallace DC et al: Diseases resulting from mitochondrial DNA point mutations. *J Inherit Metab Dis* 15:472–479, 1992.
9. Zevianni M: Nucleus-driven mutations of human mitochondrial DNA. *J Inherit Metab Dis* 15:456–471, 1992.
10. Zevianni M et al: Mitochondrial diseases. *Neurogenet Dis* 7:123–156, 1989.

Kearns-Sayre syndrome (ophthalmoplegia plus)

In 1958, Kearns and Sayre (26) described a syndrome of progressive external ophthalmoplegia, retinitis pigmentosa, and complete heart block in two unrelated patients. Alfano and Berger (1) had described a patient with retinitis pigmentosa, ophthalmoplegia, and spastic quadriplegia the year before. Jager et al. (22) reported the same disorder, but with ataxia and hearing loss, in 1960. The disorder may have been noted as early as 1878 (16).

In later reports, Kearns (24,25) added more patients, some with a complete and others with an incomplete syndrome, lacking cardiomyopathy. Drachman (13,14) proposed the term *ophthalmoplegia plus* and extended the condition to include endocrine and auditory abnormalities. Both ragged-red fibers (21,31) and bizarre mitochondria (18,26,42) were found to be part of the syndrome. Egger and Wilson (15) recognized the unique inheritance pattern, and referred to it as a "mitochondrial cytopathy syndrome." More recently, diagnostic criteria for Kearns-Sayre syndrome (KSS) have been proposed, which include (*1*) onset before 20 years, (*2*) progressive external ophthalmoplegia, (*3*) atypical pigmentary retinopathy, and (*4*) one or more of the following: ataxia, complete heart block, and elevated CSF protein (5,28). Molecular genetic studies have shown deletions or duplications of mitochondrial DNA in KSS and related mitochondrial myopathies (9,12,20,28,32,33,40). There have been many excellent reviews (4,5,9,10,12,15,18,23).

Physical findings. If onset of the syndrome occurs at an early age, patients are usually short and slightly built. Short stature has been observed in about 70% (4,8) (Fig. 10–33A,B).

Ocular system. Ptosis followed soon by progressive, generally symmetric external ophthalmoplegia is the first sign of the disorder in

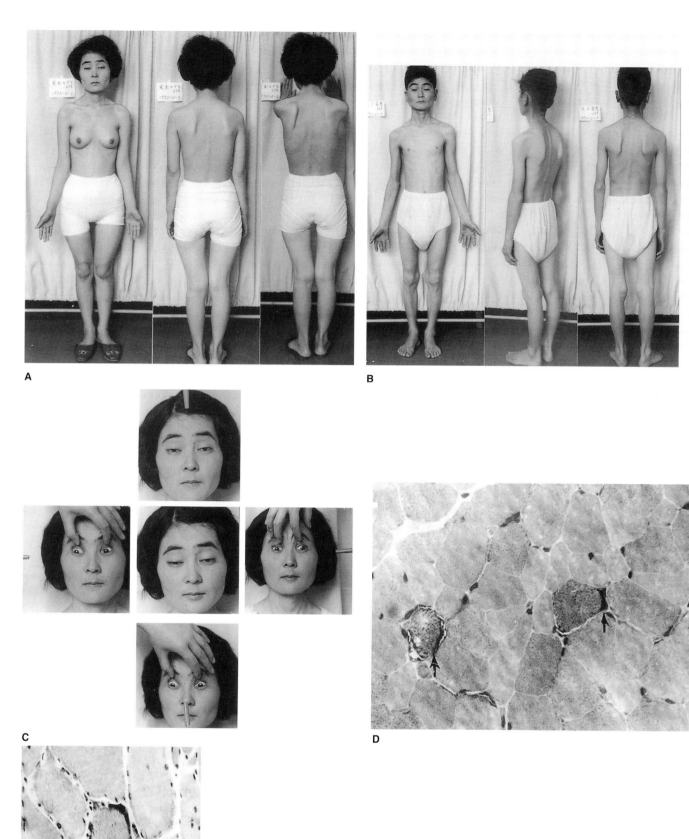

Figure 10–33. *Kearns-Sayre syndrome (ophthalmoplegia plus)*. (A,B) Moderate weakness and wasting in the shoulder and pelvic girdle muscles and the proximal muscles of the arms and legs. (C) Maximal deviation of eye in four main directions of gaze shows severe limitation of movement. (D) Excessive numbers of abnormal subsarcolemmal mitochondria (arrows) in two muscle fibers (frozen section, trichrome stain, ×470). (E) Another section of muscle showing ragged-red fibers (frozen section, trichrome stain, ×250). [(A–C) from K Tamura et al., *Brain* 97:665, 1974; (D) courtesy of Stephen A Smith, Minneapolis, Minnesota.]

about 85% of patients (Fig. 10–33C). When asymmetric, the ophthalmoplegia tends to occur on the side of the greater ptosis (10). Onset occurs in nearly all patients before age 20 (mean 10 years) (9). The disorder then progresses slowly to complete oculomotor paralysis.

Retinal pigmentary degeneration and optic atrophy usually appear soon after the ophthalmoplegia but may be the presenting sign or begin as late as 30 years. Impaired visual acuity and night vision are usually not noticed until long after the retinal changes are visible. Examination of the retina shows a scattering of fine pigment, occasionally in small clumps, throughout the retina, which often spares the area around the disc. The retinal arteries are usually not narrowed, but the retina appears thinned. These changes have been described as "atypical retinitis pigmentosa," as they are less severe than those observed in typical pigmentary retinopathy. Electroretinograms show diminished responses (5,9,10).

Cardiovascular system. Cardiac conduction defects occur in about 60% and may follow the ophthalmoplegia and retinitis from a few months to many years. The conduction defects progress through a sequence of interventricular conduction defect, incomplete bundle branch block, trifascicular disease, and, finally, complete heart block. Repeated Stokes-Adams syncopal attacks may occur and must be treated with a pacemaker because of the risk of sudden death. Congestive heart failure may also occur.

Central nervous system. Ataxia and corticospinal tract signs such as brisk tendon reflexes and extensor plantar responses occur in about 70% of patients, usually well after onset of ophthalmoplegia, and then progress slowly. Electroencephalograms show nonspecific changes in about 50%. Mental retardation or dementia has been evident in about 40% (5). Cranial CT or MRI scans may show diffuse leukoencephalopathy, cerebellar and brain stem atrophy, and calcifications in the region of the basal ganglia (6,37,38).

Peripheral nervous system and muscular system. Myopathic facial weakness, manifested in opening and closing of eyelids, has been observed in about 50% of patients. Other bulbar symptoms may include dysphonia, dysphagia, and hoarseness. The voice is weak and speech is "nasal" with incomplete closure of the epiglottis (9,10). Myopathic weakness of the neck and proximal limb muscles occurs in about 70%, but severity varies. Tendon reflexes are often decreased or absent. Some patients also have distal weakness and sensory loss, suggesting a peripheral neuropathy (16). Electromyography shows myopathic changes.

Endocrine system. Delayed sexual development occurs in about 35% (5,16,36). About 15% have either elevated blood glucose or abnormal glucose tolerance tests (7,16). Hypoparathyroidism was noted in several patients (16).

Auditory system. Sensorineural hearing loss occurs in at least 50% of patients and, rarely, may be the presenting symptom. It is most pronounced at higher frequencies and is slowly progressive (5,9,14,22,26,29,32,36,41).

Vestibular system. Caloric testing has revealed markedly diminished or absent responses to vestibular stimulation in about 85% of those tested (5).

Laboratory findings. Cerebrospinal fluid protein is often elevated to >100 mg/dl, and lactic acidosis is often present. Both are useful in distinguishing this disorder from other ocular myopathies early in the course of the disease. Recent biochemical studies have shown abnormalities of the citric acid cycle, pyruvate metabolism, and several different components of the mitochondrial respiratory chain, especially complexes I and IV (8,12,30,36). Deficiencies of complex IV seem to correlate best with severity of the clinical manifestations (11).

Pathology. The morphologic hallmark of mitochondrial myopathy in this and other mitochondrial encephalomyopathies is the presence of ragged-red fibers in muscle biopsies stained with the modified Gomori trichrome method (Fig. 10–33D,E). Affected fibers are distinguished by blotches of stain around the periphery, which result from subsarcolemmal aggregations of proliferative mitochondria. Electron microscopy shows groups of normal or enlarged mitochondria with elongated crystalline and osmiophilic inclusions and abnormally arranged cristae that are usually more abundant under the sarcolemma. Fibroblasts, hepatocytes, endothelial cells, and other cell types may show the same changes, but they are less severe. At autopsy, spongiform encephalopathy has been described (5,12,16).

Histopathological changes in the inner ear consist of severe cochleosaccular degeneration with almost complete absence of the organ of Corti in all turns. The spiral ganglia exhibit a marked reduction in cells with almost complete degeneration of nerve fibers in the long spiral lamina (27).

Heredity. While most cases are sporadic, families with multiple affected individuals have been reported. The empiric recurrence risk for sibs and children is about 5% (3). In multiplex families, Egger and Wilson (15) noted that the disorder was transmitted almost exclusively by females, consistent with maternal (mitochondrial) inheritance. However, severity of manifestations may vary greatly between relatives.

Molecular genetic studies have shown deletions, duplications, or both of mitochondrial DNA in a majority of patients with KSS. Affected individuals are usually heteroplasmic, i.e., their cells contain both normal and abnormal mitochondria. The deleted or duplicated segments often contain components of several of the respiratory chain complexes, including those in which biochemical assays have been normal. Thus, the mechanism leading from the deletion to the clinical manifestations is not known, although the ratio of normal to abnormal mitochondria in cells is thought to be important (11,28). In one patient, a mutation in the tRNALeu(UUR) gene was detected. This is the same mutation observed in most patients with MELAS syndrome (19). Another patient with a point mutation in the same gene at position 3249 and a Kearns-Sayre phenotype was described by Seneca et al. (39).

Diagnosis. Progressive external ophthalmoplegia with or without ptosis may occur as an isolated abnormality, or it may be found in association with biochemical or structural disorders affecting the oculomotor system. These have been elegantly reviewed by Drachman (13,14). Refsum syndrome may be excluded by finding normal levels of serum phytanic acid. Several other mitochondrial syndromes that should be excluded are described in this section, although patients with phenotypes overlapping with progressive external ophthalmoplegia (PEO) and mitochondrial myopathy, encephalopathy, lactic acidosis, and strokelike episodes (MELAS) have also been described, and clear distinction may be difficult (2).

Diagnosis can be made by detection of mitochondrial deletions using the PCR technique (17,34), although it should be noted that identical deletions can cause KSS, chronic progressive external ophthalmoplegia (CPEO), or Pearson syndrome (17,35). The presence of duplications in addition to deletions may help distinguish KSS from the other conditions (35).

Prognosis. The various components of the syndrome are progressive, and patients are at particular risk for death from heart block.

Summary. This disorder is characterized by (1) sporadic occurrence or maternal (mitochondrial) inheritance; (2) progressive external ophthalmoplegia and ptosis; (3) atypical pigmentary retinopathy; (4) mitochondrial myopathy with ragged-red fibers; (5) ataxia; (6) mental retardation or dementia; (7) cardiac conduction defects; (8) growth deficiency; (9) delayed sexual development; (10) vestibular abnormalities; (11) elevated CSF protein; and (12) sensorineural hearing loss.

References

1. Alfano JE, Berger JP: Retinitis pigmentosa, ophthalmoplegia, and spastic quadriplegia. *Am J Ophthalmol* 43:231–240, 1957.

2. Ashizawa T, Subramony SH: What is Kearns-Sayre syndrome after all? *Arch Neurol* 58:1053–1054, 2001.

3. Baraitser M: *The Genetics of Neurological Disorders.* Oxford University Press, Oxford, 1990, pp 380–386.

4. Bastiaensen LAK et al: Ophthalmoplegia-plus, a real nosological entity. *Acta Neurol Scand* 58:9–34, 1978.

5. Berenberg RA et al: Lumping or splitting? "Ophthalmoplegia-plus" or Kearns-Sayre syndrome? *Ann Neurol* 1:37–54, 1977.

6. Bertorini T et al: Leukoencephalopathy in oculocraniosomatic neuromuscular disease with ragged-red fibers: mitochondrial abnormalities demonstrated by computerized tomography. *Arch Neurol* 35:643–647, 1978.

7. Boltshauser E, Gauthier G: Diabetes mellitus in Kearns-Sayre syndrome. *Am J Dis Child* 132:321–322, 1978.

8. Bresolin N et al: Progressive cytochrome c oxidase deficiency in a case of Kearns-Sayre syndrome: morphological, immunological and biochemical studies in muscle biopsies and autopsy tissues. *Ann Neurol* 21:564–572, 1987.

9. Butler IJ, Gadoth N: Kearns-Sayre syndrome: a review of a multisystem disorder of children and young adults. *Arch Intern Med* 136:1290–1293, 1976.

10. Danta G et al: Chronic progressive external ophthalmoplegia. *Brain* 98:473–492, 1975.

11. Degoul F et al: Deletions of mitochondrial DNA in Kearns-Sayre syndrome and ocular myopathies: genetic, biochemical and morphological studies. *J Neurol Sci* 101:168–177, 1991.

12. DiMauro S et al: Mitochondrial myopathies. *Ann Neurol* 17:521–538, 1985.

13. Drachman DA: Ophthalmoplegia plus. The neurodegenerative disorders associated with progressive external ophthalmoplegia. *Arch Neurol* 18:654–674, 1968.

14. Drachman DA: Ophthalmoplegia plus: a classification of the disorders associated with progressive external ophthalmoplegia. In: *Handbook of Clinical Neurology, vol. 22. System Disorders and Atrophies, Part II,* Vinken PJ et al. (eds), North Holland Publishing Co., Amsterdam, 1975, pp 203–216.

15. Egger J, Wilson J: Mitochondrial inheritance in a mitochondrially mediated disease. *N Engl J Med* 309:142–146, 1983.

16. Egger J et al: Mitochondrial cytopathy. A multisystem disorder with ragged red fibers on muscle biopsy. *Arch Dis Child* 56:741–752, 1981.

17. Fischel-Ghodsian N et al: Deletion in blood mitochondrial DNA in Kearns-Sayre syndrome. *Pediatr Res* 31:557–560, 1992.

18. Gonatas NK: A generalized disorder of nervous system, skeletal muscle and heart resembling Refsum's disease and Hurler's syndrome. *Am J Med* 42:169–178, 1967.

19. Goto Y et al: A mutation in the tRNALeu(UUR) gene associated with the MELAS subgroup of mitochondrial encephalomyopathies. *Nature* 348:651–653, 1990.

20. Holt IJ et al: Mitochondrial myopathies: clinical and biochemical features of 30 patients with major deletions of muscle mitochondrial DNA. *Ann Neurol* 26:699–708, 1989.

21. Iannaccone ST et al: Familial progressive external ophthalmoplegia and ragged-red fibers. *Neurology* 24:1033–1038, 1974.

22. Jager BV et al: Occurrence of retinal pigmentation, ophthalmoplegia, ataxia, deafness, and heart block. *Am J Med* 29:888–893, 1960.

23. Joannard A et al: Syndrome de Kearns avec hypocalcémie transitore. *Pédiatrie* 32:797–806, 1977.

24. Kearns TP: External ophthalmoplegia, pigmentary degeneration of the retina, and cardiomyopathy: a newly recognized syndrome. *Trans Am Ophthalmol Soc* 63:559–625, 1965.

25. Kearns TP: Neuro-ophthalmology. *Arch Ophthalmol* 76:729–755, 1966.

26. Kearns TP, Sayre GP: Retinitis pigmentosa, external ophthalmoplegia, and complete heart block. *Arch Ophthalmol* 60:280–289, 1958.

27. Lindsay JR, Hinojosa R: Histopathologic features of the inner ear associated with Kearns-Sayre syndrome. *Arch Otolaryngol* 102:747–752, 1976.

28. Moraes CT et al: Mitochondrial DNA deletions in progressive external ophthalmoplegia and Kearns-Sayre syndrome. *N Engl J Med* 320:1293–1299, 1989.

29. Nørby S et al: Juvenile Kearns-Sayre syndrome initially misdiagnosed as a psychosomatic disorder. *J Med Genet* 31:45–50, 1994.

30. Ogasahara S et al: Improvement of abnormal pyruvate metabolism and cardiac conduction defect with co-enzyme Q10 in Kearns-Sayre syndrome. *Neurology* 35:372–377, 1985.

31. Olson W et al: Oculocraniosomatic neuromuscular disease with "ragged red fibers." *Arch Neurol* 26:475–497, 1972.

32. Petty RKH et al: The clinical features of mitochondrial myopathy. *Brain* 109:915–938, 1986.

33. Poulton J et al: Duplication of mitochondrial DNA in mitochondrial myopathy. *Lancet* 1:236–240, 1989.

34. Poulton J et al: Detection of mitochondrial DNA deletions in blood using the polymerase chain reaction: non-invasive diagnosis of mitochondrial myopathy. *Clin Genet* 39:33–38, 1991.

35. Poulton J et al: Are duplications of mitochondrial DNA characteristic of Kearns-Sayre syndrome? *Hum Mol Genet* 3:947–951, 1994.

36. Reske-Nielsen E et al: Progressive external ophthalmoplegia. Evidence for a generalized mitochondrial disease with a defect in pyruvate metabolism. *Acta Ophthalmol* 54:553–573, 1976.

37. Robertson WC Jr et al: Basal ganglia calcification in Kearns-Sayre syndrome. *Arch Neurol* 36:711–713, 1979.

38. Seigel RS et al: Computer tomography in oculocraniosomatic disease (Kearns-Sayre syndrome). *Radiology* 130:159–164, 1979.

39. Seneca S et al: A new mitochondrial point mutation in the transfer RNA(Leu) gene in a patient with a clinical phenotype resembling Kearns-Sayre syndrome. *Arch Neurol* 58:1113–1118, 2001.

40. Shanski S et al: Widespread tissue distributions of mitochondrial DNA deletions in Kearns-Sayre syndrome. *Neurology* 40:24–28, 1990.

41. Swift AC, Singh SD: Hearing impairment and the Kearns-Sayre syndrome. *J Laryngol Otol* 102:626–627, 1988.

42. Zintz R, Villiger W: Elektronenmikroskopische Befunde bei 3 Fällen von chronisch progressiver okulärer Muskeldystrophie. *Ophthalmologica* 153:439–459, 1967.

Mitochondrial encephalomyopathy, lactic acidosis, stroke-like episodes, and sensorineural hearing loss (MELAS)

MELAS is a sporadic or maternally inherited mitochondrial disorder that has been reported in over 25 patients (17). It has been separated from other mitochondrial encephalomyopathies primarily because of recurrent strokes (13).

Musculoskeletal system. Stature is normal early in life, but growth deceleration occurs, which later results in short stature. Easy fatigability and proximal weakness are observed in most patients, although it may be difficult to determine whether weakness is due to muscle disease or strokes.

Central nervous system. In most patients, early development is normal. The disease begins between 3 and 15 years of age in most patients, although later onset may occur, even in relatives of typical patients (2). The first symptoms are usually recurrent headaches or vomiting episodes, which then persist. Gradual decline in cognitive abilities follows until the often sudden onset of seizures, stroke-like episodes, or both. Seizure types include generalized or focal tonic-clonic seizures and, less frequently, myoclonic seizures.

The stroke-like episodes consist of sudden-onset hemiparesis, hemianopsia, or cortical blindness, often accompanied by other focal neurological deficits. They are often preceded by headache or vomiting and may occur repetitively. Progression of dementia is hastened by each episode. Cranial CT or MRI scans usually show areas of infarction, most commonly in the parietal and occipital lobes (Fig. 10–34A). Some patients also have bilateral basal ganglia calcifications, possibly due to pseudohypoparathyroidism (18).

Ocular system. Visual symptoms in this disorder are caused by occipital lobe and other infarcts rather than by retinal disease.

Other findings. A few patients manifest other abnormalities such as cardiomyopathy, nephrotic syndrome, and pseudohypoparathyroidism (18). Matthews et al. (9) described specific MRI changes in the cortex of the cerebrum and cerebellum.

Auditory system. Thirteen of 29 patients had sensorineural hearing loss, which was progressive and often severe (2,3,6,7,10,17). This may be the first or only symptom in some patients.

Laboratory findings. Elevation of lactate and pyruvate in both blood and CSF has been observed in all or almost all patients. Biochemical studies have shown deficiency of several different components

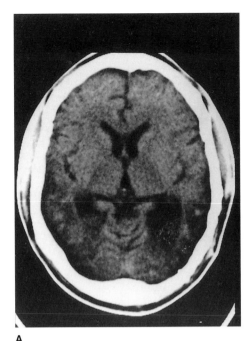

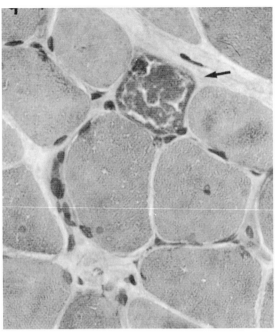

A   B

Figure 10–34. *Mitochondrial en-cephalomyopathy, lactic acidosis, stroke-like episodes, and sensorineural hearing loss (MELAS).* (A) Cranial CT scan shows bilateral strokes in parieto-occipital region and general atrophy. (B) Arrow points to ragged-red fiber. [From P Montagna et al., *Neurology* 38:751, 1988.]

of the mitochondrial respiratory chain, especially involving complex I, in some but not all patients (18).

Pathology. Ragged-red fibers and other typical mitochondrial abnormalities are observed in muscle (Fig. 10–34B) (9). Mitochondrial angiopathy in cerebral blood vessels may explain the recurrent strokes (6,12,14).

Heredity. Most cases have been sporadic. However, familial occurrence of MELAS has been reported in five families, each with vertical transmission through females (2,6,10,11,15). When combined with the recent discovery of a mitochondrial DNA mutation in many patients, it is apparent that inheritance of this disorder is maternal. Mutations in the mitochondrial tRNALeu(UUR) gene at position 3243 appear to be the cause of the disorder in a majority of patients (4,5,7,16). This corresponds to the first base of the dihydrouridine loop, which is strictly invariant across many species. The mechanism leading from the mutation to the clinical manifestations is not known. The same mutation has been found in patients with progressive external ophthalmoplegia (incomplete Kearns-Sayre syndrome) and KSS (see above). Patients with maternally inherited diabetes and deafness (MIDD) can also have this mutation. Recently a single patient with gestational diabetes, deafness, Wolff-Parkinson-White syndrome, and placenta accreta was described with this mutation (1). It is therefore specific, although not exclusive, to MELAS. Patients exhibiting combined features of both MELAS and KSS have exhibited deletions (3,20). A MERRF/MELAS overlap syndrome has been reported (19).

Diagnosis. Several other disorders, such as congenital heart disease, homocystinuria, and protein S deficiency, may present with recurrent strokes, but none has the other manifestations of MELAS. See Table 10–2.

Prognosis. Most patients experience severe disability, and early death may ensue. Patients with later onset often have a milder course.

Summary. This disorder is characterized by (*1*) sporadic occurrence or maternal inheritance; (*2*) mitochondrial myopathy with ragged-red fibers; (*3*) headache and vomiting episodes; (*4*) stroke-like episodes resulting in hemiparesis, hemianopsia, or cortical blindness; (*5*) seizures; (*6*) dementia; (*7*) growth deficiency; (*8*) lactic acidosis; and (*9*) sensorineural hearing loss.

References

1. Aggarwal P et al: Identification of mtDNA mutation in a pedigree with gestational diabetes, deafness, Wolff-Parkinson-White syndrome and placenta accreta. *Hum Hered* 51:114–116, 2001.
2. Driscoll PF et al: MELAS syndrome involving a mother and two children. *Arch Neurol* 44:971–973, 1987.
3. Förster C et al: Mitochondrial angiopathy in family with MELAS. *Neuropaediatrics* 23:165–168, 1992.
4. Goto Y et al: A mutation in the tRNALeu(UUR) gene associated with the MELAS subgroup of mitochondrial encephalomyopathies. *Nature* 348:651–653, 1990.
5. Goto Y et al: Mitochondrial myopathy, encephalopathy, lactic acidosis, and stroke-like episodes (MELAS): a correlative study of the clinical features and mitochondrial DNA mutation. *Neurology* 42:545–550, 1992.
6. Hart ZH et al: Familial poliodystrophy, mitochondrial myopathy, and lactate acidemia. *Arch Neurol* 34:180–185, 1977.
7. Inui K: Mitochondrial encephalomyopathies with the mutation of the mitochondrial tRNALeu(UUR) gene. *J Pediatr* 120:62–66, 1992.
8. Matthews PM et al: Magnetic resonance imaging shows specific abnormalities in the MELAS syndrome. *Neurology* 41:1043–1046, 1991.
9. McKelvie PA et al: Mitochondrial encephalopathies: a correlation between neuropathological findings and defects in mitochondrial DNA. *J Neurol Sci* 102:51–60, 1991 (case 2).
10. Monnens L et al: A metabolic myopathy associated with chronic lactic acidemia, growth failure, and nerve deafness. *J Pediatr* 86:983, 1975.
11. Montagna P et al: MELAS syndrome: characteristic migrainous and epileptic features and maternal transmission. *Neurology* 38:751–754, 1988.
12. Ohama E et al: Mitochondrial angiopathy in cerebral blood vessels of mitochondrial encephalomyopathy. *Acta Neuropathol* 74:226–233, 1987.
13. Pavlakis SG et al: Mitochondrial myopathy, encephalopathy, lactic acidosis, and strokelike episodes: a distinctive clinical syndrome. *Ann Neurol* 16:481–488, 1984.
14. Seyama K et al: Mitochondrial encephalopathy with lactic acidosis and stroke-like episodes with special reference to the mechanisms of cerebral manifestations. *Acta Neurol Scand* 80:561–568, 1989.
15. Shapira Y et al: Familial poliodystrophy, mitochondrial myopathy, and lactate acidemia. *Neurology* 25:614–621, 1975.
16. Tanaka M et al: Mitochondrial mutations in mitochondrial myopathy, encephalomyopathy, lactic acidosis and strokelike episodes (MELAS). *Biochem Biophys Res Commun* 174:861–868, 1991.
17. Van Hellenberg, Hubar JL et al: MELAS syndrome: report of two patients and comparison with data of 24 patients derived from the literature. *Neuropediatrics* 22:10–14, 1991.
18. Yoneda M et al: Pleiotropic molecular defects in energy-transducing complexes in mitochondrial encephalomyopathy (MELAS). *J Neurol Sci* 92:143–158, 1989.

19. Zeviani M et al: A MERRF/MELAS overlap syndrome associated with a new patient mutation in the mitochondrial DNA tRNALys gene. *Eur J Hum Genet* 1:80–87, 1993.

20. Zupanc ML et al: Deletion of mitochondrial DNA in patients with combined features of Kearns-Sayre and MELAS syndrome. *Ann Neurol* 29:680–682, 1991.

Mitochondrial encephalomyopathy, myoclonus epilepsy, ragged-red fibers, and sensorineural hearing loss (MERRF)

MERRF is a sporadic or maternally inherited mitochondrial disorder that has been reported in over 20 patients. It has been separated from other mitochondrial encephalomyopathies primarily because of myoclonic epilepsy (4). Recently, a mutation in the mitochondrial tRNALys gene has been discovered in several unrelated patients (10).

Central nervous system. Early development is usually normal. The age of onset (5–42 years) and severity may vary greatly even within a family. The most frequent presenting symptom is myoclonic jerks, sometimes preceded by ataxia and hearing loss. Both intention and action myoclonus become progressively more severe and often result in falls. They are usually accompanied by generalized tonic-clonic and other seizures. The EEG often shows a photoconvulsive response. Associated symptoms include progressive ataxia and dementia, which may be severe.

Peripheral nervous system and muscular system. Mild generalized or proximal muscle weakness and wasting of variable severity occur in most patients. Motor neuropathy has been observed in a few patients.

Ocular system. Ptosis and optic atrophy have been observed in several patients, but neither cortical blindness nor pigmentary retinopathy occurs (Fig. 10–35A,B).

Other systems. Less constant abnormalities include growth deficiency and cardiomyopathy.

Auditory system. While not emphasized in early reports, sensorineural hearing loss occurs frequently in MERRF (2). In mildly affected individuals, this may be the only symptom (7).

Laboratory findings. Elevation of lactate and pyruvate in both blood and CSF has been observed in most patients (6). Biochemical studies have shown deficiency of complexes I and IV of the respiratory chain in some, but not all, patients (12).

Pathology. Ragged-red fibers and other typical mitochondrial abnormalities are observed in muscle. In addition to variation in fiber size and ragged-red fibers, muscle cells in cross section show focal cytochrome C oxidase deficiency (5). Anti-DNA antibodies have been used to detect ragged-red fibers in muscle biopsy (1). Central nervous system abnormalities found at autopsy include (*1*) degeneration of the dentatorubral and pallidoluysian systems; (*2*) spinal cord lesions similar to those in Friedreich ataxia; and (*3*) degeneration of the substantia nigra, cerebellar cortex, inferior olivary nucleus, locus ceruleus, gracile and cuneate nuclei, and pontine tegmentum (11) (Fig. 10–35C).

Heredity. Maternal (mitochondrial) inheritance of MERRF has been demonstrated in many families (3,4,7,12). Shoffner et al. (10) initially

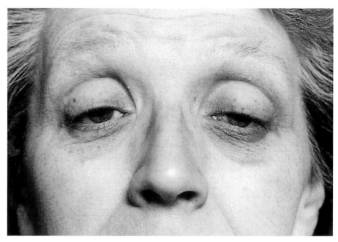

A

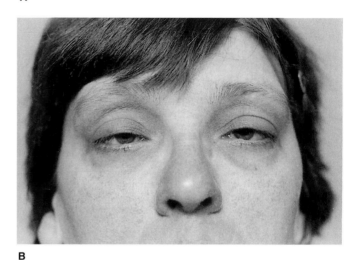

B

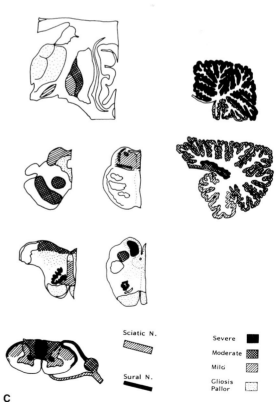

C

Figure 10–35. *Mitochondrial encephalomyopathy, myoclonus epilepsy, ragged-red fibers, and sensorineural hearing loss (MERRF).* (A,B) Bilateral ptosis in mother and daughter. (C) Line drawings of brain showing predominant areas of involvement. [(A,B) courtesy of SA Barron, Haifa, Israel; (C) from S Takeda et al., *Acta Neuropathol* 75:433, 1988.]

reported an A-to-G base substitution at nucleotide pair 8344 in the gene coding for the mitochondrial tRNALys in three unrelated patients with MERRF. Other families with this mutation were also reported (13), and Shoffner and Wallace ultimately showed that this mutation accounts for 80%–90% of those with MERRF (9). The mechanism leading from the mutation to the clinical manifestations is not known (8).

Diagnosis. Both progressive myoclonic epilepsy and hearing loss occur in several other syndromes, some or all of which might also be disorders of mitochondrial metabolism. Patients with progressive myoclonus epilepsy, ataxia, and sensorineural hearing loss (May-White syndrome) lack myopathy, and inheritance is autosomal dominant. Patients with progressive myoclonus epilepsy, dementia, and hearing loss (Latham-Munro syndrome) also lack myopathy, and inheritance is autosomal recessive. Patients with mitochondrial encephalopathy, progressive myoclonus epilepsy, ataxia, dementia, diabetes mellitus, nephropathy, and sensorineural hearing loss (Herrmann syndrome) may be differentiated by the nephropathy, but it could be a variant of MERRF because inheritance in the one family reported was probably maternal.

Summary. This disorder is characterized by (*1*) progressive myoclonus epilepsy; (*2*) mitochondrial myopathy with ragged-red fibers; (*3*) ataxia; (*4*) dementia; and (*5*) sensorineural hearing loss.

References

1. Andreetta F et al: Localization of mitochondrial DNA in normal and pathological muscle using immunological probes: a new approach to the study of mitochondrial myopathies. *J Neurol Sci* 105:88–92, 1991.
2. Bindoff LA et al: Multiple defects of the mitochondrial respiratory chain in a mitochondrial encephalopathy (MERRF): a clinical, biochemical and molecular study. *J Neurol Sci* 102:17–24, 1991.
3. Fukuhara N et al: Myoclonus epilepsy associated with ragged-red fibres (mitochondrial abnormalities): disease entity or a syndrome? *J Neurol Sci* 47:117–133, 1980.
4. Garcia Silva MT et al: The syndrome of myoclonic epilepsy with ragged-red fibers. Report of a case and review of the literature. *Neuropediatrics* 18:200–204, 1987.
5. Matsuoka T et al: Muscle histopathology in myoclonus epilepsy with ragged-red fibers (MERRF). *J Neurol Sci* 106:193–198, 1991.
6. Przyrembel H: Therapy of mitochondrial disorders. *J Inherit Metab Dis* 10:129–146, 1987.
7. Rosing HS et al: Maternally inherited mitochondrial myopathy and myoclonic epilepsy. *Ann Neurol* 17:228–237, 1985.
8. Seibel P et al: Genetic, biochemical, and pathophysiological characterization of a familial mitochondrial encephalomyopathy (MERRF). *J Neurol Sci* 105:217–224, 1991.
9. Shoffner JM, Wallace DC: Mitochondrial genetics: principles and practice. *Am J Hum Genet* 51:1179–1186, 1992.
10. Shoffner JM et al: Myoclonic epilepsy and ragged-red fiber disease (MERRF) is associated with a mitochondrial DNA tRNALys mutation. *Cell* 61:931–937, 1990.
11. Takeda S et al: Neuropathology of myoclonus epilepsy associated with ragged-red fibers (Fukuhara's disease). *Acta Neuropathol* 75:433–440, 1988.
12. Wallace DC et al: Familial mitochondrial encephalomyopathy (MERRF): genetic, pathophysiological, and biochemical characterization of a mitochondrial DNA disease. *Cell* 55:601–610, 1988.
13. Zevianni M et al: Rapid detection of the A → G(8344) mutation of mtDNA in Italian families with myoclonus epilepsy and ragged red fibers (MERRF). *Am J Hum Genet* 48:203–211, 1991.

Mitochondrial encephalomyopathy, ataxia, peripheral neuropathy, progressive myoclonus epilepsy, pigmentary retinopathy, cardiomyopathy, and sensorineural hearing loss (Borud syndrome)

In 1987, Borud et al. (1) described a complex syndrome in several individuals from two unrelated families. In both, hearing loss was the first and most important symptom. Because of the substantial overlap with other mitochondrial encephalomyopathies, this may not be a distinct clinical entity (1–3).

Clinical findings. Manifestations not described in detail included ataxia, cardiomyopathy, muscular fatigue, myoclonic jerks, peripheral neuropathy (type unspecified), and pigmentary retinopathy. Progression was apparently slow.

Auditory system. Slowly progressive hearing loss was first noticed between 18 and 26 years of age and was often the most prominent symptom. In some, it was the only recognized symptom.

Laboratory findings. Lactate and pyruvate levels were normal in blood but elevated in CSF. Biochemical studies showed mild deficiency of complex I.

Pathology. Ragged-red fibers were observed in muscle by light microscopy. Electron microscopy showed large aggregates of subsarcolemmal mitochondria of varying shapes, irregular cristae, and paracrystalline inclusions.

Heredity. Maternal (mitochondrial) inheritance was proven by very high penetrance in children born to affected women through several generations in one family.

Diagnosis. Several mitochondrial encephalomyopathies (especially MERRF) are similar, but hearing loss was more prominent in this family. See Table 10–2.

Prognosis. Details were not provided.

Summary. This disorder is characterized by (*1*) maternal (mitochondrial) inheritance; (*2*) ataxia; (*3*) cardiomyopathy; (*4*) mitochondrial myopathy; (*5*) myoclonic jerks; (*6*) peripheral neuropathy; (*7*) pigmentary retinopathy; and (*8*) sensorineural hearing loss.

References

1. Borud O et al: Increased lactate in cerebrospinal fluid from 7 siblings in a family with mitochondrial myopathy and cerebellar ataxia. *J Inherit Metab Dis* 10:400, 1987.
2. Morgan-Hughes JA et al: Mitochondrial encephalomyopathies: biochemical studies in two cases revealing defects in the respiratory chain. *Brain* 105:553–582, 1982.
3. Torbergsen T et al: Maternal inheritance in a family with mitochondrial encephalomyopathy. In: *Genetics of Neuromuscular Disorders,* Bartsocas CS (ed), Alan R. Liss, New York, 1989, pp 129–133.

Mitochondrial encephalomyopathy, progressive myoclonus epilepsy, ataxia, dementia, diabetes mellitus, nephropathy, and sensorineural hearing loss (Herrmann syndrome)

In 1964, Herrmann et al. (2) reported progressive myoclonus epilepsy, ataxia, dementia, diabetes mellitus, nephropathy, and sensorineural hearing loss in 13 individuals from three generations of a family.

Central nervous system. Light-sensitive myoclonus seizures began in the 20's and persisted, with only partial control from medications. The EEG showed a striking photomyoclonic response. Neurological examination was normal.

General health remained good until the 30's or 40's, when neurological deterioration began, consisting of ataxia, progressive organic dementia, and multiple seizure types. The latter included generalized tonic-clonic seizures in sleep, epilepsia partialis continua, and constant myoclonic jerks. Examination at this stage revealed dementia, dysarthria, dysphagia, hypotonia, diminished or absent tendon reflexes, extensor plantar responses, and eventually ataxia and nystagmus. The proband had right hemianopia, hemiparesis, and hemihypesthesia, possibly related to the seizure disorder, and died at age 43 years, which was about 6 months after onset of the terminal deterioration. The EEG of the proband during the stage of neurological deterioration showed severe generalized disorganization. Photic stimulation elicited generalized spike-and-wave activity accompanied by myoclonic jerks and interruption of consciousness (Fig. 10–36A).

Peripheral nervous system. Although no electrophysiologic studies were reported, clinical observations of ataxia and diminished or absent deep tendon reflexes suggest that neuropathy was another manifestation.

Endocrine system. One probably affected individual had juvenile diabetes mellitus. The proband and her affected cousin had mild diabetes discovered during the stage of progressive deterioration. Her younger sisters had diabetic-type glucose tolerance tests, but no glucosuria under normal conditions.

Renal system. Intravenous pyelograms showed delayed excretion of dye and marked blunting of calyces in the proband and abnormal shape of the calyces in her cousin. No affected family member had overt signs of renal disease.

Auditory system. Progressive hearing loss in the proband and her cousin began at about 35 years, which was several years after the myoclonic jerks.

Serial audiograms were described as consistent with progressive cochlear degeneration. The two affected sisters of the proband had normal hearing and audiograms at ages 28 and 40 years.

Figure 10–36. *Mitochondrial encephalomyopathy, progressive myoclonus epilepsy, ataxia, dementia, diabetes mellitus, nephropathy, and sensorineural hearing loss (Herrmann syndrome).* (A) EEG showing photomyoclonic response. (B) Microscopic appearance of parietal cortex showing diffuse neuronal loss and astrocytosis. (C) Pedigree of kindred showing 13 persons affected in three generations. [From C Herrmann et al., *Neurology* 14:212, 1964.]

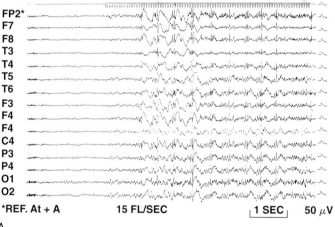

MONITOR   **PHOTIC STIM.**

FP2* F7 F8 T3 T4 T5 T6 F3 F4 F4 C4 P3 P4 O1 O2

*REF. At + A   15 FL/SEC |1 SEC| 50 μV

A

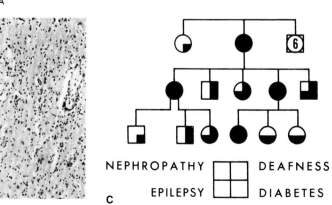

B

C

NEPHROPATHY   DEAFNESS
EPILEPSY   DIABETES

Laboratory findings. Urinalysis was normal except for glucosuria in the proband.

Pathology. Autopsy in the proband was limited to the brain and kidneys. The kidneys showed changes of low-grade glomerulonephritis and pyelonephritis, in addition to fat-filled macrophages (foam cells) and PAS-positive sudanophilic granules in the tubular epithelium. Abnormalities in the brain included (*1*) diffuse neuronal degeneration, which was particularly severe in the cerebral and cerebellar cortex; and (*4*) distension of neurons in the dentate, inferior olivary, brain stem, and other nuclei by a PAS-positive lipid (Fig. 10–36B).

Heredity. From observation of 13 affected individuals from three generations of a family, Herrmann et al. (2) presumed that inheritance was autosomal dominant. However, there is striking overlap between this disorder and several of the mitochondrial encephalomyopathies, especially MERRF, because of the myoclonic seizures. Inspection of the pedigree shows that the disease was always inherited from the mother. Thus, this syndrome probably has maternal (mitochondrial) inheritance (Fig. 10–36C).

Diagnosis. This disorder is similar to several of the mitochondrial encephalomyopathies, especially MERRF: see Table 10–2. Patients with MERRF have an earlier onset of symptoms and lack nephropathy and diabetes mellitus. Patients with progressive myoclonus epilepsy, ataxia, and sensorineural hearing loss (May-White syndrome) also lack renal disease and diabetes mellitus and have slower progression of symptoms. Patients with progressive myoclonus epilepsy, dementia, and hearing loss (Latham-Munro syndrome) lack ataxia; inheritance is autosomal recessive. In future cases, investigations for mitochondrial disorders should be done. In 1994, Feigenbaum et al. (1) described brothers with premature atherosclerosis, photomyoclonic epilepsy, diabetes mellitus, nephropathy, neurodegenerative disorder, sensorineural hearing loss, and death in the third decade. These boys did not have the PAS-positive deposits and did have atherosclerosis.

Prognosis. As in other probable mitochondrial disorders, severity appears to be variable. Complications of this disorder led to death of the two oldest patients in their 40's.

Summary. This disorder is manifested by (*1*) probable maternal (mitochondrial) inheritance; (*2*) progressive myoclonus epilepsy; (*3*) ataxia; (*4*) dementia; (*5*) diabetes mellitus; (*6*) nephropathy; (*7*) possible neuropathy; and (*8*) sensorineural hearing loss.

References

1. Feigenbaum A et al: Premature atherosclerosis with photomyoclonic epilepsy, deafness, diabetes mellitus, nephropathy, and neurodegenerative disorder in two brothers: a new syndrome? *Am J Med Genet* 49:118–124, 1994.
2. Herrmann C et al: Hereditary photomyoclonus associated with diabetes mellitus, deafness, nephropathy, and cerebral dysfunction. *Neurology* 14:212–221, 1964.

Renal tubulopathy, diabetes mellitus, and cerebellar ataxia

Rotig et al. (1) described two sisters with a rapidly progressing multisystem disorder that was found to be caused by duplication of mitochondrial DNA. Their mother was mildly affected.

Nervous system. The younger of the sisters (who lived longer) developed cerebellar ataxia, hypotonia, myoclonic jerks, and psychomotor regression during the fifth year of life.

Ocular system. At age 3 years extraocular muscle palsy, ptosis, and micropunctated pigmentary deposits developed. The electroretinogram was extinguished.

Renal system. One of the earliest manifestations of this condition was a proximal tubulopathy with polyuria and loss of potassium, sodium, calcium, and chlorine.

Skin. At approximately 1 year of age, a mottled pigmentation in photo-exposed areas developed. Erythrocyanosis in response to cold also occurred, primarily affecting digits.

Endocrine system. Anorexia occurred during the first year or so of life in both girls. The younger of the two developed insulin-dependent diabetes at age 5 years, followed by the development of major obesity.

Auditory system. Hearing loss developed around the same time as the other neurologic manifestations. The mother, who had mosaicism for the mitochondrial duplication, had hypoacusis in adulthood.

Laboratory findings. Heteroplasmy for duplication of a segment of the mitochondrial genome was detected using Southern blot analysis.

Pathology. Muscle biopsy in one child demonstrated ragged-red fibers. Metabolic assay of the biopsy suggested complex III deficiency, which was thought to be secondary to the mitochondrial genes affected by the formation of the duplication.

Diagnosis. The multisystem involvement, with progression, should clearly suggest a mitochondrial disorder.

Prognosis. This condition was rapidly progressive in the two daughters, with death occurring secondary to dehydration at ages 5 and 8 years. The mother, who had a lower level of mitochondrial duplication, had myopia, hypoacusis, and muscle weakness develop in adulthood.

Reference

1. Rotig A et al: Maternally inherited duplication of the mitochondrial genome in a syndrome of proximal tubulopathy, diabetes mellitus, and cerebellar ataxia. *Am J Hum Genet* 50:364–370, 1992.

Disorders with Mitochondrial Involvement, but Autosomal Inheritance

Mitochondrial encephalomyopathy, ataxia, amyotrophy, progressive myoclonus epilepsy, bone marrow hypoplasia, nephropathy, thyroid dysfunction, and sensorineural hearing loss (Cutler syndrome)

In 1978, Cutler et al. (1) described two sibs wth ataxia, amyotrophy, progressive myoclonus epilepsy, anemia and other signs such as bone marrow dysfunction, and nephropathy with chronic renal failure. While biochemical studies were not reported, the observation of myoclonus epilepsy and striking morphological changes of mitochondria suggests classification as a mitochondrial encephalomyopathy.

Renal system. Chronic renal failure manifested by anemia, acidosis, and azotemia was diagnosed between 1 and 3 years of age, but was probably congenital. The renal insufficiency progressed slowly thereafter, with mild elevation of creatinine, striking elevation of BUN, hyperuricemia, etc.

Hematological system. Anemia was present in infancy, probably due to the renal disease. During childhood, routine blood counts showed signs of bone marrow hypoplasia including persistent anemia, low white count, low platelet count, some megakaryocytes, and occasional giant platelets.

Central nervous system. Early development was apparently normal. Neurological abnormalities began at about 8–9 years of age, and consisted of ataxia, weakness, wasting, hemiparesis, headaches, and seizures. The initial seizures were myoclonic, but tonic-clonic seizures followed; both were refractory to treatment. One child died of complications of status epilepticus. Cranial CT scan and EMG shortly after onset of neurological symptoms were both normal in one child.

Endocrine system. Diffuse goiters were detected in childhood, also at age 8–9 years. Thyroid function studies suggested an organification defect.

Auditory system. Sensorineural hearing loss began at about the same time as the neurological symptoms, but no further description was provided.

Pathology. Pathologic changes in the kidneys at biopsy and autopsy consisted of an interstitial and tubular nephropathy with secondary glomerular sclerosis.

Immunofluorescence studies were negative. Electron microscopy showed tubular atrophy, increased numbers of tubular lysosomes, and irregular mitochondria that varied considerably in size and shape and contained numerous granules. Thyroid examination showed a simple colloid goiter.

Neuropathological abnormalities consisted of minimal periventricular gliosis and demyelination in the cerebral hemispheres with some perivascular rarefaction in the white matter and basal ganglia. The cerebellum showed striking changes consisting of severe demyelination of the white matter as well as severe neuronal loss in the dentate nuclei, granular layer, and Purkinje cell layer of the cortex, which could not be explained by edema or hypoxia. Peripheral nerves and muscle were normal.

Heredity. In this family, two sibs were affected. Although autosomal recessive inheritance is most likely, other patterns including maternal (mitochondrial) transmission cannot be excluded. The inheritance pattern is thus unknown.

Diagnosis. Patients with Alport syndrome have nephropathy, thrombocytopenia, and hearing loss, but no neurological abnormalities. Inheritance is autosomal dominant. Patients with nephropathy, macrothrombocytopathia, and hearing loss (Epstein syndrome) also lack neurological and thyroid symptoms. Patients with Pendred syndrome have goiter due to organification defect and hearing loss but lack other symptoms. Patients with mesangial IgA nephropathy, spastic paraplegia, mental retardation, and sensorineural hearing loss (Fitzsimmons syndrome) lack ataxia, myoclonus epilepsy, and thyroid disease. The syndromes with the greatest overlap are MERRF syndrome and mitochondrial encephalopathy, progressive myoclonus epilepsy, ataxia, dementia, and diabetes mellitus, nephropathy, and sensorineural hearing loss (Herrmann syndrome). The former lacks the renal, thyroid, and hematological changes. The latter lacks only thyroid disease. Both are mitochondrial encephalomyopathies; see Table 10–2.

Prognosis. The affected sibs died at 10 and 13 years of age from complications of the neurological disorder.

Summary. This disorder is characterized by (*1*) unknown, possibly autosomal recessive, inheritance; (*2*) ataxia; (*3*) amyotrophy; (*4*) progressive myoclonus epilepsy; (*5*) bone marrow hypoplasia causing anemia, leukopenia, and thrombocytopenia; (*6*) nephropathy; (*7*) thyroid disease with goiter; and (*8*) sensorineural hearing loss.

Reference

1. Cutler EA et al: A familial thyrocerebral-renal syndrome: a newly recognized disorder. *Birth Defects* 14(6B):265–274, 1978.

Mitochondrial encephalomyopathy, ataxia, ophthalmoplegia, ptosis, optic atrophy, and sensorineural hearing loss (Treft syndrome)

In 1984, Treft et al. (1) described a syndrome very similar to Kearns-Sayre syndrome but with a different pattern of inheritance in 23 individuals from a single family.

Ocular system. Visual loss was first noticed between 6 and 19 years of age and was slowly progressive. Visual acuity varied from 20/30 to 20/400 with more severe loss in older individuals. Color vision was also impaired. Central or centrocecal scotomas were found in 3 of 14 patients tested. Fundoscopy showed optic pallor that varied from mild temporal pallor in younger individuals to severe, generalized optic atrophy in their older relatives (Fig. 10–37).

Ptosis was first noticed at about age 40 years and was surgically corrected in the two oldest family members. A mild to moderate (10–20 degree) restriction of gaze, most noticeable on upward gaze, was present in older individuals.

Electroretinograms showed subnormal photopic B-waves in half of the affected individuals. The more severely affected individuals also had subnormal photopic A-wave, and scotopic A- and B-wave amplitudes. Electrooculograms and pattern shift visual-evoked responses were normal.

Central nervous system. Neurological abnormalities were reported in 9 of 17 living affected persons, including 6 with mild to moderate gait ataxia. Other abnormalities included hypoactive tendon reflexes, diminished vibratory sensation, and mild facial weakness.

Peripheral nervous system and muscular system. Several affected family members had mild facial weakness. Electromyography in three persons showed normal NCS and myopathic changes on needle exam.

Auditory system. Hearing loss was first recognized between ages 6 and 28 years, often at the same time or soon after the visual loss. Tinnitus was sometimes present. Results of pure-tone audiometry varied from normal to severe hearing loss. Specific abnormalities included positive rollover, elevated or absent acoustic reflex, positive reflex decay, and abnormal threshold tone decay. Brain stem auditory evoked responses showed either delayed and low amplitude or absent first peak. These results were interpreted as being consistent with eighth nerve (sensorineural) dysfunction.

Laboratory findings. Serum lactate was slightly increased to 1.6 mEq/L (normal 0.2–1.2 mEq/L) in one patient, but pyruvate was normal.

Pathology. Biopsy of the left lateral palpebral muscle in one patient showed numerous ragged-red fibers (some ragged-red fibers may be seen in normal extraocular muscle), while biopsy of the biceps muscle showed only 1%–2% ragged-red fibers. On electron microscopy, numerous mitochondria with increased glycogen and lipid deposition were seen in the subsarcolemmal area of the muscle fibers. Muscle biopsies were normal or showed nonspecific changes in two other patients.

Heredity. Inheritance of this disorder is clearly autosomal dominant, as demonstrated by male-to-male transmission.

Diagnosis. Patients with Kearns-Sayre syndrome (KSS) usually have pigmentary retinopathy, cardiac conduction defects, and more severe myopathy, which this syndrome lacks. Milder expression of KSS could present with identical manifestations. However, the two disorders are different because KSS has maternal inheritance, while this disorder has autosomal dominant inheritance. The ragged-red fibers and lactic acidosis extend the similarity between the two syndromes; see Table 10–2.

Prognosis. Most of the older family members were significantly disabled by the combined visual and hearing deficits. The other abnormalities were usually not severe. None of the affected members was demented.

Summary. This disorder is characterized by (1) autosomal dominant inheritance; (2) ataxia; (3) ptosis and ophthalmoplegia; (4) optic atrophy; (5) mild mitochondrial myopathy; and (6) sensorineural hearing loss.

Reference

1. Treft RL et al: Dominant optic atrophy, deafness, ptosis, ophthalmoplegia, dystaxia, and myopathy: a new syndrome. *Ophthalmology* 91:908–915, 1984.

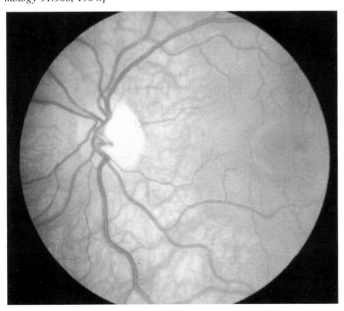

Figure 10–37. *Mitochondrial encephalomyopathy, ataxia, ophthalmoplegia, ptosis, optic atrophy, and sensorineural hearing loss (Treft syndrome).* Fundus photograph showing optic atrophy. [From RL Treft et al., *Ophthalmology* 91:908, 1984.]

Mitochondrial encephalomyopathy, gastrointestinal disease, motor and sensory neuropathy, ophthalmoplegia, and sensorineural hearing loss (MNGIE syndrome)

MNGIE (myo-, neuro-, gastrointestinal encephalopathy) syndrome, another mitochondrial encephalomyopathy, has been described in several individuals (1–5,8). Biochemical studies in three patients showed partial deficiency of cytochrome C oxidase (1).

Physical findings. Growth deficiency was common.

Gastrointestinal system. Diarrhea, malabsorption, cachexia, and weight loss, which may be intermittent or continuous, began in childhood and were the earliest and most prominent symptoms. Pancreatic function was normal. Barium X-rays late in the course of the disorder of the first patient showed inflammatory changes of the intestines, and she died at age 42. There are rare reports of individuals who do not have this manifestation (4).

Ocular system. Progressive ptosis and external ophthalmoplegia began in the 20's, well after the GI symptoms.

Central nervous system. There was no history of ataxia, dementia, seizures, or related problems. However, CT and MRI scans showed pronounced white matter hypodensity in older individuals.

Peripheral nervous system and muscular system. Generalized or proximal limb weakness and muscle atrophy began in the 30's. Tendon reflexes were diminished, but sensation remained normal. Later symptoms included paresthesias, loss of joint position (especially in the legs), and steppage gait. Electromyography showed myopathic changes. Both motor and sensory nerve conduction velocities were decreased.

Auditory system. Progressive sensorineural hearing loss was first recognized in the 30's.

Radiologic findings. Magnetic resonance imaging of the head showed diffuse white matter disease (2,9).

Laboratory findings. In one patient, CSF protein was mildly increased. In the others, blood and CSF lactate were increased. Biochemical analysis of isolated muscle mitochondria showed an isolated partial defect of complex IV of the respiratory chain (cytochrome C oxidase) in the three patients tested. Southern analysis of mitochon-drial DNA in patients showed multiple mtDNA deletions in skeletal muscle (6).

Pathology. All muscles examined showed ragged-red fibers, scattered fibers devoid of cytochrome C oxidase activity, and signs of denervation. Peripheral nerves showed mixed axonal degenerative and demyelinating features. The brain had minimal pathological changes, suggestive of an ill-defined leukoencephalopathy.

The stomach and small intestine were distended and thickened because of fibrosis of the submucosa and subserosa and because of hypertrophy of the tunica muscularis mucosae. The liver showed extensive fibrosis with focal transition to cirrhosis.

Heredity. This is an autosomal recessive trait, based on the finding of affected sibs with normal parents in some families, and consanguinity in others (5). Hirano et al. (6) subsequently mapped the MNGIE locus to 22q13.32–qter. Nishino et al. (7) identified mutations in the thymidine phosphorylase gene (*ECGFI*), which maps to this region. Suomalainen and Kaukonen (8) suggested that the gene mutation affects mitochondrial DNA stability, leading to deletions and depletion of mtDNA.

Diagnosis. The syndrome of motor and sensory neuropathy, intestinal pseudo-obstruction, leukoencephalopathy, ophthalmoplegia, and sensorineural hearing loss (POLIP syndrome) seems clinically indistinguishable, but ragged-red fibers were not described. Intestinal pseudo-obstruction also occurs without other abnormalities; see Table 10–2.

Prognosis. Severe disability and often death are the outcome.

Summary. This disorder is characterized by (*1*) autosomal recessive or maternal inheritance; (*2*) ptosis and ophthalmoplegia; (*3*) mitochondrial myopathy with ragged-red fibers; (*4*) motor and sensory neuropathy; (*5*) gastrointestinal disease; (*6*) growth deficiency; and (*7*) sensorineural hearing loss.

References

1. Bardosi A et al: Myo-, neuro-, gastrointestinal encephalopathy (MNGIE syndrome) due to partial deficiency of cytochrome C oxidase: a new mitochondrial multisystem disorder. *Acta Neuropathol* 74:248–258, 1987.
2. Blake D et al: MNGIE syndrome: report of 2 new patients. *Neurology* 40(Suppl 1):294, 1990.
3. Cervera R et al: Chronic intestinal pseudoobstruction and ophthalmoplegia in a patient with mitochondrial myopathy. *Gut* 29:544–547, 1988.
4. Gamez J et al: Phenotypic variability in a Spanish family with MNGIE. *Neurology* 59:455–457, 2002.
5. Hirano M et al: Mitochondrial neurogastrointestinal encephalomyopathy (MNGIE): clinical, biochemical, and genetic features of an autosomal recessive mitochondrial disorder. *Neurology* 44:721–727, 1994.
6. Hirano M et al: Mitochondrial neurogastrointestinal encephalomyopathy syndrome maps to chromosome 22q13.32–qter. *Am J Hum Genet* 63:526–533, 1998.
7. Nishino I et al: Thymidine phosphorylase gene mutations in MNGIE, a human mitochondrial disorder. *Science* 283:689–692, 1999.
8. Suomalainen A, Kaukonen J: Diseased caused by nuclear genes affecting mtDNA stability. *Am J Med Genet* 106:53–61, 2001.
9. Threlkeld AB et al: Ophthalmic involvement in myo-neuro-gastrointestinal encephalopathy syndrome. *Am J Ophthalmol* 114:322–328, 1992.

Atherosclerosis, deafness, nephropathy, diabetes mellitus, photomyoclonus, and degenerative neurologic disease (Feigenbaum syndrome)

Feigenbaum et al. (1) described two brothers with sensorineural hearing loss, diabetes mellitus, renal function deterioration, and progressive neurologic deterioration with photomyoclonic seizures. The first presentation of this condition is sensorineural hearing loss, which becomes manifest at age 5 years. In the late teens to early 20's, joint stiffness, decline in cognitive function, and weakness develop. The neurologic symptoms ultimately lead to spasticity, incoordination, weakness, and further cognitive decline. Anemia, insulin-dependent diabetes mellitus, nephrotic syndrome, and photomyoclonic seizures also appear around this time. Like neurologic function, renal function also deteriorates. Renal biopsy during the last part of life showed diffuse arteriolar sclerosis; skin biopsy showed reduction of some respiratory chain enzymes. Death occurred at age 31 in one brother and at 28 in the other. Autopsy findings in one brother demonstrated severe atherosclerosis, extensive and severe neuronal loss, and gliosis of brain and spinal cord. Inheritance was considered to be autosomal recessive, X-linked recessive, or mitochondrial.

Reference

1. Feigenbaum A et al: Premature atherosclerosis with photomyoclonic epilepsy, deafness, diabetes mellitus, nephropathy, and neurodegenerative disorder in two brothers: a new syndrome? *Am J Med Genet* 49:118–124, 1994.

Appendix

Other conditions with neurologic involvement, excluding mental retardation

Entity	Neurologic Finding	Chapter in this Book
Retinitis pigmentosa, nystagmus, hemiplegic migraine, SHL	Migraine	7 (eye)
Infantile Refsum syndrome	Ataxia	7 (eye)
Nucci syndrome	Spasticity	7 (eye)
Berk-Tabatznik syndrome	Spastic quadriparesis	7 (eye)
Oral-facial-digital syndrome VI	Cerebellar hypoplasia	8 (musculoskeletal)
Lemieux-Neemeh syndrome	Motor and sensory neuropathy	9 (renal)
Nephritis, myopathy, corneal crystals, and conductive hearing loss	Myopathy	9 (renal)
Fitzsimmons syndrome	Spastic paraplegia	9 (renal)
BRESHECK syndrome	Brain abnormalities	9 (renal)
Phosphoribosyl pyrophosphate synthase superactivity	Ataxia	13 (metabolic)
Levy-Chung syndrome	Congenital myopathy	14 (integumentary)
Growth retardation, mental retardation, microcephaly, seizures, dermatosis, SHL	Seizures	14 (integumentary)
Hypodontia, peg-shaped teeth, olivopontocerebellar dysplasia, hypogonadism	Olivopontocerebellar dysplasia	15 (oral and dental)

SNL, sensorineural hearing loss.

Chapter 11
Genetic Hearing Loss Associated with Cardiac Defects

ANGELA E. LIN AND HOLLY H. ARDINGER

In several hearing loss syndromes cardiac abnormalities are common or distinctive. The term *cardiac abnormality* encompasses rhythm and conduction disturbances, cardiovascular malformations (CVMs), and cardiomyopathy. All have been associated with hearing loss in genetic syndromes. The disorders discussed below were selected because they are either common conditions with frequent hearing loss and cardiac abnormalities, or uncommon, but distinctive, conditions. Disorders discussed elsewhere in this book, or disorders in which the cardiac abnormalities are uncommon and not distinctive, have been omitted.

Long-QT syndrome (LQTS) with deafness (Jervell and Lange-Nielsen syndrome, cardioauditory syndrome, surdocardiac syndrome)

Among the disorders associated with deafness and cardiac abnormalities, the Jervell and Lange-Nielsen syndrome is well known for its high morbidity and mortality and for its intriguing genetic aspects. In 1957, Jervell and Lange-Nielsen (12) described profound congenital sensorineural hearing loss, electrocardiographic abnormalities characterized by a long QT interval, repeated syncopal episodes, and sudden unexplained death in Norwegian children (Fig. 11–1A).

The Romano-Ward syndrome is also characterized by a long QT interval, syncope, and sudden death, but hearing loss does not occur. Though once considered distinct from Jervell and Lange-Nielsen syndrome, these conditions are now known to be allelic. Most recent surveys discuss them together as long-QT syndromes (LQTS). An international, prospective, longitudinal study of LQTS has systematically studied patients with deafness (Jervell and Lange-Nielsen syndrome, autosomal recessive) and without deafness (Romano-Ward syndrome, autosomal dominant) (14,21,24).

The Jervell and Lange-Nielsen syndrome is rare with an estimated incidence of 1.6 to 6 cases per million (7), which compares to the 1/10,000 to 1/15,000 incidence of all forms of LQTS (1). The frequency of Jervell and Lange-Nielsen LQTS among those with congenital profound sensorineural hearing loss is about 25/10,000 (6,7,10,16). This corresponds to roughly 1/100,000 in the general population. Conversely, Moss et al. (14) found that 7% of 328 probands with LQTS had profound sensorineural hearing loss.

Cardiovascular system. Affected children present with attacks ranging from pallor and palmar sweating to syncope (fainting with transient loss of consciousness), seizures, or aborted sudden death (cardiac arrest with resuscitation, near drowning) (1,3,14). Most present between infancy and adolescence, with a mean age of 10 years. However, the disorder may first manifest in older patients. In a study of LQTS (which included those with and without deafness), death occurred predominantly in young patients (57% by age 20 years) who were untreated (14). The types of cardiac arrhythmia include ventricular tachycardia (torsade de pointes) or fibrillation, and asystole (1). In most cases, fainting spells are precipitated by fear, excitement, exercise, loud noises, or physical exertion (14). They also vary in frequency; some patients have several syncopal attacks each month, others have only a few each year, while still others have one or two episodes their entire life. The syncopal attacks occur less frequently with age.

The hypothesis that LQTS and sudden infant death syndrome are related continues to be investigated and fiercely debated (13,17, 18,22). The Jervell and Lange-Nielsen syndrome, per se, has not been implicated.

The electrocardiographic changes include a long QT interval with usually broad T waves, which can be upright, notched, biphasic, or inverted (Fig. 12–1A). Commonly there is a resting bradycardia that fails to accelerate normally with exercise. The degree of QT prolongation varies both within and between families and from day to day in the same patient. Alternation in height or polarity of the T waves heralds imminent risk of arrhythmia. Since the QT interval varies with heart rate, the QT interval is corrected for heart rate (QTc) using the traditional Bazett's formula (prolongation beyond 460 msec is abnormal). However, recent studies (20) have used a lower limit (450 msec) if a patient is symptomatic with syncope, seizures, or aborted sudden death.

Auditory system. By definition, all patients have congenital bilateral profound sensorineural hearing loss (6–9,11,12,16). Temporal bone changes of the Scheibe type were described by Friedmann et al. (8,9). The most unique change was the accumulation of PAS-positive hyaline aggregates in an atrophic stria vascularis. There was almost complete degeneration of the organ of Corti and loss of sensory cells. The tectorial membrane was shrunken or retracted, and Reissner's membrane was adherent to the basilar membrane, practically obliterating the cochlear duct. The sensory epithelium of the utricle and saccule was atrophic, and the cristae were disorganized. There was moderate loss of spiral ganglion cells (Fig. 11–1B).

Vestibular system. Vestibular changes have not been described.

Pathology. Autopsies have been done in numerous cases. Gross and histologic examinations of the heart have exhibited no abnormalities in most cases (19). In some, special examination of the conducting system of the heart showed focal inflammatory degeneration of nerves and ganglia, the changes being most marked around the sinus and atrioventricular (AV) nodes, but other studies have not confirmed these findings (19). Bharati et al. (5) studied the conduction system and myocardium in six patients with LQTS, one of whom had Jervell and Lange-Nielsen syndrome. All had marked fatty infiltration in the approaches to the AV node and inflamed ventricular myocardium.

Heredity. The Long-QT syndromes display genetic allelism and heterogeneity (21). The Jervell and Lange-Nielsen syndrome has autosomal recessive inheritance and consanguinity is common (7,16). It is caused by homozygosity for a mutation in the *KVLQT1* gene on 11p15.5 (20) or by the *KCNE1* gene on 21q22.1 (21). In contrast, the dominant form of LQTS which lacks deafness (Romano-Ward syndrome) is caused by a heterozygous mutation in *KVLQT1* and other genes (21,24).

Accurate genetic counseling is imperative. Although the deafness in Jervell and Lange-Nielsen syndrome is caused by two genes, the potential cardiac phenotype is caused by one gene. Thus, both parents of a child with Jervell and Lange-Nielsen syndrome are obligate carriers (heterozygotes) for deafness. As such, they are also heterozygotes for the Romano-Ward long-QT interval syndrome and thus are at risk for cardiac arrhythmia (1,20).

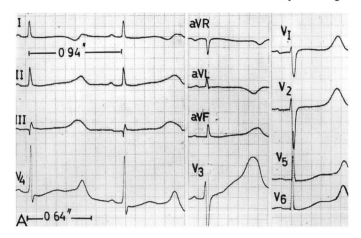

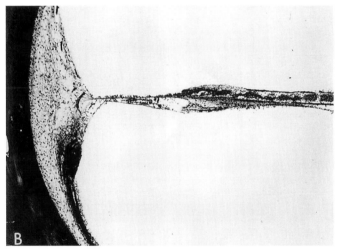

Figure 11–1. *Long-QT syndrome (LQTS) with deafness (Jervell and Lange-Nielsen syndrome, cardioauditory syndrome, surdocardiac syndrome.* (A) Electrocardiogram of a patient showing QT interval of 0.64 sec (0.41 sec is upper limit of normal). (B) Photomicrograph of cochlea showing adherent Reissner's membrane, degenerated organ of Corti, atrophic stria vascularis, and deposit of PAS-positive material. [(A) from A Jervell et al., *Am Heart J* 72:582, 1966; (B) from I Friedmann et al., *J Laryngol Otol* 80:451, 1966.]

If a sibling of the deaf proband is not deaf, then the sibling cannot have two abnormal genes (or else the sibling would be deaf). The remaining three possibilities include one abnormal gene from mother/one normal gene from father, one abnormal gene from father/one normal gene from mother, or two normal genes. Thus, the risk of having LQTS would be two out of three (66%).

The LQTS syndromes belong to the class of diseases caused by defective myocardial ion channels (2). A genotype–phenotype correlation has been suggested by Zareba et al. (24). Although measurement of the corrected QT interval remains the most commonly used (though imperfect) diagnostic test, molecular genetic testing plays a growing role (23).

Diagnosis. The diagnosis of any LQTS can be a formidable challenge. The presence of sensorineural deafness in Jervell and Lange-Nielsen syndrome facilitates recognition. As mentioned above, a long QT interval, syncopal attacks, and sudden death without hearing loss typify the autosomal dominant Romano-Ward syndrome. It is much more common than Jervell and Lange-Nielsen syndrome and symptoms are generally milder. In most studies of LQTS, Romano-Ward syndrome patients are predominant (20). In Refsum syndrome there is sensorineural hearing loss, cardiac conduction abnormalities with prolongation of the QT interval and abnormal T waves, and, occasionally, sud-

den death. The hearing loss in Refsum syndrome, however, has onset in adulthood and serum phytanic acid levels are elevated.

Fainting spells in Jervell and Lange-Nielsen syndrome may be erroneously diagnosed as epileptic seizures (12). However, the electroencephalogram is normal, whereas the electrocardiogram is grossly bizarre. Furthermore, the patients do not have profound stupor following the fainting episodes. There are several atypical cases. Furlanello et al. (10) and Athanasiou and Muller-Seydlitz (4) also described a dominant form in adults with mild hearing loss and multiple pigmented nevi. Possibly these patients had LEOPARD syndrome or multiple pigmented nevi and sensorineural hearing loss.

The reader should bear in mind that prolongation of the QT interval can be caused by a variety of drugs. Most common are diuretics that cause hypokalemia and/or some calcium channel–blocking drugs. Other drugs such quinidine, phenothiazine, imipramine, and amiodarone have been implicated, as has been hypomagnesemia. However, there is new evidence that what appears to be an "acquired" drug-induced QT prolongation may have a genetic substrate. In one Italian family, drug-induced QT prolongation was related to the presence of an otherwise clinically silent mutation of the *KVLQT1* gene (15). This introduces the tantalizing vision of prospective testing to identify individuals at risk for life-threatening arrhythmias.

Prognosis. There is little progression of the hearing loss over the years. Affected persons have a variable number of syncopal attacks. In patients with untreated LQTS (all forms), the 10-year mortality rate is at least 50% (1). Prognosis is improved by preventing syncopal attacks with beta-blocking agents, pacemaker and/or defibrillator implantation, and left cervicothoracic sympathetic ganglionectomy (1).

Summary. The major features of this syndrome include (*1*) autosomal recessive transmission; (*2*) long QT interval; (*3*) recurrent syncope or aborted sudden death beginning in early childhood and occasionally resulting in death; and (*4*) congenital severe sensorineural hearing loss.

References

1. Ackerman MJ. The QT syndrome. *Pediatr Review* 19:232–238, 1998.
2. Ackerman MJ, Clapham DE: Ion channels—basic science and clinical disease. *N Engl J Med* 336:1575–1587, 1997.
3. Ackerman MJ et al: Molecular diagnosis of the inherited long-QT syndrome in a woman who died after near-drowning. *N Engl J Med* 341:1121–1125, 1999.
4. Athanasiou DJ, Muller-Seydlitz PM: Weitere Beobachtungen zum Jervell und Lanage-Nielsen-Syndrom. *Munch Med Wochenschr* 114:1961–1965, 1972.
5. Bharati S et al: The conduction system in patients with a prolonged QT interval. *J Am Coll Cardiol* 6:1110–1119, 1985.
6. Fay JE et al: Surdo-cardiac syndrome: incidence among children in schools for the deaf. *Can Med Assoc J* 105:718–720, 1971.
7. Fraser GR et al: Congenital deafness associated with electrocardiographic abnormalities, fainting attacks, and sudden death: a recessive syndrome. *Q J Med* 33:361–385, 1964.
8. Friedmann I et al: Pathology of the ear in the cardioauditory syndrome of Jervell and Lange-Nielsen (recessive deafness with electrocardiographic abnormalities). *J Laryngol Otol* 80:451–479, 1966.
9. Friedmann I et al: Pathology of the ear in the cardioauditory syndrome of Jervell and Lange-Nielsen. Report of a third case with an appendix on possible linkage with the Rh blood group locus. *J Laryngol Otol* 82:883–896, 1968.
10. Furlanello F et al: Observation on a case of Jervell and Lange-Nielsen syndrome in an adult. *Br Heart J* 34:648–662, 1972.
11. Jervell A: The surdo-cardiac syndrome. *Eur Heart J* 6 (Suppl D):97–102, 1985.
12. Jervell A, Lange-Nielsen F: Congenital deaf-mutism, functional heart disease with prolongation of the QT interval, and sudden death. *Am Heart J* 54:59–68, 1957.
13. Lucey JF: Comments on a sudden infant death article in another journal. *Pediatrics* 103:812, 1999.
14. Moss AJ et al: The long QT syndrome. Prospective longitudinal study of 328 families. *Circulation* 84:1136–1144, 1991.
15. Napolitano C et al: Evidence for a cardiac ion channel mutation underlying drug-induced QT prolongation and life-threatening arrhythmias. *J Cardiovasc Electrophysiol* 11:691–696, 2000.

16. Sanchez Cascos A et al: Cardioauditory syndromes. Cardiac and genetic study of 511 deaf-mute children. *Br Heart J* 31:26–33, 1969.
17. Schwartz PJ et al: Prolongation of the QT interval and the sudden infant death syndrome. *N Engl J Med* 338:1709–1714, 1998.
18. Schwartz PJ et al: A molecular link between the sudden infant death syndrome and the long-QT syndrome. *N Engl J Med* 343:262–267, 2000.
19. Smith W: The long Q-T syndrome. *Aust NZ J Med* 14:700–704, 1984.
20. Splawski I et al: Molecular basis of the long-QT syndrome associated with deafness. *N Engl J Med* 336:1562–1567, 1997.
21. Splawski I et al: Spectrum of mutations in long-QT syndrome genes: *KVLQT1, HERG, SCN5A, KCNE1* and *KCNE2. Circulation* 102:1178–1185, 2000.
22. Towbin JA, Friedman RA: Prolongation of the QT interval and the sudden infant death syndrome. *N Engl J Med* 338:1760–1761, 1998.
23. Vincent GM et al: The spectrum of symptoms and QT intervals in carriers of the gene for the long-QT syndrome. *N Engl J Med* 327:846–852, 1992.
24. Zareba W et al: Influence of the genotype on the clinical course of the long-QT syndrome. *N Engl J Med* 339;960–965, 1998.

DiGeorge sequence

Angelo DiGeorge first described cases of hypoparathyroidism, thymic hypoplasia, and recurrent infection, providing the first clinical role for the thymus in immunity (7,14). DiGeorge complex (or sequence) is a heterogeneous entity considered to be related to maldevelopment of structures derived from the third and fourth pharyngeal pouches. Manifestations include absence or hypoplasia or the thymus and/or parathyroid glands (16). However, they can also include cardiovascular anomalies, particularly those of conotruncal derivation, and facial anomalies (5,17). Minimal diagnostic criteria include two of three major signs, which include (*1*) conotruncal heart defect, (*2*) T-cell deficiency, and (*3*) hypocalcemia/hypoparathyroidism (2). A significant proportion of DiGeorge sequence is caused by deletion 22q, with estimates ranging around 90% of those with DiGeorge sequence having a detectable deletion (either cytogenetically or via FISH probes that hybridize to the commonly deleted region) (8,9,22). More recently a deletion at 10p13–14 has been found in approximately 10% of those with Di George sequence (3). Other causes include teratogenic mechanisms (maternal diabetes, prenatal alcohol exposure, and retinoid embryopathy (1,12,15,28) and other chromosome anomalies (13,24,25).

Cardiovascular system. Heart defects are exceedingly common, and most involve structures considered conotruncal in origin. One of the most common is type B interrupted aortic arch, which occurs with aberrant right subclavian artery. Persistent truncus arteriosus is also a common finding, as are defects involving pulmonary arteries and tetralogy of Fallot (4,5,17,20,27).

Craniofacial findings. The most common manifestations are those associated with 22q deletion and include telecanthus with short, and often narrow, palpebral fissures; broad nasal root; prominent nose with bulbous tip and small nares; short philtrum; small mouth; micrognathia; and somewhat anomalous ears are common. Bifid uvula and highly arched or cleft palate are common oral manifestations (5,11,16,17,18).

In patients with 10p deletions common craniofacial manifestations include dysplastic or low-set ears and palatal abnormalities (6). In a recent review of DiGeorge sequence patients without 22q or 10p deletions, common craniofacial anomalies included cleft or highly arched palate and choanal atresia (2).

Other findings. Mental retardation is generally severe in those with 10p deletion, whereas cognitive development ranges from mild to no impairment in those with 22q deletion (11,26). Renal anomalies are also slightly more common in those with 10p deletion than in those with 22q deletion; they also appear to be relatively common in those with DiGeorge sequence secondary to maternal diabetes (25,29). For a more detailed discussion of 22q deletion syndrome, see Chapter 16.

Auditory system. DiGeorge patients with 22q deletions can have both external and internal ear defects. Auricular anomalies, one or more of which may be present in 80%, include small, low-set, or rotated ears, cupped or protruding ears, and helical anomalies (10). Most recent studies have found that 40%–50% of patients with hearing loss have a loss of >25 dB in at least one ear (10,21,23). The vast majority of hearing loss is conductive (70%–90%) and attributable to chronic otitis media. Palatal anomalies and velopharyngeal insufficiency are the likely causes of a high proportion of recurrent middle ear disease leading to hearing loss (10,21). Sensorineural or mixed hearing loss is seen in 5%–15% of patients, often affecting the low frequencies more severely (21,23).

DiGeorge patients with a deletion at 10p13 appear to have a higher percentage of sensorineural hearing loss (41%). The hearing loss tends to be bilateral and progressive, ranging in a loss from 40 dB to profound deafness (25).

Pathology. Temporal bone studies note a variety of defects in some DiGeorge patients, including Mondini dysplasia, shortened cochlea, and ossicular defects (19).

Laboratory. Appropriate cytogenetic evaluations and use of FISH probes can identify those with 22q or 10p deletions, as well as possibly some other cytogenetic rearrangements. Hypocalcemia and deficiency of T cells should be sought.

Heredity. As noted above, DiGeorge sequence is heterogeneous, with most cases caused by deletions in 22q.

Diagnosis. DiGeorge sequence can overlap with oculo-auriculovertebral spectrum and CHARGE association.

Summary. DiGeorge sequence is characterized by (at least two of three) (*1*) cardiac defects; (*2*) thymus hypoplasia and/or T cell–mediated immunodeficiency; and (*3*) hypocalcemia and/or absence of parathyroids. In addition, most cases are attributable to deletion of 22q11.2.

References

1. Ammann AJ et al: The DiGeorge syndrome and the fetal alcohol syndrome. *Am J Dis Child* 136:906–908, 1982.
2. Bartsch O et al: No evidence for chromosomal microdeletions at the second DiGeorge syndrome locus on 10p near D10S585. *Am J Med Genet* 83:425–426, 1999.
3. Berend SA et al: Dual-probe fluorescence in situ hybridization assay for detecting deletions associated with VCFS/DiGeorge sydnrome I and DiGeorge syndrome II loci. *Am J Med Genet* 91:313–317, 2000.
4. Carey JC et al: Spectrum of the DiGeorge "syndrome". *J Pediatr* 96:955–956, 1980.
5. Conley ME et al: The spectrum of the DiGeorge "syndrome". *J Pediatr* 94:883–890, 1979.
6. Daw SCM et al: A common region of 10p deleeted in DiGeorge and velo-cardiofacial syndromes. *Nat Genet* 13:458–460, 1996.
7. DiGeorge AM: Discussion on a new concept of the cellular basis of immunology. *J Pediatr* 67:907, 1965.
8. Driscoll D et al: A genetic etiology for DiGeorge syndrome: consistent deletions and microdeletions of 22q11. *Am J Hum Genet* 50:924–933, 1992.
9. Driscoll D et al: Deletions and microdeletions of 22q11.2 in velo-cardio-facial syndrome. *Am J Med Genet* 44:261–268, 1992.
10. Ford LC et al: Otolaryngological manifestations of velocardiofacial syndrome: a retrospective review of 35 patients. *Laryngoscope* 110:362–367, 2000.
11. Goldberg R et al: Velo-cardio-facial syndrome: a review of 120 patients. *Am J Med Genet* 45:313–319, 1993.
12. Gosseye S et al: Association of bilateral renal agenesis and DiGeorge syndrome in an infant of a diabetic mother. *Helv Paediatr Acta* 37:471–474, 1982.
13. Greenberg F et al: Prenatal diagnosis of deletion 17p13 associated with DiGeorge anomaly. *Am J Med Genet* 31:1–4, 1988.
14. Hong R: The DiGeorge anomaly (CATCH 22, DiGeorge/velocardiofacial syndrome). *Semin Hematol* 35:282–290, 1998.
15. Lammer EJ et al: Retinoic acid embryopathy. *N Engl J Med* 313:837–841, 1985.
16. Lischner HW: DiGeorge's syndrome(s). *J Pediatr* 81:1042–1044, 1972.
17. Miller MJ et al: Branchial anomalies in idiopathic hypoparathyroidism: branchial dysembryogenesis. *Henry Ford Hosp Med J* 20:3–14, 1972.

18. Muller W et al: The DiGeorge syndrome. I. Clinical evaluation and course of partial and complete forms of the syndrome. *Eur J Pediatr* 147:496–502, 1988.
19. Ohtani I, Schuknecht HF: Temporal bone pathology in DiGeorge's syndrome. *Ann Otol Rhinol Laryngol* 93:220–224, 1984.
20. Radford DJ et al: Spectrum of DiGeorge syndrome in patients with truncus arteriosus: expanded DiGeorge syndrome. *Pediatr Cardiol* 9:95–101, 1988.
21. Reyes MR et al: Hearing loss and otitis media in velo-cardio-facial syndrome. *Int J Pediatr Otorhinolaryngol* 47:227–233, 1999.
22. Scambler P et al: Microdeletions within 22q11 associated with sporadic and familial DiGeorge syndrome. *Genomics* 10:201–206, 1991.
23. Solot CB et al: Communication disorders in the 22q11.2 microdeletion syndrome. *J Commun Disord* 33:187–203, 2000.
24. Taylor MJ, Josifek K: multiple congenital anomalies, thymic dyspasia, severe congenital heart disease, and oligosyndactyly, with a deletion of the short arm of chromosome 5. *Am J Med Genet* 9:5–11, 1981.
25. Townes PL, White MR: Inherited partial trisomy 8q(22–qter). *Am J Dis Child* 132:498–501, 1971.
26. VanEsch H et al: The phenotypic spectrum of the 10p deletion syndrome versus the classical DiGeorge syndrome. *Genet Couns* 10:59–65, 1999.
27. Van Mierop LHD, Kutsche LM: Cardiovascular anomalies in DiGeorge syndrome and importance of neural crest as a possible pathogenetic factor. *Am J Cardiol* 58:133–137, 1986.
28. Wang R et al: Infants of diabetic mothers are at increased risk for the oculo-auriculo-vertebral sequence: a case-based and case-control approach. *J Pediatr* 141:611–617, 2002.
29. Wilson TA et al: DiGeorge anomaly with renal agenesis in infants of mothers with diabetes. *Am J Med Genet* 47:1078–1082, 1993.

Kabuki (Niikawa-Kuroki) syndrome

In 1981, Niikawa et al. (11) and Kuroki et al. (7) independently reported a syndrome primarily in Japanese children that was characterized by mild to moderate mental retardation, postnatal progressive growth retardation, and a strikingly unusual face reminiscent of the makeup used in Kabuki theater. Since that time, more than 300 examples have been reported in a variety of ethnic backgrounds (1–20). Wessels et al. (19) and Matsumoto and Niikawa (8) provide excellent reviews.

Craniofacial findings. The palpebral fissures are long with eversion of the lateral third of the lower eyelid. The eyebrows are arched and tend to be diminished laterally. The lashes are heavy and long. The sclerae are blue in about 30% of patients. Ptosis and strabismus are each present in one-third of patients. The nose is broad with a depressed tip. A trapezoid-shaped philtrum has been described (6) (Fig. 11–2). The teeth may be widely spaced or small in size, and some permanent teeth may be missing (9,10). Cleft lip and/or cleft palate, submucous cleft palate, or highly arched palate has been found in 70%. The occipital hairline is often low.

Musculoskeletal system. Frequent anomalies include short stature (80%), short and/or incurved fifth fingers (75%), scoliosis (25%), and various rib and vertebral malformations (20%–30%). Joint hypermobility occurs in 75% of patients, with congenital hip dislocation in 35% and in other joints such as the shoulder and knee less frequently.

Cardiovascular system. Cardiovascular malformations have been reported in about one-third of patients. Most common are coarctation of the aorta, bicuspid aortic valve, atrial septal defect, ventricular septal defect, and pulmonic stenosis; infrequent CVMs include Shone's complex, double-outlet right ventricle, and truncus arteriosus (3,4,6, 8,13,14,18–20).

Integumentary system. There is persistence of fetal fingertip pads in about 80% (6).

Auditory system. The ears are prominent with large lobules in 85%. The anthelix tends to be hypoplastic. About 40% of Japanese patients and 10% of non-Japanese patients have a pretragal pit. Otitis media is extremely frequent during childhood (70%) (6). Hearing loss is reported in 40%–50% and can be conductive, sensorineural, or mixed (5). The ossicles may be severely malformed (15) and Mondini dysplasia of the inner ear has been described (5).

Heredity. Almost all cases reported to date have been isolated examples. There is no sex predilection and no increase in consanguinity. Ten reports of affected parent and child make a new autosomal dominant mutation with variable expressivity a plausible explanation (2).

Summary. Characteristics include (*1*) occasional autosomal dominant transmission with the majority of cases being sporadic; (*2*) distinctive facial features, including elongated palpebral fissures, prominent ears; and abnormal teeth; (*3*) postnatal growth retardation; (*4*) mild to moderate mental retardation; (*5*) cardiovascular malformations; (*6*) prominent ears with frequent otitis; and (*7*) hearing loss that can be conductive, sensorineural, or mixed.

References

1. Burke LW, Jones MC: Kabuki syndrome: underdiagnosed recognizable pattern in cleft palate patients. *Cleft Palate Craniofac J* 32:77–84, 1995.
2. Courtens W et al: Further evidence for autosomal dominant inheritance and ectodermal abnormalities in Kabuki syndrome. *Am J Med Genet* 93:244–249, 2000.

Figure 11–2. *Kabuki (Niikawa-Kuroki) syndrome.* (A) Note long palpebral fissures with mild eversion of lateral third of lower lids, arched eyebrows, and outstanding ears with hypoplastic anthelix. (B,C) Similarly affected children. (D) Note the typical features in a 15-year-old Caucasian boy. [(B,C) courtesy of Y Kuroki, Yokohama, Japan; (D) courtesy of A Lin, Boston, Massachusetts.]

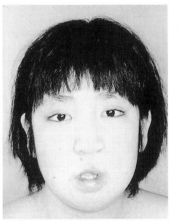
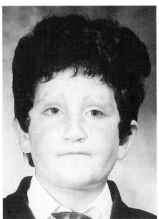

A   B   C   D

3. Galan-Gomez E et al: Kabuki make-up (Niikawa-Kuroki) syndrome in five Spanish children. *Am J Med Genet* 59:276–282, 1995.
4. Hughes HE, Davies SJ: Coarctation of the aorta in Kabuki syndrome. *Arch Dis Child* 70:512–514, 1994.
5. Igawa HH et al: Inner ear abnormalities in Kabuki make-up syndrome: report of three cases. *Am J Med Genet* 92:87–89, 2000.
6. Kawame H et al: Phenotypic spectrum and management issues in Kabuki syndrome. *J Pediatr* 134:480–485, 1999.
7. Kuroki Y et al: A new malformation syndrome of long palpebral fissures, large ears, depressed nasal tip and skeletal anomalies associated with postnatal dwarfism and mental retardation. *J Pediatr* 99:570–573, 1981.
8. Matsumoto N, Niikawa N: Kabuki make-up syndrome: a review. Am J Med Genet 117C:57–65, 2003.
9. Matsune K et al: Craniofacial and dental characteristics of Kabuki syndrome. *Am J Med Genet* 98:185–190, 2001.
10. Mhanni AA et al: Kabuki syndrome: description of dental findings in 8 patients. *Clin Genet* 56:154–157, 1999.
11. Niikawa N et al: Kabuki make-up syndrome: a syndrome of mental retardation, unusual facies, large and protruding ears and post-natal growth deficiency. *J Pediatr* 99:565–569, 1981.
12. Niikawa N et al: Kabuki make-up (Niikawa-Kuroki) syndrome: a study of 62 patients. *Am J Med Genet* 31:565–589, 1988.
13. Ohdo S et al: Kabuki make-up syndrome (Niikawa-Kuroki syndrome) associated with congenital heart disease. *J Med Genet* 22:126–127, 1985.
14. Peterson-Falzone SJ et al: Otolaryngologic manifestations of Kabuki syndrome. *Int J Pediatr Otorhinolaryngol* 38:227–238, 1997.
15. Philip N et al: Kabuki make-up (Niikawa-Kuroki) syndrome: a study of 16 non-Japanese cases. *Clin Dysmorphol* 1:63–77,1992.
16. Say B et al: Kabuki make-up syndrome and hearing impairment. *Clin Dysmorphol* 2:68–70, 1993.
17. Schrander-Stumpel C et al: The Kabuki (Niikawa-Kuroki) syndrome: further delineation of the phenotype in 29 non-Japanese patients. *Eur J Pediatr* 153:438–445, 1994.
18. Tsukahara M et al: Dominant inheritance of Kabuki-make-up syndrome. *Am J Med Genet* 73:19–23, 1997.
19. Wessels MW et al: Kabuki syndrome: a review study of three hundred patients. *Clin Dysmorphol* 11:95–102, 2002.
20. Wilson GN: Thirteen cases of Niikawa-Kuroki syndrome: report and review with emphasis on medical complications and preventive management. *Am J Med Genet* 79:112–120, 1998.

Noonan syndrome

Noonan syndrome is a relatively common condition characterized by short stature, characteristic facial features (Fig. 11–3), broad or webbed neck, and pectus carninatum superiorly and pectus excavatum inferiorly. Mild motor developmental delays related to hypotonia are common (6,8). While patients with a severe expression of Noonan syndrome may have mental retardation or learning disabilities, a detailed study of cognitive function did not find substantial deficits in the less severely affected patients. (6,8,10). The birth prevalence is approximately 1/1000 to 1/2000. Autosomal dominant inheritance with variable expression is well documented.

Cardiac anormalities are common, especially valvular pulmonic stenosis (often with a dysplastic valve), septal defects, and hypertrophic cardiomyopathy (typically asymmetric septal involvement) (6,8).

The pinnae are often thickened, posteriorly rotated, and low-set. Hearing loss is more common than thought initially. In a large series from the United Kingdom, 40% of patients reported hearing loss that was usually conductive and related to serous otitis media. Nerve deafness requiring hearing aids was noted in almost 10% of those who had been tested (3% of all patients) (8). All children with Noonan syndrome should have a complete hearing examination (6) with periodic monitoring through adulthood, as progessive sensorineural hearing loss has been reported (2,7).

Various middle and inner ear anomalies have been reported, including a temporal bone anomaly with dehiscent jugular bulb and dysplastic cochleovestibular labyrinth (4) and probable endolymphatic hydrops with central vestibular abnormalities (6).

In some families, linkage to chromosome 12q has been detected (3). The gene has recently been identified as *PTPN11* and accounts for Noonan syndrome in approximately half of the families (9). There appears to be some genotype–phenotype correlation with the presence or

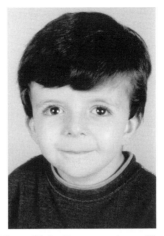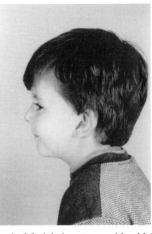

Figure 11–3. *Noonan syndrome.* Note typical facial phenotype, with widely spaced eyes, downslanting palpebral fissures, and short nose. [From J Allanson, Ottawa, Ontario, Canada.]

absence of the *PTPN11* mutation. Tartaglia et al. (9) also found that those with the *PTPN11* mutation were more likely to have pulmonic stenosis but less likely to have hypertrophic cardiomyopathy than those without the mutation. There is also clinical overlap with the LEOPARD syndrome, which is also caused by mutations in *PTPN11* (1,4). Other conditions that overlap with Noonan syndrome are the cardiofaciocutaneous and neurofibromatosis-Noonan syndromes (6).

References

1. Digilio MC et al: Grouping of multiple-lentigines/Leopard and Noonan syndromes on the *PTPN11* gene. *Am J Hum Genet* 71:389–394, 2002.
2. Foster CA, Dyhrkopp PJ: Noonan's syndrome with sensorineural hearing loss and vestibular abnormalities. *Otolaryngol Head Neck Surg* 119: 508–511, 1998.
3. Jamieson CR et al: Mapping a gene for Noonan syndrome to the long arm of chromosome 12. *Nat Genet* 8:357–360, 1994.
4. Legius E et al: *PTPN11* mutations in LEOPARD syndrome. *J Med Genet* 39:571–574, 2002.
5. Naficy S et al: Multiple temporal bone anomalies associated with Noonan syndrome. *Otolaryngol Head Neck Surg* 116:265–267, 1997.
6. Noonan JA: Noonan syndrome. An update and review for the primary pediatrician. *Clin Pediatr* 33:548–555, 1994.
7. Qiu WW et al: Audiologic manifestations of Noonan syndrome. *Otolaryngol Head Neck Surg* 118:319–323, 1998.
8. Sharland M et al: A clinical study of Noonan syndrome. *Arch Dis Child* 67:178–183, 1992.
9. Tartaglia M et al: *PTPN11* mutations in Noonan syndrome: molecular spectrum, genotype–phenotype correlation, and phenotypic heterogeneity. *Am J Hum Genet* 70:1555–1563, 2002.
10. van der Burgt I et al: Patterns of cognitive functioning in school-aged children with Noonan syndrome associated with variability in phenotypic expression. *J Pediatr* 135:707–713, 1999.

Choanal atresia, unusual face, cardiovascular malformations, and sensorineural hearing loss (Burn-McKeown syndrome)

In 1992, Burn et al. (1) described five children from three families with bilateral choanal atresia associated with CVMs, prominent pinnae, apparent hypertelorism, short palpebral fissures, deficiency of lower third of eyelids, and a characteristic facial appearance (Fig. 11–4). Sensorineural hearing loss of approximately 40 dB was noted in three of five children. The occurrence in two sib pairs raises the possibility of autosomal recessive inheritance. Toriello and Higgins (2) reported a possible sixth patient with choanal stenosis, normal hearing, and similar facial appearance. Four of the six patients had a CVM (three with ventricular septal defect, one with atrial septal defect), and two had unilateral cleft lip. Intelligence was normal in all individuals. This condition should be differentiated from the CHARGE association.

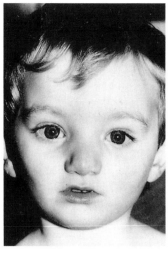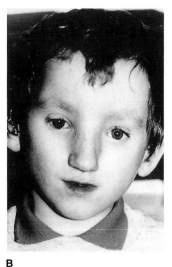

A   **B**

Figure 11–4. *Choanal atresia, unusual face, cardiovascular malformations, and sensorineural hearing loss (Burn-McKeown syndrome).* (A,B) Affected siblings showing mild ocular hypertelorism, short palpebral fissures, and abnormal outer third of lower lids. [From J Burn et al., *Clin Dysmorphol* 1:137, 1992.]

References

1. Burn J et al: New dysmorphic syndrome with choanal atresia in siblings. *Clin Dysmorphol* 1:137–144, 1992.
2. Toriello HV, Higgins JV: A boy with choanal atresia and cardiac defect: Burn-McKeown syndrome. *Clin Dysmorphol* 8:143–145, 1999.

Deafness, congenital heart defects, and posterior embryotoxon

Recently a family was described in which hearing loss, cardiac defects, and eye anomalies segregated as an autosomal dominant trait (2). Hearing loss was described as a mild to severe combined loss, predominantly affecting middle frequencies. In two individuals vestibular function was impaired, as characterized by unstable equilibrium during walking. Computed tomographic evaluation in these individuals demonstrated aplasia of the anterior semicircular canal and hypoplasia of the posterior semicircular canal. Heart defects were varied and included tetralogy of Fallot, peripheral pulmonic stenosis (most common), and septal defects. Ocular evaluation demonstrated posterior embryotoxon in all cases. No vertebral or biliary anomalies were found. Mutation analysis demonstrated that the causative gene was *JAG1*, mutations in which usually cause Alagille syndrome (1). Therefore, in any child who presents with a picture compatible with the Alagille syndrome phenotype, hearing evaluation should be performed.

References

1. Alagille D et al: Hepatic ductular hypoplasia associated with characteristic facies, vertebral malformations, retarded physical, mental, and sexual development, and cardiac murmur. *J Pediatr* 86:63–71, 1975.
2. Le Caignec C et al: Familial deafness, congenital heart defects, and posterior embryotoxon caused by cysteine substitution in the first epidermal growth factor–like domain of Jagged 1. *Am J Hum Genet* 71:180–186, 2002.

Hypertrophic cardiomyopathy and congenital deaf-mutism (Csanády syndrome)

In 1987, Csanády et al. (1) described a Hungarian family with hypertrophic cardiomyopathy (HCM) in four males over two generations, two of whom had "congenital deaf-mutism." A fifth male with deafness died from unspecified heart failure. No offspring in the third generation had HCM or deafness. The authors acknowledged possible overlap with Noonan and LEOPARD syndromes, but specifically noted the absence

of freckles or lentigines and dysmorphic features. No other families have been reported using this eponym. Cosegregation of HCM and deafness cannot be excluded as a possible explanation.

Reference

1. Csanády M et al: Hypertrophic cardiomyopathy associated with congenital deaf-mutism. *Eur Heart J* 8:528–534, 1987.

Familial bilateral blepharoptosis and left-sided obstructive cardiovascular malformations with deafness (Cornel syndrome, Bazopoulou-Kyrkanidou syndrome)

Cornel et al. (2) reported a Newfoundland father and three sons with bilateral congenital ptosis, coarctation, and deafness. In three additional relatives spanning four generations, ptosis was present. Deafness was sensorineural in two brothers and unspecified in the remainder. The narrowing of the descending aorta was not a typical discrete indentation. Instead, the authors described "complex" coarctation involving the proximal subclavian arteries. The published aortograms confirm the nearly identical appearance. The skin and musculoskeletal system were normal.

Cornel's kindred was cited by Bazopoulou-Kyrkanidou et al. (1), who reported a Greek mother and son with bilateral blepharoptosis, microcephaly, unusual facial features, peculiar voice, and mild conductive deafness. The boy had subaortic stenosis. Although there were no photographs in Cornel et al.'s study (2), photographs were reviewed by Bazopoulou-Kyrkanidou et al., who acknowledged a similar appearance. They concluded, however, that there were sufficient differences to regard them as distinct disorders. There are no other reports bearing either of these eponyms.

References

1. Bazopoulou-Kyrkanidou E et al: Familial bilateral blepharoptosis and subvalvular aortic stenosis. *Genet Couns* 6:227–232, 1995.
2. Cornel G et al: Familial coarctation of the aortic arch with bilateral ptosis: a new syndrome: *J Pediat Surg* 22:724–726 1987.

Cardiovascular malformations and deaf-mutism (Koroxenidis syndrome)

Pulmonic stenosis at either the subvalvular or valvular level and accompanied by atrial septal defect or subaortic obstruction was reported in a mother and four of her eight children (1). Two were noted to have deaf mutism, three had hypoplastic fifth digits, and one had polydactyly. This type of CVM is strongly suggestive of Noonan syndrome, which is further supported by the description of broad nasal root, hypertelorism, low-set ears, and pectus excavatum.

References

1. Koroxenidis GT et al: Congenital heart disease, deaf-mutism, and associated somatic malformations occurring in several members of one family. *Am J Med* 40:149–155, 1966.

Brachymesophalangy, hyperphalangy, cardiovascular malformation, and deafness (Camera Costa syndrome)

The most distinctive features of the Italian boy reported by Camera and Costa (1) are skeletal and include bilateral short hands, clinodactyly, radiographic brachymesophalangy, and unilateral hypersegmentation of the index finger, leading to striking ulnar deviation. He also had a membranous ventricular septal defect and bilateral sensorineural hearing loss. Further details regarding degree and onset of hearing loss were not published.

Reference

1. Camera G, Costa M. Unusual type of brachydactyly associated with intraventricular septal defect and deafness: a new condition? *Clin Dysmorphol* 6:31–33, 1997.

Appendix

Other entities with cardiac abnormalities

Entity	Cardiac Finding	Chapter in this Book
CHARGE association	Conotruncal aortic arch anomalies	6 (external ear)
Aural atresia, microtia, aortic arch abnormalities, conductive hearing loss	Aortic arch and septal defects	6 (external ear)
Axenfeld-Rieger anomaly, cardiac malformations, SHL	Septal defects, valvular insufficiency	7 (eye)
Oculo-facio-cardio-dental syndrome	Septal defects	7 (eye)
Keutel syndrome	Pulmonary stenosis	8 (musculoskeletal)
Joint fusions, mitral insufficiency, conductive hearing loss	Mitral insufficiency	8 (musculoskeletal)
Marfan syndrome	Aortic root dilatation	8 (musculoskeletal)
Prune belly syndrome with pulmonic stenosis, mental retardation, and SHL	Pulmonary stenosis	9 (renal)
Schmidley syndrome	Myocardial fibrosis	10 (neurologic)
Nathalie syndrome	Cardiac conduction defects	10 (neurologic)
LEOPARD syndrome	Pulmonary stenosis	14 (integumentary)
Woodhouse-Sakati syndrome	EKG abnormalities	14 (integumentary)
Linear band hyperpigmentation, congenital heart anomalies, moderate conductive hearing loss	Septal defects	14 (integumentary)

SHL, sensorineural hearing loss.

Chapter 12
Genetic Hearing Loss Associated with Endocrine Disorders
WILLIAM REARDON

Classifying genetic hearing loss syndromes associated with endocrine disorders in a logical and comprehensible way is probably not achievable by current approaches. This chapter summarizes conditions in which hearing loss is associated with diabetes mellitus, and thyroid, parathyroid, and gonadal dysfunction. Many other conditions addressed elsewhere in this book also have an endocrine element, and the distinction between those conditions and the ones discussed in this chapter may not always be entirely clear, or even totally logical. For the most part, however, the syndromes included here have a recognized endocrine abnormality as a fundamental and consistent feature.

Diabetes insipidus, diabetes mellitus, optic atrophy, and sensorineural hearing loss (DIDMOAD syndrome, Wolfram syndrome)

This syndrome dates from the 1938 report by Wolfram and Wagener (48) of a constellation of diabetes insipidus, diabetes mellitus, optic atrophy, and sensorineural deafness, which gave rise to the acronym DIDMOAD. Possible earlier examples have been cited (14,17,23). Gunn et al. (17) suggested that the frequency of this syndrome is between 1/150 and 1/175 among patients with juvenile diabetes. At least 200 cases have been reported (5,10,14,25,31,36).

Clinical findings. Many patients are small and underweight (29). Delayed sexual maturation and/or gonadal dysfunction have been found in about 35% of patients of both sexes (5,10,17,19,36,39,47).

Ocular system. Bilateral progressive loss of visual acuity, leading to blindness caused by primary optic atrophy (a constant feature), has been noted more often during the first decade of life and less often during the second decade (24,25,28). Fraser and Gunn (15) and Najjar et al. (30) found the average age of onset to be 10 years (Fig. 12–1A). Rarely, optic atrophy antedates the onset of diabetes mellitus (12,28). This is characterized by pale, sharply defined optic discs (29). Reduced electroretinogram (ERG) amplitudes together with the very narrow vessels of early optic atrophy suggest tapetoretinal dystrophy and retinal atrophy. Some patients exhibit mild pigment disturbance of the fundus (30,40,43). Other findings include reduction in visual fields (80%), nystagmus (40%), retinal pigmentation (20%), disturbed color vision, and bilateral cataracts (11,21).

Central nervous system. Ataxia (5,36,47,48), abnormal electroencephalogram (EEG) (10), and nystagmus (40) have been reported. On necropsy, degeneration of the geniculate bodies, pons, and cerebellum (32) as well as of the supraoptic and paraventricular nuclei (8,19) has been described. Dementia and psychiatric illness are well recorded in Wolfram syndrome. Swift et al. (45) recorded significant psychiatric findings among 60% of homozygotes and further postulated that heterozygotes have an eightfold increased risk of hospitalization for psychiatric illness or suicide compared to noncarriers (46).

Endocrine system. The diabetes mellitus, a constant feature, is variable in severity, has early onset (4–8 years), and is the first com-

ponent to appear in over 75% of cases (10) (Fig. 12–1B). Weight loss and polyuria usually become evident prior to 11 years of age (range 2–18 years). Diabetic acidosis has been found in about 10% (35,36).

Vasopressin-sensitive diabetes insipidus, found in 40%–60%, but often insidious, usually appears around 10 years of age after diabetes mellitus has become evident (10,16,19,43) (Fig. 12–1C). The polyuria may be 4–12 liters/day with a specific gravity of 1.000–1.005. The response to chlorpropamide suggests partial antidiuretic hormone deficiency.

Genitourinary system. Atonia of the urinary tract, due to progressive denervation of the bladder and manifested by hydronephrosis, hydroureters, and dilated urinary bladder, has been found in most patients (1,5,12,22,30,36) (Fig. 12–1D). Although Cremers et al. (10) and Blasi et al. (5) noted these findings in only 40% and 27% of the cases, respectively, there is a possibility of underreporting and lack of investigation.

Other findings. Intolerance to cold, delayed puberty, episodic vertigo, and dysautonomia with labile fluctuation of body temperature have been reported (5,14,26,27,42). Thiamine-responsive anemia has been reported (6). A particular feature of chromosome 4q–linked pedigrees is the propensity toward upper gastrointestinal bleeding and/or ulceration (13).

Auditory system. Hearing loss is bilateral, sensorineural, and slowly progressive, resulting in moderate to severe loss in 60%–80% of cases (10,18,19,25,30,36,43) (Fig. 12–1E). Onset is usually in the second decade (10). Although there is some variation in age of onset and severity, loss is more marked at higher frequencies (18,30,36) and, with progression, extends to lower frequencies. Auditory patterns are consistent with atrophy of the stria vascularis. In some cases, recruitment has been present; in others, it is absent (2,5,10,11). The neural lesion may be both cochlear and retrocochlear (16).

Vestibular system. Barjon et al. (2) and others cited by Cremers et al. (10) have found reduced excitability of the vestibular apparatus.

Laboratory findings. Electroencephalograms were considered abnormal in three of five cases studied by Rose et al. (40). Spinal fluid protein may also be increased (40). The ERG amplitudes are reduced. Diabetes insipidus may be demonstrated by the water deprivation test or hypertonic saline infusion test. Intravenous pyelography and voiding urethrocystography are indicated. Mutations have been established in chromosome 4p–linked families. Over 30 mutations, comprising nonsense, missense, deletions, insertions, and frame shift mechanisms, have been reported and are widely dispersed throughout the gene, which encodes a transmembrane protein (20,21,44). Most patients with a Wolfram syndrome phenotype are homozygotes for null alleles or compound heterozygotes for null allele/missense mutations (4). Khanim et al. (21) suggested that over 90% of patients with Wolfram syndrome are caused by mutation of this gene. Mutations have not been established in relation to chromosome 4q–linked families. It is also important to note the reports suggesting mitochondrial dysfunction in Wolfram syndrome (3,7,37,38,41). Rötig et al. (41) observed a heteroplasmic deletion of mtDNA of some 7.6 kb in a patient with neonatal diabetes, progressive

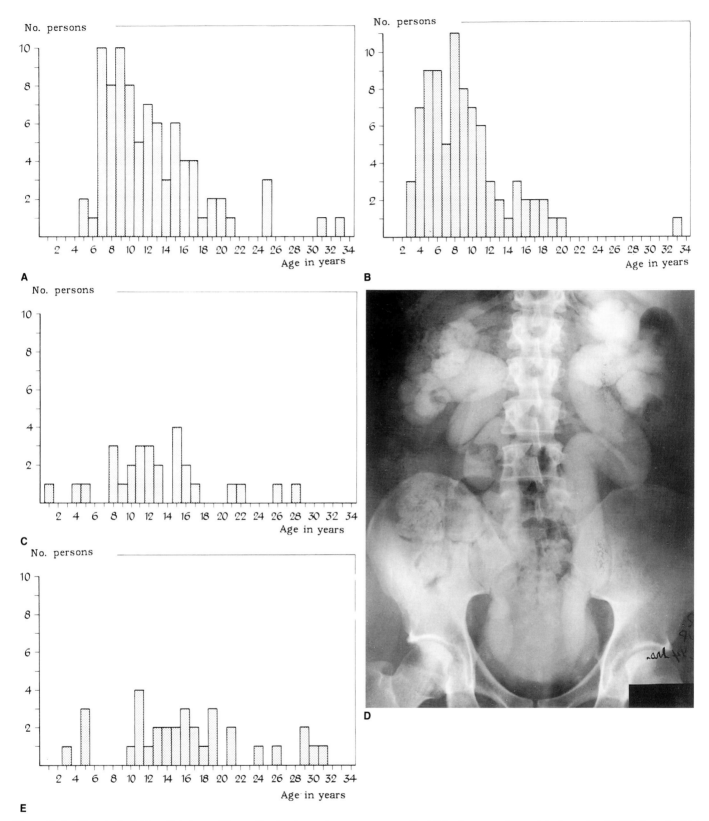

Figure 12–1. *Diabetes insipidus, diabetes mellitus, optic atrophy, and sensorineural hearing loss (DIDMOAD syndrome, Wolfram syndrome).* (A) Age at which diminished visual acuity was diagnosed in 88 patients. (B) Age at which diabetes mellitus was first diagnosed in 83 patients. (C) Age at which diabetes insipidus was first diagnosed in 28 patients. (D) Note megacystis, bilateral megaureter, and hydronephrosis. (E) Age at which hearing loss was first diagnosed in 34 patients. [(A–C,E) from C Cremers, *Acta Pediatr Scand (Suppl)* 264:3, 1977; (D) from NR Peden, *Q J Med* 58:167, 1986.]

optic atrophy and hearing loss, while Pilz et al. (37) reported a point mutation of mtDNA, position 11778, more commonly associated with Leber hereditary optic neuropathy (LHON) in a patient with Wolfram syndrome.

Heredity. Most cases are autosomal recessive, and associated with mutation of either a gene (WFS1) that maps to 4p16.1 and codes for a glycoprotein found primarily in the endoplasmic reticulum (19,20,44) or a second gene that maps to 4q22-q24 (14). Heterozygotes seem to develop diabetes mellitus with a greater than average frequency (15,34). Likewise, a predisposition to hearing loss among heterozygotes has been reported (33). Heterozygosity for missense mutation has been described in several families, segregating autosomal dominant low-frequency sensorineural hearing loss (4). In addition, mitochondrial abnormalities in several patients have been described (3,7,37,38,41). Barrientos et al. (3) described mitochondrial deletions in a family with the 4p linked form.

Diagnosis. There have been numerous examples of the binary combination of diabetes mellitus and optic atrophy in sibs, with no mention of associated hearing loss. Osei et al. (34) calculated, however, that a literature survey showed that almost 40% of cases had sensorineural loss and about 15% had diabetes insipidus. Alström syndrome, which includes diabetes mellitus, progressive sensorineural hearing loss, obesity, retinitis pigmentosa, and cortical cataracts, must be considered, as well as autosomal dominant severe optic atrophy and congenital sensorineural hearing loss. Diabetes mellitus and optic atrophy may be associated with Friedreich ataxia and Refsum syndrome. The brothers described by Codaccioni et al. (9) exhibited infantile diabetes, optic atrophy, hypogonadism, and sensorineural hearing loss. It is possible that the patient reported by Borgna-Pignatti et al. (6) actually had Rogers syndrome (see below).

Prognosis. Although visual and hearing losses become severe by middle age, life span is not reduced.

Summary. This syndrome is characterized by (*1*) autosomal recessive transmission; (*2*) onset in childhood of progressive visual loss due to optic atrophy; (*3*) diabetes mellitus and diabetes insipidus with onset in the first or second decade; and (*4*) onset of progressive sensorineural hearing loss in childhood.

References

1. Aragona F et al: Urological aspects of Wolfram's syndrome. *Eur Urol* 9:75–79, 1983.
2. Barjon P et al: Atrophie optique primitive et surdité neurogène dans le diabète juvénile (à propos de trois observations). *Presse Méd* 72:983–986, 1964.
3. Barrientos A et al: A nuclear defect in the 4p16 region predisposes to multiple mitochondrial DNA deletions in families with Wolfram syndrome. *J Clin Invest* 97:1570–1576, 1996.
4. Bespalova IN et al: Mutations in the Wolfram syndrome gene (*WFS1*) are a common cause of low frequency sensorineural hearing loss. *Hum Mol Genet* 10:2501–2508, 2001.
5. Blasi C et al: Wolfram's syndrome: a clinical, diagnostic and interpretative contribution. *Diabetes Care* 9:521–528, 1986.
6. Borgna-Pignatti C et al: Thiamine-responsive anemia in DIDMOAD syndrome. *J Pediatr* 114:405–410, 1989.
7. Bundey S et al: Mitochondrial abnormalities in the DIDMOAD syndrome. *J Inherit Metab Dis* 15:315–319, 1992.
8. Carson MJ et al: Simultaneous occurrence of diabetes mellitus, diabetes insipidus, and optic atrophy in a brother and sister. *Am J Dis Child* 131:1382–1385, 1977.
9. Codaccioni JL et al: Hypotrophie testiculaire primitive chez deux frères atteints de diabète infantile, atrophic optique familial et surdité neurogène pour l'un. *Ann Endocrinol* 30:669–676, 1969.
10. Cremers CWRJ et al: Juvenile diabetes mellitus, optic atrophy, hearing loss, diabetes insipidus, atonia of the urinary tract and bladder, and other abnormalities (Wolfram syndrome). A review of 88 cases from the literature and personal observation of 3 patients. *Acta Paediatr Scand Suppl* 264:3–16, 1977.
11. Davenport SLH, Gunn TR: Juvenile diabetes mellitus, optic atrophy, sensory nerve deafness, and diabetes insipidus—a syndrome. *J Pediatr* 90:856–857, 1977.
12. Dreyer M et al: The syndrome of diabetes insipidus, diabetes mellitus, optic atrophy, deafness and other abnormalities (DIDMOAD syndrome): two affected sibs and a short review of the literature (98 cases). *Klin Wochenschr* 60:471–475, 1982.
13. El-Shanti H et al: Homozygosity mapping identifies an additional locus for Wolfram syndrome on chromosome 4q. *Am J Hum Genet* 66:1229–1236, 2000.
14. François J: Optic-oto-diabetic syndrome. *Ophthalmologica* 173:345–351, 1976.
15. Fraser FC, Gunn T: Diabetes mellitus, diabetes insipidus and optic atrophy. *J Med Genet* 14:190–193, 1977.
16. Grosse Aldenhövel HB et al: Juvenile onset diabetes mellitus, central diabetes insipidus and optic atrophy (Wolfram syndrome)—neurological findings and prognostic implications. *Neuropediatrics* 22:103–106, 1991.
17. Gunn T et al: Juvenile diabetes mellitus, optic atrophy, sensory nerve deafness and diabetes insipidus—a syndrome. *J Pediatr* 89:565–570, 1976.
18. Higashi K: Otologic findings of DIDMOAD syndrome. *Am J Otol* 12:57–60, 1991.
19. Ikkos DG et al: Association of juvenile diabetes mellitus, primary optic atrophy, and perceptive hearing loss in three sibs, with additional idiopathic diabetes insipidus in one case. *Acta Endocrinol (Kbh)* 65:95–102, 1970.
20. Inoue H et al: A gene encoding a transmembrane protein is mutated in patients with diabetes mellitus and optic atrophy (Wolfram syndrome). *Nat Genet* 20:143–148, 1998.
21. Khanim F et al: WFS1/Wolframin mutations, Wolfram syndrome, and associated diseases. *Hum Mutat* 17:357–367, 2001.
22. Khardori R et al: Diabetes mellitus and optic atrophy in two siblings, a report on a new association and a review of the literature. *Diabetes Care* 6:67–70, 1983.
23. Kliga Y et al: Le syndrome de Wolfram. *Ann Pédiatr* 32:889–892, 1985.
24. Kocher GA et al: Progressive visual loss, diabetes mellitus, and associated abnormalites. (DIDMOAD syndrome). *J Clin Neuro-Ophthalmol* 2:241–244, 1982.
25. Labrune B, Benichou JJ: Diabéte sucréinsipide atrophie optique et surdité. *Ann Pédiatr* 38:244–297, 1991.
26. Lessell S, Rosman NP: Juvenile diabetes mellitus and optic atrophy. *Arch Neurol* 34:759–765, 1977.
27. Marquardt JL, Loriaux L: Diabetes mellitus and cystic atrophy. *Arch Intern Med* 134:32–37, 1974.
28. Mayer UM et al: Observation concerning the age of onset and the nature of optic atrophy in Wolfram's syndrome (DIDMOADS). *Ophthalmic Paediatr Genet* 5:155–158, 1985.
29. Mtanda AT et al: Optic atrophy in Wolfram syndrome. *Ophthalmic Paediatr Genet* 7:159–165, 1986.
30. Najjar SS et al: Association of diabetes insipidus, diabetes mellitus, optic atrophy, and deafness. The Wolfram or DIDMOAD syndrome. *Arch Dis Child* 60:823–828, 1985.
31. Neetens A, Verschueren C: Optico-otodiabetic syndrome. *Bull Soc Ophtalmol Fr* 203:99–107, 1982.
32. Niemeyer G, Marquardt JL: Retinal function in a unique syndrome of optic atrophy, juvenile diabetes mellitus, diabetes insipidus, neurosensory hearing loss, autonomic dysfunction, and hyperalaninuria. *Invest Ophthalmol* 11:617–624, 1972.
33. Ohata T et al: Evidence of an increased risk of hearing loss in heterozygous carriers in a Wolfram syndrome family. *Hum Genet* 103:470–474, 1998.
34. Osei K et al: Coexistence of diabetes mellitus, optic atrophy, and sensorineural deafness. *Ann Opthalmol* 18:196–198, 1986.
35. Page MM et al: Recessive inheritance of diabetes: the syndrome of diabetes insipidus, diabetes mellitus, optic atrophy and deafness. *Q J Med* 69:505–520, 1976.
36. Peden NR et al: Wolfram (DIDMOAD) syndrome: a complex long-term problem in management. *Q J Med* 58:167–188, 1986.
37. Pilz D et al: Mitochondrial mutation commonly associated with Leber's hereditary optic neuropathy observed in a patient with Wolfram syndrome (DIDMOAD). *J Med Genet* 31: 328–330, 1994.
38. Polymeropoulos MH et al: Linkage of the gene for Wolfram syndrome to markers on the short arm of chromosome 4. *Nat Genet* 8:95–97, 1994.
39. Richardson JE, Hamilton W: Diabetes insipidus, diabetes mellitus, optic atrophy and deafness: 3 cases of DIDMOAD syndrome. *Arch Dis Child* 52:796–798, 1977.
40. Rose RC et al: The association of juvenile diabetes mellitus and optic atrophy: clinical and genetic aspects. *Q J Med* 35:385–405, 1986.
41. Rötig A et al: Deletion of mitochondrial DNA in a case of early-onset diabetes mellitus, optic atrophy and deafness (DIDMOAD, Wolfram syndrome). *J Inherit Metab Dis* 16:527–530, 1993.
42. Salih MA, Tuvemo T: Diabetes insipidus, diabetes mellitus, optic atrophy and deafness (DIDMOAD syndrome). *Acta Paediatr Scand* 80:567–572, 1991.

43. Stevens PR, Macfadyen WAL: Familial incidence of juvenile diabetes mellitus, progressive optic atrophy, and neurogenic deafness. *Br J Ophthalmol* 56:496–500, 1972.
44. Strom TM et al: Diabetes insipidus, diabetes mellitus, optic atrophy and deafness (DIDMOAD) caused by mutations in a novel gene (wolframin) coding for a predicted transmembrane protein. *Hum Molec Genet* 7:2021–2028, 1998.
45. Swift RG et al: Psychiatric findings in Wolfram syndrome homozygotes. *Lancet* 336:667–669, 1990.
46. Swift RG et al: Psychiatric disorders in 36 families with Wolfram syndrome. *Am J Psychiatry* 148:775–779, 1991.
47. Tunbridge RF, Paley RG: Primary optic atrophy in diabetes mellitus. *Diabetes* 5:295–296, 1956.
48. Wolfram DJ, Wagener HP: Diabetes mellitus and simple optic atrophy among siblings: report of four cases. *Proc Mayo Clin* 13:715–718, 1938.

Diabetes mellitus, thiamine-responsive megaloblastic anemia, and sensorineural hearing loss

In 1969, Rogers et al. (12) described diabetes mellitus, thiamine-dependent megaloblastic anemia, and sensorineural hearing loss in an 11-year-old female. Subsequently, additional isolated examples and affected sibs have been reported (1,4,6,7,9–14).

The features of the thiamine-responsive anemia syndrome may be those of beriberi, and, as in that vitamin deficiency, some patients have exhibited puffiness, hoarseness, and cardiovascular and neurologic disturbances (7,8,13,15). The patients have presented before 3 months of age and have responded to high doses of thiamine.

Diabetes. The diabetes mellitus becomes manifest very early in life. It has ranged from mild glucose intolerance to clear-cut insulin-dependent diabetes. Several patients have exhibited hyperglycemia before 8 months of age (4,7).

Cardiovascular system. Congenital heart anomalies and situs inversus totalis have been found (1,14). Specific cardiac malformations include endocardial cushion defect (1) and Ebstein anomaly. Cerebral infarction and acute ischemic stroke episodes are documented in both pediatric and early adult life (8,13,15).

Hemapoietic system. The anemia is frankly megaloblastic, often with ring sideroblasts being seen (1,4,7,13). It is associated with neutropenia and thrombocytopenia (1–15). Electron microscopy has shown iron-laden mitochondria in erythroblasts (4). The anemia responds promptly (usually after 4 days) to large doses of thiamine for as long as it is administered. Typically, the anemia becomes evident during early childhood (range 3 months–13 years). Poggi et al. (9,10) correctly forecast that the disorder results from an inherited defect in thiamine transport across biological membranes. This hypothesis has now been confirmed (see Heredity).

Auditory system. Sensorineural hearing loss develops early, having been identified in a 3-month-old child (7). The age of onset is from 3 months to 6 years and the loss is usually profound (1–15). Rindi et al. (11) suggested that early recognition and treatment with a lipophilic form of thiamine results in a better outcome in terms of anemia and hearing disturbance.

Heredity. The occurrence of several affected sibs with normal but consanguineous parents indicates autosomal recessive inheritance. The gene is located at 1q23.3 and the condition is caused by mutations in the *SLC19A2* gene. This gene encodes a transmembrane protein whose functional characteristics indicate that it is a high-affinity transporter of thiamine (2,3,5,13).

Diagnosis. Thiamine-dependent anemia may be found in DID-MOAD syndrome. Diabetes with hearing loss and cerebrovascular events may be reminiscent of MELAS. Scarfe et al. (13), citing respiratory chain complex I abnormality (specifically reduced pyruvate dehydrogenase complex) emphasize the scope of clinical overlap between

this condition and mitochondrial disorders. Other clinical features observed in this disorder, including optic/retinal anomalies, aminoaciduria, short stature, and bundle branch block, may also show a clinical overlap with mitochondrial disorders.

Of the mutations described in this disorder, almost all involve loss of function, there being only one missense mutation of *SLC19A2* to date (2,3,6,13). These result in a depletion of intracellular thiamine and enzymes dependent on thiamine, including pyruvate dehydrogenase complex and α-ketoglutarate dehydrogenase may be reduced.

Summary. Characteristics include (*1*) autosomal recessive inheritance; (*2*) diabetes mellitus in childhood; (*3*) thiamine-responsive megaloblastic anemia; (*4*) variable heart anomalies; (*5*) sensorineural hearing loss; and (*6*) mutations of the *SLC19A2* gene.

References

1. Abboud MR et al: Diabetes mellitus, thiamine-dependent megaloblastic anemia, and sensorineural deafness associated with deficient α-ketoglutarate dehydrogenase deficiency. *J Pediatr* 107:537–541, 1985.
2. Diaz GA et al: Mutations in a new gene encoding thiamine transporter cause thiamine-responsive megaloblastic anaemia syndrome. *Nat Genet* 22: 309–312, 1999.
3. Fleming JC et al: The gene mutated in thiamine-responsive megaloblastic anaemia with diabetes and deafness (TRMA) encodes a functional thiamine transporter. *Nat Genet* 22:305–308, 1999.
4. Haworth C et al: Thiamine-responsive anaemia: a study of two further cases. *Br J Haematol* 50:549–561, 1982.
5. Labay V et al: Mutations in *SLC19A2* cause thiamine-responsive megaloblastic anaemia associated with diabetes mellitus and deafness. *Nat Genet* 22:300–304, 1999.
6. La Grutta A et al: Anemia megaloblastica tramino sensible associata a diabete mellito a sordità. *Rev Ital Pediatr* 6:65–70, 1980.
7. Mandel H et al: Thiamine-dependent beriberi in the "thiamine-responsive anemia syndrome." *N Engl J Med* 311:836–838, 1984.
8. Morimoto A et al: A case of thiamine responsive megaloblastic anaemia syndrome with nystagmus, cerebral infarction, and retinal degeneration. *J Jpn Pediatr Socico* 100:2137–2145, 1996.
9. Poggi V et al: Thiamin-responsive megaloblastic anaemia: a disorder of thiamin transport? *J Inherit Metab Dis* 7 (Suppl 2):153–154, 1984.
10. Poggi V et al: Studies on thiamine metabolism in thiamine-responsive megaloblastic anemia. *Eur J Pediatr* 148:307–311, 1989.
11. Rindi G et al: Thiamine transport by erythrocytes and ghosts in thiamine-responsive megaloblastic anaemia. *J Inherit Metab Dis* 15:231–242, 1992.
12. Rogers LE et al: Thiamine-responsive megaloblastic anemia. *J Pediatr* 74:494–504, 1969.
13. Scharfe C et al: A novel mutation in the thiamine responsive megaloblastic anaemia gene *SLC19A2* in a patient with deficiency of respiratory chain complex I. *J Med Genet* 37:669–673, 2000.
14. Viana MB, Carvalho RI: Thiamine-responsive megaloblastic anemia, sensorineural deafness, and diabetes mellitus: a new syndrome? *J Pediatr* 93: 235–238, 1978.
15. Villa V et al: Acute ischaemic stroke in a young woman with the thiamine-responsive megaloblastic anaemia syndrome. *J Clin Endocr Metab* 85: 947–949, 2000.

Maternally-transmitted diabetes mellitus and hearing loss

Several reports have cited families in which diabetes mellitus and sensorineural hearing loss are transmitted through the female line, consistent with mitochondrial inheritance (Fig. 12–2A) (1–4,7,9,10,13–15). The specific mtDNA mutations have varied from one reported pedigree to the next, as has the clinical profile, but the most frequently recorded mutation is the A3243G point mutation. This mutation is most commonly associated with the MELAS phenotype (*M*itochondrial *E*ncephalopathy, *L*actic *A*cidosis and *S*troke-like *E*pisodes), approximately 90% of patients with that presentation having the A3243G mutation in the leucine tRNA (Fig. 12–2B) (5). While hearing impairment is a well-characterized clinical component of the MELAS phenotype (8), the association with hearing impairment is more universal in patients with the diabetes/hearing loss presentation than in any of the alternative clinical presentations of the A3243G mutation. Other mtDNA mutations de-

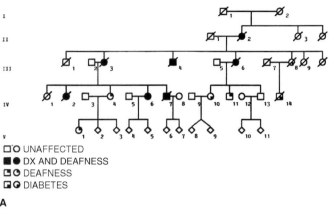

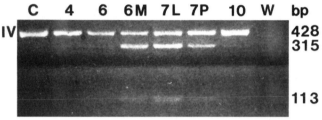

A

□○ UNAFFECTED
■● DX AND DEAFNESS
◧◔ DEAFNESS
◪◑ DIABETES

B

Figure 12–2. *Maternally transmitted diabetes mellitus and hearing loss.* (A) Pedigree demonstrating maternal transmission of the diabetes mellitus/hearing loss phenotype associated with mitochondrial DNA mutation. (B) Illustration of the mtDNA 3243 mutation described in Reardon and Harding (8). Amplification of DNA has been followed by cleavage with restriction enzyme *Apa1*. *Apa1* cuts the 428 base pair (bp) amplification product into two, 315 and 113 bp, in the presence of the 3243 mutation. Samples from generation IV are shown. C, control; W, water; case numbers correspond to pedigree. DNA is lymphocyte derived in all samples except M (muscle), L (liver), and P (pancreas). Mutant (315 bp) fragments are too faint to be seen in IV₄. [(A) reproduced with permission from W Reardon and AE Harding, *J Audiol Med* 4:40–51, 1995.]

scribed in association with the diabetes/hearing loss phenotype include cotransmission of a mtDNA deletion and duplication (2), cosegregation of a tRNA lysine mutation (8334) with the 3243 in tRNA leucine (13), a partial tandem triplication associated with duplication of mtDNA (7), and a large mitochondrial deletion of 7 kb (12).

Diabetes mellitus. Reduced levels of circulating insulin are reported (9). Glucose tolerance profiles range from normal to impaired to non–insulin-dependent diabetes mellitus (15). Usually the clinical onset of diabetes is in the third or fourth decade and is often preceded by clinically documented hearing deficit (1,8,10).

Auditory system. Sensorineural loss is very common in this condition (4), with 61% of diabetic patients with the 3243 mutation having a hearing loss in one survey (6). The hearing loss is often progressive with onset in early adult life.

Associated clinical features. Several clinical features are recorded (1–15), as might be expected of a mitochondrially transmitted disease, notably retinopathy, macular pattern dystrophy (said to be specific for this disorder), myopathy and rapidly progressive cardiomyopathy (4,11).

Summary. Characteristics of this disorder include (*1*) maternal transmission; (*2*) non–insulin-dependent diabetes mellitus; (*3*) progressive sensorineural hearing loss.

References

1. Ballinger SW et al: Maternally transmitted diabetes and deafness associated with a 10.4 kb mitochondrial DNA deletion. *Nat Genet* 1:11–15, 1992.
2. Ballinger SW et al: Mitochondrial diabetes revisited [letter]. *Nat Genet* 7:458–459, 1994.
3. Chinnery PF et al: Nonrandom tissue distribution of mutant mtDNA. *Am J Med Genet* 85:498–501, 1999.
4. Guillausseau P-J et al: Maternally inherited diabetes and deafness: a multicenter study. *Ann Intern Med* 134:721–728, 2001.
5. Hammans SR et al: The mitochondrial DNA transfer RNA^Leu(UUR)A-G(3243) mutation: a clinical and genetic study. *Brain* 118:721–734, 1995.
6. Kadowaki T et al: A subtype of diabetes mellitus associated with a mutation of mitochondrial DNA. *N Engl J Med* 330:962–968, 1994.
7. Negrier M-LM et al: Partial triplication of mtDNA in maternally transmitted diabetes mellitus and deafness [letter]. *Am J Hum Genet* 63:1227–1232, 1998.
8. Reardon W, Harding AE: Mitochondrial genetics and deafness. *J Audiol Med* 4:40–51, 1995.
9. Reardon W et al: Diabetes mellitus associated with a pathogenic point mutation in mitochondrial DNA. *Lancet* 340:1376–1379, 1992.
10. Schulz JB et al: Mitochondrial gene mutations and diabetes mellitus [letter]. *Lancet* 341:438–439, 1993.
11. Silveiro SP et al: Myocardial dysfunction in maternally inherited diabetes and deafness. *Diab Care* 26:1323–1324, 2003.
12. Souied EH et al: Macular dystrophy, diabetes, and deafness associated with a large mitochondrial DNA deletion. *Am J Ophthalmol* 125:100–103, 1998.
13. Sue CM et al: Mitochondrial gene mutations and diabetes mellitus [letter]. *Lancet* 341:437–438, 1993.
14. van den Ouweland JMW et al: Mutation in mitochondrial tRNALeu (UUR) gene in a large pedigree with maternally transmitted type II diabetes mellitus and deafness. *Nat Genet* 1:368–371, 1992.
15. Velho G et al: Clinical phenotypes, insulin secretion, and insulin sensitivity in kindreds with maternally inherited diabetes and deafness due to mitochondrial tRNA Leu(UUR) gene mutation. *Diabetes* 45:478–487, 1996.

Lipodystrophic diabetes and conductive hearing loss (Seip-Berardinelli syndrome)

Van Leeuwen (13) described a combination of conductive hearing loss with lipodystrophy of the face and arms, bone "cysts," and mild mental retardation in three adult sisters. Numerous other examples have been reported but rarely has mention been made of hearing loss or bone radiolucencies.

Physical findings. The face is striking; the gaunt look is due to loss of subcutaneous fat, especially the buccal fat pad (Fig. 12–3A–E).

Integumentary system. Lipodystrophy is generalized and usually congenital. In the clinically overlapping condition of Lawrence syndrome, the lipodystrophy develops later (8). At birth there may be generalized lanugo-like hirsutism, which increases with age. The scalp hair may become excessively curly and thick. Acanthosis nigricans of the axillae, wrists, and ankles is a common feature.

Musculoskeletal system. Adult short stature (57–59 inches) is usual. Small bony defects or radiolucencies filled with red marrow may be scattered throughout the tibia, ilium, humerus, and fibula (1–6,9,15,16) (Fig. 12–3F,G). This represents failure of red marrow to be replaced by fat (2).

Endocrine system. Breast development is poor, and menses are delayed and irregular. There is enlarged penis or clitoris. An association with polycystic ovaries is noted (1,14). The diabetes is insulin-resistant and nonketotic. Hyperlipemia is a constant feature.

Nervous system. About 50% of patients have mild mental retardation.

Auditory system. All three sisters described by Van Leeuwen (13) manifested conductive hearing loss at about 5–6 years of age. Although

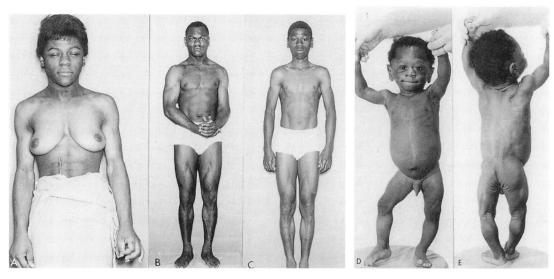

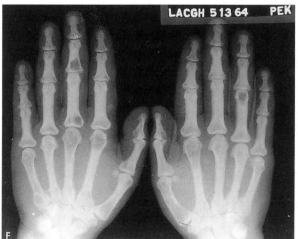
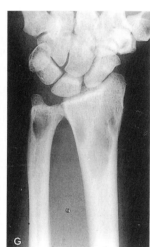

Figure 12–3. *Lipodystrophic diabetes and conductive hearing loss (Seip-Berardinelli syndrome).* (A–C) Patients at ages 22, 20, and 14, respectively. (D,E) Six-month-old affected sib. (F) Cystic angiomatosis of phalanges and metacarpals. (G) Similar lesions of distal radius and ulna. [From JD Brunzell et al., *Ann Intern Med* 69:501, 1968.]

the degree of hearing loss was not stated, it was implied that it was severe. Hearing loss has also been reported by Kawamura et al. (6).

Vestibular system. No studies were reported.

Heredity. Inheritance is autosomal recessive. There is genetic heterogeneity, with two known loci on chromosomes 9q34 and 11q13 (10). Mutations in the chromosome 11–linked families have been identified (10). The nature of the mutations, mainly insertion/deletion events, are predicted to result in severe disruption of the protein with resultant loss of function.

Diagnosis. To be excluded is partial lipodystrophy, in which the face is spared; onset of lipodystrophy is between 5 and 15 years of age and it affects females more commonly (F:M = 4:1). Associated nephropathy is seen in 25%–50% of cases about 5–20 years after appearance of the lipodystrophy (7,11,12,16). Senior and Gellis (12) noted unilateral sensorineural hearing loss in 2 of their 14 patients.

Summary. The syndrome is characterized by (*1*) autosomal recessive inheritance; (*2*) lipodystrophy usually present from birth or possibly developing in later childhood in the Lawrence form; (*3*) hyperlipemia; (*4*) acanthosis nigricans; (*5*) insulin-resistant diabetes mellitus;

(*6*) occasionally multiple bone radiolucencies; and (*7*) severe conductive hearing loss.

References

1. Brunzell JD et al: Congenital generalized lipodystrophy accompanied by systemic cystic angiomatosis. *Ann Intern Med* 69:501–576, 1968.
2. Fleckenstein JL et al: The skeleton in congenital, generalized lipodystrophy: evaluation using whole-body radiographic surveys, magnetic resonance imaging and technetium-99m bone cintigraphy. *Skeletal Radiol* 21:381–386, 1992.
3. Griffiths HJ, Rossini AA: A case of lipoatrophic diabetes. *Radiology* 114:329–330, 1975.
4. Güell-Gonzalez JR et al: Bone lesions in congenital generalized lipodystrophy. *Lancet* 2:104–105, 1971.
5. Huseman C et al: Congenital total lipodystrophy: an endocrine study in three siblings. *J Pediatr* 93:221–226, 1978.
6. Kawamura T et al: Congenital generalized lipodystrophy. *Jpn J Dermatol* 82:73–79, 1972.
7. Kraai EJ, van Son W: Partial lipodystrophy (facies Voltarien) and hypocomplementaemic nephritis. *Br J Dermatol* 18:115–116, 1983.
8. Lawrence RD: Lipodystrophy and hepatomegaly with diabetes, lipaemia and other metabolic disturbances. *Lancet* 1:724–741, 1946.
9. Lejeune E, Tourniaire J: Altérations osseuses et diabète lipo-atrophique. *Lyon Méd* 222:789–800, 1969.
10. Magre J et al: Identification of the gene altered in Berardinelli-Seip congenital lipodystrophy on chromosome 11q13. *Nat Genet* 28:365–370, 2001.

11. Piscatelli RL et al: Partial lipodystrophy: metabolic studies in three patients. *Ann Intern Med* 73:963–970, 1970.

12. Senior B, Gellis SS: The syndromes of total lipodystrophy and of partial lipodystrophy. *Pediatrics* 33:593–612, 1964.

13. Van Leeuwen HC: Über familiäres Vorkommen von Lipodystrophia progressiva zusammen mit Otosklerose, Knochencysten und geistiger Debilität. *Z Klin Med* 123:534–547, 1933.

14. Van Maldergem L et al: Total lipodystrophy, polycystic ovaries and cystic angiomatosis of bones (Brunzell syndrome): confirmation of a separate entity. *Am J Hum Genet* 51(Suppl);A109, 1992.

15. Westenberg RL et al: The roentgenographic findings in total lipodystrophy. *AJR Am J Roentgenol* 103:154–164, 1968.

16. Zafarulla MYM: Lipodystrophy: a case of partial lipodystrophy. *Br J Oral Maxillofac Surg* 23:52–57, 1985.

Goiter and profound congenital sensorineural hearing loss (Pendred syndrome)

Although the first recorded case may well be that of Mondini in 1791 (25,32), the syndrome is eponymously named for Pendred's report in 1896 of a pair of sisters with goiter and profound congenital hearing loss (44). The syndrome received little attention until 1927 when Brain (6) collected 12 examples, 5 of them familial. Further important milestones in assisting the recognition of the syndrome came from Morgans and Trotter (41) in 1958, who demonstrated partial failure of organification of iodine in affected individuals, and from Fraser et al. (20), in 1960 for their demonstration of the diagnostic value of the perchlorate discharge test; affected individuals showed a >10% discharge of iodide following perchlorate challenge. More recently, the recognition by Phelps (45) that dilatation of the vestibular aqueduct is seen in almost all cases of Pendred syndrome on computed tomography (CT) scan of the petrous temporal bone has provided an important avenue of patient identification.

Estimates of prevalence vary; Fraser's large-scale study in the British Isles suggests a rate of 7.5 cases per 100,000 births in the British Isles (19), and an estimate of about 1/100,000 births was proposed by a Scandinavian study (42). Pendred syndrome accounts for possibly 5% of cases of congenital hearing loss (19) but is certainly more common than previously credited.

Several authors have highlighted the absence of the classical clinical presentation of goiter and sensorineural hearing loss, thus making diagnosis less likely in individual cases (9,36,47,48). Two main patient categories having emerged: those with a classical goiter/hearing loss presentation, and those with hearing loss but no goiter, the hearing loss being associated with dilatation of the vestibular aqueduct on CT scanning (11,12,40,50,62).

Endocrine system. Goiter is a feature in approximately 80% of cases (49), noted prepubertally in 33% (Fig. 12–4A,B). The development of goitre as a new clinical feature has not been observed beyond the age of 35 years. Most are diffuse and soft without a bruit. Progressive enlargement of goiter is occasionally observed. Long-standing goiters tend to be nodular, especially in females. About 50% of patients are euthyroid and 50% are hypothyroid (33,49). After thyroidectomy, most goiters recur, even if thyroid therapy is instituted (19,49). However, spontaneous resolution of goiter has been recorded (21). Congenital hypothyroidism in Pendred syndrome is very rarely reported (9,22).

Since the original definition of the syndrome and its diagnosis relied on the presence of goiter, most studies will have an overrepresentation of the true prevalence of goiter. In this context it should be noted that among patients with sensorineural hearing loss ascertained radiologically with detection of dilatation of the vestibular aqueduct, only 20% had evidence of thyroid enlargement on examination (50). Scott et al. (56) have reported that mutations associated with classical Pendred syndrome have complete loss of pendrin-induced chloride and iodide transport and that mutations associated with a deafness/dilated vestibular aqueduct phenotype retain some degree of ion transport. These observations are not echoed by clinical practice findings among patients sharing the same underlying mutation (40).

Ocular system. Gomez-Pan et al. (23) and Howe and Crombie (27) reported an unusual deposition of pigment in the retina in three sibs, but there have been no other similar reports.

Auditory system. Although variations occur, audiometric testing reports show a congenital bilateral 40 to 100 dB sensorineural hearing loss that is more severe in higher frequencies (35). Hearing loss is severe in over 50% of patients. The age at detection may be variable (33). Luxon (39) did not observe a similar degree of variability, reporting a uniform profound symmetrical sensorineural hearing loss in all of the 33 cases examined. Fluctuation in hearing thresholds is common during childhood. Acute deterioration in hearing threshold without subsequent recovery has been observed on several occasions in patients with dilated vestibular aqueduct and is sometimes provoked by head injury, diving, or flying (31,39). Progressive hearing impairment is a feature of one-third of younger patients with the condition (39). Speech development is generally poor because of the early severe hearing loss.

Vestibular system. Formal evaluation of vestibular function has shown inconsistent results, some investigators reporting normal responses (14,30,64). Caloric tests, however, have shown depressed vestibular function in about 40% of patients with classical Pendred syndrome (3,19,33,35,37). Evidence of bilateral vestibular hypofunction was observed in one-third of cases in one study (39), while unilateral vestibular disturbance was present in a further third. Moreover, vestibular dysfunction is well established in patients with sensorineural hearing loss/dilated vestibular aqueduct (26,31,39,54).

Laboratory findings. In vitro studies of pendrin function have demonstrated that wild-type protein enhances transmembraneous transport of iodide and chloride. In contrast, defective transport of these anions is observed in the presence of mutations (55,56). Immunolocalization studies show that pendrin is localized to the apical membrane of thyrocytes (52). It appears that the consequence of mutation in the gene is defective transport of iodide from the thyrocyte into the colloid for incorporation into thyroglobulin. Uptake of iodide at the basal membrane of the thyrocyte is mediated by the Na/I symporter and is therefore not disrupted. The effects of perchlorate challenge are to cause discharge of unincorporated iodide from the thyrocyte—hence the basis of the perchlorate discharge test as a diagnostic tool. In situ hybridization studies of *PDS* expression in the murine inner ear show that the gene is expressed in several discrete areas and is thought to have a major function in regulation of endolymphatic fluid composition, consistent with its known anion transport role (17). Targeted disruption of the mouse *Pds* gene has been reported (18) and *Pds*$^{-/-}$ mice show significant hearing loss, with vestibular disturbance also being observed in about 50% of cases. Anatomical ear abnormalities comprising enlarged endolymphatic duct and sac are observed. Ultrastructural changes are multiple, and the degenerative process is progressive. No thyroid disease is observed in *Pds*$^{-/-}$ mice.

PDS is also expressed in the kidney. In keeping with the known ion transport function, studies of *PDS* activity in the kidney demonstrate a role in the cortical collecting duct and proximal tubule in which pendrin appears to mediate Cl^-/base exchange, including OH^-, HCO_3^-, and formate (52,58).

Radiology. The association with Mondini malformation is well established (2,25,32–34). However, a full Mondini malformation, with deficiency of the interscalar septum in the distal coils of the cochlea, is seen in only 20% of patients with Pendred syndrome (46) (Fig. 12–4C). In contrast, dilatation of the vestibular aqueduct was seen in most (>80%) patients on CT scan (Fig. 12–4D), and in 20 of 20 patients surveyed by MRI scan, enlargement of the endolymphatic sac and duct was noted (46) (Fig. 12–4C). These findings have been confirmed by several authors (1,12,62). Additionally, there were reports of siblings with dilatation of the vestibular aqueduct. This occurrence probably indicates Pendred syndrome presenting in the nonclassical form without goiter (24,53,60).

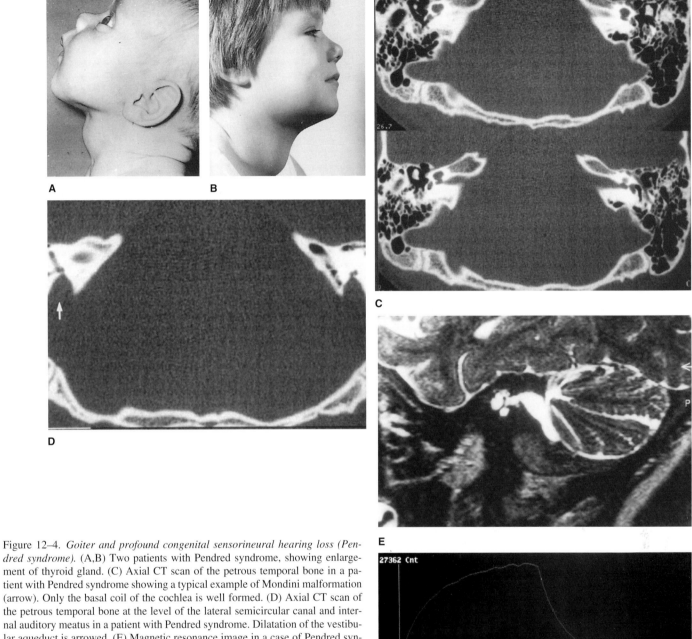

Figure 12–4. *Goiter and profound congenital sensorineural hearing loss (Pendred syndrome).* (A,B) Two patients with Pendred syndrome, showing enlargement of thyroid gland. (C) Axial CT scan of the petrous temporal bone in a patient with Pendred syndrome showing a typical example of Mondini malformation (arrow). Only the basal coil of the cochlea is well formed. (D) Axial CT scan of the petrous temporal bone at the level of the lateral semicircular canal and internal auditory meatus in a patient with Pendred syndrome. Dilatation of the vestibular aqueduct is arrowed. (E) Magnetic resonance image in a case of Pendred syndrome showing dilatation of the endolymphatic sac. (F) A typical perchlorate discharge test in a patient with Pendred syndrome. The radiolabelled iodide is concentrated in the thyroid following administration. Perchlorate stimulates discharge of the incompletely bound iodide, resulting in a 60% discharge of iodide in this patient. [(B) Courtesy of R Sacrez, Strasbourg, France; (C,F) from W Reardon et al., *Q J Med* 90:443–447, 1997; (D) from W Reardon et al., *Q J Med* 93:99–104, 2000; (E) from W Reardon and PD Phelps, Dublin, Ireland.]

Pathology. Grossly, the thyroid is nodular and variable in size. Microscopically, the cells lining the follicles are tall and active with scanty colloid production. At times, nuclear pleomorphism and papillary infoldings are noted, and adenocarcinoma has been erroneously diagnosed (5,15,25,29,51,59,65).

Changes in the inner ear are bilaterally symmetric and correspond closely to Mondini malformation in some cases (28). The endolymphatic duct is usually dilated (22). Occasionally, supporting cells in the organ

of Corti are noted, and rarely hair cells are seen. There are few spiral ganglion cells and no fibers in the lamina spiralis. The vestibular nerve and facial nerve appear normal.

Heredity. Inheritance is autosomal recessive (19). The syndrome was mapped to chromosome 7q31 in an inbred family initially thought to have a nonsyndromic form of hearing loss (4). The recognition that this locus represented Pendred syndrome awaited mapping studies in families with a more classical presentation (10,57). More recently, the identification of the gene defect by Everett et al. (16) as mutations of a transmembranous ion transport protein, now named pendrin, has facilitated molecular diagnosis. Over 30 mutations in the causative gene *PDS* have been published (7,11,16,38,50,63), comprising nucleotide substitutions in most instances. There are four recurrent mutations that make up the majority of mutant alleles (11,63).

Diagnosis. Several complementary approaches to diagnosis exist. Neuroradiology of the petrous temporal bone is probably the investigation of choice in that it offers the likelihood of identifying those patients whose hearing loss might otherwise be classified as nonsyndromic. Dilatation of the vestibular aqueduct may also be seen in branchio-otorenal syndrome, but is not the sole radiological feature in such patients; the clinical features should enable differentiation between the two entities (8). Mondini malformation is not specific to Pendred syndrome and has also been recorded in Wildervanck syndrome, Johanson-Blizzard syndrome, DiGeorge syndrome, Kabuki syndrome, and trisomy 13. The perchlorate discharge test (Fig. 12–4F) may still have a place in the goitrous presentation, although this infrequently undertaken test probably requires adherence to a set protocol and intravenous (IV) administration of the perchlorate if results are to be optimized (47). False-positive results and false-negative results are known to occur (43,47,48,50). Ultimately, mutation analysis of the *PDS* gene may be pursued. To date, 38 mutations have been published (7,11,16,38,50,63), comprising nucleotide substitutions in most instances. There are four recurrent mutations that make up the majority of mutant alleles (11,63).

About 20% of children with endemic hypothyroidism exhibit sensorineural hearing loss (13), and differentiation from Pendred syndrome can be difficult. However, in congenital hypothyoidism there is a negative perchlorate test. Moreover, congenital hypothyroidism is uncommon in Pendred syndrome. Toomey et al. (61) reported autosomal recessive inheritance of agenesis of the thyroid and sensorineural hearing loss.

Prognosis. The hearing loss can progress acutely during childhood, especially in the nonclassical presentation with dilated vestibular aqueduct associated with sensorineural hearing loss. Life span is normal.

Summary. Characteristics of this syndrome include (*1*) autosomal recessive transmission; (*2*) postpubertal development of goiter in most cases; (*3*) positive perchlorate discharge test; (*4*) symmetric, generally severe, congenital sensorineural hearing loss; (*5*) frequent disturbance of vestibular function; (*6*) characteristic radiological malformations of dilatation of the vestibular aqueduct and endolymphatic sac +/− Mondini malformation; and (*7*) mutation of the *PDS* gene.

References

1. Abe S et al: Fluctuating sensorineural hearing loss associated with enlarged vestibular aqueduct maps to 7q31, the region containing the Pendred gene. *Am J Med Genet* 82:322–328, 1999.
2. Andersen PE: Radiology of Pendred's syndrome. *Adv Otorhinolaryngol* 21:9–18, 1974 (same patients as in ref. 25).
3. Arnvig J: Vestibular function in deafness and severe hardness of hearing. *Acta Otolaryngol (Stockh)* 45:283–288, 1955.
4. Baldwin CT et al: Linkage of congenital, recessive deafness (*DFNB4*) to chromosome 7q and evidence for genetic heterogeneity in the Middle Eastern Druze population. *Hum Mol Genet* 4:1637–1642, 1995.
5. Batsakis JG, Nishiyama RH: Deafness with sporadic goiter. Pendred's syndrome. *Arch Otolaryngol* 76:401–406, 1962.
6. Brain WR: Heredity in simple goiter. *Q J Med* 20:303–319, 1927.
7. Campbell C et al: Pendred syndrome, DFNB4, and PDS/SLC26A4 identification of eight novel mutations and possible genotype–phenotype correlations. *Hum Mutat* 17:403–411, 2001.
8. Chen A et al: Phenotypic manifestations of branchiootorenal syndrome. *Am J Med Genet* 82:322–328, 1995.
9. Coakley JC et al: The association of thyroid dyshormonogenesis and deafness (Pendred syndrome): experience of the Victorian neonatal screening programme. *J Paediatr Child Health* 28:398–401, 1992.
10. Coyle B et al: Pendred syndrome (goitre and sensorineural hearing loss) maps to chromosome 7 in the region containing the nonsyndromic deafness gene *DFNB4*. *Nat Genet* 12:421–423, 1996.
11. Coyle B et al: Molecular analysis of the *PDS* gene in Pendred syndrome (sensorineural hearing loss and goitre). *Hum Mol Genet* 7:1105–1112, 1998.
12. Cremers CWRJ et al: Progressive sensorineural hearing loss and a widened vestibular aqueduct in Pendred syndrome. *Arch Otolaryngol Head Neck Surg* 124:501–505, 1998.
13. Debruyne F et al: Hearing in congenital hypothyroidism. *Audiology* 22:404–409, 1983.
14. Deraemaeker R: Congenital deafness and goiter. *Am J Hum Genet* 8:253–256, 1956.
15. Elman DS: Familial association of nerve deafness with nodular goiter and thyroid carcinoma. *N Engl J Med* 259:219–223, 1958.
16. Everett LA et al: Pendred syndrome is caused by mutations in a putative sulphate transporter gene (*PDS*). *Nat Genet* 17:411–422, 1997.
17. Everett LA et al: Expression pattern of the mouse ortholog of the Pendred syndrome gene (*Pds*) suggests a key role for Pendrin in the inner ear. *Proc Natl Acad Sci USA* 96:9727–9732, 1999.
18. Everett LA et al: Targeted disruption of mouse *Pds* provides insight about the inner-ear defects encountered in Pendred syndrome. *Hum Mol Genet* 10:153–161, 2001.
19. Fraser GR: Association of congenital deafness with goiter (Pendred's syndrome). A study of 207 families. *Ann Hum Genet* 28:201–249, 1965.
20. Fraser GR et al: The syndrome of sporadic goiter and congenital deafness. *Q J Med* 29:279–295, 1960.
21. Friis J et al: Thyroid function in patients with Pendred's syndrome. *J Endocrinol Invest* 11:97–101, 1988.
22. Gill H et al: Histopathological findings suggest the diagnosis in an atypical case of Pendred syndrome. *Clin Otolaryngol* 24:523–526, 1999.
23. Gomez-Pan A et al: Pituitary-thyroid function in Pendred's syndrome. *BMJ* 2:152–153, 1974.
24. Griffith AJ et al: Familial large vestibular aqueduct syndrome. *Laryngoscope* 106:960–965, 1996.
25. Hartley GJ, Phelps PD: Minor works of Carlo Mondini: the anatomical section of a boy born deaf. *Am J Otol* 18:288–293, 1996.
26. Hill JH et al: Enlargement of the vestibular aqueduct. *Am J Otolaryngol* 5:411–414, 1984.
27. Howe JW, Crombie AL: Fundus changes in Pendred's syndrome. *J Pediatr Ophthalmol* 12:178–179, 1975.
28. Hvidberg-Hansen J, Jorgensen M: The inner ear in Pendred's syndrome. *Acta Otolaryngol (Stockh)* 66:129–135, 1968.
29. Illum P: Thyroid carcinoma in Pendred's syndrome. *J Laryngol Otol* 92:435–439, 1978.
30. Illum P et al: Fifteen cases of Pendred's syndrome. *Arch Otolaryngol* 96:297–304, 1972.
31. Jackler RK, De La Cruz A: The large vestibular aqueduct syndrome. *Laryngoscope* 99:1238–1243, 1989.
32. Johnsen T et al: Mondini cochlea in Pendred's syndrome. A histological study. *Acta Otolaryngol (Stockh)* 102:239–247, 1986.
33. Johnsen T et al: Pendred's syndrome. Acoustic, vestibular and radiological findings in 17 unrelated patients. *J Laryngol Otol* 101:1187–1192, 1987.
34. Johnsen T et al: CT-scanning of the cochlea in Pendred's syndrome. *Clin Otolaryngol* 14:389–393, 1989.
35. Kabakkaya Y et al: Pendred's syndrome. *Ann Otorhinolaryngol* 102:285–288, 1993.
36. Kopp P et al: Phenocopies for deafness and goiter development in a large inbred Brazilian kindred with Pendred's syndrome associated with a novel mutation in the *PDS* gene. *J Clin Endocrinol Metab* 84:336–341, 1999.
37. Kraft E et al: Diagnose und Therapie des Pendred-Syndromes. *Sprache Stimme Gehör* 15:45–47, 1991.
38. Krawczak M, Cooper DN: The human gene mutation database. http://archiveuwcm.ac.uk.
39. Luxon LM: Neuro-otological findings in Pendred syndrome. *Int J Audiol* 42:82–88, 2003.
40. Masmoudi S et al: Pendred syndrome: phenotypic variability in two families carrying the same *PDS* missense mutation. *Am J Med Genet* 90:38–44, 2000.
41. Morgans ME, Trotter WR: Association of congenital deafness with goitre; the nature of the thyroid defect. *Lancet* 1:607–609, 1958.
42. Nilsson LR et al: Nonendemic goitre and deafness. *Acta Paediatr Scand* 53:117–131, 1964.
43. O Mahoney CF et al: When the triad of congenital hearing loss, goitre and perchlorate positive is not Pendred syndrome. *J Audiol Med* 5:157–165, 1996.
44. Pendred V: Deafmutism and goitre. *Lancet* 2:532, 1896.
45. Phelps PD: Large vestibular aqueduct: large endolymphatic sac? *J Laryngol Otol* 110:1103–1104, 1996.
46. Phelps PD et al: Radiological malformations of the ear in Pendred syndrome. *Clin Radiol* 53:268–273, 1998.

47. Reardon W et al: Pitfalls in practice—diagnosis and misdiagnosis in Pendred syndrome. *J Audiol Med* 6:1–9, 1997.
48. Reardon W et al: Pendred syndrome—100 years of underascertainment? *Q J Med* 90:443–447, 1997.
49. Reardon W et al: Prevalence, age of onset and natural history of thyroid disease in Pendred syndrome. *J Med Genet* 36:595–598, 1999.
50. Reardon W et al: Enlarged vestibular aqueduct: a radiological marker of Pendred syndrome, and mutation of the *PDS* gene. *Q J Med* 93:99–104, 2000.
51. Roberts KD: Thyroid carcinoma in childhood in Great Britain. *Arch Dis Child* 32:58–60, 1957.
52. Royaux IE et al: Pendrin, encoded by the Pendred syndrome gene, resides in the apical region of renal intercalated cells and mediates bicarbonate secretion. *Proc Natl Acad Sci USA* 98:4221–4226, 2001.
53. Satoh H et al: Four cases of familial hearing loss with large vestibular aqueducts. *Eur Arch Otorhinolaryngol* 256:83–86, 1999.
54. Schessel DA, Nedzelski JM. Presentation of large vestibular aqueduct syndrome to a dizziness unit. *J Otolaryngol* 21:265–269, 1992.
55. Scott DA et al: The Pendred syndrome gene encodes a chloride/iodide transport protein. *Nat Genet* 21:440–443, 1999.
56. Scott DA et al: Functional differences of the PDS gene product are associated with phenotypic variation in patients with Pendred syndrome and non-syndromic hearing loss (DFNB4). *Hum Mol Genet* 9:1709–1715, 2000.
57. Sheffield VC et al: Pendred syndrome maps to chromosome 7q21–34 and is caused by an intrinsic defect in thyroid iodine organification. *Nat Genet* 12:424–426, 1996.
58. Soleimani M et al: Pendrin: an apical Cl⁻/OH⁻/HCO3⁻ exchanger in the kidney cortex. *Am J Physiol Renal Physiol* 280:356–364, 2001.
59. Thieme ET: Report of the occurrence of deaf-mutism and goiter in four of six siblings of a North American family. *Ann Surg* 146:941–948, 1957.
60. Tong KA et al: Large vestibular aqueduct syndrome: a genetic disease? *AJR Am J Roentgenol* 168:1097–1101, 1997.
61. Toomey KE et al: Autosomal recessive sensorineural deafness and congenital absence of the thyroid. Abstract 788, 8th International Congress Human Genetics, October 6–11, 1991, Washington, DC.
62. Usami S et al: Non-syndromic hearing loss associated with enlarged vestibular aqueduct is caused by *PDS* mutations. *Hum Genet* 104:188–192, 1999.
63. Van Hauwe P et al: Two frequent missense mutations in Pendred syndrome. *Hum Mol Genet* 7:1099–1104, 1998.
64. von Harnack GA et al: Das erbliche Syndrom: Innenohrschwerhörigkeit und Jodfehlverwertung mit Kropf. *Dtsch Med Wochenschr* 86:2421–2428, 1961.
65. Wildner GP, Wittig G: Zur Histomorphologie der Schilddruse beim Pendredschen Kropf-Taubheits-Syndrom. *Zentralbl Allg Pathol* 109:52–61, 1966.

Johanson-Blizzard syndrome

In 1971, Johanson and Blizzard (12) reported three unrelated children with characteristic hypoplasia of nasal alae, severe mental and somatic retardation, malabsorption due to pancreatic insufficiency, and sensorineural hearing loss. Earlier examples are those of Morris and Fisher (19) and Lumb and Beautyman (15). Over 35 patients have been reported (1–31).

Physical findings. Birth weight has been low in about 55% of patients (18,24).There is failure to thrive; somatic retardation is usually severe. At least 70% remain well below the third centile for height, weight, and head circumference, with true microcephaly occurring in 35% (20,24).

Craniofacial findings. Hypoplasia of nasal alae, producing a beak-like nose, is striking and appears to be a constant feature (Fig. 12–5A, B). Aplasia of lacrimal puncta or cutaneolacrimal fistula has been noted (6,19,25). The anterior fontanel often exhibits delayed closure (19). Midline skin dimples and/or defects over the anterior and posterior fontanels have been noted in 90% of patients (9,10,12,17,25). The scalp hair is often blond, sparse, dry, and coarse. In the frontal area, the hair nearly always has a marked upsweep with extension of the lateral hairline onto the forehead. Cranial radiology has shown a reduction in facial, skeletal, and cranial base measurements, especially the length of the maxilla (20).

Musculoskeletal system. Severe hypotonia with hyperextensibility of joints is noted in 80% (11,18,19,25). Pitting edema of the hands and feet due to protein losing enteropathy may be striking (19,20). Bone age is delayed in about 80% (20,26).

Genitourinary and gastrointestinal systems. Single urogenital orifice with infantile ovaries and double or septate vagina and bicornuate uterus, clitoromegaly, micropenis, cryptorchidism, or urethrovaginal fistula are found in 30% of patients. There is imperforate or anteriorly placed anus in about 35% (4,6,7,9,10,12,16,17,24,26,29). Kristjansson et al. (14) suggested that some examples of genital hypoplasia are secondary to hypopituitarism. Pancreatic insufficiency and malabsorption are constant features (18). The malabsorption caused by the multiple enzyme deficiencies leads to hypoproteinism, anemia, and failure to thrive.

Central nervous system. Speech is rudimentary both from hearing loss and psychomotor retardation. At least 60% of affected individuals are mentally retarded (IQ 35–50), but intelligence may be normal (17,23,24,28) or only mildly delayed (6,11,20,29).

Endocrine findings. Hypothyroidism has been documented in about 30% (9,11,17,18,24,31) and there were several other possible examples of thyroid dysfunction (5,6,12,21). Hurst and Baraitser (11) suggested that the hypothyroidism may be of pituitary origin. Exocrine pancreatic dysfunction is well described (5,9,18) and is ascribed to a primary defect in acinar formation (13). Diabetes is rare but documented (27).

Integumentary system. Nipples and areolae may be hypoplastic (24).

Cardiovascular system. Atrial and ventricular septal defects and situs inversus have been reported in 15% (10,11). W Reardon has witnessed an affected individual die of dilated cardiomyopathy at age 6 months.

Dental findings. There is severe microdontia in both dentitions. The permanent dentition may be entirely absent except for first permanent molars (31). Roots of deciduous teeth are short, irregular, and deformed. Crowns of the few secondary teeth are frequently reduced in form, incisors being conical, and maxillary molars having only three cusps. The tooth pulps are large. Permanent first molars are somewhat taurodont (21,23).

Auditory system. Bilateral severe to profound sensorineural hearing loss due to Mondini-type malformation has been noted in about 65% of patients (6–8,11,12,17,18,24,26). Braun et al. (3) described cystic dilatation of the cochlea and vestibule (Fig. 12–5C,D).

Vestibular system. Absent vestibular function is reported (26), although most reported cases have not had formal vestibular assessment.

Laboratory findings. Iron deficiency, low hemoglobin, fatty, foul, bulky stools, hypocalcemia, and low total serum proteins are evident in early infancy (29). Combined proteolytic, lipolytic, and amylolytic defects are manifested by complete absence of trypsin, chymotrypsin, amylase, carboxypeptidase, and lipase activities.

Pathology. Pancreatic changes include dramatic fibrous connective tissue or fatty replacement (5,9,18). The brain exhibits abnormal gyral formation and cortical neuronal disorganization (4,5).

Heredity. Parental consanguinity (2,16,25,26) and affected sibs (6,10,17,23) clearly indicate autosomal recessive inheritance.

Diagnosis. Johanson-Blizzard syndrome shares proteolytic deficiency with other disorders: cystic fibrosis, Schwachman syndrome, cartilage-hair hypoplasia, trypsinogen deficiency disease, and intestinal enterokinase deficiency. Their differentiation and the use of electrophoretic studies of pancreatic enzymes have been discussed at length by Townes (29). Prenatal diagnosis by ultrasonographic findings has been reported (1,30).

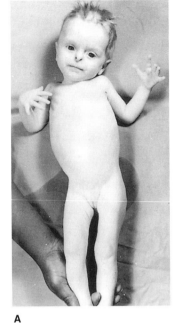

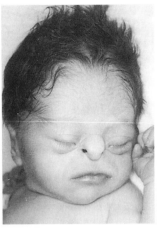

A   B

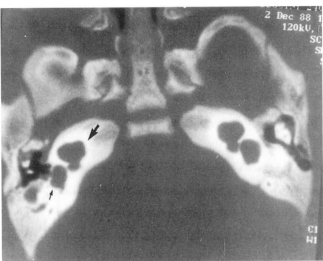

C

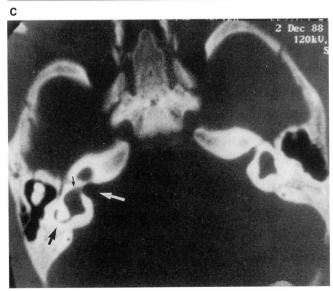

D

Signs and symptoms manifested by the sisters described by Reichart et al. (23) are similar to those of Johanson-Blizzard syndrome, but they probably represent another disorder. Several other syndromes are characterized by varying degrees of hypoplasia of nasal alae: trichorhinophalangeal syndrome, oculodentoosseous dysplasia, craniocarpotarsal dysplasia, and Roberts pseudothalidomide syndrome. Aplasia cutis congenita usually occurs as an isolated finding but may be seen with trisomy 13, focal dermal hypoplasia, and Sakati syndrome, among others. Aplasia cutis congenita of the scalp is associated with a plethora of disorders (8).

Prognosis. The disorder is life threatening. The mental retardation is often marked, although there is a report of normal intelligence (17). Many affected children have died despite full medical treatment.

Summary. This syndrome is characterized by (1) autosomal recessive inheritance; (2) hypoplasia of nasal alae; (3) exocrine pancreatic insufficiency; (4) somatic and mental retardation; (5) hypothyroidism; (6) single urogenital orifice, double vagina, and bicornuate uterus; (7) absence of permanent teeth; (8) congenital profound sensorineural hearing loss; and (9) absent vestibular function.

References

1. Auslander R, et al: Johanson-Blizzard syndrome: a prenatal ultrasonographic diagnosis. *Ultrasound Obstet Gynecol* 13:450–452, 1999.
2. Baraitser M, Hodgson SV: The Johanson-Blizzard syndrome. *J Med Genet* 19:302–303, 1981.
3. Braun J et al: The temporal bone in the Johanson-Blizzard syndrome. A CT study. *Pediatr Radiol* 21:580–583, 1991.
4. Bresson JL et al: Le syndrome de Johanson-Blizzard. Une autre cause de lipomatose pancreatique. *Arch Fr Pédiatr* 37:21–24, 1980.
5. Daentl DL et al: The Johanson-Blizzard syndrome: case report and autopsy findings. *Am J Med Genet* 3:129–135, 1979.
6. Day DW, Israel JN: Johanson-Blizzard syndrome. *Birth Defects* 14(6B): 275–287, 1978.
7. Gershoni-Baruch R et al: Johanson-Blizzard syndrome: clinical spectrum and further delineation of the syndrome. *Am J Med Genet* 35:546–551, 1990.
8. Gorlin RJ et al: *Syndromes of the Head and Neck,* 4th ed. Oxford University Press, New York, 2001.
9. Gould NS et al: Johanson-Blizzard syndrome: clinical and pathological findings in 2 sibs. *Am J Med Genet* 33:194–199, 1989.
10. Helin I, Jödal U: A syndrome of congenital hypoplasia of the alae nasi, situs inversus, and severe hypoproteinemia in two siblings. *J Pediatr* 99:932–934, 1981.
11. Hurst JA, Baraitser M: Johanson-Blizzard syndrome. *J Med Genet* 26:45–48, 1989.
12. Johanson A, Blizzard R: A syndrome of congenital aplasia of the alae nasi, deafness, hypothyroidism, dwarfism, absent permanent teeth and malabsorption. *J Pediatr* 79:982–987, 1971.
13. Jones NL et al: Pathophysiology of the pancreatic defect in Johanson-Blizzard syndrome: a disorder of acinar development. *J Pediatr* 125:406–408, 1994.
14. Kristjansson K et al: Johanson-Blizzard syndrome and hypopituitarism. *J Pediatr* 113:851–853, 1988.
15. Lumb G, Beautyman W: Hypoplasia of the exocrine tissue of the pancreas. *J Pathol Bacteriol* 64:679–685, 1952.
16. Mardini MK et al: Johanson-Blizzard syndrome in a large inbred kindred with three involved members. *Clin Genet* 14:247–250, 1978.
17. Moeschler JB, Lubinsky MS: Johanson-Blizzard syndrome with normal intelligence. *Am J Med Genet* 22:69–73, 1985.

Figure 12–5. *Johanson-Blizzard syndrome.* (A,B) Note striking facies marked by aplasia of nasal alae. (C) High-resolution CT at level of oval window. Cochlea is replaced by cystic cavity (big arrow). Note cystic dilatation of vestibular (small arrow). Picture is consistent with Mondini-type malformation. (D) CT at level of internal acoustic canals. Note marked dilatation of the vestibule (small arrow), normal lateral semicircular canal (big arrow). Internal acoustic canals are widened, shortened, and anteverted (white arrow). [(A) from A Johanson and R Blizzard, *J Pediatr* 79:982, 1971; (B) from R Gershoni-Baruch et al., *Am J Med Genet* 35:546, 1990; (C,D) courtesy of R Gershoni-Baruch and J Brown, Haifa, Israel.]

18. Moeschler JB et al: The Johanson-Blizzard syndrome: a second report of full autopsy findings. *Am J Med Genet* 26:133–138, 1987.
19. Morris MD, Fisher DA: Trypsinogen deficiency disease. *Am J Dis Child* 114:203–208, 1967.
20. Motohashi N et al: Roentgenocephalometric analysis of craniofacial growth in the Johanson-Blizzard syndrome. *J Craniofac Genet Dev Biol* 1:57–72, 1981.
21. Ono K et al: Oral findings in Johanson-Blizzard syndrome. *J Oral Med* 42:14–16, 1987.
22. Park IJ et al: Special female hermaphroditism associated with multiple disorders. *Obstet Gynecol* 39:100–106, 1972.
23. Reichart P et al: Ektodermale Dysplasie und exokrine Pankreasinsuffizienz–ein erblich bedingtes Syndrom. *Dtsch Zahnärztl Z* 34:263–265, 1979.
24. Rudnik-Schöneborn S et al: Johanson-Blizzard-Syndrom. *Klin Pädiatr* 203:33–38, 1991.
25. Schussheim A et al: Exocrine pancreatic insufficiency with congenital anomalies. *J Pediatr* 89:782–784, 1976.
26. Sismanis A et al: Rare congenital syndrome associated with profound hearing loss. *Arch Otolaryngol* 105:222–224, 1979.
27. Steinbach WJ, Hintz RL. Diabetes mellitus and profound insulin resistance in Johanson-Blizzard syndrome. *J Pediatr Endocrinol Metab* 13:1633–1636, 2000.
28. Swanenburg de Veye HFN et al: A child of high intelligence with the Johanson-Blizzard syndrome. *Genet Couns* 2:21–25, 1991.
29. Townes PL, White MR: Identity of two syndromes: proteolytic, lipolytic and amylolytic deficiency of the exocrine pancreas with congenital anomalies. *Am J Dis Child* 135:248–250, 1981.
30. Vanlieferinghen P et al: Prenatal ultrasonographic diagnosis of a recurrent case of Johanson-Blizzard syndrome. *Genet Couns* 14:105–107, 2003.
31. Zerres K, Holtgrave EA: The Johanson-Blizzard syndrome: report of a new case with special reference to the dentition and review of the literature. *Clin Genet* 30:177–183, 1986.

Lingual thyroid and sensorineural hearing loss

An association between sensorineural hearing loss and lingual thyroid has been recorded on only a couple of occasions. Elidan et al. (1) described a female patient with lingual thyroid, mental retardation, and severe sensorineural hearing loss. However, at birth there was an asphyxic episode. An intrauterine infection due to cytomegalovirus or toxoplasmosis might have been responsible for the mental retardation and sensorineural hearing loss, but perinatal TORCH tests were not done. Wetke (2) noted a female patient with lingual thyroid and bilateral 50–60 dB sensorineural hearing loss that first became evident at approximately 8 years of age. Intelligence was normal. In view of the scarcity of reports, it seems unlikely that this association represents a true syndromic observation and a chance association seems more likely.

References

1. Elidan J et al: Lingual thyroid, sensorineural hearing loss and mental retardation: a coincidental association. *J Laryngol Otol* 97:539–542, 1983.
2. Wetke R: Struma baseos linguae og bilateral perceptiv h renedsaettelse. *Ugeskr Laeger* 151:2734–2735, 1989.

Congenital absence of thyroid and sensorineural hearing loss

Congenital absence of the thyroid has a prevalence of 1 per 3000 to 4000 births (4), although striking racial differences have been observed by some authors, who drew attention to the higher prevalence among whites (2,3). While familial aggregation is described (1,6,8), most cases are not associated with deafness.

Toomey et al. (9) described the association between sensorineural hearing loss and congenital absence of the thyroid in a 3-year-old male, offspring of a consanguineous union. The absence of thyroid was documented by technetium 99 scan. The child exhibited microcephaly with slightly delayed development, hypotelorism, hypogenitalism, and moderate to severe sensorineural hearing loss. The paternal grandparents were also first cousins and had three children with late-onset progressive sensorineural hearing loss.

The case reported by Peters and Bankier (7) should also be noted for the observation of agenesis of the thyroid gland with sensorineural hearing loss in a male patient, offspring of a nonconsanguineous union. Initially confined to the middle frequencies, the hearing defect progressed to involve loss of high-frequency acuity. This patient additionally had a lipomatous myelomeningocoele.

Debruyne et al. (5), in reporting a 20% prevalence of sensorineural hearing loss among congenitally hypothyroid children, specifically identified three hearing-impaired individuals whose hypothyroidism was due to thyroid agenesis.

References

1. Ainger LE, Kelley VC: Familial athyreotic cretinism: report of 3 cases. *J Clin Endocrinol* 15:469–475, 1955.
2. Brown AL et al: Racial differences in the incidence of congenital hypothyroidism. *J Pediatr* 99:934–936, 1981.
3. Childs B, Gardner LI: Etiologic factors in sporadic cretinism: an analysis of 90 cases. *Ann Hum Genet* 19:90–96, 1954.
4. Clifton-Bligh RJ et al: Mutation of the gene encoding human TTF-2 associated with thyroid agenesis, cleft palate and choanal atresia. *Nat Genet* 19:399–401, 1998.
5. DeBruyne F et al: Hearing in congenital hypothyroidism. *Audiology* 22:404–409, 1983.
6. Greig WR et al: Thyroid dysgenesis in two pairs of monozygotic twins and in a mother and child. *J Clin Endocrinol* 26:1309–1316, 1966.
7. Peters HL, Bankier A: Lipomatous myelomeningocele, athyrotic hypothyroidism and sensorineural deafness: a new form of syndromal deafness? *J Med Genet* 35:948–950, 1998.
8. Sutherland JM, et al: Familial nongoitrous cretinism apparently due to maternal antithyroid antibody. *N Engl J Med* 263:336–341, 1960.
9. Toomey KE et al: Autosomal recessive sensorineural deafness and congenital absence of the thyroid. Abstract 788, Proceedings of the 8th International Congress on Human Genetics, October 6–11, 1991, Washington, DC.

Generalized resistance to thyroid hormone (GRTH) and sensorineural hearing loss

The full-blown clinical syndrome of generalized resistance to thyroid hormone (GRTH), comprising goiter, stippled epiphyses, delayed bone age, and severe congenital sensorineural hearing loss, dates from the report of Refetoff et al. (12) in 1967. This kindred is now known to have a homozygous deletion of the thyroid hormone receptor beta (TRHB) locus on chromosome 3 (19,20). The observation of affected siblings, offspring of a consanguineous union, gave rise to a supposition that the condition was of an autosomal recessive nature (12). Clinically overlapping families in whom goiter and delayed bone maturation were identified segregating in an autosomal dominant manner have also been shown to have mutations of the *TRHB* gene (12,13,19–23). Most such mutations are missense and likely through a dominant negative mode of action result in a presumed loss of receptor-binding function (20). Deafness has been a feature of at least eight families (13), comprising about 4% of affected individuals (23).

Physical findings. As emphasized by Refetoff et al. (13), there are no pathognomic signs associated with GRTH. Hearing loss, nystagmus, neonatal jaundice, delayed bone maturation, stippled epiphyses in the recessive form, learning disability, and attention deficit hyperactivity disorder (ADHD) are all well described.

Endocrine system. Goiter is the single most common finding, being recorded in over 90% of cases (13). Thyroid enlargement is usually diffuse and recurred in several cases after surgical resection. Typically there is elevated T_4, with nonsuppressed thyroid-stimulating hormone (TSH) levels, but without evidence of thyrotoxicosis. Tissue resistance to thyroid hormone represents a heterogeneous group of disorders. The thyroid gland elaborates excessive levels of thyroid hormone. The defect in peripheral resistance to thyroid hormone is due to defective thyroid hormone feedback regulation, i.e., thyrotropin (TSH) is nonsuppressed.

Radiographic findings. Radiographs of the autosomal recessive form showed stippling throughout the ossification centers, most prominently in the proximal and distal femoral and proximal tibial and humeral epiphyses (Fig. 12–6A). Bone age was mildly retarded. In time, the stippling disappeared, but the epiphyseal heads of the humerus and femur became flattened; all three sibs showed varus deformity of the femoral necks. Laminograms of the petrous bones showed decreased length of the internal auditory canals. In the more common autosomal dominant form, delayed bone age is a feature of approximately 50% of cases (13). Stippled epiphyses have also been an occasional observation in other cases, probably of autosomal dominant form (13).

Auditory system. Congenital severe bilateral sensorineural hearing loss was present in all three siblings manifesting the recessive form (12). The hearing loss was more marked in the higher frequencies (Fig. 12–6B). The degree of hearing impairment in autosomal dominant forms is variable, but very limited data are available (6,13,16,18). Four percent of affected individuals are thought to have sensorineural hearing impairment (23).

Heredity. Both autosomal dominant (13) and autosomal recessive (12,19,20) forms are described and mutation of the THRB locus is established in both forms (11,14,19–23). In excess of 38 different point mutations have been reported (11), generally clustered in the hormone-binding domain. In the consanguineous family on which the original syndrome description is based (12), a homozygous deletion of the *THRB* gene at 3p24.3 has been demonstrated (19,20). While autosomal dominant inheritance is the rule, about 10% of case are thought to be autosomal recessively determined (19).

Diagnosis. Resistance to the action of thyroid hormone in peripheral tissues has been described in over 300 cases (1–4,6–10,12, 13,15–18,23). In only a few cases did patients have hearing loss (6,16,18). Stippled epiphyses may occur in a number of disorders: chondrodysplasia punctata, Zellweger syndrome, multiple epiphyseal dysplasia, warfarin embryopathy, and many other conditions (5).

Prognosis. There appeared to be no progression of any aspect of the disorder in the recessively described cases (12). The stippled epiphyses cleared and, although the femoral heads were flattened, the patients experienced no difficulty in ambulation.

Summary. This is a clinically heterogeneous syndrome characterized by (*1*) goiter with abnormally high T$_4$ in the presence of normal levels of TSH; (*2*) bony abnormalities comprising delayed bone age, occasionally with stippled epiphyses; (*3*) moderate to severe congenital sensorineural hearing loss in the recessive form, but with generally normal or only mildly impaired sensorineural hearing loss in the dominant form; and (*4*) evidence of developmental delay or ADHD in many patients.

References

1. Bode HH et al: Partial target organ resistance to thyroid hormone. *J Clin Invest* 52:776–782, 1973.
2. Brooks MH et al: Familial hormone resistance: *Am J Med* 71:414–421, 1981.
3. Elewaut A et al: Familial partial target organ resistance to thyroid hormones. *J Clin Endocrinol Metab* 43:575–581, 1976.
4. Gershengorn MC, Weintraub BD: Thyrotropin-induced hyperthyroidism caused by selective pituitary resistance to thyroid hormone. *J Clin Invest* 56:633–642, 1975.
5. Gorlin RJ et al: *Syndromes of the Head and Neck,* 4th ed. Oxford University Press, New York, 2001.
6. Kaplowitz PB et al: Peripheral resistance to thyroid hormone in an infant. *J Clin Endocrinol Metab* 53:958–963, 1981.
7. Lamberg BA: Congenital euthyroid goitre and partial peripheral resistance to thyroid hormones. *Lancet* 1:854–857, 1973.
8. Mäenpä J, Liewendahl K: Peripheral insensitivity to thyroid hormones in a euthyroid girl with goitre. *Arch Dis Child* 55:207–212, 1980.
9. Novogroder M et al: Juvenile hyperthyroidism with elevated thyrotropism (THS) and normal 24 hour FSH, LH, GH and prolactin secretory rates. *J Clin Endocrinol Metab* 45:1053–1059, 1977.
10. Ohzeki T et al: Thyroid hormone unresponsiveness in two siblings with intrauterine growth retardation and exophthalmos. *Eur J Pediatr* 141:181–183, 1984.
11. Pohlenz J et al: New point mutation (R243W) in the hormone binding domain of the c-erbA beta-1 gene in a family with generalised resistance to thyroid hormone. *Hum Mutat* 7:79–81, 1996

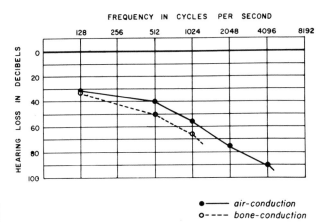

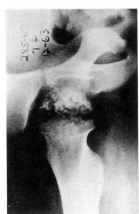

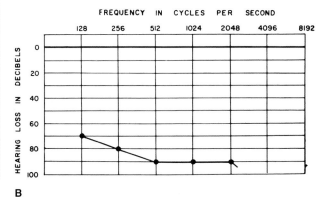

Figure 12–6. *Generalized resistance to thyroid hormone (GRTH) and sensorineural hearing loss.* (A,B) Twelve- and 8-year-old sibs with sharp facies, pectus carinatum, and winged scapulae. (A) Radiograph showing stippled epiphysis of femoral head. Similar changes were present at the knees and in the proximal humerus. (B) Pure-tone audiograms of two sibs showing similar hearing loss, more marked in the higher frequencies. [From S Refetoff et al., *J Clin Endocrinol Metab* 27:279, 1967.]

A   B

12. Refetoff S et al: Familial syndrome combining deaf-mutism, stippled epiphyses, goiter and abnormally high PBI: possible target organ refractoriness to thyroid hormone. *J Clin Endocrinol* 27:279–294, 1967.

13. Refetoff S et al: The syndromes of resistance to thyroid hormone. *Endocrine Rev* 14:348–399, 1993

14. Sakurai A et al: Generalized resistance to thyroid hormone associated with a mutation in the ligand-binding domain of the human thyroid hormone receptor beta. *Proc Natl Acad Sci* 86:8977–8981, 1989.

15. Salazar A et al: Studies on a new case of resistance to the action of thyroid hormone. *Endocrinology* 208(Suppl):265, 1981.

16. Salmerón De Diego J et al: Syndrome of "inappropriate secretion of thyroid-stimulating hormone" by partial target organ resistance to thyroid hormones. *Acta Endocrinol* 99:361–368, 1981.

17. Schneider G et al: Peripheral resistance to thyroxine: a cause of short stature in a boy without goiter. *Clin Endocrinol* 4:111–118, 1975.

18. Seif FJ et al: Syndrome of elevated thyroid hormone and SSH blood levels. *Ann Endocrinol (Paris)* 87(Suppl 215):81–82, 1978.

19. Takeda K et al: Screening of nineteen unrelated families with generalized resistance to thyroid hormone for known point mutations in the thyroid hormone receptor β gene and the detection of a new mutation. *J Clin Invest* 87:486–502, 1991.

20. Takeda K et al: Recessive inheritance of thyroid hormone resistance caused by complete deletion of the protein coding region of the thyroid hormone receptor-B gene. *J Clin Endocrinol Metab* 74:49–55, 1992.

21. Usala SJ et al: A base mutation of the C-erbA-beta thyroid hormone receptor in a kindred with generalized thyroid hormone resistance: molecular heterogeneity in two other kindreds. *J Clin Invest* 85:93–100, 1990.

22. Usala SJ et al: Diverse abnormalities of the C-ERBAB thyroid hormone receptor gene in generalised thyroid hormone resistance. *Adv Exp Med Biol* 299:251–258, 1991

23. Vassart G et al: Thyroid disorders. In: *The Metabolic and Molecular Bases of Inherited Disease*, 7th ed., Scriver CR et al (eds), McGraw-Hill, New York, 1995, Vol. II, pp 2883–2928.

Sensorineural hearing loss associated with iodine deficiency and/or congenital hypothyroidism

In addition to the specific syndromes outlined above, it has long been recognized that endemic cretinism is associated with hearing loss (10,15). Reports from specific geographical areas known to be iodine-deficient have established widespread neurological and developmental sequelae among affected individuals (4,7,11), including sensorineural deafness in perhaps 50% of cases (8). Ill understood at present, it is speculated that these clinical findings are the consequence of restricted availability of iodine to the fetus during critical phases of CNS development. In general support of this hypothesis are observations of spatiotemporal variation in thyroid hormone receptor expression in the rat brain during development (2,3) and the likely importance of transcription factors such as thyroid hormone receptors in development of the mammalian cochlea (5). Moreover, thyroid hormone beta receptor has been shown to be essential to normal auditory development in the mouse, although, in view of the reported widespread expression pattern throughout the developing CNS, it is interesting that no other neurological deficits have been observed in thyroid hormone beta receptor knockout mice (9). It is also worth observing that in the autosomal recessive form of GRTH described by Refetoff et al. (12), patients who have a homozygous deletion of the thyroid hormone receptor beta locus have no other structural CNS disturbance apart from hearing loss, although ADHD has been observed. Likewise, organ of Corti abnormalities have been recorded in congenitally hypothyroid rat models, and a time- or developmental stage–specific response to thyroxine treatment is suggested by the rescuing action of thyroxine from these morphogenetic effects of congenital hypothyroidism (16,17).

Hearing impairment associated with successfully treated congenital hypothyroidism is well reported (1,6,13,14). The prevalence and degree of sensorineural hearing impairment among reported cohorts vary and not all reported patient groups are comparable. The highest rate of hearing loss was that observed by Anand et al. (1) at 80%, in a cohort of 20 patients ranging in age from 15 to 50 years. In contrast, a more recent study of 75 children identified through newborn thyroid-screening programs and investigated longitudinally indicated hearing problems in

20%, of which two-thirds were sensorineural and one-third, conductive (13).

References

1. Anand VT et al: Auditory investigations in hypothyroidism. *Acta Otolaryngol (Stockh)* 108:83–87, 1989.

2. Bradley DJ et al: Spatial and temporal expression of alpha and beta thyroid hormone receptor mRNAs, including the beta2 subtype, in the developing mammalian nervous system. *J Neurosci* 12:2288–2302, 1992.

3. Bradley DJ et al: Alpha and beta thyroid hormone receptor (TR) gene expression during auditory neurogenesis: evidence for TR isoform-specific transcriptional regulation in vivo. *Proc Natl Acad Sci USA* 91:439–443, 1994.

4. Choufoer JC et al: Endemic goiter in western New Guinea. II: clinical picture, incidence and pathogenesis of endemic cretinism. *J Clin Endocrinol Metab* 25:385–402, 1965.

5. Corey DP, Breakefield XO: Transcription factors in inner ear development. *Proc Natl Acad Sci USA* 91:433–436, 1994.

6. Crifo S et al: A retrospective study of audiological function in a group of congenital hypothyroid patients. *Intl J Pediatr Otorhinolaryngol* 2:347–355, 1980.

7. Delange FM et al: A survey of the clinical and metabolic patterns of endemic cretinism. *Adv Exp Med Biol* 30:175–187, 1972.

8. DeLong GR et al: Neurological signs in congenital iodine-deficiency disorder (endemic cretinism). *Dev Med Child Neurol* 27:317–324, 1985.

9. Forrest D: Thyroid hormone receptor beta is essential for development of auditory function. *Nat Genet* 13:354–357, 1996.

10. McCarrison R: Observations on endemic cretinism in the Chitral and Gilgit valleys. *Lancet* 2:1275–1280, 1908.

11. Pharoah POD et al: Neurological damage to the fetus resulting from severe iodine deficiency during pregnancy. *Lancet* 1:308–310, 1971.

12. Refetoff S et al: Familial syndrome combining deaf-mutism, stippled epiphyses, goiter and abnormally high PBI: possible target organ refractoriness to thyroid hormone. *J Clin Endocrinol* 27:279–294, 1967.

13. Rovet J et al: Long-term sequelae of hearing impairment in congenital hypothyroidism. *J Pediatr* 128:776–783, 1996.

14. Rubenstein M et al: Hearing dysfunction associated with congenital sporadic hypothyroidism. *Ann Otol* 83:814–819, 1974.

15. Trotter WR: The association of deafness with thyroid dysfunction. *Br Med Bull* 16:92–98, 1960.

16. Uziel A: Effects of hypothyroidism on the structural development of the organ of Corti in the rat. *Acta Otolaryngol* 92:469–480, 1981.

17. Uziel A: Periods of sensitivity to thyroid hormone during the development of the organ of Corti. *Acta Otolaryngol (Stockh) Suppl* 429:23–27, 1986.

Hypoparathyroidism, deafness, and renal disease (HDR syndrome)

A phenotypic overlap between patients identified with 10p13–14 deletions and DiGeorge syndrome was recognised because of the shared clinical features including hypoparathyroidism, congenital heart malformations, immunodeficiencies, sensorineural hearing loss, and renal malformations (4,5,7–10,12). The term *HDR syndrome* dates from the 1997 report of Hasegawa et al. of this triad of clinical features associated with a de novo 10p deletion (5). Bilous et al. (2) recorded renal dysplasia, hypoparathyroidism, and sensorineural hearing loss in eight members of two generations of the same family. Although the features were variable, four individuals had all three clinical components. A further two individuals had renal dysplasia as the sole feature. Functional haploinsufficiency of the *GATA3* gene has now been established as the molecular basis of the disorder (11,14).

Endocrine system. Hypocalcemia and/or hypoparathyroidism are the essential characteristics. Muroya et al. (11) reported these findings in 11 of 13 biochemically examined cases. Ten of these cases had afebrile convulsions, irritability, or tetany and were shown to have low parathyroid hormone (PTH) levels. Other features consistent with hypocalcemia include cataracts, enamel hypoplasia, and basal ganglia calcification (1,11,16). The other case was clinically asymptomatic but neonatal hypocalcaemia was recorded and PTH assay indicated a low level of hormone.

Auditory system. Sensorineural hearing loss was a consistent feature in 9 of 11 cases examined by audiometry or by brain stem auditory evoked response (11). The degree of hearing loss was variable, embracing mild to profound impairment, but was generally symmetrical. Hearing loss was clinically suspected in other cases for whom formal audiological evaluation was not available in view of speech delay or other suggestive clinical observations. Reporting on individuals with hypoparathyroidism, Ikeda et al. (6) identified several with different degrees of sensorineural hearing loss. A proportion of these cases may have had unrecognized HDR syndrome.

Renal findings. Bilous et al. (2) recorded large renal cysts in two of the individuals reported. Abnormal serum creatnine concentrations and reduction in glomerular filtration rate were seen in individuals with the full-blown syndrome. Intravenous urography was consistent with renal dysplasia in that the kidneys were small and irregular with compressed collecting systems, while renal biopsy demonstrated both normal and dysplastic areas. Muroya et al. (11) reported likely or confirmed renal lesions in 13 of 16 cases identified. These lesions, requiring a range of complementary investigations for their demonstration, comprised renal aplasia, hypoplasia, pelvicalyceal malformations, vesicoureteric reflux, and extensive renal scarring. Six cases progressed to chronic renal failure.

Heredity. Most cases have been identified in the context of cytogenetically visible or molecularly proven deletions (3,8,11,14). Several such cases have also had developmental delay in addition to the other clinical problems. Heterozygous whole gene deletions, intragenic deletions, and other forms of mutation, including missense mutations, have been identified in the *GATA3* gene in affected individuals and families (11,14). On the basis of DNA-binding studies, these mutations are thought to result in functional haploinsufficiency of *GATA3* (14). A history consistent with autosomal dominant transmission should be sought.

Diagnosis. Establishing the diagnosis by molecular means should remove much of the diagnostic uncertainty that has surrounded this condition. It is clear from those cases reported that a high index of clinical suspicion, careful evaluation of family history, and detailed investigation both clinically and cytogenetically have been the mainstays of diagnosis.

Barakat et al. (1) reported two brothers with sensorineural deafness, hypoparathyroidism, and steroid resistant nephrosis, leading to renal failure and death at ages 5 and 8 years. Autopsy findings showed absence of the parathyroid glands in one brother and hypoplastic glands in the other. These authors also described a second family in which male twins had a similar clinical profile and autopsy showed fibrotic parathyroid glands and thickened glomerular basement membranes. The likelihood that this report represents the original description of HDR syndrome has been addressed by Hasegawa et al. (5), who emphasize the likelihood of autosomal dominant inheritance in the Barakat report, since the paternal grandmother and her three siblings all had degrees of hearing loss.

Further possible reports of this syndrome include those of Shaw et al. (13) and Yumita et al. (16). Shaw et al. (13) described hypoparathyroidism and renal insufficiency in four cousins, two of whom had sensorineural hearing loss. Yumita et al. (16) reported two families with idiopathic hypoparathyroidism and progressive sensorineural deafness. It is more difficult to classify the report from Watanabe et al. (15) of a three-generational family ascertained through hypocalcemic seizures in a male infant. Five individuals were found with hypoparathyroidism and sensorineural hearing loss. Renal investigations were normal and there was no evidence of impaired renal function.

Summary. The syndrome is characterized by a clinically variable presentation embracing (*1*) hypoparathyroidism that need not be symptomatic; (*2*) renal anomalies; (*3*) hearing impairment; and (*4*) autosomal dominant inheritance.

References

1. Barakat AY et al: Familial nephrosis, nerve deafness, and hypoparathyroidism. *J Pediatr* 91:61–64, 1977.
2. Bilous RW et al: Autosomal dominant familial hypoparathyroidism, sensorineural deafness, and renal dysplasia. *N Engl J Med* 327:1069–1074, 1992.
3. Daw SCM et al: A common region of 10p deleted in DiGeorge and velocardiofacial syndromes. *Nat Genet* 13:458–460, 1996.
4. Greenberg F et al: Hypoparathyroidism and T cell immune defect in a patient with 10p deletion syndrome. *J Pediatr* 109:489–492, 1986.
5. Hasegawa T et al: HDR syndrome (hypoparathyroidism, sensorineural deafness, renal dysplasia) associated with del(10)(p13). *Am J Med Genet* 73:416–418, 1997.
6. Ikeda K et al: Sensorineural hearing loss associated with hypoparathyroidism. *Laryngoscope* 97:1075–1079, 1987.
7. Kato Z et al: Interstitial deletion of the short arm of chromosome 10: report of a case and review of the literature. *Jpn J Hum Genet* 41:333–338, 1996.
8. Lichtner P et al: An HDR (hypoparathyroidism, deafness, renal dysplasia) syndrome locus maps distal to the DiGeorge syndrome region on 10p13–14. *J Med Genet* 37:33–37, 2000.
9. Lipson A et al: Velo-cardio-facial and partial DiGeorge phenotype in a child with interstitial deletion at 10p13—implications for cytogenetics and molecular biology. *Am J Med Genet* 65:304–308, 1996.
10. Lynch S et al: Comparison of facial features of DiGeorge syndrome (DGS) due to deletion 10p13–10pter with DGS due to 22q deletion. *J Med Genet* 32:149, 1995.
11. Muroya K et al: GATA3 abnormalities and the phenotypic spectrum of HDR syndrome. *J Med Genet* 38:374–380, 2001.
12. Schuffenhauer S et al: DiGeorge syndrome and partial monosomy 10p: case report and review. *Ann Genet* 38:162–167, 1995.
13. Shaw NJ et al: Autosomal recessive hypoparathyroidism with renal insufficiency and developmental delay. *Arch Dis Child* 66:1191–1194, 1991.
14. Van Esch H et al: GATA3 haplo-insufficiency causes human HDR syndrome. *Nature* 406:419–422, 2000.
15. Watanabe T et al: Autosomal dominant familial hypoparathyroidism and sensorineural deafness without renal dysplasia. *Eur J Endocrinol* 139:631–634, 1998.
16. Yumita S et al: Familial idiopathic hypoparathyroidism and progressive sensorineural deafness. *Tohoku J Exp Med* 148:135–141, 1986.

Hyperparathyroidism, nephropathy, and sensorineural hearing loss

Edwards et al. (1) described renal failure, parathyroid hyperplasia with hyperparathyroidism, and sensorineural hearing loss in a consanguineous Pakistani family. A sister and brother had the full-blown syndrome, while a sister had hearing loss and hyperparathyroidism only, a brother had hearing problems and renal failure, and a further brother had hearing loss in the absence of other features. The renal failure did not show evidence of hematuria. This factor as well as the parathyroid hyperplasia and presumed autosomal recessivity led the authors to differentiate between the condition and Alport syndrome. The possibility that the family may represent an example of HDR syndrome (see above) cannot be excluded.

Summary. This syndrome is characterised by (*1*) apparent autosomal recessive inheritance; (*2*) progressive nephropathy with renal failure; (*3*) variable occurrence of hyperparathyroidism; and (*4*) variable sensorineural hearing loss.

Reference

1. Edwards BD et al: A new syndrome of autosomal recessive nephropathy, deafness and hyperparathyroidism. *J Med Genet* 26:289–293, 1989.

Pseudohypoparathyroidism and sensorineural hearing loss

Pseudohypoparathyroidism (PHP) encompasses a heterogeneous syndrome group caused by a deficit in the G-protein system, proteins responsible for transduction of biological signals through the outer cell membrane. Pseudohypoparathyroidism can be caused by multiple pre-

and post-receptor defects. There is decreased parathormone (PTH) effect in all body tissues despite normal secretion by the parathyroid glands. The organ resistance leads to hypocalcemia and hyperphosphatemia and occasional tetanic seizures, paresthesias, laryngeal spasm, and ectopic calcification in the eye, subcutaneous tissues, and brain. Following intravenous PTH infusion there is usually no urinary increase in cAMP.

Clinical features include short stature, round facies, obesity, and, at times, mental retardation.

Auditory system. Koch et al. (1) noted sensorineural hearing loss in 14 of 22 patients. The loss was bilateral and involved the higher frequencies. La Rouere et al. (2) reported malleus head fixation with associated conductive hearing loss. Wilson and Trembath (3) drew attention to the high prevalence of secretory middle ear disease in young children, resulting in surgical insertion of grommets in a high proportion of their cases. In view of the many case reports of PHP and the paucity of audiologic findings, these reports need substantiation.

References

1. Koch T et al: Sensorineural hearing loss owing to deficient G proteins in patients with pseudohypoparathyroidism: results of a multicentre study. *Eur J Clin Invest* 20:416–421, 1990.
2. La Rouere MJ et al: Malleus head fixation: association with pseudohypoparathyroidism. *Am J Otol* 11:354–356, 1990.
3. Wilson LC, Trembath RC: Syndrome of the month: Albright's hereditary osteodystrophy. *J Med Genet* 31:779–784, 1994.

Hypopituitary dwarfism and sensorineural hearing loss (Winkelmann syndrome)

Winkelmann et al. (1) reported two sisters with hypothalamohypophyseal dwarfism and sensorineural hearing loss.

Physical findings. Birth weight and size were normal. Proportionate growth retardation was first noted at the time of school registration. Adult height was 139 cm in one sister and 146 cm in the other (Fig. 12–7).

Endocrine system. Neither girl achieved sexual maturity, i.e., neither developed pubic hair or breasts, and both had primary amenorrhea. The external and internal genitalia were infantile.

Auditory system. At the age of approximately 6–8 years, rapidly progressive hearing loss was noted. By 12 years of age, both sisters were totally deaf.

Vestibular system. No studies were reported.

Laboratory findings. Radiographic examination of the sisters as adults showed generalized retarded bone age (open cranial sutures and absence of epiphyseal fusion).

Radioimmunologic assays of plasma levels of human growth hormone (HGH) were 3.0 ng/ml (normal levels are 30.0 ± 10.0 ng/ml), rising no higher than 5.0 ng/ml on insulin stimulation. Follicle-stimulating hormone (FSH) and luteinizing hormone (LH) assays were at prepubertal levels. Radioactive iodine uptake, cortisol, and corticosterone excretion were normal. Urinary 17-hydroxy- and 11-hydroxy-corticosteroid levels were normal, even after corticotropin stimulation. Serum cholesterol and triglycerides were elevated in one girl but were normal in the other.

Heredity. The parents and one sister of the patients were normal. There was no known parental consanguinity. Inheritance appears to be autosomal recessive.

Diagnosis. There are several types of pituitary dwarfism, but none has been associated with sensorineural hearing loss.

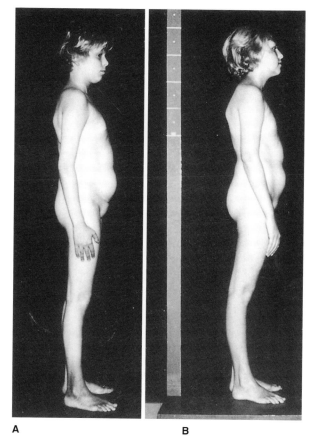

A   B

Figure 12–7. *Hypopituitary dwarfism and sensorineural hearing loss (Winkelman syndrome).* (A,B) Sisters at 22 and 19 years of age, respectively, exhibiting reduced height and lack of sexual maturity. [From W Winkelmann et al., *Internist* 13:52, 1972.]

Summary. Characteristics of the syndrome include (*1*) autosomal recessive inheritance; (*2*) somatic and sexual infantilism due to deficiency of growth hormone and gonadotropins; (*3*) normal intelligence; and (*4*) sensorineural hearing loss, appearing at about 6–8 years of age and progressing rapidly to complete hearing loss.

Reference

1. Winkelmann W et al: Hypothalamohypophysärer Minderwuchs mit Innenohrschwerhörigkeit bei zwei Schwestern. *Internist* 13:52–56, 1972.

Prenatal dwarfism, elevated growth hormone levels, mental retardation, and congenital hearing loss

In 1969, Van Gemund et al. (4) reported two male sibs with prenatal dwarfism, elevated serum immunoreactive growth hormone and end-organ unresponsiveness, mental retardation, and congenital hearing loss.

Physical findings. Birth weight at term was <1900 grams. Both sibs were proportionately short. Head circumference was reduced. Pubertal signs, even under therapy, did not appear until 20 years of age. The midface was underdeveloped (Fig. 12–8).

Central nervous system. Both sibs had IQs of less than 40.

Auditory system. Both sibs were congenitally profoundly deaf, and neither achieved any facility of speech. The hearing loss was not otherwise described.

Vestibular system. No studies were reported.

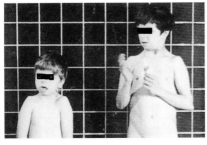
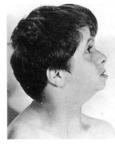

A   **B**

Figure 12–8. *Prenatal dwarfism, elevated growth hormone levels, mental retardation, and congenital hearing loss.* (A) Sibs at 12 years of age (height, 97 cm) and 22 years of age (height, 117 cm). (B) Note hypoplasia of midface. [From JJ Van Gemund et al., *Maandschr Kindergeneeskd* 37:372, 1969.]

Laboratory findings. Radiographic study showed severely delayed skeletal maturation. Insulin-induced hypoglycemia evoked markedly high levels of immunoreactive HGH. Exogenous HGH induced normal responses of serum insulin, glucose, and free fatty acids but failed to increase nitrogen retention and urinary hydroxyproline excretion. Unresponsiveness to the somatotropic effects of HGH was postulated.

Heredity. The normal parents of the two affected males were consanguineous. The disorder probably has autosomal recessive inheritance. A maternal uncle had dwarfism and mental retardation. Thus, X-linked inheritance cannot be excluded.

Diagnosis. Laron-type pituitary dwarfism is characterized by high-serum immunoreactive HGH levels but mental retardation or hearing loss is not present. Defective growth hormone receptor binging, usually as a result of mutation in the growth hormone receptor gene (1–3), is found in Laron-type dwarfism.

Prognosis. Although the disorder was not life-threatening, prognosis for growth was poor since treatment was ineffective.

Summary. Characteristics of this syndrome include (*1*) autosomal or X-linked recessive inheritance; (*2*) prenatal dwarfism; (*3*) elevated serum immunoreactive growth hormone and end-organ unresponsiveness; (*4*) mental retardation; and (*5*) profound congenital hearing loss, probably sensorineural.

References

1. Berg MA et al: Diverse growth hormone receptor gene mutations in Laron syndrome. *Am J Hum Genet* 52:998–1005, 1993.
2. Daughaday WH, Trevedi B: Absence of serum growth hormone binding protein in patients with growth hormone receptor deficiency (Laron dwarfism). *Proc Natl Acad Sci USA* 84:4636–4640, 1987.
3. Goddard AD et al: Mutations of the growth hormone receptor in children with idiopathic short stature. *N Engl J Med* 333:1093–1098, 1995.
4. Van Gemund JJ et al: Familial prenatal dwarfism and elevated serum-immunoreactive growth hormone levels and end-organ unresponsiveness. *Maandschr Kindergeneeskd* 37:372–382, 1969.

Hypogonadotrophic hypogonadism, anosmia, and sensorineural hearing loss (Kallmann syndrome)

Although attributed eponymously to Kallmann et al.'s 1944 report (13), the syndrome of hypogonadism and anosmia appears to have been first recorded by Maestre de San Juan in 1856 (17). The hypogonadism is consequent on reduced hypothalamic secretion of gonadotropin-releasing hormone (GnRH), which can be partial or complete. The estimated prevalence of the condition is 1/10,000 males and 1/50,000 females (12).

Genitourinary system. Arising from the hypogonadism, the typical profile of affected adult males includes small genitalia and sparse sexual hair. About 60% have gynecomastia and eunuchoid habitus. Cryptorchidism and infantile testes have been reported (30). Clinical presentation is usually in the teenage years with delayed appearance of secondary sexual charactristics.

Microscopically there are decreased numbers of germ cells and aspermia. Leydig cells are absent. Manifesting females range in signs from irregular to absent menses, scanty pubic and axillary hair, and failure of breast development. In some cases, the ovaries appear fetal (18). Other carrier females are normal. Unilateral renal aplasia is well described (9,10,31).

Craniofacial findings. About 15% of patients have cleft lip and/or cleft palate (6,16,25–27,29,32).

Anosmia. The anosmia, which can require formal evaluation, is secondary to agenesis of olfactory lobes, the patient frequently being unaware of the sensory deficit. Although MRI scanning has been used to demostrated the absence of the olfactory bulbs (24), it is not as reliable as a thorough assessment of olfactory function in identifying affected individuals. Some females can show partial or complete anosmia (18).

Auditory findings. Hearing loss is an occasional finding, though not a cardinal feature of the disorder. Lieblich et al. (16) found 5 of 23 patients to have decreased hearing. Bardin et al. (3) noted hearing loss in 2 of 7 patients, and Hill et al. (11) found it in 2 of 11 patients. There are several isolated examples (13,26,27). In most cases it has been mild, bilateral, and sensorineural, but Hill et al. (11) found moderate to severe mixed loss more marked at middle frequencies. Levy and Knudtzon (15) noted unilateral hearing loss. Radiologic studies have shown abnormal morphology of semicircular canals and internal auditory meatus (11).

Vestibular findings. Absence of response to caloric and rotational chair testing is recorded (11).

Other clinical findings. The most important of other clinical findings is that of mirror movements, thought to result from absence of neural fibers within the corpus callosum that normally cross and inhibit the contralateral pyramidal tract (21). This hypothesis is supported by MRI findings from Krams et al. (14) identifying thickened corticospinal tracts in affected individuals. Pes cavus, eye movement disorders, cerebellar ataxia, and mental retardation are all recorded, although it is important to note that in the X-linked form, mental retardation is almost exclusively a feature of patients with deletions on Xp22.3 (22). Patients with contiguous gene deletions of this region can manifest additional clinical features of ichthyosis, chondrodysplasia punctata, short stature, and ocular albinism (1,2,4).

Laboratory findings. Urinary gonadotropins are low. There is a lack of postnatal rise of LH and testosterone in early infancy and blunted response to LHRH and HCG stimulation tests (7). In older cases, levels of FSH and LH are low and testosterone levels are much reduced in males, paralleled by low estradiol in females.

Heredity. Most cases are X-linked. The X-linked gene is at Xp22.3 (19), adjacent to the genes for ichthyosis and chondrodysplasia punctata (2,4). Mutations within the coding sequence of the gene have been established in several individuals and families with the nondeletion form of Kallman syndrome (5,24). Kallman syndrome represents a neuronal migration defect, with the KAL protein being responsible for synaptogenesis between the olfactory bulb and the incoming axons. Autosomal forms of Kallman syndrome are also reported, both dominant (15,20,27) and recessive pedigrees (8,25,28,32) have been described.

Diagnosis. Among male patients with hypogonadism, about 2.5% have Kallmann syndrome (23). This disorder should be differentiated from hypogonadism and severe congenital mixed hearing loss and Richards-Rundle syndrome.

Summary. This syndrome is characterized by (*1*) hypopituitary hypogonadism; (*2*) anosmia; (*3*) occasional other malformations such as cleft lip or palate and renal agenesis; and (*4*) additional neurological findings, characteristically mirror movements and, in rare instances, hearing loss.

References

1. Ballabio A et al: X-linked ichthyosis due to steroid sulphatase deficiency associated with Kallmann syndrome (hypogonadrophic hypogonadism and anosmia): linkage relationships with Xg and cloned DNA sequences from the distal short arm of the X chromosome. *Hum Genet* 72:237–740, 1986.
2. Ballabio A et al: Contiguous gene syndromes due to deletions in the distal short arm of the human X chromosome. *Proc Natl Acad Sci USA* 86:10001–10005, 1989.
3. Bardin CW et al: Studies of the pituitary–Leydig cell axis in young men with hypogonadotropic hypogonadism and hyposmia: comparison with normal men, prepubertal boys, and hypopituitary patients. *J Clin Invest* 48:2046–2056, 1969.
4. Bick D et al: Male infant with ichthyosis, Kallmann syndrome, chondrodysplasia punctata, and an Xp chromosome deletion. *Am J Med Genet* 33:100–107, 1989.
5. Bick D et al: Intragenic deletion of the *KALIG-1* gene in Kallmann's syndrome. *N Engl J Med* 326:1752–1755, 1992.
6. Christian JC et al: Hypogonadotropic hypogonadism with anosmia. The Kallmann syndrome. *Birth Defects* 7(6):166–171 (case 4).
7. Evain-Brion D et al: Diagnosis of Kallmann's syndrome in early infancy. *Acta Paediatr Scand* 71:937–940, 1982.
8. Floret D et al: Association d'un hypogonadisme hypogonadotrophinurique et d'une surdité familiale. Variante du syndrome de Kallmann? *J Génét Hum* 24(Suppl):207–214, 1976.
9. Hardelin J-P et al: Heterogeneity in the mutstions responsible for X chromosome–linked Kallmann syndrome. *Hum Mol Genet* 2:373–377, 1993.
10. Hermanussen M, Sippell WG: Heterogeneity of Kallmann's syndrome. *Clin Genet* 28:106–111, 1985.
11. Hill J et al: Audiological, vestibular and radiological abnormalities in Kallmann's syndrome. *J Laryngol Otol* 106:530–534, 1992.
12. Jones J, Kemman E: Olfacto-genital dysplasia in the female. *Obstet Gynecol Annu* 5:443, 1976.
13. Kallmann FJ et al: The genetic aspects of primary eunuchoidism. *Am J Ment Defic* 48:203–236, 1944.
14. Krams M et al: Kallmann's syndrome: mirror movements associated with bilateral corticospinal tract hypertrophy. *Neurology* 52:816–822, 1999.
15. Levy CM, Knudtzon J: Kallmann syndrome in two sisters with other developmental anomalies also affecting the father. *Clin Genet* 43:51–53, 1992.
16. Lieblich JM et al: Syndrome of anosmia with hypogonadotropic hypogonadism (Kallmann syndrome): clinical and laboratory studies in 23 cases. *Am J Med* 73:506–519, 1982.
17. Maestre de San Juan A: Teratologia: Falta total de los nervios olfactorios con anosmian en un individuo en quien exista un atrofia congenita de los testiculos y miembro viril. *El Siglo Med* 3:211, 1856.
18. Males JL et al: Hypogonadotropic hypogonadism with anosmia—Kallmann's syndrome: A disorder of olfactory and hypothalamic function. *Arch Intern Med* 131:501–507, 1973.
19. Meitinger T et al: Definitive localization of X-linked Kallmann syndrome (hypogonadotropic hypogonadism and anosmia) to Xp22.3: close linkage to the hypervariable repeat sequence CRI-5232. *Am J Hum Genet* 47:664–669, 1990.
20. Merriam GR et al: Father-to-son transmission of hypogonadism with anosmia. *Am J Dis Child* 131:1216–1219, 1977.
21. Naas R: Mirror movement asymmetries in congenital hemiparesis : the inhibition hypothesis revisited. *Neurology* 35:1059–1062, 1985.
22. Nagata K et al: A novel interstitial deletion of *KAL1* in a Japanese family with Kallman syndrome. *J Hum Genet* 45:237–240, 2000.
23. Pawlowitzki IH et al: Estimating frequency of Kallman syndrome among hypogonadic and among anosmic patients. *Am J Med Genet* 26:473–479, 1987.
24. Quinton R et al: The neuroradiology of Kallmann's syndrome: a genotypic and phenotypic analysis. *J Clin Endocrinol Metab* 81:3010–3017, 1996.
25. Rosen SW: The syndrome of hypogonadism, anosmia and midline cranial anomalies. In: Proceedings of the 47th Meeting of the Endocrinology Society, 1965.
26. Santen RJ, Paulsen CA: Hypogonadotropic eunuchoidism: I. Clinical study of the mode of inheritance. *J Clin Endocrinol* 36:47–54, 1973.
27. Schwankhaus JDD et al: Neurologic findings in men with isolated hypogonadotropic hypogonadism. *Neurology* 39:223–226, 1989.
28. Sparkes RS et al: Familial hypogonadotropic hypogonadism and anosmia. *Arch Intern Med* 121:534–538, 1968.
29. Tagatz G et al: Hypogonadotropic hypogonadism associated with anosmia in the female. *N Engl J Med* 283:1326–1329, 1970.
30. Turner RC et al: Cryptorchidism in a family with Kallmann's syndrome. *Proc R Soc Med* 67:33–35, 1974.
31. Wegenke JD et al: Familial Kallman syndrome with unilateral renal aplasia. *Clin Genet* 7:368–381, 1976.
32. White BJ et al: The syndrome of anosmia with hypogonadotropic hypogonadism: a genetic study of 18 new families and a review. *Am J Med Genet* 15:417–435, 1983.

Autosomal recessive ovarian dysgenesis and congenital sensorineural hearing loss (Perrault syndrome)

In 1951, Perrault et al. (14) described a syndrome of gonadal dysgenesis and severe sensorineural hearing loss in two sisters. In 1963, Josso et al. (8) reexamined the sisters and found a normal 46, XX chromosome constitution. Reviewing the entity in 1998, Gardiner et al. (5) identified 34 reported cases and emphasized the inconstancy of associated clinical findings among affected individuals, specifically mental retardation, lower limb weakness, ataxia, and short stature.

Physical findings. Short stature has been a feature of several individuals (11).

Mental status. Mild mental retardation was noted by Christakos et al. (3). Gardiner at al. (5) observed mental retardation in two of three new families reported. Likewise, Gottschalk et al. (6) emphasized the high prevalence of neurological abnormalities, including mental retardation, among reported cases. It is pertinent to observe that most reported cases are of normal intelligence.

Genitourinary system. XX gonadal dysgenesis refers to primary amenorrhea, with streak gonads observed on laparoscopy. Generally the breasts are underdeveloped, and pubic and axillary hair is sparse (Fig. 12–9). The fallopian tubes and uterus are hypoplastic.

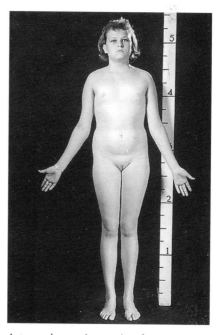

Figure 12–9. *Autosomal recessive ovarian dysgenesis and congenital sensorineural hearing loss (Perrault syndrome).* Seventeen-year-old patient was one of three sisters affected with this syndrome. Note normal height and lack of sexual development. [Courtesy of RB Greenblatt, Augusta, Georgia.]

Affected males have normal genitalia and exhibit normal testicular function.

Other findings. Nishi et al. (11) drew attention to associated features of ataxia, pes equinovarus, nystagmus, and limitation of extraocular movements. These associated features do not conform to a consistent pattern among published families. Similarly, in reporting cerebellar hypoplasia in an affected case, Gottschalk et al. (6) noted the high prevalence of neurological abnormalities among reported cases. Amor et al. (1) have discussed the condition in the context of cerebellar ataxia and ovarian dysgenesis in female siblings with progressive adult-onset hearing loss, hypergonadotropic hypogonadism, normal secondary sexual development, streak ovaries, and small uterus. There is striking clinical overlap between patients described by neurologists with cerebellar ataxia and hypogonadism (1) and some of the associated findings in cases described as examples of Perrault syndrome (2–15). Further possible phenotypic differences are introduced by the family reported by Linssen et al. (9), in whom amelogenesis imperfecta is also a feature. The possibility of heterogeneity arises.

Auditory system. Congenital profound (2,8,11,14) to moderate to severe (10,12,13) sensorineural hearing loss appears to be the general experience in females and is the only finding in affected males. Only one female has not exhibited hearing loss (11). Pallister and Opitz (12) have observed progressive hearing loss. Adult onset of progressive hearing impairment was reported in the siblings studied by Amor et al. (1). Polytomography has shown no abnormality (2).

Vestibular system. No nystagmus was seen following caloric stimulation (2). Diminished vestibular function was also noted by Amor et al. (1) in a somewhat atypical family.

Laboratory findings. Urinary gonadotropins (LH and FSH) are markedly elevated. Estrogen excretion is diminished.

Heredity. Parental consanguinity (3,8,14,15) and affected sibs (8–11,13,14) clearly indicate autosomal recessive inheritance. Hearing loss appears to be the sole manifestation in most affected males. Most reported cases are female, the syndrome being unrecognizable in males. McCarthy and Opitz (10) argued the case for underascertainment.

Diagnosis. The diagnosis rests upon the exclusion of Turner syndrome, Noonan syndrome, and endocrinopathy coincidental to the hearing impairment. Clinicians may wish to consider possible overlap with Richards and Rundle syndrome in ataxic individuals.

Summary. Characteristics include (*1*) autosomal recessive inheritance; (*2*) primary amenorrhea and streak gonads; (*3*) deficiency of breast and pubic hair; (*4*) elevated urinary gonadotropins; (*5*) sensorineural hearing loss as the only expression in males; and (*6*) possibly diminished vestibular function.

References

1. Amor DJ et al: New variant of familial cerebellar ataxia with hypergonadotropic hypogonadism and sensorineural deafness. *Am J Med Genet* 99:29–33, 2001.
2. Bösze P et al: Perrault's syndrome in two sisters. *Am J Med Genet* 16:237–241, 1983.
3. Christakos AC et al: Gonadal dysgenesis as an autosomal recessive condition. *Am J Obstet Gynecol* 104:1027–1030, 1969.
4. Cruz OLM et al: Sensorineural hearing loss associated with gonadal dysgenesis in sisters. *Am J Otol* 13:82–83, 1992.
5. Gardiner CA et al: The Perrault syndrome: report of three families with different phenotypic features and a review of the literature. Presented at the 8th Manchester Birth Defects Conference, 1998.
6. Gottschalk M et al: Neurologic anomalies of Perrault syndrome. *Am J Med Genet* 65:274–276, 1996.
7. Granat M et al: 46,XX gonadal dysgenesis associated with congenital nerve deafness. *Int J Gynaecol Obstet* 17:231–233, 1979.
8. Josso N et al: Le syndrome de Turner familial. Étude de deux familles avec caryotypes XO et XX. *Ann Pédiatr* 10:163–167, 1963.
9. Linssen WHJP et al: Deafness, sensory neuropathy, and ovarian dysgenesis: a new syndrome or a broader spectrum of Perrault syndrome? *Am J Med Genet* 51:81–82, 1994.
10. McCarthy DJ, Opitz JM: Perrault syndrome in sisters. *Am J Med Genet* 22:629–631, 1985.
11. Nishi Y et al: The Perrault syndrome: clinical report and review. *Am J Med Genet* 31:623–629, 1988.
12. Pallister PD, Opitz JM: The Perrault syndrome: autosomal recessive ovarian dysgenesis with facultative, non sex-linked sensorineural deafness. *Am J Med Genet* 4:239–246, 1979.
13. Perez-Ballester B et al: Familial gonadal dysgenesis. *Am J Obstet Gynecol* 107:1262–1263, 1970.
14. Perrault M et al: Deux cas de syndrome de Turner avec surdi-mutité dans une meme fratrie. *Bull Mem Soc Méd Hop Paris* 16:79–84, 1951.
15. Simpson JL et al: Gonadal dysgenesis in individuals with apparently normal chromosomal complements. Tabulation of cases and compilation of genetic data. *Birth Defects* 7(6):215–228, 1971.

Hypogonadism and severe congenital mixed hearing loss

In 1982, Myhre et al. (4) described a syndrome of primary hypogonadism and congenital severe mixed hearing loss in six males in two kindreds.

Endocrine system. All individuals had delayed onset of puberty ranging from mild to severe. Adults appeared to be sterile.

Musculoskeletal system. Four of six males had thickened calvaria, especially in the frontal, parietal, and occipital areas. All had delayed bone age.

Central nervous system. All patients performed below their intellectual potential because of lack of emotional and social maturity. However, only the proband had a reduced intelligence quotient (IQ = 65).

Auditory system. Hearing loss became evident soon after birth. Hearing loss by air conduction was >70 dB for all frequencies in all six patients. Bone conduction was reduced at all frequencies, indicating an air–bone gap and an increment of conductive hearing loss coupled with the sensorineural component. Fixation of the stapes was found. Female heterozygotes had normal hearing.

Laboratory findings. Primary hypogonadism was shown by low levels of plasma testosterone in adults, and there was low plasma testosterone response to HCG stimulation in prepubertal males. Testicular biopsy showed a combination of immaturity and aberrant germ cell maturation with arrest at the spermatogonial or early spermatocyte stage. Plasma FSH was elevated in all patients.

Heredity. Inheritance was clearly X-linked recessive with normal female heterozygotes. The maternal line was traced back to Ireland. There is strong reason to consider that this syndrome may be representative of a contiguous gene deletion syndrome, and that the hearing deficit may be the result of deletion of the *POU3F4* gene on Xq21 (1–3) (Fig. 12–10A,B). Other patients with hearing abnormality resulting from deletion of this region have been shown to have the characteristic radiological appearance of gusher-associated hearing loss (5,6) (Fig. 12–10C) and hypogonadism has been a described feature in at least one such case (1). It should also be noted that a significant sensorineural element to the hearing impairment may obscure the conductive element, making diagnosis on the basis of audiological characteristics difficult (7).

Diagnosis. This syndrome differs from congenital adrenal hypoplasia, gonadotrophin deficiency, and progressive high-frequency

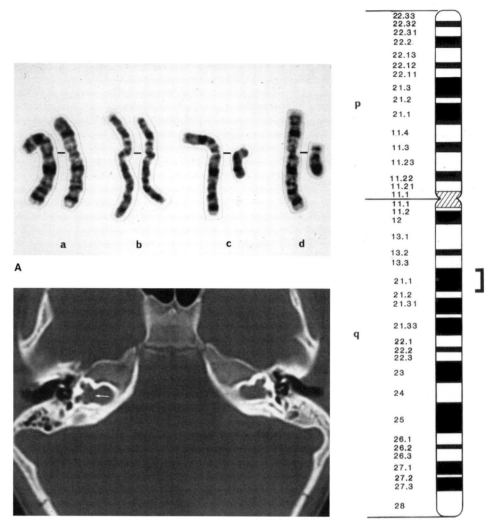

Figure 12–10. *Hypogonadism and severe congenital mixed hearing loss.* (A,B) GTG-banded sex chromosomes showing deletion of Xq21.1 in two related carrier females (a,b) and from two affected males (c,d). The deleted X is on the right in the heterozygotes and the Y chromosome is pictured on right in the males. The diagram of the X chromosome indicates the location of the deleted segment. (C) High-resolution CT scan of the cochlea in an affected male with Xq21.1 deletion. The arrow indicates the dilated facial nerve canal. The normal distinction between the basal coil of the cochlea and the internal auditory meatus has been lost. [From W Reardon et al., *Am J Med Genet* 44:513–517, 1992, reprinted by permission of Wiley-Liss, Inc., a subsidiary of John Wiley & Sons, Inc.]

sensorineural hearing loss. It also should be differentiated from Kallmann syndrome in which there is anosmia.

Summary. Characteristics include (*1*) X-linked recessive inheritance; (*2*) primary hypogonadism; (*3*) thickened calvaria; (*4*) emotional and social immaturity; and (*4*) severe congenital sensorineural hearing loss.

References

1. Bach I et al: Microdeletions in patients with gusher-associated X-linked mixed deafness (DFN3). *Am J Hum Genet* 50:38–44, 1992.
2. Cremers FPM et al: The ins and outs of X-linked deafness type 3. In: Kitamura K, Steel KP (eds) *Genetics in Otorhinolaryngology.* Basel, Karger, 2000, pp 184–195.
3. De Kok YJM et al: Association between X-linked mixed deafness and mutations in the POU domain gene *POU3F4. Science* 267:685–688, 1995.
4. Myhre SA et al: Congenital deafness and hypogonadism. A new X-linked recessive disorder. *Clin Genet* 22:299–307, 1982.
5. Phelps PD et al: X-linked deafness, stapes "gusher" and a distinctive defect of the inner ear. *Neuroradiology* 33:326–330, 1991.
6. Reardon W et al: Phenotypic evidence for a common pathogenesis in X-linked deafness pedigrees and in Xq13–21 deletion related deafness. *Am J Med Genet* 44:513–517, 1992.
7. Reardon W et al: Neuro-otological function in X-linked hearing loss: a multipedigree assessment and correlation with other clinical parameters. *Acta Otolaryngol (Stockh)* 113:706–714, 1993.

Congenital adrenal hypoplasia, gonadotrophin deficiency, and progressive high-frequency sensorineural hearing loss

Familial gonadotropin deficiency as a feature of adrenocortical failure in males dates from the 1973 report of Brook et al. (1) and subsequent affirmation by Zachmann et al. (6). An X-linked form of congenital adrenal hypoplasia had been reported earlier (5), but recognition of gonadotropin deficiency as an integral element of that disorder awaited the 1991 review of Kletter et al. (3). Mutations in the *DAX1* gene cause X-linked congenital adrenal hypoplasia and hypogonadotropic hypogonadism (4).

In 1992, Zachmann et al. (7) noted progressive sensorineural hearing loss that began at about 14 years of age in three brothers with X-linked congenital adrenal hypoplasia and hypogonadotropic hypogonadism. Initially involving high tones, it progressed to affect lower frequencies and to become severe (80–95 dB loss) with age. As hearing impairment associated with this disorder seems to be unusual, the possibility that the hypogonadism in the family reported by Zachmann et al. (6,7) represents Kallmann syndrome has to be considered.

It should be noted that X-linked adrenal hypoplasia may be associated with glycerol kinase deficiency myopathy and mental retardation, representing a contiguous gene deletion syndrome of Xp21 (2). This syndrome differs from hypogonadism and severe congenital mixed hearing loss, which is also a contiguous gene deletion syndrome of the X chromosome, but in which the hearing impairment dates from birth. The significant clinical overlap with adrenoleukodystrophy should also be kept in mind.

References

1. Brook CGD et al: Familial congenital adrenal hypoplasia. *Helv Paediatr Acta* 28:277, 1973.
2. Goonewardena P et al: Molecular Xp deletion in a male: suggestion of a locus for hypogonadotropic hypogonadism distal to the glycerol kinase and adrenal hypoplasia loci. *Clin Genet* 35:5–12, 1989.
3. Kletter GB et al: Congenital adrenal hypoplasia and isolated gonadotropin deficiency. *Trends Endocrinol Metab* 2:123–128, 1991.
4. Muscatelli F et al: Mutations in the *DAX-1* gene give rise to both X-linked adrenal hypoplasia congenita and hypogonadotropic hypogonadism. *Nature* 372:672–676, 1994.
5. Weiss L, Mellinger RC: Congenital adrenal hypoplasia—an X-linked disease. *J Med Genet* 7:27–32, 1970.
6. Zachmann M et al: Gonadotropin deficiency and cryptorchidism in three prepubertal brothers with congenital adrenal hypoplasia. *J Pediatr* 97:255–257, 1980.
7. Zachmann M et al: Progressive high frequency hearing loss: an additional feature of the syndrome of congenital adrenal hypoplasia in gonadotrophin deficiency. *Eur J Pediatr* 151:167–169, 1992.

Unusual face, cleft palate, pseudohermaphroditism, mental retardation, and conductive hearing loss

In 1986, Ieshima et al. (1) described male and female sibs with intrauterine growth retardation and failure to thrive, severe mental retardation, microcephaly, hypotonia, repeated respiratory infections, pulmonary hypertension with PDA, and cleft palate. Conduction hearing loss was documented in one sibling.

The face was characterized by asymmetry, arched eyebrows, hypertelorism, broad nasal bridge, small nose with anteverted nostrils, microtia, and micrognathia.

The male had hypospadias, micropenis, cryptorchidism, and shawl scrotum. Inheritance is probably autosomal recessive.

Reference

1. Ieshima A et al: Peculiar facies, deafness, cleft palate, male pseudo-hermaphroditism, and growth and psychomotor retardation: a new autosomal recessive syndrome? *Clin Genet* 30:136–141, 1986.

Appendix

Other entities with endocrine dysfunction

Entity	Endocrine Finding	Chapter in this Book
Alstrom syndrome	Diabetes, obesity	7 (eye)
Edwards syndrome	Diabetes, hypogonadism	7 (eye)
Reinstein syndrome	Hypogonadism	7 (eye)
Jan syndrome	Hyperinsulinemia	7 (eye)
Schaap syndrome	Hypogonadism	7 (eye)
Total color blindness, liver degeneration, endocrine dysfunction, and SHL	Hypothyroidism, ACTH abnormalities	7 (eye)
Hansen syndrome	Hypothyroidism, diabetes	7 (eye)
Kumar-Masel syndrome	Müllerian dysgenesis	8 (musculoskeletal)
Renal failure, severe hypertension, abnormal steroidogenesis, hypogenitalism, and SHL	Hypogenitalism	9 (renal)
Richards-Rundle syndrome	Hypogonadotrophic hypogonadism	10 (neurologic)
Wells-Jankovic syndrome	Hypogonadotrophic hypogonadism	10 (neurologic)
Nathalie syndrome	Hypogonadism	10 (neurologic)
Dyck syndrome	Adrenocortical deficiency	10 (neurologic)
Herrmann syndrome	Diabetes	10 (neurologic)
Cutler syndrome	Thyroid dysfunction	10 (neurologic)
Feigenbaum syndrome	Diabetes mellitus	10 (neurologic_
Johnson-McMillin syndrome	Hypogonadism	14 (integumentary)
Woodhouse-Sakati syndrome	Hypogonadism	14 (integumentary)
Hypodontia, peg-shaped teeth, olivopontocerebellar dysplasia, hypogonadism, and hearing loss	Hypogonadism	15 (oral and dental)

SHL, sensorineural hearing loss.

Chapter 13
Genetic Hearing Loss Associated with Metabolic Disorders

MICHAEL L. NETZLOFF, SARAH H. ELSEA, AND RACHEL A. FISHER

In this chapter we have included metabolic diseases that are known to be associated with genetic hearing loss but have omitted some extremely rare metabolic diseases that may, by chance alone, be seen with hearing loss. Because of the relative frequency of nonsyndromic hearing loss, with an increasing number of defined genes inherited not only in a monogenic fashion but also via mitochondrial mechanisms, chance associations of these conditions with metabolic disease have likely occurred.

Mucopolysaccharidoses

The mucopolysaccharidoses (MPS) are a group of lysosomal storage diseases caused by deficiency in various enzymes catalyzing the degradation of glycosaminoglycans (older term, *mucopolysaccharides*). The various enzyme deficiencies block the catabolism of the acid glycosaminoglycans, dermatan sulfate, heparan sulfate, keratan sulfate, chondroitin sulfate, or hyaluronan, either singly or in various combinations. Clinical and biochemical findings can differentiate seven distinct mucopolysaccharidoses designated MPS-I through MPS-IX (MPS-V and MPS-VIII are no longer used). The types of mucopolysaccharidoses have in common several clinical features, although to varying degrees. These include a chronic, unremitting progressive course, a particular skeletal dysplasia known as dysostosis multiplex, abnormal face, organomegaly, and multisystem involvement. Deficits include the areas of hearing, vision, cardiac function, airway obstruction, and restricted joint mobility. The diseases can cause profound mental retardation as is found in patients with MPS-IH (Hurler syndrome), the severe form of MPS-II (Hunter syndrome), and all enzymatic types of Sanfilippo syndrome (MPS-III), frequently leading to death in childhood. Normal intellect can be retained in the remaining mucopolysaccharidoses; typically patients with the mild form of MPS-II (mild Hunter syndrome), MPS-IS (Scheie syndrome), MPS-IH/S (Hurler-Scheie syndrome), MPS-IV (Morquio syndrome), the mild form of MPS-VI (Maroteaux-Lamy syndrome), and the mild form of MPS-VII (Sly syndrome) survive into adulthood (2,7,9,18,21,33,37).

Although the features that the various conditions have in common allow provisional clinical diagnosis, there is often marked heterogeneity among and even within each of these diseases.

MPS-IH (Hurler syndrome)

Hurler syndrome (OMIM 252800) has been suggested as the prototype for the mucopolysaccharidoses, but this is true for only the most severely affected patients with this condition. As such, Hurler syndrome is usually recognized early during infancy, when the patients may be unusually large, but growth later decelerates beginning at about 16 to 18 months. Early diagnosis is facilitated by the finding of inguinal and umbilical hernias and the development of coarse facial features, the characteristic skeletal malformations, recurrent otitis media, hepatosplenomegaly, and macroglossia (Fig. 13–1A,B). Cardiac failure may occur prior to the recognition of the storage disorder and the cardiomyopathy that develops secondary to endocardial fibroelastosis may

be fatal. Delay in development is usually recognized between 12 and 24 months of age and becomes progressive. Clouding of the cornea, though obvious in the established disease, is not so apparent in the early stages when photophobia may be a more noteworthy ocular feature.

Confirmation of the clinical diagnosis is aided by the excessive urinary excretion of dermatan and heparan sulfate, and enzymatic confirmation of the diagnosis is possible using synthetic substrates. Despite interventions, death often occurs before 10 years of age and is usually caused by respiratory infection and cardiac failure (2,7,18,21,37).

MPS-IS (Scheie syndrome)

Scheie syndrome (OMIM 252800) is a mild form of MPS-I that is never recognized clinically during infancy and rarely identified during childhood. The face is described as normal later in life, during adolescence and adulthood, but the patient may have hypertrichosis during adolescence. The picture does not suggest Hurler syndrome, although there is mandibular prominence with a broad nose and wide nares. Patients often have joint contractures, which can become quite debilitating later in life along with carpal tunnel syndrome. Umbilical and inguinal hernias can be present during childhood. Corneal clouding is progressive and, during adulthood, along with glaucoma and retinal degeneration, can contribute to significant loss of vision. Patients typically have a normal to low normal stature and normal intelligence. The neck appears shorter and the trunk appears somewhat shorter than the limbs. There may be hepatosplenomegaly, and most adults with this disorder have aortic valvular disease that can be improved by valve replacement. Life expectancy is normal, with the exception of those patients with significant cardiac disease (2,7,18,21,37).

MPS-IH/S (Hurler-Scheie syndrome)

This designation is used for a clinical entity (OMIM 252800) in which there are features of both Hurler and Scheie syndromes as well as a deficiency of the enzyme α-L-iduronidase. Most of these patients, except for some reported Japanese, do not appear to be a genetic compound between MPS-IH and MPS-IS alleles. Rather, patients seem to be an expression of another homozygous mutant allele at the same locus. Clinical signs are observable by 2 years of age but can be as late as 3 to 8 years of age. These patients are markedly short and have dysostosis multiplex, significant organomegaly, umbilical and/or inguinal hernias, and progressive corneal clouding. Hypertrichosis has been reported along with thickening of the skin and carpal tunnel syndrome. Survival to adulthood is common, with the cause of death most often being cardiac or upper airway obstruction. Intelligence is entirely normal (2,4,7,9,18,37).

MPS II (Hunter syndrome)

Hunter syndrome (OMIM 309900) presents as both a mild and a severe disease form that results from allelic mutations. The severe disease appears to be more frequent than the mild disease, which is compatible with survival to adulthood. The severe disease results in rapid intellectual deterioration and progression of the dysostosis multiplex, with death occurring usually between the ages of 10 and 15 years.

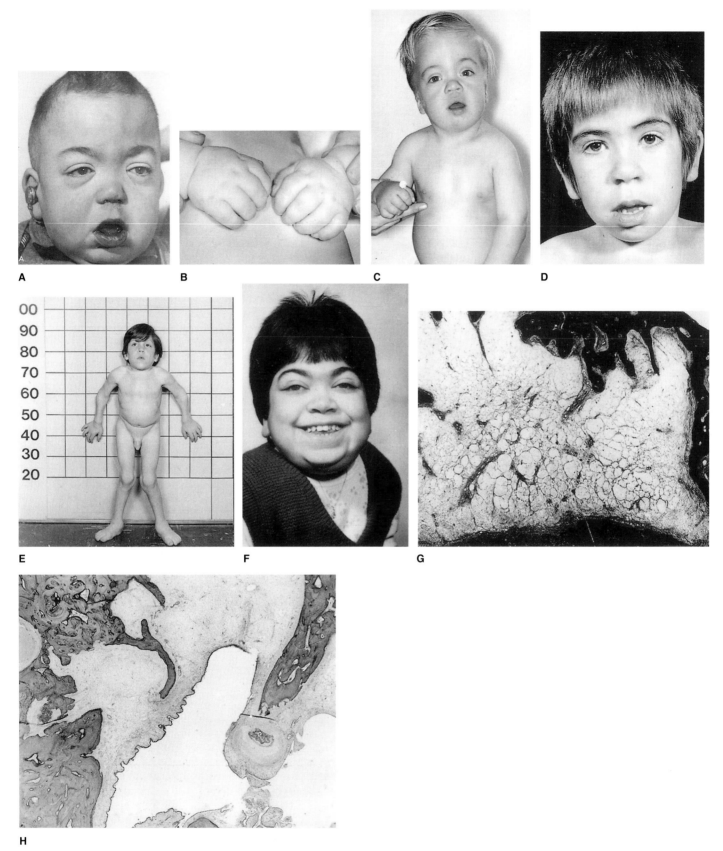

H

Figure 13–1. *Mucopolysaccharidoses.* (A) Patient with Hurler syndrome. (B) Hands showing joint contractures. (C) Patient with Hunter syndrome. (D) Patient with Sanfilippo syndrome. (E) Patient with Morquio syndrome. Note short stature, short trunk, pectus carinatum, enlarged joints, genua valga, and flat feet. (F) Patient with Maroteaux-Lamy syndrome. (G) Pneu- matic cells of tegmen filled by reticular tissue. (H) Tympanic mucous membrane is high and papillomatous. Long process of incus is disintegrated. [(D) courtesy of P Harper, Cardiff, Wales; (E) courtesy of SL Levin, Baltimore, Maryland; (G,H) from G Kelemen, *J Laryngol* 80:791, 1968.]

In the severe Hunter form, the facial features are comparable to those of Hurler syndrome. There is some coarsening in the mild Hunter syndrome as well. In patients with the severe Hunter form, the neck appears short; abdominal hernia with a protruding abdomen is frequent (Fig. 13–1C). Claw-hand deformity with reduced joint mobility occurs. Intelligence may be only slightly reduced or unimpaired in the mild form of disease, but in the severe disease form there is progressive deterioration. The younger severe-form patients present with chronic diarrhea, a suggestive symptom in these patients. Gross corneal clouding does not occur in either form (2,7,9,18,37).

MPS III (Sanfilippo syndrome)

Sanfilippo syndrome is a similar group of disorders caused by deficiency in one of four enzymes responsible for the degradation of heparan sulfate. The four nonallelic forms are not distinguishable clinically, although overall type A (OMIM 252900) is the most severe, is associated with an earlier onset, progresses more rapidly, and has a shorter survival than the other forms. Type B (OMIM 252920) patients frequently can remain functional to the third or even fourth decade; however, these are generalizations. Type C (OMIM 252930) and D (OMIM 252940) Sanfilippo syndromes also appear to be clinically heterogeneous. Onset of clinical features typically occurs in a previously well-appearing child between 2 and 6 years of age, often at the time the child is ready to start school. Presenting features are frequently behavioral with hyperactivity and aggressive behavior and some delay in development. Although physical signs are present, including hypertrichosis, coarsening of hair, mild hepatosplenomegaly, which later disappears as the patients age, height is frequently normal and there may be limited joint mobility at the elbows and knees without hand involvement. Older children may develop mild facial coarseness suggestive of MPS IH (Hurler syndrome) (Fig. 13–1D).

Severe intellectual deterioration occurs from 6 to 10 years of age and this in combination with normal physical development and strength results in treatment difficulties. The disease progresses to complete loss of function and death between 10 and 20 years of age (2,7,11,18,37).

MPS IVA and MPS IVB (Morquio syndrome)

Two forms of Morquio syndrome have been described with different enzyme deficiencies. While initially type A (OMIM 253000) was considered to be the severe form and type B (OMIM 253010) the mild form, subsequent reports have indicated that there is a wide spectrum of severity in both of these conditions. Mild forms thus occur in both the type A and type B conditions and are characterized by normal stature and relatively mild skeletal abnormalities, mild corneal clouding, and the absence of the typical urinary excretion of keratan sulfate. Typically the more severe condition is characterized by short trunk dwarfism, progressive deformity of the spine, a short neck with hyperextension, odontoid hypoplasia that can be life threatening, and normal intelligence (Fig. 13–1E). These skeletal abnormalities are atypical for the mucopolysaccharidoses and patients show a marked pectus carinatum with kyphosis and kyphoscoliosis of the thorax beginning in the second year. The lumbar spine frequently has a gibbus-like kyphosis. There may be excessive wrist joint mobility, but decreased joint mobility of the large joints, particularly of the hips and knees, sometimes occurs, an observation that may sometimes apply to the elbows. The wrists tend to become enlarged and there is an ulnar deviation to the fingers and hands. The corneas have diffuse opacification. The type A patients with the *N*-acetylgalactosamine 6-sulfatase deficiency have dental abnormalities with discolored crowns and pitted enamel that is thin and tends to flake off. This may predispose them to dental caries. Type II patients with the enzyme deficiency β-galactosidase, by contrast, have no dental abnormalities. This feature may allow clinical differentiation of the two conditions (2,7,9,18,37).

MPS VI (Maroteaux-Lamy syndrome)

MPS VI (OMIM 253200) presents in widely varying forms of severity. In the severe form, macrocephaly and chest prominence may present at birth, although most signs are recognized by 1–3 years of age in the severe type, by late childhood in the intermediate type, and by the second decade in the mild type. Patients with the severe form of disease have remarkably short stature and the disease progression is rapid, resulting in severe disability, coarse facial features, a typical "crouched" stance posture with hyperextended head and flexed hips and knees, severe skeletal abnormalities, corneal clouding, hearing loss, and prominent cardiac abnormalities that often lead to death in adolescence (Fig. 13–1F). Hepatomegaly is always present after 6 years of age, and splenomegaly occurs in about one-half of patients. Mental retardation is not a feature of Maroteaux-Lamy syndrome. Patients with the mild form may occasionally attain normal adult stature, but most are shorter than patients with the Scheie syndrome, which may allow differentiation. In many patients, growth in height virtually comes to a stop after the age of 7–8 years (2,7,9,18,37).

MPS VII (Sly syndrome)

The severe neonatal form of Sly syndrome (type I) (OMIM 253220) is one of the few lysosomal storage diseases, including the mucopolysaccharidosis, which is recognizable immediately at birth. Patients present with hepatosplenomegaly and hydrops fetalis and expire within the first few months of life. In this mucopolysaccharidosis, as in many others, there is a wide variability in phenotypic presentation. The first patient described with this condition had a milder phenotype (infantile form) and presented with features suggesting the diagnosis of Hurler or the more severe type of Hunter syndromes. The face resembles that of Hurler syndrome, with a depressed nasal bridge but full lips, hypertelorism, anteverted nares, and prominent alveolar processes. The corneas can appear grossly cloudy to inspection in the neonatal form but are less obvious in the milder types. The milder varieties appear to include mental retardation, which is nonprogressive. The severe neonatal form shows regression and may be the most common type of Sly syndrome. There is heterogeneity among the neonatal forms as well, ranging from death in utero to mild or no hydrops fetalis. Mothers of MPS VII patients have an increased number of spontaneous abortions.

In patients presenting beyond the infantile period (juvenile form), as in the other mucopolysaccharidoses, there is variation in presentation. Many with the severe form have the typical Hurler-like features with hepatomegaly, inguinal and/or umbilical hernias, developmental delay, moderate skeletal abnormalities, and repeated episodes of pneumonia early in life. Corneal clouding has been variable and patients presenting in the juvenile period apparently have little or no dysostosis multiplex, in contrast to the other more severe forms. Patients with mild juvenile form presenting after 4 years of age can have normal intelligence, (2,7,9,18,37).

MPS IX (hyaluronidase deficiency)

Only a single patient has been described with this enzyme deficiency (OMIM 601492). This patient had acquired short stature, normal joint movement, and normal intelligence. She presented with bilateral nodular soft tissue masses in the joints, which periodically swelled and resolved within 3 days. She had mild facial dysmorphic features, and radiographs revealed multiple intraarticular soft tissue masses and acetabular erosions, apparently due to the hyaluronan normally found in high concentration in cartilage and synovial fluid (20).

All forms of mucopolysaccharidoses

Auditory system. It is likely that in all of the forms of mucopolysaccharidoses representative patients have conductive hearing loss caused by recurrent upper respiratory infections and frequent serous otitis media (31). However, many patients also have sensorineural loss. With the accumulating glycosaminoglycans, the auditory brain stem responses have been described as abnormal in a nonspecific way, thought due to a combination of middle ear, cochlear, eighth nerve, and lower brain stem pathology (18). Intervention with pressure-equalizing (PE) tubes, particularly those designed to remain more permanently implanted, can have significant benefit on the conductive hearing loss in these individuals. Hearing aids will help both conductive and sensorineural loss (18,37).

Most patients with the most severe mucopolysaccharidoses, for example, MPS-IH (Hurler syndrome), have some form of conductive hearing loss secondary to frequent episodes of serous otitis media. Komura et al. (13) described pathologic findings almost exclusively limited to the middle ear. Except for some hyperplasia of the arachnoid in the internal auditory canal, the investigators concluded that the conductive component was due almost exclusively to otitis media and poor connection of the ossicles. Kelemen (10) described pneumatic cells of the tegmen filled with reticular mesenchymal tissue and mucous membrane of the middle ear, which is high and papillomatous (Fig. 13–1G,H). Some patients, however, also have sensorineural hearing loss. Friedmann et al. (5) and Schachern et al. (29) described temporal bone pathology in Hurler syndrome patients with glycosaminoglycan-containing cells. The blood vessels were surrounded with osteoid tissue similar to that seen in otosclerosis. The stapes was deformed and covered with a thickened mucosa and granulation tissue. There was degeneration of the organ of Corti and the Reissner's and tectorial membranes were covered with hemorrhagic material. The vestibulocochlear nerves were disrupted by large, vacuolated cells. This pathology suggests the etiology for combined conductive and sensorineural hearing loss in cases of Hurler syndrome. Hair cell dysfunction has also been implicated (2,5,8,12,29,32).

Similar otolaryngological findings were described by Ruckenstein et al. (26) in patients with the Hurler-Scheie syndrome (MPS-IH/S).

In MPS IS (Scheie syndrome), the hearing loss may be partially due to a cochlear lesion, but the loss is probably a mixed conductive and sensorineural disease, unlikely to be profound (8,15,19,23).

Hearing loss occurs in one-quarter to one-half of patients who have Hunter syndrome (MPS II), though the loss is usually not severe (8,39–41). Hayes et al. (8) reported that the hearing loss associated with MPS II was sensorineural in type; however, in subsequent reports a conductive component more often than a mixed hearing loss was described. Fujitani et al. (6) describe the accumulation of glycosaminoglycans in the pharyngeal tonsil leading to a conductive hearing impairment. Adenoidectomies were recommended for these patients. Peck (22) reported that the conductive component of hearing loss may persist even after myringotomies. Wolff (38) demonstrated absence of the joint cavity between the malleus and incus bones but did not describe features typical of otosclerosis. She found irregular bone nodules in the round window, as well as alterations, which were suggestive of those reported by Keleman (10) in the Hurler syndrome. Zechner et al. (41,42) found the middle ear mucosa to be edematous and to contain a foamy PAS-positive cytoplasm. The shape of the malleus and incus was retained, but they contained large hyperemic marrow spaces, the stapes appearing normal. Clear evidence of otosclerotic foci were found near the oval and round windows and the organ of Corti was normal. The cytoplasm of the spiral and vestibular ganglia were also involved with foamy PAS-positive material. This pathology would clearly suggest a cause for both a conductive and a sensorineural component of hearing loss in these patients.

In earlier reports, MPS III and hearing loss have only rarely been associated. Spranger et al. (33,34) found this condition in only 1 of 10 patients and it was found in only 2–3 of 8 patients in a study by Rampini (23) and in 2 patients examined by Ruckenstein et al. (26). More recent suggestions are that the hearing impairment may be fairly common in the moderately to severely affected patients (21). It appears at approximately the age of 6–7 years and is progressive, similar to the mental retardation. Difficulties in studying these patients, who are both aggressive and uncooperative, make audiometry difficult.

In patients with Morquio syndrome, hearing impairment usually begins during adolescence and is progressive and is almost universally found in those patients who survive beyond the second decade. Hearing loss may be conductive, mixed, or sensorineural. The conductive component is not surprising because of the chronic middle ear disease in these patients (2,11,24,26,28,36,37).

Patients with MPS VI (Maroteaux-Lamy syndrome) demonstrate conductive or mixed conductive sensorineural hearing loss in approximately 25%. Onset is between the ages of 6 and 8 years and appears to result primarily from episodes of recurrent otitis media (2,21,34,35).

The more mildly affected patients with MPS VII (Sly syndrome) survive into adolescence and develop a mild sensorineural hearing deficit (37). The pathology of the ear in MPS VII has been better studied in a murine model of the disease. Berry et al. (1) showed external auditory canal obstruction, severe otitis media, and alterations in the articulation of the ossicles, which cause a conductive hearing loss. In addition, there was hair cell damage and lysosomal storage, which may contribute to the sensorineural hearing loss. Using this animal model, Kyle et al. (16) were able to demonstrate that a complete β-glucuronidase deficiency could be completely corrected using a gene transfer. Furthermore, in the same animal model, bone marrow transplantation was used to demonstrate reduction in the hearing loss associated with the murine MPS VII using the auditory-evoked brain stem response technique. Treatment resulted in less thickening of the tympanic membrane of the middle ear mucosa and decreased distortion of the ossicles in the cochlear bone. Treatment appears to result in long-term improvement in auditory function (27). Finally, using adeno-associated virus (AAV)–mediated neonatal gene transfer, Daly et al. (3) demonstrated improvement in survival and auditory function in treated mice compared to the untreated mutant siblings.

The experience with MPS IX (hyaluronidase deficiency) consists of only one patient. At age 14 years, she had a history of developing hearing loss following frequent episodes of otitis media (20).

Vestibular system. Vestibular function was reduced bilaterally in one patient studied with MPS II (Hunter syndrome). Electronystagmographic findings were also reported in another patient with MPS IV (Morquio syndrome) (28).

Radiographic findings. Radiographs in all the mucopolysaccharidoses except MPS IV (Morquio syndrome) and MPS IX demonstrate a typical pattern of skeletal anomalies called "dysostosis multiplex." This is most severe in Hurler and Maroteaux-Lamy syndromes and is minimal in Scheie and Sanfilippo syndromes, with Hunter syndrome being intermediate in severity. The dysostosis is characterized by the development of macrocephaly with skull deformities and a J-shaped deep, elongated sella. The ribs are broad and oar-shaped (canoe paddle-shaped in Maroteaux-Lamy syndrome), and vertebrae have biconvex end-plates and the lower thoracic and upper lumbar vertebral bodies are hook shaped after 12–18 months of age. There are pelvic dysplasia, short tubular bones with widened diaphyses, and an epiphyseal dysplasia. The coarse irregular bone structure and abnormalities worsen with age.

The hands assume a claw-like position of the fingers, which are foreshortened. The hands remain normal in Sanfilippo syndrome, but a characteristic thickening of the posterior occiput develops, along with ovoid-shaped vertebral bodies.

The skeletal findings in Morquio syndrome, in contrast, consist of a distinctive spondyloepiphyseal dysplasia with involvement of the femoral head, platyspondly, and odontoid hypoplasia, which can lead to life-threatening complications, genu valgum, and shortening of the tubular bones. Enamel hypoplasia of the teeth occurs in type A Morquio syndrome.

Enzyme deficiencies. Specific lysosomal enzyme deficiencies have been described for each of the distinct mucopolysaccharide disorders and are summarized in Table 13–1.

Urinary glycosaminoglycans. The different enzyme deficiencies lead to excretion of various forms and quantities of glycosaminoglycan

Table 13–1. The mucopolysaccharidoses

Type	Eponym	Clinical Dysmorphism	Skeletal Dysplasia	Corneal Opacities	Mental Retardation	Excessive Urinary GAGs	Defective Mode of Enzyme	Gene Inheritance	Locus
IH	Hurler	Severe	Severe	Yes	Yes	DS and HS	α-L-iduronidase	AR	4p16.3
IH/S	Hurler-Scheie	Intermediate	Moderate	Yes	No	DS and HS	α-L-iduronidase	AR	4p16.3
IS	Scheie	Mild	Mild	Yes	No	DS and HS	α-L-iduronidase	AR	4p16.3
IIA	Hunter (severe)	Early (moderate)	Moderate	No	Yes	DS and HS	Iduronate 2-sulfatase	XR	Xq27.3
IIB	Hunter (mild)	Late (moderate)	Moderate	No	No	DS and HS	Iduronate 2-sulfatase	XR	Xq27.3
IIIA	Sanfilippo A	Mild	Minimal	No	Yes	HS	Heparan-N-sulfatase	AR	17q.25.3
IIIB	Sanfilippo B	Mild	Minimal	No	Yes	HS	α-N-acetyl glucosaminidase	AR	17q21
IIIC	Sanfilippo C	Mild	Minimal	No	Yes	HS	Acetyl-CoA: α-glucosaminide N-acetyl-transferase	AR	Chromosome 14
IIID	Sanfilippo D	Mild	Minimal	No	Yes	HS	N-acetylglucos-amine-6-sulfatase	AR	12q14
IVA	Morquio A	Severe	Severe	Yes	No	KS	Galactose-6-sulfatase	AR	16q24
IVB	Morquio B	Severe	Severe	Yes	No	KS	β-galactosidase	AR	3p14–21
VIA	Maroteaux-Lamy (mild)	Mild to moderate	Moderate	Yes	No	DS	Arylsulfatase B	AR	5q11–q13
VIB	Maroteaux-Lamy (severe)	Severe	Severe	Yes	Mild	DS	Arylsulfatase B	A R	5q11–q13
VII	Sly	Severe	Severe	No	Late	DS amd HS	β-glucuronidase	AR	7q11.2–q22

AR, autosomal recessive; DS, dermatan sulfate; GAGs, glycosaminoglycans; HS, heparan sulfate; KS, keratan sulfate; XR, X-linked recessive.

(GAG) products of degradation. In general, the failure to degrade heparin sulfate and its accumulation more often leads to mental retardation and skeletal affects. Mesenchymal effects result from impaired degradation of dermatan, chondroitin, and keratan sulfate. Keratan sulfate impairs skeletal growth but has other tissue effects and is excreted singly in Morquio syndrome, especially during childhood (33,37). The urinary GAG excretion of the various mucopolysaccharidoses is summarized in Table 13–1.

Heredity. All MPS enzyme deficiencies are autosomal recessive, except for MPS II (Hunter syndrome), which is X-linked. The inheritance of MPS IX is presumed to be autosomal recessive. Each gene has been mapped, prenatal diagnoses of several mucopolysaccharidoses have been accomplished, and all are potentially amenable to DNA diagnosis.

Diagnosis. Confirmation of the clinical impression is possible for each of these disorders by specific enzyme testing using leukocytes from peripheral blood, skin biopsy fibroblasts, or lymphoid cells. Prenatal diagnosis is possible using amniocytes and, in some cases, chorionic villi have been used.

Clinical differentiation among the classic mucopolysaccharidoses is relatively easy. Patients with MPS IH (Hurler syndrome) and MPS II (Hunter syndrome) are normal at birth but develop mental retardation, short stature, coarse face, organomegaly, restricted joint mobility, and, in MPS IH, corneal clouding. Hunter syndrome patients frequently develop profuse diarrhea and the corneas remain grossly clear. They also can develop nodular skin lesions over the back, upper arms, thorax, and lateral thighs, which are likely unique among the MPS syndromes (18,33). Patients with MPS VI (Maroteaux-Lamy syndrome) have normal intellect but corneal opacity. The nonlethal infantile form of MPS VII (Sly syndrome) resembles Hurler syndrome with short stature, visceromegaly, dysostosis, and mental delays, especially with regard to speech (37).

The oligosaccharidoses are most often clinically confused with the mucopolysaccharidoses. Oligosaccharides, however, rather than acid glycosaminoglycans, are stored in excess in these conditions and glycosaminoglycans are not excreted in excess.

Summary. The mucopolysaccharidoses represent a varied group of lysosomal enzyme deficiencies with increased glycosaminoglycan excretion and excessive storage, resulting in organ and tissue pathology that is incremental. All mucopolysaccharidoses except MPS II (Hunter syndrome, X-linked) are inherited as autosomal recessive conditions and are chemically distinct, with storage and excretion of specific glycosaminoglycans and different degradatory enzyme deficiencies. Hearing loss of varying types and degrees occur in all the enzyme categories of the mucopolysaccharidoses.

References

1. Berry CL et al: Pathology of the ear in murine mucopolysaccharidosis type VII. Morphologic correlates of hearing loss. *Lab Invest* 71:438–445, 1994.
2. Bredenkamp JK et al: Otolaryngologic manifestations of the mucopolysaccharidoses. *Ann Otol Rhinol Laryngol* 101:472–478, 1992.
3. Daly TM et al: Prevention of systemic clinical disease in MPS VII mice following AAV-mediated neonatal gene transfer. *Gene Ther* 8:1291–1298, 2001.
4. Fallis N et al: A case of polydystrophic dwarfism with urinary excretion of dermatan sulfate and heparan sulfate. *J Clin Endocrinol* 28:26–33, 1968.
5. Friedmann I et al: Histopathologic studies of the temporal bone in Hurler's disease. *J Laryngol Otol* 99:29–42, 1985.
6. Fugitani T et al: Pathological and biochemical study in the adenoid of mucopolysaccharidosis II. *Int J Pediatr Otorhinolaryngol* 10:205–212, 1985.
7. Gorlin RJ et al: *Syndromes of the Head and Neck,* 4th ed. Oxford University Press, New York, 2001, pp. 119–139.
8. Hayes E et al: The otologic manifestations of mucopolysaccharidoses. *Am J Otol* 2:65–69, 1980.
9. Hopwood JJ, Morris CP: The mucopolysaccharidoses: diagnosis, molecular genetics and treatment. *Mol Biol Med* 7:381–404, 1990.
10. Kelemen G: Hurler's syndrome and the hearing organ. *J Laryngol* 80:791–803, 1966.
11. Kelemen G: Morquio's disease and the hearing organ. *ORL* 39:233–240, 1977.
12. Kittel G: Pfaundler-Hurlersche Krankheit oder Gargoylismus unter HNO-ärztlicher Sicht. *Z Laryngol Rhinol Otol* 42:206–217, 1963.
13. Komura Y et al: ABR and temporal bone pathology in Hurler's disease. *Int J Pediatr Otorhinolaryngol* 43:179–188, 1998.
14. Konigsmark B, Gorlin RJ: *Genetic and Metabolic Deafness.* W.B. Saunders, Philadelphia, 1976.
15. Koskenoja M, Suvanto E: Gargoylism. Report of adult form with glaucoma in two sisters. *Acta Ophthalmol (Kbh)* 37:234–240, 1959.
16. Kyle JW et al: Correction of murine mucopolysaccharidosis VII by a human beta-glucuronidase transgene. *Proc Natl Acad Sci USA* 87:3914–3918, 1990.

17. LeGuern E et al: More precise localization of the gene for Hunter syndrome. *Genomics* 7:358–362, 1990.

18. Leroy JG, Crocker AC: Clinical definition of Hunter-Hurler phenotypes. A review of 50 patients. *Am J Dis Child* 112:518–530, 1966.

19. Murray JF: Pulmonary disability in the Hurler syndrome. *N Engl J Med* 261:378–382, 1959.

20. Natowicz MR et al: Clinical and biochemical manifestations of hyaluronidase deficiency. *N Engl J Med* 335:1029–1033, 1996.

21. Neufeld EF, Muenzer J: The mucopolysaccharidoses. In: *The Metabolic and Molecular Bases of Inherited Disease,* 8th ed., Scriver CR et al (eds), McGraw-Hill, New York, 2001, pp 3421–3452.

22. Peck JE: Hearing loss in Hunter's syndrome—mucopolysaccharidosis II. *Ear Hear* 5:243–246, 1984.

23. Rampini S: Das Sanfilippo-Syndrome. *Helv Paediatr Acta* 24:55–91, 1969.

24. Riedner ED, Levin LS: Hearing pattern in Morquio's syndrome (mucopolysaccharidosis IV). *Arch Otolaryngol* 103:518–520, 1977.

25. Robins MM et al: Morquio's disease: an abnormality of mucopolysaccharide metabolism. *J Pediatr* 62:881–889, 1963.

26. Ruckenstein MJ et al: The management of otolaryngological problems in the mucopolysaccharidoses: a retrospective view. *J Otolaryngol* 20:177–183, 1991.

27. Sands MS et al: Syngeneic bone marrow transplantation reduces the hearing loss associated with murine mucopolysaccharidosis type VII. *Blood* 86:2033–2040, 1995.

28. Sataloff RT et al: Morquio's syndrome. *Am J Otol* 8:443–449, 1987.

29. Schachern P et al: Mucopolysaccharidosis I-H (Hurler's syndrome) and human temporal bone histopathology. *Ann Otol Rhinol* 93:65–69, 1980.

30. Scheie HG et al: A newly recognized forme fruste of Hurler's disease (gargoylism). *Am J Ophthalmol* 53:753–769, 1962.

31. Schleier E, Streubel HG: Phoniatrische Aspekte bei Kindern mit Mukopolysaccharidose. *Folia Phoniat* 28:65–72, 1976.

32. Schuknecht HG: *Pathology of the Ear,* 2nd ed. Harvard University Press, Cambridge, MA, 1993.

33. Spranger J: Mucopolysaccharidoses. In: *Principles and Practice of Medical Genetics* 3rd ed. Rimoin DL et al (eds), Churchill Livingstone, New York, 1996, pp 2071–2079.

34. Spranger JW et al: Die HS-Mukopolysaccharidose von Sanfilippo (Polydystrophic Oligophrenie). Bericht uber 10 Patienten. *Z Kinderheilkd* 101:71–84, 1967.

35. Vogler C et al: Murine mucopolysaccharidosis type VII: the impact of therapies on the clinical course and pathology in a murine model of lysosomal storage disease. *J Inherit Metab Dis* 21:575–586, 1998.

36. Von Noorden GK et al: Ocular findings in Morquio-Ullrich's disease. *Arch Ophthalmol* 64:585–591, 1960.

37. Whitley CB: The mucopolysaccharidoses. In: *Heritable Disorders of Connective Tissue,* Beighton P (ed), C.V. Mosby, St. Louis, 1993, pp 367–499.

38. Wolff D: Microscopic study of temporal bones in dysostosis multiplex (gargoylism). *Laryngoscope* 52:218–222, 1942.

39. Young ID, Harper PS: Long-term complications of Hunter's syndrome. *Clin Genet* 16:125–132, 1979.

40. Young ID, Harper PS: Mild form of Hunter's syndrome. Clinical delineation based on 31 cases. *Arch Dis Child* 57:826–836, 1982.

41. Zechner G, Altmann F: The temporal bone in Hunter's syndrome (gargoylism). *Arch Klin Exp Ohren Nasen Kehlkopfheilkd* 192:137–144, 1968.

42. Zechner G, Moser M: Otosclerosis and mucopolysaccharidosis. *Acta Otolaryngol* 103:384–386, 1987.

Oligosaccharidoses, Gangliosidoses, and Lipidoses

α-Mannosidosis

Since the first description by Öckerman in 1967 (27), at least 90 cases of α-mannosidosis (OMIM 248500) have been reported in the medical literature (12,21,35).

Clinical features. As is the case with the other lysosomal storage diseases, wide variation in severity is seen in patients with α-mannosidosis (6,7,12,14,22,27). The severe form seen during infancy has been referred to as type I, while the milder form in children and adults is type II (4–6). Nearly all patients have some degree of mental retardation, which is very slowly progressive in type II patients, as is the dysostosis multiplex and facial coarsening. The latter consists of a broad nose with flat bridge, hypertelorism, prominent supraorbital ridges, prominent jaw and forehead, and enlarged tongue, suggestive of but milder than MPS-IH (12) (Fig. 13–2). The skeletal dysplasia (34) has thickening of the calvaria in most patients, ovoid vertebral bodies with flattening and beaking, and sometimes a gibbus. Hepatomegaly and hernias occur, and in 25%, distinctive ocular findings occur as spoke-like cataracts and corneal opacities (1,2,16,17). Recurrent bacterial infections (thought to be a leukocyte chemotactic defect) can begin even in the first year of life. In type I patients, the progression of mental deterioration, hepatosplenomegaly, and dysostosis is rapid, resulting in death often between 3 and 10 years of age (6–8,34).

The milder juvenile-adult onset (type II) form may have more normal early development with milder findings, which appear to be almost imperceptibly progressive, and the patients often survive into adulthood (6,25,34). Additional findings may include pancytopenia (32), hydrocephalus, spastic paraplegia, and destructive synovitis (9). Head magnetic resonance imaging (MRI) studies have demonstrated bony changes, cerebellar atrophy, and white matter signal changes. Decreases in IgG levels can occur, and PR interval decreases have been reported on the electrocardiogram (ECG) (34).

Auditory findings. High-frequency sensorineural deafness occurs in both type I and II patients and is nearly constant and more often severe in type II α-mannosidosis (2,3,7–10,15,18,19,24,25,28,35).

Laboratory findings. A useful laboratory finding is the occurrence of vacuoles in peripheral and bone marrow lymphocytes in almost all patients with α-mannosidosis (3,34). Increased urinary excretion of several mannose-rich oligosaccharides can be demonstrated by thin-layer

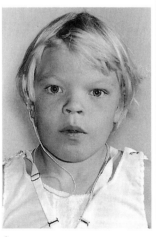
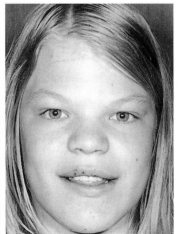
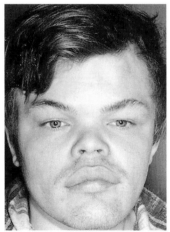

A   **B**   **C**

Figure 13–2. *Mannosidosis.* (A–C) Note gradual coarsening of features with age in 6-year-old, 11-year-old, and 18-year-old sibs.

chromatography (2,6). Demonstration of elevated serum levels of dolichol may be a useful screening method, but it is not specific and may occur in patients with aspartylglycosaminuria (34). Diagnosis is made by demonstrating decreased α-mannosidase levels in leukocytes, fibroblasts, and cultured amniotic fluid cells. Prenatal diagnosis is possible using the latter method, as well as chorionic villi (29,30).

Heredity. Autosomal recessive inheritance has been demonstrated with parental consanguinity in 25% of couples. As indicated earlier, clinical presentation is heterogeneous and intrafamilial variation can be considerable (21). The gene maps to 19cen–q12 (13,23).

Differential diagnosis. Other storage disorders, especially the mucopolysaccharidoses and other oligosaccharidoses and aspartyl-glycosaminuria, should be considered.

References

1. Arbisser AE et al: Ocular findings in mannosidosis. *Am J Ophthalmol* 82:465–471, 1976.
2. Autio S et al: Mannosidosis: clinical, fine-structural and biochemical findings in three cases. *Acta Paediatr Scand* 62:555–565, 1973.
3. Autio S et al: The clinical course of mannosidosis. *Ann Clin Res* 14:93–97, 1982.
4. Aylesworth AS et al: Mannosidoses: phenotype of a severely affected child and characterization of α-mannosidase activity in cultured fibroblasts from the patient and his parents. *J Pediatr* 88:814–818, 1976.
5. Bach G et al: A new variant of mannosidosis with increased residual enzymatic activity and mild clinical manifestations. *Pediatr Res* 12:1010–1015, 1978.
6. Bennett JK et al: Clinical and biochemical analysis of two families with type I and type II mannosidosis. *Am J Med Genet* 55:21–26, 1995.
7. Booth CW et al: Mannosidosis: clinical and biochemical studies in a family of affected adolescents and adults. *J Pediatr* 88:821–824, 1976.
8. Desnick RJ et al: Mannosidosis: clinical, morphologic, immunologic and biochemical studies. *Pediatr Res* 10:985–996, 1976.
9. Eckhoff DG, Garlock JS: Severe destructive polyarthropathy in association with a metabolic storage disease. *J Bone Joint Surg* 74A:1257–1261, 1992.
10. Farriaux JP, Fontaine G: La mannosidose: un diagnostic simple. *Arch Fr Pediatr* 33:11–22, 1976.
11. Gorlin RJ: Genetic hearing loss associated with endocrine and metabolic disorders. In: *Hereditary Hearing Loss and Its Syndromes,* Gorlin RJ et al (eds), Oxford University Press, New York, 1995, pp 322–324.
12. Jansen PH et al: Mannosidosis: a study of two patients presenting clinical heterogeneity. *Clin Neurol Neurosurg* 89:185–192, 1987.
13. Kaneda Y et al: Regional assignment of five genes on human chromosome 19. *Chromosoma* 95:8–12, 1987.
14. Kistler JP et al: Mannosidosis—new clinical presentation, enzyme studies and carbohydrate analysis. *Arch Neurol* 34:45–51, 1977.
15. Kraft E, Zorowka P: Pädaudiologisch-phoniatrische Aspekte der Mannosidose. *HNO* 38:99–101, 1990.
16. Kuellman B et al: Mannosidosis: a clinical and histopathologic study. *J Pediatr* 75:366–370, 1969.
17. Letson RD, Desnick RJ: Punctate lenticular opacities in type II mannosidosis. *Am J Ophthalmol* 85:218–224, 1978.
18. Loeb H et al: Clinical, biochemical and ultrastructural studies of an atypical form of mucopolysaccharidosis. *Acta Paediatr Scand* 58:220–228, 1969.
19. Michelakakis H et al: Phenotypic variability of mannosidosis type II: report of two Greek siblings. *Genet Couns* 3:195–199, 1992.
20. Milla PJ et al: Mannosidosis: clinical and biochemical study. *Arch Dis Child* 52:937–942, 1977.
21. Mitchell ML et al: Mannosidosis: two brothers with different degrees of disease severity. *Clin Genet* 20:191–202, 1981.
22. Montgomery TR et al: Mannosidosis in an adult. *Johns Hopkins Med J* 151:113–117, 1982.
23. Nebes VL, Schmidt MC: Human lysosomal alpha-mannosidosis: isolation and nucleotide sequence of the full length cDNA. *Biochem Biophys Res Commun* 200:239–245, 1994.
24. Noll RB et al: Follow-up language and cognitive development in patients with mannosidosis. *Arch Neurol* 43:157–159, 1986.
25. Noll RB et al: Long-term follow-up biochemical and cognitive functioning in patients with mannosidosis. *Arch Neurol* 46:507–509, 1989.
26. Öckerman PA: A generalized storage disorder resembling Hurler's syndrome. *Lancet* 2:239–241, 1967.
27. Patton MA et al: Mannosidosis in two brothers: prolonged survival in the severe phenotype. *Clin Genet* 22:284–289, 1982.
28. Perelman R et al: Mannosidose associée à l'absence d'alpha-L-antitrypesine. *Ann Pédiatr* 22:385–396, 1975.
29. Petushkova NA: First-trimester diagnosis of an unusual case of α-mannosidosis. *Prenat Diagn* 11:279–283, 1991.
30. Poenaru L et al: Antenatal diagnosis in three pregnancies at risk for mannosidosis. *Clin Genet* 16:428–432, 1979.
31. Poenaru L et al: Evaluation of possible first-trimester prenatal diagnosis in lysosomal diseases by trophoblast biopsy. *Pediatr Res* 18:1032–1034, 1984.
32. Press OW et al: Pancytopenia in mannosidosis. *Arch Intern Med* 143:1266–1268, 1983.
33. Spranger J et al: The radiographic features of mannosidosis. *Radiology* 119:401–407, 1976.
34. Thomas GH: Disorders of glycoprotein degradation: α-mannosidosis, β-mannosidosis, fucosidosis and sialidosis. In: *The Metabolic and Molecular Bases of Inherited Disease*, 8th ed. Scriver CR et al (eds), McGraw-Hill, New York, 2001, pp 3507–3533.
35. Vidgoff J et al: Mannosidosis in three brothers—a review of the literature. *Medicine* 57:335–348, 1977.

β-Mannosidosis

Clinical features. Jones and Dawson (6) first described deficiency of β-mannosidase in goats, resulting in severe neurologic disease, profound hearing loss, and early death from central nervous system dysmyelination. Discovered later, the human equivalent (OMIM 248510) has proven to be a milder disease than any of the animal models despite complete deficiency of β-mannosidase in all patients (15). Most such patients are reported to be normal during early infancy. However, all but 2 of the 13 patients thus far reported have developed mental retardation, the most consistent clinical feature (9,13,15). Respiratory infections and hearing loss are common and reported in over 60% of the patients (15). Features suggesting a lysosomal storage disease such as facial coarsening rarely occur, and hepatosplenomegaly, corneal clouding, and dysostosis multiplex and vacuolated lymphocytes have not been reported in β-mannosidosis patients (15) except one, who also coincidentally had Sanfilippo A mucopolysaccharidosis. The mild, atypical phenotype probably results in underdiagnosis of β-mannosidosis. The most severely affected patient died at 15 months after developing status epilepticus at 12 months and had severe quadriplegia (3). Two brothers with a milder form have lived to adulthood and have few other clinical findings besides mental retardation and angiokeratomas, resembling those seen in Fabry disease (2). Another similar adult female patient had normal intelligence but an introverted personality (13). An adolescent male with normal intellect had progressive dysmyelinating peripheral neuropathy and clinical depression (9). Other behavioral traits include aggression and emotional instability (11).

Mildly dysmorphic facial features have been described but are not usually as severe or typical as that of the mucopolysaccharidoses. Bony malformations but not dysostosis multiplex and recurrent skin and respiratory infections were described in a severely retarded female with β-mannosidase deficiency who died at age 20 years from bronchopneumonia (7). Brain CT scans are usually normal, but atrophy was reported in the most severely affected patient (3). The small number of patients described and the heterogeneity of clinical findings both between and within families preclude accurate description of the β-mannosidosis phenotype. Recent descriptions of specific mutations suggest partial genotype–phenotype correlations, especially with regard to the associated deafness. For example, homozygosity for the human null mutation in particular is associated with hearing loss (KH Friderici, personal communication).

Auditory system. Light- and electron-microscopic otic alterations have been described in the more severe Nubian goat model (12) of the milder human β-mannosidosis. Patients with β-mannosidosis often tend to have infections of not only the upper and lower respiratory tract but also of the ear (15). Deafness occurs in 62% of reported cases, is sensorineural, and is reported to be mild to moderate (2,4,7,9–11,15–17).

Laboratory findings. In contrast to the utility of finding vacuolated lymphocytes in a patient suspected of having α-mannosidosis, only cytoplasmic vacuoles have been reported in a skin biopsy in one patient with β-mannosidosis (2), but not vacuolated lymphocytes or bone marrow cells. Another single patient had slight vacuolization and granulation of the bone marrow cells.

Urinary oligosaccharides in an abnormal pattern can be demonstrated by thin-layer chromatography in β-mannosidosis patients (5). Standard oligosaccharide screening methods may yield false-negative results in β-mannosidosis patients, but a new high-performance liquid chromatography (HPLC) method has demonstrated abnormalities (14). A single β-mannosidosis patient was shown to have elevated ethanolamine in plasma and urine, the significance of which remains obscure (7).

Assay of β-mannosidase in leukocytes and fibroblasts provides a more definitive diagnosis (11,15). Prenatal diagnosis using cultured amniotic fluid cells and chorionic villi should be possible according to two reports of normal and heterozygotic levels in unaffected fetuses at risk (8,16). Alkhayat et al. (1) identified β-mannosidase gene mutations in association with human β-mannosidosis.

Heredity. β-mannosidosis is an autosomal recessive disorder (OMIM 248510). The gene has been mapped to chromosome 4q21–q25 (1).

References

1. Alkhayat AH et al: Human beta-mannosidase cDNA characterization and first identification of a mutation associated with human beta-mannosidosis. *Hum Mol Genet* 7:75–83, 1998.
2. Cooper A et al: Human β-mannosidase deficiency. *N Engl J Med* 315:1231, 1986.
3. Cooper A et al: β-mannosidase deficiency in a female infant with epileptic encephalopathy. *J Inherit Metab Dis* 14:18–22, 1991.
4. Dorland L et al: β-mannosidosis in two brothers with hearing loss. *J Inherit Metab Dis* 11(Suppl2):255–258, 1988.
5. Hommes FA, Varghese M: High-performance liquid chromatography of urinary oligosaccharides in the diagnosis of glycoprotein degradation disorders. *Clin Chim Acta* 203 211–224, 1991.
6. Jones MZ, Dawson G: Caprine beta-mannosidosis: inherited deficiency of beta-D-mannosidase. *J Biol Chem* 256:5185–5188, 1981.
7. Kleijer WJ et al: β-mannosidase deficiency: heterogeneous manifestations in the first female patient and her brother. *J Inherit Metab Dis* 13:867–872, 1990.
8. Kleijer WJ et al: Prenatal analyses in a pregnancy at risk for β-mannosidosis. *Prenat Diagn* 12:841–843, 1992.
9. Levade T et al: Human β-mannosidase deficiency associated with peripheral neuropathy. *Ann Neurol* 35:116–119, 1994.
10. Michelakakis H et al: Phenotypic variability of mannosidosis type II: report of two Greek siblings. *Genet Couns* 3:195–199, 1992.
11. Poenaru L et al: Human β-mannosidosis. A 3-year-old boy with speech impairment and emotional instability. *Clin Genet* 41:331–334, 1992.
12. Render JA et al: Otic pathology of caprine beta-mannosidosis. *Vet Pathol* 25:437–442, 1988.
13. Rodriguez-Serna M et al: Angiokeratoma corporis diffusum associated with β-mannosidase deficiency. *Arch Dermatol* 132:1214–1222, 1996.
14. Sewell AC: Urinary oligosaccharides. In: *Techniques in Diagnostic Human Biochemical Genetics,* Hommes FA (ed), Wiley-Liss, New York, 1991, p 219.
15. Thomas, GH: Disorders of glycoprotein degradation: α-mannosidosis, β-mannosidosis, fucosidosis and sialidosis. In: *The Metabolic and Molecular*
16. Wenger DA et al: Human β-mannosidase deficiency. *N Engl J Med* 315:1201–1205, 1986.
17. Wijburg H et al: β-mannosidosis and ethanolaminuria in female patients. *Eur J Pediatr* 151:311, 1992.

Bases of Inherited Disease, 8th ed., Scriver CR et al (eds), McGraw-Hill, New York 2001, pp 3507–3533.

Aspartylglucosaminuria [aspartylglucosaminidase (AGA) deficiency]

In 1967, Jenner and Pollitt (15) first described aspartylglucosaminuria (OMIM 208400), an oligosaccharidosis in which glycoprotein-derived aspartyl-glucosamine accumulates in various tissues. Autio et al. (5,6) carried out detailed studies on 57 Finnish patients. In eastern Finland, Mononen et al. (17,18) estimated a frequency of 1/3643 children. Aspartylglucosaminuria is a lysosomal storage disease caused by deficiency of *N*-aspartyl-β-glucosaminidase due to mutations in the *AGU* gene and resulting in defective degradation of asparagine-linked glycoproteins (4).

Infancy and childhood are usually characterized by recurrent diarrhea and frequent respiratory infections. There is early onset of splenomegaly with abdominal protrusion. Progressive mental retardation to an IQ of 40 or less in the second decade is a constant feature. It usually first becomes evident around 5 years of age. Speech is severely delayed. In about 35%, the voice becomes raspy and adult-like. Periodic hyperactivity, hyperirritability, and/or aggressive reactions have been noted in about 50%. Clumsy gait and poor coordination of the hands are observed early in life (4,10).

There is remarkable resemblance among affected individuals (Fig. 13–3A,B). The features gradually become coarse during childhood, the nasal bridge being short, broad, and low. The nostrils are anteverted and the lips thickened. There are mild hypertelorism, epicanthal folds, and crystal-like lens opacities in about 50% of patients. The facial skin, particularly that of the eyelids and cheeks, has a tendency to sag with age. The teeth are often spaced, and the gingiva and tongue are enlarged in about one-half the patients.

Inguinal and/or, more often, umbilical hernias have been found in about 35% of affected individuals before the age of 3 months. Muscular hypotonia has been noted in about 20%. Genua valga is present in at least 75%. The calvaria is characteristically thickened and the head is brachycephalic. The frontal sinuses are absent or poorly developed. There is mild dysostosis multiplex in the spine. The long bones, metacarpals, and phalanges have thin cortices. Kyphosis or scoliosis and protuberant abdomen have been frequently reported. Growth retardation is seen only after 15 years of age, and short stature is common (4). Chronic arthritis is fairly common; not just in affected patients, but also carriers of the *AGU* gene (1).

Mild to moderate hearing loss has been found in 50% of adults with this disorder although the degree of mental retardation has often made estimation difficult. Both conductive and sensorineural hearing loss have been noted (5,6).

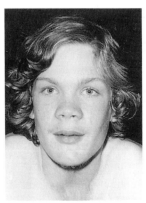
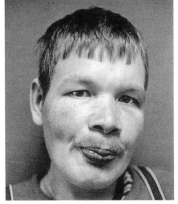
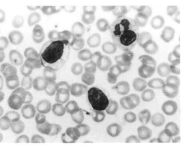

A   **B**   **C**

Figure 13–3. *Aspartylglucosaminuria.* (A,B) Coarse facies in two unrelated patients. (C) Vacuolated lymphocytes in peripheral blood smear. [(A) courtesy of R Stevenson, Greenwood, South Carolina; (B) courtesy of S Autio, Helsinki, Finland; (C) from JN Isenberg and H Sharp, *J Pediatr* 86:713,1975.]

From 5% to 20% of the blood lymphocytes are vacuolated in 75% of the patients, and about 50% exhibit neutropenia and decreased prothrombin time (Fig. 13–3C).

Inheritance is autosomal recessive. Although the disorder has been found in various groups (4,7,9,12,21–23), most patients are Finnish (20). In eastern Finland, about 1/40 is a heterozygote (17,18). Heterozygotes may be identified and prenatal detection is possible (3,4). The gene, *AGA* (aspartylglucosaminidase), is located at 4q32–q35 (2,4,8,11,19). The definitive diagnosis is made by finding markedly decreased aspartylglucosaminidase in the plasma, leukocytes, or cultured skin fibroblasts (13,14) or by finding aspartylglucosaminuria by chromatographic or electrophoretic methods (6,16).

References

1. Arvio M et al. Carriers of the aspartylglucosaminuria genetic mutation and chronic arthritis. *Ann Rheum Dis* 61:180–181, 2002.
2. Aula P et al: Assignment of the structural gene encoding human aspartylglucosaminuria to the long arm of chromosome 4 (4q21–4qter). *Am J Hum Genet* 36:1215–1224, 1984.
3. Aula P et al: Prenatal diagnosis and fetal pathology of aspartylglucosaminuria. *Am J Med Genet* 19:359–367, 1984.
4. Aula et al: Aspartylglucosaminuria. In: *The Metabolic and Molecular Bases of Inherited Disease,* 8th ed., Scriver CR et al. (eds). McGraw-Hill, New York, 2001, pp 3535–3550.
5. Autio S: Aspartylglycosaminuria. Analysis of thirty-four patients. *J Ment Defic Res Monogr Ser* 1:1–93, 1972.
6. Autio S et al: Aspartylglucosaminuria (AGU). Further aspects of its clinical picture, mode of inheritance, and epidemiology based on a series of 57 patients. *Ann Clin Res* 5:149–155, 1973.
7. Chitayat D et al: Aspartylglycosaminuria in a Puerto Rican family: additional features of a panethnic disorder. *Am J Med Genet* 31:527–532, 1988.
8. Engelen J et al: Assignment of the aspartylglucosaminuria gene (*AGA*) to 4q33–q35 based on decreased activity in a girl with a 46,XX,del(4)(q33) karyotype. *Cytogenet Cell Genet* 60:208–209, 1992.
9. Gehler J et al: Aspartylglycosaminuria in an Italian family: clinical and biochemical characteristics. *J Inherit Metab Dis* 4:229–230, 1981.
10. Gorlin RJ et al: *Syndromes of the Head and Neck,* 4th ed. Oxford University Press, New York, 2001, pp. 141–143.
11. Gron K et al: Linkage of aspartylglucosaminuria to marker loci on the long arm of chromosome 4. *Hum Genet* 85:233–236, 1990.
12. Hreidarsson S et al: Aspartylglucosaminuria in the United States. *Clin Genet* 23:427–435, 1983.
13. Isenberg JN, Sharp HL: Aspartylglycosaminuria: psychomotor retardation masquerading as a mucopolysaccharidosis. *J Pediatr* 86:713–718, 1975.
14. Isenberg JN, Sharp HL: Aspartylglucosaminuria: unique biochemical and ultrastructural characteristics. *Hum Pathol* 7:469–481, 1976.
15. Jenner FA, Pollitt RJ: Large quantities of 2-acetamido-1-(beta-L-aspartamido)-1,2-dideoxyglucose in the urine of mentally retarded siblings. *Biochem J* 103:48–49, 1967.
16. Maury CP, Palo J: *N*-Acetylglucosamine-asparagine levels in tissues of patients with aspartylglucosaminuria. *Clin Chem Acta* 108:293–299, 1980.
17. Mononen I et al: Aspartylglucosaminuria in the Finnish population. *Proc Natl Acad Sci USA* 88:2941–2945, 1991.
18. Mononen I et al: High prevalence of aspartylglycosaminuria among school-age children in eastern Finland. *Hum Genet* 87:266–268, 1991.
19. Morris C et al: Chromosomal localization of the human glycoasparaginase gene to 4q32–q33. *Hum Genet* 88:295–297, 1992.
20. Palo J, Mattsson K: Eleven new cases of aspartylglycosaminuria. *J Ment Defic Res* 14:168–173, 1970.
21. Stevenson RE et al: Aspartylglucosaminuria. *Proc Greenwood Genet Ctr* 1:69–72, 1982.
22. Yoshida K et al: Two Japanese with aspartylglycosaminuria: clinical and morphological features. *Clin Genet* 40:318–325, 1991.
23. Ziegler R et al: Aspartylglucosaminurie. Klinische Beschreibung von zwei deutschen Patienten. *Monatsschr Kinderheilkd* 137:454–457, 1989.

Sialidosis (neuraminidase 1 deficiency, mucolipidosis I; sialidase 1 deficiency)

Sialidosis (OMIM 256550) is an autosomal recessive lysosomal storage disease that results from neuraminidase (sialidase) deficiency. The type I form (also called "cherry red spot myoclonus syndrome") presents within the first two to three decades of life with cherry red macular spots, progressive myoclonus, ataxia, visual loss, and normal in-

telligence (1–3,6–14). The type I form does not have dysmorphic features, but the myoclonus is poorly controlled by medication and very debilitating. Onset may occur in late childhood or may not occur until the second or third decade of life when ataxia may be the presenting symptom (1–3,6–14).

The type II form involves myoclonus, cherry red spots, visual loss, ataxia, cataracts, course facies, hepatosplenomegaly, kyphosis, and mental retardation (Fig. 13–4). The type II form has been subdivided into congenital and infantile (or childhood), depending on the time of onset of symptoms (1,4,5,7–14). There is a broad spectrum of severity in the type II category; however, the disease is progressive and involves a mucopolysaccharidosis-like phenotype, and survival may go to the second decade (1,4,5,7–14).

Vacuolated lymphocytes and bone marrow and placental foam cells are prominent in the type II form but are lacking in the type I form. There is tissue storage of sialyloligosaccharides, increased urinary excretion of sialic acid containing oligosaccharides, and marked elevation of individual oligosaccharides due to defective sialidase (neuraminidase) (1).

Several patients with the type II childhood disease have had impaired hearing (2–14). Conductive (13,14) or mixed (3,6,8) hearing loss has been reported.

References

1. d'Azzo A et al: Galactosialidosis. In: *The Metabolic and Molecular Bases of Inherited Disease,* 8th ed. Scriver CR et al. (eds), McGraw-Hill, New York, 2001, pp 3811–3826.
2. Goldberg MF et al: Macular cherry red spot, corneal clouding and beta-galactosidase deficiency. *Arch Intern Med* 128:387–398, 1971.
3. Kelly TE: Mucolipidosis I (acid neuraminidase deficiency). *Am J Dis Child* 135:703–708, 1981.
4. King M et al: Infantile type 2 sialidosis in a Pakistani family—a clinical and biochemical study. *J Inherit Metab Dis* 7:91–96, 1984.
5. Laver J et al: Infantile lethal neuraminidase deficiency (sialidosis). *Clin Genet* 23:97–101, 1983.
6. Louis JJ et al: Une observation de mucolipidose de type 1 par déficit primaire en alpha D neuraminidase. *J Génét Hum* 31:79–91, 1983.

Figure 13–4. *Sialidosis, type 2.* Two affected Pakistani sibs, aged 13 and 12 years, with mother and normal 15-year-old sib. [From M King et al., *J Inherit Metabol Dis* 7:91, 1984.]

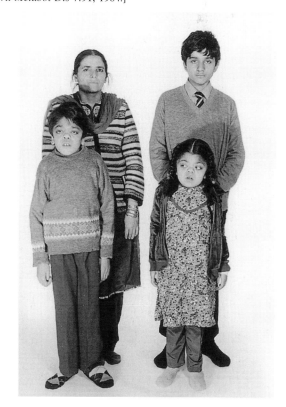

7. Lowden JA, O'Brien JS: Sialidosis: a review of human neuraminidase deficiency. *Am J Hum Genet* 31:1–18, 1979.
8. Maroteaux P et al: Sialidose par déficit en alpha (2–6) neuraminidase sans atteinte neurologique. Mucolipidose de type I? *Arch Fr Pédiatr* 35:286–291, 1978.
9. Spranger J: Mucolipidosis I: Phenotype and nosology. *Perspect Inherit Metab Dis* 4:303–315, 1981.
10. Spranger J et al: Lipomucopolysaccharidose. *Z Kinderheilkd* 103:285–306, 1968.
11. Spranger J et al: Mucolipidosis I—a sialidosis. *Am J Med Genet* 1:21–29, 1977.
12. Staalman CR, Bakker HD: Mucolipidosis I: roentgenographic follow-up. *Skeletal Radiol* 12:153–161, 1984.
13. Winter RM et al: Sialidosis type 2 (acid neuraminidase deficiency): clinical and biochemical features of a further case. *Clin Genet* 18:203–210, 1980.
14. Young ID et al: Neuraminidase deficiency: case report and review of the phenotype. *J Med Genet* 24:283–290, 1987.

Fabry disease (α-galactosidase A deficiency)

Fabry disease (OMIM 301500) is an X-linked recessive disorder with variable clinical expression that results from deficiency of α-galactosidase A, a lysosomal enzyme. Mutations in the *GLA* gene result in an enzymatic defect that leads to the systemic accumulation of the glycosphingolipids, ceramide trihexoside, particularly in the plasma and lysosomes of the vascular endothelium and smooth muscle cells (2). The single most debilitating symptom consists of excruciating episodic burning pain in fingers and toes, which begins in childhood.

In affected males, progressive endothelial glycolipid deposition results in ischemia and infarction and leads to major clinical manifestations. Other cardiac findings may include hypertension, anginal chest pain, myocardial ischemia or infarction, mitral insufficiency, and various cerebrovascular manifestations (6). Diminished caloric and rotatory responses are found in nearly all affected men (4).

Cutaneous vascular lesions (angiokeratomas) are typically present and are telangiectases that cluster in superficial layers of the skin (Fig. 13–5). They appear during childhood and become progressive with age, being most dense between the umbilicus and the knee. Hypohidrosis is common (2).

Aneurysmal dilatation and tortuosity of conjunctival and retinal vessels are seen as well as a characteristic keratopathy. The corneal haziness and whorled streaks are noted in all hemizygous males and in about 80% of female carriers. Fabry cataracts occur in hemizygous males and in some heterozygous females (2,5).

Early in the course of the disease, casts, red cells, and lipid inclusions with characteristic birefringent "Maltese crosses" appear in the urinary sediment. Proteinuria, isosthenuria, and gradual deterioration of renal function as well as development of azotemia occur in the second to fourth decades.

Auditory findings. Hearing impairment is relatively common. Morgan et al. (4) described nonsymptomatic hearing loss in seven affected men and four obligate female carriers. The hearing loss was more marked at higher frequencies in three of five patients older than 30 years.

Hearing loss was also noted by Bird and Lagunoff (1). Schachern et al. (7) described the otologic histopathology in two patients with Fabry disease and sensorineural hearing loss, indicating hair cell loss and strial and spiral ligament atrophy.

Heredity. The disease has X-linked recessive inheritance with variable expression.

In carrier females, features are largely limited to keratopathy, but a few manifesting heterozygotes have been described. The gene has been mapped to Xq22 (3).

References

1. Bird TD, Lagunoff D: Neurological manifestations of Fabry disease in female carriers. *Ann Neurol* 4:537–540, 1978.
2. Desnick RJ et al: α-galactosidase deficiency: Fabry disease. In: *The Metabolic and Molecular Bases of Inherited Disease,* 8th ed., Scriver CR et al (eds). McGraw-Hill, New York, 2001, pp 3733–3774.
3. Gorlin RJ et al: *Syndromes of the Head and Neck,* 4th ed. Oxford University Press, New York, 2001, pp. 154–157.
4. Morgan SH et al: The neurological complications of Anderson-Fabry disease (α-galactosidase A deficiency)—investigation of symptomatic and presymptomatic patients. *Q J Med* 75:491–504, 1990.
5. O'Brien BD et al: Pathophysiologic and ultrastructural basis for intestinal symptoms in Fabry's disease. *Gastroenterology* 82:957–960, 1982.
6. Sakuraba H et al: Cardiovascular manifestations in Fabry's disease: a high incidence of mitral valve prolapse in hemizygotes and heterozygotes. *Clin Genet* 29:276–283, 1986.
7. Scharchern, PA et al: Otologic histopathology of Fabry's disease. *Ann Otol Rhinol Laryngol* 98: 359–363, 1989.

Gaucher-like disease (glucosylceramide-β-glucosidase deficiency, pseudo-Gaucher disease)

Gaucher-like disease (OMIM 231005) was first described by Uyama et al. (4) when three adult sibs with glucosylceramide-β-glucosidase deficiency were reported. Since that time, several additional cases have been described (1–3,5). The usual stigmata of Gaucher disease were not evident, but the disorder is caused by the same enzymatic defect as seen in Gaucher disease: a deficiency of lysosomal β-glucosidase (1,3).

The presenting feature of this disorder is typically a supranuclear gaze palsy during childhood, but the other manifestations do not become evident until young adulthood. Hydrocephalus, corneal opacities, valvular heart disease, sensorineural hearing loss, deformed toes, and leptomeningeal fibrous thickenings, calcification of the aorta, aortic stenosis, and mitral stenosis have been described on autopsy (1–5).

Homozygosity for the D409H mutation in the acid β-glucosidase gene (*GBA*) is thought to result in this specific phenotype (3,5).

References

1. Abrahamov A et al: Gaucher's disease variant characterized by progressive calcification of heart valves and unique genotype. *Lancet* 346: 1000–1003, 1995.
2. Beutler E et al: 1342C mutation in Gaucher's disease. *Lancet* 346:1637, 1995.
3. Chabas A et al: Unusual expression of Gaucher's disease: cardiovascular calcifications in three sibs homozygous for the D409H mutation. *J Med Genet* 32:740–742, 1995.
4. Uyama E et al: Hydrocephalus, corneal opacities, deafness, valvular heart disease, deformed toes and leptomeningeal fibrous thickening in adult siblings: a new syndrome associated with beta-glucocerebrosidase deficiency and a mosaic population of storage cells. *Acta Neurol Scand* 86:407–420, 1992.
5. Uyama E et al: D409H/D409H genotype in Gaucher-like disease [letter]. *J Med Genet* 34:175, 1997.

Neuraminidase deficiency with β-galactosidase deficiency (Goldberg syndrome, galactosialidosis)

Galactosialidosis, due to a combined neuraminidase and β-galactosidase deficiency (OMIM 256540), results from mutations in the β-galactosidase protective protein gene (cathepsin A, *PPGB*) (8). It is an au-

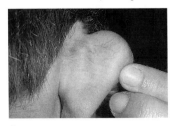

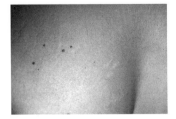

Figure 13–5. *Fabry disease.* (A) Note telangiectases on ear of 6-year-old patient. (B) Note angiomas in older patient. [From D Shelley et al., *Pediatr Dermatol* 12:216, 1995.]

A   B

tosomal recessive condition that results in dwarfism, coarse face, conjunctival telangiectases, corneal clouding, macular cherry red spot, hearing loss, mental retardation, seizures, dysostosis multiplex, and, in Japanese patients, angiokeratomas (1–7) (Fig. 13–6). Organomegaly is typically not present. This disorder may present in one of three forms: (*1*) neonatal hydropic, (*2*) late infantile, and (*3*) juvenile or adult.

Electron microscopy of skin biopsies and peripheral blood lymphocytes shows membrane-bound fibrillogranular inclusions. Elevated urine sialyloligosaccharides but not free sialic acid is seen.

References

1. Chitayat D et al: Juvenile galactosialidosis in a white male: a new variant. *Am J Med Genet* 31:887–901, 1988.
2. Gorlin RJ et al: *Syndromes of the Head and Neck,* 4th ed. Oxford University Press, New York, 2001, pp. 145–147.
3. Ishibashi A et al: Beta-galactosidase and neuraminidase deficiency associated with angiokeratoma corporis diffusum. *Arch Dermatol* 120:1344–1346, 1984.
4. Kuriyama M et al: Adult mucolipidosis with betagalactosidase and neuraminidase deficiencies. *J Neurol Sci* 46:245–254, 1980.
5. Maire I, Nivelon-Chevallier A: Combined deficiency of beta-galactosidase and neuraminidase: three affected siblings in a French family. *J Inherit Metab Dis* 4:221–223, 1981.
6. Petit C et al: Hereditary hearing loss. In: *The Metabolic and Molecular Bases of Inherited Disease,* 8th ed. Scriver CR et al. (eds), McGraw-Hill, New York, 2001, p 6292.
7. Suzuki Y et al: Beta-galactosidase deficiency—juvenile and adult patients. *Hum Genet* 36:219–229, 1977.
8. Zhou XY et al: A mutation in a mild form of galactosialidosis impairs dimerization of the protective protein and renders it unstable. *EMBO J* 10:4041–4048, 1991.

Multiple sulfatase deficiency (mucosulfatidosis)

The clinical features of multiple sulfatase deficiency (OMIM 272200) are those found in steroid sulfatase deficiency (ichthyosis), mu-

Figure 13–6. *Galactosialidosis.* (A) Mild coarseness of facial features. Muscular upper body. (B) Mild irregularities in vertebral bodies. [From D Chitayat et al., *Am J Med Genet* 31:887, 1988.]

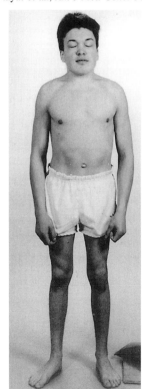
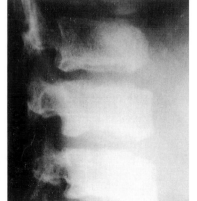

A   **B**

copolysaccharidoses (dysostosis multiplex, psychomotor delay, coarse facial features, hepatosplenomegaly, and hearing loss), and late infantile metachromatic leukodystrophy (motor weakness, psychomotor delay, demyelinization, and gliosis of white matter of the brain) (1–11). With the condition presenting during the first 2 years of life, the children gradually lapse into a vegetative state, and death is usually during the first decade (7).

Hearing loss has been briefly described (4,10,11) but not otherwise characterized. Using auditory brain stem evoked response, it has been demonstrated that the retrocochlear auditory system becomes involved.

An increase in cerebrospinal fluid protein has been demonstrated. Alder-Riley granules are found in leukocytes. The disorder is an autosomal recessive condition and is most often confused with MPS II (7).

References

1. Austin J: Multiple sulfatase deficiency. *Arch Neurol* 28:258–264, 1973.
2. Burch M et al: Multiple sulphatase deficiency presenting at birth. *Clin Genet* 30:409–415, 1986.
3. Burk RD et al: Early manifestations of multiple sulfatase deficiency. *J Pediatr* 104:574–578, 1984.
4. Couchat J et al: La mucosulfatidose: Étude de trois cas familaux. *Arch Fr Pédiatr* 31:775–795, 1974.
5. Crawfurd M d'A: Genetics of steroid sulphatase deficiency and X-linked ichthyosis. *J Inherit Metab Dis* 5:153–163, 1982.
6. Gorlin RJ et al: *Syndromes of the Head and Neck,* 4th ed. Oxford University Press, New York, 2001, pp. 153–154.
7. Hopwood JJ, Ballabio A: Multiple sulfatase deficiency and the nature of the sulfatase family. In: *The Metabolic and Molecular Bases of Inherited Disease,* 8th ed., Scriver CR et al (eds), McGraw-Hill, New York, 2001, pp 3725–3732.
8. Perlmutter-Cremer N et al: Unusual early manifestation of multiple sulfatase deficiency. *Ann Radiol* 24:43–48, 1981.
9. Rampini S et al: Die Kombination von metachromatischer Leukodystrophie und Mukopolysaccharidose als selbständiges Krankeitsbild (Mukosulfatidose). *Helv Paediatr Acta* 5:436–461, 1970.
10. Soong BW et al: Multiple sulfatase deficiency. *Neurology* 28:1273–1275, 1988.
11. Vamos E et al: Multiple sulphatase deficiency with early onset. *J Inherit Metab Dis* 4:103–104, 1981.

Gangliosidoses

GM₁ gangliosidosis

GM_1 gangliosidosis is an autosomal recessive oligosaccharidosis caused by lysosomal accumulation of the ganglioside asialo-GM_1 ganglioside and galactose-containing oligosaccharides due to a functionally deficient acid-β-D-galactosidase. The disease was first recognized in 1964 by Landing et al (5).

There are three major forms: infantile (type I, OMIM 230500), juvenile (type II, OMIM 230600), and adult (type III, OMIM 230650). The infantile form is manifest shortly after birth. In its full expression, it is characterized by hypotonia, poor suck and swallow, failure to thrive, and progressive cerebral deterioration, with death usually occurring between 6 months and 2 years of age from bronchopneumonia. The facial features are coarse at birth, in contrast to the face in MPS IH, which is normal for the first 6 months (Fig. 13-7). Approximately 60% of patients have mild macrocephaly with frontal bossing. The nasal bridge is depressed, the philtrum is prominent, the cheeks are full, and the eyelids puffy. Cherry red macular spots are detected in about 50% of cases. The tongue and alveolar processes are enlarged. The hands are short and stubby, and there are multiple flexion contractures, especially at the knees and elbows. Kyphoscoliosis is an early finding. X-ray changes typical of dysostosis multiplex are more severe and appear earlier than those in MPS IH. In addition to gross motor delay, patients exhibit seizures, blindness, generalized hyperreflexia, and spastic quadriplegia. Hepatomegaly is present after 6 months of age.

The juvenile form (type II) is characterized by age of onset at 6–20 months, with death occurring at 3–10 years. There is mental and motor retardation, but the face is not coarse and the dysostosis multiplex is mild.

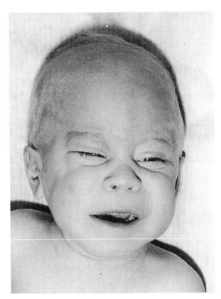

Figure 13–7. *GM₁ gangliosidosis, infantile form (type 1)*. Note coarse face, frontal bossing, full cheeks. [Courtesy of R Scott, Seattle, Washington.]

Locomotor ataxia is first noted at approximately 1 year of age. This is associated with loss of coordinated hand movements, choreoathetosis, moderate muscular weakness of extremities, and loss of speech. Internal strabismus is common. Progressive spasticity follows. Seizures appear during the second year of life. Patients are subject to recurrent infections, especially bronchopneumonia, from which they usually succumb.

In the adult form (type III), gait disturbance and dysarthria begin during adolescence. There is slowly progressive dystonia involving the face and limbs, eventually incapacitating the patient. However, intellectual impairment is not marked. Onset occurs during adolescence, with most patients dying after the second decade of life.

Hearing loss has been often noted in some juvenile patients. Suzuki et al. (7) found that three of six patients exhibited hearing loss. No note has been made regarding hearing loss in the infantile form (1–6,8).

Between 10% and 80% of peripheral lymphocytes are vacuolated, with foam cells being found in the marrow and viscera. Neurons of the central nervous system and retina have a granular appearance because of GM_1 ganglioside-loaded lysosomes. In the juvenile and adult forms, the changes in the lymphocytes and marrow are less marked. Under electron microscopy, these appear as whorled and striped "zebra bodies" identical to those seen in Tay-Sachs disease. Urinary excretion of galactose-containing oligosaccharides is markedly elevated.

β-Galactosidase deficiency also causes Morquio B disease (a mild phenotype of Morquio A disease), which has skeletal dysplasia, corneal clouding, and no central nervous system involvement (8).

References

1. Babarik A et al: Corneal clouding in GM₁-generalized gangliosidosis. *Br J Ophthalmol* 60:565–567, 1976.
2. Benson PF et al: GM₁-generalized gangliosidosis variant with cardiomegaly. *Postgrad Med J* 52:159–165, 1976.
3. Gorlin RJ et al: *Syndromes of the Head and Neck*, 4th ed. Oxford University Press, New York, 2001, pp. 139–140.
4. Hooft C et al: The GM₁ gangliosidosis (Landry disease). *Eur Neurol* 2:225–241, 1969.
5. Landing BH et al: Familial neurovisceral lipidosis. *Am J Dis Child* 18:503–528, 1964.
6. O'Brien JS et al: Juvenile GM₁ gangliosidosis: clinical, pathological, chemical and enzymatic studies. *Clin Genet* 3:411–434, 1972.
7. Suzuki Y et al: Beta-galactosidase deficiency in juvenile and adult patients—report of six Japanese cases and review of the literature. *Hum Genet* 36:219–226, 1977.
8. Suzuki Y et al: Beta-galactosidase deficiency (β-galactosidosis): Gm₁ gangliosidosis and Morquio B disease. In: *The Metabolic and Molecular Bases of Inherited Disease*, 8th ed. Scriver CR et al. (eds), McGraw-Hill, New York, 2001, pp 3775–3809.

Tay-Sachs disease (type I GM₂ gangliosidosis)

Tay (11), in 1881, and Sachs (10), in 1887, independently described a new disorder, with Tay concentrating on the eye changes and Sachs, the clinical features, diagnostic signs, and pathology. An excellent historical review is that of Evans (2).

Tay-Sachs disease (OMIM 272800) is an autosomal recessive neurodegenerative disorder resulting from the deficiency of β-hexosaminidase A and due to mutations in the *HEXA* gene (3). The disease is characterized by macrocephaly, paralysis, dementia, blindness, and significant developmental delay, with onset typically in infancy (3).

The infant is ostensibly normal for the first couple months of life, but between 3 and 6 months, irritability, voluntary muscle weakness, and visual inattention become apparent. There is an exaggerated startle reflex to sudden sounds. Most affected infants learn to smile and reach for objects, but there is poor head control. Some crawl and sit unaided and even pull to a standing position, but never achieve the ability to walk. After 1 year of age, marked mental and motor retardation, apathy, and loss of developmental milestones are apparent. There may be episodes of laughter (gelastic seizures). After 18 months, seizures (often myoclonic) and spasticity become marked and death often occurs by age 5 (3,6).

Blindness becomes apparent before 1 year of age. Examination of the retina reveals a cherry red spot in at least 90%, which represents involvement of the ganglion cells of the retina. Since they are concentrated at the macula, the normal reddish color is lost and the macule appears gray. Since the fovea contains no ganglion cells, it remains red, which contrasts with the grayish macula. During the late stages of the disease, probably all infants experience severe hearing impairment, but the cause is uncertain (1,3,4). Boies (1) noted the frequent occurrence of otitis media.

The disorder results from accumulation of GM_2 ganglioside in neurons due to deficiency of the lysosomal enzyme, hexosaminidase A (from mutations in the *HEXA* gene). Tay-Sachs disease is most prevalent in the Ashkenazi Jewish and French-Canadian populations (7). Identification of heterozygotes has led to reduction in frequency of the disorder. The enzyme deficiency can be detected in serum, skin fibroblasts, or amniocytes (3).

The neuronal cell bodies of ganglion cells become ballooned out by the stored ganglioside. These changes are also seen in ganglion cells of the inner ear (1). On electron microscopy, one can see numerous membrane-bound concentrically laminated structures in the cytoplasm.

Electroencephalographic studies are grossly abnormal, often showing hypsarrhythmia. A later-onset form of Tay-Sachs disease or GM_2 gangliosidosis that results in ataxia, dementia, motor neuron disease, depression, and/or schizophrenia has also been reported (3,8,9). Sandhoff disease (OMIM 268800) is similar in clinical presentation to infantile Tay-Sachs, but onset is earlier and progression is more rapid. Biochemically, there is deficiency of both hexosaminidase A and B in Sandhoff disease. Hepatosplenomegaly is common. The cherry red spot is not specific for Tay-Sachs disease. It may be seen in other forms of GM_2 gangliosidosis, types A and C Niemann-Pick disease, infantile Gaucher disease, metachromatic leukodystrophy, sialidosis, and other conditions (5).

References

1. Boies LR Jr: Tay-Sachs disease in its relation to otolaryngology. *Arch Otolaryngol* 77:166–173, 1963.
2. Evans PR: Tay-Sachs disease: a centenary. *Arch Dis Child* 62:1056–1059, 1987.
3. Gravel RA: The GM₂ gangliosidoses. In: *The Metabolic and Molecular Bases of Inherited Disease*, 8th ed., Scriver CR et al (eds), McGraw-Hill, New York, 2001, pp 3827–3876.
4. Kelemen G: Tay-Sachs-Krankheit und Gehörorgan. *Z Laryngol Rhinol Otol* 44:728–738, 1965.
5. Kivlin JD et al: The cherry-red spot in Tay-Sachs and other storage diseases. *Ann Neurol* 17:356–360, 1985.
6. Kolodny EH: Tay-Sachs disease. In: *Genetic Diseases Among Ashkenazi Jews*, Goodman RM, Molutsky AG (eds), Raven Press, New York, 1979, pp 217–229.

7. Myerowitz R, Hogikyan ND: Different mutations in Ashkenazi Jewish and non-Jewish French Canadians with Tay-Sachs disease. *Science* 232:1646–1648, 1986.
8. Navon, R et al: Hexosaminidase A deficiency in adults. *Am J Med Genet* 24:179–196, 1986.
9. Parnes S et al: Hexosaminidase—a deficiency presenting as atypical juvenile-onset spinal muscular atrophy. *Arch Neurol* 42:1176–1180, 1985.
10. Sachs B: On arrested development, with special reference to its cortical pathology. *J Nerv Ment Dis* 14:541–543, 1887.
11. Tay W: Symmetrical changes in the region of the yellow spot in each eye of an infant. *Trans Ophthalmol Soc UK* 1:55–57, 1881.

Krabbe disease (globoid cell leukodystrophy)

Krabbe disease or globoid cell leukodystrophy (OMIM 245200) due to deficiency of galactocerebrosidase was first described by Krabbe (2) in 1916. The reader is referred to Wenger et al. (3) and Aicardi (1) for excellent summaries of this group of leukodystrophies.

Onset of Krabbe disease typically occurs between 3 and 8 months of age. Early signs are nonspecific and include retardation in motor development, hyperirritability, episodic fever, feeding difficulties, vomiting, spasticity of limbs and back, and seizures. By the first year, markedly hyperactive tendon reflexes are noted. There is severe spasticity, scissoring of legs, and flexion of arms. As the disease progresses, the hyperactive reflexes are lost and replaced by diminished or absent reflexes. There is also reduced nerve conduction velocity. Macrocephaly, reflecting the brain storage of galactosylceramide in the brain, is only occasionally seen. Optic atrophy and sluggish pupillary reflexes are usually seen. Cherry red spots are rarely noted. Terminally, the patients are often blind. In the late phase of the disorder, most patients become profoundly deaf. Death usually occurs by age 3.

Computed tomography scans initially show discrete symmetric dense areas in the gray matter of the cerebral hemispheres, thalamus, and cerebellum, and in periventricular encapsular white matter. In later stages, there is diffuse atrophy of both white and gray matter. Microscopically, varying degrees of deterioration of neurons in the pons, thalamus, and dentate nucleus and many globoid cells in the white matter, lack of myelin, and presence of severe gliosis have been noted. The cytoplasm of the globoid cells stains positive with PAS. Leukocytes, serum, cultured fibroblasts, amniocytes, or chorionic villi of affected and carriers are deficient in galactocerebrosidase.

Inheritance of Krabbe disease is autosomal recessive and is due to mutations in the *GALC* gene at 14q31 (3). The disorder involves all ethnic groups but appears to be somewhat more prevalent in Scandinavia, where the incidence has been calculated at 2–4/1000 births. In Israel, among a large inbred Druze isolate, the remarkably high frequency of 6/1000 births was reported. Patients usually die before the end of the second year of life.

References

1. Aicardi J: The inherited leukodystrophies. *J Inherit Metab Dis* 16:733–743, 1993.
2. Krabbe K: A new familial infantile form of diffuse brain sclerosis. *Brain* 39:74–114, 1916.
3. Wenger D et al: Galactosylceramide lipidosis: globoid cell leukodystrophy (Krabbe disease). In: *The Metabolic Basis of Inherited Disease,* 8th ed. Scriver CR et al (eds), McGraw-Hill, New York, 2001, pp 3669–3694.

Lipidoses

Niemann-Pick type C disease

In 1989, Fink et al. (2) expansively described the clinical spectrum of Niemann-Pick type C disease (OMIM 257220), dividing it into three phenotypes based on onset, severity, and progression. As with other forms of Niemann-Pick disease, the common features of type C include hepatosplenomegaly and the accumulation of various amounts of sphingomyelin and other lipids in liver, spleen, and bone marrow. Ataxia and athetosis are also observed, with onset in mid-childhood, and death usually during the second decade of life. It is an autosomal recessive condition due to mutations in the *NPC1* gene at 18q11-q12 (4).

The organomegaly and the progressive neurologic deterioration are predicated on a defect in the esterification of exogenously supplied cholesterol. Sphingomyelinase deficiency is not observed in type C disease. It is inherited in an autosomal recessive fashion with mutations in the *NPC1* gene leading to disease (1,3,6,7)

Among 28 patients of ages 2–37 years, 21 were found to have high-frequency auditory deficit with varying degrees of severity (5). Hearing loss progressed with increasing severity of somatic signs and symptoms. An early disturbance of an acoustic reflex function was found in 23 of 27 patients studied. Pure-tone studies showed that about 75% were affected. Auditory brain stem response was abnormal in 53%.

References

1. Carstea ED et al: Niemann-Pick C1 disease gene: homology to mediators of cholesterol homeostasis. *Science* 277:228–231, 1997.
2. Fink JK et al: Clinical spectrum of Niemann-Pick disease type C. *Neurology* 39:1040–1049, 1989.
3. Greer WL et al: The Nova Scotia (type D) form of Niemann-Pick disease is caused by a 3097G-T transversion in NPC1. *Am J Hum Genet* 63: 52–54, 1998.
4. Patterson MC et al: Niemann-Pick disease type C. A lipid trafficking disorder. In: *The Metabolic and Molecular Bases of Inherited Disease,* 8th ed., Scriver CR et al (eds), McGraw-Hill, New York, 2001, pp 3611–3634.
5. Pikus A: Audiologic profile in Niemann-Pick C. *Ann NY Acad Sci* 630:313-314, 1991.
6. Yamamoto T et al: *NPC1* gene mutations in Japanese patients with Niemann-Pick disease type C. *Hum Genet* 105:10–16, 1999.
7. Yamamoto T et al: Genotype–phenotype relationship of Niemann-Pick disease type C: a possible correlation between clinical onset and levels of NPC1 protein in isolated skin fibroblasts. *J Med Genet* 37: 707–711, 2000.

Peroxisomal Disorders

Peroxisomes are membrane-bound organelles found in the cytoplasm of nucleated cells (5). They contain enzymes for the β-oxidation of a number of complex compounds including very long straight-chain fatty acids, compounds with a branched carbon chain such as pristanic acid derived from dietary phytanic acid, and a number of long-chain bile acid intermediates. Defects in peroxisomal metabolism result in increased levels of some or all of these substrates (9). The combined incidence of peroxisomal disorders in the western European population is estimated at 1–2/10,000.

Classification. Peroxisomal disorders are categorized into two groups according to their pathophysiological origin. The first group involves defective biogenesis of the organelle itself. The second group encompasses defects in individual peroxisome-associated enzymes (1–3) (Table 13–2).

The biogenesis disorders may be further subdivided into those in which no peroxisomes are formed, resulting in multiple peroxisomal en-

Table 13–2. Peroxisomal disorders

Group 1. Disorders of Biogenesis

Zellweger syndrome (MIM 214100)
Neonatal adrenoleukodystrophy (MIM 202370)
Infantile Refsum disease (MIM 266510)
Rhizomelic-type chondroplasia punctata (MIM 215100)
Zellweger-like syndrome (MIM 170993)

Group 2. Single Enzyme Deficits

X-linked adrenoleukodystrophy (MIM 300100)
Refsum disease (MIM 266500)
Acatalasemia (MIM 115500)
Acyl CoA oxidase deficiency (MIM 264470)
   β-Methylacyl CoA racemase deficiency (MIM 604489)
   3-Ketoacyl CoA thiolase deficiency (MIM 261510)
D-bifunctional protein deficiency (MIM 261515)
Dihydroxyacetonephosphate acyltransferase deficiency (MIM 222765)
Alkyl dihydroxyacetonephosphate synthase deficiency (MIM 600121)
Hyperoxaluria type 1 (MIM 259900)

zyme deficits, and those in which the organelles are present but fail to import subsets of the peroxisomal enzymes. By analogy with yeast peroxisomes (4), it is thought that at least 20 and perhaps as many as 50 genes are required for human peroxisome biogenesis. Eleven human genes have been identified, designated *PEX* and a number, indicating homology with a yeast gene (6). Mutations in *PEX* genes 1, 2, 3, 5, 6, 10, 12, 13, 16, and 19 give rise to defects in peroxisome biogenesis, causing (in order of severity) Zellweger syndrome (ZS), neonatal adrenoleukodystrophy (NALD), and infantile Refsum disease (IRD). Rhizomelic-type chondroplasia punctata (RCDP), caused by failure to import a subset of the peroxisomal enzymes, is associated with mutations in the *PEX7* gene (1,3,7,12).

Clinical features. The peroxisomal biogenesis disorders represent a spectrum of disease ranging from the severe early lethal forms of ZS to quite mild syndromes with patients surviving well into adulthood. The range of phenotypic expression can be caused by mutations in different genes and by different mutations in the same gene, so that a specific syndrome cannot, by clinical exam alone, be easily attributed to a specific genetic defect. Thus, the labeling of a patient with a particular peroxisomal syndrome serves more to indicate the severity of the disease than to identify the specific genetic cause.

The neuropathology of ZS, NALD, and IRD involves both defects in migration of neural crest cells and demyelination. Classical ZS is characterized by hypotonia and global retardation from birth. The liver is enlarged and almost all patients develop seizures. Dysmorphology includes a high forehead and large fontanelle. There is calcific stippling of the patella. In addition, there may be congenital heart disease and renal dysfunction associated with cortical microcysts. Zellweger infants have neuronal deafness and retinal degeneration. The majority of do not survive their first year. The NALD phenotype is less severe and the infants may develop slowly and then regress. All have impaired hearing. The average age at death is about 2 years. As with Zellweger patients there is often microscopic evidence of both disordered neural cell migration and defective myelination. Patients with IRD survive on average to about age 6 years. Over 90% have impaired hearing and retinopathy. Milder atypical cases of peroxisomal biogenesis including Zellweger-like disorders have been reported with no or slight hearing loss (7,13). All the peroxisomal biogenesis disorders have essentially the same biochemical abnormalities consisting of increased levels of very long-chain fatty acids, bile acid intermediates, and phytanic acid and deficiencies of plasmalogen and docosahexanoic acid.

Rhizomelic-type chondroplasia punctata is a severe phenotype and average survival is about 1 year. There is severe psychomotor delay and hearing loss is reported in about 70% of cases.

In the second group of peroxisomal disorders, deficiencies in 10 isolated peroxisomal enzymes have been recognized. The individual peroxisomal enzyme deficiencies demonstrate a wide spectrum of phenotypes, presumably due to different effects of different mutations (7,10–12). In general, they mimic the range of phenotypes seen in the biogenesis disorders. The least severely affected individuals have normal hearing and may survive into adulthood.

In childhood X-linked adrenoleukodystrophy, the most common disorder in this group, children are normal at birth. The onset of symptoms is usually between 3 and 10 years of age and involves changes in intellect, perception, and behavior accompanied by progressive spastic paraparesis. Most patients develop signs of adrenal insufficiency. Hearing loss is progressive and characterized by poor speech perception. Auditory brain stem responses have been reported as abnormal both in presymptomatic cases and in adult carriers (8).

Classic Refsum disease is characterized by retinitis pigmentosa, chronic polyneuropathy, and signs of cerebellar dysfunction. A proportion of patients have sensorineural deafness and some may develop ichthyosis.

Heredity. With the exception of X-linked adrenoleukodystrophy (X-linked recessive), all the peroxisomal disorders are autosomal recessive.

References

1. Cavaletti G et al: Adrenoleukodystrophy. Report of a case with extremely slow progression of symptoms. *Acta Neurol* 12:109–114, 1990.
2. Clayton PT: Clinical consequences of defects in peroxisomal β-oxidation. *Biochem Soc Trans* 29:298–305, 2001.
3. de Duve C: Functions of microbodies (peroxisomes). *J Cell Biol* 27:25a–26a, 1965.
4. Distel B et al: A unified nomenclature for peroxisome biogenesis factors. *J Cell Biol* 135:1–3, 1996.
5. MacCollin M et al: Ataxia and peripheral neuropathy: a benign variant of peroxisome dysgenesis. *Ann Neurol* 28:833–836, 1990.
6. Moser HW: Genotype–phenotype correlations in disorders of peroxisome biogenesis. *Mol Genet Metab* 68:316–327, 1999.
7. Moser HW: Molecular genetics of peroxisomal disorders. *Front Biosci* 5:298–306, 2000.
8. Moser HW, Raymond GV: Genetic peroxisomal disorders: why, when, and how to test. *Ann Neurol* 44:713–715, 1998.
9. Raymond GV: Peroxisomal disorders. *Curr Opin Neurol* 14:783–787, 2001.
10. Shimizu H et al: Auditory brainstem response and audiologic findings in adrenoleukodystrophy: its variant and carrier. *Otolaryngol Head Neck Surg* 98:215–220, 1988.
11. Steinberg SJ et al: Peroxisomal disorders: clinical and biochemical studies in 15 children and prenatal diagnosis in 7 families. *Am J Med Genet* 85:502–510, 1999.
12. Suzuki Y et al: Clinical, biochemical and genetic aspects and neuronal migration in peroxisome biogenesis disorders. *J Inherit Metab Dis* 24:151–165, 2001.
13. van der Klei VM: Yeast peroxisomes: function and biogenesis of a versatile cell organelle. *Trends Microbiol* 5:502–509, 1997.

Fatty Acid Disorders

Triglyceride storage disease with impaired long-chain fatty acid oxidation (neutral lipid storage disease, Chanarin-Dorfman syndrome)

A syndrome of congenital ichthyosis, cataracts, lipid droplets in the cytoplasm of many types of cells, and sensorineural hearing loss was first reported in 1966 by Rozenszajn et al. (9). Members of the same kindred were later studied by Dorfman et al. (5) in 1975.

Triglyceride storage disease with impaired long-chain fatty acid oxidation is characterized by widespread cellular accumulation of triglycerides (4). The triglyceride deposits in viable epidermal cells and alkanes in the stratum corneum lead to clinical manifestations of ichthyosis. The specific enzyme defect has not yet been identified.

Congenital ichthyosis with generalized scaling of the face and flexures and mild erythroderma are characteristic (1–14) (Fig. 13–8A). Involvement of the face, in turn, produces tautness and/or ectropion. Nuclear cataracts, which may appear in infancy, have been found in about 45% (5,6,11,13). Ectropion (5,11,14) and retinal dysfunction (5,9) have been noted. Strabismus, ptosis, and nystagmus have also been reported (10,13). Ataxia, developmental delay, and growth retardation are also characteristic (2).

The liver shows severe fatty metamorphosis, and hepatosplenomegaly is often seen (1–5,8,9). Gluten-sensitive enteropathy (7) and lipid inclusions within the epithelial cells of the entire gastrointestinal tract are described (1,3,8,10). Myopathy with weakness and abnormal electromyograms have been reported in about 65% of cases (1,3,8). Muscle biopsy has shown lipid droplets and atrophy, both in type I and type II fibers, the former being more severely affected. Cultured myoblasts exhibit non–membrane-bound lipid droplets (1). Ataxia and nystagmus (9) and developmental delay (11,13) have been described. Mild growth retardation has also been noted (1,12).

Childhood-onset sensorineural hearing loss, probably progressive, has been reported in 60% of patients. Hearing loss is bilateral and most severe at higher frequencies with mixed ranges from 30 to 80 dB loss (2,5,7,9,11,13).

Peripheral blood smears show prominent cytoplasmic vacuoles in virtually all granulocytes and monocytes but not in lymphocytes (Fig. 13–8B). Histochemical studies have demonstrated that this represents

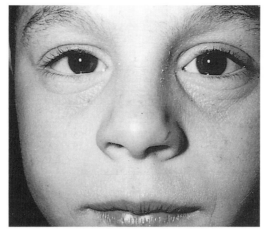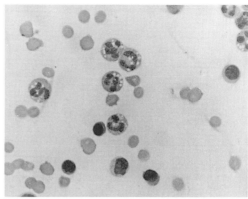

Figure 13–8. *Neutral lipid storage disease.* (A) Note ichthyotic changes of facial skin. (B) Virtually all granulocytes exhibit prominent cytoplasmic vacuoles. [From ML Williams et al., *Am J Med Genet* 20:711, 1985.]

A **B**

neutral lipid (3,8,9). Similar non–membrane-bound lipid droplets are found in various epithelial cells, hepatocytes, and striated muscle cells. Defective lamellar body components have been described (6). Heterozygotes may be identified by the presence of similar vacuoles in circulating eosinophils (11,12). Elevated creatinine phosphokinase has been found in some patients (1,3,8,13). Liver and muscle enzymes (alkaline phosphatase, lactic dehydrogenase, alanine aminotransferase) were also elevated (11).

Lipid droplets in the basal and granular cell layers of the skin are characteristic but have also been noted in Refsum syndrome. Ichthyosis and neurological abnormalities are found in several additional disorders (CHIME syndrome, Sjögren-Larsson syndrome, multiple sulfatase deficiency, trichothiodystrophy, among others), but in none is there neutral lipid storage.

The disorder clearly has autosomal recessive inheritance. Consanguinity has been found in over 40% (2,5,9,11,13). The gene maps to 3p21.

References

1. Angelini C et al: Multisystem triglyceride storage disease with impaired long-chain fatty acid oxidation. *Ann Neurol* 7:5–10, 1980.
2. Assmann G, Seedorf U: Acid lipase deficiency: Wolman disease and cholesterol ester storage disease. In: *The Metabolic and Molecular Bases of Inherited Disease,* 8th ed., Scriver CR et al (eds), McGraw-Hill, New York, 2001, pp 3551–3574.
3. Chanarin I et al: Neutral-lipid storage disease: a new disorder of lipid metabolism. *BMJ* 1:553–555, 1975.
4. DiDonato S et al: Multisystem triglyceride storage disease is due to specific defect in the degradation of endocellularly synthesized triglycerides. *Neurology* 38:1107–1110, 1988.
5. Dorfman ML et al: Ichthyosiform dermatosis with systemic lipidosis. *Arch Dermatol* 110:261–266, 1975.
6. Elias PM, Williams ML: Neutral lipid storage disease with ichthyosis. Defective lamellar body contents and intercellular dispersion. *Arch Dermatol* 121:1000–1008, 1985.
7. Masumeci S et al: Ichthyosis and neutral lipid storage disease. *Am J Med Genet* 29:377–382, 1988.
8. Miranda A et al: Lipid storage, myopathy, ichthyosis and steatorrhea. *Muscle Nerve* 2:1–13, 1979.
9. Rozenszajn L et al: Jordan's abnormality in white blood cells. *Blood* 28:258–265, 1966.
10. Slavin G et al: Morphologic features in a neutral lipid storage disease. *J Clin Pathol* 28:701–710, 1975.
11. Srebrnik A et al: Dorfman-Chanarin syndrome. *J Am Acad Dermatol* 17:801–808, 1987.
12. Venicie PY et al: Ichthyosis and neutral lipid storage disease (Dorfman-Chanarin syndrome). *Pediatr Dermatol* 5:173–177, 1988.
13. Williams ML et al: Ichthyosis and neutral lipid storage disease. *Am J Med Genet* 20:711–726, 1985.
14. Williams ML et al: Neutral lipid storage disease with ichthyosis: lipid content and metabolism of fibroblasts. *J Inherit Metab Dis* 11:131–143, 1988.

Organic Acid and Amino Acid Disorders

Biotinidase deficiency (late-onset multiple carboxylase deficiency)

Biotinidase deficiency is an autosomal recessive condition (OMIM 253260) characterized by multiple carboxylase deficiency of late onset (4,8,13,15,17,22,25). Clinical symptoms are variable both within and between families. Newborn screening for biotinidase deficiency occurs in at least 24 states in the United States (5). The disease incidence estimated from newborn screening is 1/140,000 for complete deficiency (17,18).

Clinical symptoms rarely occur before 3 months of age, although infants have presented as young as 3 weeks. Cutaneous and neurologic symptoms usually occur with mild to moderate depletion of biotin. Breast milk contains less biotin than cow's milk and may contribute to earlier presentation (25). Hyperventilation (20%), seizures (65%), ataxia (60%), hypotonia (85%), developmental delay (65%), optic atrophy (45%), conjunctivitis (40%), and skin rash (65%) occur between 3 months and several years of age (23,26–28). The rash is a dry, erythematous, scaly eruption. About 80% have alopecia. Oral moniliasis is seen in 25% (3). The developmental delay may progress to mental retardation in untreated patients.

Hearing loss has been described in approximately 15%–50% of patients (2,11,12,17,24,25). It has not been well characterized but has been described as sensorineural or mixed and has been reported as early as 3 months of age.

Affected children may have metabolic acidosis (65%), lactic acidemia (65%), hyperammonemia (40%), and organic aciduria (85%). The underlying biochemical defect is deficient activity of the enzyme biotinidase. Metabolic acidosis, organic aciduria, and hyperammonemia occur late in the disease and may be absent in both presymptomatic and asymptomatic cases (13,16).

Biotin is a cofactor for several carboxylase enzymes. Although biotin is available in the diet, biotin levels are maintained in the body by the action of biotinidase, which liberates biotin from partially degraded carboxylase enzymes (3,4,10). Affected individuals are unable to recycle endogenous biotin and to completely degrade biotin-dependent carboxylases (22). They are thus dependent upon dietary biotin. Biotin levels may be normal or low.

Measurement of biotinidase activity can be done by a colorimetric method or radioassay (20,27). Affected individuals have less than 1% of normal activity in serum, leukocytes, fibroblasts, and liver (21). Obligate heterozygotes have about half the normal biotinidase activity. Urinary organic acid excretion includes β-hydroxyisovaleric acid, β-methylcrotonylglycine, β-hydroxypropionic acid and methyl citric, and lactic acid (20). Ketolactic acidemia may be marked.

There are several alleles, with mutations in the biotinidase gene (*BTD*) at 3p25 (1,9). Profound biotinidase deficiency refers to less than 10% of mean normal activity. A partial deficiency state is described as 10%–30% of mean activity (7). The diagnosis should be suspected in children with suggestive neurologic or cutaneous findings of unknown cause. Measurement of the urine organic acids will usually establish the diagnosis.

Biotinidase deficiency is treated with daily biotin supplement, and with early diagnosis and treatment virtually all symptoms can be prevented (5,17), although there is evidence that the hearing loss tends to be irreversible (6).

References

1. Cole H et al: Human serum biotinidase: cDNA cloning, sequence, and characterization. *J Biol Chem* 269:6566–6570, 1994.
2. Diamantopoulos N et al: Biotinidase deficiency: accumulation of lactate in the brain and response to physiologic doses of biotin. *Neurology* 36:1107–1109, 1986.
3. Fisher A et al: Biotin-responsive immunoregulatory dysfunction in multiple carboxylase deficiency. *J Clin Immunol* 2:35–38, 1981.
4. Gaudry M et al: Deficient liver biotinidase activity in multiple carboxylase deficiency. *Lancet* 2:397, 1983.
5. Genetics in Primary Care, newborn screening education web site: http://genes-r-us.uthscsa.edu/resources/newborn/screenstatus.htm.
6. Heller AJ et al: Localization of biotinidase in the brain: implications for its role in hearing loss in biotinidase deficiency. *Hear Res* 173:62–68, 2002.
7. McVoy JR et al: Partial biotinidase deficiency: clinical and biochemical features. *J Pediatr* 116:78–83, 1990.
8. Nieto-Barrera M et al: Biotinidase deficiency. *Int Pediatr* 4:285–288, 1989.
9. Pomponio RJ: Mutational hotspot in the human biotinidase gene causes profound biotinidase deficiency. *Nat Genet* 11:96–98, 1995.
10. Schubiger G et al: Biotinidase deficiency: clinical course and biochemical findings. *J Inherit Metab Dis* 7:129–130, 1984.
11. Strausserg RE et al: Reversible deafness caused by biotinidase deficiency. *Pediatr Neurol* 23(3):269–270, 2000.
12. Suormala TM et al: Comparison of patient with complete and partial biotinidase deficiency: biochemical studies. *J Inherit Metab Dis* 13:76–92, 1990.
13. Sutherland SJ et al: Screening for biotinidase deficiency in children with unexplained neurologic or developmental abnormalities. *Clin Pediatr* 30:81–84, 1991.
14. Taitz LS et al: Long-term auditory and visual complications of biotinidase deficiency. *Early Hum Dev* 11:325–331, 1985.
15. Thoene J, Wolf B: Biotinidase deficiency in juvenile multiple carboxylase deficiency. *Lancet* 2:398, 1983.
16. Wallace SJ: Biotinidase deficiency: presymptomatic treatment. *Arch Dis Child* 60:574–575, 1985.
17. Wolf B: Disorders of biotin metabolism. In: *The Metabolic and Molecular Bases of Inherited Disease,* 8th ed. Scriver CR et al (eds), McGraw-Hill, New York, 2001, pp 3935–3964.
18. Wolf B, Feldman GL: The biotin-dependent carboxylase deficiencies. *Am J Hum Genet* 34:699–716, 1982.
19. Wolf B, Heard GS: Screening for biotinidase deficiency in newborns: worldwide experience. *Pediatrics* 85:512–517, 1990.
20. Wolf B, McVoy JS: A sensitive radioassay for biotinidase activity: deficiency activity in tissues of serum biotinidase-deficient individuals. *Clin Chim Acta* 135:275–281, 1983.
21. Wolf B et al: Biotinidase deficiency: the enzymatic defect in late-onset multiple carboxylase deficiency. *Clin Chim Acta* 131:273–281, 1983.
22. Wolf B et al: Deficient biotinidase activity in late-onset multiple carboxylase deficiency. *N Engl J Med* 308:161, 1983.
23. Wolf B et al: Phenotypic variation in biotinidase deficiency. *J Pediatr* 103:233–237, 1983.
24. Wolf B et al: Hearing loss in biotinidase deficiency. *Lancet* 2:1365–1366, 1983.
25. Wolf B et al: Biotinidase deficiency: a novel recycling defect. *J Inherit Metab Dis* 8 (Suppl 1):53–58, 1985.
26. Wolf B et al: Clinical findings in four children with biotinidase deficiency detected through a statewide neonatal screening program. *N Engl J Med* 313:16–19, 1985.
27. Wolf B et al: Biotinidase deficiency: initial clinical features and rapid diagnosis. *Ann Neurol* 18:614–617, 1985.
28. Wolf B et al: Biotinidase deficiency. *Ann NY Acad Sci* 447:252–262, 1985.

Canavan disease (*N*-acetylaspartic aciduria)

Canavan disease (OMIM 271900), a spongy degeneration of the brain, is characterized by megalencephaly, leukodystrophy, severe progressive psychomotor retardation, optic atrophy, hypotonia, and death typically by 18 months of age (1–10). It is associated with elevated *N*-acetylaspartic acid in the urine resulting from *N*-aspartoacylase deficiency and is due to mutations in the *ASPA* gene at 17pter-p13x (2).

Macrocephaly appears at about 3 months. By the end of the first year there is a general demyelinating process characterized by severe axial hypotonia with peripheral hypertonicity and hyperreflexia (1–10). Rapid onset of seizures and opisthotonic crises are characteristic. Computed tomography scan reveals demyelination. The children soon become blind and deaf and die of intercurrent illness in a vegetative state.

Inheritance is autosomal recessive (2,3,6,7). It is especially prevalent in Ashkenazi Jews from eastern Poland, Lithuania, and western Russia (10), as well as in Middle Eastern populations.

References

1. Adachi M et al: Spongy degeneration of the central nervous system (van Bogaert and Bertrand type; Canavan disease). *Hum Pathol* 4:331–347, 1973.
2. Beaudet AL: Aspartoacylase deficiency. In: *The Metabolic and Molecular Bases of Inherited Disease,* 8th ed., Scriver CR et al (eds), McGraw-Hill, New York, 2001, pp 5700–5806.
3. Divry P et al: *N*-acetylaspartic aciduria: report of three new cases in children with a neurologic syndrome associating macrocephaly and leukodystrophy. *J Inherit Metab Dis* 11:307–308, 1988.
4. Echenne B et al: Spongy degeneration of the neuraxes (Canavan–van Bogaert disease) and *N*-acetylaspartic aciduria. *Neuropaediatrics* 20:79–81, 1989.
5. Elpeleg ON et al: Canavan disease and *N*-acetylaspartic aciduria. *Neuropaediatrics* 20:238, 1989.
6. Hagenfeldt L et al: *N*-acetylaspartic aciduria due to aspartoacylase deficiency. A new aetiology of childhood leukodystrophy. *J Inherit Metab Dis* 10:135–141, 1987.
7. Kvittingen EA et al: *N*-acetylaspartic aciduria in a child with progressive cerebral atrophy. *Clin Chim Acta* 158:217–227, 1986.
8. Matalon R: Aspartocyclase deficiency and N-acetylaspartic aciduria in patients with Canavan disease. *Am J Med Genet* 29:463–471, 1988.
9. Ozand PT et al: Aspartocyclase deficiency and Canavan disease in Saudi Arabia. *Am J Med Genet* 35:266–268, 1990.
10. Ungar M, Goodman RM: Spongy degeneration of the brain in Israel. *Clin Genet* 23:23–29, 1983.

3-Methylglutaconic aciduria

3-Methylglutaconic aciduria (OMIM 250950, type I or 3-methylglutaconyl-CoA hydratase deficiency) is a metabolic error involving the amino acid leucine and is characterized by infantile progressive encephalopathy. Choreoathetosis, spastic paraparesis, dementia, seizures, optic atrophy, and sensorineural hearing loss can result (3–7,9). Onset is noted soon after birth with life-threatening metabolic acidosis. Episodes of vomiting, seizures, hypotonia, somnolence, and acidosis are precipitated by infections, large protein intake, or surgery. Sensorineural hearing loss has been reported in ~20% (3–7). 3-Methylglutaconic acid and 3-methylglutaric acid are found in increased amounts in the urine (8).

Defects in all eight enzymes involved in the degradation of leucine have been reported to result in 3-methylglutaconic aciduria. Type I involves deficiency of 3-methylglutaconyl coenzyme A hydratase, whereas the other forms have normal activity for this enzyme (Fig. 13–9). Type II or Barth syndrome is due to mutations in the *TAZ* gene (*tafazzin*) (2). Type III is due to mutations in the *OPA3* gene (1,8).

Inheritance is autosomal recessive for type I, X-linked recessive for type II or Barth syndrome (OMIM 302060), autosomal recessive for type III (OMIM 258501), and unknown for type IV (OMIM 250951).

References

1. Anikster Y et al: Type III 3-methylglutaconic aciduria (optic atrophy plus syndrome, or Costeff optic atrophy syndrome): identification of the *OPA3* gene and its founder mutation in Iraqi Jews. *Am J Hum Genet* 69:1218–1224, 2001.
2. Bione S et al: A novel X-linked gene, G4.5.(sic) is responsible for Barth syndrome. *Nat Genet* 12:385–389, 1996.

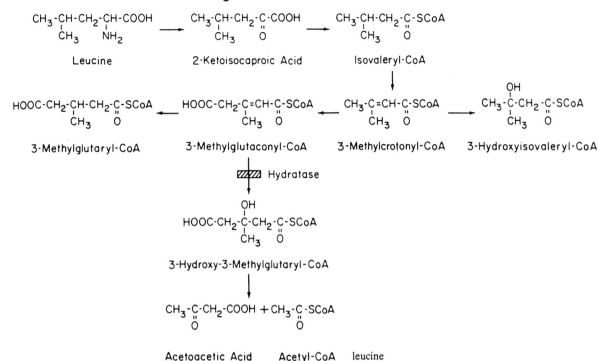

Figure 13–9. *3-Methylglutaconic aciduria.* 3-MG-CoA hydratase and its place in the catabolic pathway for leucine. [From KM Gibson, *Eur J Pediatr* 148:76, 1988.]

3. Chitayat D et al: 3-Methylglutaconic aciduria: a marker for as yet unspecified disorders and the relevance of prenatal deafness in a new type (type 4). *J Inherit Metabol Dis* 15:204–212, 1992.
4. Duran M et al: Inherited 3-methylglutaconic aciduria in two brothers—another defect of leucine metabolism. *J Pediatr* 101:551–554, 1982.
5. Gibson KM: 3-Methylglutaconic aciduria: a phenotype in which activity of 3-methylglutoconyl-coenzyme A hydratase is normal. *Eur J Pediatr* 148:76–82, 1988.
6. Gibson KM et al: Variable clinical presentation in three patients with 3-methylglutaconyl-coenzyme A hydratase deficiency. *J Inherit Metab Dis* 21:631–638, 1998.
7. Greter J et al: 3-Methylglutaconic aciduria: report in a sibship with infantile progressive encephalopathy. *Eur J Pediatr* 129:231–238, 1978.
8. Sweetman L, Williams JC: Branched chain organic acidurias. In: *The Metabolic and Molecular Bases of Inherited Disease,* 8th ed., Scriver CR et al (eds), McGraw-Hill, New York, 2001, pp 2137–2140.
9. Zeharia A et al: 3-Methylglutaconic aciduria: a new variant. *Pediatrics* 89:1080–1082, 1992.

Histidinuria

Histidinuria (OMIM 235830), without histidinemia, due to a renal tubular defect is associated with mental retardation, myoclonic seizures, a long and shallow philtrum, large and protuberant ears with simple auricles, broad nasal bridge, brachydactyly, and hypoplastic toenails.

One report associated histidinuria with bilateral sensorineural hearing loss of moderate degree (3); however, four additional individuals in three families have been reported (1,2,4) with no mention of hearing loss. All reported patients have been male.

References

1. Holmgren G et al: Histidinuria and normal-histidinemic histinuria. *Acta Paediatr Scand* 63:220, 1974.
2. Kamoun PP et al: Renal histidinuria. *J Inherit Metab Dis* 4:217–219, 1981.
3. Nyhan WL, Hilton S: Histidinuria: defective transport in histidine. *Am J Med Genet* 44:558–561, 1992.
4. Sabater J et al: Histidinuria: a renal and intestinal histidine transport deficiency found in two mentally retarded children. *Clin Genet* 9:117–124, 1976.

Other Disorders

X-linked hypophosphatemia (familial hypophosphatemic rickets or osteomalacia, vitamin D–resistant rickets or osteomalacia)

The association of impaired hearing and X-linked hypophosphatemic osteomalacia (OMIM 307800) in adolescents and adults was described by Davies et al. in 1984 (3). Other investigators confirmed the association (2,8,9,11,22).

Clinical findings. A marked reduction in renal tubular reabsorption of phosphate results in hypophosphatemia, leading to rickets in children and osteomalacia in adults with X-linked hypophosphatemia. Frequent daily supplementation of phosphate, plus treatment with vitamin D compounds substantially corrects the short stature and bowing of long bones seen in the untreated condition (5,6,13). In some adult patients, ankylosis of the spine resembling ankylosing spondylitis occurs (10) and bony overgrowth can narrow the spinal canal with resultant spinal cord compression (1). The male hemizygotes often respond more poorly to therapy than related female heterozygotes (13), evidence of gene dosage effect in the expression of this disorder.

Auditory system. In their assessment of 25 adolescent and adult patients with X-linked hypophosphatemic osteomalacia, Davies et al. (3) reported that 12 patients had subjective hearing loss and 2 had episodic tinnitus, vertigo, and deafness resembling Ménière's disease. More objective pure-tone audiometry showed 19 with sensorineural loss, 3 of whom had an additional conductive element. Differentiation of sensory (cochlear) from neural deafness by means of stapedius reflex threshold, percentage speech discrimination score, tone decay, and loudness recruitment indicated cochlear dysfunction, confirmed by Jonas et al. (8).

Generalized osteosclerosis and thickening of the petrous bone with some narrowing of the internal auditory meatus have been reported in 11 patients with X-linked hypophosphatemic osteomalacia and hearing loss (12).

In audiometry studies by Meister et al. (9) on 19 subjects with hypophosphatemic bone disease, no hearing loss or significant auditory findings were noted among children or young adult patients. However, sensorineural hearing loss was noted in the three oldest subjects (40–58 years of age), although a history of noise exposure in two of them could explain the observations. Since the hearing loss appeared to be age-dependent and was more frequent at higher frequencies (22), presbycusis could have been the explanation. These studies suggest that if an association exists between hypophosphatemic bone disease and hearing impairment, auditory signs will not develop until adulthood in treated patients.

Vestibular system. Of 19 patients with X-linked hypophosphatemic osteomalacia and documented sensorineural hearing loss, 10 had depressed caloric response in one or both ears, and two had Ménière's disease (3).

Heredity. X-linked dominant inheritance of hypophosphatemic rickets/osteomalacia is known (15–17,23). The gene has been mapped to Xp22.2–p22.1 (14) and codes for an endopeptidase referred to as PEX (for "phosphate-regulating gene with homologies to endopeptidases on the X chromosome") (7), also abbreviated PHEX (4). In 1987, Boneh et al. (2) suggested genetic heterogeneity in the human disease based on a mouse model. The initial genetic data and phenotypic differences suggested that two different mouse genes were mutated, but later cloning studies demonstrated that the mouse *Hyp* (the model for the human disease) and *Gy* are allelic mutations (19). The human equivalent of the mouse Gy mutation has not yet been definitely identified.

Differential diagnosis. Hypophosphatemia occurs as part of autosomal dominant hypophosphatemic bone disease (17) responsive to vitamin D analog treatment alone, and autosomal recessive hypophosphatemic rickets with hypercalciuria (20), responsive to phosphate therapy alone. Neither disorder has reported deafness.
Weir (21) reported two pairs of siblings with apparent autosomal recessive hypophosphatemic rickets, three of which had 50–80 dB sensorineural deafness and all of whom had marked narrowing of the internal auditory canal.
Stamp and Baker (18) noted two of three adult children of a first-cousin marriage who presented with severe rickets in infancy, resistant to treatment with vitamin D. They reported early fusion of the cranial sutures, increased bone density, nerve deafness, and lifelong hypophosphatemia unaffected by treatment.

References

1. Adams JE, Davies M: Intraspinal new bone formation and spinal cord compression in familial hypophosphataemic vitamin D resistant osteomalacia. *Q J Med* 61:1117–1129, 1986.
2. Boneh A et al: Audiometric evidence for two forms of X-linked hypophosphatemia in humans, apparent counterparts of Hyp and Gy mutations in mouse. *Am J Med Genet* 27:997–1003, 1987.
3. Davies M et al: Impaired hearing in X-linked hypophosphataemic (vitamin D–resistant) osteomalacia. *Ann Intern Med* 100:230–232, 1984.
4. Dixon PH et al: Mutational analysis of *PHEX* gene in X-linked hypophosphatemia. *J Clin Endocrinol Metab* 83:3615–3623, 1998.
5. Glorieux FH: Rickets, the continuing challenge. *N Engl J Med* 325: 1875–1877, 1991.
6. Glorieux FH et al: Use of phosphate and vitamin D to prevent dwarfism and rickets in X-linked hypophosphatemia. *N Engl J Med* 287:481–487, 1972.
7. HYP Consortium: A gene (*Hyp*) with homologies to endopeptidases is mutated in patients with X-linked hypophosphatemic rickets. *Nat Genet* 11:130–156, 1995.
8. Jonas AJ et al: Hearing deficits associated with hypophosphatemic rickets. *Pediatr Res* 20:266A, 1986.
9. Meister M et al: Audiologic findings in young patients with hypophosphatemic bone disease. *Ann Otol Rhinol Laryngol* 95:415–420, 1986.
10. Moser CR, Fessel WJ: Rheumatic manifestations of hypophosphatemia. *Arch Intern Med* 134:674–678, 1974.
11. O'Malley S et al: Electrocochleographic changes in the hearing loss associated with X-linked hypophosphatemic osteomalacia. *Acta Otolaryngol (Stockh)* 100:13–18, 1985.
12. O'Malley SP et al: The petrous temporal bones and deafness in X-linked hypophosphataemic osteomalacia. *Clin Radiol* 39:528–530, 1988.
13. Petersen DJ et al: X-linked hypophosphatemic rickets: a study (with literature review) of linear growth response to calcitriol and phosphate therapy. *J Bone Miner Res* 7:583–597, 1992.
14. Rowe PSN et al: Three DNA markers for hypophosphataemic rickets. *Hum Genet* 89:539–542, 1992.
15. Scriver CR, Tenenhouse HS: On the heritability of rickets, a common disease. *Johns Hopkins Med J* 149:179–187, 1981.
16. Scriver CR et al: X-linked hypophosphatemia: an appreciation of a classic paper and a survey of progress since 1958. *Medicine* 70:218–228, 1991.
17. Scriver CR et al: Hypophosphatemic nonrachitic bone disease: an entity distinct from X-linked hypophosphatemia in the renal defect, bone involvement, and inheritance. *Am J Med Genet* 1:101–117, 1977.
18. Stamp TB, Baker CRI: Recessive hypophosphataemic rickets and possible aetiology of the vitamin D–resistant syndrome. *Arch Dis Child* 51:360–365, 1976.
19. Strom TM et al: *Pex* gene deletions in Gy and Hyp mice provide mouse models for X-linked hypophosphatemia. *Hum Mol Genet* 6:165–171, 1997.
20. Tieder M et al: Hereditary hypophosphatemic rickets with hypercalciuria. *N Engl J Med* 312:611–617, 1985.
21. Weir N: Sensorineural deafness associated with recessive hypophosphataemic rickets. *J Laryngol Otol* 91:717–722, 1977.
22. Whyte M et al: Audiologic abnormalities are common in mice and men with sex-linked hypophosphatemic bone disease. *J Bone Mineral Res* 1:195A, 1986.
23. Winters RW et al: A genetic study of familial hypophosphatemia and vitamin D–resistant rickets with a review of the literature. *Medicine* 37:97–142, 1958.

Phosphoribosylpyrophosphate synthetase superactivity (ataxia and sensorineural hearing loss with hyperuricemia)

Phosphoribosylpyrophosphate synthetase 1 (PRPS1, OMIM 311850) catalyzes the phosphoribosylation of ribose 5-phosphate to 5-phosphoribosyl-1-pyrophosphate and is necessary for the de novo and salvage pathways of purine, pyrimidine, and pyridine biosynthesis. Rosenberg et al. (15) reported a large family in which five persons had hyperuricemia, renal failure, ataxia, and sensorineural hearing loss. Urate levels were elevated in other family members without renal insufficiency, suggesting the latter did not cause the hyperuricemia. The pedigree suggested X-linked inheritance with some females showing partial and others complete expression. Later studies have associated this disorder with overactivity of phosphoribosylpyrophosphate synthetase, resulting from resistance to nucleotide feedback inhibition (2,4,7,8,12) (Fig. 13–10A).

Clinical features. PRPS1 superactivity is expressed in two clinical phenotypes. The milder form, which presents as a late juvenile to early adult disease, is restricted to males without neurologic deficits or hearing loss, but with gout or uric acid urolithiasis (4,7). The more severe form is characterized by symptoms beginning in early childhood (the deafness sometimes begins in infancy) (16) in hemizygous males. Signs of uric acid overproduction, including gout, occur in association with impairment of neural development (ataxia, slurred speech, and proximal muscle weakness) (12,17,18), often including sensorineural hearing loss (7). Heterozygous females may develop gout during the age period of reproduction and some may develop hearing loss (3,18). Six such families have been studied, five of which had only defective down-regulation of PRPS1 from the allosteric effectors of PRPS1 activity, or this lack of normal feedback inhibition in combination with PRPS1 catalytic overactivity (3,5,7,18). The sixth family showed only isolated PRPS1 superactivity, no more severe than that seen in all the other cases associated with the later-onset phenotype without neurologic deficits (1). In addition, all families with inhibitor-resistant PRPS1 did not have neurologic disease or presentation during childhood (20). Neurologic features in the single family presented much later in childhood (15). Ataxia, slurred speech, and proximal weakness had onset in the teens or 20's for the male probands, and in the 30's for their mother. Examination showed proximal weakness and muscle wasting, hyperactive deep tendon reflexes, ataxia of gait and limbs, and mild loss of vibra-

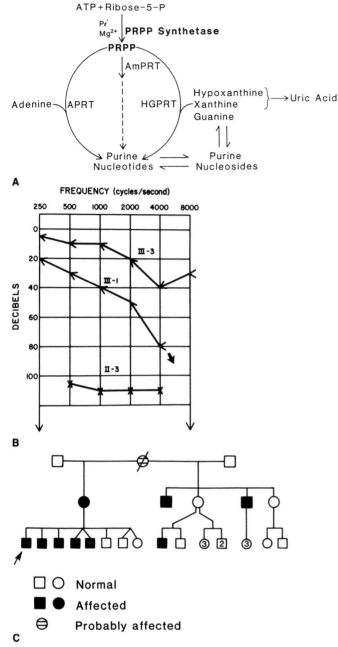

A

B

C

□ ○ **Normal**

■ ● **Affected**

⊖ **Probably affected**

Figure 13–10. *Phosphoribosylpyrophosphate synthetase superactivity (ataxia and sensorineural hearing loss with hyperuricemia).* (A) Schematic diagram of the synthesis of phosphoribosylpyrophosphate (PRPP) and the utilization of this compound in the 10-step pathway of purine synthesis de novo (dashed arrow) and in the single-step reactions of purine base salvage catalyzed by adenine phosphoribosyltransferase (APRT) and hypoxanthinephosphoribosyltransferase (HPRT). The sequence by which purines are degraded to the end product, uric acid, is also shown. Inherited superactivity of PRPP synthetase is associated with excessive rate of purine nucleotide and uric acid synthesis, presumably as a consequence of increased synthesis of the rate-limiting substrate, PRPP. ATP, adenosine triphosphate; Pi, inorganic phosphate; AmPRT, amidophosphoribosyltransferase. (B) Composite audiogram showing progression of hearing loss. III-3, age 18; III-1, age 22; II-3, age 38. (C) Pedigree of family showing X-linked recessive inheritance with partial expression in females. [(A) from MA Becker et al., *Arthritis Rheum* 29:880, 1986; (B,C) from AL Rosenberg et al., *N Engl J Med* 282:992, 1970.]

tory sensation. Motor nerve conduction studies were normal (15). Dysmorphic features may also be present, including triangular face, prominent forehead, epicanthus, and hypotelorism described in two boys (11).

Auditory system. Simmonds et al. (16) described hyperuricemia in a 3-year-old boy and his mother, both of whom had high-frequency hearing loss from infancy. The child was hypotonic and had locomotor delay. Two male siblings who died in early childhood probably had the same disorder. Biochemical evidence of PRS superactivity was presented (18). In a later-onset family reported by Rosenberg et al. (15), five boys, including twins, had hyperuricemia, ataxia, renal insufficiency, and hearing loss, and their mother also had reduced hearing. Abnormal purine metabolism and neurologic features presented in late childhood and hearing loss began in the second to fourth decades (Fig. 13–10B). Unilateral hearing loss has also been reported (12).

Vestibular system. Electronystagmograms have shown abnormalities suggesting a disturbance central to the labyrinth.

Laboratory findings. In the first two families reported, biochemical abnormalities consisted of elevated plasma and urine uric acid and urine hypoxanthine (4). Some individuals also had metabolic acidosis and intermittent hyperammonemia. The urine purine/creatinine ratio confirmed gross purine overproduction. Erythrocyte hypoxanthine-guanine phosphoribosyltransferase activities were normal. Phosphoribosylpyrophosphate (PRPP) synthetase levels in lymphoblasts were increased well above control range (18). Renal function tests, especially creatinine and insulin clearance, were usually decreased without clinical evidence of renal disease. PRPP synthetase 1 has been mapped to Xq26, just centromeric to the HPRT locus (2,9).

Heredity. Inheritance is X-linked semidominant (Fig. 13–10C), with more severe clinical and biochemical expression in hemizygous males than in heterozygous females. Genetic heterogeneity suggested by differences in phenotypic expression and mechanisms leading to excessive enzyme activity has been proven. Defects in allosteric regulation of PRPS1 are the result of point mutations in the PRPS1 gene (6). In contrast, PRPS1 catalytic superactivity results from altered regulation of the expression of the normal PRS isoform, apparently by increasing intracellular concentration of normal PRPS1 (14).

Prognosis. Some affected boys have died in infancy of pneumonia (15). Most other males have become severely disabled. The disease in affected females has later onset and is less severe than in affected males.

Differential diagnosis. Sensorineural hearing loss and ataxia can occur as autosomal dominant (13) and recessive (10) traits without hyperuricemia. Determination of plasma uric acid will differentiate the PRPS1 overactivity/hearing loss syndrome.

References

1. Becker MA: Hyperuricemia and gout. In: *The Metabolic and Molecular Bases of Inherited Disease,* 8th ed., Scriver CR et al (eds), McGraw-Hill, New York, pp 2526–2528, 2001.
2. Becker MA et al: Regional localization of the gene for human phosphoribosylpyrophosphate synthetase on the X chromosome. *Science* 203: 1016–1019, 1979.
3. Becker MA et al: Variant human phosphoribosylpyrophosphate synthetase altered in regulatory and catalytic functions. *J Clin Invest* 65:109–120, 1980.
4. Becker MA et al: Phosphoribosylpyrophosphate synthetase superactivity. A study of five patients with catalytic defects in the enzyme. *Arthritis Rheum* 29:880–888, 1986.
5. Becker MA et al: Superactivity of human phosphoribosyl pyrophosphate synthetase due to altered regulation by nucleotide inhibitors and inorganic phosphate. *Biochim Biophys Acta* 882:168–176, 1986.
6. Becker MA et al: Overexpression of the normal phosphoribosylpyrophosphate synthetase 1 isoform underlies catalytic superactivity of human phosphoribosylpyrophosphate synthetase. *J Biol Chem* 271:19894–19899, 1986.

7. Becker MA et al: Inherited superactivity of phosphoribosylpyrophosphate synthetase: association of uric acid overproduction and sensorineural deafness. *Am J Med* 85:383–390, 1988.

8. Becker MA et al: Neurodevelopmental impairment and deranged PRPP and purine nucleotide synthesis in inherited superactivity of PRPP synthetase. *Adv Exp Med Biol* 253A:15–22, 1989.

9. Becker MA et al: Cloning of cDNAs for human phosphoribosylpyrophosphate synthetases 1 and 2 and X chromosome localization of PRPS1 and PRPS2 genes. *Genomics* 8:555–561, 1990.

10. Berman W et al: A new familial syndrome with ataxia, hearing loss, and mental retardation. Report of three brothers. *Arch Neurol* 29:258–261, 1973.

11. Christen HJ et al: Distinct neurological syndrome in two brothers with hyperuricaemia. *Lancet* 340:1167–1168, 1992.

12. Mavrikakis ME et al: Gout and neurological abnormalities associated with cardiomyopathy in a young man. *Ann Rheum Dis* 49:942–943, 1990.

13. Nicolaides P et al: Cerebellar ataxia, areflexia, pes cavus, optic atrophy, and sensorineural hearing loss (CAPOS): a new syndrome. *J Med Genet* 33:419–421, 1996.

14. Roessler BJ et al: Human X-linked phosphoribosylpyrophosphate synthetase superactivity is associated with distinct point mutations in the PRPS1 gene. *J Biol Chem* 268:26476–26481, 1993.

15. Rosenberg AL et al: Hyperuricemia and neurologic deficits. A family study. *N Engl J Med* 282:992–997, 1970.

16. Simmonds HA et al: An X-linked syndrome characterized by hyperuricaemia, deafness, and neurodevelopmental abnormalities. *Lancet* 2:68–70, 1982.

17. Simmonds HA et al: Evidence of a new syndrome involving hereditary uric acid overproduction, neurological complications and deafness. *Adv Exp Med Biol* 165:97–102, 1984.

18. Simmonds HA et al: An inborn error of purine metabolism, deafness and neurodevelopmental abnormality. *Neuropediatrics* 16:106–108, 1985.

19. Sperling O et al: Altered kinetic property of erythrocyte phosphoribosylpyrophosphate synthetase in excessive purine production. *Rev Eur Etud Clin Biol* 17:703–706, 1972.

20. Sperling O et al: Human erythrocyte phosphoribosylpyrophosphate synthetase mutationally altered in regulatory properties. *Biochem Med* 7:389–395, 1973.

Appendix

Other entities with a metabolic dysfunction

For an additional entity with a metabolic dysfunction, see Congenital cataracts, hypercholesterolemia, spasticity of lower limbs, and sensorineural hearing loss, in Chapter 7.

Chapter 14
Genetic Hearing Loss Associated with Integumentary Disorders
HELGA V. TORIELLO

Some syndromes associated with integumentary disorders are extremely rare, having been recorded in only a few families, while others are relatively common. For example, Waardenburg syndrome, the best known of this group of over 55 disorders, is present in at least 2%–5% of those affected with congenital hearing loss.

Waardenburg syndrome

The most characteristic features of Waardenburg syndrome (WS) are widely spaced medial canthi (dystopia canthorum), broad nasal root, and confluent eyebrows (synophrys). Patients frequently have variably colored irides as well as a white forelock. Although certain aspects of this disorder were described by Hammerschlag (42) in 1905, van der Hoeve (118) in 1916, and Mende (77) in 1926, the syndrome was first well defined by Waardenburg in 1948 (121,122). Waardenburg (122) estimated that 1.4% of those with profound hearing loss in The Netherlands had this syndrome. DiGeorge et al. (24) suggested that about 2.3% of those with congenital hearing loss have Waardenburg syndrome. It is possible that the actual frequency is twice this estimate, since only about 50% have ocular and/or pigmentation anomalies. Waardenburg syndrome has been divided into four types, depending on the phenotype and presence of additional features. Types I and II (4,39,40) are distinguished from each other by the presence of dystopia canthorum (type I) or its absence (type II). In addition, the frequency of sensorineural hearing loss is higher in type I than in type II. Type III is characterized by the presence of limb defects and is also referred to as Klein-Waardenburg syndrome. It was first described by Klein in 1950 (64) in a female patient with primary telecanthus, synophrys, partial albinism of skin and hair, and blue irides. However, she also had osseous dysplasia, aplasia of the first two ribs and carpal bones, and cystic alteration of the sacrum. She exhibited cutaneous union of the thorax and upper arm as well as syndactyly (Fig. 14–1L). Other somewhat similarly affected patients have been described (33,75,83,105,108,110,123) and, based on the presence of this condition in three members of one family and three generations in another, autosomal dominant inheritance was postulated (65,108,110). Shah et al. (109) described what they considered another possible variant of Waardenburg syndrome, which included pigmentary anomalies of hair, eye, and skin as well as Hirschsprung disease in the phenotype. They suggested this was a new autosomal recessive variant of the Waardenburg syndrome. This has become known as the Shah-Waardenburg syndrome, or WS4. Similar cases (i.e., affected sibs with normal consanguineous parents) have been described by others (1,14,26,66,68,72,76,124). Hearing loss appears to be rare in WS4.

Type I is 1.5–2 times more common than type II (18,40) (Table 14–1), and both are more common than types III and IV. At least 1600 cases have been reported (18).

Craniofacial findings. The facial findings in individuals with Waardenburg syndrome type I (WS1) and type III (WS3) are similar, with one common manifestation being laterally displaced medial canthi (dystopia canthorum), which produce an appearance of widely spaced eyes, although the interpupillary distance is usually within normal limits (110). The maximal normal inner canthal distance in children up to 16 years of age is 34 mm; in adult women, 37 mm; in adult

men, 39 mm (24,100). About 85% of patients with WS1 have inner canthal distances exceeding these measurements. True ocular hypertelorism occurs in only approximately 10% (93), and 50%–75% have thick eyebrows that tend to be confluent (synophrys) (18,21). This characteristic may be less evident in women because they tend to pluck glabellar hairs.

The nasal root is high and broad in most cases, whereas the nasal alar cartilages are hypoplastic to some degree. A somewhat smooth nasolabial philtrum is present in almost 50% of patients (18,21); cleft lip/palate and facial asymmetry are found in about 3% (23,32,35,122) (Fig. 14–1A–D). Extensive craniofacial anthropometric studies were carried out in WS1 by da Silva et al. (19). Head circumference, clivus length, and facial depth were smaller than in controls. The nose was narrow, the nasal bone was hypoplastic, and the philtrum was short. The maxilla was short and retropositioned.

In Waardenburg syndrome type II (WS2), dystopia canthorum is almost never present (although see 104) and the frequencies of synophrys and broad nasal root are lower (6%–23% and 29%, respectively) (70). However, pigmentary disturbances of the iris are more common, occurring in 42% (70) (Fig. 14–1E–H).

An interesting family was described by Pierpont et al. (98). Two of the individuals had phenotypes that were consistent with WS1, in that dystopia canthorum was present (in addition, the proband had cleft lip/palate). However, the maternal great-uncle had white forelock and iris pigmentary anomalies only. Linkage analysis did not demonstrate linkage to *PAX3*, thus ruling out WS1 as the condition in this family. It may therefore be possible to have dystopia canthorum occur in rare individuals with WS2.

Integumentary system. In both Waardenburg syndromes types I and II, white forelock (poliosis), originating at the hairline in the middle of the forehead and continuing posteriorly, is found in 20%–40%, varying from the width of only a few hairs to a large white forelock. In females, poliosis may not be evident as a result of dyeing of hair. Premature graying of hair, eyebrows, and eyelashes has been noted in several kindreds (24,122). The frequency has ranged from 10% to 35% (18,23,40). A black forelock has been reported in types I and II (3,23) (Fig. 14–1I).

In about 15%–20%, skin pigmentary changes ranging from small piebald areas to depigmentation with patchy areas of pigmentation have been observed (18,23). In several patients (26), the arms and face showed a patchy or freckled hyperpigmentation. Several African-American patients described by DiGeorge et al. (24) showed large areas of vitiligo.

Gastrointestinal system. Hirschsprung disease, a disorder of intestinal motility characterized by absence of parasympathetic plexuses of the gut, is an associated feature of WS4. However, Hirschsprung disease has also been reported in both WS1 (1,8,14,26,90,101,109) and WS2 (17,30,61,72,76).

Musculoskeletal system. Skeletal anomalies occur in WS3, and usually affect the upper limbs. Most common are hypoplastic arms with decreased muscle mass and camptodactyly (110). Winging of the scapulae (Sprengel shoulder) also occurs (23,93). A few indivuals have had more severe limb defects, but the genetic basis of their Waardenburg

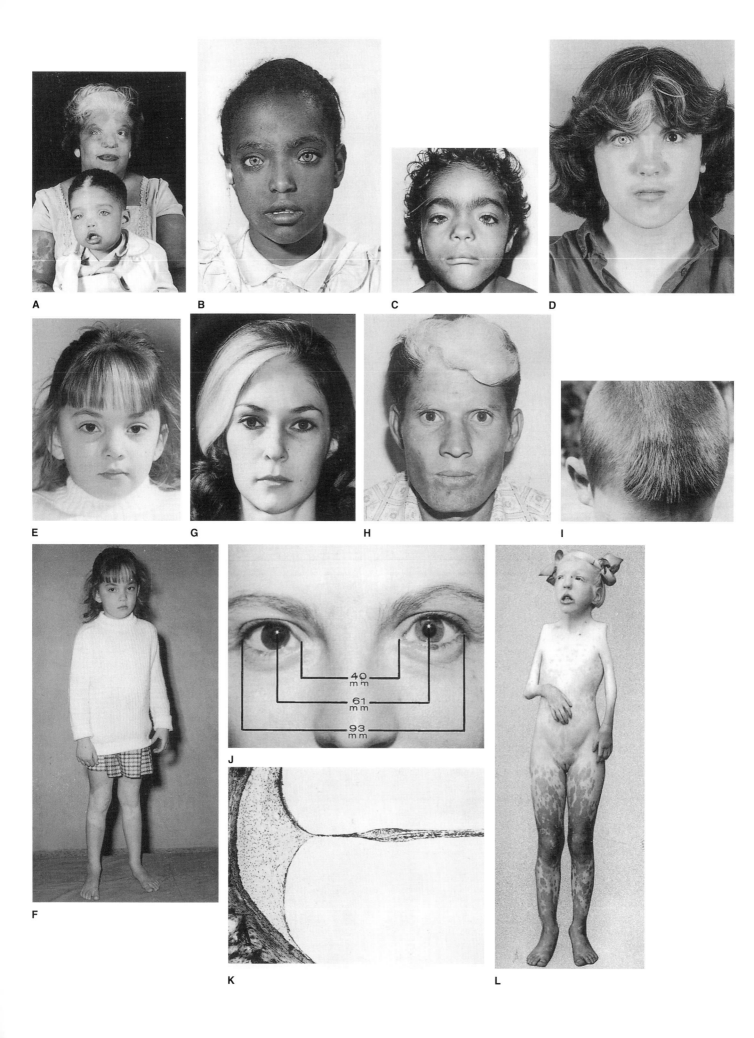

A B C D

E G H I

F J K L

Table 14–1. Waardenburg syndrome

	Type I (with dystopia) %	Type II (without dystopia) %
Dystopia canthorum	100	0
High broad nasal root	90	30
Synophrys	85	25
Heterochromia irides	35	30
Hypoplastic blue irides	10	15
Hypopigmented ocular fundi	25	?
White forelock	30	40
Early graying	20	5
Partial albinism	20	15
Hearing loss, bilateral	20	55
Hearing loss, unilateral	15	5
Hypoplastic nasal alae	50	0
Smooth nasolabial frenum	40	0

Adapted from MJ Hageman and JW Delleman, *Am J Hum Genet* 29:468, 1977; EO da Silva, *Am J Med Genet* 40:65, 1991.

syndrome is different from that in those with a more typical WS3 (see Heredity section). These were thought to represent examples of contiguous gene deletion (63,95,96).

Ocular system. Iridal pigmentary changes are common, and various terms have been used to describe these changes. The term *heterochromia* refers to eyes of different colors (e.g., one blue, one brown), whereas *segmental heterochromia* or *bicolor irides* refers to segments of different colors within the same eye. *Hypoplastic irides* describe the brilliant blue eyes found in some. Iridal pigmentary changes occur in fewer than 20% of those with WS1 but in over 40% of those with WS2 (69). Those with WS3 can also have isochromia irides (light brown irides with a mosaic pattern) (109). Liang et al. (68) have suggested that those with WS3 are more likely to have bicolor irides (Fig. 14–1J). The ocular pigmentary findings in this condition may be a function of the underlying molecular defect (see Heredity). Norkl et al. (89) presented evidence that the pigmentation pattern in the dark eye was abnormal, contrary to previous belief that the light (or blue) eye was abnormal and the dark eye was normal (21). They found that the pigment is limited to the anterior border layer of the iris, thus producing a monotonous color and texture.

Fundus pigmentation may vary as much as iris pigmentation in this disorder. A relationship between the pigmentation pattern of the iris and that of the fundus has been found (32,89). In all cases in which a blue iris was present, the corresponding fundus was blond or albinoid. In patients having a brown iris, the fundus was normal with brunette coloration. The fundus corresponding to bicolored irides was mottled, the

←

Figure 14–1. *Waardenburg syndrome, type I.* (A) Mother and son exhibiting white forelock; mother displays heterochromia irides; son has blue irides. Eyes appear widely spaced. Mother has widespread piebaldism. (B) Note that white forelock is absent but medial portion of eyebrows is white. Irides are bilaterally blue in this profoundly deaf girl. (C) Note marked synophrys. (D) Girl with white forelock. (E–H) *Waardenburg syndrome, type II.* Note normal eyes and white forelock and piebald legs of girl. (I) Black forelock in Waardenburg syndrome, type I. (J) Note heterochromia irides, increased inner canthal distance but normal interpupillary and outer canthal distances; patient plucks glabellar hairs. (K) Section of cochlea showing absence of organ of Corti. (L) *Klein-Waardenburg syndrome.* Affected female shows hypoplasia of shoulder girdle due to contiguous gene deletion. [(A) from V Penchaszadeh and F Char, *Birth Defects* 7(4):129, 1971; (B) from AM DiGeorge et al., *J Pediatr* 57:649, 1960; (C) courtesy of EO da Silva, Pernambuco, Brazil; (D) courtesy of MJ Hageman, Haarlem, The Netherlands; (H,I) from S Arias, *Birth Defects* 7(4):87,1971; (K) from L Fisch, *J Laryngol Otol* 73:355, 1959; (L) from D Klein, *Helv Paediatr Acta* 5:38, 1950.]

pigment sector of the iris corresponding to that of the fundus. Visual acuity was normal in all cases, although the frequency of amblyopia and strabismus is higher than in a normal population (19). Glaucoma has been reported in a few patients (38,57,89) and congenital cataracts in one (84). Ocular albinism has also been described in a few individuals (11,82) (but see Heredity).

In type I, the inferior lacrimal points are displaced laterally, in most cases as far as the cornea. There is an increased susceptibility to dacryocystitis (86,125).

Neurologic system. One child with WS4 had a hypomyelinating neuropathy in addition to WS4 (52); three other children have been described with a peripheral and autonomic neuropathy in addition to WS4 (116). All of these children had mutations of *SOX10*, and it was postulated that the nature of the mutation was responsible for the variant phenotype.

Other findings. There have been occasional case reports of spina bifida/meningomyelocele (16,18,47,93), mental retardation and electroencephalographic (EEG) abnormalities (15), severe mental retardation and peripheral neuropathy (60), cerebellar infarction (86), Dandy-Walker malformation (120), atrial septal defect (10), multicystic dysplastic kidney (54), absent vagina (34), and pituitary tumor (62). The significance of these findings is unknown but some may well be coincidental (but see above).

Auditory system. Hageman and Delleman (40) reported the frequency of hearing loss to be 36% and 57% in WS1 and WS2, respectively; more recent reports have suggested that the frequency of hearing loss in WS1 is 58%–75% and in WS2, 78%–91% (70,88,92). The extent of loss is quite variable, ranging from no measurable clinical loss to severe congenital unilateral or bilateral sensorineural loss (28,39, 45,88). Bilateral loss is more common (88).

Audiogram shapes vary, in that some individuals have unilateral or bilateral residual hearing at lower frequencies; some have uniform hearing loss in the lower and middle frequencies, but with some improvement in the higher tones; yet others have a U-shaped audiogram with hearing loss more severe between 1000 and 4000 Hz (28,88,91). The hearing loss in type 2 has been found to be progressive in 70% (45). Oysu et al. (91) recommended using distortion-product otoacoustic emissions (DPOAEs) to investigate hearing in children with Waardenburg syndrome.

Vestibular system. Although some authors (12,20,125) described vestibular findings in Waardenburg syndrome, the most complete surveys of vestibular function were done by Marcus (73), Hageman (39,41), and Black et al. (13), who evaluated 22, 25, and 20 patients, respectively. Marcus (73) found that 21 of 22 individuals had vestibular function abnormalities, some of whom had normal hearing. Rotation or caloric testing showed variable vestibular response in one or both ears. Of four children with mild to moderate sensorineural hearing loss, a vestibular function abnormality was found in rotation testing, in caloric testing, or in both. Sometimes only one side showed vestibular abnormalities. Six members of the family had no response to the vestibular function test, whereas one had completely normal function except for slightly reduced response to cold caloric stimulation. Hageman (39) found that of his 25 patients, 5 had significant caloric asymmetry and hearing loss; 6 had pathologic positional nystagmus but with hearing loss only in 2; and 2 had optokinetic asymmetry with normal hearing in both. Black et al. (13) did extensive testing in their subjects and found vestibular symptoms in 18 of 20. The most common symptoms reported included dizziness, tinnitus, disequilibrium, vertigo, and aural pressure. The authors felt the clinical pattern was consistent with secondary endolymphatic hydrops, which was supported by the fact that symptoms were often provoked by dietary fluid and electrolyte changes, hormonal fluctuations, and changes in barometric pressure.

Although most tomographic studies of the inner ear have shown normal findings (31,43,74,87), a few investigators (44,55,58,73) have found abnormal development of semicircular canals, especially in type 2.

Laboratory findings. Tomograms on two patients described by Marcus and Valvassori (74) showed hypoplasia of the cochlea and of the superior and horizontal semicircular canal walls as well as complete absence of the posterior semicircular canal. Galich (31), however, did not find any such abnormalities. Oysu et al. (92) reviewed the literature and found that regardless of the type of Waardenburg syndrome, only 17% had a radiological abnormality of the inner ear, usually involving the semicircular canal; in only 3 of 36 studied was a cochlear abnormality found.

Pathology. The inner ear pathology has been described only in a few children, one presumed with WS1 (28) and two with WS4 (85,101,112). Merchant et al. (78) provided a detailed description of otopathologic findings in an adult with WS1. In the child with WS1, the organ of Corti was found to be absent in all coils. The stria vascularis and cochlear neurons were atrophic. (Fig. 14–1K). In the adult, Merchant et al. (78) demonstrated a correlation between degree of hearing loss and absence of melanocytes and hair cells. They suggested that the hearing loss in WS1 is the result of abnormal migration of melanocytes, which in turn leads to abnormal development of the stria vascularis and other cochlear structures. The two children with WS4 had atrophy of the organ of Corti, stria vascularis, and saccular macula; one also had diminished cells in the cochlear spiral ganglion and degeneration of vestibular sense organs. Evidence of massive hemorrhage in the perilymphatic and endolymphatic fluid spaces at the hook portion of the cochlea was present in the other child with WS4. Similar findings have been observed in white cats, dogs, horses, mice, mink, and other laboratory animals (5,22,46,49,51), although the pathogenesis may be somewhat different in the various species.

Heredity. A variation in the *Hup2* gene, the human homologue of the mouse *Pax-3* (a mutation that causes *Splotch*), was found in a family with WS type 2 (9,25,29). WSI therefore is caused by mutations in the *PAX3* gene, which maps to 2q35 (9,27,53,81,113,114). This syndrome exhibits autosomal dominant transmission with striking variation in the degree of expressivity of the various components (99). The mutant gene appears to affect the neural crest from which the melanocytes and ganglionic primordia are derived (6,9,29,37,53,63,80,103). However, mice with Splotch mutations have normal hearing (111). WS2 is heterogeneous, with genes at four or more loci, although this too appears to be an autosomal dominant trait. The microphthalmia-associated transcription factor (*MITF*), which maps to 3p14.1–p12.3, is the cause of approximately 10% of WS2 cases (50,102). Recently, homozygous deletions in *SLUG* (*SNAI2*), which maps to 8q11, were described in two individuals considered to have WS2 (106). In addition, there are other, as yet unidentified, genes that map to 1p21–p13.3 (67) or 8p23 (107). It is also unknown whether there are still other loci responsible for the WS2 phenotype. Van Camp et al. (117) described an individual with WS2 and Hirschsprung disease in which an interstitial deletion of 13q occurred. Some of the individuals who also have ocular albinism have in addition to the *MITF* mutation homozygosity or heterozygosity for a polymorphism in the *TYR* gene, which in turn leads to reduced tyrosinase activity (82).

WS3 is also caused by *PAX3* mutation (79). Some individuals with a WS3 phenotype have also been found to have small deletions of 2q35–36, thus the WS3 phenotype was originally considered to be part of a contiguous gene deletion syndrome (95,96). However, there have also been reports of individuals with WS3 having very small deletions in one copy of the *PAX3* gene (115) or point mutations (48), thus the situation is more complex than previously realized, and the phenotype may be dependent on modifying genes at other loci (7). There has also been a description of an individual with a severe WS3 phenotype in whom the cause was homozygosity for *PAX3* (127).

WS4 is also heterogeneous and is caused by homozygosity for *EDN3* or *EDNRB* mutations or heterozygosity for *SOX10*. WS4 can therefore be inherited as either an autosomal recessive or autosomal dominant trait, depending on the molecular basis for the phenotype (102). See Table 14–2.

Diagnosis. Several individuals or families with either variant forms of Waardenburg syndrome or similar conditions have been reported. These include two families who likely had piebaldism with associated Hirschsprung disease (59,71); a family with white forelock, premature graying, defective neutrophil mobility, and sensorineural hearing loss in an autosomal dominant pattern (43); a black male with hypopigmentation, hearing loss, cataracts, small head size, hypogonadism, restricted joint motility, and osteosarcoma (94); and sibs with congenital sensorineural hearing loss, mental retardation, and hyperkeratosis of the palms and soles with possible autosomal recessive inheritance (2).

Dystopia canthorum and hypertelorism may be seen in a variety of conditions (97). Synophrys is a feature of de Lange syndrome and may also occur with pilonidal cyst (36). Poliosis, vitiligo, and dysacousia may be seen in combination with alopecia, uveitis, and meningoencephalitis in the Vogt-Koyanagi-Harada syndrome (56). Heterochromia irides may be acquired, may be inherited as an autosomal dominant trait, or may be associated with Romberg syndrome (28). Cases of heterochromia in combination with congenital hearing loss but without blepharophimosis have been reviewed (18). One must exclude dominant piebaldism and sensorineural hearing loss. Piebaldism may occur with Hirschsprung disease without Waardenburg syndrome (69). The ABCD (*A*lbinism, *B*lack lock, *C*ell migration disorder of the gut, and *D*eafness) syndrome is similar to WS4 and has been shown to be caused by mutations in the *EDNRB* gene (119).

Prognosis. The hearing loss may be progressive, at least in WS2 (45).

Summary. Waardenburg syndrome is actually a heterogeneous group of conditions caused by mutations in related genes. WS1 is the most common and is characterized by a typical facial appearance, sensorineural hearing loss, and pigmentary changes of the skin, hair, and irides. WS3 is similar to WS1 with the additional manifestation of upper limb defects. WS2 has few, if any, facial manifestations, but does include more frequent pigmentary changes and hearing loss. WS4 is associated with Hirschsprung disease. WS1, WS2, and WS3 are autosomal dominant conditions, whereas WS4 can occur as an autosomal dominant or autosomal recessive trait.

References

1. Ambani LM: Waardenburg and Hirschsprung syndromes. *J Pediatr* 102:802, 1983.
2. Amini-Elihou S: Une famille Suisse atteinte du syndrome de Klein-Waardenburg associé à une hyperkératose palmo-plantaire et à une oligophrénie grave. *J Génét Hum* 18:307–363, 1970.

Table 14–2. Molecular basis for Waardenburg syndrome phenotypes and related conditions

Condition	Causative genes	Other conditions caused by gene	Mode of inheritance
WS1	*PAX3*	Craniofacial-deafness-hand (Sommer) syndrome, WS3	Autosomal dominant
WS2	*MITF*	Tietz albinism-deafness	Autosomal dominant
WS2	*SLUG*		Autosomal recessive
WS2	Other, unidentified		
WS3	*PAX3*		Autosomal dominant
WS4	*EDNRB*	Hirschsprung disease	Autosomal recessive
WS4	*SOX10*	Yemenite deaf-blind syndrome	Autosomal dominant

3. Arias S: Genetic heterogeneity in the Waardenburg syndrome. *Birth Defects* 7(4):87–101, 1971.

4. Arias S: Letter to the editor. Waardenburg syndrome: two distinct types. *Am J Med Genet* 6:99–100, 1981.

5. Asher JH Jr et al: Mouse and hamster mutants as models for Waardenburg syndrome in humans. *J Med Genet* 27:618–626, 1990.

6. Asher JH Jr et al: Waardenburg syndrome (WS): the analysis of a single family with a WSI mutation showing linkage to RFLP markers on human chromosome 2q. *Am J Hum Genet* 48:43–52, 1991.

7. Asher JH Jr et al: Effects of *PAX3* modifier genes on craniofacial morphology, pigmentation, and viability: a murine model of Waardenburg syndrome variation. *Genomics* 34:285–298, 1996.

8. Badner JA, Chakravarti A: Waardenburg syndrome and Hirschsprung disease: evidence for pleiotropic effects of a single dominant gene. *Am J Med Genet* 35:100–104, 1990.

9. Baldwin CT et al: An exonic mutation in the *HuP2* paired domain gene causes Waardenburg's syndrome. *Nature* 355:637–638, 1992.

10. Banerjee AK: Waardenburg's syndrome associated with ostium secundum atrial septal defect. *J R Soc Med* 79:677–678, 1986.

11. Bard LA: Heterogeneity and Waardenburg's syndrome. *Arch Ophthalmol* 96:1193–1198, 1978.

12. Bellotto R et al: Cochleo-vestibular features in Waardenburg's syndrome. *Adv Audiol* 3:75–83, 1985.

13. Black FO et al: A vestibular phenotype for Waardenburg syndrome? *Otol Neurotol* 22:188–194, 2001.

14. Branski D et al: Hirschsprung's disease and Waardenburg's syndrome. *Pediatrics* 63:803–805, 1979.

15. Cantani A et al: Mental retardation and EEG abnormalities in Waardenburg's syndrome: two case reports (EEG anomalies in Waardenburg's syndrome). *Pädiatr Pädol* 24:137–140, 1989.

16. Carezani-Gavin M et al: Waardenburg syndrome associated with meningomyelocele. *Am J Med Genet* 42:135–136, 1992.

17. Currie ABM, Boddy SAM: Associated developmental abnormalities of the anterior end of the neural crest: Hirschsprung's disease–Waardenburg's syndrome. *J Pediatr Surg* 21:248–250, 1986.

18. da Silva EO: Waardenburg I syndrome: a clinical and genetic study of two large Brazilian kindreds, and literature review. *Am J Med Genet* 40:65–74, 1991.

19. da Silva EO et al: Craniofacial anthropometric studies in Waardenburg syndrome type I. *Clin Genet* 44:20–25, 1993.

20. DeHaas EBH, Tan KE: Waardenburg's syndrome. *Doc Ophthalmol* 21:239–282, 1966.

21. Delleman JW, Hageman MJ: Ophthalmological findings in 34 patients with Waardenburg's syndrome. *J Pediatr Ophthalmol* 15:341–345, 1978.

22. Deol MS: Inherited diseases of the inner ear in light of studies in the mouse. *J Med Genet* 5:137–157, 1968.

23. De Saxe M et al: Waardenburg's syndrome in South Africa. *S Afr Med J* 66:256–261, 1984.

24. DiGeorge AM et al: Waardenburg's syndrome. *J Pediatr* 57:649–669, 1960.

25. Epstein DJ et al: *Splotch* (*Sp2H*), a mutation affecting development of the mouse neural tube, shows a deletion within the paired homeodomain of Pax-3. *Cell* 67:767–774, 1991.

26. Farndon PA, Bianchi A: Waardenburg's syndrome associated with total aganglionosis. *Arch Dis Child* 58:932–933, 1983.

27. Farrer LA et al: Waardenburg syndrome (WS) type I is caused by defects at multiple loci, one of which is near ALPP on chromosome 2. *Am J Med Genet* 50:902–913, 1992.

28. Fisch L: Deafness as part of anhereditary syndrome. *J Laryngol Otol* 73:355–383, 1959.

29. Foy C et al: Assignment of the locus for Waardenburg syndrome type I to human chromosome 2q37 and possible homology to the Splotch mouse. *Am J Hum Genet* 46:1017–1023, 1990.

30. Fried K, Beer S: Waardenburg's syndrome and Hirschsprung's disease in the same patient. *Clin Genet* 18:91–92, 1980.

31. Galich R: Temporal bone involvement in Waardenburg's syndrome. *Ear Nose Throat J* 64:441–445, 1985.

32. Goldberg MF: Waardenburg's syndrome with fundus and other anomalies. *Arch Ophthalmol* 76:797–810, 1966.

33. Goodman RM et al: Upper limb involvement in the Klein-Waardenburg syndrome: evidence for further genetic heterogeneity. *Am J Med Genet* 11:425–433, 1982.

34. Goodman RM et al: Absence of the vagina and right sided adnexa uteri in the Waardenburg syndrome: a possible clue to the embryological defect. *J Med Genet* 25:355–357, 1988.

35. Gorlin RJ: Facial clefting and its syndromes. *Birth Defects* 7(7):3–49, 1971.

36. Gorlin RJ et al: *Syndromes of the Head and Neck,* 3rd ed. Oxford University Press, New York, 1990.

37. Grundfast KM, San Augustin TB: Finding the gene(s) for Waardenburg syndrome(s). *Otolaryng Clin North Am* 25:935–952, 1992.

38. Gupta V, Aggarwal HC: Open anle glaucoma as a manifestation of Waardenburg's syndrome. *Indian J Ophthalmol* 48:49–50, 2000.

39. Hageman MJ: Audiometric findings in 34 patients with Waardenburg's syndrome. *J Laryngol Otol* 91:575–584, 1977.

40. Hageman MJ, Delleman JW: Heterogeneity in Waardenburg syndrome. *Am J Hum Genet* 29:468–485, 1977.

41. Hageman MF, Oosterveld WJ: Vestibular findings in 25 patients with Waardenburg's syndrome. *Arch Otolaryngol* 103:648–652, 1977.

42. Hammerschlag V: Demonstration eines congenitalen taubstummen Jungen mit hell-blauen Augen, weissem Haarstreifen und rotatorischem Nystagmus. *Monatsschr Ohrenheilkd* 39:554–555, 1905.

43. Hayward AR et al: Defect of neutrophil mobility with dominant inheritance in a family with Waardenburg's syndrome. *Arch Dis Child* 56:279–282, 1981.

44. Higashi K et al: Aplasia of posterior semicircular canal in Waardenburg syndrome type II. *J Otolaryngol* 21:262–264, 1992.

45. Hildesheimer M et al: Auditory and vestibular findings in Waardenburg's type II syndrome. *J Laryngol Otol* 103:1130–1133, 1989.

46. Hilding DA et al: Deaf white mink: electron microscopic study of the inner ear. *Ann Otol* 76:647–663, 1967.

47. Hol FA et al: A frameshift mutation in the gene for *PAX3* in a girl with spina bifida and mild signs of Waardenburg syndrome. *J Med Genet* 32:52–56, 1995.

48. Hoth CF et al: Mutations in the paired domain of the human *PAX3* gene cause Klein-Waardenburg syndrome (WS-III) as well as Waardenburg syndrome type I (WS-I). *Am J Hum Genet* 52:455–462, 1993.

49. Hudson WR, Ruben RJ: Hereditary deafness in the Dalmatian dog. *Arch Otolaryng* 75:213–219, 1962.

50. Hughes AE et al: A gene for Waardenburg syndrome type 2 maps close to the human homologue of the microphthalmia gene at chromosome 3p12–p14.1. *Nat Genet* 7:509–512, 1994.

51. Inoue K et al: Congenital hypomyelinating neuropathy, central dysmyelination, and Waardenburg-Hirschsprung disease: phenotypes linked by *SOX10* mutation. *Ann Neurol* 52:836–842, 2002.

52. Innes JRM, Saunders LZ: Diseases of the central nervous system of domesticated animals and comparisons with human neuropathology. *Adv Vet Sci* 3:33–196, 1957.

53. Ishikiriyama S: Gene for Waardenburg syndrome type 1 is located at 2q35, not at 2q37.3. *Am J Med Genet* 46:608, 1993.

54. Jankauskiene A et al: Multicystic dysplastic kidney associated with Waardenburg syndrome type 1. *Pediatr Nephrol* 11:744–745, 1997.

55. Jensen J: Tomography of inner ear in case of Waardenburg's syndrome. *AJR Am J Roentgenol* 101:828–833, 1967.

56. Johnson WC: Vogt-Koyanagi-Harada syndrome. *Arch Dermatol* 88:146–149, 1963.

57. Kadoi C et al: Branch retinal vein occlusion in a patient with Waardenburg syndrome. *Ophthalmologica* 210:354–357, 1996.

58. Kanzaki J et al: Vestibular function and radiological findings in Waardenburg's syndrome. *Pract Otorhinolaryngol (Basel)* 64:1439–1444, 1971.

59. Kaplan P, de Chaderevian JP: Piebaldism-Waardenburg syndrome: histopathologic evidence for a neural crest syndrome. *Am J Med Genet* 31:679–688, 1988.

60. Kawabata E et al: Waardenburg syndrome: a variant with neurological involvement. *Ophthalmic Paediatr Genet* 8:165–170, 1987.

61. Kelley RI, Zackai EH: Congenital deafness, Hirschsprung's and Waardenburg's syndrome. *Am J Med Genet* 33:65A, 1981.

62. Kimura H et al: Waardenburg's syndrome and pituitary tumor. *Acta Ophthalmol* 72:642–644, 1994.

63. Kirkpatrick SJ et al: Waardenburg syndrome type 1 in a child with deletion (2)(q35q36.2). *Am J Med Genet* 44:699–700, 1992.

64. Klein D: Albinisme partiel (leucisme) avec surdí-mutité, blépharophimosis et dysplasie myo-ostéo-articulaire. *Helv Paediatr Acta* 5:38–58, 1950.

65. Klein D: Historical background and evidence for dominant inheritance of the Klein-Waardenburg syndrome (type III). *Am J Med Genet* 14:231–239, 1980.

66. Kuolkarni ML et al: Genetic heterogeneity in Waardenburg's syndrome. *J Med Genet* 26:411–412, 1989.

67. Lalwani AK et al: A locus for Waardenburg syndrome type II maps to chromosome 1p13.3–2.1. *Am J Hum Genet* 55(suppl):A14, 1994

68. Liang JC et al: Bilateral bicolored irides with Hirschsprung disease. *Arch Ophthalmol* 101:69–73, 1983.

69. Liu XZ et al: Hearing loss and pigmentary disturbances in Waardenburg syndrome with reference to WS type II. *J Laryngol Otol* 109:96–100, 1995.

70. Liu XZ et al: Waardenburg syndrome type II: phenotypic findings and diagnostic criteria. *Am J Med Genet* 55:95–100, 1995.

71. Mahakrishnan A, Srinivasan MS: Piebaldness with Hirschsprung's disease. *Arch Dermatol* 116:1102, 1980.

72. Mallory SB et al: Waardenburg's syndrome with Hirschsprung's disease: a neural crest defect. *Pediatr Dermatol* 3:119–124, 1986.

73. Marcus RE: Vestibular function and additional findings in Waardenburg's syndrome. *Acta Otolaryngol (Stockh) Suppl* 229:5–30, 1968.

74. Marcus RE, Valvassori G: Cochleovestibular apparatus: radiologic studies in hereditary and familial hearing loss. *Int Audiol* 9:95–102, 1970.

75. Marx P, Bertrand J: Une cas de syndrome de Waardenburg-Klein. *Bull Soc Ophtalmol Fr* 68:444–447, 1968.

76. Meire F et al: Waardenburg syndrome. Hirschsprung megacolon and Marcus Gunn ptosis. *Am J Med Genet* 27:683–686, 1987.

77. Mende I: Über eine Familiehereditär-degenerativer Taubstummheit mit mongoloidem Einschlag und teilweisen Leukismus der Haut und Haare. *Arch Kinderheilkd* 79:214–222, 1926.

78. Merchant SN et al: Otopathology in a case of type I Waardenburg's syndrome. *Ann Otol Rhinol Laryngol* 110:875–882, 2001.

79. Milunsky A et al: A mutation in the Waardenburg syndrome (WS-I) gene in a family with WS-III. *Am J Hum Genet Suppl* 51:A222, 1992 (same cases as in ref. 80).

80. Moase CE, Trasler DG: Splotch locus mouse mutants: models for neural tube defects and Waardenburg syndrome type I in humans. *J Med Genet* 29:145–151, 1992.

81. Morrell R et al: A plus-one frameshift mutation in *PAX3* alters the entire deduced amino-acid sequence of the paired box in a Waardenburg syndrome type I (WSI) family. *Hum Mol Genet* 2:1487–1488, 1993.

82. Morrell R et al: Apparent digenic inheritance of Waardenburg syndrome type 2 (WS2) and autosomal recessive ocular albinism (AROA). *Hum Mol Genet* 6:659–664, 1997.

83. Mossallam J et al: Waardenburg's syndrome in Egypt. *Ain Shams Med J* 25:43–48, 1974.

84. Mullaney PB et al: Clinical and morphological features of Waardenburg syndrome type II. *Eye* 12:353–357, 1998.

85. Nakashima S et al: Temporal bone histopathologic findings of Waardenburg's syndrome. *Laryngoscope* 102:563–567, 1992.

86. Narod SA et al: Cerebellar infarction in a patient with Waardenburg syndrome. *Am J Med Genet* 31:903–907, 1988.

87. Nemansky J, Hageman MJ: Tomographic findings in Waardenburg's syndrome. *AJR Am J Roentgenol* 124:250–255, 1975.

88. Newton V: Hearing loss and Waardenburg's syndrome: implication for genetic counselling. *J Laryngol Otol* 104:97–103, 1990.

89. Norkl TM et al: Pigment distribution in Waardenburg's syndrome: a new hypothesis. *Graefes Arch Klin Exp Ophthalmol* 224:487–492, 1986.

90. Omenn GS, McKusick VA: The association of Waardenburg syndrome and Hirschsprung megacolon. *Am J Med Genet* 3:217–223, 1979.

91. Oysu C et al: Audiometric manifestations of Waardenburg's syndrome. *ENT Ear Nose Throat J* 79:704–709, 2000.

92. Oysu C et al: Temporal bone imaging findings in Waardenburg's syndrome. *Int J Pediatr Otorhinol* 58:215–221, 2001.

93. Pantke OA, Cohen MM Jr: The Waardenburg syndrome. *Birth Defects* 7(7):147–152, 1971.

94. Parry DM et al: Waardenburg-like features with cataracts, small head size, joint abnormalities, hypogonadism and osteosarcoma. *J Med Genet* 15:66–69, 1978.

95. Pasteris NG et al: A chromosome deletion of 2q35–36 spanning loci HuP2 and COL4A3 results in Waardenburg syndrome type III (Klein-Waardenburg syndrome). Abstract 884, *Am J Hum Genet* 41:A224, 1992.

96. Pasteris NG et al: Discordant phenotype of two overlapping deletions involving the *PAX3* gene in chromosome 2q35. *Hum Mol Genet* 2:953–959, 1993.

97. Peterson MA et al: Comments on frontonasal dysplasia, ocular hypertelorism and dystopia canthorum. *Birth Defects* 7(7):120–124, 1971.

98. Pierpont JW et al: A family with unusual Waardenburg syndrome type 1 (WS1), cleft lip (palate), and Hirschsprung disease is not linked to *PAX3*. *Clin Genet* 47:139–143, 1995.

99. Preus M et al: Waardenburg syndrome: penetrance of the major signs. *Am J Med Genet* 15:383–388, 1983.

100. Pryor HB: Objective measurement of interpupillary distance. *Pediatrics* 44:973–977, 1969.

101. Rarey KE, Davis LE: Inner ear anomalies in Waardenburg's syndrome associated with Hirschsprung's disease. *Int J Pediatr Otolaryngol* 8:181–189, 1984.

102. Read AP: Waardenburg syndrome. *Adv Otorhinolaryngol (Basel)* 56:32–38, 2000.

103. Read AP et al: Assignment of Waardenburg syndrome type 1 to 2q37. *J Med Genet* 27:652–653, 1990.

104. Reynolds JE et al: Analysis of variability of clinical manifestations in Waardenburg syndrome. *Am J Med Genet* 57:540–547, 1995.

105. Sachs R: Dystopie du canthus interne associée a une forme fruste du syndrome de Rocher-Sheldon. *Ann Ocul (Paris)* 197:672–683, 1964.

106. Sanchez-Martin M et al: SLUG (SNAI2) deletions in patients with Waardenburg disease. *Hum Mol Genet* 11:3231–3236, 2002.

107. Selicorni A et al: Cytogenetic mapping of a novel locus for type II Waardenburg syndrome. *Hum Genet* 110:64–67, 2002.

108. Senrui H: Congenital clasped thumbs with Waardenburg syndrome in generations of one family: an undescribed congenital anomalies complex. *J Pediatr Orthoped* 4:472–476, 1984.

109. Shah KN et al: White forelock, pigmentary disorder of irides and log segment Hirschsprung disease: possible variant of Waardenburg disease. *J Pediatr* 99:432–434, 1981.

110. Sheffer R, Zlotogora J: Brief clinical report: autosomal dominant inheritance of Klein-Waardenburg syndrome. *Am J Med Genet* 42:320–322, 1992.

111. Steel KP, Smith RJH: Normal hearing in Splotch (Sp+); The mouse homologue of Waardenburg syndrome type 1. *Nat Genet* 2:75–79, 1992.

112. Takasaki K et al: Histopathologic findings of the inner ears with Alport, Usher, and Waardenburg syndromes. *Adv Otorhinolaryngol (Basel)* 56:218–222, 2000.

113. Tassabehji M et al: Waardenburg's syndrome patients have mutations in the human homologue of the *PAX-3* paired box gene. *Nature* 355:635–636, 1992.

114. Tassabehji M et al: Mutations in the *PAX3* gene causing Waardenburg syndrome type 1 and type 2. *Nat Genet* 3:26–30, 1993.

115. Tekin M et al: Waardenburg syndrome type 3 (Klein-Waardenburg syndrome) segregating with a heterozygous deletion in the paired box domain of *PAX3*: a simple variant or a true syndrome? *Clin Genet* 60:301–304, 2001.

116. Touraine RI et al: Neurological phenotype in Waardenburg syndrome type 4 correlates with novel *SOX10* truncating mutations and expression in developing brain. *Am J Hum Genet* 66:1496–1503, 2000.

117. Van Camp G et al: Chromosome 13q deletion with Waardenburg syndrome: further evidence for a gene involved in neural crest function on 13q. *J Med Genet* 32:531–536, 1995.

118. van der Hoeve J: Abnorme Lange der Tränenröhrchen mit Ankyloblepharon. *Klin Monatsbl Augenheilkd* 56:232–238, 1916.

119. Verheij JB et al: ABCD syndrome is caused by a homozygous mutation in the *EDNRB* gene. *Am J Med Genet* 108:223–225, 2002.

120. Yoder BJ, Prayson RA: Shah-Waardenburg syndrome and Dandy-Walker malformation: an autopsy report. *Clin Neuropathol* 21:236–240, 2002.

121. Waardenburg PJ: Dystopia punctorum lacrimalium, blepharophimosis, enpartiele irisatrophia bij een doofstomme. *Ned Tijdschr Geneeskd* 92:3463–3466, 1948.

122. Waardenburg PJ: A new syndrome combining developmental anomalies of the eyelids, eyebrows, and nose root with pigmentary defects of the iris and head hair and congenital deafness. *Am J Hum Genet* 3:195–253, 1951.

123. Wilbrandt HR, Ammann F: Nouvelle observation de la forme grave du syndrome de Klein-Waardenburg. *Arch Klaus Stift Vererbungsforsch* 39:80–92, 1964.

124. Woodyear LL et al: Waardenburg syndrome associated with Hirschsprung disease and other abnormalities. *Pediatrics* 65:368–369, 1980.

125. Zelig S et al: Waardenburg syndrome with associated multiple anomalies. *ORL* 46:34–37, 1984.

126. Zlotogora J et al: Homozygosity for Waardenburg syndrome. *Am J Hum Genet* 56:1173–1178, 1995.

Forelocks, backlocks, and sensorineural hearing loss

White forelock is seen in Waardenburg syndromes 1 and 2. Very rarely a black forelock has been noted. However, RJ Gorlin has seen patients who clearly did not have Waardenburg syndrome but who had sensorineural hearing loss and various pigmentary hair anomalies: yellow forelock, brown backlock (Fig. 14–2A,B), and black forelock. In 1992 a mother, daughter, and son were noted. It is likely that other researchers have observed the association but we have not found any cases cited in the literature. For a related subject, the reader is referred to the section on BADS and ermine phenotype.

Through the courtesy of Dr. Ursula Froster (Lübeck, Germany), one editor (RJ Gorlin) became aware of a child with trisomy 21 with cleft lip, white scalp hair except for the hair in the occipital area, aganglionic megacolon, and congenital profound sensorineural hearing loss (Fig. 14–2C,D). The ABCD (Albinism, Black lock, Cell migration disorder of the neurocytes of the gut, and Deafness) syndrome was described by Gross et al. (1) in a Kurdish kindred. The proband had a black lock at the right temporal occipital region and retinal depigmentation. Bilateral congenital deafness was present, as was a total lack of sympathetic and parasympathetic

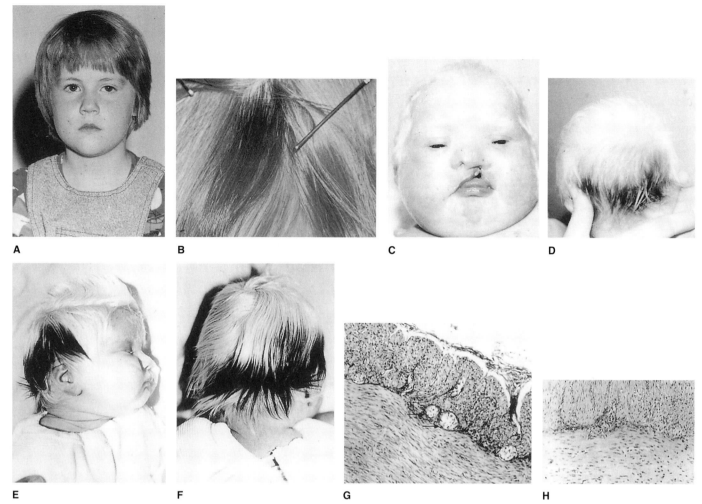

Figure 14–2. *Forelocks, backlocks, and sensorineural hearing loss.* (A) Six-year-old female with profound hearing loss. There is mild ptosis of the left eyelid. (B) Brown backlock. (C,D) Child with Down syndrome, cleft lip, white hair with black backlocks, total aganglionosis, and profound sensorineural hearing loss. (E,F) One of five affected siblings with white hair, black back-locks, total aganglionosis, and profound sensorineural hearing loss (ABCD syndrome). (G) Section of intestine showing normal ganglion cells. (H) Absence of ganglion cells in patient shown in (E) and (F). [(A,B) courtesy of W Lenz, Münster, Germany; (C,D) courtesy of Ursula Froster, Lübeck, Germany; (E–H) from A Gross et al., *Am J Med Genet* 56:322–326, 1999.]

innervation of the large and small intestine. Death occurred at 5 weeks; four prior affected sibs all died a few days after birth. Verheij et al. (4) described another patient with the ABCD syndrome, in whom a homozygous mutation in the *EDNRB* gene was found. This indicates that ABCD syndrome is likely a variant expression of Shah-Waardenburg syndrome.

Probable models in the mouse and horse, respectively, have been described by Lane (2) and McCabe et al. (3).

References

1. Gross A et al: Autosomal-recessive neural crest syndrome with albinism, black lock, cell migration disorder of the neurocytes of the gut, and deafness: ABCD syndrome. *Am J Med Genet* 56:322–326, 1995.
2. Lane PW: Association of megacolon with two recessive spotting genes in the mouse. *J Hered* 57:29–31, 1966.
3. McCabe L et al: Avero lethal white foal syndrome: equine model of aganglionic megacolon (Hirschsprung syndrome). *Am J Med Genet* 36:336–340, 1990.
4. Verheij JB et al: ABCD syndrome is caused by a homozygous mutation in the *EDNRB* gene. *Am J Med Genet* 108:223–225, 2002.

X-linked pigmentary abnormalities and congenital sensorineural hearing loss (Ziprkowski-Margolis syndrome)

A Moroccan Jewish family having 14 males with congenitally profound hearing loss and a unique pigmentary disorder in three generations was described by Ziprkowski et al. (7) and Margolis (4,5) in 1962. Four of the affected individuals were studied in detail and all showed similar clinical features. An isolated example was reported by Campbell et al. (1).

Integumentary system. At birth, the skin was albinotic except for areas of light pigmentation over the gluteal and scrotal areas. Pigmentation gradually increased, particularly involving the arms, legs, buttocks, and face. Only a few spots appeared on the scalp. The hair remained completely white even when growing in the pigmented areas (Fig. 14–3A).

The skin changes ultimately involved the entire body and were characterized by large, leopard-like spots of hypopigmentation and hyperpigmentation. Areas of the skin were sharply demarcated with rather symmetric distribution of pigmentary change. Nonpigmented areas were whitish-pink, whereas brown or pleomorphic hyperpigmented areas were mottled with shades of color varying from light brown to deep brown-black. The pigmented areas measured from a few millimeters to several centimeters in size (Fig. 14–3B,C).

Ocular system. Campbell et al. (1) described partly albinotic retinas, myopia, and strabismus in their patient.

Auditory system. All affected individuals had profound congenital hearing loss. Otologic examination showed normal auricles, audi-

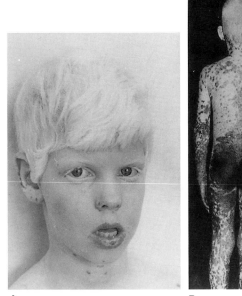
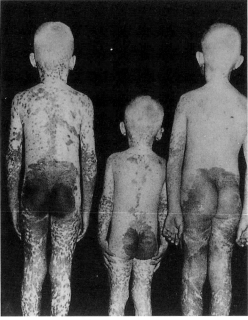
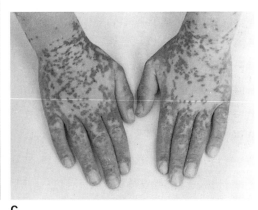

A   B   C

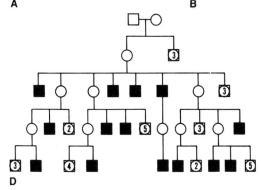

D

Figure 14–3. *X-linked pigmentary abnormalities and congenital sensorineural hearing loss (Ziprkowski-Margolis syndrome).* (A) Affected male. (B) Three affected sibs exhibiting characteristic pigmentary pattern. Greatest pigment intensity is over the buttocks and gradually extends with age. Scalp hair is albinoid. (C) Hands of affected male. (D) Pedigree showing 14 affected males in three generations of a family. [(A,C) courtesy of RM Goodman, Tel Aviv, Israel; (B) courtesy of L Ziprkowski, Tel Hashomer, Israel; (D) adapted from L Ziprkowski et al., *Arch Dermatol* 86:530, 1962.]

tory canals, and ear drums. Pure-tone audiometry showed no response to frequencies above 500 Hz. No other audiometric tests were described. Female heterozygotes exhibited reduced hearing detectable on audiometry (2).

Vestibular system. In three patients tested, caloric vestibular tests showed no vestibular responses. A fourth showed moderate depression of vestibular response, more marked on the left side (7).

Laboratory findings. A series of skull radiographs in one patient showed apparently normal cochleas, semicircular canals, and internal acoustic meatus. Bone age was normal. Electrocardiographic (ECG) tests performed on five patients were normal except for bundle branch block in one patient. Other examinations were within normal limits.

Pathology. Histologically, the skin manifested areas of hypopigmentation and hyperpigmentation. The melanocytes in hypopigmented areas were only weakly dopa-positive, whereas those in hyperpigmented areas were strongly dopa-positive.

Heredity. Fourteen cases have been described in males in three generations of a single kindred (Fig. 14–3D). Transmission occurred through clinically unaffected mothers to 50% of their sons, a pattern characteristic of X-linked inheritance (7). The gene has been localized to Xq26.3–q27.1 by Litvak et al. (3) and Shiloh et al. (6).

Diagnosis. This syndrome shows pigmentary skin changes somewhat similar to those found in recessive piebaldism and congenital sen-

sorineural hearing loss. The melanotic pigmentary changes differ, however, in that there are large symmetric areas of depigmentation filled by small flecks of hyperpigmentation in the latter syndrome. This pattern of pigmentation is in contrast to the general lack of pigmentation over the entire body with large confluent pigmented areas appearing in certain sites in Ziprkowski-Margolis syndrome. Furthermore, depressed vestibular response has been noted in Ziprkowski-Margolis syndrome, whereas normal responses have been elicited in recessive piebaldness and congenital sensorineural hearing loss (DA Dolowitz, personal communication, 1970).

Prognosis. There is little evidence that the hearing loss is progressive. Pigmentary changes with increasing spotty pigmentation continue from infancy through the second decade of life but change little thereafter.

Summary. Characteristics of this syndrome include (*1*) X-linked inheritance; (*2*) pigmentary changes of the skin beginning in infancy and characterized by large irregular spots of hypopigmentation and hyperpigmentation; (*3*) depressed vestibular responses; and (*4*) congenital profound sensorineural hearing loss.

References

1. Campbell B et al: Waardenburg's syndrome. *Arch Dermatol* 86:718–724, 1962.
2. Fried K et al: Hearing impairment in female carriers of the sex-linked syndrome of deafness with albinism. *J Med Genet* 6:132–134, 1969.
3. Litvak G et al: Localization of X-linked albinism-deafness syndrome (ADFN) to Xq by linkage with DNA markers. *Cytogenet Cell Genet* 46:652, 1987.

4. Margolis E: A new hereditary syndrome–linked deaf-mutism associated with total albinism. *Acta Genet (Basel)* 12:12–19, 1962.
5. Margolis E: Sex-linked albinism associated with deafness. *Ala J Med Sci* 3:479–482, 1966.
6. Shiloh Y et al: Genetic mapping of X-linked albinism-deafness syndrome (ADFN) to Xq26.3–q27.1. *Am J Hum Genet* 47:20–27, 1990.
7. Ziprkowski L et al: Partial albinism and deaf mutism due to a recessive sex-linked gene. *Arch Dermatol* 86:530–539, 1962.

White hair, joint contractures, defective chemotaxis, and sensorineural hearing loss (Davenport syndrome)

In 1979, Davenport et al. (1) reported a previously undescribed constellation of hearing loss, white hair, skin changes, and altered chemotaxis. The condition affected individuals in three generations of a family.

Integumentary system. Two of three affected individuals had strikingly light hair (the third had light brown hair), and all three had fair skin (Fig. 14–4A). Numerous other skin changes were noted, including squamous papillomas and psoriasiform rash. These did not appear until a few months of age and ultimately affected all parts of the body. Candidiasis was noted on several occasions. Nails showed leukonychia and spooning.

Musculoskeletal system. All affected individuals were described as having tight heel cords from infancy, which generally necessitated Achilles tendon lengthening (Fig. 14–4B). Other joint contractures occurred over time, variably affecting elbows, shoulders, wrists, hips, knees, and ankles. Body habitus was described as thin.

Other findings. Dysmorphic facial features included prominent nasal tip, long philtrum, thin upper lip, and pointed chin. It is unknown whether these are part of the phenotype or a variant familial pattern. Intellect was unaffected by this condition.

Figure 14–4. *White hair, joint contractures, defective chemotaxis, and sensorineural hearing loss (Davenport syndrome).* (A) White hair in mother and son. Note that tight heel cords cause son to walk on toes. (B) Picture of mother as a child shows tight heel cords. [From SLH Davenport, *Birth Defects* 15(5B):227, 1979.]

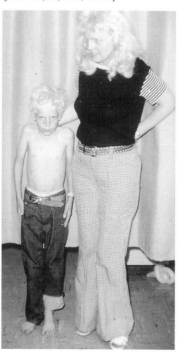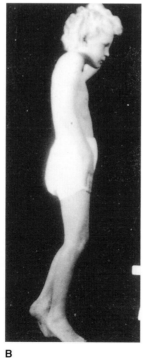

A **B**

Auditory system. Hearing was assessed in only two affected individuals. The child had moderately severe sensorineural hearing loss above 1500 Hz, specific tests determining a cochlear lesion as the cause. The mother had profound generalized loss. However, she had also been given dihydrostreptomycin, which may have led to more severe hearing loss. The hearing loss in both was diagnosed in early childhood.

Vestibular system. Vestibular function was normal.

Laboratory findings. Immunologic studies demonstrated depression of granulocyte and monocyte chemotaxis. Tests for autoantibodies were negative.

Pathology. Skin biopsy of a hyperkeratotic papilloma showed papillomatosis, acanthosis, hyperkeratosis, and focal parakeratosis.

Heredity. The presence of this condition in mother and son, with probable presence in the mother's mother as well, is consistent with autosomal dominant inheritance.

Diagnosis. Other conditions with hyperkeratosis and hearing loss need to be ruled out.

Prognosis. The hearing loss as well as the joint contractures appeared to be slowly progressive. Intellect and life span were unimpaired.

Summary. The major phenotypic features include (*1*) autosomal dominant inheritance; (*2*) hypopigmentation of skin, hair, and eyes; (*3*) joint contractures; (*4*) psoriasiform lesions of the skin; (*5*) abnormal chemotaxis; and (*6*) sensorineural hearing loss with onset in early childhood.

Reference

1. Davenport SLH et al: Dominant hearing loss, white hair, contractures, hyperkeratotic papillomata, and depressed chemotaxis. *Birth Defects* 15(5B): 227–237, 1979.

Autosomal dominant piebaldism and sensorineural hearing loss (Telfer syndrome)

Although possibly described earlier by Hammerschlag (4) in 1908, this syndrome was well defined by Telfer et al. (10) in 1971 in two Pennsylvania kindreds. In the first family, 11 persons in four generations were affected; in the second, a father and daughter manifested this disorder. Spritz and Beighton (7) described a single case, but in which there might have been a positive family history that could not be substantiated.

Integumentary system. All affected persons had congenital absence of pigmentation, consisting of white forelock, white pubic hair, and variable patterns of absent pigmentation of the forehead, trunk, arms, and legs (Fig. 14–5A–C).

Central nervous system. In two individuals, IQs ranged from 56 to 68. Four had low normal intelligence (IQs, mid-80s). The rest were of average intelligence. Finucane et al. (2) reported that some of the individuals in one of the original families reported by Telfer et al. had fragile X segregating as a coincidental trait, thus explaining the mental retardation in some of the individuals. All patients with retardation were stated to have ataxia of gait of uncertain onset. This also could have been attributable to fragile X. Dobyns (personal communication, 1992), on follow-up of some affected individuals, was not able to substantiate any neurologic findings. It is unknown whether the individuals examined by Dobyns had fragile X.

Auditory system. Hearing loss was variable, in some being normal in one ear with moderate loss in the other, whereas others exhibited mild loss in one ear and profound loss in the other. Of 10 patients ex-

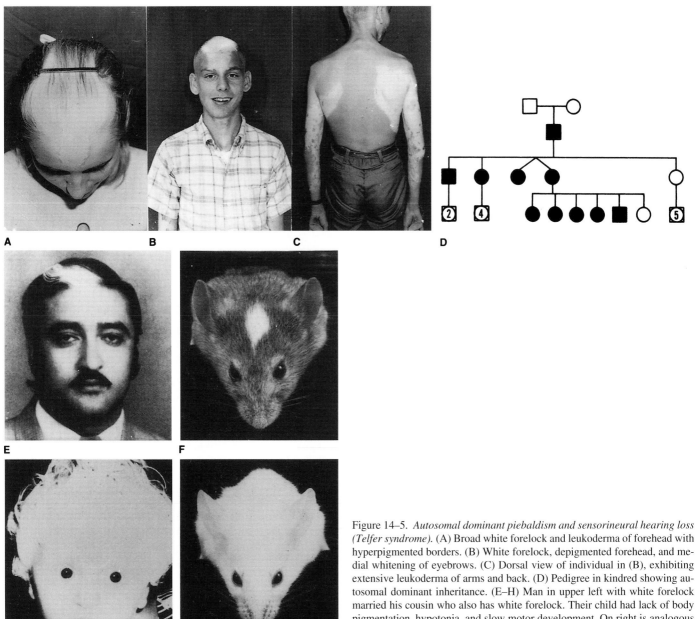

Figure 14–5. *Autosomal dominant piebaldism and sensorineural hearing loss (Telfer syndrome).* (A) Broad white forelock and leukoderma of forehead with hyperpigmented borders. (B) White forelock, depigmented forehead, and medial whitening of eyebrows. (C) Dorsal view of individual in (B), exhibiting extensive leukoderma of arms and back. (D) Pedigree in kindred showing autosomal dominant inheritance. (E–H) Man in upper left with white forelock married his cousin who also has white forelock. Their child had lack of body pigmentation, hypotonia, and slow motor development. On right is analogous situation in mouse model, the result of homozygosity for the gene. [(A–D) from MA Telfer et al., *Am J Hum Genet* 23:383, 1971; (E–H) from MA Hultén et al., *J Med Genet* 24:568, 1987.]

amined, 6 had hearing loss ranging from mild high-frequency to profound sensorineural loss that appeared to be progressive.

Vestibular system. Vestibular testing was not described.

Heredity. Inheritance is clearly autosomal dominant (Fig. 14–5D). Piebald trait, by itself, is autosomal dominant and has been mapped to 4q12 (5,8,9). Mutations in the *KIT* proto-oncogene are thought to be responsible. The patient of Spritz and Beighton (7) was shown to have a mutation in the *KIT* proto-oncogene. There may therefore be certain mutations that are associated with deafness in addition to the piebaldism, whereas other mutations are associated with piebaldism alone.

Diagnosis. Autosomal dominant piebaldism as an isolated trait is well known. It is characterized by congenital patches of white skin and white hair. Melanocytes are absent from these areas. The condition is thought to result from malmigration of melanoblasts from the neural crest (1,3).

Several other syndromes show pigmentary abnormalities and hearing loss. In the syndrome of X-linked pigmentary abnormalities and congenital sensorineural hearing loss (Ziprkowski-Margolis syndrome), the skin lacks pigment at birth but exhibits progressive pigmentation thereafter. The hearing loss is congenital and profound, differing markedly from the congenital piebaldism and variable hearing loss in the present syndrome. Waardenburg syndrome type 2 exhibits piebaldism and sensorineural hearing loss. If the neurologic signs were absent, as noted by Dobyns (personal communication, 1992), perhaps this family really represents that condition.

Recessive piebaldism and congenital sensorineural hearing loss (Woolf syndrome) differs in inheritance pattern. In addition, ataxia and mental retardation have not been noted in that disorder. Vitiligo appears later in life.

Hultén et al. (6) reported homozygosity for the piebald trait in the offspring of first-cousin Pakistani parents. The child was profoundly deaf with hypotonia and slow motor development (Fig. 14–5E–H). His sib as well as their parents and several close relatives had only the piebald trait.

Prognosis. The hearing loss is progressive, whereas the pigment loss is not. The course of neurologic impairment has not been described.

Summary. This syndrome is characterized by (*1*) autosomal dominant inheritance; (*2*) congenital piebaldism; (*3*) ataxia or coordination difficulties in about 80%; (*4*) mental retardation in about 80%; and (*5*) variable, sometimes asymmetric, sensorineural hearing loss in about 60%.

References

1. Cooke JV: Familial white skin spotting (piebaldness) ("partial albinism") with white forelock. *J Pediatr* 41:1–12, 1952.
2. Finucane B et al: Concurrence of dominant piebald trait and fragile X syndrome [letter]. *Am J Hum Genet* 48:815, 1991.
3. Frogatt P: An outline with bibliography of human piebaldism and white forelock. *Isr J Med Sci* 398:86–94, 1951.
4. Hammerschlag V: Zur Kenntnis der hereditär-degenerativen Taubstummheit. VI. Über einen mutmasslichen Zusammenhang zwischen "hereditärer Taubheit" und "hereditärer Ataxie." *Z Ohrenheilkd* 56:126–138, 1908.
5. Hoo JJ et al: Tentative assignment of piebald trait gene to chromosome band 4q12. *Hum Genet* 73:230–231, 1986.
6. Hultén MA et al: Homozygosity in piebald trait. *J Med Genet* 24:568–571, 1987.
7. Spritz RA, Beighton P: Piebaldism with deafness: molecular evidence for an expanded syndrome. *Am J Med Genet* 75:101–103, 1998.
8. Spritz RA et al: Deletion of the *KIT* and *PDGFRA* genes in a patient with piebaldism. *Am J Med Genet* 44:492–495, 1992.
9. Spritz RA et al: Dominant negative and loss of function mutations of the c-*kit* (mast stem cell growth factor receptor) proto-oncogenes in human piebaldism. *Am J Hum Genet* 50:261–269, 1992.
10. Telfer MA et al: Dominant piebald trait (white forelock and leukoderma) with neurologic impairment. *Am J Hum Genet* 23:383–389, 1971.

Autosomal recessive piebaldism and congenital sensorineural hearing loss (Woolf syndrome)

Piebaldism and congenital sensorineural hearing loss were reported in two of three Hopi Indian brothers by Woolf et al. (9) in 1965.

Integumentary system. The boys, 8 and 12 years of age, showed a similar pattern of depigmentation. Although the major part of their bodies (including the back and legs) showed normal pigmentation, the entire head and hair as well as a strip across the upper chest and over both arms were depigmented. Numerous small spots of hypopigmentation and hyperpigmentation were within these depigmented areas (Fig. 14–6A,B).

Ocular system. The irides were blue with a pattern of very fine clumps of pigment closely and uniformly spaced throughout the retina. Vision was normal.

Auditory system. The brothers had marked congenital hearing loss. They attended a school for the deaf but had not learned to speak. Audiograms showed a bilateral 60–100 dB sensorineural hearing loss. Hearing was normal in an affected male sib and in both parents.

Vestibular system. Caloric vestibular tests were normal.

Laboratory findings. No radiographs, blood tests, or urine tests were described.

Pathology. Skin biopsies were not reported.

Heredity. The parents were nonconsanguineous. There was no history of pigmentary defects or of hearing loss in either parent's family. The syndrome has either autosomal or X-linked recessive inheritance.

Diagnosis. This syndrome should be easily differentiated from X-linked pigmentary abnormalities and congenital sensorineural hearing loss, in which large leopard-like spots of varying intensity of pigmen-

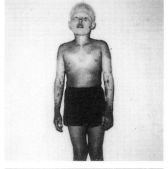
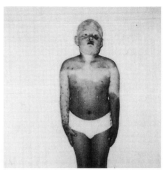
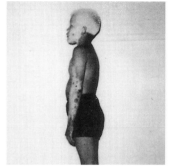
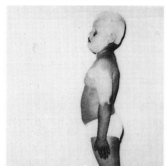

A

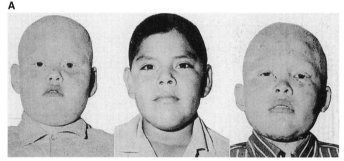

B

Figure 14–6. *Autosomal recessive piebaldism and congenital sensorineural hearing loss (Woolf syndrome).* (A) Two Hopi Indian brothers showing similarity in depigmentation involving head, arms, and chest. (B) Facies of the two affected sibs (8 and 12 years old) and their normal 10-year-old brother. [From CM Woolf et al., *Arch Otolaryngol* 82:244, 1965.]

tation are found. Further, vestibular responses are depressed or absent. In contrast, the caloric responses are normal in the syndrome considered here. Recessive vitiligo and sensorineural hearing loss can be excluded (7,8) by its later onset.

Piebaldism may have isolated autosomal dominant inheritance (5,6). Isolated cases of piebaldism and "profound deafness" were briefly mentioned by Reed et al. (4). The patients, a 6-year-old girl and a 21-year-old man, had broad white forelocks and symmetric white spots over the arms, legs, and abdomen. Their condition was not otherwise documented.

Authors (1–3) who have cited examples of piebaldism and hearing loss did not document the cases sufficiently for us to judge whether they were examples of this syndrome. Probably several of the cases were isolated examples of persons having Waardenburg syndrome type II.

Prognosis. Neither the pigmentary loss nor the hearing loss was progressive.

Summary. Characteristics of this syndrome include (*1*) probable autosomal or X-linked recessive inheritance; (*2*) pigmentary changes, including depigmentation of head and arms, and hyperpigmented spots in depigmented areas; (*3*) normal vestibular responses; and (*4*) congenital sensorineural hearing loss.

References

1. Fisch L: Deafness as part of an hereditary syndrome. *J Laryngol Otol* 73:355–382, 1959.
2. Houghton NI: Waardenburg's syndrome with deafness as the presenting symptom. Report of two cases. *N Z Med J* 63:83–89, 1964 (case 1).
3. Mounier-Kuhn P et al: Albinisme partiel et surdimutité. *J Fr Otorhinolaryngol* 7:915–919, 1958.
4. Reed WB et al: Pigmentary disorders in association with congenital deafness. *Arch Dermatol* 95:176–186, 1967.
5. Smith NG, Schulz H: Partial albinism. *Arch Dermatol* 71:468–470, 1955.
6. Sundfor H: A pedigree of skin-spotting in man. *J Hered* 30:66–77, 1939.
7. Thurman TF et al: Deafness and vitiligo. *Birth Defects* 12(5):315–320, 1976.
8. Tosti A et al: Deafness and vitiligo in an Italian family. *Dermatologica* 172:178–179, 1986.
9. Woolf CM et al: Congenital deafness associated with piebaldness. *Arch Otolaryngol* 82:244–250, 1965.

Linear band hyperpigmentation, congenital heart anomalies, and moderate conductive hearing loss

In 1979, Alimurung et al. (1) reported an infant who developed symmetric, largely linear bands of truncal hyperpigmentation at 2 weeks of age, which gradually faded overtime. Birth weight was less than the third centile. Additional anomalies included left auricular atresia with concomitant moderate hearing loss and cardiac defects (atrial septal defect and dextrocardia). It is possible that the skin changes represent mosaicism.

Reference

1. Alimurung FM et al: Zebra-like hyperpigmentation in an infant with multiple congenital defects. *Arch Dermatol* 115:878–881, 1979.

Oculocutaneous albinism and congenital sensorineural hearing loss, autosomal dominant (Tietz-Smith syndrome)

In 1963, Tietz (6) described a large kindred with oculocutaneous albinism and congenital sensorineural hearing loss. Fourteen individuals (6 males, 8 females) were affected in six generations. Reed et al. (2) reexamined the kindred and cast doubt upon the validity of the findings. However, in 1993, Smith et al. (3) ascertained a branch of the family, which included 19 affected members (11 females, 8 males). Tassabehji et al. (5) and later Amiel et al. (1) also described an affected mother and son (Fig. 14–7).

Ocular findings. The irides are blue and there is no nystagmus or photophobia. The fundi were stated to be normal by Tietz (6) but exhibited ocular albinoidism according to Smith et al. (3,4).

Integumentary findings. Albinism is manifest in hair and skin, but as noted above, the irises are normal. Smith et al. (3,4) indicated that in their family, the hair becomes somewhat darker with age and those affected can become freckled and tan mildly. The eyebrows and eyelashes do not darken but remain blond. The mother and son reported by Tassabehji et al. (5) and Amiel et al. (1) had reddish hair.

Audiologic findings. All affected family members had congenital profound sensorineural hearing loss. Audiometry revealed at least a 100 dB loss with no evidence of progression.

Vestibular findings. Vestibular function was thought to be abnormal, according to Smith et al. (4).

Heredity. Autosomal dominant inheritance seems evident, although there has been no male-to-male transmission. Preliminary linkage studies gave no evidence of linkage studies with Waardenburg syndrome on chromosome 2, piebaldism on chromosome 4, tyrosinase on chromosome 11, or oculocutaneous albinism 2 on chromosome 15 (2). Re-

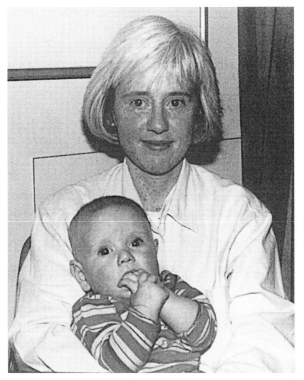

Figure 14–7. *Oculocutaneous albinism and congenital sensorineural hearing loss, autosomal dominant (Tietz-Smith syndrome).* Note oculocutaneous albinism in mother and son. [From R Winter, London, UK.]

cently mutations in the same region of the *MITF* gene have been found to be responsible for the findings in all reported families. *MITF* mutations can also cause some cases of Waardenburg syndrome type 2.

Summary. Characteristics include (*1*) autosomal dominant inheritance; (*2*) albinism of skin and scalp hair; (*3*) normal irides but mild albinoid changes of fundi; (*4*) congenital profound sensorineural hearing loss; and (*5*) altered vestibular function.

References

1. Amiel J et al: Mutation of the *MITF* gene in albinism-deafness syndrome (Tietz syndrome). *Clin Dysmorphol* 7:17–20, 1998.
2. Reed WB et al: Pigmentary disorders in association with congenital deafness. *Arch Dermatol* 95:176–186, 1967.
3. Smith SD et al: Gene localization studies in a unique dominant syndrome of hypopigmentation and congenital deafness. Presented at the Association for Research in Otolaryngology, St. Petersburg, Florida, February, 1993.
4. Smith SD et al: Tietz syndrome (hypopigmentation/deafness) caused by mutation of *MITF*. *J Med Genet* 37:446–448, 2000.
5. Tassabehji M et al: The mutational spectrum in Waardenburg syndrome. *Hum Mol Genet* 4:213–217, 1995.
6. Tietz W: A syndrome of deaf-mutism associated with albinism showing dominant autosomal inheritance. *Am J Hum Genet* 15:259–263, 1963.

Oculocutaneous albinism and congenital sensorineural hearing loss, autosomal recessive

A syndrome characterized by total oculocutaneous albinism and congenital severe hearing loss was found in four children in two sibships in a kindred and described by Ziprkowski and Adam (5) in 1964. However, only one sibship was examined.

Integumentary system. Two sibs exhibited classic albinism with totally white skin. The hair was white and the irides were translucent blue. Lacking pigment, the optic fundus was pink. The sibs had nystagmus and photophobia. In both sibs the medial portion of the eyebrows was absent (Fig. 14–8A).

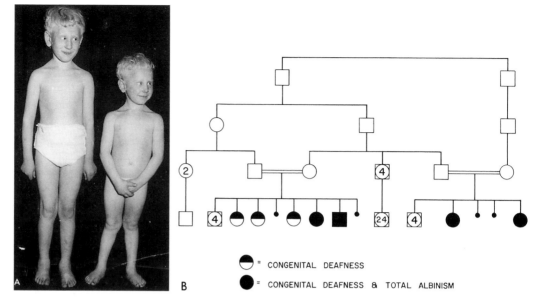

Figure 14–8. *Oculocutaneous albinism and congenital sensorineural hearing loss, autosomal recessive.* (A) Deaf-mute sibs exhibiting total albinism. (B) Pedigree of affected inbred kindred. (From L Ziprkowski and A Adam, *Arch Dermatol* 89:151, 1964.]

= CONGENITAL DEAFNESS

= CONGENITAL DEAFNESS & TOTAL ALBINISM

Auditory system. Audiometric tests on two sibs showed a response only at 500 Hz at 90 dB in one ear. There was a history of congenital severe hearing loss in two albino cousins. Audiograms of the parents were normal.

Vestibular system. No vestibular function tests were described.

Pathology. Skin biopsy from an older affected sib showed no evidence of pigment in the basal layer of the epithelium. The dopa reaction was positive.

Heredity. From the pedigree it is obvious that the parents in both sibships were closely related. The family was of Moroccan Jewish extraction. There were nine children, two of whom exhibited total albinism and hearing loss. Three children had congenital sensorineural hearing loss but no skin pigmentation abnormality, and four sibs were normal (Fig. 14–8B). Whether two genes are involved—one producing congenital severe sensorineural hearing loss and the other producing hearing loss and albinism—or whether the syndrome was the pleiotropic effect of a single gene cannot be determined from this single sibship. When we consider the second sibship in which two of six sibs were affected with albinism and hearing loss, whereas the other four were completely normal, it would appear most likely that an autosomal recessive gene is responsible.

Diagnosis. Reed et al. (2) reported male sibs with oculocutaneous albinism and sensorineural hearing loss. The brothers were also partially blind from hypoplasia of the fovea. Both were severely mentally retarded. Autosomal dominant oculocutaneous albinism and congenital hearing loss were reported by Tietz (4). On reexamination of several members of the kindred, Reed et al. (2) cast doubt upon the validity of the findings. However, Smith et al. (3) have examined the kindred once again and attest to the validity of a condition now termed oculocutaneous albinism and congenital sensorineural hearing loss, autosomal dominant. In all other syndromes that include hearing loss and pigmentary abnormalities, areas of hypo- and hyperpigmentation have been found, clearly separating the oculocutaneous albinism and congenital sensorineural hearing loss syndrome. Hultén et al. (1) described oculocutaneous albinism and profound hearing loss as homozygous expression of the piebald trait.

Prognosis. There is no apparent change in the albinism or hearing loss throughout the life span of affected persons.

Summary. The characteristics of this syndrome include (*1*) autosomal recessive inheritance; (*2*) albinism of the entire body, including the optic fundi and irides; (*3*) deficient medial eyebrows; and (*4*) congenital severe sensorineural hearing loss.

References

1. Hultén MA et al: Homozygosity in the piebald trait. *J Med Genet* 24:568–571, 1987.
2. Reed WB et al: Pigmentary disorders in association with congenital deafness. *Arch Dermatol* 95:176–186, 1967.
3. Smith SD et al: Gene localization studies in a unique dominant syndrome of hypopigmentation and congenital deafness. Presented at the Association for Research in Otolaryngology, St. Petersburg, Florida, February, 1993.
4. Tietz W: A syndrome of deaf-mutism associated with albinism showing dominant autosomal inheritance. *Am J Hum Genet* 15:259–264, 1963.
5. Ziprkowski L, Adam A: Recessive total albinism and congenital deaf-mutism. *Arch Dermatol* 89:151–155, 1964.

BADS and similar phenotypes

Witkop (3) first reported a pair of sibs who had the combination of black locks, oculocutaneous albinism, and sensorineural deafness and coined the mnemonic BADS.

Integumentary system. Skin and hair were stark white with the exception of congenital black tufts of hair and brown macules on the skin.

Ocular system. The ocular features were similar to those of individuals with tyrosine-negative oculocutaneous albinism, in that nystagmus, photophobia, absent fundal pigment and foveal pit, transparently gray irides, and myopia were present.

Auditory system. Hearing loss was congenital and sensorineural, profound in one sib and moderate in the other.

Pathology. Melanocytes were absent in the white hair and skin but present in pigmented areas. White hair bulbs were tyrosinase-negative, whereas black hair bulbs had normal tyrosinase activity.

Heredity. Inheritance is most likely autosomal recessive, in that affected sibs of each sex were described. An obligate heterozygote had a white streak of hair and a fundal lesion.

Diagnosis. There are likely at least two other conditions with a similar phenotype. However, differences exist among these conditions that help distinguish them from each other. The Witkop-King syndrome (2) is characterized by acquired, progressive black hair tufting, severe congenital sensorineural hearing loss, and no visual defects, whereas the patient described by O'Doherty and Gorlin (3) had black scalp hair at birth, which was shed and replaced by white hair with black locks; sensorineural hearing loss, which did not occur until late childhood; and trunk skin with brown and vitiliginous patches (Fig. 14–9). Hopkin et al. (1) described a similar case who also had mildly delayed development.

Prognosis. This condition is not progressive, although individuals may be socially delayed.

Summary. The characteristics of this syndrome include (1) autosomal recessive inheritance; (2) white skin with congenital brown macules; (3) white hair with congenital black locks; and (4) sensorineural hearing loss.

References

1. Hopkin RJ et al: Ermine phenotype: further characterization of neurologic and pigmentary features. Presented at the 23rd Annual DW Smith Workshop on Malformations and Morphogenesis, Greenville, SC 2002.
2. O'Doherty NJ, Gorlin RJ: The ermine phenotype: pigmentary–hearing loss heterogeneity. *Am J Med Genet* 30:945–952, 1988.
3. Witkop CJ Jr: Inherited disorders of pigmentation. *Clin Dermatol* 3:70–134, 1985.

Yemenite-type hypopigmentation, blindness, and sensorineural hearing loss

A Yemenite brother and sister, aged 9 and 11 years, with patchy hypopigmentation, hearing loss, and eye abnormalities were described by Warburg et al. (4) in 1990. Hennekam and Gorlin (2) and Lewis (3) each noted an isolated example.

Integumentary system. Both children described by Warburg et al. (4) had areas of gray hair, at the midline in the boy and at the temples in the girl. The remainder of the hair was reddish-blond or blond. Eyelashes and eyebrows were white. Skin, in general, was lighter toned than that of parents or unaffected sibs, and there were several areas of depigmentation, with some of these having darkly pigmented areas within them (Fig. 14–10A–C).

Ocular system. Both sibs described by Warburg et al. (4) had nystagmus, microcornea, unilateral iridal coloboma, bilateral choroidal colobomata, and visual impairment (Fig. 14–10D). The children described by Hennekam and Gorlin (2) and Lewis (3) did not have coloboma or microcornea.

Other findings. The oral mucosa was pale, and dental eruption was delayed. Taurodontism was present in one child; some also had delayed tooth eruption (2,3). Hennekam's patient had an uncertain gait and mild learning difficulties.

Auditory system. Hearing loss was thought to be congenital. Brain stem audiometry demonstrated sensorineural hearing loss with a threshold of 70 dB at 2000 Hz in the girl and 60 dB at 2000 Hz in the boy (4). The boy also had a 40 dB conductive component to his hearing loss. Hennekam's patient had congenital severe hearing loss.

Pathology. Skin biopsies demonstrated absent melanocytes in hypopigmented areas but normal melanocytes in pigmented and hyperpigmented areas.

Heredity. The presence of this condition in sibs with normal parents is highly suggestive of autosomal recessive inheritance; however, Bondurand et al. (1) recently demonstrated a heterozygous *SOX10* mutation in the individual reported by Hennekam and Gorlin (2). They did not find this alteration in the patients described by Warburg et al. (4), therefore suggesting that these patients have different syndromes, one (the severe form, as described by Warburg et al.) inherited as an autosomal recessive trait, the second (mild form, as described by Hennekam and Gorlin) inherited as an autosomal dominant trait.

Diagnosis. This syndrome can be distinguished from other albinism–hearing loss syndromes by the patchy pigmentation. Waardenburg syndrome can also be distinguished by mode of inheritance and lack of ocular findings. Individuals with vitiligo, muscle wasting, achalasia, and congenital sensorineural hearing loss lack hyperpigmentation, and those with piebaldism and sensorineural hearing loss, both dominant and recessive forms, do not have ocular anomalies.

Prognosis. Intelligence is unimpaired and life span is probably not affected.

Figure 14–9. *Ermine phenotype.* (A–D) A 35-year-old female with ermine phenotype. Notice black streaks in otherwise white hair, normal-colored irises, and vitiligo of skin. BADS has similar clinical changes. [From NJ O'Doherty and RJ Gorlin, *Am J Med Genet* 30:945, 1988.]

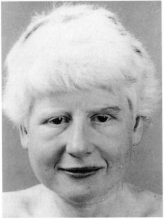
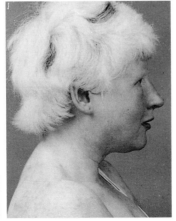
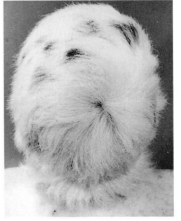
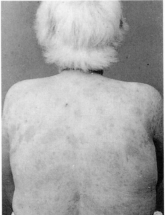

A   B   C   D

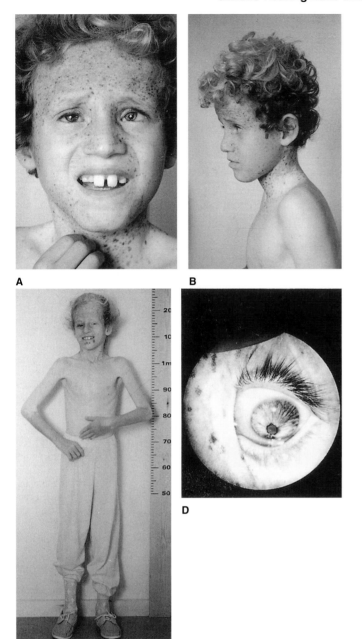

C

Figure 14–10. *Yemenite-type hypopigmentation, blindness, and sensorineural hearing loss.* (A–C) Affected male and female sibs with hypomelanotic hair, skin patches, freckles, microcornea, and monocular coloboma. (D) Iridal coloboma. [Courtesy of M Warburg, Gentofte, Denmark.]

Summary. The condition is characterized by (*1*) probable autosomal dominant inheritance; (*2*) hypopigmentation with areas of hyperpigmentation; (*3*) microcornea and colobomata; and (*4*) congenital or early infantile onset of bilateral hearing loss.

References

1. Bondurand N et al: *SOX10* mutation in a mild form of the Yemenite deaf-blind hypopigmentation syndrome. *Eur J Hum Genet* 7(Suppl):95, 1999.
2. Hennekam RCM, Gorlin RJ: Confirmation of the Yemenite (Warburg) deaf-blind hypopigmentation syndrome. *Am J Med Genet* 65:146–148, 1996.
3. Lewis RA: Ocular albinism and deafness. *Am J Hum Genet* 30:57A, 1978.
4. Warburg M et al: The Yemenite deaf-blind hypopigmentation syndrome. *Ophthalmic Paediatr Genet* 11:201–207, 1990.

Universal dyschromatosis, small stature, and sensorineural hearing loss

In 1977, Rycroft et al. (1) reported a syndrome of melanotic hyper- and hypopigmentation in a 6-year-old daughter of normal consanguineous parents. Dark reticulate skin pigmentation and depigmentation first appeared at about 6 months of age. Height and weight were below the third centile. Intelligence was normal, but she first walked at 2 years. Vision and fundi were normal. Shono and Toda (2) described a female with photosensitivity and hyper- and hypopigmented macules.

High-frequency sensorineural hearing loss was noted with speech delay but was not otherwise characterized by Rycroft et al. (1). Mild high-tone loss was also found by Shono and Toda (2). Universal dyschromatosis usually has autosomal dominant inheritance, but both of these patients were isolated examples.

References

1. Rycroft RJG et al: Universal dyschromatosis, small stature, and high-tone deafness. *Clin Exp Dermatol* 2:45–48, 1977.
2. Shono S, Toda K: Universal dyschromatosis associated with photosensitivity and neurosensory hearing defect. *Arch Dermatol* 126:1659–1660, 1990.

Recessive vitiligo and sensorineural hearing loss

A kindred from an isolated Lousiana village has been described. In 1976, Thurmon et al. (1) reported five children in one sibship with congenital hearing loss, three of whom also had vitiligo. Two more remote cousins had only vitiligo. Nonprogressive congenital hearing loss varied from profound to high-frequency to mild flat loss. The vitiligo began around the waist and flexion creases of the limbs at 6–8 years and slowly spread.

In a second kindred, Tosti et al. (2), in 1986, noted three affected brothers in an Italian family. The vitiligo appeared at less than 20 years of age and was variable in expression among the three brothers. Sensorineural hearing loss appeared between 10 and 16 years of age. The loss was symmetric, bilateral, and severe.

The conditions are likely heterogeneous. To be excluded are various reports on congenital piebaldism and sensorineural hearing loss.

References

1. Thurmon TF et al: Deafness and vitiligo. *Birth Defects* 12(5):315–320, 1976.
2. Tosti A et al: Deafness and vitiligo in an Italian family. *Dermatologica* 172:178–179, 1986.

Hypopigmentation, muscle wasting, achalasia, and congenital sensorineural hearing loss

In 1971, Rozycki et al. (1) described a brother and sister with congenital depigmented areas on the neck and torso, marked muscle wasting in the hands, feet, and legs, achalasia, and congenital severe sensorineural hearing loss.

Physical findings. Height was reduced below the third centile.

Integumentary system. Both patients had depigmented areas over the neck and torso. There were no hyperpigmented spots in these areas (Fig. 14–11A).

Nervous system. Marked muscle wasting was evident in the hands, feet, and legs (Fig. 14–11A,B). Both sibs had hyperreflexia with flexor plantar responses and normal sensation. A history of frequent vomiting and dysphagia was noted for both patients.

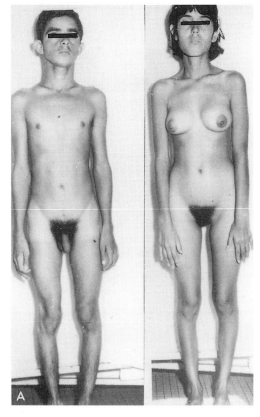

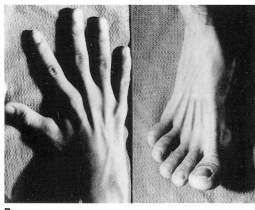

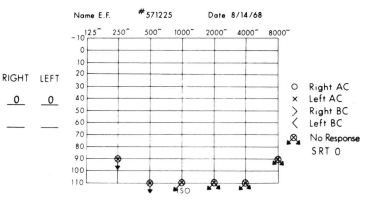

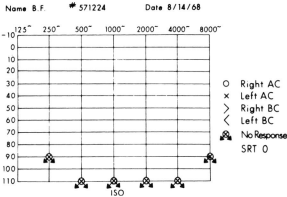

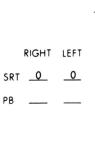

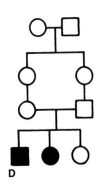

Figure 14–11. *Hypopigmentation, muscle wasting, achalasia, and congenital sensorineural hearing loss.* (A) Sibs having short stature and muscle wasting. (B) Muscle wasting of hands and feet. (C) Audiogram of the two sibs. (D) Pedigree of affected sibs. [From DA Rozycki et al., *Arch Otolaryngol* 93:194, 1971.]

Auditory system. Both sibs had congenital severe sensorineural hearing loss (Fig. 14–11C).

Vestibular system. Caloric vestibular tests were normal.

Laboratory findings. An anterior tibialis muscle biopsy in the male revealed grouped muscle atrophy, indicating neuropathy that was confirmed by electromyography in both patients. A barium swallow, esophageal pressure studies, and responses to methacholine indicated achalasia in both sibs. Extensive laboratory studies were essentially normal except for elevated thymol turbidity and possible cephalin-cholesterol flocculation.

Heredity. Since the parents were first cousins and clinically normal, the syndrome probably has autosomal recessive inheritance (Fig. 14–11D).

Diagnosis. In recessive piebaldism and congenital sensorineural hearing loss (Woolf syndrome), there are small hyperpigmented spots in areas of depigmentation. Musculature and esophageal motility is normal, however, in contrast to hypopigmentation, muscle wasting, and achalasia seen in the syndrome described here.

Prognosis. The syndrome is not life threatening. The hearing loss is not progressive.

Summary. The syndrome is characterized by (*1*) autosomal recessive inheritance; (*2*) mild pigment loss; (*3*) short stature; (*4*) distal neuropathic muscle wasting, more marked in the legs; (*5*) abnormal esophageal motility; and (*6*) congenital severe sensorineural hearing loss.

Reference

1. Rozycki DL et al: Autosomal recessive hearing loss associated with short stature, vitiligo, muscle wasting, and achalasia. *Arch Otolaryngol* 93:194–197, 1971.

Congenital myopathy, secretory diarrhea, bullous skin eruption, microcephaly, and deafness (Levy-Chung syndrome)

Levy et al. (4) described three sibs with the combination of congenital myopathy, secretory diarrhea with secondary zinc deficiency, bullous skin eruption that resolved during infancy, microcephaly, and sensorineural hearing loss.

Craniofacial findings. All children had normal head circumferences at birth, with microcephaly not noted until the second year of life. The palpebral fissures were downslanting, but otherwise facial features were unremarkable.

Integumentary system. All three sibs had congenital blisters primarily on the hands and feet. These resolved during early infancy, but during early childhood, a diffuse erythroderma developed. The erythroderma in turn evolved into skin hyperpigmentation with areas of hypopigmentation.

Musculoskeletal system. These children had hypotonia at birth, as well as multiple contractures affecting several joints. The joint contractures resolved during childhood, and although the hypotonia showed improvement, it was still present in the oldest child at age 4 years.

Other findings. All children had secretory diarrhea that developed during the first 1–2 months of life. Preceding infections often triggered attacks of diarrhea.

Auditory system. Sensorineural hearing loss was diagnosed by age 2 in the two older children. The youngest child, who was 2 months at the time of the report, was not known to have hearing loss. However, subsequent follow-up has demonstrated that this child also has hearing loss (Dr. Anyane-Yeboa, personal communication, 2003). The hearing loss was otherwise not characterized.

Vestibular findings. None were reported.

Pathology. A muscle biopsy done on the youngest child demonstrated abnormally small myofibers, predominantly type 2. Skin biopsy was not consistent with epidermolysis bullosa, but was indicative of a nutritional deficiency state.

Heredity. The presence of this condition in three sibs with normal parents suggests that autosomal recessive inheritance is most likely, although mitochondrial inheritance could not be ruled out.

Diagnosis. This condition can be distinguished from epidermolysis bullosa muscular dystrophy (1), type 1 carbohydrate-deficient glycoprotein syndrome (3), and the syndrome of intractable diarrhea-dysmorphic features (2).

Prognosis. Long-term prognosis is unknown; the oldest child was 4 years at the time of the report.

Summary. This condition is characterized by (*1*) likely autosomal recessive inheritance; (*2*) congenital myopathy; (*3*) congenital skin blistering; (*4*) later-onset skin hyperpigmentation with areas of hypopigmentation; (*5*) postnatal-onset microcephaly; and (*6*) postnatal-onset sensorineural hearing loss.

References

1. Fine JD et al: Autosomal recessive epidermolysis bullosa simplex: generalized phenotypic featues suggestive of junctional or dystrophic epidermolysis bullosa, and association with neuromuscular disease. *Arch Dermatol* 125:931–938, 1989.
2. Girault D et al: Intractable infant diarrhea associated with phenotypic abnormalities and immunodeficiency. *J Pediatr* 125:36–42, 1994.
3. Jaeken J et al: Phosphomannose isomerase deficiency: a carbohydrate-deficient glycoprotein syndrome with hepatic-intestinal presentation. *Am J Hum Genet* 62:1535–1539, 1998.
4. Levy J et al: Congenital myopathy, recurrent secretory diarrhea, bullous eruption of skin, microcephaly, and deafness: a new genetic syndrome? *Am J Med Genet* 116A:20–25, 2003.

Multiple lentigines (LEOPARD) syndrome

In 1969, Gorlin et al. (8) coined the term *LEOPARD syndrome* as an acronym from the following phenotypic features: *L*entigines, *E*lectrocar-diographic defects, *O*cular hypertelorism, *P*ulmonary stenosis, *A*bnormalities of genitalia, *R*etardation of growth, and sensorineural *D*eafness (7,21). Earlier case reports were thoroughly reviewed by Gorlin et al. (8), Voron et al. (30), and Colomb and Morel (4). More recently Coppin and Temple (5) have reviewed the findings from over 80 reported patients.

Craniofacial findings. The face is usually triangular in shape and shows biparietal bossing, ocular hypertelorism, ptosis of upper eyelids, epicanthal folds, broad flat nose, low-set ears, and short neck with occasional webbing (5).

Integumentary system. When present, dark-brown lentigines are striking. They are numerous, small (1–5 mm), and spare only the mucosal surfaces. Most highly concentrated over the neck and upper trunk, they may appear over the face, scalp, palms, soles, and genitalia (10) (Fig. 14–12A,B). They usually appear during childhood (but may be present at birth), and increase in number until puberty. Larger spots have been termed "café noir" patches (9). The lentigines differ from freckles in appearing at an earlier age, having no relation to sun exposure, and microscopically having a greater number of melanocytes per unit of skin area and prominent rete ridges. Some individuals also have café-au-lait spots and axillary freckling (30); localized hypopigmentation can also occur (5). Some patients may lack lentigines (9). One must then base identification of the syndrome upon the presence of other characteristics and/or familial occurrence. Approximately 20% of individuals have café-au-lait spots (30). There is also an increased incidence of granular cell schwannomas of the skin.

Cardiovascular system. Valvular pulmonary stenosis, usually mild, appears to be the most common cardiac abnormality, occurring in 40% of patients. In others, there is an unusual alteration in the pulmonary valve, which has been termed "pulmonary valvular dysplasia" (12). The pulmonary valve reveals three distinct cusps but no commissural fusion. The obstruction is based on thickening of the pulmonary valvular leaflets by disorganized myxomatous tissue that renders the valve leaflets immobile. Clinically, patients with this type of valvular anomaly have a pulmonary systolic ejection murmur but no ejection click. Similar changes have been seen much less commonly in the aortic valves. Some patients have hypertrophic cardiomyopathy, involving primarily the interventricular septum, which results in both subaortic and subpulmonic stenosis (6,21,24). In other reports, associated atrial septal defect, infundibular or supravalvular pulmonary stenosis, or muscular subaortic stenosis has been described (12,13,15). There is a unique and frequently present electrocardiographic anomaly that tends to characterize this syndrome regardless of the type of cardiac malformation. This feature is a superiorly oriented mean QRS axis in the frontal plane, generally located between 60 and 120 degrees (S1, S2, S3 pattern) (16,22,23) (Fig. 14–12C). This may not be demonstrable in every patient, but it may be present in others with the syndrome in whom no structural abnormality of the heart has been demonstrated. Electrocardiograms in several patients have revealed complete heart block, hemiblock, complete bundle branch block, or endocardial fibroelastosis (23).

Musculoskeletal system. Growth retardation is common, with 85% of patients being below the 25th centile for both height and weight, and 20% below the third centile for both parameters (11,19,30).

Pectus carinatum or excavatum, dorsal kyphosis, and hyperflexibility of metacarpophalangeal joints of fingers and thumbs as well as winging of the scapulae have been commonly observed. Spina bifida occulta, cubitus valgus, limited motion at the elbows, and deficient outer table of the temporal bone have also been described (8,20,24).

Genitourinary system. Genital hypoplasia in males, including small penis and small, cryptorchid testes, is the most common finding. Hypospadias has been present in about 50% of the male patients (9). In females absence or hypoplasia of an ovary and/or late menarche may occur (5). On the basis of published cases and unpublished material, it appears that more cases have been transmitted through females; thus the gonadal hypoplasia has been of greater significance in the male.

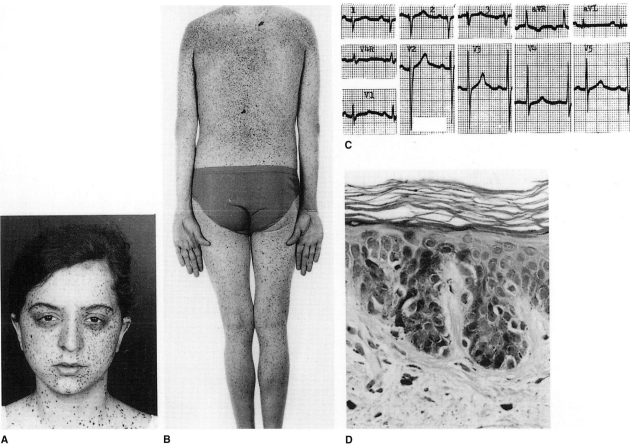

Figure 14–12. *Multiple lentigines (LEOPARD) syndrome.* (A) Lentigines involving entire body but more marked over upper thorax and face. (B) Numerous lentigines on dorsal surface of body. (C) Electrocardiographic anomalies including S1, S2, S3 abnormality. (D) Skin lesion showing elongated rete ridges and increased pigment in basal cells. There are numerous melanocytes (clear cells) in the basal layer of the epithelium. [(A,C,D) from AJ Capute et al., *Arch Dermatol* 100:207, 1969; (B) courtesy of K Thestrup-Pedersen, Aarhus, Denmark.]

Central nervous system. Mild mental retardation has been noted in about 20% (17,19,29); electroencephalographic abnormalities have also been noted (20).

Auditory system. Sensorineural hearing loss has been observed in 15%–25% (5,19). There is marked variation in the degree of hearing loss in different affected persons, but in most it is mild. In contrast, both the mother and daughter described by Capute et al. (3) had congenital severe sensorineural hearing loss with very poor speech development. Because of the severity of hearing loss, special audiometric tests could not be done. Lassonde et al. (13) noted profound hearing loss in their patient. Hearing loss is usually of childhood onset, but can develop during adulthood (5).

Vestibular system. Vestibular testing was described by Capute et al. (3). Caloric tests in these two patients showed no abnormalities.

Pathology. Skin biopsy taken from an area of hyperpigmentation shows elongated rete ridges and increased pigment cells in the basal layer (Fig. 14–12D).

Heredity. The syndrome has autosomal dominant inheritance with variable expressivity (9). The most clinically evident feature of this condition is the lentigines, usually absent at birth, but appearing progressively thereafter. Ease of diagnosis is obviously enabled by their presence. Recently, mutations in the *PTPN11* gene (which is responsible for some cases of Noonan syndrome) have been found in individuals with LEOPARD syndrome, indicating that Noonan and LEOPARD are allelic (7,14).

Diagnosis. Noonan syndrome (18) has many features in common with LEOPARD syndrome, including hypertelorism, eyelid ptosis, small stature, pulmonary stenosis without an ejection click, abnormal QRS axis (frequently S1, S2, S3), undescended testes and delayed development of secondary sex characteristics, skeletal anomalies of the chest, and autosomal dominant inheritance with incomplete penetrance. Patients with Noonan syndrome may occasionally show webbing of the neck, but they lack lentigines and hearing loss. There are at least two genes responsible for the Noonan syndrome phenotype (27,28); LEOPARD syndrome is allelic with one of those genes, *PTPN11*.

Watson (31) described a syndrome of short stature, mild mental retardation, pulmonary valvular stenosis, and café-au-lait spots. The gene for Watson syndrome has been mapped to the region of the NF gene, representing intralocus heterogeneity (1,2).

Sutton et al. (25) described 11 patients with multiple lentigines and hypertrophic obstructive cardiomyopathy; however, hearing, genitalia, and growth were normal. In the review by Coppin and Temple (5), these patients are included as examples of LEOPARD syndrome. Whether they exhibit variable manifestation of LEOPARD syndrome or have a distinct condition is as yet unknown. Halal et al. (10) described a dominantly inherited disorder of multiple lentigines, café-au-lait spots, hypertelorism, myopia, and hiatal hernia or peptic ulcer. One can also find numerous lentigines in Carney syndrome. Swanson et al. (26) described a male with unilateral sensorineural hearing loss; nevi and freckles on his back, chest, and face; lack of sexual hair; anosmia; small penis; and renal anomalies—a type of Kallmann syndrome.

Prognosis. Apparently the only progressive feature in this syndrome is the increasing number of lentigines throughout the first two decades of life. Some patients with severe obstructive cardiomyopathy meet early death (24), but most experience a normal life span.

Summary. Characteristics of the syndrome include (*1*) autosomal dominant inheritance with variable expressivity; (*2*) lentigines developing after birth; (*3*) electrocardiographic defects exhibiting some combination of block in the bundle branch system; (*4*) pulmonary stenosis and/or hypertrophic cardiomyopathy; (*5*) ocular hypertelorism; (*6*) abnormalities of genitalia, including cryptorchidism and hypospadias; (*7*) somatic and occasionally mild mental retardation; (*8*) winged scapulae and various minor skeletal abnormalities; (*9*) sensorineural hearing loss, variable in severity; and (*10*) normal vestibular function.

References

1. Allanson JE, Watson GH: Watson syndrome: nineteen years on. *Proc Greenwood Genet Ctr* 6:733, 1987.
2. Allanson JE et al: Watson syndrome: is it a subtype of neurofibromatosis? *Proc Greenwood Genet Ctr* 9:63, 1990.
3. Capute AJ et al: Congenital deafness and multiple lentigines. A report of cases in a mother and daughter. *Arch Dermatol* 100:207–213, 1969.
4. Colomb D, Morel JP: Le syndrome des lentigines multiples. *Ann Dermatol Venereol* 111:371–381, 1984.
5. Coppin BD, Temple IK: Multiple lentigines syndrome (LEOPARD syndrome or progressive cardiomyopathic lentiginosis). *J Med Genet* 34:582–586, 1997.
6. Csanady M et al: Hypertrophic cardiomyopathy associated with congenital deaf-mutism. *Eur Heart J* 8:525–534, 1987.
7. Digilio MC et al: Grouping of multiple-lentigines/LEOPARD and Noonan syndromes on the *PTPN11* gene. *Am J Hum Genet* 71:389–394, 2002.
8. Gorlin RJ et al: The multiple lentigines syndrome—a complex comprising multiple lentigines, electrocardiographic conduction abnormalities, ocular hypertelorism, pulmonary stenosis, abnormalities of genitalia, retardation of growth, sensorineural deafness, and autosomal dominant hereditary pattern. *Am J Dis Child* 17:652–662, 1969.
9. Gorlin RJ et al: The LEOPARD (multiple lentigines) syndrome revisited. *Birth Defects* 7(4):110–115, 1971.
10. Halal F et al: Gastro-cutaneous syndrome: peptic ulcer/hiatal hernia, multiple lentigines/café-au-lait spots, hypertelorism, and myopia. *Am J Med Genet* 11:161–176, 1982.
11. Hopkins BE et al: Familial cardiomyopathy and lentiginosis. *Aust NZ J Med* 5:359–364, 1975.
12. Koretzky ED et al: Congenital pulmonary stenosis resulting from dysplasia of valve. *Circulation* 40:43–53, 1969.
13. Lassonde M et al: Generalized lentigines associated with multiple congenital defects (LEOPARD syndrome). *Can Med Assoc J* 103:293–294, 1970.
14. Legius E et al: *PTPN11* mutations in LEOPARD syndrome. *J Med Genet* 39:571–574, 2002.
15. Lynch PJ: LEOPARD syndrome. *Arch Dermatol* 101:119, 1970.
16. Matthews NL: Lentigo and electrocardiographic changes. *N Engl J Med* 278:780–781, 1968.
17. Moynahan EJ: Multiple symmetrical moles, with psychic and somatic infantilism and genital hypoplasia. First male case of a new syndrome. *Proc R Soc Med* 55:959–960, 1962.
18. Noonan J, Ehmke O: Associated noncardial malformations in children with congenital heart disease. *J Pediatr* 63:469–470, 1963.
19. Pickering D et al: Little LEOPARD syndrome. Description of 3 cases and review of 24. *Arch Dis Child* 46:85–90, 1971.
20. Polani PE, Moynahan EJ: Progressive cardiomyopathic lentiginosis. *Q J Med* 41:205–225, 1972.
21. Ruiz-Maldonado R et al: Progressive cardiomyopathic lentiginosis: report of six cases and one autopsy. *Pediatr Dermatol* 1:146–153, 1983.
22. Seuanez H et al: Cardio-cutaneous syndrome (the LEOPARD syndrome). Review of the literature and a new family. *Clin Genet* 9:266–276, 1976.
23. Smith RF et al: Generalized lentigo, electrocardiographic abnormalities, conduction disorders, and arrhythmias in three cases. *Am J Cardiol* 25:501–506, 1970.
24. Somerville J, Bonham-Carter RE: The heart in lentiginosis. *Br Heart J* 34:58–66, 1972.
25. Sutton MG St J et al: Hypertrophic obstructive myopathy and lentiginosis: a little known neural ectodermal syndrome. *Am J Cardiol* 47:214–217, 1981.
26. Swanson SL et al: Multiple lentigines syndrome. New findings of hypogonadotrophism, hyposmia and unilateral renal agenesis. *J Pediatr* 78:1037–1039, 1971.
27. Tartaglia M et al: Mutations in *PTPN11*, encoding the protein tyrosine phosphatase SHP-2, cause Noonan syndrome. *Nat Genet* 29:465–468, 2001.
28. Tartaglia M et al: *PTPN11* mutations in Noonan syndrome: molecular spectrum, genotype–phenotype correlation, and phenotypic heterogeneity. *Am J Hum Genet* 70:1555–1563, 2002.
29. Vickers HR, Macmillan D: Profuse lentiginosis, minor cardiac abnormality, and small stature. *Proc R Soc Med* 62:1011–1012, 1969.
30. Voron DA et al: Multiple lentigines syndrome: case report and review of the literature. *Am J Med* 60:447–456, 1976.
31. Watson GH: Pulmonary stenosis, café-au-lait spots, and dull intelligence. *Arch Dis Child* 42:303–307, 1967.

Multiple pigmented nevi and sensorineural hearing loss

In 1981, Peserico et al. (1) described a four-generation, 17-member family with a combination of multiple pigmented nevi and sensorineural hearing loss (Fig. 14–13A). Six members had nevi only, and 11 had both (Fig. 14–13B). The hearing loss was initially high frequency but later involved middle frequencies, and we would categorize it as autosomal dominant late-onset progressive type. There is, of course, the possibility that the two conditions were independently inherited.

Reference

1. Peserico A et al: Familial multiple pigmented naevi and sensorineural deafness. A new autosomal dominant syndrome? *Int J Pediatr Otorhinolaryngol* 3:269–272, 1981.

Figure 14–13. *Multiple pigmented nevi and sensorineural hearing loss.* (A) Numerous pigmented nevi. (B) Pedigree of family with multiple pigmented nevi and sensorineural hearing loss. [From A Peserico et al., *Int J Pediatr Otorhinolaryngol* 3:269, 1981.]

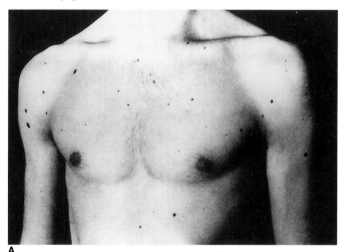

A

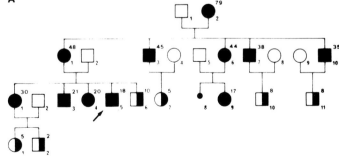

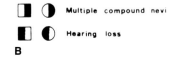

Multiple compound nevi

Hearing loss

B

Scant hair, camptodactyly, and sensorineural hearing loss

In 1970, Mikaelian et al. (1) described a syndrome characterized by congenital alopecia with later scant and brittle hair, flexion contractures of the little fingers, and moderately severe sensorineural hearing loss in a brother and sister.

Integumentary system. The boy had alopecia until 10 years of age when sparse and brittle hair developed on his scalp. The authors did not state whether pili torti was present. The girl had sparse hair from early childhood.

Musculoskeletal system. Since birth, the girl had not been able to extend her little fingers, and her brother had some difficulty in full extension of all fingers. Examination showed soft tissue contractures producing a constant flexion at the first interphalangeal joints. The girl had moderate kyphoscoliosis, but her brother had a normal spine. Both were markedly retarded in height and the boy met his milestones late.

Auditory system. Hearing loss, which was probably congenital, was similar in both sibs. It was first noticed in early childhood, and although it was suggested that it was slowly progressive, this point was not documented. Recent hearing tests showed a 45–80 dB sensorineural hearing loss, more marked at higher frequencies with speech reception at thresholds of about 60 dB bilaterally. A threshold tone-decay test showed no fatigue, and the SISI test was positive bilaterally, suggesting a cochlear locus for the hearing loss.

Vestibular system. Vestibular tests were normal.

Laboratory findings. A battery of laboratory tests was normal. Radiographs showed the head of the proximal phalanx of the little finger to be rotated slightly forward. No bony changes other than kyphoscoliosis in the girl were noted.

Heredity. The affected individuals (2 among 10 sibs) were the product of a first-cousin mating. There was no family history of hearing loss or digital or hair abnormalities. Inheritance appears to be autosomal recessive.

Diagnosis. These sibs may have had the syndrome of pili torti and sensorineural hearing loss. However, no microscopic description of the hair was presented. Moreoever, camptodactyly had not been reported in that syndrome (2).

Prognosis. There is possibly documented evidence that the hearing loss is slowly progressive.

Summary. Characteristics include (*1*) autosomal recessive inheritance; (*2*) short stature; (*3*) sparse scalp hair; (*4*) camptodactyly; and (*5*) sensorineural hearing loss.

References

1. Mikaelian DO et al: Congenital ectodermal dysplasia with hearing loss. *Arch Otolaryngol* 92:85–89, 1970.
2. Robinson GC, Johnston MM: Pili torti and sensory neural hearing loss. *J Pediatr* 70:621–623, 1967.

Rapp-Hodgkin syndrome

Rapp-Hodgkin syndrome is an autosomal dominant condition (9,10). Phenotypic features include sparse and coarse hair (pili torti), high forehead, narrow nose, maxillary hypoplasia, hypodontia and teeth with conical crown form, cleft lip/palate, dysplastic nails, hypohidrosis, and normal development. Hearing loss has been described, presumably due to chronic otitis media secondary to cleft palate (3). However, very narrow ear canals have been reported (3,4,6,8).

The condition has some similarity to Hay-Wells syndrome. Ankyloblepharon filiforme adnatum is a prominent feature in that disorder. Indeed, a case was reported in which the mother had apparent Rapp-Hodgkin syndrome, whereas her child had features of both EEC (*E*ctrodactyly, *E*ctodermal dysplasia, *C*lefting) syndrome and Hay-Wells syndrome (7). Since the latter two conditions are caused by *p63* mutations (2,5) this would not be surprising and suggests Rapp-Hodgkin may also be caused by *p63* mutations. This has recently been shown to be the case (1).

References

1. Bougeard G et al.: The Rapp-Hodgkin syndrome results from mutations of the TP63 gene. *Eur J Hum Genet* 11:700–704, 2003.
2. Celli J et al: Heterozygous germline mutations in the p53 homolog p63 are the cause of EEC syndrome. *Cell* 99:143–153, 1999.
3. Felding IB, Björklund LJ: Rapp-Hodgkin ectodermal dysplasia. *Pediatr Dermatol* 7:126–131, 1990.
4. Lavrijsen APM, Breslau-Siderius EJ: Pili torti as a marker of Rapp-Hodgkin ectodermal dysplasia syndrome in three generations. *Br J Dermatol* 121:812–813, 1989.
5. McGrath JA et al: Hay-Wells syndrome is caused by heterozygous missense mutations in the SAM domain of p63. *J Hum Mol Genet* 10:221–229, 2001.
6. Meyerson MD: The effect of syndrome diagnosis on speech remediation. *Birth Defects* 21(2):47–68, 1985.
7. Moerman P, Fryns J-P: Ectodermal dysplasia, Rapp-Hodgkin type in a mother and severe ectrodactyly–ectodermal dysplasia–clefting syndrome (EEC) in her child. *Am J Med Genet* 63:479–481, 1996.
8. Salinas CF, Marcos Montes G: Rapp-Hodgkin syndrome: observation on 10 cases and characteristic hair changes. *Birth Defects* 24(2):149–168, 1988.
9. Schroeder HW Jr, Sybert VP: Rapp-Hodgkin ectodermal dysplasia. *J Pediatr* 110:72–75, 1987.
10. Silengo MC et al: Distinctive hair changes (pili torti) in Rapp-Hodgkin ectodermal dysplasia syndrome. *Clin Genet* 21:297–300, 1982.

Hay-Wells syndrome (AEC syndrome)

Hay-Wells syndrome is an autosomal dominant syndrome (caused by *p63* mutation) that includes ankyloblepharon, ectodermal defects, and cleft lip and/or palate (1–4). Ectodermal defects include coarse, sparse, wiry hair (pili torti), mild hypohidrosis, hypodontia, and nail dystrophy. Palmoplantar hyperkeratosis can also occur, generally after the age of 10 years. All affected individuals have had cleft palate or velopharyngeal incompetence; cleft lip appears to be a more variable feature. The maxilla is hypoplastic. Hearing loss, when it occurs, is conductive (1,3,4).

References

1. Greene SL et al: Variable expression in ankyloblepharon–ectodermal defects–cleft lip and palate syndrome. *Am J Med Genet* 27:207–212, 1987.
2. McGrath JA et al: Hay-Wells syndrome is caused by heterozygous missense mutations in the SAM domain of p63. *J Hum Mol Genet* 10:221–229, 2001.
3. Shwayder T et al: Hay-Wells syndrome. *Pediatr Dermatol* 3:399–402, 1986.
4. Spiegel J, Colton A: AEC syndrome: ankyloblepharon, ectodermal defects, and cleft lip and palate. *J Am Acad Dermatol* 12:810–815, 1985.

Tsakalakos ectodermal dysplasia and sensorineural hearing loss

In 1986, Tsakalakos et al. (2) described a mother and daughter with an unusual ectodermal dysplasia and sensorineural hearing loss.

Integumentary system. The proband had sparse hair affecting the scalp, axillary, and pubic areas, but sparing the eyebrows and eyelashes. The mother, in addition, had sparse eyebrows and eyelashes. Several teeth were missing and those that were present had conical crown form and were widely spaced. Nails were variably affected and had ridges and leukonychia punctata, and/or were dystrophic. Skin lesions were varied and included dermal hypoplasia on the tip of the nose, scar-like lesions around the mouth and chin, areas of hyperpigmentation, lentigines, seborrheic keratoses, and small skin tags. Sweating was apparently normal.

Other findings. Both mother and daughter had no breast development; the daughter had absent nipples as well.

Auditory system. Bilateral sensorineural hearing loss was present in both females. Audiograms demonstrated a 15 dB loss in the daughter, while the mother had total hearing loss on the right and 15–35 dB loss on the left.

Pathology. Microscopic examination of hair demonstrated node-like swellings on the shafts. Skin biopsy taken from a hyperpigmented area showed a normal epidermis with areas of atrophy and increased pigmentation.

Heredity. The presence of this condition in mother and daughter, as well as in two of the mother's sibs and three of her paternal aunts and uncles, is highly suggestive of autosomal dominant inheritance with variable expressivity.

Diagnosis. Other conditions of the tricho-odonto-onychial subgroup of ectodermal dysplasia can be distinguished by the overall phenotypic pattern and mode of inheritance (1).

Prognosis. Life span and intellectual function are not affected.

Summary. Features of this condition include (*1*) autosomal dominant inheritance; (*2*) amastia with or without athelia; (*3*) sparse hair; (*4*) numerous skin tags; and (*5*) bilateral sensorineural hearing loss.

References

1. Pinheiro M et al: A previously undescribed condition: tricho-odonto-onychodermal syndrome. A review of the tricho-odonto-onychial subgroup of ectodermal dysplasias. *Br J Dermatol* 105:371–372, 1981.
2. Tsakalakos N et al: A previously undescribed ectodermal dysplasia of the tricho-odonto-onychial subgroup in a family. *Arch Dermatol* 122:1047–1053, 1986.

Tricho-odonto-onychial dysplasia

Pinheiro et al. (1) described four sisters with a new ectodermal dysplasia. Physical features included variable alopecia, enamel hypoplasia leading to loss of teeth, numerous pigmented nevi, dystrophic nails, bony deficiency of the frontoparietal region, and supernumerary nipples. One girl had unilateral mixed hearing loss associated with meatal atresia. Inheritance is likely autosomal recessive.

Reference

1. Pinheiro M et al: Trichoodontoonychial dysplasia—a new meso-ectodermal dysplasia. *Am J Med Genet* 15:67–70, 1983.

Keratitis-ichthyosis-deafness (KID) syndrome

KID syndrome is a disorder (or possibly a heterogeneous group of disorders) that includes congenital (or early-onset) erythrokeratoderma, hyperkeratosis of palms and/or soles, and sensorineural hearing loss as component manifestations. Numerous patients have been described (2,11,18,21–58). The mnemonic KID syndrome (*K*eratitis, *I*chthyosis, *D*eafness) was proposed by Skinner et al. (50) in 1981. Other cited cases have different metabolic disturbances (25,53). Some of these are listed as distinct syndromes in this text.

We object to the "I" in KID syndrome, because the changes are not those of an ichthyosis but an erythrokeratoderma; however, we suspect that the acronym is too entrenched to be changed. Recently, however, Caceres-Rios et al. (7) have suggested changing the name to KED, for *K*eratodermatous *E*ctodermal *D*ysplasia.

Integumentary system. The condition is characterized by congenital cutaneous alterations, which are described as dry, red, rough skin; erythematous and scaly skin; erythroderma; and erythrokeratoderma (7). There have been reports of some affected children developing these skin changes during the first weeks of life. These skin changes are then followed by the permanent cutaneous changes that develop during the first year. They are characterized as verrucous or hyperkeratotic plaques. The skin is affected bilaterally, although not necessarily symmetrically. The plaques are most common on the face, but can also develop on the knees, elbows, buttocks, and scalp (Fig. 14–14A–D). The margins of the reddish patches change slowly, becoming more extensive with time. The dorsa of the feet have hyperkeratotic plaques. The palms exhibit a dry "orange-peel" change (30,34) (Fig. 14–14D). Positive response to treatment with aromatic retinoids has been reported (45).

The nails are dystrophic, thickened, and yellow. Variable degrees of alopecia are common, especially affecting scalp hair, eyebrows, and eyelashes. Some cases of alopecia are congenital, so are not secondary to the skin changes. Hyperplastic lesions about the mouth have been described. Defective dentition and reduced sweating have also been noted (7).

Squamous cell carcinomas have been reported (2,18,22,29,32,36,50) as well as malignant fibrous histiocytoma (8) and multiple trichilemmal tumors (27).

Ocular system. Severe photophobia followed by vascularizing keratitis has been described in most patients. Leukoma, opacity, and corneal abrasion have also been described. The eye changes tend to be progressive, and blindness may result (10,11,25,44,50,54). One group has suggested that topical cyclosporin may reduce the neovascularizations that occur, but these findings are preliminary (13).

Central nervous system. Mild mental retardation may be seen (29). Some patients have exhibited tight heel cords (6,8,29). Others have diminished or absent tendon reflexes of the lower extremities. Two patients have had cerebellar hypoplasia on CT scan (9,24).

Immune system. These children are susceptible to a variety of infections, including those that are viral, mycotic, bacterial, and candidial (2,14,16,18,22,30,32,33). The basis for this apparent susceptibility is unknown, although Pincus et al. (41) described increased IgE and IgG levels and decreased chemotaxis in an affected child. Others have also reported elevated serum IgE levels (20,30,39). One affected infant died of overwhelming septicemia (17).

Auditory system. The hearing loss is generally congenital sensorineural and severe and may be bilateral or unilateral (1,2,4,7,18,34,36,44,47,48,50) (Fig. 14–14E). Temporal bone study (52) has shown cochleosaccular abnormality with immaturity of the organ of Corti, degeneration of the stria vascularis, and poor innervation of the saccule. The utricle and semicircular canals were normal.

Laboratory findings. Histologic study of the skin showed a "basket-weave" hyperkeratosis and a mild chronic inflammatory infiltrate around blood vessels in the upper dermis. Follicular plugging of the epidermis is common. The oral mucosa exhibits marked epithelial edema. Probable heterogeneity is demonstrated by various metabolic disorders described by different authors. Jurecka et al. (25) noted glycogen storage in their patient; Wilson et al. (58) found normal glycogen stores, but abnormal copper accumulation, in the liver of their patient. Histologic studies of the inner ear have found cochlear alteration and atrophy of the organ of Corti (12,39).

Heredity. Most patients have been isolated examples, although cases of parent-to-child transmission (18,35,38,43,50) as well as instances of affected sibs with normal parents (14,31) are known. It is likely that this is an autosomal dominant trait with the cases of affected sibs born to normal parents being examples of gonadal mosaicism. The report of affected half-sibs supports this hypothesis (28); however, a rare recessive form of the condition cannot be ruled out. It was found recently that heterozygosity for mutations in *GJB2* (the connexin-26 gene) cause KID, at least in 10 of 10 patients analyzed (43). Van Steensel et al. (56) also described a case and suggested that digenic inheritance may be a factor in KID syndrome.

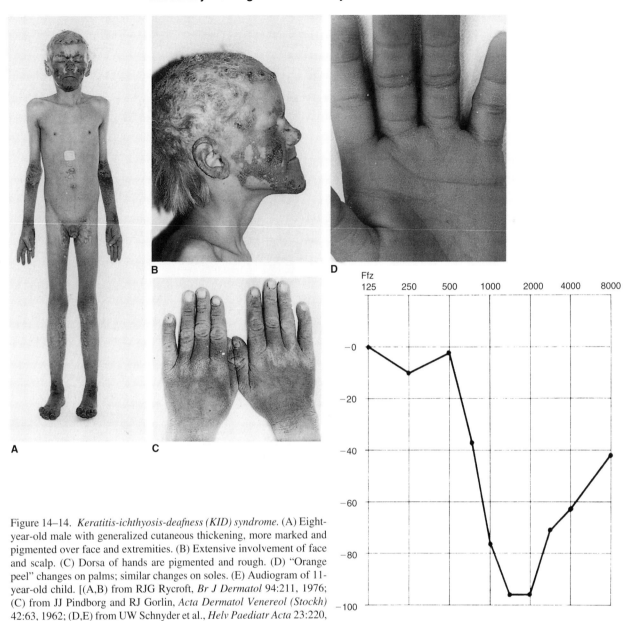

Figure 14–14. *Keratitis-ichthyosis-deafness (KID) syndrome.* (A) Eight-year-old male with generalized cutaneous thickening, more marked and pigmented over face and extremities. (B) Extensive involvement of face and scalp. (C) Dorsa of hands are pigmented and rough. (D) "Orange peel" changes on palms; similar changes on soles. (E) Audiogram of 11-year-old child. [(A,B) from RJG Rycroft, *Br J Dermatol* 94:211, 1976; (C) from JJ Pindborg and RJ Gorlin, *Acta Dermatol Venereol (Stockh)* 42:63, 1962; (D,E) from UW Schnyder et al., *Helv Paediatr Acta* 23:220, 1968.]

Diagnosis. Caceres-Rios et al. (7) have recommended diagnostic criteria for KID, which includes erythrokeratoderma, sensorineural hearing loss, vascularizing keratitis, reticulated palmoplantar hyperkeratosis, and alopecia as obligatory features. Supportive criteria include susceptibility to infection, dental dysplasia, hypohidrosis, and growth delay. The KID syndrome shares several features with the syndrome of generalized spiny hyperkeratosis, universal alopecia, and congenital sensorineural hearing loss. Whether the conditions are the same disorder cannot be determined at this time, but we suspect they are. Based on molecular analysis, ichthyosis, hystrix-like, with deafness (HID) and KID syndromes have been shown to be the same entity (55).

The skin lesions most closely resemble those of erythrokeratoderma variabilis, which has autosomal dominant inheritance. However, the erythematous patches in that disorder, erratically outlined, change in size and shape from day to day. The hyperkeratotic patches have a striking geographic outline. In contrast to the erythematous patches, however, they tend to be site-specific, involving particularly the face, buttocks, and extensor surface of limbs.

In KID syndrome, the skin lesions are typical in appearance, but they fail to exhibit the marked fluctuation in size, location, and shape.

Desmons et al. (14) described congenital ichthyosiform erythroderma, hepatomegaly, and congenital sensorineural hearing loss in three of six children of consanguineous parents. There was mild growth retardation.

Other erythrokeratodermas have been reviewed by Beare et al. (3), but none were associated with hearing loss. Patients with ichthyosiform erythroderma and hearing loss have been briefly mentioned by Fraser (15). Inheritance was not known. A rare X-linked condition called IFAP (*I*chthyosis *F*ollicularis, *A*lopecia, *P*hotophobia) syndrome has phenotypic resemblance to KID, although deafness is not reported as a manifestation of IFAP, and herniae and normal teeth and nails are not manifestations of KID (5).

An autosomal dominantly inherited syndrome of ichthyosis congenita, mental retardation, and congenital sensorineural hearing loss was reported by Gryczynska and Omulecki (19) in 22 members in three generations. Documentation, however, was so scant that we are uncertain as to the nature of the disorder.

As noted above, the child described by Wilson et al. (58) and the patient reported by Jurecka et al. (25) likely have distinct conditions that include keratitis, ichthyosis, and hearing loss in the phenotype but have an underlying metabolic cause. We are uncertain whether the child reported by Mallory et al. (33) has KID syndrome.

Prognosis. There is no evidence that the hearing loss or skin lesions are progressive. However, squamous cell carcinomas affected approximately 11% of patients.

Summary. The characteristics of this syndrome include (*1*) autosomal dominant inheritance; (*2*) atypical erythrokeratoderma; and (*3*) congenital sensorineural hearing loss.

References

1. Anton-Lamprecht I et al: Progressive erythrokeratoderma and cochlear impairment. *Int J Pediatr Otorhinolaryngol* 15:279–289, 1988.
2. Baden HP, Alper JC: Ichthyosiform dermatosis, keratitis, and deafness. *Arch Dermatol* 113:1701–1704, 1977.
3. Beare JM: Familial annular erythema. An apparently new dominant mutation. *Br J Dermatol* 78:59–68, 1966.
4. Beare JM et al: Atypical erythrokeratoderma with deafness, physical retardation, and peripheral neuropathy. *Br J Dermatol* 87:308–314, 1972.
5. Boente MDC et al: Atrichia, ichthyosis, follicular hyperkeratosis, chronic candidiasis, keratitis, seizures, mental retardation and infuinal hernia: a severe manifestation of IFAP syndrome? *Eur J Dermatol* 10:98–102, 2000.
6. Burns FS: A case of generalized congenital keratoderma with unusual involvement of the eyes, ears, and nasal and buccal mucous membranes. *J Cutan Dis* 33:255–260, 1915.
7. Caceres-Rios H et al: Keratitis, ichthyosis, and deafness (KID syndrome): review of the literature and proposal of a new terminology. *Pediatr Dermatol* 13:105–113, 1996.
8. Carey AB et al: Malignant fibrous histiocytoma in keratitis, ichthyosis, and deafness syndrome. *J Am Acad Dermatol* 19:1124–1126, 1988.
9. Chia LG, Li WM: Clinical and electrophysiological studies in a patient with keratitis, ichthyosis, and deafness (KID) syndrome. *J Neurogenet* 4:57–64, 1987.
10. Cram DL et al: A congenital ichthyosiform syndrome with deafness and keratitis. *Arch Dermatol* 115:467–471, 1979.
11. Cremers CWRJ et al: Deafness, ichthyosiform erythroderma, corneal involvement, photophobia and dental dysplasia. *J Laryngol Otol* 91:585–590, 1977.
12. DeBerker D et al: Fatal keratitis, ichthyosis and deafness syndrome (KIDS). Aural, ocular, and cutaneous histopathology. *Am J Dermatopathol* 15:64–69, 1993.
13. Derse M et al: Successful topical cyclosporin A in the therapy of progressive vascularising keratitis in keratitis-ichthyosis-deafness (KID) syndrome (Senter syndrome). *Klin Monatsbl Augenheilkd* 219:383–386, 2002.
14. Desmons F et al: Erythrodermie ichthyosiforme congénitale seche, surdi-mutité, hepatomegalie de transmission recessive autosomique. *Bull Soc Fr Dermatol Syph* 78:585–591, 1971.
15. Fraser GR: The role of genetic factors in the causation of human deafness. *Audiology (Basel)* 10:212–221, 1971.
16. Frings G: Erythrokeratodermia progressiva partim symmetrica mit Innenohrschwerhörigkeit und endogenem Ekzem. *Z Hautkrankh* 63:151–152, 1988.
17. Gilliam A, Williams ML: Fatal septicemia in an infant with keratitis, ichthyosis, and deafness (KID) syndrome. *Pediatr Dermatol* 19:232–236, 2002.
18. Grob JJ et al: Keratitis, ichthyosis, and deafness (KID) syndrome. Vertical transmission and death from multiple squamous cell carcinomas. *Arch Dermatol* 123:777–782, 1987.
19. Gryczynska D, Omulecki A: Syndrome of deafness, ichthyosis congenita and mental retardation with dominant inheritance. *Otolaryngologia Polska* 27:647–652, 1973 (in Polish).
20. Harms M et al: KID syndrome (keratitis, ichthyosis, and deafness) and chronic mucocutaneous candidiosis: case report and review of the literature. *Pediatr Dermatol* 2:1–7, 1984 (same case as ref. 13).
21. Haxthausen H: Hyperkeratosis ichthyosiformis? Acanthosis nigricans in a 4-year-old girl with congenital deafness. *Acta Dermatol Venereol (Stockh)* 35:191–192, 1955.
22. Hazen PG et al: Keratitis, ichthyosis and deafness syndrome with development of multiple cutaneous neoplasms. *Int J Dermatol* 28:190–191, 1989.
23. Helm K et al: Systemic cytomegalovirus in a patient with the keratitis, ichthyosis, and deafness (KID) syndrome. *J Am Acad Dermatol* 23:385–388, 1990.
24. Hsu H-C et al: Keratitis, ichthyosis, and deafness (KID) syndrome with cerebellar hypoplasia. *Int J Dermatol* 27:695–697, 1988.
25. Jurecka W et al: Keratitis, ichthyosis, and deafness syndrome with glycogen storage. *Arch Dermatol* 121:799–801, 1985.
26. Kiesewetter F et al: Progressive symmetric erythrokeratoderma with deafness: histological and ultrastructural evidence for a subtype distinct from Schnyder's syndrome. *Dermatology* 186:222–225, 1993.
27. Kim K-H et al: Keratitis, ichthyosis and deafness syndrome with development of multiple hair follicle tumours. *Br J Dermatol* 147:139–143, 2002.
28. Kone-Paut I et al: Keratitis, ichthyosis, and deafness (KID) syndrome in half sibs. *Pediatr Dermatol* 15:219–221, 1998.
29. Lancaster L Jr, Fournet LF: Carcinoma of the tongue in a child: report of case. *J Oral Surg* 27:269–270, 1969.
30. Langer K et al: Keratitis, ichthyosis, and deafness (KID) syndrome: report of three cases and a review of the literature. *Br J Dermatol* 122:689–697, 1990.
31. Legrand J et al: Un syndrome rare oculo-auriculo-cutanée. *J Fr Ophtalmol* 5:441–445, 1982.
32. Madariaga J et al: Squamous cell carcinoma in congenital ichthyosis with deafness and keratitis. *Cancer* 57:2026–2029, 1986.
33. Mallory SB et al: Ichthyosis, deafness, and Hirschsprung's disease. *Pediatr Dermatol* 6:24–27, 1989.
34. Marghescu S et al: Kongenitale Erythrokeratodermie mit Taubheit Schnyder. *Hautarzt* 33:416–419, 1982.
35. McCrae JD Jr: Keratitis, ichthyosis, and deafness (KID) syndrome. *Int J Dermatol* 29:89–93, 145–146, 1990.
36. Morris MR et al: The keratitis, ichthyosis and deafness syndrome. *Otolaryngol Head Neck Surg* 104:526–528, 1991.
37. Muramatou F et al: KID syndrome: congenital ichthyosiform dermatosis with keratitis and deafness. *J Dermatol* 14:158–162, 1987.
38. Nazzaro V et al: Familial occurrence of KID (keratitis, ichthyosis, deafness) syndrome. *J Am Acad Dermatol* 23:385–388, 1990.
39. Ochs HD et al: Ichthyosiform keratoderma and congenital neurosensory deafness. *J Pediatr* 93:331, 1978.
40. Oikarenen A et al: A congenital ichthyosiform syndrome with deafness and elevated steroid disulfate levels. *Acta Dermatol Venereol (Stockh)* 60:503–507, 1980.
41. Pincus SH et al: Defective neutrophil chemotaxis with variant ichthyosis, hyperimmunoglobulinemia E and recurrent infections. *J Pediatr* 87:908–911, 1975.
42. Pindborg JJ, Gorlin RJ: Oral changes in acanthosis nigricans (juvenile type). *Acta Dermatol Venereol (Stockh)* 42:63–71, 1962.
43. Richard G, et al: Missense mutations in *GJB2* encoding connexin-26 cause the ectodermal dysplasia keratitis-ichthyosis-deafness syndrome. *Am J Hum Genet* 70:1341–1348, 2002.
44. Rycroft RJG et al: Atypical ichthyosiform erythroderma, deafness and keratosis. A report of two cases. *Br J Dermatol* 94:211–218, 1976.
45. Sahoo B et al: KID syndrome: response to acitretin. *J Dermatol* 29:499–502, 2002.
46. Schnyder UW et al: Eine weitere Form von atypischer Erythrokeratodermie mit Schwerhörigkeit und cerebraler Schädigung. *Helv Paediatr Acta* 23:220–230, 1968.
47. Senter TP et al: Atypical ichthyosiform erythroderma and congenital neurosensory deafness—a distinct syndrome. *J Pediatr* 92:68–72, 1978.
48. Silvestri DL: Ichthyosiform dermatosis and deafness. *Arch Dermatol* 114:1243–1244, 1978.
49. Singh K: Keratitis, ichthyosis, and deafness (KID syndrome). *Australas J Dermatol* 28:38–41, 1987.
50. Skinner BA et al: The keratitis, ichthyosis, and deafness (KID) syndrome. *Arch Dermatol* 117:285–289, 1981.
51. Stalder JF, Litoux F: Cas pour diagnostic. *Ann Dermatol Venereol* 115:357–358, 1988.
52. Tsuzuku T et al: Temporal bone findings in keratosis, ichthyosis and deafness syndrome. *Ann Otol Rhinol Laryngol* 101:413–416, 1992.
53. Tuppurainen K et al: The KID syndrome in Finland. *Acta Ophthalmol* 66:692–698, 1988.
54. Van Everdingen JJE et al: Normal sweating and tear production in congenital ichthyosiform erythroderma with deafness and keratitis. *Acta Dermatol Venereol (Stockh)* 62:76–78, 1982. [Same case as Cremers (11)]
55. Van Geel et al: HID and KID syndromes are associated with the same connexin 26 mutation. *Br J Dermatol* 146:938–942, 2002.
56. Van Steensel MAM et al: A novel connexin 26 mutation in a patient diagnosed with keratitis-ichthyosis-deafness syndrome. *J Invest Dermatol* 118:724–727, 2002.
57. Voigtländer V: Hereditäre Verhornungsstörungen und Taubheit. *Z Hautkrankh* 52:1017–1025, 1977.

58. Wilson GN et al: Keratitis, hepatitis, ichthyosis and deafness: report and review of KID syndrome. *Am J Med Genet* 40:255–259, 1991.

Congenital ichthyosiform dermatosis, mental retardation, dysmorphic appearance, retinal colobomas, and conductive hearing loss (CHIME syndrome)

In 1983–85, Zunich and coworkers (3–5) reported two unrelated children with a distinctive syndrome involving the brain, eyes, and skin. In 1988, Zunich et al. (5) noted a similarly affected sib and was informed of another isolated case. The authors now use the acronymic mnemonic CHIME syndrome (*C*oloboma, *H*eart defect, *I*chthyosis, *M*ental retardation, *E*ar) (Zunich et al. 3–6). Another case, as well as follow-up of the original patients, was described by Shashi et al. (2). Schnur et al. (1) reported the sixth case.

Craniofacial findings. A recognizable facial appearance was noted, consisting of brachycephaly, hypertelorism, epicanthal folds, broad nasal root, cupped ears with rolled helices, short philtrum, and full lips. The teeth were small and irregularly placed with an occasional duplicated or bifid tooth. One child had cleft palate, another had submucous cleft palate.

Central nervous system. Global developmental delay was manifest during the first year. Mental retardation was apparent in early childhood. One child had a developmental level of about 1 year at age 3 years, and the other had a developmental level of 1.5–2 years at age 6.5 years. Examination showed autistic behavior and a wide-based gait. Generalized tonic-clonic seizures began during the first year. These seizures generally became more severe following puberty and appear to have been poorly controlled by medication. Cranial CT scans showed mild cerebral atrophy in some. In addition, affected individuals have tended to have outbursts of violent behavior.

Musculoskeletal system. Brachydactyly and broad second toes and, in one child, radial deviation of some fingers and ulnar deviation of others were noted.

Ocular system. Bilateral retinal colobomas were noted in 5 of 6 patients; the sixth child had choroidal colobomas. One had unilateral ptosis and strabismus. Another had slight corneal clouding. Visual acuity was not described.

Integumentary system. A pruritic migratory ichthyosiform eruption was observed during the first month of life and persisted thereafter. Examination in childhood showed an erythematous scaly eruption over most of the trunk and limbs that appeared as sharply demarcated plaques with figurate borders that measured 1–10 cm. Uninvolved skin appeared normal. Over time, the skin dryness and rash tended to wax and wane. The face was red with parallel lamellar scales, and the hair fine, sparse, and blond. The palms and soles were thickened. Small and low-set nipples seemed to be a constant feature. Dermatoglyphics showed increased arches.

Cardiovascular system. Three children had congenital heart anomalies.

Auditory system. Moderate conductive hearing loss that resulted from marked exfoliation of the external auditory canal and tympanic membrane was evident. Auditory-evoked response was abnormal (5).

Laboratory findings. Electroencephalogram, bone marrow preparation, chromosome analysis, and immune function studies were normal.

Pathology. The skin was thickened with hyperplastic epidermis and exaggerated rete ridges, which often penetrated the upper portion of the dermis. All layers of the skin had increased cells, especially in the spinous and granular cell layers. Dark basal cells and scattered inflammatory cells were also seen.

Heredity. Zunich et al. (6) reported autosomal recessive inheritance.

Diagnosis. The KID syndrome consists of keratitis, ichthyosis, and sensorineural hearing loss without neurological abnormalities. Rud syndrome consists of mental retardation, seizures, congenital ichthyosis, hypogonadism, short stature, and sensorineural hearing loss. Neither has similar eye abnormalities or conductive hearing loss. Refsum syndrome comprises ataxia, retinitis pigmentosa, sensorineural hearing loss, and sometimes ichthyosis. It is associated with elevated levels of serum phytanic acid. Rud syndrome differs by also including hypogonadism, sensorineural hearing loss, and retinitis pigmentosa.

Prognosis. In general, individuals have good health but severe mental retardation, seizures that worsen after puberty, and markedly delayed or absent speech. The patient of Schnur et al. developed leukemia at $4\frac{1}{2}$ years, however.

Summary. This disorder is characterized by (*1*) possible autosomal recessive inheritance; (*2*) congenital migratory ichthyosiform dermatosis; (*3*) mental retardation; (*4*) seizures; (*5*) abnormal facial appearance including hypertelorism; (*6*) retinal colobomas; (*7*) brachydactyly; and (*8*) conductive hearing loss related to the skin abnormality.

References

1. Schnur RE et al: Acute lymphoblastic leukemia in a child with the CHIME neuroectodermal dysplasia syndrome. *Am J Med Genet* 72:24–29, 1997.
2. Shashi V et al: Neuroectodermal (CHIME) syndrome: an additional case with long-term follow-up of all reported cases. *J Med Genet* 32:465–469, 1995.
3. Zunich J, Kaye CI: New syndrome of congenital ichthyosis with neurologic abnormalities. *Am J Med Genet* 15:331–333, 1983.
4. Zunich J, Kaye CI: Additional case report of new neuroectodermal syndrome. *Am J Med Genet* 17:707–710, 1984.
5. Zunich J et al: Congenital migratory ichthyosiform dermatosis with neurologic and ophthalmologic abnormalities. *Arch Dermatol* 121:1149–1156, 1985.
6. Zunich J et al: Autosomal recessive transmission of neuroectodermal syndrome. *Arch Dermatol* 124:1188–1189, 1988.

Congenital ichthyosiform erythroderma, hepatomegaly, and congenital sensorineural hearing loss (Desmons syndrome)

In 1971, Desmons et al. (2) described three adult siblings with what may be a unique condition (3). There are many phenotypic similarities between this condition and KID syndrome.

Integumentary system. All affected individuals had congenital ichthyosiform erthryoderma, which primarily affected palms and soles. Hair and eyelashes were described as abundant and, in a 46-year-old female, they were white. Teeth and nails were normal.

Musculoskeletal system. Short stature was pronounced, with adult height of 141 cm in the female and 165 cm in the males.

Other findings. Hepatomegaly was marked in all three sibs and was diagnosed by age 4.

Auditory system. All sibs had profound, bilateral congenital sensorineural hearing loss.

Laboratory findings. Skin biopsy verified the clinical impression of ichthyosiform erythroderma. Liver biopsies revealed moderate glycogen storage, with cirrhosis in one individual. Connexin studies should be carried out.

Heredity. The condition was found in three sibs (one female and two males) who had unaffected parents and children. Inheritance is probably autosomal recessive.

Diagnosis. There are many similarities to KID syndrome but, as noted above, the metabolic derangements help distinguish this condition. Britton et al. (1) described a single male infant with hyperkeratosis, congenital hearing loss, and hepatomegaly, but the presence of total alopecia and recurrent infections and the transient nature of the hepatomegaly help distinguish this condition.

Prognosis. Although two sibs were still alive at the time of the report and were 57 and 41 years of age, a third sib had died at 41 years of liver failure. Intellectual function appeared to be normal.

Summary. The main characteristics of this condition include (*1*) autosomal recessive inheritance; (*2*) ichthyosiform erythroderma primarily affecting palms and soles; (*3*) short stature; (*4*) hepatomegaly; and (*5*) congenital sensorineural hearing loss.

References

1. Britton H et al: Keratosis follicularis spinulosa decalvans. *Arch Dermatol* 114:761–764, 1978.
2. Desmons F et al: Erythrodermie ichthyosiforme congenitale seche, surdi-mutité, hepatomegalie, de transmission recessive autosomique. *Bull Soc Fr Dermatol Syph* 78:585–591, 1971.
3. Wilson GN et al: Keratitis, hepatitis, ichthyosis, and deafness: report and review of KID syndrome. *Am J Med Genet* 40:255–259, 1991.

Generalized spiny hyperkeratosis, universal alopecia, and congenital sensorineural hearing loss

In 1969, Morris et al. (3) reported a syndrome of generalized hyperkeratosis, universal alopecia, and sensorineural hearing loss. In 1971, Myers et al. (4) reviewed the same patient and described another infant with the same disorder. Britton et al. (1), Salomon et al. (5), and Freire-Maia et al. (2) reported other examples of this condition.

Integumentary system. At or soon after birth, the skin became thick and the few scalp hairs were lost. There were markedly diminished sweating and frequent episodes of hyperthermia in warm weather.

The skin exhibited marked, generalized hyperkeratosis, some sites having spine-like projections of heaped keratin, whereas other places, such as the periorbital, perioral, and groin areas, were less hyperkeratinized (Fig. 14–15A,B). Follicular plugging was evident on the extremities (Fig. 14–15C). The palms and soles were uniformly hyperkeratotic. Universal alopecia with the exception of the eyelids having an occasional eyelash was noted. Acanthosis nigricans and nail involvement were documented (6).

Auditory system. Congenital bilateral moderately severe sensorineural hearing loss, more marked in the high tones, was evident (Fig. 14–15D). The external auditory canals were filled with hard, thick debris. When this was removed, the tympanic membranes were noted to be thickened. The temporal bones in one case showed Scheibe's cochleosaccular abnormality (4).

Vestibular system. Vestibular testing was not mentioned.

Laboratory findings. Salomon et al. (5) found low urinary levels of cystine, lysine, histidine, and arginine.

Pathology. Histopathologic study of the skin revealed basketweave hyperkeratosis. The dilated orifices of the pilar units were plugged, and the hair follicles were atrophied (Fig. 14–15E–H). None of the affected individuals had a positive family history. This may represent an autosomal dominant entity with each reported case representing a new mutation.

Diagnosis. This syndrome most closely resembles keratitis-ichthyosis-deafness (KID) syndrome. There are several shared features. Whether these represent separate entities is not known. Ichthyosis in its many forms can be excluded on clinical and histologic grounds.

Ichthyosiform erythroderma can also be excluded, since it is not associated with universal alopecia. Connexin studies are indicated

Prognosis. One child died in infancy from aspiration. Whether this death resulted from the child's having the syndrome cannot be ascertained from the limited number of examples.

Summary. Characteristics of this syndrome include (*1*) generalized spiny hyperkeratosis; (*2*) universal alopecia; (*3*) hypohidrosis; (*4*) obstruction of lacrimal punctae; and (*5*) congenital sensorineural hearing loss.

References

1. Britton H et al: Keratosis follicularis spinulosa decalvans. *Arch Dermatol* 114:761–764, 1978.
2. Freire-Maia N et al: An ectodermal dysplasia syndrome of alopecia, onychodysplasia, hypohidrosis, hyperkeratosis, deafness, and other manifestations. *Hum Hered* 27:127–133, 1977.
3. Morris J et al: Generalized spiny hyperkeratosis, universal alopecia, and deafness. *Arch Dermatol* 100:692–698, 1969.
4. Myers EN et al: Congenital deafness, spiny hyperkeratosis, and universal alopecia. *Arch Otolaryngol* 93:68–74, 1971.
5. Salomon T et al: Erythrodermia ichthyosiformis congenita, mit Hypotrichose, Anhidrose, Taubstummheit und verminderten Ausscheidung einiger Aminosäuren im Harn. *Hautarzt* 25:448–453, 1974.

Ichthyosis, hystrix-like, with deafness (HID)

Heinz-Wilhelm (4) and Gülzow and Anton-Lamprecht (3) described patients with ichthyosis hystrix and bilateral deafness (Fig. 14–15G,H). Other sporadic patients were subsequently described (1,2); Konig et al. (5) described an affected parent and child, leading to the suggestion that this is an autosomal dominant trait. The skin abnormalities appear soon after birth and resemble an erythema. Soon thereafter, hyperkeratotic masses appear and involve most of the skin. Palms and soles are mildly affected, thus differentiating this condition from KID syndrome. Sweating is decreased, and head hair may be scant secondary to scarring alopecia. Eyelashes also tend to be absent, whereas beard, pubic, and axillary hair can be present, but scanty. Hearing loss is moderately severe and is likely congenital. Retinas in one patient (1) were described as albinoid. Pes cavus and hypoactive reflexes were also present in this patient. Mental retardation does not occur in this condition.

Nousari et al. (6) described a patient with ichthyosis hystrix and deafness, but with other features that were more consistent with a diagnosis of KID syndrome. They suggested that HID and KID syndromes are variants of the same disorder. Others have noted that there are differences observed on electron microscopy (7), therefore these two conditions could also be distinct. However, it has been shown that both conditions are caused by identical mutations in connexin 26, thus they are indeed the same disorder (8).

References

1. Baden HP, Bronstein BR: Ichthyosiform dermatosis and deafness. *Arch Dermatol* 124:102–106, 1988.
2. Badillet C et al: Ichtyosiform dermatosis and deafness: report of a case and review of the literature. *Arch Dermatol* 124:102–106, 1988.
3. Gülzow J, Anton-Lamprecht I: Ichthyosis hystrix gravior typus Rheydt: ein otologisch-dermatologisches Syndrome. *Laryngol Rhinol Otol (Stuttg)* 56:949–955, 1977.
4. Heinz-Wilhelm B: Ichthosis hystrix Typus Rheydt (Ichthyosis hystrix gravior mit praktischer Taubheit). *Z Hautkrankheit* 52:763–766, 1977.
5. Konig A et al: Autosomal dominant inheritance of HID syndrome (hystrix-like ichthyosis with deafness). *Eur J Dermatol* 7:554–555, 1997.
6. Nousari H et al: KID syndrome associated with features of ichthyosis hystrix. *Pediatr Dermatol* 17:115–117, 2000.
7. Traupe H: *The Genetic Ichthyoses, in Texbook of Pediatric Dermatology.* Harper J, Oranje A, Prose N (eds), Blackwell Science, 2000.
8. Van Geel M et al: HID and KID syndromes are associated with the same connexin 26 mutation. *Br J Dermatol* 146:938–942, 2002.

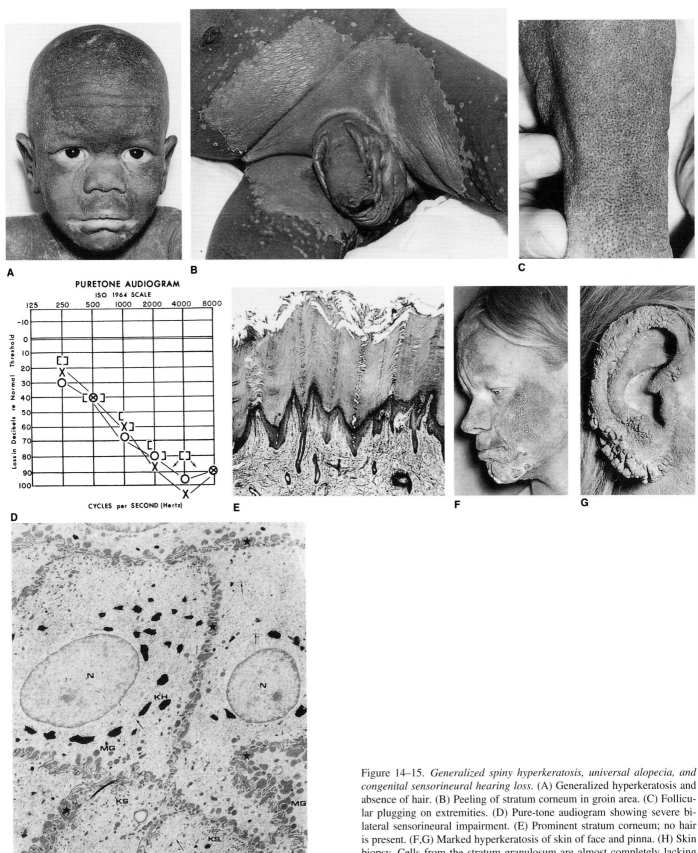

Figure 14–15. *Generalized spiny hyperkeratosis, universal alopecia, and congenital sensorineural hearing loss.* (A) Generalized hyperkeratosis and absence of hair. (B) Peeling of stratum corneum in groin area. (C) Follicular plugging on extremities. (D) Pure-tone audiogram showing severe bilateral sensorineural impairment. (E) Prominent stratum corneum; no hair is present. (F,G) Marked hyperkeratosis of skin of face and pinna. (H) Skin biopsy. Cells from the stratum granulosum are almost completely lacking tonofibrils, normal keratohyaline granules (KH), numerous keratinosomes (KS), and unusual production of mucous granules (MG). [(A–C) from J Morris et al., *Arch Dermatol* 100:692, 1969; (D–E) from EN Myers et al., *Arch Otolaryngol* 93:68, 1971; (F–H) from J Gülzow and I Anton-Lamprecht, *Laryngol Rhinol Otol* 56:949, 1977.]

Keratopachydermia, digital constrictions, and sensorineural hearing loss (Vohwinkel-Nockemann syndrome)

The term *Vohwinkel syndrome* refers to the combination of hyperkeratosis involving the palms, soles, knees, and elbows, and ring-like furrows developing on the fingers and toes. These features in conjunction with congenital sensorineural hearing loss affecting four members of a kindred were described by Nockemann (15) in 1961. Similarly involved individuals have been reported by other authors (1,7–10,14,16,18,20).

Integumentary system. By about 2 years of age, thickening of the palmar and plantar skin begins, followed by involvement of the skin of the elbows and knees (Fig. 14–16A–D). At about 5 years of age, ring-shaped furrows develop in the skin and soft tissues of the middle phalanx of fingers and toes (Fig. 14–16A). This condition has been severe enough to require digital amputation in several affected persons (15) (Fig. 14–16C). The patients of Drummond (9) developed constricting bands around three fingers of each hand. The bands were about 1/8 to 1/4 inch in width and encircled each affected finger. Marked hyperker-

atosis of the palms and a thickening of the epidermis over the knuckles and knees were evident. In some patients, the hyperkeratoses of the dorsa of the hands and feet were starfish-shaped; those on the knees and elbows tended to be linear (10) (Fig. 14–16B,C). Diffuse alopecia of the scalp began at about 15 years of age. Ainhum-like constriction of all toes appeared near the posterior nail fold.

Histologic examination of one of the digits, which had been removed because of severe pain, showed marked thickening of the stratum corneum of the skin (15). In the area of the groove this layer was reduced to half this thickness. The remaining layers of the epithelium were normal but somewhat thinner in the area of constriction. Elastic fibers were more abundant and interconnected in the area of the grooves.

Auditory system. All individuals reported by Nockemann (15) and Drummond (9) manifested congenital profound hearing loss. No other audiometric information was presented. Other patients have had bilateral high-frequency sensorineural hearing loss (1,2,8,10,20). Ocaña Sierra et al. (16) noted progressive sensorineural hearing loss. However, none of the individuals reported by Camisa and Rossana (7) had hearing loss (but however, see Heredity).

Figure 14–16. *Keratopachydermia, digital constrictions, and sensorineural hearing loss (Vohwinkel-Nockermann syndrome).* (A–D) Sharply marginated hyperkeratosis of palms and soles. Note digital contrictions, which, in one case, have led to amputation of a toe. Also note starfish-

like alterations of dorsum of hand and linear lesions of knees. (E) Pedigree of family. [(A–D) from F Aksu and C Mietens, *Pädiatr Prax* 23:303, 1980; (E) modified from PF Nockemann, *Med Welt* 56:1894, 1961.]

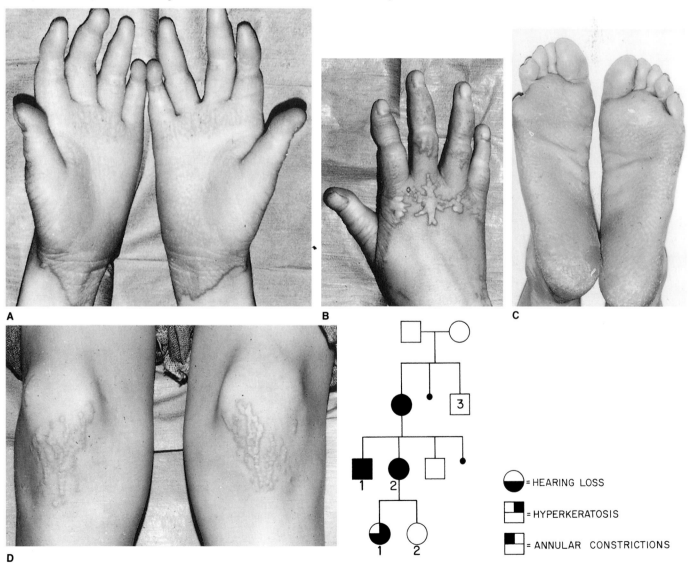

Vestibular system. No mention was made of vestibular tests by any author.

Radiographic findings. Radiographs of the feet of the proband described by Gibbs and Frank (10) showed constriction of the shaft of the distal phalanx of the right fourth toe.

Heredity. Pedigrees have shown dominant transmission (10,15, 16,20) (Fig. 14–16E). The patients presented by Drummond (9) and Chang Sing Pang et al. (8) represented isolated cases. Maestrini et al. (12) studied the family reported by Camisa and Rossana (7) and mapped the gene to 1q21. They subsequently identified a mutation in the loricrin gene; loricrin is a major component of the cornified cell envelope. Korge et al. (11) also found mutations in loricrin, but only in those individuals who did not have deafness. In some of the patients who also had deafness (16,18), Maestrini et al. (13) found a missense mutation in the connexin 26 gene. Vohwinkel syndrome is clearly heterogeneous, with the form associated with ichthyosis caused by loricrin mutations, and the form associated with deafness caused, at least in part, by connexin 26 mutations.

Diagnosis. Ainhum-like constriction of the digits and hyperkeratosis of the palms and soles as a binary combination (Vohwinkel syndrome) have been described by many authors (7,17,19,21), but hearing loss was not mentioned. This is clearly a distinct entity, as noted above. It has been described as an autosomal recessive disorder as well (3). Ring-like constriction of the digits, seen with a plethora of hereditary and nonhereditary conditions, has been extensively reviewed by Gibbs and Frank (10). Bhatia et al. (4) reported an autosomal recessively inherited disorder of Vohwinkel syndrome and congenital alopecia universalis. However, in none of these conditions was there associated hearing loss. The hearing loss syndrome reported by Bititci (5) involved a circumscribed palmoplantar keratoderma (vide infra).

The syndrome of keratopachydermia, digital constrictions, and hearing loss can be distinguished from other isolated cases of annular constrictions of the fingers and toes because of the marked hearing loss and dominant transmission of the disorder.

Prognosis. There is no apparent change in hearing loss with age. The prognosis for the involved digits is poor, since there is usually continuing constriction of the phalanges and eventual loss of some digits, although oral etretinate seems to reverse this process (6,8,20).

Summary. Characteristics of this syndrome include (1) dominant transmission, probably autosomal; (2) hyperkeratosis of the palms, soles, elbows, and knees; (3) ring-like constrictions of the soft tissues of the middle phalanges of the fingers and toes; and (4) congenital mild to severe sensorineural hearing loss.

References

1. Aksu F, Mietens C: Keratopachydermie mit Schnurfürchen an Fingern und Zehen und Innenohrschwerhörigkeit. *Pädiatr Prax* 23:303–310, 1980.
2. Bell M et al: Pseudo-Ainhum bei Morbus Vohwinkel. *Hautarzt* 44:738–741, 1993.
3. Bergman R et al: Mal de Maleda keratoderma with pseudoainhum. *Br J Dermatol* 128:207–212, 1993.
4. Bhatia KK et al: Keratomahereditaria mutilans (Vohwinkel's disease) with congenital alopecia universalis (atrichia congenita). *J Dermatol* 16:231–236, 1989.
5. Bititci OO: Familial hereditary progressive sensorineural hearing loss with keratosis palmaris and plantaris. *J Laryngol Otol* 89:1143–1146, 1975.
6. Brambilla L et al: Unusual case of Meleda keratoderma treated with aromatic retinoid etretinate. *Dermatologica* 168:283–286, 1984.
7. Camisa C, Rossana C: Variant of keratoderma hereditaria mutilans (Vohwinkel's syndrome). *Arch Dermatol* 120:1323–1328, 1984.
8. Chang Sing Pang AFI et al: Successful treatment of keratoderma hereditaria mutilans with an aromatic retinoid. *Arch Dermatol* 117:225–228, 1981.
9. Drummond MA: A case of unusual skin disease. *Irish J Med Sci* 8:85–86, 1939.
10. Gibbs RC, Frank SB: Keratomahereditaris mutilans (Vohwinkel). *Arch Dermatol* 94:619–625, 1966.
11. Korge BP et al: Loricrin mutation in Vohwinkel's keratoderma is unique to the variant with ichthyosis. *J Invest Dermatol* 109:604–610, 1997.
12. Maestrini E et al: A molecular defect in loricrin, the major component of the cornified cell envelope, underlies Vohwinkel's syndrome. *Nat Genet* 13:70–77, 1996.
13. Maestrini E et al: A missense mutation in connexin26, D66H, causes mutilating keratoderma with sensorineural deafness (Vohwinkel's syndrome) in three unrelated families. *Hum Mol Genet* 8:1237–1243, 1999.
14. McGibbon DH, Watson RT: Vohwinkel's syndrome and deafness. *J Laryngol Otol* 91:853–857, 1977.
15. Nockemann PF: Erbliche Hornhautverdickung mit Schnurfürchen an Fingern und Zehen und Innenohrschwerhörigkeit. *Med Welt* 56:1894–1900, 1961.
16. Ocaña Sierra J et al: Syndrome de Vohwinkel. *Ann Dermatol Syph* 102: 41–45, 1975.
17. Piers F: Hereditary keratodermia and ainhum. *Br J Dermatol* 79:693–698, 1967.
18. Sensi A et al: Vohwinkel syndrome (mutilating keratoderma associated with craniofacial anomalies). *Am J Med Genet* 50:201–203, 1994.
19. Vohwinkel KH: Keratomahereditarium mutilans. *Arch Dermatol Syph* 158:354–364, 1929.
20. Wereide K: Mutilating palmoplantar keratoderma successfully treated with etretinate. *Acta Dermatovenereol* 64:566–569, 1984.
21. Wigley JEM: A case of hyperkeratosis palmaris et plantaris associated with ainhum-like constriction of the fingers. *Br J Dermatol* 41:188–191, 1929.

Palmoplantar hyperkeratosis and sensorineural hearing loss

A number of authors have described individuals or families with palmoplantar hyperkeratosis and sensorineural hearing loss as a binary syndrome. This is a heterogeneous group, which has only recently begun to be sorted out. Families with autosomal dominant progressive sensorineural hearing loss were described by Bititci (1), Hatamochi et al. (4), and Sharland et al. (10) (Fig. 14–17). In most cases, ultimate hearing loss has been severe. Sevior et al. (9) described another family with apparent autosomal dominant inheritance of palmoplantar hyperkeratosis and deafness. They identified in this family and the one reported by Hatamochi et al. (4) an A75445G mitochondrial mutation which they believed was responsible for the phenotype. They also pointed out that in the family reported by Bititci (1) there was no male-to-male inheritance, a finding also consistent with mitochondrial inheritance. Martin et al. (7) also described a family with this mutation and the combination of palmoplantar hyperkeratosis and deafness. Heathcote et al. (6) studied the family reported by Sharland et al. (10) and found a missense mutation (G59A) in the connexin 26 gene. In addition, Richard et al. (8) described a family with profound prelingual deafness and palmoplantar keratoderma in which an R75W missense mutation in the connexin 26 gene was found. Uyguner et al. (12) reported a family with an R75Q mutation in the connexin 26 gene. The reader is referred back to the previous entry in which D66H mutations of the connexin 26 gene occur. Blanchet-Bardon et al. (2) reported an isolated example. Two patients, reported as examples of Papillon-Lefèvre syndrome (palmoplantar hyperkeratosis with periodontopathia) with hearing loss, are those of Thorel (11) and Hübner and Menzel (5). The case of Thorel (11) appears to be a legitimate example. The parents were consanguineous. However, that of Hübner and Menzel (5) does not appear to represent Papillon-Lefèvre syndrome. The description of the periodontal disorder, appearing in the 20's, is certainly not typical of that syndrome. Gloor et al. (3) described sibs with circumscripted palmoplantar keratoses and hearing loss. An additional sib had CHILD syndrome, but they suspected that this was adventitious.

References

1. Bititci OO: Familial hereditary progressive sensorineural hearing loss with keratosis palmaris and plantaris. *J Laryngol Otol* 89:1143–1146, 1975.
2. Blanchet-Bardon C et al: Clinically specific type of focal palmoplantar keratoderma with sensorineural deafness. *Dermatologica* 175:148–151, 1987.
3. Gloor M et al: Familiäre zirkumscripte Plantarkeratose mit Schallempfindungsschwerhörigkeit. *Hautarzt* 440:304–307, 1989.
4. Hatamochi A et al: Diffuse palmoplantar keratoderma with deafness. *Arch Dermatol* 118:605–607, 1982.

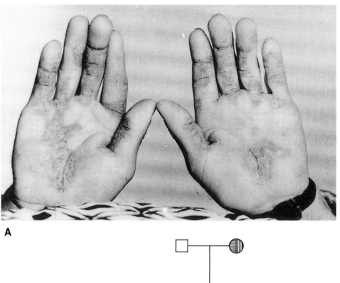

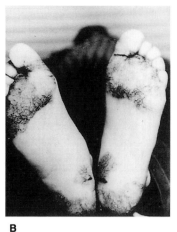

A

B

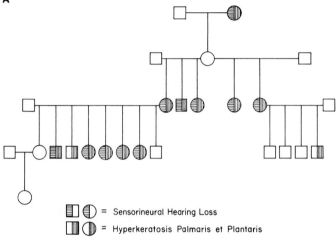

C

□╫ ◖╫ = Sensorineural Hearing Loss

▥ ◖╫▥ = Hyperkeratosis Palmaris et Plantaris

Figure 14–17. *Palmoplantar hyperkeratosis and sensorineural hearing loss.* (A,B) Focal hyperkeratosis of palms and soles. (C) Modified pedigree of family. [(A,B) from OO Bititci, *J Laryngol Otol* 89:1143, 1975.]

5. Hübner U, Menzel V: Keratosis palmoplantaris mit Periodontopathie (Papillon-Lefèvre-Syndrom) und Innenohrschwerhörigkeit. *Dermatol Monatsschr* 174:267–271, 1988.

6. Heathcote K et al: A connexin 26 mutation causes a syndrome of sensorineural hearing loss and palmoplantar hyperkeratosis (MIM 148350). *J Med Genet* 37:50–51, 2000.

7. Martin L et al: Inherited palmoplantar keratoderma and sensorineural deafness associated with A7445G point mutation in the mitochondrial genome. *Br J Dermatol* 143:876–883, 2000.

8. Richard G et al: Functional defects of Cx26 resulting from a heterozygous missense mutation in a family with dominant deaf-mutism and palmoplantar keratoderma. *Hum Genet* 103:393–399, 1998.

9. Sevior KB et al: Mitochondrial A7445G mutation in two pedigrees with palmoplantar keratoderma and deafness. *Am J Med Genet* 75:179–185, 1998.

10. Sharland M et al: Autosomal dominant palmoplantar hyperkeratosis and sensorineural deafness in three generations. *J Med Genet* 29:50–52, 1992.

11. Thorel F: Un cas de maladie de Méléda variété Papillon-Lefévre avec surdité. *Bull Soc Fr Dermatol Syph* 71:707–708, 1964.

12. Uyguner O et al: The novel R75Q mutation in the *GJB2* gene causes autosomal dominant hearing loss and palmoplantar keratoderma in a Turkish family. *Clin Genet* 62:306–309, 2002.

Palmoplantar hyperkeratosis, leukonychia, and sensorineural hearing loss

In 1983, Crosti et al. (3) reported two brothers with hyperkeratosis of the palms and soles, total leukonychia, and sensorineural hearing loss. The leukonychia as an isolated finding in fingers and toes involved this family for three generations. It began in early childhood and affected four other members.

The scalp hair of the two boys was rough, bristly, and dark in color. Ultrastructural study revealed dysplasia with changes such as complete and incomplete twisting (pili torti) and longitudinal grooves.

Palmoplantar hyperkeratosis appeared by the age of 5 years. The teeth of both sibs had transverse linear hypoplasia of the enamel.

Hearing loss was congenital, but not otherwise described.

Total congenital leukonychia as an isolated finding is inherited as an autosomal dominant trait. It has also been seen in association with knuckle pads, leukonychia, and mixed hearing loss, with total alopecia (4) and multiple sebaceous cysts (1,2). Pili torti has been described with sensorineural hearing loss and with hyperkeratosis palmaris, tooth anomalies, and sensorineural hearing loss.

References

1. Bauer AW: Beiträge zur klinischen Konstitutionpathologie. V. Heredofamiliäre Leukonychie und multiple Atherombildung der Kopfhaut. *Z Ang Anat* 5:47–58, 1920.

2. Bushkill L et al: Leukonychia totalis, multiple sebaceous cysts and renal calculi. A syndrome. *Arch Dermatol* 111:899–900, 1975.

3. Crosti C et al: Leuconychie totale et dysplasie ectodermique. Observations de deux cas. *Ann Dermatol Venereol* 110:617–622, 1983.

4. Darier J, Le Sourd L: Pelade décalvante avec des lesions des ongles. *Ann Dermatol Syph* 9:1009–1013, 1898.

Palmoplantar hyperkeratosis, short stature, unusual facial appearance, hypodontia, and sensorineural hearing loss

In 1989, Seow (1) described 18 members of a four-generation family with a syndrome comprising palmoplantar hyperkeratosis, proportionate short stature, unusual face, clinodactyly, epilepsy, hypodontia, and sensorineural hearing loss. Among five family members examined, the facies was characterized by frontal bossing and ocular hypertelorism (Fig. 14–18A). Abnormal hair whorls and a low posterior hairline were also observed.

Integumentary system. Moderate diffuse hyperkeratosis of the palms and soles was noted at birth. Hypoplasia of the nails ranged from severe hypoplasia in the fifth finger to mild hypoplasia in other fingers (Fig. 14–18B–D).

Musculoskeletal system. The patients were of proportionate short stature (less than third centile). Clinodactyly of the fifth fingers was noted, and bone age was grossly retarded. Three of five members examined exhibited epilepsy of petit mal type.

Dental findings. Four of five individuals had missing teeth, most often the lower lateral incisors. One had taurodontism, two had enamel hypoplasia, and one had fused maxillary incisors (Fig. 14–18E).

Heredity. Inheritance was clearly autosomal dominant.

References

1. Seow WK: Palmoplantar hyperkeratosis with short stature, facial dysmorphism, and hypodontia—a new syndrome? *Pediatr Dent* 11:145–150, 1989.

Figure 14–18. *Palmoplantar hyperkeratosis, short stature, unusual facial appearance, hypodontia, and sensorineural hearing loss.* (A) Hypertelorism, frontal bossing, and low hairline. (B–D) Palmoplantar hyperkeratosis, clinodactyly, and hypoplasia of nail of fifth finger. [From WK Seow, *Pediatr Dent* 11:145, 1989.]

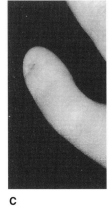
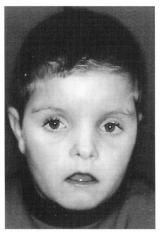
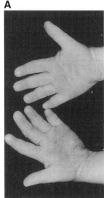
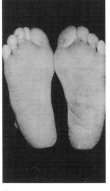

A

B   C   D

Mutilating keratopachydermia, hypotrichosis, acrodermatitis enteropathica-like lesions, and sensorineural hearing loss (Olmsted syndrome)

In 1927, Olmsted (7) described a syndrome of infantile onset of progressive hyperkeratosis of palmar and plantar surfaces and flexor areas of extremities. Over 20 cases have subsequently been reported, including several recent reports and reviews (1–6, 8–10).

Hyperkeratosis is noted around body orifices, periorally, in the groin, and on the inner thighs. Oral and perioral hyperkeratosis can be marked (6) (Fig. 14–19A,B). The keratoses are diffuse, symmetric, and sharply marginated. They lead to flexion contractures of the fingers (Fig. 14–19C,D). There is associated hypohidrosis. Linear papules are observed at friction sites. Nail dystrophy is present. The distal phalanges of the extremities undergo dissolution (Fig. 14–19E,F). Hypotrichosis or generalized alopecia is evident from birth. The joints are excessively lax (Fig. 14–19G). There appears to be an association with malignant epithelial tumors, and in one case, malignant melanoma (3). Various histopathologic studies have been done, and have found hyperproliferation of the epidermis (6,9). Immunoreactivity studies found abnormal expression of keratins 5 and 14 (4). Although some have found improvement after treatment with retinoids (3,10), others have not (5).

Hearing loss has been noted at higher frequencies. Most patients represent sporadic occurrences, although autosomal dominant inheritance has been suggested (1). Other mutilating keratopachydermias and acrodermatitis enteropathica must be considered in the differential diagnosis.

References

1. Atherton DJ et al: Mutilating palmoplantar keratoderma with periorificial keratotic plaques (Olmsted's syndrome). *Br J Dermatol* 122:245–252, 1990.
2. Bergonse FN et al: Olmsted syndrome: the clinical spectrum of mutilating palmoplantar keratoderma. *Pediatr Dermatol* 20:323–326, 2003.
3. Dessureault J et al: Olmsted syndrome-palmoplantar and periorificial keratodermas: associated with malignant melanoma. *J Cutan Med Surg* Apr 22 [Epub ahead of print], 2003
4. Fonseca E et al: Olmsted syndrome. *J Cutan Pathol* 28:271–275, 2001.
5. Frias-Iniesta J et al.: Olmsted syndrome: report of a new case. *Br J Dermatol* 136:935–939, 1997.
6. Larregue M et al: Olmsted syndrome:report of two new cases and literature review. *J Dermatol* 27:557–568, 2000.
7. Olmsted HC: Keratoderma palmaris et plantaris congenitalis: report of a case showing associated lesions of unusual location. *Am J Dis Child* 33:757–764, 1927.
8. Poulin Y et al: Olmsted syndrome–congenital palmoplantar and peri-orificial keratoderma. *J Am Acad Dermatol* 10:600–610, 1984
9. Requena L et al: Olmsted syndrome: report of a case with study of the cellular proliferation in keratoderma. *Am J Dermatopathol* 23:514–520, 2001.
10. Ueda M et al: Partial improvement of Olmsted syndrome with etretinate. *Pediatr Dermatol* 10:376–381, 1993.

Knuckle pads, leukonychia, and mixed hearing loss (Schwann syndrome, Bart-Pumphrey syndrome)

A syndrome consisting of leukonychia, knuckle pads, and mixed hearing loss was first described by Schwann (5) in 1963. Bart and Pumphrey (1), Crosby and Vidurrizaga (2), and Ramer et al. (4) confirmed the association.

Integumentary system. In two kindreds, firm, thickened skin or knuckle pads appeared over the interphalangeal joints of the fingers and toes from early childhood. All fingernails and toenails exhibited leukonychia (white nails) obscuring the lunula. Hyperkeratosis of the palms and soles appeared in middle life (Fig. 14–20A–E). In one family (1), spoon-nails (koilonychia) also developed. A 13-year-old male proband had hyperkeratosis of the palms and soles as well as leukonychia (2).

Auditory system. Audiometric findings in the patients were variable. Bart and Pumphrey (1) noted a 10–100 dB hearing loss, most marked in

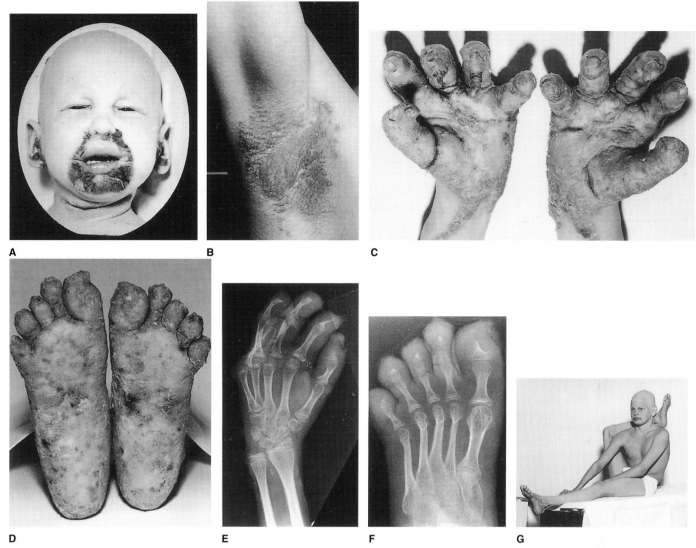

Figure 14–19. *Mutilating keratopachydermia, hypotrichosis, acrodermatitis enteropathica-like lesions, and sensorineural hearing loss (Olmstead syndrome).* (A) Acrodermatitis enteropathica–like changes around mouth, nose, ears at 2 years of age. (B–D) Involvement of hands, feet, and axilla at 21 years. Thick keratoderma with marked destruction of digits. Note sharp margination at wrists with linear extension to forearms. (E,F) Severe osteoporosis with osteolysis of terminal phalanges and soft tissue swellings. (G) Large joints exhibit striking laxity. [(C–G) from Y Poulin et al., *J Am Acad Dermatol* 10:600, 1984.]

the higher frequencies (Fig. 14–20F). In two cases, a pure sensorineural hearing loss was present. In the remaining three cases, mixed hearing loss was present in at least one ear. In another case, one ear showed a 10–70 dB sensorineural hearing loss while the other ear had a 70–90 dB mixed hearing loss. The left middle ear of one patient showed such disorganization that the ossicles and facial nerve could not be identified. In the second family, three members had sensorineural defect that was severe in one and moderate in two; the fourth family member had a minor sensorineural loss and slight conductive defect bilaterally. Schwann (5) noted congenital severe hearing loss, otherwise unspecified. Radiographs of the temporal bones showed normal cochlear and labyrinthine structures. Ramer et al. (4) suggested that affected females have greater hearing loss.

Vestibular system. Caloric vestibular tests were described in three individuals. One showed normal response, while another showed no response, indicating vestibular paresis. The third patient had a hypoactive response on one side and a normal response on the other (1).

Heredity. Bart and Pumphrey (1) found a total of 21 affected persons in six generations with autosomal dominant transmission (Fig.

14–20G). Nine had only hearing loss, whereas the others had both hearing loss and leukonychia. It is possible that leukonychia was not noted in those not carefully examined. Crosby and Vidurrizaga (2) described a father and three children.

Diagnosis. Leukonychia, by itself, is inherited as an autosomal dominant trait. It may be associated with a plethora of syndromes. Three other syndromes exhibiting abnormalities of the nails and hearing loss, namely, dominant onychodystrophy, coniform teeth, and sensorineural hearing loss, DOOR syndrome, and palmoplantar hyperkeratosis, leukonychia, and sensorineural hearing loss, must be excluded.

The combination of knuckle pads with leukonychia and palmoplantar keratoderma is seen most often without hearing loss (3).

Prognosis. The hearing loss was not progressive.

Summary. Characteristics of the syndrome include (*1*) autosomal dominant inheritance; (*2*) knuckle pads overfingers and toes; (*3*) leukonychia; (*4*) hyperkeratosis of palms and soles; and (*5*) mild to severe mixed hearing loss.

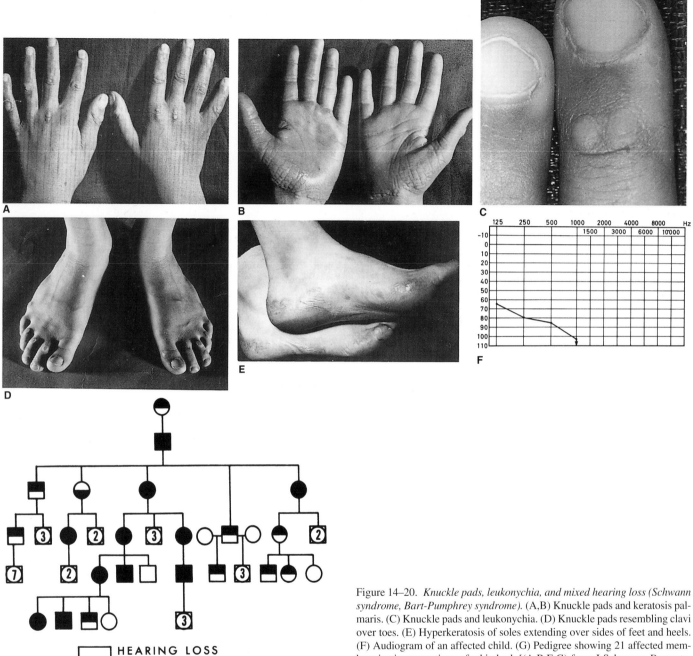

Figure 14–20. *Knuckle pads, leukonychia, and mixed hearing loss (Schwann syndrome, Bart-Pumphrey syndrome).* (A,B) Knuckle pads and keratosis palmaris. (C) Knuckle pads and leukonychia. (D) Knuckle pads resembling clavi over toes. (E) Hyperkeratosis of soles extending over sides of feet and heels. (F) Audiogram of an affected child. (G) Pedigree showing 21 affected members in six generations of a kindred. [(A,B,E,G) from J Schwann, *Dermatologica* 126:335, 1963; (C,D,F) from RS Bart and RE Pumphrey, *N Engl J Med* 276:202, 1967.]

References

1. Bart RS, Pumphrey RE: Knuckle pads, leukonychia, and deafness: a dominantly inherited syndrome. *N Engl J Med* 276:202–207, 1967.
2. Crosby EF, Vidurrizaga RH: Knuckle pads, leukonychia, deafness,and keratosis palmoplantaris. Report of a family. *Johns Hopkins Med J* 129(Suppl):90–92, 1976.
3. Paller AS, Hebert AA: Knuckle pads in children. *Am J Dis Child* 140:915–917, 1986.
4. Ramer JC et al: Familial leukonychia, knuckle pads, hearing loss, and palmoplantar hyperkeratosis: an additional family with Bart-Pumphrey syndrome. *J Med Genet* 31:68–71, 1994.
5. Schwann J: Keratosis palmaris et plantaris cum surditate congenita et leukonychia totale unguium. *Dermatologica* 126:335–353, 1963.

Hyperkeratosis palmoplantaris striata, pili torti, hypohidrosis, oligodontia, and sensorineural hearing loss

In 1982, Egelund and Frentz (2) reported a 14-year-old female with lusterless coarse terminal scalp hair, sparse eyebrows and lashes, hyperkeratosis of palms and soles, generalized hypohidrosis (except for palms), oligodontia, and moderate nonprogressive mid-frequency sensorineural hearing loss. A paternal grandmother was noted to have similar hair, eyebrows, and palmoplantar hyperkeratosis. The intervening parent was apparently unaffected, however.

Braun-Falco and Landthaler (1) described an 18-year-old female with ichthyosis vulgaris, pili torti, hypodontia, and sensorineural hearing loss. Both parents had hearing loss but none of the other stigmata.

References

1. Braun-Falco O, Landthaler M: Ichthyosis vulgaris, Taubheit, Pili torti und Zahnanomalien. *Hautarzt* 29:276–280, 1978.
2. Egelund E, Frentz G: Case of hyperkeratosis palmoplantaris combined with pili torti, hypohidrosis, hypodontia and hypacusis. *Acta Otolaryngol* 94:571–573, 1982.

Pili torti and sensorineural hearing loss (Björnstad syndrome)

A syndrome characterized by pili torti (flat, twisted hair) and sensorineural hearing loss was described by Björnstad (2) in 1965. A number of other authors have recognized this combination (4,6,7,9–16,18,19).

Integumentary system. The hair is untidy in appearance, being short, dry, lusterless, and brittle. Scalp hair, eyebrows, and eyelashes are usually affected (Fig. 14–21A,B). Pili torti is often present at birth but occasionally develops during childhood. The teeth, nails, and skin are generally normal, although one patient described by Porters (11) had greenish, fragile teeth with no evidence of enamel dysplasia.

Auditory system. Although approximately 50% of patients reported had a 20–80 dB hearing loss that was more severe at high tones (2,4,9,11,12,15,19), the patient described by Robinson and Johnston (14) had severe bilateral sensorineural hearing loss. Onset of hearing loss ranges from being congenital to developing in adulthood. Scott et al. (15) found profound hearing deficit over the entire hearing range.

No other audiometric tests were described.

Other findings. Because one of the original patients described by Björnstad had genital hypoplasia, it has been suggested that hypogo-

nadism is an occasional manifestation of this condition. This would therefore suggest that the sibs reported by Reed et al. (12) and later Crandall et al. (3) had Björnstad syndrome, rather than a distinct condition.

Vestibular system. Vestibular tests were not reported.

Pathology. Microscopic examination of the hair show markedly flattened, moderately twisted hairs (Fig. 14–21C,D).

Heredity. Although evidence suggests that the syndrome is hereditary, the mode of transmission is not clear. Björnstad (2) reported five patients with this disorder. Two had affected sibs and one had an affected aunt. The two other patients were isolated examples. Of the four patients described by Reed et al. (3,12), three were thought later to have another syndrome (see Crandall syndrome), and the fourth boy had a deaf mother who was not examined. Audiograms and physical examinations of the three sibs of the 5-year-old girl described by Robinson and Johnston (14) were normal. There was no family history of hearing loss or hair defect. The only parent with possible involvement described by Reed et al. (12) was not examined by the authors. Cremers and Geerts (4) described two families with an apparently dominant mode of inheritance with low penetrance for hearing loss, whereas Porters (11) described affected sibs with normal parents. Voigtländer (19) reported two affected sibs with normal parents. Lubianca Neto et al. (7) described a large kindred that appeared consistent with autosomal recessive inheritance. They mapped the causative gene to 2q34–36. Petit et al. (9) and Richards and Mancini (13) found autosomal dominant inheritance. This is therefore likely a heterogeneous entity with both dominant and recessive forms, with hearing loss being a more infrequent sign in the autosomal dominant form.

Diagnosis. Pili torti without hearing loss inherited as a dominant trait has been described. Björnstad (2) presented eight patients, only five of whom had sensorineural hearing loss. Whether all had the same syndrome with variable hearing loss or there were two separate conditions (genetic heterogeneity)—both with pili torti but only one with hearing loss—is not yet clear. A number of conditions associated with short, brittle hair must be excluded (Menke disease, monilethrix, pseu-

Figure 14–21. *Pili torti and sensorineural hearing loss (Björnstad syndrome).* (A) Twenty-year-old female with short, sparse, easily breakable hair. Note hearing aid. (B) Hair of 23-year-old affected brother showing irregular reflection of light. (C) Twisted hair shaft. (D) Note band-like hair shaft showing torsion on its own axis and marked cuticular defects. [(A,B,D) from V Voigtländer, *Dermatologica* 159:50, 1979; (C) courtesy of CWRJ Cremers, Nijmegen, The Netherlands.]

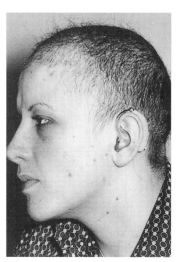
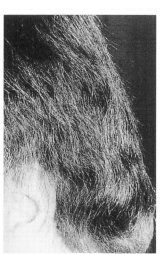
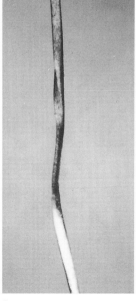
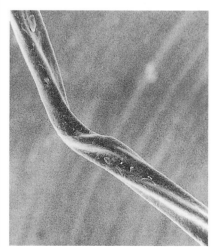

A   **B**   **C**   **D**

domonilethrix, Netherton disease, trichorrhexis nodosa, argininosuccinic aciduria, etc.) but none has associated hearing loss (1,5,8,10,16). Differential diagnosis has been well discussed by Scott et al. (15).

The syndrome of hyperkeratosis palmoplantaris striata, pili torti, hypodontia, and sensorineural hearing loss appears to be a distinct entity.

Prognosis. There is no evidence that the hearing loss is progressive. Mental retardation is a fairly infrequent complication (11,17).

Summary. Characteristics of this disease include (*1*) probable autosomal recessive inheritance; (*2*) congenital pili torti; and (*3*) congenital moderate to severe sensorineural hearing loss.

References

1. Bentley-Phillips B, Bayles MAN: A previously undescribed hereditary hair anomaly (pseudo-monilethrix). *Br J Dermatol* 89:159–167, 1973.
2. Björnstad R: Pili torti and sensory-neural loss of hearing. In: Proceedings of the 17th Meeting of Combined Scandinavian Dermatology Association, Copenhagen, May, 1965.
3. Crandall BF et al: A familial syndrome of deafness, alopecia and hypogonadism. *J Pediatr* 82:461–465, 1973.
4. Cremers CWRJ, Geerts SJ: Sensorineural hearing loss and pili torti. *Ann Otol Rhinol Laryngol* 88:100–104, 1979 [family 3 is same as that of Porters (11)].
5. Levin B: Arginosuccinic aciduria. *Am J Dis Child* 113:162–165, 1967.
6. Loche F et al: Pili torti with congenital deafness (Björnstad syndrome): a case report. *Pediatr Dermatol* 16:220–221, 1999.
7. Lubianca Neto et al: The Björnstad syndrome (sensorineural hearing loss and pili torti) disease gene maps to chromosome 2q34–36. *Am J Hum Genet* 62:1107–1112, 1998.
8. Michalowski R et al: Netherton-Syndrom mit Alopezie und Prolinurie. *Hautarzt* 29:205–208, 1978.
9. Petit A et al: Pili torti with congenital deafness (Björnstad's syndrome)—review of three cases in one family suggesting autosomal dominant inheritance. *Clin Exp Dermatol* 18:94–95, 1993.
10. Pollitt RJ et al: Sibs with mental and physical retardation and trichorrhexis nodosa with abnormal amino acid composition of the hair. *Arch Dis Child* 43:211–216, 1968.
11. Porters JE: Pili torti met neurologische doofheid. *Ned Tijdschr Geneeskd* 120:311, 1976.
12. Reed WB et al: Hereditary syndromes with auditory and dermatological manifestations. *Arch Dermatol* 95:456–461, 1967.
13. Richards KA, Mancini AJ: Three members of a family with pili torti and sensorineural hearing loss: the Björnstad syndrome. *J Am Acad Dermatol* 46:301–303, 2002.
14. Robinson GC, Johnston MM: Pili torti and sensory neural hearing loss. *J Pediatr* 70:621–623, 1967.
15. Scott MJ et al: Björnstad syndrome and pili torti. *Pediatr Dermatol* 1:45–50, 1983.
16. Selvaag, E: Pili torti and sensorineural hearing loss. A follow-up of Björnstad's original patients and a review of the literature. *Eur J Dermatol* 10:91–97, 2000.
17. Singh S, Bresman MJ: Menkes' "kinky hair syndrome" (trichopoliodystrophy). *Am J Dis Child* 125:572–578, 1973.
18. Van Buggenhout G et al: Björnstad syndrome in a patient with mental retardation. *Genet Couns* 9:201–204, 1998.
19. Voigtländer V: Pili torti with deafness (Björnstad syndrome). *Dermatologica* 159:50–54, 1979.

Alopecia, hypogonadism, anosmia, malformed pinnae, and conductive hearing loss (Johnson-McMillin syndrome)

In 1983, Johnson et al. (4) reported 16 members of a three-generation kindred with alopecia, malformed ears, anosmia, hypogonadism, and conductive hearing loss of varying severity. Johnston et al. (5) reported an unrelated male child with alopecia, oligodontia, hypohidrosis, mild developmental delay, unilateral microtia and atresia of the external auditory canal, and mild unilateral conductive hearing loss.

Craniofacial findings. Facial asymmetry was evident in six individuals. Cleft palate was present in one patient. Six family members

had micrognathia. Complete anosmia was noted in two males and partial anosmia in one female. The nose was prominent with a small mandible. Several had severe dental caries. One patient of Johnston et al. (5) had oligodontia.

Integumentary system. All 16 family members from one kindred had alopecia (4) (Fig. 14–22A–D). In 13, alopecia was total and congenital. No alopecia was found by Hennekam and Holties (3). Sweating appeared to be normal in the large family. However, hypohidrosis was noted in the nonfamilial case. No nail anomalies were reported. Hyperpigmented spots were noted in one family (3).

Genitourinary system. Three males exhibited hypogonadism, secondary to LH/FSH deficiency (4) (Fig. 14–22E).

Figure 14–22. *Alopecia, hypogonadism, anosmia, malformed pinnae, and conductive hearing loss (Johnson-McMillin syndrome).* (A–D) Four members of original family showing alopecia and minor ear malformation. (E) Hypoplastic genitalia. [From VP Johnson et al., *Am J Med Genet* 15:497, 1983.]

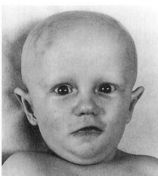
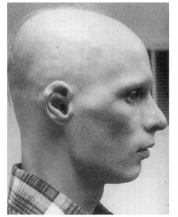

A   B

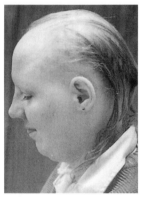
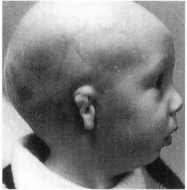

C   D

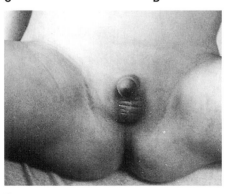

E

Other findings. Mild mental retardation was present in some cases (3–5). Two had congenital heart disease: one ventriculoseptal defect, the second a complex structural abnormality. About 50% of patients have been short (5).

External ear. The auricles in the 19 affected individuals varied in formation and placement from severe unilateral microtia with atresia of the external auditory canal, protuberant or cupped ears, prominent ears, and ears with small lobules, to normally formed but low-set ears. Atresia of the external auditory canal was found in four patients. Malformations appeared to be more severe in males than in females.

Auditory system. Seven family members had conductive hearing loss, often unilateral, which was moderate to severe. In two persons the impairment appeared to be secondary to otitis media (4). Tympanograms performed on one family member revealed bony sclerosis of the tympanic membrane with secondary reduction in size of the middle ear cavity. The malleus was identifiable but the small ossicles were difficult to visualize. Reconstructive surgery on one family member revealed a malleus described as a "deformed ball of bone with a small spicule sticking from it." It was attached to a normally shaped incus. The stapes was normally set in the oval window.

Laboratory findings. Endocrinological studies on the three males with hypogonadism demonstrated LH and FSH deficiency.

Heredity. Two case reports (3,4) clearly document autosomal dominant transmission, with variable expression.

The unrelated affected patient may represent a new dominant mutation. As he lacked some characteristics of the original kindred, and since he had hypohidrosis, not present in the original family, it is unclear whether he had the same condition.

Diagnosis. A number of neuroectodermal or neuroendocrine conditions have been described. Kallmann syndrome has the association of hypogonadotropic hypogonadism, anosmia, and hearing loss (7). Generalized alopecia, hypogonadism, and sensorineural hearing loss were noted in three brothers with normal parents, suggesting autosomal recessive or X-linked inheritance (Crandall syndrome) (2). Familial hypogonadotropic hypogonadism with alopecia but without anosmia has also been reported (9). Björnstad syndrome involves alopecia and sensorineural hearing loss (1). Although similar to Crandall's patients, the syndrome described here includes conductive hearing loss, alopecia with microscopically normal, albeit narrow, hair shafts, pinna anomalies, anosmia or hyposmia, marked dental caries, micrognathia or retrognathia, and facial nerve palsy. Other variable findings include cleft palate, cardiac defects, and mental retardation. Virtually all of the facial and branchial arch structures are derived from the neural crest (6). The first and second branchial arches contribute to the hillocks of His, ossicles, and trigeminal and facial nerves. The mesoderm that invades the palatal shelves is neuroectoderm from the lateral and ventral aspects of the neural crest (10). The olfactory bulb consists of epithelium from the nasal placodes, and neural extension from the telencephalon (8). The pituitary–hypothalamic axis arises from an outpouching of the ventral neural ridge, Rathke's pouch, and the infundibular portion of the diencephalon. By invoking the ectodermal/neuroectodermal origin, disparate clinical findings involving hair, ears, palate, facial nerve, olfactory bulb, and hypothalamic–pituitary axis find common ground.

Prognosis. The defects are congenital with no evidence of progression. With the exception of one girl with complex congenital heart disease who died of heart failure early in life, there were no life-threatening complications (4).

Summary. Characteristics of this syndrome include (*1*) autosomal dominant inheritance; (*2*) variable malformations of the external ear; (*3*) alopecia; (*4*) anosmia or hyposmia; (*5*) hypogonadotropic hypogonadism; (*6*) excessive dental caries; (*7*) occasional facial asymmetry, mental retardation, and congenital heart disease; and (*8*) variable degrees of conductive hearing loss.

References

1. Björnstad R: Pili torti and sensorineural loss of hearing. In: Proceedings of the 17th Meeting, Northern Dermatological Society, Copenhagen, 1965.
2. Crandall BF et al: A familial syndrome of deafness, alopecia and hypogonadism. *J Pediatr* 82:461–465, 1973.
3. Hennekam RCM, Holties FJAM: Johnson-McMillin syndrome: report of another family. *Am J Med Genet* 47:714–716, 1993.
4. Johnson VP et al: A newly recognized neuroectodermal syndrome of familial alopecia, anosmia, deafness and hypogonadism. *Am J Med Genet* 15:497–506, 1983.
5. Johnston K et al: Alopecia-anosmia-deafness-hypogonadism syndrome revisited. *Am J Med Genet* 26:925–927, 1987.
6. Johnston MC: The neural crest in abnormalities of the face and brain. *Birth Defects* 11(7):1–18, 1975.
7. Kallmann FJ et al: The genetic aspects of primary eunuchoidism. *Am J Ment Defic* 48:203–236, 1944.
8. Remnick, H: *Embryology of the Face and Oral Cavity.* Fairleigh Dickinson University Press, Teaneck, NJ, 1970, pp 18–19.
9. Satti IS, Salem Z: Familial hypogonadotropic hypogonadism with alopecia. *Can Med Assoc J* 121:428–434, 1979.
10. Stark RB: Mesodermal deficiency as a pathogenic factor in facial anomalies. In: *Craniofacial Anomalies,* Longacre JB (ed), Lippincott, New York, 1968, pp 91–94.

Alopecia, hypogonadism, diabetes mellitus, mental retardation, ECG abnormalities, and sensorineural hearing loss (Woodhouse-Sakati syndrome)

In 1983, Woodhouse and Sakati (2) reported two Saudi Arabian families in which there were multiple sibs with hypogonadism, alopecia, mental retardation, ECG abnormalities, diabetes mellitus, and sensorineural hearing loss. Gul et al. (1) reported an additional family.

Clinical findings. Height was normal but body proportions were eunuchoid. There was complete absence of breast tissue and pubic hair in females but moderate growth of pubic hair and genital development in males.

Integumentary system. The scalp hair was short, sparse, and fine without pili torti. Variable loss of eyebrow and scalp hair was more severe in older affected members. Beard growth in males was also absent.

Cardiovascular system. Electrocardiographic findings in four of the sibs showed S-T segment depression and flattened T waves.

Central nervous system. Mental retardation varied from mild to severe.

Endocrine system. Primary amenorrhea and failure of sexual maturation (absence of breast tissue and sexual hair) were evident in females. Laparotomy demonstrated hypoplastic uterus, rudimentary fallopian tubes, and streak gonads. Affected males had some pubic hair and genital development. All had mild diabetes mellitus.

Auditory system. Among four patients tested, sensorineural hearing loss ranged from mild (20–40 dB) to severe (55–70 dB).

Laboratory findings. Hyperglycemia and abnormal glucose tolerance tests were noted in most cases. Hypogonadism was demonstrated by markedly decreased testosterone and estradiol levels. Luteinizing hormone and FSH were elevated in two patients.

Pathology. Testicular biopsy showed moderately severe depression of spermatogenesis, prominent Sertoli cells, few Leydig cells, and some atrophic tubules with thickening of the basement membrane. Histology of the streak gonads showed fibrous stroma with small calcified deposits but no oogonia.

Heredity. Affected were two sibs and sib first cousins in one family and three sibs in another two families each. Consanguinity was noted in all families. Autosomal recessive inheritance is apparent.

Diagnosis. Although hypogonadism, diabetes mellitus, and mental retardation can be seen in several syndromes, for example, Laurence-Moon syndrome and Alström syndrome, the patients clearly do not fit these syndromes. Alopecia and hypogonadism are also seen in Crandall syndrome (generalized alopecia, hypogonadism, and sensorineural hearing loss), but diabetes and ECG anomalies were not found in that disorder. Patients with Richards-Rundle syndrome have slowly progressive ataxia and lack the skin changes. The syndrome of congenital alopecia, mental retardation, and sensorineural hearing loss must also be excluded.

Prognosis. Most of the patients live into adult life.

Summary. The syndrome is characterized by (*1*) autosomal recessive inheritance; (*2*) mental retardation; (*3*) alopecia; (*4*) diabetes mellitus; (*5*) hypogonadism; (*6*) ECG abnormalities; and (*7*) sensorineural hearing loss.

References

1. Gul D et al: Woodhouse and Sakati syndrome (MIM 241080): report of a new patient. *Clin Dysmorphol* 9:123–125, 2000.
2. Woodhouse NJY, Sakati NA: A syndrome of hypogonadism, alopecia, diabetes mellitus, mental retardation, deafness, and ECG abnormalities. *J Med Genet* 20:216–219, 1983.

Generalized alopecia, hypogonadism, and sensorineural hearing loss (Crandall syndrome)

Crandall et al. (2) reported three brothers affected with short stature. Two had secondary hypogonadism, alopecia, and sensorineural hearing loss. A third brother was similarly involved but exhibited only minimal hypogonadism. They had been reported earlier by Reed et al. (6) as having Björnstad syndrome before they were recognized as having hypogonadism. However, Selvaag (7) has suggested that this is still consistent with a variable phenotype associated with Björnstad syndrome.

Integumentary system. The boys exhibited lanugo hair at birth but lost this and never developed body, axillary, or pubic hair. They had only very sparse head hair, which was broken about 0.5 cm from the scalp. Eyelashes were short, curled, and deficient, and eyebrows were absent (Fig. 14–23A).

Genitourinary system. Infrequent erections and/or ejaculations were experienced. In two of the sibs, the testes were markedly reduced in size.

Musculoskeletal system. Height ranged between the third and 25th centiles. The upper-to-lower segment ratio ranged from normal in two brothers to 1.22 in the other brother. Bone age was slightly decreased. The carrying angle was increased in two of the boys. Muscular development was generally poor.

Other findings. Mental development was slightly retarded in two brothers. A high-pitched voice noted in all three boys was attributed to a prepubertal larynx.

Auditory system. Sensorineural hearing loss was detected at time of schooling. The hearing loss was described as being slowly progressive and ranged from 65 to 85 dB at 18–21 years. The monotonous voice, however, suggests earlier onset.

Vestibular system. No studies were reported.

Laboratory findings. Plasma LH and testosterone levels were significantly reduced in two boys. Normal response to human chorionic

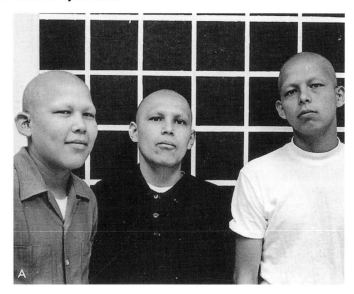

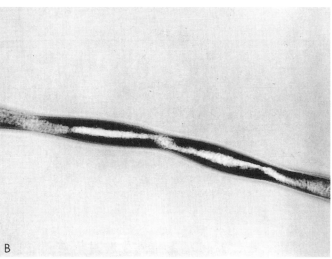

Figure 14–23. *Generalized alopecia, hypogonadism, and sensorineural hearing loss (Crandall syndrome).* (A) Three male sibs affected with hearing loss and alopecia. The two brothers on the left also exhibit growth hormone deficiency and luteinizing hormone deficiency. (B) Scalp hair exhibiting characteristic twisting of hair shaft (pili torti). [From BF Crandall et al., *J Pediatr* 82:461, 1973.]

gonadotropin indicated gonadotropin insufficiency. There was also diminished release of growth hormone. Microscopic examination of the head hair showed twisting of the hair shaft, which was characteristic of pili torti (Fig. 14–23B). Dermatoglyphic analysis exhibited low total ridge counts in two of the boys.

Heredity. The occurrence of the syndrome in three sons of normal parents suggests autosomal recessive inheritance. X-linkage cannot be completely ruled out, but there were none affected among seven children from the mother's second marriage, and she did not exhibit any stigmata of a possible carrier.

Diagnosis. Pili torti as an isolated entity may be sporadic or may exhibit autosomal recessive inheritance (1). This disorder must be differentiated from the syndrome of pili torti and sensorineural hearing loss (Björnstad syndrome). Growth hormone deficiency (4,5) and LH deficiency (3) occur as separate disorders, but they are not associated with hearing loss or with a total lack of body hair as in the syndrome considered here.

Alopecia and hypogonadism have been associated with hearing loss in the syndromes of alopecia, hypogonadism, diabetes mellitus, mental retardation, ECG abnormalities, and sensorineural hearing loss (Wood-house-Sakati syndrome). One should also rule out the syndrome of congenital alopecia, mental retardation, and sensorineural hearing loss.

Summary. The syndrome is characterized by (*1*) recessive inheritance, probably autosomal; (*2*) generalized alopecia with pili torti; (*3*) growth retardation; (*4*) hypogonadism; and (*5*) severe sensorineural hearing loss.

References

1. Appel B, Messina SJ: Pili torti hereditaria. *N Engl J Med* 226:912–915, 1942.
2. Crandall B et al: A familial syndrome of deafness, alopecia, and hypogonadism. *J Pediatr* 82:461–465, 1973.
3. Ewer RW: Familial monotropic pituitary gonadotropin insufficiency. *J Clin Endocrinol Metab* 28:783–788, 1968.
4. Goodman HG et al: Isolated growth hormone and multiple pituitary-hormone deficiencies. *N Engl J Med* 278:57–68, 1968.
5. Poskitt EM, Rayner PH: Isolated growth hormone deficiency: two families with autosomal dominant inheritance. *Arch Dis Child* 49:55–59, 1974.
6. Reed WB et al: Hereditary syndromes with auditory and dermatologic manifestations. *Arch Dermatol* 95:456–461, 1967.
7. Selvaag E: Pili torti and sensorineural hearing loss: a follow-up of Bjornstad's original patients and a review of the literature. *Eur J Dermatol* 10:91–97, 2000.

Congenital alopecia, mental retardation, and sensorineural hearing loss

Perniola et al. (2) described male and female sibs with congenital alopecia and mental retardation. Seizures were first observed in both children at 3 months, but improved with time. Height was at the 10th to 25th centile. Intelligence quotients ranged from 35 to 45. A sensorineural hearing loss of 40–50 dB was found in the male sib at 3 years of age. Penchazadeh (personal communication, 1992) described a male child with this combination (Fig. 14–24).

The parents were first cousins. Baraitser et al. (1) described three cousins from an inbred Middle Eastern family, who had congenital alopecia and severe mental retardation. Hearing loss was not reported. Inheritance is probably autosomal recessive.

To be excluded are the syndromes of generalized alopecia, hypogonadism, and sensorineural hearing loss (Crandall syndrome) and alope-

Figure 14–24. *Congenital alopecia, mental retardation, and sensorineural hearing loss.* Male child with alopecia, triangular shape of skull, mild hypertelorism, heterochromia irides, and mixed hearing loss. [Courtesy of VB Penchaszadeh, New York, New York.]

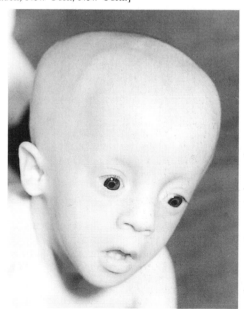

cia, hypogonadism, diabetes mellitus, mental retardation, ECG abnormalities, and sensorineural hearing loss (Woodhouse-Sakati syndrome).

References

1. Baraitser M et al: A new alopecia/mental retardation syndrome. *J Med Genet* 20:64–75, 1983.
2. Perniola T et al: Congenital alopecia, psychomotor retardation, convulsions in two sibs of a consanguineous marriage. *J Inherit Metab Dis* 3:49–53, 1980.

DOOR (*d*eafness, *o*nycho-*o*steodystrophy, *r*etardation) syndrome

In 1970, Walbaum et al. (16) reported a syndrome characterized by mental retardation, congenital severe sensorineural hearing loss, rudimentary fingernails and toenails, and dysplastic terminal phalanges in male and female sibs. Several similar cases have been described (1,2,5–16). The sibs reported by Feinmesser and Zelig (4) are considered to have the same syndrome. DOOR syndrome seems to be identical with Eronen syndrome (3,6,17).

Craniofacial findings. Characteristic facial findings include broad nasal bridge and alae, square nasal tip, long upper lip, and skin-vermilion border (9) (Fig. 14–25A,B). Downslanting palpebral fissures, ptosis, large nostrils, micrognathia, facial asymmetry, and low-set ears (9,10) are also noted.

Integumentary system. The nails are absent or severely hypoplastic on all fingers and toes. Dermatoglyphic studies have shown almost all finger and toe prints to have arches (1,2,16).

Dental findings. The enamel has been described as yellow or hypoplastic.

Musculoskeletal system. The thumbs are long and have an extra phalanx and two flexion creases. In a few patients, the little fingers were short and clinodactylous (Fig. 14–25C–F). Radiographic examination showed an extra phalanx or greatly enlarged terminal phalanx in the thumbs and halluces. The terminal phalanx was hypoplastic in the remaining fingers and toes. In some patients, there were only two phalanges in the little fingers and fusion of the middle and distal phalanges of the third to fifth toes (Fig. 14–25G,H). Thomas and Nevin (15) noted some generalized osteoporosis as well.

Ocular system. Occasional ocular anomalies include cataracts (3) and optic atrophy (3,5,6,8,9,15).

Neurologic system. All patients are mentally retarded and most exhibit grand mal seizures from infancy.

Auditory system. Severe congenital sensorineural hearing loss is evident in all those affected.

Vestibular system. Vestibular function was found to be abnormal in one of two patients tested (4).

Laboratory findings. Patton et al. (9) reported increased levels of 2-oxoglutarate in plasma and urine of three unrelated patients, including one reported previously by Nevin et al. (8). However, the patient of Lin et al. (7) had normal urinary 2-oxoglutarate excretion. Rajab et al. (12) described four severely affected children who also had progressive blindness. They had significantly elevated levels of 2-oxoglutarate excretion, which led Rajab et al. to postulate that there is heterogeneity within the autosomal recessive DOOR syndrome, with the more severely affected cases being associated with elevated excretion of 2-oxoglutarate.

Heredity. Inheritance is clearly autosomal recessive.

Diagnosis. This syndrome shares many features with dominant onychodystrophy, triphalangeal thumbs, and congenital sensorineural

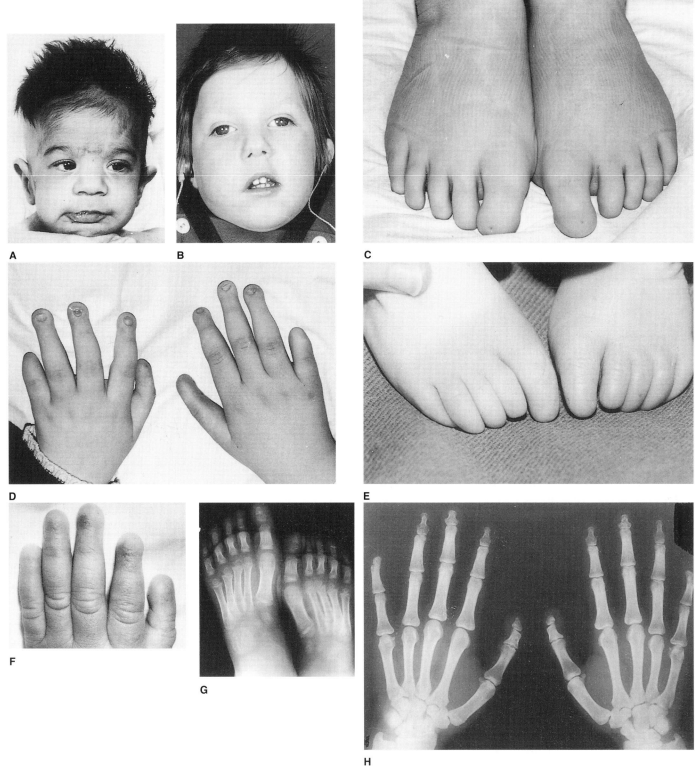

Figure 14–25. *DOOR (deafness, onycho-osteodystrophy, retardation) syndrome.* (A) Typical facies showing broad nasal bridge and alae, relatively long upper lip and thin vermilion border, epicanthal folds, and micrognathia. (B) Another patient with normal facies. Note exotropia. (C) Same patient showing absence of toenails. (D) Fingers of another patient. (E) Toes of same patient. (F) Close-up of hands showing agenesis of fingernails. (G) Triphalangy of halluces and agenesis of terminal phalanges of others toes. (H) Radiograph showing triphalangeal thumbs and blunting of terminal phalanges of third and fifth fingers. [(A,F) from MA Patton et al., *Am J Med Genet* 26:207, 1987; (C) from PS Thomas and NC Nevin, *Ann Radiol,* 25:54, 1982; (B,D,E) courtesy of NC Nevin, Belfast, Northern Ireland; (G) from QH Qazi and EM Smithwick, *Am J Dis Child* 120:255, 1970; (H) from R Walbaum et al., *J Génét Hum* 18:101, 1970.]

hearing loss (Goodman-Maghadam syndrome) but differs in that it is associated with mental retardation and seizures. Eronen et al. (3) and LeMerrer et al. (6) described children with absent distal phalanges and nails, unusual facial features, seizures, and optic atrophy. The presence of renal cystic dysplasia and absence of hearing loss or triphalangeal thumbs led to the suggestion that this was a distinct condition. We agree with Winter (17) that the Eronen syndrome is the same as DOOR syndrome.

The combination of mental retardation and absence of nails and terminal phalanges may be seen in a plethora of disorders such as fetal hydantoin syndrome, fetal alcohol syndrome, Coffin-Siris syndrome, and dup(9p) syndrome.

Prognosis. The hearing loss and mental retardation were profound.

Summary. This syndrome is characterized by (1) autosomal recessive inheritance; (2) rudimentary fingernails and toenails; (3) digital abnormalities, including triphalangeal thumbs and halluces and hypoplastic terminal phalanges of the remaining digits; (4) mental retardation; (5) grand mal seizures; and (6) congenital profound sensorineural hearing loss.

References

1. Bos CJM et al: DOOR syndrome: additional case and literature review. *Clin Dysmorphol* 3:15–20, 1994.
2. Cantwell RJ: Congenital sensorineural deafness associated with onycho-osteo-dystrophy and mental retardation (D.O.O.R. syndrome). *Humangenetik* 26:261–265, 1975.
3. Eronen M et al: New syndrome: a digito-reno-cerebral syndrome. *Am J Med Genet* 22:281–285, 1985.
4. Feinmesser M, Zelig S: Congenital deafness associated with onychodystrophy. *Arch Otolaryngol* 74:507–508, 1969.
5. Hess RO, Pecotte JK: Additional case report of the DOOR syndrome. *Am J Med Genet* 19:401–405, 1984.
6. LeMerrer M et al: Digito-reno-cerebral syndrome: confirmation of Eronen syndrome. *Clin Genet* 42:196–198, 1992.
7. Lin HJ et al: DOOR syndrome (deafness, onycho-osteodrystrophy, and mental retardation): a new patient and delineation of neurologic variability among recessive cases. *Am J Med Genet* 47:534–539, 1993.
8. Nevin NC et al: Deafness, onycho-osteodystrophy, mental retardation (DOOR) syndrome. *Am J Med Genet* 13:325–332, 1982.
9. Patton MA et al: DOOR syndrome (deafness, onychosteodystrophy, and mental retardation): elevated plasma and urinary 2-oxoglutarate in three unrelated patients. *Am J Med Genet* 26:207–215, 1987.
10. Qazi QH, Nangia BS: Abnormal distal phalanges and nails, deafness, mental retardation, and seizure disorder: a new familial syndrome. *J Pediatr* 104:391–394, 1984.
11. Qazi QH, Smithwick EM: Triphalangy of thumbs and great toes. *Am J Dis Child* 120:255–257, 1970.
12. Rajab A et al: Further delineation of the DOOR syndrome. *Clin Dysmorphol* 9:247–251, 2000.
13. Sadoun E et al: Onychodystrophie déficits, sensoriels et mental, convulsions néonatales (DOOR syndrome). *Arch Fr Pédiatr* 46:465–466, 1989.
14. Sanchez O et al: The deafness, onycho-osteo-dystrophy, mental retardation syndrome. *Hum Genet* 58:228–230, 1981.
15. Thomas PS, Nevin NC: Radiological findings in the DOOR syndrome. *Ann Radiol* 25:54–58, 1982.
16. Walbaum R et al: Surdité familiale avec osteo-onycho-dysplasie. *J Génét Hum* 18:101–108, 1970.
17. Winter RM: Eronen syndrome identical with DOOR syndrome. *Clin Genet* 43:167, 1993.

Dominant onychodystrophy, triphalangeal thumbs, and congenital sensorineural hearing loss (Goodman-Moghadam syndrome)

A syndrome characterized by rudimentary fingernails and toenails and congenital severe sensorineural hearing loss was described by Goodman et al. (1) and Moghadam and Statten (2).

Integumentary system. Affected individuals had very similar abnormalities of fingernails and toenails. The nails were rudimentary (about one-fourth normal size) but otherwise apparently normally formed (Fig. 14–26A). Hair and skin pigmentation and teeth were normal.

Musculoskeletal system. Triphalangeal thumbs were a characteristic finding. Bulbous swellings of the soft tissue about the terminal phalanges were evident in all affected individuals but varied in severity.

Auditory system. Both mother and father in the family studied by Goodman et al. (1) had congenital severe sensorineural hearing loss. Otologic examination showed no abnormalities of the canals or drums. In the family examined by Moghadam and Statten (2), the son had severe congenital sensorineural hearing loss, whereas the mother exhibited a bilateral low-tone moderate (30–40 dB) sensorineural hearing loss.

Vestibular system. Vestibular findings were not reported by either group of investigators.

Laboratory findings. In the family reported by Goodman et al. (1), radiographs of the mother's hands and feet showed an extra phalanx in the right thumb, an absence of a phalanx in both little fingers, and underdevelopment of the tufts of the distal phalanges of the hands. There was also absence in the second, third, and fourth toes of the left foot (Fig. 14–26B,C). Findings on the right foot were not noted, nor were radiographic findings described in the son. Other skeletal structures were normal. In the family described by Moghadam and Statten (2), each thumb had three phalanges and the fingers and toes showed pointed or rudimentary phalanges.

Heredity. Since this syndrome was found in a mother and son in two kindreds, the disorder appears to be transmitted by a dominant gene. Since there was no male-to-male transmission, X-linked dominant inheritance cannot be excluded.

Diagnosis. This syndrome can be differentiated from DOOR syndrome of rudimentary nails, dysplastic terminal phalanges, mental retardation, and sensorineural hearing loss because of its dominant hereditary transmission. Although genetic heterogeneity is possible, the syndrome presented here may be transmitted via a dominant gene that may be incompletely penetrant. This syndrome can also be distinguished from dominant onychodystrophy, coniform teeth, and sensorineural hearing loss (Robinson syndrome) since the teeth in affected individuals were normal.

Sensorineural hearing loss and triphalangeal thumbs may also be seen in the syndrome of lop ears, imperforate anus, triphalangeal thumbs, and sensorineural hearing loss (Townes-Brocks syndrome).

Prognosis. The onychodystrophy and hearing loss are both congenital. There is no evidence of progression of the disease in later life.

Summary. The major characteristics of this syndrome include (1) autosomal dominant transmission; (2) onychodystrophy of fingernails and toenails; (3) triphalangeal thumbs; and (4) congenital severe sensorineural hearing loss.

References

1. Goodman RM et al: Hereditary congenital deafness with onychodystrophy. *Arch Otolaryngol* 90:474–477, 1969.
2. Moghadam H, Statten P: Hereditary sensorineural hearing loss associated with onychodystrophy and digital malformations. *Can Med Assoc J* 107:310–312, 1972.

Dominant onychodystrophy, type B brachydactyly, and ectrodactyly

A dominantly inherited condition consisting of nail and hand defects was described by Kumar and Levick (1) in 1986. All six affected individuals had absence of terminal phalangeal creases, hypoplastic and absent nails, and "stiffness" of digits on the hands. All but one individual had similarly affected toes. Two had missing digits. One had bilateral sensorineural hearing loss as well.

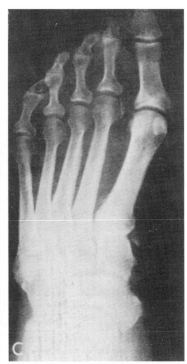

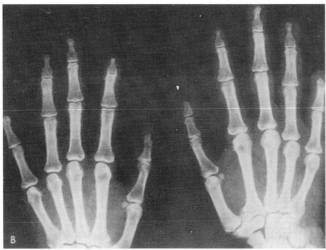

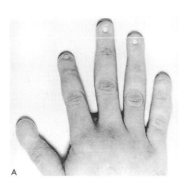

Figure 14–26. *Dominant onychodystrophy, triphalangeal thumbs, and congenital sensorineural hearing loss (Goodman-Moghadam syndrome).* (A) Right hand of the proband's affected son showing nail and terminal digital changes. (B) Radiograph of the proband's hands showing underdevelopment of the tufts of the distal phalanges, especially of the index fingers and thumbs. In addition, there is an extra phalanx of the right thumb and absence of a phalanx in both little fingers. (C) Radiograph of the proband's left foot showing only two distal phalanges in all digits. The terminal tuft of the large toe is also underdeveloped. [From RM Goodman et al., *Arch Otolaryngol* 90:474, 1969.]

The pedigree did not allow us to rule out X-linked dominant inheritance.

Reference

1. Kumar D, Levick RK: Autosomal dominant onychodystrophy and anonychia with type B brachydactyly and ectrodactyly. *Clin Genet* 30:219–225, 1986.

Dominant onychodystrophy, coniform teeth, and sensorineural hearing loss (Robinson syndrome)

A syndrome consisting of small, fissured nails, malformed teeth, and sensorineural hearing loss was described by Robinson et al, in 1962 (4). Four of five affected family members were studied by the authors. Kondoh et al. (3) reported another family. A third family was reported by Bonioli et al. (1), although this is likely not an example of Robinson syndrome.

Dental findings. Each of those affected had coniform crowned teeth, many of which were missing (oligodontia) (Fig. 14–27A).

Integumentary system. Fingernails and toenails were absent or small and fissured, apparently being affected from birth (Fig. 14–27B,C). Hair and skin were normal.

Musculoskeletal system. In one kindred, one affected individual had ulnar hexadactyly of one hand, whereas another of the kindred exhibited soft tissue syndactyly of toes 1–2 and 3–4 of one foot.

Auditory system. A generally symmetric sensorineural hearing loss of 10–100 dB was found in all affected persons. Higher frequencies were more strikingly involved, particularly in one patient whose hearing was normal to 4000 Hz but showed profound hearing loss at all higher frequencies. One sib had sensorineural hearing loss of over 70 dB in all frequencies, whereas another sib had almost normal hearing at very low frequencies but a 60 dB loss in higher frequencies. Apparently the hearing loss was congenital. No progression was noted to develop in later years. Other audiometric tests were not described.

Vestibular system. No vestibular tests were reported.

Laboratory findings. Sweat electrolyte concentrations were elevated in two cases and nearly normal in the other two.

Heredity. Since individuals in at least three generations in both families were affected, inheritance is probably autosomal dominant.

Diagnosis. The syndrome of recessive onychodystrophy and congenital sensorineural hearing loss differs from this syndrome in that the teeth are not affected, the nails do not exhibit the striking fissuring, and transmission is autosomal recessive. Oligodontia and/or coniform crowned teeth may be seen in a number of syndromes: hypohidrotic ectodermal dysplasia, chondroectodermal dysplasia, Rieger syndrome, incontinentia pigmenti, and others (2).

Prognosis. The nail and tooth anomalies and the hearing loss did not change with time.

Summary. Characteristics of this syndrome include (*1*) autosomal dominant transmission; (*2*) onychodystrophy; (*3*) teeth with coniform crowns and oligodontia; (*4*) elevated sweat electrolyte concentrations; and (*5*) moderate to severe sensorineural hearing loss.

References

1. Bonioli E et al: La sindrome di Robinson (onico-odontodisplasia e sordità percettiva). *Minerva Pediatr* 36:421–424, 1984.
2. Gorlin RJ et al: *Syndromes of the Head and Neck,* 4th ed. Oxford University Press, New York, 2001.
3. Kondoh T et al: Autosomal dominant onychodystrophy and congenital sensorineural deafness. *J Hum Genet* 44:60–62, 1999.
4. Robinson GC et al: Familial ectodermal dysplasia with sensorineural deafness and other anomalies. *Pediatrics* 30:797–802, 1962.

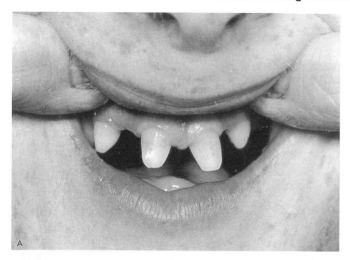

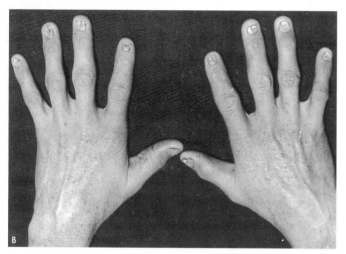

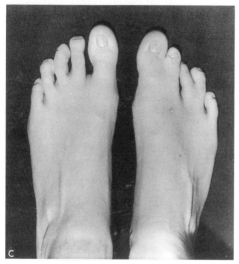

Figure 14–27. *Dominant onychodystrophy, coniform teeth, and sensorineural hearing loss (Robinson syndrome).* (A) Absent and misshapen coniform crowned teeth. (B) Small dystrophic fingernails having furrows and cracks. (C) Syndactyly and toenail hypoplasia. [From GC Robinson et al., *Pediatrics* 30:797, 1962.]

Atopic dermatitis and sensorineural hearing loss

Four families have been reported in which individuals had atopic dermatitis and sensorineural hearing loss. Clinical and hereditary differences suggest heterogeneity.

Integumentary system. Konigsmark et al. (2) described two brothers and a sister who had dermatitis with onset at about age 10. The skin lesions consisted of mild ichthyosis with lichenified, excoriated erythematous areas involving the forearms, elbows, antecubital fossae, wrists, hands, and waist but sparing the legs (Fig. 14–28A,B). Schultz Larsen et al. (3) reported a four-generation family in which 4 of 11 affected persons had typical atopic dermatitis affecting hands, wrists, forearms, ankles, and legs. Onset was during infancy. Verbov (4) noted a three-generation family of four affected members. Two members of this family had atopy, one had eczema affecting the trunk, and all four had palmoplantar keratoderma. Frentz et al. (1) described two brothers with atopic dermatitis of infantile onset. Both had palmoplantar keratoderma. The paternal family history was suggestive of autosomal dominant palmoplantar keratoderma, whereas there were individuals with atopic dermatitis on the mother's side of the family.

Auditory system. In the family of Konigsmark et al. (2), hearing loss was first noted at 3–5 years of age. In no case was impairment severe enough to cause difficulty in school. Hearing tests at 5 or 6 years showed bilateral symmetric sensorineural hearing loss of 15–55 dB for both air and bone conduction. The speech reception threshold corresponded to the expected hearing loss. Speech discrimination was over 90% in all three sibs. The SISI test was 100% at 2000 to 4000 Hz, and tone decay tests were negative. Otologic examination showed no abnormalities except for hearing loss. Hearing tests repeated over a 10-year period showed no progression of hearing loss. In the second family (3), 10 of 11 members had bilateral sensorineural hearing loss of middle frequencies with onset between infancy and 10 years. The amount of loss was 35–55 dB. It is unknown whether the hearing loss was progressive. In the third family (4), the hearing loss was described as congenital and involved the high tones. Those in the fourth family (1) had nonprogressive bilateral sensorineural hearing loss of middle frequencies with onset between the ages of 4 and 6.

Vestibular system. Testing done on only three sibs of one family showed normal function (2).

Laboratory findings. In three of four families, IgE levels were found to be elevated (1,3,4). Skin tests carried out in two families were positive for numerous allergies (1,3).

Pathology. In one family (2), biopsy of an active skin plaque in the antecubital fossa of the proband showed moderate acanthosis, hyperkeratosis, and a patchy lymphocytic infiltrate in the upper dermis (Fig. 14–28C).

Heredity. The inheritance pattern is consistent with autosomal recessive in the family described by Konigsmark et al. (2), and autosomal dominant in the families described by Verbov (4) and Schultz Larsen et al. (3). It is possible that in the fourth family (1) atopy and palmoplantar keratosis were segregating as autosomal dominant traits and the sensorineural hearing loss was an autosomal recessive condition affecting only the two brothers.

Diagnosis. The autosomal recessive disorder seems to be characterized by atypical dermatitis, whereas the disorder in the autosomal dominant condition is more typical atopic dermatitis for both age of onset and distribution on the body.

Prognosis. The hearing loss was apparently nonprogressive, and intelligence was normal.

Summary. The major characteristics are (*1*) unknown hereditary pattern; (*2*) atopic dermatitis; and (*3*) nonprogressive sensorineural hearing loss.

References

1. Frentz G et al: Congenital perceptive hearing loss and atopic dermatitis. *Acta Otolaryngol* 82:242–244, 1976.
2. Konigsmark BW et al: Familial neural hearing loss and atopic dermatitis. *JAMA* 204:953–957, 1968.

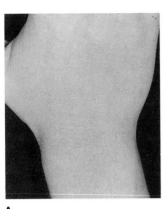
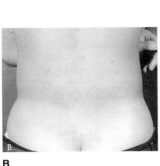
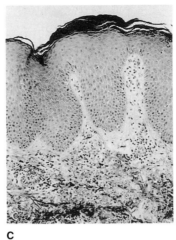

A   B   C

Figure 14–28. *Atopic dermatitis and sensorineural hearing loss.* (A) Dermatitis involving dorsum of wrist in proband. (B) Similar changes at waist. (C) Antecubital skin biopsy showing acanthosis, hyperkeratosis,and lymphocytic infiltrate in dermis. [From BW Konigsmark et al., *JAMA* 204:953, 1968.]

3. Schultz Larsen F et al: Atopic dermatitis and congenital deafness. *Br J Dermatol* 99:325–328, 1978.
4. Verbov JC: Palmoplantar keratoderma, deafness, and atopy. *Br J Dermatol* 116:881–882, 1987.

Hidrotic ectodermal dysplasia, Halal type

Halal et al. (1) described a provisionally unique family in which affected individuals had the combination of absent scalp hair, eyelashes, and eyebrows; small dysplastic nails; mild mental retardation; and in one individual, unilateral mixed hearing loss. Sweating was normal, thus distinguishing it from many of the other ectodermal dysplasias. Inheritance is likely autosomal recessive.

Reference

1. Halal F et al: A distinct type of hidrotic ectodermal dysplasia. *Am J Med Genet* 38:552–556, 1991.

Xeroderma pigmentosum

Xeroderma pigmentosum (XP) is a group of disorders characterized by hypersensitivity of the skin to sunlight, which results in atrophy of the exposed skin and development of pigmentation, telangiectasia, keratoses, and cutaneous malignancy in childhood. These changes result from defective DNA repair of damage done by ultraviolet radiation. Various other abnormalities such as growth retardation, mental retardation, microcephaly, ataxia, dysarthria, choreoathetosis, corticospinal tract involvement, peripheral neuropathy, and hypogonadism may occur. These abnormalities are more common in those of complementation group D in the United States and Europe (vide infra).

Currently, there are nine excision-repair complementation groups (A through I) and one excision-proficient form. Ethnic differences are apparent, groups A, C, D and the variant being common in the United States, Europe, and Egypt, while group A is common in Japan. Most group A children manifest neurologic signs by age 7 years while group D exhibits changes between 7 and 20 years of age (5,10,11). The reader should consult Cockayne syndrome for patients manifesting overlap with that disorder.

Auditory findings. Progressive sensorineural hearing loss primarily affecting higher tones appears to have cochlear origin (2–8). Mimaki et al. (8) noted that 22 of 34 patients with group A XP had sensorineural hearing loss, whereas in their review of 830 XP cases, Kraemer et al. (5) noted hearing loss in only 28. It seems likely that there is a predisposition to hearing loss in one of the XPA subclasses, that being the group of patients with reduced nerve conduction, difficulty walking, and occasional microcephaly as occasional manifestations (1). Therefore,

the presence of deafness appears to be limited to those with the severe form of XPA.

Heredity. Inheritance is autosomal recessive. A gene for XPA has been mapped to 9q34.1 (12). The other complementation groups all map to different loci [for review, see Cleaver et al. (1)].

Prognosis. The frequency of neurodegenerative symptoms is dependent on the type of XP group. Skin cancers are extremely common, appearing on average 50 years earlier than in the general population. Avoidance of unnecessary ultraviolet (UV) exposure and use of sunblocks are strongly recommended (9).

References

1. Cleaver JE et al: A summary of mutations in the UV-sensitive disorders: xeroderma pigmentosum, Cockayne syndrome, and trichothiodystrophy. *Hum Mutat* 14:9–22, 1999.
2. Kanda T et al: Peripheral neuropathy in xeroderma pigmentosum. *Brain* 113:1025–1044, 1990.
3. Kenyon GS et al: Neuro-otological abnormalities in xeroderma pigmentosum with particular reference to deafness. *Brain* 108:771–784, 1985.
4. Kraemer KH, Slor H: Xeroderma pigmentosum. *Clin Dermatol* 3:33–69, 1985.
5. Kraemer KH et al: Xeroderma pigmentosum: cutaneous, ocular, and neurologic abnormalities in 830 published cases. *Arch Dermatol* 123:241–250, 1987.
6. Longridge NS: Audiological assessment of deafness associated with xeroderma pigmentosum. *J Laryngol Otol* 90:539–551, 1976.
7. Mamada A et al: Delayed sensorineural deafness and skin carcinogenesis in a Japanese xeroderma pigmentosum group D patient. *Photodermatology* 5:83–91, 1988.
8. Mimaki T et al: EEG and CT abnormalities in xeroderma pigmentosum. *Acta Neurol Scand* 80:136–141, 1989.
9. Moriwaki S-I, Kraemer KH: Xeroderma pigmentosum—bridging a gap between clinic and laboratory. *Photoderm Photoimmun Photomed* 17:47–54. 2001.
10. Reed WB et al: Xeroderma pigmentosum. Clinical and laboratory investigation of its basic defect. *JAMA* 207:2073–2079, 1969 (case 2).
11. Robbins JH et al: Neurological disease in xeroderma pigmentosum. *Brain* 114:1335–1362, 1991.
12. Tanaka K et al: Analysis of the human DNA excision repair gene involved in group A xeroderma pigmentosum and containing a zinc-finger domain. *Nature* 348:73–76, 1990.

Premature aging, microcephaly, unusual face, multiple nevi, and sensorineural hearing loss (Shepard-Elliot-Mulvihill syndrome)

Shepard (7), in 1971, and Elliot (4) and Mulvihill and Smith (5), in 1975, described a male with somatic retardation, multiple pigmented nevi, micropenis, and hypospadias. Other examples have been reported (1–3,6,8).

Clinical findings. Stature was below the third centile (1,2,5,6,8). Mental retardation was found in most cases (1,2,5–7), with normal mentation found in others (3,8).

Craniofacial findings. The craniofacial phenotype was characterized by microcephaly, broad forehead, fine scalp hair, sparse facial hair, disproportionately small face with reduced lower facial height, flared protruded maxillary incisors, and small pointed chin. Facial subcutaneous fat became deficient. The ears were lobeless (Fig. 14–29). Oligodontia was a constant feature. The voice was high-pitched and hoarse.

Integumentary system. There were numerous pigmented nevi of the face, neck, upper arms, and trunk.

Genitourinary system. Micropenis (1,2,4,5), cryptorchidism (4), and hypospadias (1,4,5,7) and hypogonadism (2) were reported.

Other findings. Miscellaneous observations included incomplete right bundle branch block (2) and reduced T cells and T-helper cells with an increase in natural killer cells (2,6). The liver was enlarged in a few cases.

Auditory system. There was moderate progressive hearing loss, with both sensorineural hearing loss and conductive hearing loss having been observed (1,2,6–8).

Laboratory findings. Despite liver enlargement, liver function tests were normal. Some patients had low IgG levels. Ohashi et al. (6) and Bartsch et al. (2) found severe T-cell deficiency.

Heredity. All reported patients have been male and family history in all three was negative for similarly affected individuals. None of the parents were consanguineous. The inheritance pattern, therefore, is unknown.

Diagnosis. The appearance of premature aging may suggest the diagnosis of Cockayne syndrome or progeria, but the presence of nevi in this condition helps distinguish it. The facial appearance may be suggestive of oculodentoosseous dysplasia, but mental retardation, short stature, and pigmented nevi are not part of that phenotype. Pigmented nevi are a feature of LEOPARD syndrome, as are short stature and genital defects, but the presence of cardiac findings and autosomal dominant inheritance in the latter suggests it is a separate entity.

Prognosis. Mild to moderate mental retardation may be present; life span is apparently unaffected, but the oldest affected individual was 17 years at the time of the report (2).

Summary. This condition is characterized by (*1*) unknown inheritance; (*2*) prematurely aged appearance; (*3*) slow growth following intrauterine growth retardation; (*4*) nevi or lentigines appearing in late infancy; (*5*) genital anomalies; (*6*) mild to moderate mental retardation; and (*7*) sensorineural hearing loss.

References

1. Baraitser M et al: A recognisable short stature syndrome with premature aging and pigmented naevi. *J Med Genet* 25:53–56, 1988.
2. Bartsch O et al: Progeroid syndrome with short stature and pigmented naevi. *Am J Hum Genet* 53:398A, 1993.
3. De Silva DC et al: Mulvihill-Smith progeria-like syndrome: a further report with delineation of phenotype, immunologic deficits, and novel observation of fibroblast abnormalities. *Am J Med Genet* 69:56–64, 1997.
4. Elliot DE: Undiagnosed syndrome of psycho-motor retardation, low birthweight, dwarfism, skeletal, dental, dermal and genital anomalies. *Birth Defects* 11(2):364–367, 1975.
5. Mulvihill JJ, Smith DW: Another disorder with shortness of stature and premature aging. *Birth Defects* 11(2):368–371, 1975.
6. Ohashi H et al: Premature aging and immunodeficiency: Mulvihill-Smith syndrome? *Am J Med Genet* 45:597–600, 1993.
7. Shepard MK: An unidentified syndrome with abnormality of skin and hair. *Birth Defects* 7(8):353–354, 1971.
8. Wong W et al: Case report for syndrome identification. *Cleft Palate J* 16:286–2990, 1979.

Figure 14–29. *Premature aging, microcephaly, unusual face, multiple nevi, and sensorineural hearing loss (Shepard-Elliot-Mulvihill syndrome).* (A,B) Microcephaly, broad forehead, sparse facial hair, disproportionately small facies with reduced lower facial height, and numerous pigmented nevi of face and neck. (C,D) Note other patient similarly affected. [(A,B) courtesy of O Bartsch, Lübeck. Germany; (C,D) from M Baraitser et al., *J Med Genet* 25:53, 1988.]

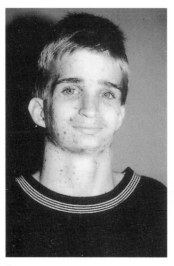

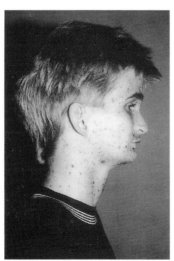

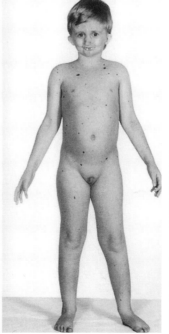

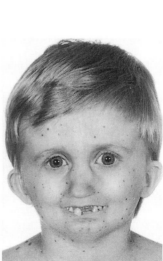

A   B   C   D

Anhidrosis and progressive sensorineural hearing loss (Helweg-Larsen and Ludvigsen syndrome)

Congenital anhidrosis is one of many ectodermal dysplasias. It may be an isolated finding, but usually it is associated with other skin defects—most frequently, oligodontia and hypotrichosis. In 1946, Helweg-Larsen and Ludvigsen described a syndrome characterized by congenital anhidrosis and progressive sensorineural hearing loss (2). They examined six affected family members and diagnosed eight other cases by history.

Integumentary system. Patients exhibited a marked inability to sweat; onset was at about 1 year of age. During heavy exertion or hot weather, patients felt very uncomfortable and frequently were unable to work because of headache, dyspnea, and palpitation. Instead of sweat, granules of salt appeared on the skin of the axillae, neck, and nasal bridge. A starch-iodine test performed on one patient showed little evidence of sweating except on the bridge of the nose, axillae, forearms, neck, and pectoral regions. In each of these areas 6 to 28 sweat spots appeared (Fig. 14–30A). During muscular work, no increase in the number of sweat points was noted. The proband was placed in a hot room (52° C) for 50 minutes, and in another test was given 0.3 mg of pilocarpine subcutaneously. In this individual, sweating was limited to only a few sweat points. By contrast, a normal control individual sweated profusely in both tests.

Auditory system. Five individuals with impaired sweat secretion also suffered with progressive sensorineural hearing loss, which had been noticed first at 35–45 years of age. Audiograms obtained on two members showed severe high-tone sensorineural hearing loss. No further description of hearing loss was made.

Vestibular system. Vestibular tests were not mentioned.

Laboratory findings. Complete blood count and urinalysis were normal in the proband.

Pathology. Skin biopsies from the forearms showed normal hair follicles and blood vessels but no sweat glands or sebaceous glands. Skin biopsy from the axilla of one patient showed a marked lack of sweat glands and sebaceous glands.

Heredity. The diagnosis of anhidrosis was well established in six persons tested. Eight additional cases were diagnosed by history. Five affected with anhidrosis also had progressive hearing loss, which was confirmed by audiometric tests (Fig. 14–30B).

The pedigree of the family showed 14 affected persons in five generations, a pattern compatible with autosomal dominant inheritance.

Diagnosis. Several types of anhidrosis have been described. An autosomal recessively transmitted form characterized by anhidrosis but without abnormalities of teeth, face, or brain was presented by Mahloudji and Livingston (3). Both X-linked and the rare autosomal recessive types of hypohidrotic ectodermal dysplasia include anodontia and hypotrichosis (1). While hearing loss has been reported, it is rare (4,5,7). Anhidrosis also occurs in association with congenital sensory neuropathy (6). These types of hereditary anhidrosis differ in mode of transmission and in associated defects from that described here.

Prognosis. More persons need to be studied to define clearly the progression of the hearing loss, which, apparently, is slowly progressive.

Summary. Characteristics of this syndrome include (1) autosomal dominant transmission; (2) congenital anhidrosis; and (3) onset of progressive sensorineural hearing loss in middle age.

References

1. Gorlin RJ et al: Hypohidrotic ectodermal dysplasia in females. A critical analysis and argument for genetic heterogeneity. *Z Kinderheilkd* 108:1–11, 1970.
2. Helweg-Larsen HF, Ludvigsen K: Congenital familial anhidrosis and neurolabyrinthitis. *Acta Dermatol Venereol* 26:489–505, 1946.
3. Mahloudji M, Livingston KE: Familial and congenital simple anhidrosis. *Am J Dis Child* 113:477–479, 1967.
4. Passarge E et al: Anhidrotic ectodermal dysplasia as autosomal recessive trait in an inbred kindred. *Humangenetik* 3:181–185, 1966.
5. Reich H, Kumpf W: Nase, Nasennebenhöhlen und Innenohr bei anhidrotischer ektodermaler Dysplasie. *HNO* 22:284–286, 1974.
6. Vassella F et al: Congenital sensory neuropathy with anhidrosis. *Arch Dis Child* 43:124–130, 1968.
7. Wesser DW, Vistnes LM: Congenital ectodermal dysplasia, anhidrotic, with palatal paralysis and associated chromosome abnormality. *Plast Reconstr Surg* 44:396–398, 1969.

Figure 14–30. *Anhidrosis and progressive sensorineural hearing loss (Helweg-Larsen and Ludvigsen syndrome).* (A) Scattered sweat points in pectoral area indicated by starch-iodine test. (B) Pedigree showing 14 affected persons in five generations. [From HF Helweg-Larsen and K Ludvigsen, *Acta Dermatol Venereol (Stockh)* 26:489, 1946.]

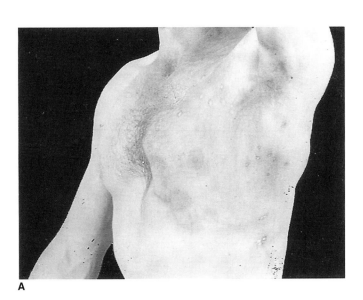

A

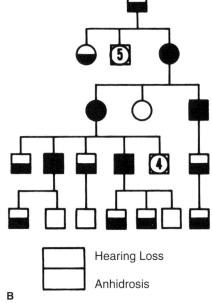

B

Cylindromatosis

Cylindromatosis is a condition characterized by multiple tumors involving the nasolabial folds, face, eyelids, ears, scalp, and upper trunk, although 90% occur on the head and neck (1–5). Tumors generally do not appear before puberty and are either cylindromas (basophilic cells surrounded by hyaline) or tricho-epitheliomas (horn cells). There has been one report of parotid gland involvement (4). Inheritance is autosomal dominant with more marked variability of expression and decreased penetrance in males, thus leading to an apparently altered sex ratio. Hearing loss, if present, is usually secondary to tumors in the ear canals. Gene mapping studies have shown that the gene maps to 16q12–13 in all affected families studied, indicating there is no evidence of genetic heterogeneity (5). The gene (*CYLD*) has recently been identified as a tumor-suppressor gene (2).

References

1. Anderson DE, Howell JB: Epithelioma adenoides, cysticum genetic update. *Br J Dermatol* 95:225–232, 1976.
2. Bignell GR et al: Identification of the familial cylindromatosis tumour-suppressor gene. *Nat Genet* 25:160–165, 2000.
3. Blandy JP et al: Turban tumours in brother and sister. *Br J Surg* 49:136–140, 1961.
4. Jungehulsing M et al: Turban tumour with involvement of the parotid gland. *J Laryngol Otol* 113:779–783, 1999.
5. Takahashi M et al: Linkage and LOH studies in 19 cylindromatosis families show no evidence of genetic heterogeneity and refine the CYLD locus on chromosome 16q12–q13. *Hum Genet* 106:58–65, 2000.

Symmetrical lipomatosis and sensorineural hearing loss

In 1984, Stevenson et al. (3) described an extensive family in which 21 individuals in four generations had a condition characterized by symmetrical lipomatosis, stiff skin, systemic manifestations, and hearing loss of variable degrees.

Craniofacial findings. All examined individuals were described as having midface hypoplasia. Proptosis was common and ocular findings such as divergent squint and conjunctivitis were noted. The skin was tight around the perioral area, thus limiting facial expression.

Integumentary system. The skin was tight and stiff, particularly in the perioral area and extremities. Subcutaneous tissues of hands and feet were decreased, and lipomatous hypertrophy of subcutaneous tissues, primarily of the chest and upper abdomen, was noted.

Musculoskeletal system. The small joints appeared enlarged, and most joints had stiffness and/or decreased movement. Arthralgia, muscle cramps, and muscle atrophy were also common.

Cardiovascular system. Hypertension and arteriosclerosis were present in more than 50% of the examined patients.

Renal system. Most affected individuals had hematuria and nephrolithiasis. One examined stone had a composition of 99% calcium oxalate and 1% hydroxyapatite.

Gastrointestinal system. Gastrointestinal complaints were common and included peptic ulcer, duodenal ulcer, and dysphagia.

Auditory system. Sensorineural hearing loss, usually bilateral, was variable, in some cases preceding onset of other symptoms.

Laboratory findings. Many individuals had elevated blood glucose, hyperlipemia, hyperuricemia, elevated urea nitrogen, elevated testosterone in females, and proteinuria.

Pathology. Muscle biopsies were normal, but skin biopsy showed hyalinization of dermal collagen. Radiographs demonstrated swelling of interphalangeal joints.

Heredity. Inheritance is autosomal dominant.

Diagnosis. Although this condition shares some features with scleroderma and the "stiff skin" syndromes, involvement of internal organs and the presence of hearing loss help differentiate this condition. Stevenson et al. (3) believe this condition is the same as symmetric lipomatosis (Lanois-Bensuade syndrome) (1,2), but no other individuals with this condition have had hearing loss or renal or gastrointestinal disorders, so this may represent a unique condition among the heterogeneous lipomatoses.

Prognosis. This condition has onset in early childhood. It is progressive and causes debilitation, but apparently no decrease in life span.

Summary. Characteristics of this provisionally unique condition include (*1*) autosomal dominant inheritance; (*2*) stiff skin; (*3*) lipomatosis of chest and upper abdomen; (*4*) joint stiffness; (*5*) peptic ulcer; (*6*) arteriosclerosis; (*7*) kidney stones; and (*8*) sensorineural hearing loss.

References

1. Enzi G: Multiple symmetric lipomatosis: an updated clinical report. *Medicine* 63:56–64, 1984.
2. Enzi G et al: Sensory, motor and autonomic neuropathy in patients with multiple symmetric lipomatosis. *Medicine* 64:388–392, 1986.
3. Stevenson RE et al: Symmetrical lipomatosis associated with stiff skin and systemic manifestations in four generations. *Proc Greenwood Genet Ctr* 3:56–64, 1984.

Aplasia cutis-ear malformations

In 1979, Anderson et al. (1) described a four-generation Mexican-American family in which affected family members had aplasia cutis, lop ears, facial paresis, and preauricular and/or sternal pits. One individual had unilateral conductive loss associated with meatal atresia on the same side. Inheritance was autosomal dominant.

Reference

1. Anderson CE et al: Autosomal dominantly inherited cutis aplasia congenita, ear malformations, right-sided facial paresis, and dermal sinuses. *Birth Defects* 15(5B):265–270, 1979.

Focal dermal hypoplasia (Goltz-Gorlin syndrome)

Focal dermal hypoplasia is characterized by atrophy and linear hypo- and hyperpigmentation of skin, localized cutaneous deposits of superficial fat, multiple papillomas of mucous membranes or perioral skin, atrophy of nails, and a host of ocular and skeletal abnormalities (Fig. 14–31). These have been reviewed by Goltz et al. (7) and Ginsburg et al. (5), and exhaustively by Goltz (6).

Inheritance is X-linked dominant, with male lethality. A few instances of mother-to-daughter transmission have been documented (1,12), as well as mosaicism in a father with transmission to his daughter (9). Skewed X-inactivation has been demonstrated, but this does not occur universally (12). About 95% of the cases are sporadic (6,16,17). It has been suggested that MIDAS, Aicardi, and Goltz-Gorlin syndromes are all caused by involvement of the same genes (12), but this was refuted by Mucke et al. (13) on the basis that MIDAS and Goltz-Gorlin have never occurred in the same family. Perhaps 5%–10% of patients with this syndrome have hearing loss. No study has been carried out on the temporal bone. Holden and Akers (10) reported mixed hearing deficit, noted at 3 years of age, in their patient. Stollman (15) made brief note of sensorineural hearing loss in his patients. Goltz (6) and Reber et al. (14) also found mixed hearing loss. Daly (3), Ginsburg et al. (5), and Ferrara

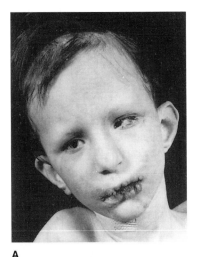

A

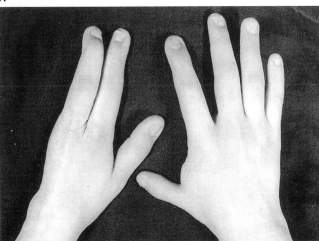

B

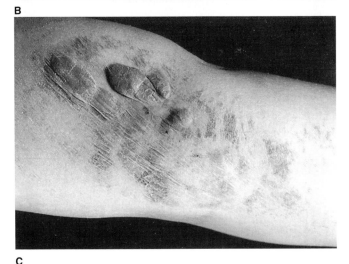

C

Figure 14–31. *Focal dermal hypoplasia (Goltz-Gorlin syndrome).* (A) Note multiple frambesiform lesions on lips, coloboma of iris, strabismus, and thin hair. (B) Note postsurgical correction of hands. Note small thumb, reduction of digits postaxially on one hand, and hypoplastic nails. (C) Multiple saccular growths presenting in antecubital area.

(4) described narrowed external auditory meatus. Cholesteatomas of the middle ear have also been reported (2,15). Gordjani et al. (8) described obstructive papillomatosis of the larynx in a 14-year-old girl, and Irvine et al. (11) described intestinal malrotation in a patient.

References

1. Bellosta M et al: Focal dermal hypoplasia: report of a family with 7 affected women in 3 generations. *Eur J Dermatol* 6:499–500, 1996.
2. Büchner SA, Itin P: Focal dermal hypoplasia syndrome in a male patient. *Arch Dermatol* 128:1078–1082, 1992.
3. Daly JG: Focal dermal hypoplasia. *Cutis* 4:1354–1359, 1968.
4. Ferrara A: Goltz's syndrome. *Am J Dis Child* 123:263, 1972.
5. Ginsburg LD et al: Focal dermal hypoplasia syndrome. *AJR Am J Roentgenol* 110:561–571, 1970.
6. Goltz RW: Focal dermal hypoplasia syndrome: an update. *Arch Dermatol* 128:1108–1111, 1992.
7. Goltz RW et al: Focal dermal hypoplasia syndrome. *Arch Dermatol* 101:1–11, 1970.
8. Gordjani N et al: Focal dermal hypoplasia (Goltz-Gorlin syndrome) associated with obstructive papillomatosis of the larynx and hypopharynx. *Eur J Dermatol* 9:618–620, 1999.
9. Gorski JL: Father-to-daughter transmission of focal dermal hypoplasia associated with nonrandom X-inactivation: support for X-linked inheritance and paternal X chrmosome mosaicism. *Am J Med Genet* 40:332–337, 1991.
10. Holden JD, Akers HA: Goltz's syndrome: focal dermal hypoplasia combined mesoectodermal dysplasia. *Am J Dis Child* 114:292–300, 1967.
11. Irvine AD et al: Focal dermal hypoplasia (Goltz syndrome) associated with intestinal malrotation and mediastinal dextroposition. *Am J Med Genet* 62:213–215, 1996.
12. Lindsay EA et al: Microphthalmia with linear skin defects (MLS) syndrome: Clinical, cytogenetic, and molecular characterization. *Am J Med Genet* 49:229–234,1994.
13. Mucke J et al: Letter to the editor: MIDAS syndrome respectively MLS syndrome: a separate entity rather than a particular lysonization pattern of the gene causing Goltz syndrome. *Am J Med Genet* 57:117–118, 1998.
14. Reber T et al: Goltz-Gorlin-Syndrom bei einem Mann. *Hautarzt* 38:218–224, 1987.
15. Stollman K: Bisher noch nicht beschriebene Befunde bei Incontinentia pigmenti. *Dermatol Wochenschr* 153:489–496, 1967.
16. Temple IK et al: Focal dermal hypoplasia (Goltz syndrome). *J Med Genet* 27:80–97, 1990.
17. Wechsler MA et al: Variable expression in focal dermal hypoplasia. *Am J Dis Child* 142:297–300, 1988.

Ruzicka syndrome

Ruzicka et al. (1) described a 15-year-old girl with congenital ichthyosis, brachydactyly, clinodactyly, and accessory cervical ribs. Bilateral high-frequency sensorineural hearing loss was diagnosed soon after birth. Thyroid cancer was diagnosed at age 14. Development was retarded, even taking into consideration the hearing loss.

Reference

1. Ruzicka T et al: Syndrome of ichthyosis congenita, neurosensory deafness, oligophrenia, dental aplasia, brachydactyly, clinodactyly, accessory cervical ribs and carcinoma of the thyroid. *Dermatologica* 162:124–136,1981.

Epidermolysis bullosa, type Nielsen-Sjölund

Neilsen and Sjölund (1) reported two sisters with epidermolysis bullosa simplex, partial anodontia, and other ectodermal defects. The blistering of the skin appeared between age 3 months and 1 year and was limited to the feet in both girls and to the hands in one. The hair became sparse and brittle after 4 months but eventually regrew. The nails were curved and/or thickened. Profound hearing loss was found in one ear of one girl at age 5 years. Intellectual development appeared normal. Inheritance was likely autosomal recessive.

Reference

1. Nielsen PG, Sjölund E: Epidermolysis bullosa simplex localisata associated with anodontia, hair and nail disorders: a new syndrome. *Acta Dermatol Venereol (Stockh)* 65:526–530, 1985.

Hairy ears and Y-linked sensorineural hearing loss

There are large numbers of Indian pedigrees in which affected males have long hairs growing from the helix of the pinnae (1–5) (Fig. 14–32). In these kindreds, the affected male gives the trait of hairy ears to all his sons but to none of his daughters. It therefore has been proposed that the trait is Y-linked. Rao (2–4) proposed that hairy ears result from the interaction of two loci, one on the homologous segment of the X and Y chromosomes and one on the nonhomologous segment of the Y chromosome. Tarantino et al. (6) reported seven affected males in four generations. All had hairy ears. The hearing loss affected all tones at 40–60 dB loss.

References

1. Dronamraju KR: Y-linkage in man. *Nature* 201:424–425, 1964.
2. Rao DC: A contribution to the genetics of hypertrichosis of the ear rims. *Hum Hered* 20:486–492, 1970.
3. Rao DC: Two-gene hypothesis for hairy pinnae. *Acta Genet Med Gemellol* 19:448–453, 1970.
4. Rao DC: Hypertrichosis of the ear rims: two remarks on the two-gene hypothesis. *Acta Genet Med Gemellol* 21:216–220, 1972.
5. Stern C et al: New data on the problem of Y-linkage of hairy pinnae. *Am J Hum Genet* 16:455–471, 1964.
6. Tarantino V et al: Sorditaá ereditaria legata al cromosome Y? Studio di un gruppo famigliare. *Otorinolaringologia* 40:107–109, 1990.

Histiocytic dermatoarthritis

This condition has been described in two kindreds by Zayid and Farraj (2) and Valente et al. (1). Manifestations include cutaneous nodules, early-onset seronegative arthritis, particularly of the hands and feet, and ocular lesions consisting of glaucoma, uveitis, and/or cataracts. Inheritance pattern in both families was consistent with an autosomal dominant gene. Hearing deficit, a moderate sensorineural loss, was present in only one individual.

References

1. Valente M et al: Familial histiocytic dermatoarthritis: histologic and ultrastructural findings in two cases. *Am J Dermatopathol* 9:491–496, 1987.
2. Zayid I, Farraj S: Familial histiocytic dermatoarthritis: a new syndrome. *Am J Med* 54:793–800, 1973.

Elastic connective tissue nevi, osteopoikilosis, and conductive hearing loss (Buschke-Ollendorff syndrome)

Herzberg et al. (1) described dizygotic twin brothers with multiple painless nonpruritic subcutaneous yellow nodules, mostly on the trunk,

Figure 14–32. Hairy ears Y-linked and sensorineural hearing loss. Hairy ears.

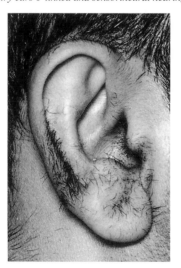

which had been present for at least 2 years. The paternal grandmother had similar skin lesions and hearing difficulties reported to be otosclerosis. The father had congenital spinal stenosis with disc herniation at L5–S1 and nerve root compression. He had two palpable subcutaneous nodules on one calf and thigh. Both brothers were below the fifth centile in height. Skin biopsy of a nodule from one twin showed thickened elastic fibers deep within the reticular dermis. The fibers were clumped and associated with increased mucin. The grandmother's biopsy also showed increased elastic fibers in the dermis, which had irregular orientation and fragmentation. X-rays of the father's knees showed multiple osteopoikilotic areas. Otosclerosis of the petrous bone with hearing loss has been reported in several other cases of Buschke-Ollendorff syndrome (2,3). Short stature has occasionally been found in the condition.

References

1. Herzberg A et al: Buschke-Ollendorff syndrome, otosclerosis and congenital spinal stenosis. Annual meeting of American Society of Human Genetics. *Am J Hum Genet* 51(Suppl):Abst. 377, 1992.
2. Piette-Brion B et al: Dermatofibromes, élastomes et surdité. Un nouveau cas de syndrome de Buschke-Ollendorff. *Dermatologica* 168:255–258, 1984.
3. Strosberg J, Adler RG: Otosclerosis associated with osteopoikilosis. *JAMA* 246:2030–2031, 1982.

IBIDS syndrome

The term *IBIDS syndrome* refers to a combination of *I*chthyosis, *B*rittle hair, *I*mpaired intelligence, *D*ecreased fertility, and *S*hort stature, which is a form of trichothiodystrophy. Its association with axial osteosclerosis and peripheral osteopenia has also been noted (1). Among approximately 10 cases that have been reported, 2 have been associated with mixed hearing loss. These reports were not well documented audiologically (2,3).

References

1. Civitelli R et al: Central osteosclerosis with ectodermal dysplasia: clinical, laboratory, radiologic, and histopathologic characterization with review of the literature. *J Bone Min Res* 4:863–875, 1989.
2. Dowd PM, Munro DD: Ichthyosis and osteopetrosis. *J R Soc Med* 76:423–426, 1983.
3. Johnson F et al: Case report 50. *Skeletal Radiol* 2:185–186, 1978.

Coarse face, mental retardation, skin granulomata, and profound congenital sensorineural hearing loss (Fountain syndrome)

In 1974, Fountain (1) reported four mentally retarded sibs who exhibited massive swelling of the lips and profound congenital sensorineural hearing loss. Fryns et al. (2,3) described another pair of sibs and an isolated patient. Van Buggenhout et al. (5) reported two additional cases and provided follow-up on the three patients reported by Fryns et al. (2,3).

Physical findings. Birth weight and length are normal, but adult height is less than 153 cm. Head size ranges from normal to macrocephalic. The face is "coarse" with swelling of the subcutaneous tissue of the cheeks. The palpebral fissures are narrow, and nasal tip is broad and fleshy. The lips can be initially normal, but become progressively fuller over time, so that by adulthood they are quite full and prominent. Three of four sibs in one kindred had granulomatous swelling of the lips (1) (Fig. 14–33). The hands and feet were short and plump with short, broad terminal phalanges (2,3).

Musculoskeletal system. Radiographic changes included thickening of the calvaria and poor modeling of the distal femur and distal radius (1,2). The acetabula were shallow (1).

Integumentary system. One patient had buccal mucosal tags and gingival enlargement at 15 years of age (1). At 22 years, the lower lip

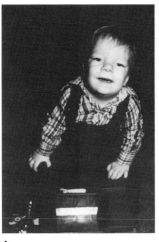

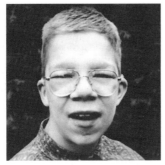

B

A

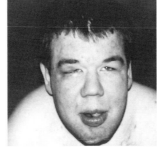

D

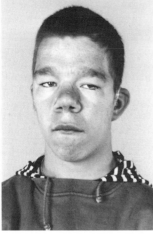

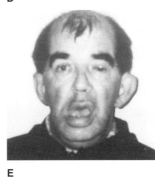

C   E

Figure 14–33. *Fountain syndrome.* (A) Child at age 2¹/₂ years. (B) Same child at 5 years. (C) Same individual at age 17 years. (D) Another individual at 26 years. (E) Third affected individual at age 44 years. Note "coarse" face and full lips. [From GJCM Van Buggenhout et al., *Genet Couns* 7:177–183, 1996. Reprinted with permission of JP Fryns, ed, *Genetic Counseling.*]

became progressively swollen and granulomatous. Her brother had inguinal hernia repair, followed by a foreign body granulomatous reaction. At age 22 years, he experienced enlargement of the upper lip. A third sib exhibited no granulomata. The other patients were not reported to have granulomata, so this may be just an occasional finding in this condition.

Central nervous system. All affected sibs were mentally retarded, ranging from mild to severe (2), with generalized hypotonia (2). This resulted in mild scoliosis in adult years. Infantile seizures were manifest in two sibs (3) and childhood-onset seizures occurred in a third child (5). Speech tends to be absent. The personality is described as friendly (5).

Auditory system. All patients exhibited profound congenital sensorineural hearing loss with rudimentary hearing at the lowest frequencies (2). Tomography of the temporal bones showed absence of cochlear windings (Mondini anomaly) (2).

Vestibular system. Vestibular studies were not carried out.

Pathology. Gingival biopsy showed a granulomatous infiltrate marked by large, foamy cells that did not contain fat. The PAS stain was mildly positive and diastase-resistant (1).

Heredity. Inheritance appears to be autosomal recessive, although it is interesting that the male:female ratio is 7:1.

Diagnosis. The syndrome most closely resembles aspartylglucosaminuria, an autosomal recessive disease characterized by mental retardation, coarse facial features, sagging cheeks, frequent infections, diarrhea, and vacuolated lymphocytes. However, in Fountain syndrome, biochemical studies have been normal (1,2).

The edematous facial changes are similar to those of Melkersson-Rosenthal syndrome (4), however, mental retardation and deafness are not found in that syndrome.

Prognosis. Although the disorder is not life-threatening, the general outlook is poor.

Summary. The syndrome is characterized by (*1*) probably autosomal recessive inheritance; (*2*) mental retardation; (*3*) somewhat reduced height; (*4*) occasional skin granulomata; (*5*) thickened calvaria and poor modeling of bones; and (*6*) severe congenital sensorineural hearing loss.

References

1. Fountain RB: Familial bone abnormalities, deaf mutism, mental retardation, and skin granulomas. *Proc R Soc Med* 67:878–879, 1974.
2. Fryns JP: Fountain's syndrome: mental retardation, sensorineural deafness, skeletal abnormalities, and coarse facies with full lips. *J Med Genet* 26:722–724, 1989.
3. Fryns JP et al: Mental retardation, deafness, skeletal abnormalities and coarse face with full lips: confirmation of the Fountain syndrome. *Am J Med Genet* 26:551–556, 1987.
4. Gorlin RJ et al: *Syndromes of the Head and Neck,* 4th ed. Oxford University Press, New York, 2001, pp. 751–752.
5. Van Buggenhout GJCM et al: Fountain syndrome: further delineation of the clinical syndrome and follow-up data. *Genet Couns* 7:177–186, 1996.

Growth retardation, mental retardation, microcephaly, seizures, dermatosis, and sensorineural hearing loss

In 1990, Boudhina et al. (1) described a syndrome of significant growth retardation, mental retardation, microcephaly, seizures, scaly dermatosis, and sensorineural hearing loss in three sibs. The epilepsy was of the grand mal type. Other features seen in the siblings include hyperpigmentation of the skin, genua valga, hallux valgus, and cubitus valgus. The sensorineural hearing loss was not otherwise documented. Inheritance appears to be autosomal recessive.

Reference

1. Boudhina T et al: Syndrome famial associant: nanisme, microcéphalie, oligophrenie, epilepsie, surdité et dermatose. Un nouveau syndrome. *Ann Pédiatr* 37:400–403, 1990.

Kassutto syndrome

In 1987, Kassutto et al. (1) reported on a father and daughter with frontal bossing, facial asymmetry, temporal alopecia, broad nasal root, small nasal alae, and short lingual frenulum producing a mild bifid tongue.

Hearing loss was bilateral with onset in infancy; while the degree was unknown in the child, it was severe enough to warrant hearing aids. The father had nonprogressive moderate sensorineural hearing loss with onset in infancy but milder in degree than that of his daughter.

Inheritance appears to be autosomal dominant.

References

1. Kassutto S et al: A new autosomal dominant craniofacial deafness syndrome. *Clin Genet* 32:355–359, 1987.

Finucane hearing loss–hypopigmentation–skeletal defects syndrome

In 1992, Finucane et al. (1) described two unrelated children with unusual facial appearance, mental retardation, hypopigmented areas of skin, skeletal defects, and sensorineural hearing loss. Both children attended the same special education class and were referred because of striking physical and behavioral similarities. The first child, a female, exhibited developmental delay and self-stimulating behaviors from infancy. She rolled over at 8 months, sat alone at 11 months, and walked independently at 15 months. At 15 months, global delay and growth retardation with delayed bone age were evident. Mild to moderate sensorineural hearing loss was documented at 6 years. She had bilateral epicanthi, a broad fleshy nose, depressed nasal bridge, anteverted nares, deep nasolabial folds, and broad mouth (Fig. 14–34). Multiple hypopigmented areas were noted over the back and lower abdominal, inguinal, and axillary areas. At age 8 years, carpal centers appeared grossly delayed with phalangeal ossification centers being focally dysplastic. At 15 years of age, she was essentially nonverbal and exhibited delayed puberty.

The second patient also had delayed developmental milestones, first sitting alone at 9 months and walking independently at 4 years. A facies similar to that of the first patient was evident. Multiple hypopigmented spots were apparent over the torso and extremities. Audiologic evaluation of the second patient revealed severe bilateral sensorineural hearing loss.

Skeletal abnormalities seen in both children included scoliosis, abnormally placed thumbs, brachydactyly V, and dysplastic carpal bones.

Reference

1. Finucane B et al: A new mental retardation syndrome with deafness, distinctive facies, and skeletal anomalies. *Am J Med Genet* 43:844–847, 1992.

Radial aplasia, hyperkeratosis, enterocolitis

Hilhorst-Hofstee et al. (1) described a child with the combination of cleft palate, micrognathia, radial aplasia, three fingers and hypoplastic thumb, hip dysplasia, small or absent patellae, and imperforate anus. Postnatally she developed communicating hydrocephalus that was shunted; bilateral hearing loss was detected at that time. At 8 months she developed erythema of the knees and extensor surfaces, and at 9

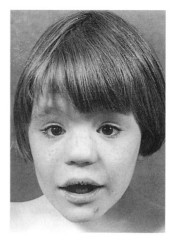

Figure 14–34. *Finucane hearing loss–hypopigmentation–skeletal defects syndrome.* Broad fleshy nose, broad mouth, almond-shaped ears. [From B Finucane et al., *Am J Med Genet* 43:844, 1992.]

months a rash resembling poikiloderma appeared on her face. She had early-onset diarrhea; biopsies revealed partial villous atrophy. Growth was markedly delayed. The CT scan demonstrated normal cochlea, but with shorted semicircular canals. The authors suggested that she (as well as the two other nondeaf patients in the report) had either a provisionally unique syndrome or a severe form of Rothmund-Thomson syndrome. Rothmund-Thomson syndrome has recently been reviewed by Wang et al. (2) in 41 patients; only 1 had deafness (but interestingly also had hydrocephalus). Hearing loss is therefore not a major component of Rothmund-Thomson syndrome, but whether the hearing loss in this patient is sufficient to suggest that she has a unique syndrome is uncertain.

References

1. Hilhorst-Hofstee Y et al: Radial aplasia, poikiloderma and auto-immune enterocolitis—new syndrome or severe form of Rothmund-Thomson syndrome? *Clin Dysmorphol* 9:79–86, 2000.
2. Wang LL et al: Clinical manifestations in a cohort of 41 Rothmund-Thomson syndrome patients. *Am J Med Genet* 102:11–17, 2001.

Appendix

Other entities with integumentary anomalies

Entity	Integumentary Finding	Chapter in this Book
Aural atresia, microtia, skin mastocytosis, short stature, conductive hearing loss	Mastocytosis	6 (external ear)
Retinitis pigmentosa, vitiligo, SHL	Vitiligo	7 (eye)
Oral-facial-digital syndrome I	Milia	8 (musculoskeletal)
EEC syndrome	Ectodermal dysplasia	8 (musculoskeletal)
Trichorhinophalangeal syndromes	Sparse hair	8 (musculoskeletal)
Muckle-Wells syndrome	Urticaria	9 (renal)
Renal disease, hyperprolinemia, ichthyosis, SHL	Ichthyosis	9 (renal)
BRESHECK syndrome	Ectodermal dysplasia	9 (renal)
Chanarin-Dorfman syndrome	Ichthyosis	13 (metabolic)
Bocian-Rimoin syndrome	Ectodermal dysplasia	15 (oral and dental)

SHL, sensorineural hearing loss.

Chapter 15
Genetic Hearing Loss Associated with Oral and Dental Disorders
ROBERT J. GORLIN

The number of genetic disorders of hearing loss associated with oral and dental disorders is small, but placing them in a separate group seems worthwhile.

Otodental syndrome

In 1972, Levin and Jorgenson (7) described a syndrome of dental anomalies and sensorineural hearing loss. To date, several unrelated families have been described (1–11,13,15,16); one case is doubtful (12). An early example is that of Denes and Csiba (4).

Dental findings. The incisors of both dentitions are spared. The crowns of the canines and posterior teeth are enlarged, bulbous, and malformed with multiple prominent lobules (Fig. 15–1A,B). The deciduous dentition is more severely involved. The relationship between cusps and major grooves is eliminated (Fig. 15–1C); hence the use of the term *globodontia* (11). An enamel defect is frequently noted on the facial surface of the canine teeth. Premolar teeth are frequently missing or small in size (1–5,10,11). There is often delayed eruption of the deciduous malformed teeth or even of the permanent posterior teeth (1,2,15). One can observe duplicated pulp chambers with denticle formation, a longitudinal dental septum, and early pulpal obliteration. The molar teeth have a tendency toward conical or taurodont root form. Complex and/or compound odontomas have also been described in the posterior maxilla and mandible (1,10,15). The enamel may be somewhat hypoplastic (8,10,15,16).

Auditory system. Progressive bilateral sensorineural hearing loss to about 65 dB is found at all frequencies but is more pronounced at about 1000 Hz. It usually plateaus by the fourth decade (3). The age of onset of the hearing loss ranges from early childhood to middle age, which may complicate making diagnosis of the disorder (3,6,8).

Eyes. Iris colobomas were reported in one family (15).

Laboratory findings. Radiologic examination of the teeth has demonstrated taurodontism of molar teeth with large calcifications in pulp chambers and root canals. In some individuals, the deciduous molar appears to have two separate pulp chambers, the extra one distolingually.

Vestibular system. Caloric testing has been normal.

Pathology. No pathological studies have been described.

Heredity. Inheritance is clearly autosomal dominant with variable expressivity (2). Studies on the family with ocular abnormalities (15) showed linkage to 20q13.1 (14). It is unknown whether this gene also causes otodental syndrome without ocular defects.

Diagnosis. Premolars are absent in about 5% of the general population. Taurodontism may occur as an isolated finding or part of a syndrome.

Summary. This syndrome is characterized by (1) autosomal dominant inheritance; (2) dental changes, which include globoid canines and posterior teeth and taurodontism; and (3) bilateral high-tone sensorineural hearing loss.

References

1. Beck-Mannagetta J et al: Odontome und pantonale Hörstörung bei otodentalem Syndrom. *Dtsch Zahnärtzl Z* 39:232–241, 1984.
2. Chen RJ et al: "Otodental" dysplasia. *Oral Surg Oral Med Oral Pathol* 66:353–358, 1988.
3. Cook RA et al: Otodental dysplasia: a five-year study. *Ear Hear* 2:90–94, 1981.
4. Denes J, Csiba A: An unusual case of hereditary developmental anomalies of cuspids and molars. *Fogorv Sz* 62:208–212, 1969.
5. Gundlach KKH, Witkop CJ Jr: Globodontie—eine neue erbliche Zahnformanomalie. *Dtsch Zahnärztl Z* 21:194–196, 1977.
6. Jorgenson RJ et al: Otodental dysplasia. *Birth Defects* 11(5):115–119, 1975.
7. Levin LS, Jorgenson RJ: Familial otodental dysplasia: a "new" syndrome. *Am J Hum Genet* 24:A61, 1972.
8. Levin LS et al: Otodental syndrome. A "new" ectodermal dysplasia. *Clin Genet* 8:136–144, 1975.
9. Mesaros AJ Jr, Basden JW: Otodental syndrome. *Gen Dent* 44:427–429, 1996 (one case, same as ref. 15).
10. Salmeron JI et al: Odontogenic tumours and dental anomalies in children. *Craniomaxillofac Surg Suppl* 1:151, 1996.
11. Santos-Pinto L et al: Otodental syndrome: three familial case reports. *Pediatr Dent* 20:208–211, 1998.
12. Stewart DJ, Kinirons MJ: Globodontia. *Br Dent J* 152:287–288, 1982.
13. Van Doorne L et al: Otodental syndrome. *Int J Oral Maxillofac Surg* 27:121–124, 1998.
14. Vieira H et al: First genomic localization of oculo-oto-dental syndrome with linkage to chromosome 20q13.1. *Invest Ophthal Vis Sci* 43:2540–2545, 2002.
15. Winter GB: The association of ocular defects with the otodental syndrome. *J Int Assoc Dent Child* 14:83–87, 1983.
16. Witkop CJ Jr.: Globodontia in the otodental syndrome. *Oral Surg* 41:472–483, 1976.

Amelogenesis imperfecta, leukonychia, and sensorineural hearing loss

A syndrome characterized by sensorineural hearing loss, amelogenesis imperfecta, and leukonychia was described in a pair of sibs by Heimler et al. (1) in 1991. Tischkowitz et al. (3) and Pollak et al. (2) added two new cases.

Dental changes. Primary teeth were oddly normal, but the permanent teeth exhibited amelogenesis imperfecta. The teeth were discolored and, in addition, the molars and premolars were hypoplastic in both children (Fig. 15–2A).

Integumentary system. The nails in some children had transverse lines proximally (Beau's lines) and punctate leukonychia (Fig. 15–2B,C).

Auditory system. Profound bilateral sensorineural hearing loss was diagnosed at 18 months in one child, at $2^{1}/_{2}$ years in two others, and unilaterally at 7 years in still another. Hearing was normal for the first 2 years in one child, so the loss was not congenital.

Laboratory findings. Urinalysis, serum calcium, phosphorus, and creatinine were all normal.

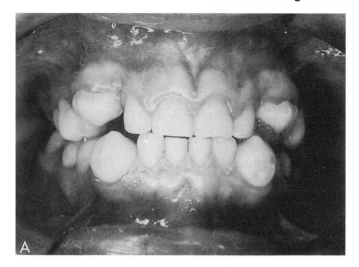

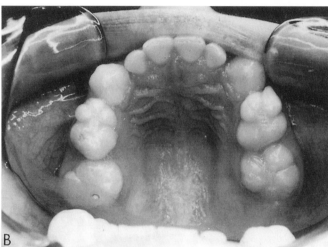

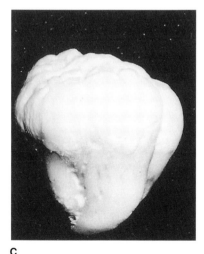

C

Figure 15–1. *Otodental syndrome.* (A,B) Note normal central and lateral incisors. Canines and deciduous molars are enormous in size. (C) Extracted 6-year molar. [(A,B) courtesy of CJ Witkop Jr, Minneapolis, Minnesota; (C) from J Beck-Mannagetta et al., *Dtsch Zahnärztl Z* 39:232, 1984.]

Heredity. The presence of this condition in sibs of each sex (1,2) and unaffected parents suggest autosomal recessive inheritance, but in no case was there parental consanguinity.

Diagnosis. The differential diagnosis includes Robinson syndrome, which is inherited as an autosomal dominant trait and includes

syndactyly and/or polydactyly in addition to nail and tooth anomalies.

Prognosis. Intelligence is normal. Life span is likely to be unaffected.

Summary. This condition consists of (*1*) possible autosomal recessive inheritance; (*2*) enamel hypoplasia of permanent teeth; (*3*) minor nail anomalies; and (*4*) bilateral sensorineural hearing loss.

References

1. Heimler A et al: Sensorineural hearing loss, enamel hypoplasia and nail abnormalities in sibs. *Am J Med Genet* 39:192–195, 1991.
2. Pollak C et al: Sensorineural hearing loss and enamel hypoplasia with subtle nail findings: Another family with Heimler's syndrome. *Clin Dysmorphol* 12:55–58, 2003.
3. Tischkowitz M et al: Amelogenesis imperfecta, sensorineural hearing loss, and Beau's lines: a second case report of Heimler's syndrome. *J Med Genet* 36:940–943, 1999.

Multiple anterior dens invaginatus and sensorineural hearing loss

A female child seen by Kantaputra and Gorlin (1) had double dens invaginatus of maxillary central incisors combined with premolarization of maxillary lateral incisors and first deciduous molars. She was missing two lower right permanent incisors. There was dens invaginatus of the lower left central and lateral incisors (Fig. 15–3A–C).

Figure 15–2. *Amelogenesis imperfecta, leukonychia, and sensorineural hearing loss.* (A) Severe enamel hypoplasia. (B) Leukonychia. (C) Beau's lines on toenail. [From A Heimler et al., *Am J Med Genet* 39:192, 1991.]

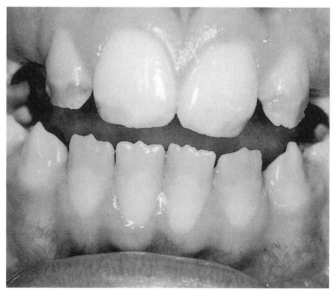

A

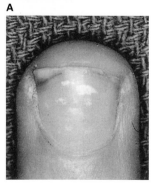

B

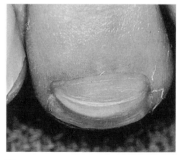

C

Facial appearance was normal except for some fullness at the bridge of the nose and somewhat dilated nostrils (Fig. 15–3D). She had bilateral, moderately severe sensorineural hearing loss. Although estimate of IQ was approximately 75, this may well have been in error due to a combination of hearing loss and shyness.

Reference

1. Kantaputra PN, Gorlin RJ: Double dens invaginatus of molarized maxillary central incisors, premolarization of maxillary lateral incisors, multituberculism of the mandibular incisors, canines and first premolar, and sensorineural hearing loss. *Clin Dysmorphol* 1:128–136, 1992.

Natal teeth, bifid tongue, and profound sensorineural hearing loss

An apparently unique association of natal teeth, bifid tongue, and profound sensorineural hearing loss was reported in a Saudi Arabian male child by Darwish et al. (1).

The natal teeth were lower central incisors. The tongue tip was bifid. The lingual frenum was in normal position without undue traction on the tongue. Hearing loss was profound without additional description.

While the association of the three anomalies may be one of chance, odds against this would appear great.

Reference

1. Darwish S et al: Natal teeth, bifid tongue and deaf mutism. *J Oral Med* 42:49–56, 1987.

Oligodontia and congenital sensorineural hearing loss

Two pair of sibs with sensorineural hearing loss and oligodontia have been reported by Lee et al. (2) in 1978 and by Glass and Gorlin (1) in 1979.

Dental findings. In one family (2), both children lacked permanent maxillary lateral incisors; one was missing the permanent canines as well. In the second family (1), at least 10 permanent teeth were missing, with several diastemas present (Fig. 15–4).

Other findings. Both children in the first family (2) experienced episodes of dizziness beginning at age 2. Projectile vomiting accompanied the dizzy spells at age 6.5 in one child. This finding was not present in the other family.

Auditory system. In all four children, profound bilateral sensorineural hearing loss was diagnosed by 11 months of age. Tympanograms were normal in all the children.

Vestibular system. In the first family (2), vestibular examination showed normal caloric responses.

Laboratory findings. Routine blood chemistries, urinalysis, blood cell count, serum electrolytes, ECG, and computed tomography were all normal.

Heredity. The inheritance of this condition is most likely autosomal recessive. However, it is possible that the two sib pairs have similar,

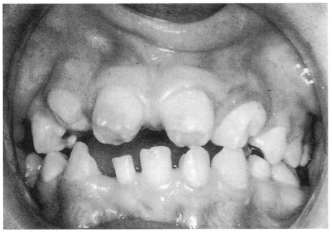

A

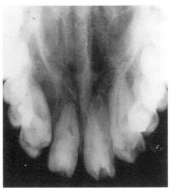

B

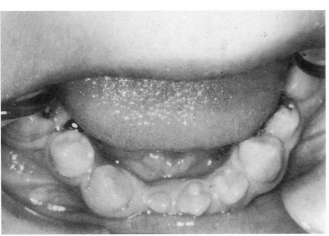

C

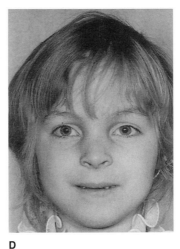

D

Figure 15–3. *Multiple anterior dens invaginatus and sensorineural hearing loss.* (A) Molarized maxillary central incisors having three cusps labially, two cusps lingually, and one cusp mesially. Premolarized maxillary lateral incisor with one cusp labially and lingually. (B) Radiograph reveals both maxillary central and lateral incisors with two root canals. Double dens invaginatus is observed in the maxillary central incisors. (C) Multituberculism of the mandibular left incisors, canines, and first premolars. (D) Seven-year-old female with broad nasal bridge, dilated nostrils, and sensorineural hearing loss. [From PN Kantaputra and RJ Gorlin, *Clin Dysmorphol* 1:128, 1992.]

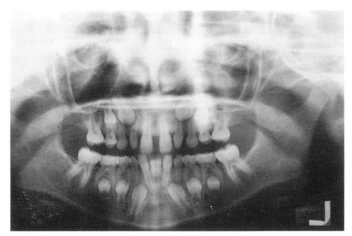

A

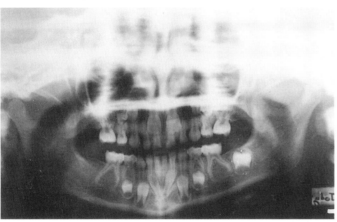

B

Figure 15–4. *Oligodontia and congenital sensorineural hearing loss.* (A,B) Absence of numerous permanent teeth in siblings. [From L Glass and RJ Gorlin, *Arch Otolaryngol* 105:621, 1979.]

yet distinct, conditions. The sibs reported by Glass and Gorlin (1) did not have dizziness and did have more severe oligodontia.

Diagnosis. This condition should be distinguished from other various ectodermal dysplasias that have associated hearing loss.

Prognosis. Life span and intellectual function were not impaired.

Summary. The main features of this condition are (*1*) autosomal recessive inheritance; (*2*) hypodontia; and (*3*) profound bilateral sensorineural hearing loss. Dizziness may be a distinguishing feature, as noted above.

References

1. Glass L, Gorlin RJ: Congenital profound sensorineural deafness and oligodontia: a new syndrome. *Arch Otolaryngol* 105:621–622, 1979.
2. Lee M et al: Autosomal recessive sensorineural hearing impairment, dizziness, and hypodontia. *Arch Otolaryngol* 104:292–293, 1978.

Compound odontomas, maxillary hypoplasia, rectal stenosis, and sensorineural hearing loss

In 1982, Seinsch (2) described a boy with several anomalies including multiple compound odontomas, marked hypoplasia of the maxilla, submucous cleft palate, persistent buccal pharyngeal membrane, high rectal stenosis, and sensorineural hearing loss. Although Gorlin et al. (1) described several multiple odontoma-intestinal stenosis syndromes, none was associated with hearing loss.

References

1. Gorlin RJ et al: *Syndromes of the Head and Neck,* 4th ed. Oxford University Press, New York, 2001.
2. Seinsch W: Missbildungssyndrome mit Schallenempfindungsschwerhörigkeit und Sprachenentwicklungsstörung. *Laryngol Rhinol Otol* 61:314–315, 1982.

Hypodontia and peg-shaped teeth, olivopontocerebellar dysplasia, hypogonadism, and hearing loss

Rushton and Genel (1) described two sibs born to consanguineous parents. The sibs had olivopontocerebellar degeneration, hypogonadotrophic hypogonadism, and hypodontia (1). Neurologic features included hyperreflexia and ataxia. Despite normal growth hormone levels, stature was below the third centile in both sibs, suggesting tissue nonresponsiveness to growth hormone. The teeth were described as peg-shaped with enamel hypoplasia; some teeth were also missing. Unilateral hearing loss of 60 dB above 2000 Hz of unspecified type was noted in one sib. Skin and hair were normal. Inheritance is likely autosomal recessive.

Reference

1. Rushton AR, Genel M: Hereditary ectodermal dysplasia, olivopontocerebellar degeneration, short stature and hypogonadism. *J Med Genet* 18:335–339, 1981.

Gingival fibromatosis and sensorineural hearing loss

Jones et al. (5), in 1977, Hartsfield et al. (3), in 1985, and Wynne et al. (7), in 1995, reported families with multiple members having generalized gingival fibromatosis and sensorineural hearing loss. The family described by Jorgenson and Crocker (6) also manifested allergy.

Oral findings. Changes were limited to teeth and gingiva. Dental eruption was described as delayed in one family (1) with the first primary tooth erupting at 13 months in the proband. Eruption of permanent teeth was delayed as well. The proband in another family (2) had only eight permanent teeth at 12 years. The gingivae were described as hypertrophied, with stippled and nodular areas (Fig. 15–5). Supernumerary teeth were described in one family.

Auditory system. Hearing loss became evident in the second decade. Audiometric testing revealed a sloping, moderate (30–70 dB)

Figure 15–5. *Gingival fibromatosis and sensorineural hearing loss.* Gingival fibromatosis has buried many teeth.

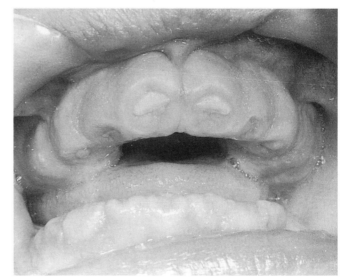

sensorinueral loss, which was greater at high frequencies. This loss was usually bilateral but varied between ears.

Vestibular system. Testing was not done.

Pathology. Histologic examination of the gingiva demonstrated areas of increased fibroblasts and evidence of continuous, active production of collagen.

Heredity. This condition has autosomal dominant inheritance. A gene for sensorineural hearing loss has been mapped to 2p21–p22, while a gene for gingival fibromatosis has been mapped to the same location (2,4).

Diagnosis. Gingival hyperplasia can occur as an isolated hereditary trait or can be associated with other anomalies in other syndromes (1). However, no other conditions with hearing loss as a component manifestation have been described.

Summary. This syndrome is characterized by (1) autosomal dominant inheritance; (2) generalized gingival fibromatosis; and (3) sensorineural hearing loss.

References

1. Chaib H et al: A gene responsible for a sensorineural nonsyndromic recessive deafness maps to chromosome 2p22-23. *Hum Mol Genet* 5:155–158, 1996.
2. Gorlin RJ et al: *Syndromes of the Head and Neck,* 4th ed. Oxford University Press, New York, 2001.
3. Hartsfield JK et al: Gingival fibromatosis with sensorineural hearing loss. An autosomal dominant trait. *Am J Med Genet* 22:623–627, 1985.
4. Hartsfield JK et al: Genetic linkage of hereditary gingival fibromatosis to chromosome 2p21. *Am J Hum Genet* 62:876–883, 1998.
5. Jones G et al: Familial gingival fibromatosis associated with progressive deafness in five generations of a family. *Birth Defects* 13(13B):195–201, 1977.
6. Jorgenson R, Crocker ME: Variations in the inheritance and expression of gingival fibromatosis. *J Periodontol* 45:472–477, 1974.
7. Wynne SE et al: Hereditary gingival fibromatosis associated with hearing loss and supernumerary teeth—a new syndrome. *J Periodontol* 66:75–79, 1995.

Neuroendocrine carcinoma of salivary glands, sensorineural hearing loss, and enamel hypoplasia

Michaels et al. (1) described four sibs from the Isle of Man with low-grade neuroendocrine carcinoma of salivary glands, severe sensorineural hearing loss, and enamel hypoplasia.

The submandibular glands were involved in three cases, and the minor salivary glands of the nasal cavity and maxillary sinuses in one. The tumors manifested when the patients were in their 30's. The tumors consisted of well-differentiated neoplastic ducts surrounded by neoplastic myoepithelial cells, together with sheets of epithelial cells expressing neuroendocrine markers by immunohistochemistry (Fig. 15–6). Metastasis to the cervical neck nodes occurred in all four individuals.

In the two male patients, there was severe sensorineural hearing loss which developed in adult life, unilateral in one brother and bilateral in the other. In the brother with the bilateral sensorineural hearing loss, a vestibular schwannoma was noted on one side.

Amelogenesis imperfecta was seen in three of the four siblings and in four of their offspring. The teeth were described as having a brown-yellow surface with vertical bands suggestive of the X-linked hypoplastic type.

Reference

1. Michaels L et al: Family with low-grade neuroendocrine carcinoma of salivary glands, severe sensorineural hearing loss, and enamel hypoplasia. *Am J Med Genet* 83:183–186, 1999.

Unusual face, digital anomalies, and supernumerary teeth

Ravine et al. (personal communication, 1995) corresponded regarding a syndrome of supernumerary teeth and tracheal subglottic hypoplasia predisposing to recurrent group in childhood.

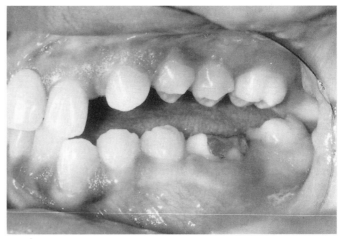

Figure 15–6. *Ankylosed teeth, maxillary hypoplasia, and fifth finger clinodactyly.* Note failure of premolars and molars to meet at the occlusal plane. [From MZ Pelias and MC Kinnebrew, *Clin Genet* 27:496, 1985.]

The hands appeared unusual with prominent distal and proximal interphalangeal joints, clinodactyly of the fifth fingers, brachydactyly of fingers and toes, club feet, and external rotation of hips.

The face is unusual due to prominent forehead and prominent widow's peak. Progressive conductive hearing loss and supernumerary teeth were noted.

Four generations were involved with male-to-male transmission. Autosomal dominant inheritance is evident.

Unusual face and autosomal dominant hypohidrotic ectodermal dysplasia (Bocian-Rimoin syndrome)

In 1979, Bocian and Rimoin (1) reported an autosomal dominant form of ectodermal dysplasia characterized by hypohidrosis; sparse body hair, scalp hair, eyebrows, and eyelashes; thin, slow-growing nails; hypoplastic nasal bridge; hypoplastic nasal alae; anteverted nostrils; long philtrum; and thin inverted upper lip. Tooth eruption was somewhat delayed. Oligodontia resulted in a number of deciduous teeth being maintained. The enamel was hypoplastic.

Somewhat similar findings are seen in the autosomal dominantly inherited disorder(s) described by Harrod et al. (2), Saihan and Warin (4), and Jorgenson et al. (3). However, unusual facies was not noted.

We wonder if this is not Hay-Wells syndrome.

References

1. Bocian M, Rimoin DL: A new autosomal dominant syndrome of hypohidrotic ectodermal dysplasia and unusual facies. *Birth Defects* 15(5B):239–251, 1979.
2. Harrod MJ et al: Dominantly inherited hypohidrotic ectodermal dysplasia with dental anomalies. *Birth Defects* 13(3C):236, 1976.
3. Jorgenson RJ et al: Autosomal dominant ectodermal dysplasia. *J Craniofac Genet Dev Biol* 7:403–412, 1987.
4. Saihan E, Warin RP: Ectodermal dysplasia. *Br J Dermatol* 97(Suppl 15):34–36, 1977.

Sensorineural hearing loss, retinal pigment epithelium lesions, and discolored teeth

Innis et al. (1) described a sibship with the combination of ocular, dental, and auditory abnormalities. Eye findings consisted of creamy white lesions that accumulated at the level of the retinal pigment epithelium. These lesions usually developed after age 2 years. Dental findings consisted of brown discoloration of molars and/or canines only. Deciduous teeth were affected; the permanent teeth had not yet erupted in any of the children at the time of the report, so it is unknown whether they too would be affected. Hearing loss developed between the ages of 2 and 4 years and was sensorineural. Loss was more severe in the higher than in the lower frequencies. Because of the age of the children at the time of the report, it is not known whether the hearing loss is progressive.

There is some superficial similarity to otodental syndrome, but in the one family that had eye anomalies as a component manifestation of oto-dental syndrome, the eye defects were iridal colobomas (2).

References

1. Innis JW et al: Apparently new syndrome of sensorineural hearing loss, retinal pigment epithelium lesions, and discolored teeth. *Am J Med Genet* 75:13–17, 1998.
2. Winter GB: The association of ocular defects with the otodental syndrome. *J Int Ass Dent Child* 14:83–87, 1983.

Appendix

Other entities with dental abnormalities

Entity	Dental Finding	Chapter in this Book
Oculo-facio-cardio-dental syndrome	Oligodontia, canine gigantism	7 (eye)
Carpal and tarsal anomalies, cleft palate, oligodontia, conductive hearing loss	Oligodontia	8 (musculoskeletal)
Temtamy preaxial brachydactyly syndrome	Microdontia, talon cusp formation	8 (musculoskeletal)
Palmoplantar hyperkeratosis, short stature, unusual face, hypodontia, SHL	Oligodontia	14 (integumentary)
Hyperkeratosis palmoplantaris striata, pili torti, hypohidrosis, oligodontia, SHL	Oligodontia	14 (integumentary)

SHL, sensorineural hearing loss.

Chapter 16
Genetic Hearing Loss Associated with Chromosome Disorders

ANNE B.S. GIERSCH AND CYNTHIA MORTON

Cytogenetics is the study of chromosomes and the disorders associated with rearrangements, duplications, or deletions of their parts or of complete chromosomes. For example, one of the most commonly occurring genetic syndromes in humans, Down syndrome, is caused by the presence of an extra chromosome number 21. The recent completion of the human genome sequence has illustrated the density of genes on human chromosomes and has revealed that even submicroscopic regions of chromosomes can encode dozens of genes.

As might be expected, gene dosages are tightly regulated. Too many or two few genes can have lethal consequences to a developing organism, especially one as complex as *Homo sapiens*. Approximately a third of all human conceptions end in miscarriage, and half of these are due to chromosome aberrations, either numerical or structural (6). As illustrated in the sections below, a human born with a chromosome imbalance or rearrangement can have a host of clinical features, from subtle to severe, depending on the size of the imbalance or the particular gene(s) disrupted.

Cytogenetics is not a classical method for studying hearing loss. Patients with chromosome defects, especially the more severe cases such as trisomies, are often so severely compromised both physically and mentally that hearing status is not adequately addressed. But for proper clinical management it is crucial to assess the hearing of patients with chromosome aberrations. Individuals facing mental and/or physical hurdles may have their intellectual development even further impaired by the burden of undiagnosed hearing loss. In a recent report on the etiology of hearing loss at a school for the deaf in The Netherlands, 7% of the student population was found to have a chromosome anomaly (1). That is in contrast to the less than 1% of the general population that has some form of chromosome abnormality. Cytogenetics has also proven to be an invaluable tool for disease gene identification in auditory disorders, as illustrated in certain cases below.

Methodology

Humans normally have 46 chromosomes in each cell; 22 pairs of autosomes and one pair of sex chromosomes. In conventional cytogenetics, chromosomes are visualized in the light microscope at $1000\times$ magnification after being arrested in metaphase by specific mitotic inhibitors. Each has a short arm (p) and a long arm (q) separated by a centromere. A *karyotype* is a display of chromosomes from largest to smallest with the chromosomes oriented so that the p arm is on top (Fig. 16–1). For conventional cytogenetic analysis, chromosome preparations are stained to produce a dark–light banding pattern that is characteristic for each chromosome. The most common staining method is G-banding. This technique consists of proteolytic digestion with trypsin followed by staining with Giemsa. Each band is numbered according to an international system of nomenclature (11). For illustrative purposes, chromosomes are often displayed in a schematic standardized format called an *ideogram* (Fig. 16–2).

In the past several years, new molecular techniques such as fluorescent in situ hybridization (FISH) have been developed that augment conventional cytogenetic analysis. Fluorescently labeled molecular probes hybridized to chromosomes have the advantage of being able to detect deletions, duplications, or rearrangements that are too small or subtle to be observed by light microscopy. In certain instances, molec-ular probes can be used directly on interphase cells without requiring growth and mitotic arrest of a cell sample in metaphase. In these cases, the chromosomes per se are not analyzed, only the presence or absence of the unique molecular marker. For example, a rapid test for a suspected trisomy can be performed on fetal cells after amniocentesis, or a gene rearrangement typical of certain cancers can be rapidly detected in a bone marrow sample.

Cytogenetic Disorders due to Aneuploidy

Aneuploidy is a numerical aberration of a whole chromosome, either an extra (trisomy) or missing (monosomy) copy. In general, additional genetic material is better tolerated during development than chromosome loss. Indeed, monosomy of any autosome is lethal; only loss of a sex chromosome can result in a live-born human. Only three autosomal trisomies can survive to term: trisomies 21, 18, and 13. All other full autosomal trisomies are usually lethal during development.

The increasing incidence of chromosome trisomies with advanced maternal age is well documented (6), although the mechanism for this phenomenon is unknown. For example, the risk of having a child with an autosomal trisomy at age 25 is approximately 1:1300 live births, at age 35 the risk is 1:350, and at age 45 the risk is 1:20 (6).

Down syndrome (trisomy 21)

Down syndrome, with an incidence of 1:600 live births, is the most common chromosome defect in humans. The collection of congenital anomalies associated with this well-known syndrome is caused by the presence of an extra copy of chromosome number 21. Since 21 is the smallest chromosome with the fewest number of genes, the gene dosage imbalance resultant from the extra chromosome is one of the few autosomal trisomies tolerated during development, although only about 30% of Down syndrome fetuses survive to term (5). Trisomies 13 and 18, illustrated below, have a much more dire clinical picture for the small percentage of babies that are live born; all other full autosomal trisomic conceptions end in miscarriage.

Physical findings. The combination of mildly dysmorphic features of Down syndrome, while not invariably present, comprise the characteristic physical phenotype of this familiar syndrome (Fig. 16–3). The most common among these findings are upslanting palpebral fissures, loose skin on the nape of the neck, brachycephaly, narrow palate, hyperflexibility, flat nasal bridge, "sandal" gap between the first and second toes, short, broad hands, short neck, epicanthal folds, abnormal teeth, short, incurved fifth finger, furrowed protruding tongue, and transverse palmar crease (5). Clearly none of these findings are life-threatening, nor would they be expected to affect development in any meaningful way. Hypotonia is often the most obvious physical finding in Down syndrome newborns. Muscle tone improves with age but tends to remain below average. More serious for the Down syndrome patient are neurologic abnormalities, including mental retardation, and congenital malformations that can affect long-term health and development.

Mental retardation and developmental delay are universal hallmarks of Down syndrome, although quite variable in presentation. Develop-

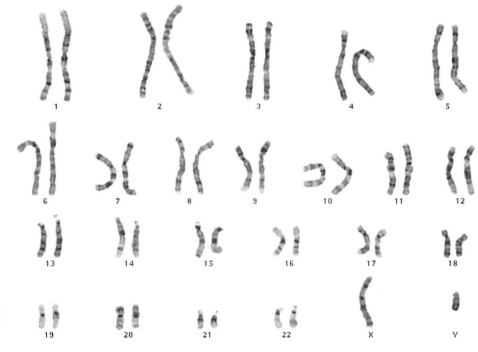

Figure 16–1. G-banded human male karyotype (46,XY), consisting of the normal complement of 46 chromosomes including one X and one Y.

mental landmarks tend to become increasingly delayed with age, such that a 5-year-old lags further behind normal peers than does a 1-year-old. Although IQs decrease with age, there is a wide range of attainable IQs, likely due to genetic background and environmental factors. The average IQ for a 2-year-old is around 60 while that for a 10-year-old is 35. Individuals with a mosaic karyotype (see Cytogenetics) may be less severely retarded and occasionally achieve near-normal IQs but may also be indistinguishable in phenotype from individuals with full trisomy. Ultimately, however, most adults with Down syndrome display dementia with an Alzheimer disease (AD)–like phenotype beginning some time around age 30 or 40, with very similar brain pathology to that observed in AD.

Congenital heart disease is the most frequent major physical abnormality in Down syndrome patients. An average of 40% of Down syndrome patients are affected by some form of potentially life-threatening heart defect, most commonly atrioventricular canal, ventricular septal defect, atrial septal defect, patent ductus arteriosus, or tetralogy of Fallot (listed in order of most common). Gastrointestinal tract abnormalities are also more common among individuals with Down syndrome than in the general population, although not nearly as frequent as cardiac defects. Most common is duodenal stenosis or atresia, imperforate anus, and Hirschsprung disease. The incidence of leukemia is also elevated 10- to 15-fold above that in the normal population. Males with Down syndrome are nearly always infertile; females have reduced fertility (5,8).

Individuals with Down syndrome are more susceptible to a variety of infectious diseases. This is likely due in part to thymus abnormalities with a concomitant reduction in the numbers of circulating T lymphocytes. Infection constitutes a leading cause of morbidity and mortality among Down syndrome patients. It also has a bearing on conductive hearing loss due to chronic otitis media in trisomic individuals (see below).

Auditory system. The external ears of Down syndrome patients tend to be small, low-set, and slightly posteriorly rotated. In about half of individuals with Down syndrome, the upper helices are overfolded or the ears are dysplastic (8). Temporal bones of Down syndrome patients show both middle and inner ear defects in some studies, and only middle ear abnormalities in other studies [reviewed in Bilgin et al. (2)]. Cochlear defects include Mondini dysplasia and overall shortened cochlear length in a percentage of ears. Stapes malformations, residual

mesenchyme obstructing the round window, and otitis media comprise most middle ear structural abnormalities.

Most studies cite a 40%–80% incidence of hearing loss in children with Down syndrome (7,9,10,12,13). The variation in incidence is likely due to a combination of measurement factors, such as age of evaluation, technique used (ABR vs. behavioral testing), and definition of hearing loss (15 dB loss vs. 25 dB loss). Hearing loss can be conductive, sensorineural, or mixed, although most studies agree that the largest component is conductive. Although conductive hearing loss in Down syndrome individuals can be due to congenital middle ear anomalies such as stapes malformations, it appears that a significant proportion of conductive hearing loss is acquired through recurrent middle ear infections.

Otitis media with effusion is a chronic problem in children with Down syndrome, 50% to 80% of whom have recurrent ear infections (9,13). Insertion of tympanostomy tubes is 17 times more frequent than that of the general population (9), with more than half the children in one study requiring multiple tube placements (13). Early data from one longitudinal study show that aggressive medical and surgical management of chronic otitis media can drastically reduce the incidence of hearing loss in the Down syndrome population (13). Other studies advocate a more conservative approach, finding the cure rate of otitis media with effusion in individuals with Down syndrome to be less than that of normal controls (7). The cause of chronic ear infections in Down syndrome is likely due to a combination of physiological defects. Children with Down syndrome tend to have stenotic ear canals, a small nasopharynx, and dysfunctional eustachian tubes (4), possibly due to hypotonia of the velopharyngeal muscles (10). Each of these conditions can facilitate fluid buildup and trap infectious agents in the middle ear. Combined with the immune system deficits caused by thymus hypoplasia, it becomes obvious why otitis media with effusion is a chronic condition in such a high percentage of these individuals.

Management of otitis media with effusion in the Down syndrome population could have a significant impact, both medically and developmentally. Evidence from several studies [reviewed in Mazzoni et al. (10)] suggests that individuals with Down syndrome with significant hearing loss have poorer language acquisition, lower IQs, and more delayed developmental milestones than those with better hearing, although others have found no correlation between hearing loss and language quotient (12). Audiological evaluations should occur in all infants with Down syndrome and be followed up annually into the school-aged years (3).

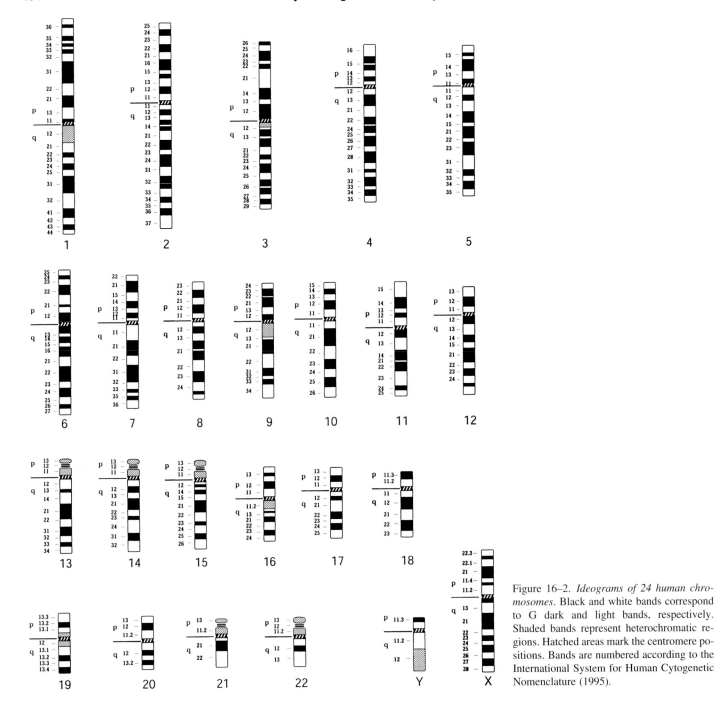

Figure 16–2. *Ideograms of 24 human chromosomes.* Black and white bands correspond to G dark and light bands, respectively. Shaded bands represent heterochromatic regions. Hatched areas mark the centromere positions. Bands are numbered according to the International System for Human Cytogenetic Nomenclature (1995).

Cytogenetics. The vast majority (95%) of Down syndrome cases are due to an extra copy of a normal chromosome 21, such that the individual has a total of 47 chromosomes with three 21s (47,+21) in all cells. Two to four percent of cases are mosaic for the extra 21—that is, not all cells are trisomy 21. This can be the result of either meiotic or mitotic nondisjunction. In <5% of Down syndrome cases, the additional 21 is due to the presence of a chromosome rearrangement that results in the additional 21 being translocated to another chromosome. Most often, this occurs as a Robertsonian translocation, where the short arm of the 21 is translocated to the short arm of one of the other acrocentric chromosomes (13, 14, 15, 21 or 22). These cases are significant in that the translocation can be inherited from a phenotypically normal parent, who is a balanced translocation carrier. If the mother is the Robertsonian translocation carrier, the risk for a second trisomy 21 pregnancy is 10%–15%; if the father is the carrier, the risk is <2% (6). The fact that the chromosome rearrangement is inherited can also have reproductive consequences for other family members. Genetic counseling is recommended.

References

1. Admiraal RJ, Huygen PL: Causes of hearing impairment in deaf pupils with a mental handicap. *Int J Pediatr Otorhinolaryngol* 51:101–108, 1999.
2. Bilgin H et al: Temporal bone study of Down's syndrome. *Arch Otolaryngol Head Neck Surg* 122:271–275, 1996.
3. Carey JC: Health supervision and anticipatory guidance for children with genetic disorders (including specific recommendations for trisomy 21, trisomy 18, and neurofibromatosis I). *Pediatr Clin North Am* 39:25–53, 1992.
4. Dahle AJ, McCollister FP: Hearing and otologic disorders in children with Down syndrome. *Am J Ment Defic* 90:636–642, 1986.

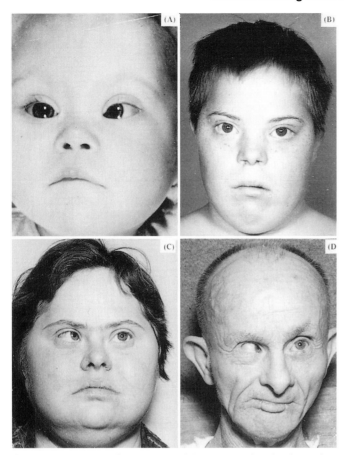

Figure 16–3. *Down syndrome (trisomy 21).* (A–D) Facies of patients of various ages.

5. Epstein CJ: Down syndrome (trisomy 21). In: *The Molecular and Metabolic Basis of Inherited Disease*, Scriver CR et al (eds), McGraw-Hill, New York, 2001, pp 1223–1256.
6. Gardner R, Sutherland G: *Chromosome Abnormalities and Genetic Counseling.* 2nd ed. Oxford University Press, New York, 1996.
7. Iino Y et al: Efficacy of tympanostomy tube insertion for otitis media with effusion in children with Down syndrome. *Int J Pediatr Otorhinolaryngol* 49:143–149, 1999.
8. Jones KL: *Smith's Recognizable Patterns of Human Malformation*, 5th ed. W.B. Saunders, Philadelphia, 1997, p 857.
9. Leonard S et al: Medical aspects of school-aged children with Down syndrome. *Dev Med Child Neurol* 41:683–688, 1999.
10. Mazzoni D et al: Abnormal pinna type and hearing loss correlations in Down's syndrome. *J Intell Disabil Res* 38:549–560, 1994.
11. Mitelman F (ed): *ISCN 1995. An International System for Cytogenetic Nomenclature (1995).* S. Karger, Basel, 1995.
12. Roizen N et al: Hearing loss in children with Down syndrome. *J Pediatrics* 123:S9–S12, 1993.
13. Shott SR et al: Hearing loss in children with Down syndrome. *Int J Pediatr Otorhinolaryngol* 61:199–205, 2001.

Trisomy 13 (Patau syndrome)

Trisomy 13 incidence at birth is only about 1 in 12,000 (2), as the majority of such conceptions are inviable and do not survive to term. The presence of an extra chromosome 13 results in a collection of physical anomalies first described by Patau (4) in 1960.

Clinical findings. Babies born with trisomy 13 rarely survive more than a few days and only 5% survive to 6 months of age. Severe mental retardation is universal due to various forebrain defects, most notably holoprosencephaly. Other very characteristic findings of trisomy

13 include eye defects ranging from microphthalmia to anophthalmia, cleft lip and/or palate, microcephaly, postaxial polydactyly of hands and feet, seizures, and cardiac defects (most commonly ventral septal defect, atrial septal defect, and patent ductus arteriosus) (Fig. 16–4A–C). Dozens of other physical abnormalities have also been noted (3). In the mosaic state, the phenotype can vary from mild to severe, depending on the level of mosaicism and organs affected by the trisomic cells. A review of 32 mosaic trisomy 13 cases reports detection of trisomy 13 in 4% to 87% of blood cells. Severity of the phenotype did not always correspond with mosaicism level (1).

Auditory system. The ears of an individual with trisomy 13 often have abnormal helices and tend to be low-set. Temporal bone studies show multiple abnormalities of the cochlea and vestibular systems, including semicircular canal and utricular, saccular, and macular anomalies, shortened cochlear length, widened cochlear aqueduct, and abnormalities of the modiolus (Fig. 16–4D–F). Middle ear deformities were also occasionally present (6,7). Considering the reported temporal bone findings, most patients are probably hearing impaired or deaf, but because of the combined clinical and neurological impairments, hearing ability is often not evaluated. Delatycki and Gardner (1) noted at least two cases of documented hearing loss in mosaic trisomy 13 cases.

Cytogenetics. The majority of trisomy 13 cases are full free-lying trisomies, i.e., 47 chromosomes. Robertsonian translocation of a chromosome 13 onto another acrocentric chromosome has also been reported (1,5) (see Down syndrome, Cytogenetics, for a description of Robertsonian translocations.)

References
1. Delatycki M, Gardner R: Three cases of trisomy 13 mosaicism and a review of the literature. *Clin Genet* 51:403–407, 1997.
2. Hook E, Hammerton J: The frequency of chromosome abnormalities detected in consecutive newborn studies—differences between studies—results by sex and severity of phenotyic involvement. In: *Population Cytogenetics*, Hook E, Porter I (eds), Academic Press, New York, 1997, pp 63–79.
3. Jones KL: *Smith's Recognizable Patterns of Human Malformation*, 5th ed., W.B. Saunders, Philadelphia, 1997.
4. Patau K: Multiple congenital anomaly caused by an extra chromsome. *Lancet* 1:790, 1960.
5. Robinson WP et al: Molecular studies of translocations and trisomy involving chromosome 13. *Am J Med Genet* 61:158–163, 1996.
6. Sando I et al: Temporal bone histopathological findings in trisomy 13 syndrome. *Ann Otol Rhinol Laryngol* 84:1–20, 1975.
7. Schuknecht HF: *Pathology of the Ear*, 2nd ed. Lea & Febiger, Philadelphia, 1993.

Trisomy 18 (Edwards syndrome)

In 1960 Edwards et al. (2) described this pattern of malformation in babies with an extra chromosome 18. The incidence is 1 in 5000 births. There is a marked preponderance of females (3:1), possibly due to a higher miscarriage rate of male fetuses with trisomy 18.

Clinical findings. Trisomy 18 pregnancies are marked by polyhydramnios, intrauterine growth retardation, and a two-vessel umbilical cord. Babies are characteristically hypotonic with underdeveloped skeletal muscle. Half of the newborns with trisomy 18 die within the first week; 90% die within the first year of life (8). Those that survive have profound mental retardation and seizures. The occiput is often prominent and the bifrontal diameter is narrow. The mouth is small with a high arched palate (Fig. 16–5A,B). A very characteristic finding is clenched hands with the index and fifth fingers overlapping the third and fourth (Fig. 16–5C). So-called rocker-bottom feet with syndactyly of second and third toes is also a common finding. The sternum tends to be short and umbilical hernias are common. Ventricular septal defect, atrial septal defect, or patent ductus arteriosus are frequent cardiac anomalies and often the cause of death. Dozens of other clinical find-

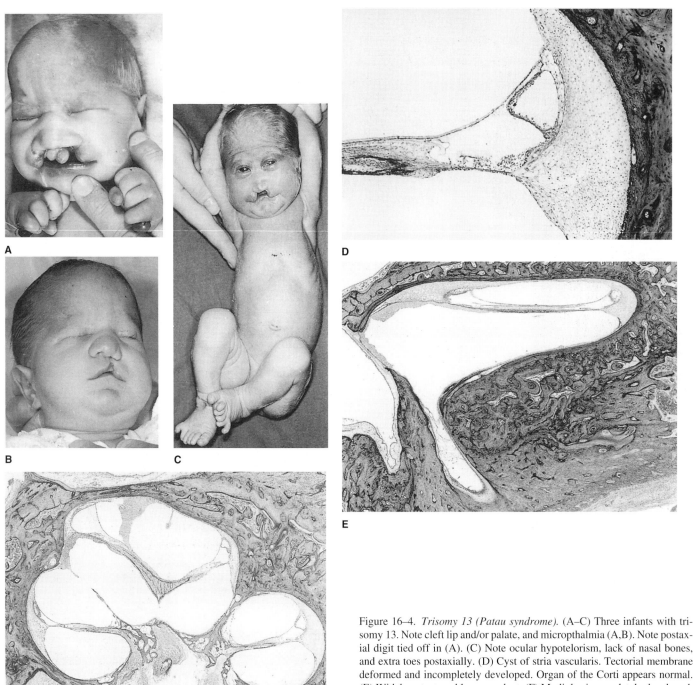

Figure 16–4. *Trisomy 13 (Patau syndrome)*. (A–C) Three infants with trisomy 13. Note cleft lip and/or palate, and micropthalmia (A,B). Note postaxial digit tied off in (A). (C) Note ocular hypotelorism, lack of nasal bones, and extra toes postaxially. (D) Cyst of stria vascularis. Tectorial membrane deformed and incompletely developed. Organ of the Corti appears normal. (E) Widely patent cochlear aqueduct. (F) Modiolus incompletely developed. Most cochlear neurons lie within the internal auditory canal. Stria vascularis is aplastic and cystic. [(D–F) from HF Schuknecht, *Pathology of the Ear*, Harvard University Press, 1974.]

ings observed less often than those listed above have been reported (3). Mosaicism for trisomy 18 may lead to partial expression of the phenotype from mild to almost full expression (5,7).

Auditory system. Ears are low-set, posteriorly rotated, and malformed and can have atresia of the external auditory canal. Temporal bone studies from fetuses and young children with trisomy 18 show abnormalities of the middle and inner ear, including failed ossification of the malleus, incus, and stapes and retarded development of the cochlea (1,4,6) (Fig. 16–5D). Given the temporal bone findings, it is likely that most babies with trisomy 18 are deaf or severely hearing impaired; however, audiometric analysis has not been reported.

Cytogenetics. Full trisomy 18 is the norm. A handful of mosaic cases have been reported (5,7). Like all trisomies, incidence of trisomy 18 increases with advanced maternal age.

References

1. Chrobok V, Simakova E: Temporal bone findings in trisomy 18 and 21 syndromes. *Eur Arch Otorhinolaryngol* 254:15–18, 1997.
2. Edwards J et al: A new trisomic syndrome. *Lancet* 1:787, 1960.
3. Jones KL: *Smith's Recognizable Patterns of Human Malformation*, 5th ed. W.B. Saunders, Philadelphia, 1997.
4. Miglets AW et al: Trisomy 18. A temporal bone report. *Arch Otolaryngol* 101:433–437, 1975.
5. Plessis G et al: Trisomy 18 mosaicism in a mildly retarded boy with postnatal overgrowth. *Ann Genet* 40:235–237, 1997.

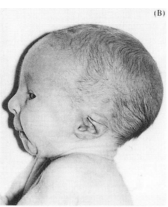
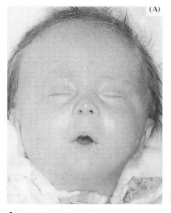
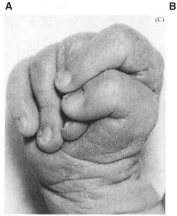

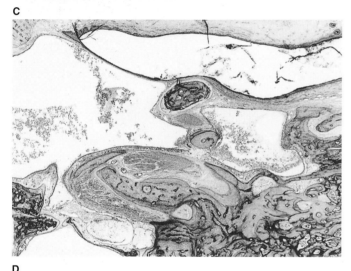

Figure 16–5. *Trisomy 18 (Edwards syndrome)*. (A,B) Infants with trisomy 18. Note small mouth, narrow bifrontal diameter, micrognathia, prominent occiput, and malformed pinna. (C) Note typical clenched hand with overlapping fingers. (D) Temporal bone section from 3.5-year-old male with trisomy 18. Middle ear anomalies consist of a large cochleariform process, abnormal course of the facial nerve, bifurcated tensor tympani muscle, and ossicular deformities. [From HF Schuknecht, *Pathology of the Ear*, Harvard University Press, 1974.]

6. Sando I et al: Temporal bone findings in trisomy 18 syndrome. *Arch Otolaryngol* 91:552–559, 1970.
7. Schubert R et al: Clinical, cytogenetic, and molecular findings in 45,X/47,XX,+18 mosaicism: clinical report and review of the literature. *Am J Med Genet* 110:278–282, 2002.
8. Weber WW et al: Trisomy 17-18(E): studies in long-term survival with reports of two autopsied cases. *Pediatrics* 34:533–541, 1964.

Turner syndrome

The features of Turner syndrome were first described in 1938 (10) and five decades later were determined to be caused by loss of a sex chromosome (2). Although the phenotype of individuals with Turner syndrome is not particularly severe, 99% of conceptuses abort spontaneously. The incidence of Turner syndrome at birth is around 1 in 2000.

Clinical features. Turner syndrome patients are phenotypically female. Classical features are short stature (average adult height is 56 inches), thick or webbed neck, and streak gonads (Fig. 16–6). Patients are almost invariably infertile. Growth hormone therapy typically improves height; estrogen therapy aids secondary sexual development. Other common clinical findings are a wide chest with broadly spaced nipples, low posterior hairline, and edema in the neonatal period. Approximately 60% of patients experience renal problems such as horseshoe kidney, cleft renal pelvis, or other minor kidney problems. Cardiac anomalies, which affect only about 20% of patients, can include bicuspid aortic valve, coarctation of the aorta, and valvular aortic stenosis. Mild facial anomalies include a narrow palate and small mandible (5). A girl with Turner syndrome may manifest an X-linked recessive disorder because only one X chromosome is present (8). Some individuals with Turner syndrome have difficulty with social adjustments. The IQ can be slightly below normal, with problems arising particularly in math and spatial reasoning (11). As a result, nonverbal IQ in Turner syndrome girls tends to be lower than verbal IQ.

Audiologic findings. Auricular anomalies including low-set ears, narrow external auditory canal, cupped auricles, and/or protruding ears are found in 20% to 45% of individuals [reviewed in Barrenas et al. (1)]. Chronic otitis media, frequently leading to conductive hearing loss, is a very common finding among girls with Turner syndrome. Various reports cite 50% to 90% of patients having recurrent ear infections, often requiring tympanostomy tube placement for drainage (1,3,4,6,7,9). Because of the recognized high incidence of otitis media and hearing loss in girls with Turner syndrome, the American Academy of Pediatrics recommends an otologic evaluation for otitis media at every pediatric visit and, if present, aggressive treatment for it (8).

Cytogenetics. Unlike the autosomal aneuplodies, Turner syndrome is not associated with advanced maternal age. In fact, in 80% of cases

Figure 16–6. *Turner syndrome*. (A,B) Note pterygium colli, eyelid ptosis, protruding ears, broad chest with widely spaced nipples, and small aerolae. In (B), note diminished height in adult. [Courtesy of G Tagatz, Minneapolis, Minnesota.]

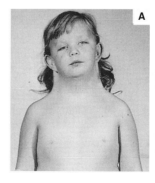
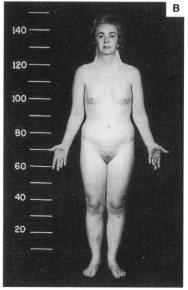

the paternal sex chromosome is absent. The most frequent chromosome constitution is 45,X in all cells, however, about half of Turner syndrome cases have other karyotypes. Approximately 25% of Turner patients have a mosaic karyotype, with only a proportion of the cells being 45,X. In the remaining cases, the second X chromosome is structurally abnormal, most frequently an isochromosome Xq (11). Y chromosome mosaicism can also be present and poses an increased risk for development of gonadoblastoma in the dysgenic gonads (8).

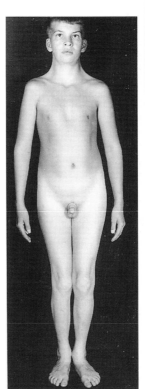
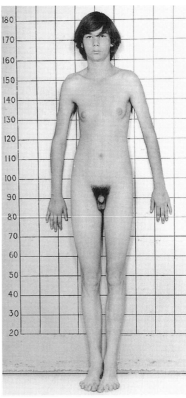

References

1. Barrenas ML et al: The influence of karyotype on the auricle, otitis media and hearing in Turner syndrome. *Hear Res* 138:163–170, 1999.
2. Ford CE et al: A sex chromosome anomaly in a case of gonadal dysgenesis (Turner's syndrome). *Lancet* 1:711, 1959.
3. Gungor N et al: High frequency hearing loss in Ullrich-Turner syndrome. *Eur J Pediatr* 159:740–744, 2000.
4. Hultcrantz M, Sylven L: Turner's syndrome and hearing disorders in women aged 16–34. *Hear Res* 103:69–74, 1997.
5. Jones KL: *Smith's Recognizable Patterns of Human Malformation*, 5th ed. W.B. Saunders, Philadelphia, 1997.
6. Roush J et al: Early-onset sensorineural hearing loss in a child with Turner syndrome. *J Am Acad Audiol* 11:446–453, 2000.
7. Sculerati N et al: Hearing loss in Turner syndrome. *Laryngoscope* 106:992–997, 1996.
8. Seashore MR et al: Health supervision for children with Turner syndrome. *Pediatrics* 96:1166–1173, 1995.
9. Stenberg AE et al: Otological problems in children with Turner's syndrome. *Hear Res* 124:85–90, 1998.
10. Turner HH: A syndrome of infantilism, congenital webbed neck and cubitus valgus. *Endocrinology* 23:566–578, 1938.
11. Willard H: The sex chromsomes and X chromosome inactivation. In: *The Molecular and Metabolic Basis of Inherited Disease*, Scriver CR et al (eds), McGraw-Hill, New York, 2001.

Klinefelter syndrome (XXY syndrome)

Klinefelter syndrome affects 1 in 500 to 1 in 1000 males. It is the single most common cause of male infertility.

Clinical findings. Klinefelter males tend to be tall and thin with disproportionately long legs. Development is relatively normal until puberty when hypogonadism becomes more evident. Testes are small and testosterone production is low. Gynecomastia and a feminine body habitus can become pronounced, beginning at puberty (Fig. 16–7). Patients are almost always infertile. Testosterone replacement therapy beginning in adolescence can help bring about a more normal pattern of secondary sexual development and body habitus, but it does nothing to aid fertility (3,5). The IQ is in the low–normal range, with verbal comprehension being more compromised than performance. Behavioral and psychosocial problems such as poor attention span, poor judgment, and insecurity are often noted (2,4).

Auditory system. Defects of the external or middle ear are not often noted. One study found sensorineural hearing loss in 19% of boys and men with a 47,XXY karyotype (1). No conductive loss was noted. In a study of Danish teenage boys, poor auditory discrimination and delayed speech development were common among individuals with Klinefelter syndrome. Hearing was not tested, but the above findings suggest undetected hearing loss may be present (4).

Cytogenetics. The vast majority (80%) of Klinefelter syndrome patients have a 47,XXY karyotype. Mosaic karyotypes of 46,XY/47,XXY are less frequently detected. Klinefelter variants, with three or more Xs, also exist. The phenotype tends to be more severe, including heart defects and mental retardation, with a higher number of X chromosomes. As would be expected when more than one X chromsome is present, cells from individuals with Klinefelter syndrome are Barr body positive due to X inactivation (5).

References

1. Anderson H et al: Hearing defects in males with sex chromosome anomalies. *Acta Otolaryngol* 72:55–58, 1971.

Figure 16–7. *Klinefelter syndrome (XXY syndrome).* Left: Sixteen-year-old male with XXYY Klinefelter syndrome. Note pterygium colli, sparse pubic hair, and small testicular size. Right: Note gynecomastia and female pubic escutcheon.

2. Jones KL: *Smith's Recognizable Patterns of Human Malformation*, 5th ed. W.B. Saunders, Philadelphia, 1997.
3. Smyth CM, Bremner WJ: Klinefelter syndrome. *Arch Intern Med* 158:1309–1314, 1998.
4. Sorensen K: Physical and mental development of adolescent males with Klinefelter syndrome. *Horm Res* 37:55–61, 1992.
5. Willard H: The sex chromsomes and X chromosome inactivation. In: *The Molecular and Metabolic Basis of Inherited Disease*, Scriver CR et al (eds), McGraw-Hill, New York, 7th ed., 1995, pp 719–737.

Unbalanced 11/22 translocation

This disorder, caused by unbalanced segregation of a translocation rcp(11;22)(q23;q11), is the most frequent non-Robertsonian balanced rearrangement in humans.

Physical findings. The clinical features partly overlap with those of cat eye syndrome (tetrasomy for 22(pter–q11)) and (mosaic) trisomy 22. The face is characterized by a broad and flat nose, long and well-marked philtrum, receding mandible (very marked in the first years of life), and abnormal auricles (Fig. 16–8). There is male genital hypoplasia with micropenis, small scrotum, and cryptorchidism. Congenital malformations include cleft palate (more than 50%), heart defects (at least 50%), anal atresia with fistula, renal malformations, hypoplasia of the diaphragm, intestinal malrotation, 13 pairs of ribs, bipartite clavicles, and cerebral malformations. In contrast to the cat eye syndrome and trisomy 22, coloboma of the iris does not occur in this disorder. Mental deficiency is severe to profound. Survival is reduced with at least 50% of live-born patients not surviving the first 3 years. There is a tendency toward stereotypic movement, seizures, and autistic behavior (1,3,6). Causes for early death include cardiac failure, the consequences of brain malformations, seizure disorders, and fatal infections.

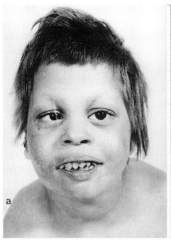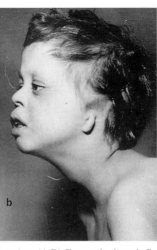

Figure 16–8. *Unbalanced 11/22 translocation.* (A,B) Esotropia, broad, flat nose, prominent upper lip, everted lower lip, preauricular tag. Other ear was microtic. [From A Schinzel et al., *Hum Genet* 56:269, 1981.]

Auditory system. The external ears exhibit preauricular pits, tags, or both, the most consistent finding of the syndrome. The pinnae are relatively long and narrow, often protruding and misshapen. Less commonly there is severe microtia with atresia or absence of the external ear canals (1,6). Some patients have severe conductive hearing loss (1–3,6) while others exhibit sensorineural hearing loss (1,4,6). Ohtani et al. (5) identified Mondini dysplasia of the bony and membranous labyrinth in one patient. The true incidence of hearing loss of both types, however, is unknown because most patients do not undergo hearing tests and/or cannot be tested with subjective methods because of their severe mental retardation.

Cytogenetic findings. Karyotypes reveal an extra marker chromosome smaller than a 22 and with different staining qualities of the distal long arm. In one parent, almost always the mother, the identical marker replaces a 22 and an abnormal 11 with an elongated long arm. The translocation is reciprocal, with breakpoints probably at 11q23 and 22q11, and thus the unbalanced products are trisomic for a segment of 11(q23–qter) and a centromere-containing segment of 22 (pter–q11). Unbalanced 2:2 segregations obviously do not survive in utero. The translocation is frequent and occurs in all populations and races. Family studies following the detection of a chromosomally unbalanced patient usually disclose multiple balanced carriers in several generations. There is also an excess of reproductive loss in these families.

Etiology, pathogenesis, and heredity. Nonfamilial occurrence has so far not been reported. However, this might be impossible without molecular studies. At least 90% of patients have the extra chromosome material from maternal translocations. Fertility of translocation carrier males is not grossly reduced; thus there is either sperm selection, or unbalanced paternally derived embryos are more likely to spontaneously abort. The risk to a female carrier is as high as 10% for producing a chromosomally unbalanced offspring (7).

Summary. Hearing loss is probably frequent in patients who are partially trisomic for 11 and 22 because of unbalanced segregation of 11/22 translocations. Conductive hearing loss in patients with or without obstruction of the external ear canals has more frequently been reported than sensorineural hearing loss, but the exact incidences are poorly known, as is their etiology.

References

1. Fraccaro M et al.: The 11q;22q translocation: a European collaborative analysis of 43 cases. *Hum Genet* 56:21–51, 1980.
2. Gustavson KH et al: Three non-mongoloid patients of similar phenotype with an extra G-like chromosome. *Clin Genet* 3:135–146, 1072.
3. Iselius L et al: The 11q;22q translocation: a collaborative study of 20 new cases and analysis of 110 families. *Hum Genet* 64:343–355, 1983.
4. Najafzadeh TM, Dumars KW: Duplication of distal 11q and 22q. Occurrence in two unrelated families. *Am J Med Genet* 8:341–347, 1981.
5. Ohtani I et al: Temporal bone histopathology in trisomy 22. *Int J Pediatr Otorhinolaryngol* 59:137–141, 2001.
6. Schinzel A et al: Incomplete trisomy 22. I. Familial 11/22 translocation with 3:1 meiotic disjunction. Delineation of a common clinical picture and report of nine new cases from six families. *Hum Genet* 56:249–261, 1981.
7. Zackai EH, Emanuel BS: Site-specific reciprocal translocation, t(11;22) (q23;q11), in severeal unrelated families with 3:1 meiotic disjunction. *Am J Med Genet* 7:507–521, 1980.

Cytogenetic Deletion Syndromes and Hearing Loss

Deletion syndromes, or contiguous gene syndromes, are disorders caused by deletion of one or more genes in a chromosomal region. The responsible chromosome segment is usually small on a cytogenetic scale (<5 Mb) but can contain multiple dosage-sensitive genes which each contribute to the phenotype independently (6). Terminal deletions, such as in 1p– syndrome and Wolf-Hirschhorn syndrome, can occur at multiple breakpoints that result in heterogeneity in deletion size. In contrast, interstitial deletions like those observed in DiGeorge and Smith-Magenis syndromes often occur at recombination "hotspots." They are the result of illegitimate recombination of low copy number repeats that are conserved in the chromosomal regions deleted (2); these disorders have recently been designated "genomic diseases."

Monosomy 1p syndrome

Monosomy 1p syndrome arises from deletion of the very terminal portion of the short arm of one chromosome 1. The incidence of this deletion is estimated to be 1:5000 to 1:10,000 (5,9), making it the one of the most common microdeletion syndromes.

Clinical findings. Patients with distal 1p deletions show a variety of clinical features (7,9). Developmental delay and mental retardation are nearly universal. The degree of mental deficiency is quite variable and in some instances has been noted to correlate with the size of the deletion. Children have growth delay and failure to thrive. Microcephaly is common. Dysmorphic features most often include a large anterior fontanelle, prominent forehead, deep-set eyes, short or slanting palpebral fissures, and flat nasal bridge with midface hypoplasia (Fig. 16–9). Cleft lip/palate or other palatal anomalies are also frequently seen. Various cardiac abnormalities have been noted. Central nervous system problems include hypotonia, usually noted at birth, seizures, and a variety of brain malformations. Self-abusive behavior including head banging and hand biting has been noted in several cases (4).

Auditory system. The external ears of patients with 1p terminal deletions can be dysplastic, small, low-set, and/or asymmetrical (9) with thickened helices (7). Sensorineural or conductive hearing loss occurs in approximately 50%–60% of patients whose hearing has been carefully evaluated. In the largest study to date, 44% of patients had bilateral high-frequency hearing loss, 11% had conductive hearing loss, and 5% had mild sensorineural hearing loss (3). Unilateral severe hearing loss was also noted in several patients (1,8). Wu et al. (10) studied the deleted interval in 30 patients and defined a minimal deletion interval in which hearing loss was present. The authors speculate that a hearing loss gene may reside distal to marker D1S2845.

Cytogenetics. The deletion is usually terminal, with breakpoints ranging from 1p36.13 to 1p36.33, but interstitial deletions have also been noted (9). A majority of cases are de novo and occur on the maternal chromosome 1 (10), although there seem to be no consistent clinical differences in children with deletions originating from either parent (5). Inherited cases are usually the result of one parent being the carrier of a balanced translocation involving 1p36 and segregating an

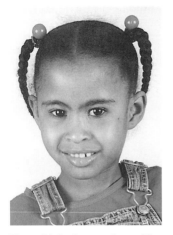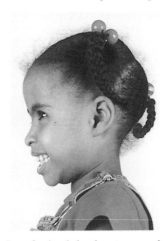

Figure 16–9. *1p– syndrome.* Note prominent forehead, deeply set eyes, and mild midface hypoplasia. [Courtesy of M Rush, Detroit, Michigan.]

unbalanced chromosomal complement to their offspring (1,9). For this reason, whenever a 1p36 deletion is detected, parental chromosomes should also be analyzed. Although it is possible to visualize the 1p terminal deletion on high-resolution G-banded chromosomes, most cases are confirmed using fluorescently labeled molecular probes that hybridize to the region. The mechanism for chromosome breakage in this area is unknown.

References

1. Barbi G et al: Reciprocal translocation t(1;15)(p36.2;p11.2): confirmation of a suggestive cytogenetic diagnosis by in situ hybridization and clinical case report on resulting monosomy (1p). *Am J Med Genet* 43:722–725, 1992.
2. Emanuel BS, Shaikh TH: Segmental duplications: an 'expanding' role in genomic instability and disease. *Nat Rev Genet* 2:791–800, 2001.
3. Heilstedt HA et al: Bilateral high frequency hearing loss is commonly found in patients with the 1p36 deletion syndrome. *Am J Hum Genet* 63:A106, 1998.
4. Reish O et al: Partial monosomy of chromosome 1p36.3: characterization of the critical region and delineation of a syndrome. *Am J Med Genet* 59:467–475, 1995.
5. Shaffer LG, Heilstedt HA: Terminal deletion of 1p36. *Lancet* 358(Suppl):S9, 2001.
6. Shaffer LG et al: Molecular cytogenetics of contiguous gene syndromes: mechanisms and consequences of gene dosage imbalance. In *The Molecular and Metabolic Basis of Inherited Disease*, Scriver CR et al. (eds), McGraw-Hill, New York, 2001, pp 1291–1324.
7. Shapira S et al: Chromosome 1p36 deletions: the clinical phenotype and molecular characterization of a common newly delineated syndrome. *Am J Hum Genet* 61:642–650, 1997.
8. Slavotinek A et al: Screening for submicroscopic chromosome rearrangements in children with idiopathic mental retardation using microsatellite markers for the chromosome telomeres. *J Med Genet* 36:405–411, 1999.
9. Slavotinek A et al: Monosomy 1p36. *J Med Genet* 36:657–663, 1999.
10. Wu Y et al: Molecular refinement of the 1p36 deletion syndrome reveals size diversity and a preponderance of maternally derived deletions. *Hum Mol Genet* 8:313–321, 1999.

Wolf-Hirschhorn syndrome (4p– syndrome)

Wolf-Hirschhorn syndrome is a malformation syndrome caused by deletion of the terminal portion of the chromosome 4 short arm, usually at band 4p16.3. The incidence of this relatively rare disorder is reported to be about 1 in 50,000 births. Two good reviews have recently been published (2,11).

Clinical findings. Individuals with Wolf-Hirschhorn syndrome are recognized by their characteristic dysmorphic features, described as a "Greek helmet" face. This finding includes a prominent glabella, hypertelorism, a broad, beaked nose, and frontal bossing (Fig. 16–10). Infants have intrauterine growth retardation and microcephaly. Develop-

mental and mental retardation are typically profound. Other frequent findings include cleft lip/palate, down-turned "fishlike" mouth, and posterior scalp defects. Cardiac atrial septal defects are also common (6). The mortality rate within the first 2 years is 21% (11). Survival also correlates with the presence or absence of an unbalanced translocation: those with de novo deletions had a median survival time of 34 years; those with unbalanced translocations had median survival of 18 years. (11).

Auditory system. External ear anomalies, such as preauricular pits and skin tags, and helix hypoplasia are common (7,9). Variable degrees of conductive hearing loss have been reported in up to a third of Wolf-Hirschhorn patients in one study (1). Other reports include a high percentage of patients with chronic otitis media, without any comments on possible subsequent conductive hearing loss (5,7). The high incidence of palatal defects likely contributes to otitis media. Bilateral sensorineural deafness has been reported in several patients (1,7) but is not a common finding.

The recessive disorder Wolfram syndrome (*WFS1*) also maps to 4p16. Wolfram syndrome presents as juvenile-onset diabetes mellitus, progressive optic atrophy, and profound deafness. Mutations in the *WFS1* gene were recently implicated in the autosomal dominant nonsyndromic hearing disorder DFNA6/14/38 (3,12), a low-frequency sensorineural hearing loss that does not progress to profound deafness. It was postulated that the few Wolf-Hirschhorn patients with severe to profound deafness might have deletions of 4p16 that also encompass the *WFS1* locus. However, given the different hearing loss phenotypes in the two patient populations and the fact that the nonsyndromic low-frequency hearing loss mutations in *WFS1* are point mutations and not deletions or truncations (4), this seems unlikely to be true.

Cytogenetics. Most 4p deletions causing Wolf-Hirschhorn syndrome occur de novo; however, about 15% of cases are the result of a structural rearrangement in one of the parents (8). A terminal deletion from 4p16.3–pter is the most frequent finding, but larger terminal deletions, or interstitial deletions, have also been noted. Most deletions are large enough to be seen by conventional cytogenetic methods. FISH may be required to detect small deletions or cryptic rearrangements (10).

References

1. Battaglia A et al: Natural history of Wolf-Hirschhorn syndrome: experience with 15 cases. *Pediatrics* 103:830–836, 1999.
2. Battaglia A et al: Wolf-Hirschhorn (4p–) syndrome. *Adv Pediatr* 48:75–113, 2001.
3. Bespalova IN et al: Mutations in the Wolfram syndrome 1 gene (*WFS1*) are a common cause of low frequency sensorineural hearing loss. *Hum Mol Genet* 10:2501–2508, 2001.
4. Cryns K et al: Mutations in the *WFS1* gene that cause low-frequency sensorineural hearing loss are small non-inactivating mutations. *Hum Genet* 110:389–394, 2002.

Figure 16–10. *Wolf-Hirschhorn syndrome (4p– syndrome).* (A,B) Note hypertelorism and prominent nasal bridge. [From W Smith, Portland, Maine.]

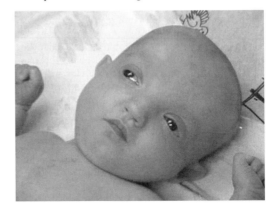

5. Estabrooks LL et al: Summary of the 1993 ASHG ancillary meeting "recent research on chromosome 4p syndromes and genes". *Am J Med Genet* 55:453–458, 1995.
6. Jones KL: *Smith's Recognizable Patterns of Human Malformation*, 5th ed. W.B. Saunders, Philadelphia, 1997.
7. Lesperance MM et al: Otologic manifestations of Wolf-Hirschhorn syndrome. *Arch Otolaryngol Head Neck Surg* 124:193–196, 1998.
8. Lurie IW et al: The Wolf-Hirschhorn syndrome. I. Genetics. *Clin Genet* 17:375–384, 1980.
9. Opitz JM: Twenty-seven-year follow-up in the Wolf-Hirschhorn syndrome. *Am J Med Genet* 55:459–461, 1995.
10. Shaffer LG et al: Molecular cytogenetics of contiguous gene syndromes: mechanisms and consequences of gene dosage imbalance. In: *The Molecular and Metabolic Basis of Inherited Disease*, Scriver CR et al. (eds), Mc-Graw-Hill, New York, 2001, pp 1291–1324.
11. Shannon NL et al: An epidemiological study of Wolf-Hirschhorn syndrome: life expectancy and causes for mortality. *J Med Genet* 38:674–679, 2001.
12. Young TL et al: Non-syndromic progressive hearing loss DFNA38 is caused by heterozygous missense mutation in the Wolfram syndrome gene *WFS1*. *Hum Mol Genet* 10:2509–2514, 2001.

Smith-Magenis syndrome

First described in 1986 (8), Smith-Magenis syndrome is a contiguous gene deletion syndrome that displays characteristic physical, mental, and behavioral abnormalities. The deletion is typically 5 Mb on the short arm of chromosome 17 at band p11.2. The incidence of Smith-Magenis syndrome is approximately 1 in 25,000 (7).

Clinical findings. The clinical picture of Smith-Magenis syndrome includes minor craniofacial dysmorphisms (brachycephaly, prominant forehead, epicanthal folds, broad nasal bridge, prognathism, and synophrys) that give patients a very characteristic appearance (Fig. 16–11A,B). Significant clinical findings include anomalies of the eye (85% of patients, mostly myopia), skeletal system (Fig. 16–11C) (65% of patients; mild scoliosis, radial-ulnar defects), brain (52% of patients; ventriculomegaly, enlarged cisterna magna, enlarged foramen magnum), heart (37% of patients; pulmonic stenosis, ventricular septal defect, atrial septal defect, mitral valve prolapse), and urinary tract (35% of patients; duplication of the collecting system, renal agenesis, ectopic kidneys) [reviewed in Greenberg et al. (3)]. No patients are expected to have all of these defects, but a combination of two or more findings is frequent. The IQ ranges from 20 to 80, with most patients in the 40–55 range, which is considered moderate mental retardation. Presence of a deep, hoarse voice is common and may be due to laryngeal defects in some patients.

Among the more notable findings in Smith-Magenis syndrome are characteristic behavioral abnormalities. Sleep disturbances are common, especially difficulty in falling asleep and staying asleep at night, followed by frequent napping during the day. Abnormalities in circadian rhythms of melatonin levels are likely to underlie this unusual sleep pattern (5). Smith-Magenis patients also have a tendency toward self-injurious behavior, including head-banging, wrist-biting, and sticking foreign objects under their nails or in their noses or ears (2).

Auditory system. About 70% of Smith-Magenis patients are hearing impaired, with approximately two-thirds showing conductive loss and one-third having sensorineural hearing loss (3). Otitis media is frequent and may be due partly to velopharyngeal incompetence. Hearing loss is generally mild to moderate, although more profound hearing loss has also been noted.

Interestingly, a form of nonsyndromic autosomal recessive deafness, DFNB3, maps to the 5 Mb region of 17p11.2 typically deleted in Smith-Magenis patients (1). Mutations in the unconventional myosin gene *MYO15A* cause DFNB3 in humans and a deafness and vestibular phenotype called *shaker-2* in mice (6,9). *MYO15A* is usually hemizygous in Smith-Magenis patients. Liburd et al. showed that in at least one Smith-Magenis patient with severe sensorineural hearing loss, the *MYO15A* allele that was not deleted was in fact mutated (4). A highly conserved threonine in the tail region of the protein was changed to an isoleucine. The authors speculate that one deleted *MYO15A* and one mutated *MYO15A* are the underlying cause of this particular patient's severe hearing loss.

Cytogenetic findings. Many of the deletions at 17p11.2 that cause Smith-Magenis syndrome are visible by routine high-resolution cytogenetic banding. Fluorescent in situ hybridization with molecular probes that hybridize in the Smith-Magenis deletion region is commonly performed to confirm a cytologically visible deletion or diagnose a cryptic rearrangement.

References

1. Friedman TB et al: A gene for congenital, recessive deafness DFNB3 maps to the pericentromeric region of chromosome 17. *Nat Genet* 9:86–91, 1995.
2. Greenberg F, et al: Molecular analysis of the Smith-Magenis syndrome: a possible contiguous-gene syndrome associated with del(17)(p11.2). *Am J Hum Genet* 49:1207–1218, 1991.

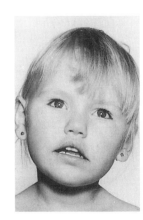 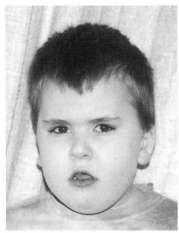 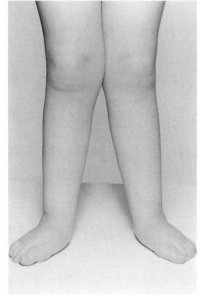

Figure 16–11. *Smith-Magenis syndrome* [del(17p11.2)]. (A,B) Children with global delay, hypotonia, frontal bossing, broad nasal bridge, short philtrum, prominent upper lip, and carp-shaped mouth. (C) Note genua valga and flat feet. [(A,C) from MA Hamill et al., *Ann Génét* 31:36, 1988; (B) courtesy of SR Patil, Iowa City, Iowa.] **A** **B** **C**

3. Greenberg F et al: Multidisciplinary clinical study of Smith-Magenis syndrome (deletion 17p11.2) [see comments]. *Am J Med Genet* 62:247–254, 1996.

4. Liburd N et al: Novel mutations of *MYO15A* associated with profound deafness in consanguineous families and moderately severe hearing loss in a patient with Smith-Magenis syndrome. *Hum Genet* 109:535–541, 2001.

5. Potocki L et al: Circadian rhythm abnormalities of melatonin in Smith-Magenis syndrome. *J Med Genet* 37:428–433, 2000.

6. Probst FJ et al: Correction of deafness in *shaker-2* mice by an unconventional myosin in a BAC transgene. *Science* 280:1444–1447, 1998.

7. Shaffer LG et al: Molecular cytogenetics of contiguous gene syndromes: mechanisms and consequences of gene dosage imbalance. In: *The Molecular and Metabolic Basis of Inherited Disease*, Scriver CR et al (eds), McGraw-Hill, New York, 2001, pp 1291–1324.

8. Smith AC et al: Interstitial deletion of (17)(p11.2p11.2) in nine patients. *Am J Med Genet* 24:393–414, 1986.

9. Wang A et al: Association of uncoventional myosin *MYO15* mutations with human nonsyndromic deafness DFNB3. *Science* 280:1447–1451, 1998.

Del18p (18p−) syndrome

The del(18p) syndrome is the pattern of congenital anomalies caused by deletion of the entire short arm of chromosome 18 with breakpoint at 18p11 to 18q11.

Physical findings. The del(18p) syndrome is characterized by growth retardation, mental deficiency of usually moderate degree, and a relatively nonspecific combination of congenital major and minor anomalies. The phenotype most resembles that of Turner syndrome. The pattern of dysmorphic features is not striking at birth but becomes more distinct with age. It includes brachycephaly, broad face with ptosis of upper eyelids, broad nose, downturned corners of mouth, malocclusion, and a tendency to develop dental caries (Fig. 16–12). Broad and short neck with low posterior hairline, pectus excavatum, kyphoscoliosis, genital hypoplasia (especially in males), broad hands with short fingers and short and incurved fifth fingers, and partial 2–3 syndactyly of toes are also found (Fig. 16–12A,B). Approximately 10% to 20% have holoprosencephaly ranging from agenesis of the olfactory bulbs and tracts to cyclopia. These infants either die perinatally or later and, if they survive with milder forms of the malformation, are severely to profoundly mentally deficient. As holoprosencephaly may overshadow all other findings of the syndrome, it is important for later genetic counseling to karyotype all patients with this disorder, especially the lethal forms. Other malformations are far less important and comprise a large spectrum: heart defects, various eye anomalies, kidney malformations, and rarely others (3). There is also a tendency to develop autoimmune disorders (thyroiditis, Graves disease, rheumatoid arthritis, and eczema). Occasional patients have congenital alopecia and/or growth hormone deficiency. Most patients are moderately retarded, but sometimes mental capacity can be normal or near normal (11,12). Dystonia may be a relatively common later-onset complication in these patients (7) At least 120 cases have been reported (6).

Other findings. Similar to the del(18q) syndrome, serum IgA is absent or markedly decreased in about 35% of patients (12).

Auditory system. The external ears in del(18p) syndrome patients are large, posteriorly angulated, and protruding. Rudimentary auricles with atresia of outer auditory canals and presumably conductive hearing loss have rarely been reported (2,8). While several case reports have mentioned hearing loss in del(18p) patients, the true incidence is not known. In some, moderate to severe hearing loss has not been further specified (9,10); in others there has been conductive hearing loss of mild degree (4). Finally, profound hearing loss was found in an 18-year-old female with moderate mental retardation (2), indicating that sensorineural hearing loss may also occur. Adache and Hayashi (1) also noted sensorineural hearing loss.

Cytogenetic findings. Diagnosis is based on finding deletion of the entire short arm of one chromosome 18, most having a breakpoint at 18p11. In about 10% of cases the deletion is due to an unbalanced de novo translocation and, in the latter, breakpoints may be at the proximal long arm. The other chromosome involved most often is an acrocentric and includes its centromeric region in the translocation. Finally, unbalanced segregation of familial translocations or inversions occur, with duplication–deletions rarely being found (5,9). In rare cases the deletion is inherited from a parent (13).

Etiology, pathogenesis, and heredity. Del(18p) usually occurs de novo and in only an estimated 10% or less is it familial (13). The pathogenesis of the hearing loss is unknown, with the exception of the cases where it is secondary to recurrent otitis.

Prognosis. Hearing loss in the del(18p) syndrome is mostly not progressive and rarely leads to profound loss. Hearing aids will generally provide a reasonable hearing capacity. Survival of individuals is variable and depends on whether severe malformations are present.

Summary. Hearing loss occurs in del(18p) syndrome, but its incidence is not known. Conductive hearing loss has been established. Sensorineural hearing loss is less common. Whether malformations of the middle and inner ear may also occur is not known.

References

1. Adache K, Hayashi M: An 18p− syndrome doe to 15/18 translocation with facial palsy and deafness. *Tohoku J Exp Med* 133:307–311, 1981.

2. Ayraud N et al: Syndrome 18p−. Une nouvelle observation. *Ann Genet (Paris)* 12:122–125, 1969.

3. Buffoni L et al: Nanismo ipofisario e sindrome malformativa multipla "tipo Goldenhar" in soggetto condelezione del braccio corto del chromosoma 18. *Minerva Pediatr* 28:716–729, 1976.

4. Dolan LM et al: 18p− syndrome with a single central maxillary incisor. *J Med Genet* 19:396–398, 1981.

5. Fraccaro M et al: Structural aberrations of chromosome 18. III. Two G/18 translocations, one identified as 22/18. *Ann Génét (Paris)* 15:93–98, 1972.

6. Gorlin RJ et al: *Syndromes of the Head and Neck,* 4th ed. Oxford University Press, New York, 2001

7. Klein C et al: Genetic analysis of three patients with an 18p− syndrome and dystonia. *Neurology* 52:649–651, 1999.

8. Lurie IW, Lazjuk GI: Partial monosomies 18. *Humangenetik* 15:203–222, 1972.

9. Malpuech G et al: Délétion du bras court du 18 par translocation t(G−;18p+). Une étude en fluorescence par la moutarde de quinacrine. *Ann Génét (Paris)* 14:213–218, 1971.

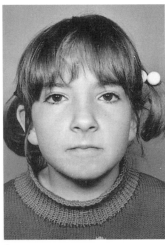 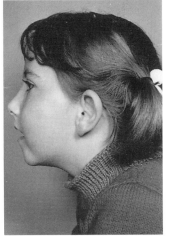

Figure 16–12. *Del(18) syndrome.* (A,B) Essentially normal face, but mild hypertelorism, wide mouth, and outstanding ears. [From A Schinzel, *Arch Genet* 52:1, 1979.]

A   **B**

10. Nishikawa M et al: A case of familial cystathioninuria with goiter and some anomalies. *Endocrinol Jpn* 17:57–63, 1970.
11. Schinzel A: Partielle Monosomien von Chromosom 18. I. Partielle Monosomie für den kurzen Arm, 18p− Syndrome. *Arch Genet (Zurich)* 52:125–130, 1979.
12. Schinzel A: *Catalogue of Unbalanced Chromosome Aberrations in Man.* Walter de Gruyter and Co., Berlin, 1983.
13. Tsukahara M et al: Familial del(18p) syndrome. *Am J Med Genet* 99:67–69, 2001.

Del18q (18q−) syndrome

The del(18q) syndrome is defined as the pattern of congenital anomalies caused by terminal deletion of the long arm of chromosome 18 with breakpoint at 18q21.2 to 18q22.2.

Physical findings. The del(18q) syndrome is characterized by a very specific combination of major and minor congenital anomalies. The pattern of dysmorphic features is striking and often allows for clinical recognition. It includes midface hypoplasia with prominent forehead and mandibular overbite, everted lower lip, short upper lip with poorly formed philtrum, downturned corners of mouth, small teeth, narrow and small nose, epicanthic folds, strabismus, nystagmus with pale optic discs, and external ear anomalies (Fig. 16–13).

Kyphoscoliosis and vertebral anomalies are common. Limb anomalies include proximally placed thumbs, tapering fingers, clubfeet, irregular position and proximal 2–3 syndactyly of toes, and multiple dimples over major joints. Frequent malformations include congenital heart anomalies (20%), cleft palate (10%), cleft lip (10%), cataract, glaucoma, coloboma and other eye malformations (including microphthalmia), hernias, and various renal malformations. Hypospadias and cryptorchidism are frequent in males. Most patients have short stature, in large part attributable to growth hormone insufficiency (3), and almost all are mentally retarded. The IQs range from rarely normal to severely retarded (5,10–13). More than 100 cases have been reported.

Auditory system. The external ears in del(18q) syndrome patients are low-set, mostly exhibiting hypoplastic helix, prominent anthelix, and prominent antitragus. The external ear canal is narrow in at least 35% of cases. Bilateral atresia can be seen, as well as unilateral narrowness and contralateral atresia. A preauricular tag was observed only once (8); a pit, never. Conductive hearing loss was reported in about 15% of pa-

tients, but it is obviously more frequent than this percentage would indicate (1,8,12–15); a number were newborns and hearing loss was not tested. Thus hearing impairment is frequent in del(18q) syndrome, usually being caused by atresia of the auditory canals and rarely being due to the sequelae of cleft palate (6,7). Malformations of the middle ear were not found in any patients examined. Possible additional sensorineural loss was reported in single cases of the syndrome with conductive hearing impairment, but this has never been convincingly documented (4,9).

Other findings. Serum IgA is absent or markedly decreased in about 35% (5). This finding does not seem to correlate with clinical findings.

Cytogenetic findings. The diagnosis is based on finding terminal deletion of the long arm of one chromosome 18, with breakpoint at 18q21 or 18q22. More distal deletions result in milder clinical findings, and interstitial deletions cause a different pattern of anomalies. Until 1998, investigators had not found a strong correlation between phenotype and size of deletion (8,11); however, Brkanac et al. (2) found that among 35 patients diagnosed as having del(18q) via karyotypic means, 5 actually had either interstitial deletions or more complex, cryptic rearrangements, thus providing at least a partial explanation for the previous findings.

The deletion occurs de novo in at least 80% of cases. The rest of the aberrations are due to either parental translocations or inversions, or to direct transmission from mother to child. A proportion of ring 18 chromosome carriers exhibit the del(18q) syndrome and hearing loss with narrow auditory canals.

Prognosis. Hearing loss in del(18q) is rarely progressive. Approximately 10% of those affected die within the first few months; however, most have a normal life expectancy (8).

Summary. Conductive hearing loss is frequent in the del(18q) syndrome; most patients have very narrow or atretic external ear canals that contribute significantly to the occurrence of hearing loss.

References

1. Bergstrom L et al: External auditory atresia and the deleted chromosome. *Laryngoscope* 11:1905–1917, 1974.
2. Brkanac Z et al: Identification of cryptic rearrangements in patients with 18q− deletion syndrome. *Am J Hum Genet* 62:1500–1506, 1998.
3. Cody JD et al: Growth hormone insufficiency associated with haploinsufficiency at 18q23. *Am J Med Genet* 71:420–425, 1997.
4. Corney MJ, Smith S: Early development of an infant with 18q− syndrome. *J Ment Defic Res* 28:303–307, 1984.
5. Henrot B et al: Délétion du bras long du chromosome 18, hypothyroidie primaire, anémie de Biermer et hypogammaglobulinémie de type IgM. *Arch Fr Pédiatr* 46:729–732, 1968.
6. Kushnick T, Matsushita G: Partial deletion of long arms of chromosome 18. *Pediatrics* 42:729–732, 1989.
7. Martin AO et al: Clinical implications of chromosomal inversions. A pericentric inversion in No. 18 segregating in a family ascertained through an abnormal proband. *Am J Perinatol* 1:81–88, 1983.
8. Miller G et al: Neurologic manifestations in 18q− syndrome. *Am J Med Genet* 37:128–132, 1990.
9. Nance WE et al: Partial E-18 long-arm deletion. *Lancet* 1:303, 1968.
10. Schinzel A: Partielle Monosomien von Chromosom 18. Partielle Monosomie für das distale Segment des langen Armes, 18q− Syndrome. *Arch Genet* 52:130–136, 1979.
11. Strathdee G et al: Analysis of clinical variation seen in patients with 18q terminal deletions. *Am J Med Genet* 59:476–483, 1995.
12. Sulzer M, Zierler H: 18q− Deletion bei Mutter und Tochter. *Wien Klin Wochenschr* 88:571–575, 1976.
13. Wertelecki W, Gerald PS: Clinical and chromosomal studies of the 18q− syndrome. *J Pediatr* 78:44–52, 1971.
14. Wilson MG et al: Syndromes associated with deletion of the long arm of chromosome 18 [del(18q)]. *Am J Med Genet* 3:155–174, 1979.
15. Wolf JW et al: Atlanto-occipital rotatory fixation associated with the 18q− syndrome. *J Bone Joint Surg* 62A:295–297, 1980.

Figure 16–13. *Del(18q) syndrome.* (A,B) Note midface hypoplasia, and deep-set eyes. [(A) from JD Mürken, *Zkinderheikld* 109:1, 1970, (B) courtesy of H. Toriello, Grand Rapids, MI.]

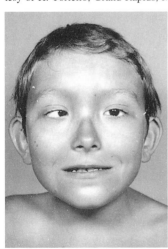
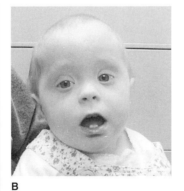

A

B

Deletion 22q11 spectrum (velocardiofacial syndrome, Shprintzen syndrome, DiGeorge complex, conotruncal anomaly face syndrome, Cayler asymmetric crying facies syndrome)

Shprintzen et al. (21,22) described a syndrome with a distinctive facial appearance, prominent nose, cardiovascular malformations, cleft palate, and learning disabilities that became known as the velocardiofacial syndrome. The overlap between DiGeorge sequence and velocardiofacial syndrome was observed by Stevens et al. (25). Shortly after a deletion of chromosome 22q11 was reported in patients with velocardiofacial syndrome and the DiGeorge sequence (7,19), the same chromosome abnormality was found in conotruncal anomaly face syndrome (3), Cayler syndrome (10), and in some patients with Opitz G/BBB syndrome (13). To date, over 150 different characteristics have been described as part of the deletion 22q11 spectrum, attesting to the highly variable phenotype (11,14,15,18). The incidence of 22q11 deletions has been estimated to be approximately 1 per 4000 (4).

Craniofacial findings. Approximately 10% of cases are microcephalic (6). The face becomes more distinctive past infancy and is described as long with malar flatness and retrognathia. A prominent and squared nasal root, bulbous nasal tip, and hypoplastic alae nasi are usually present, and the mouth is often small and kept open (9,14,21,22) (Fig. 16–14A–C). A dimpled or bifid nasal tip may be seen (12). Asymmetric crying face and facial nerve palsy have both been reported (10,18). About 15% of patients have the Robin sequence (11).

Ocular system. Palpebral fissures tend to be narrow with hooded upper lids or ptosis. Tortuous retinal vessels, coloboma, small optic discs, and posterior embryotoxon have been observed (11,14).

Cardiovascular system. A cardiovascular malformation (CVM) is present in ~80% of patients. While a wide variety of defects has been reported, certain conotruncal defects are more common in this condition, including tetralogy of Fallot (22%) (especially when associated with pulmonary atresia and aortopulmonary collateral vessels), interrupted aortic arch–type B (15%), and truncus arteriosus (7%) (15). Evaluation for DiGeorge sequence (including absent or hypoplastic thymus and parathyroids) should be considered, especially in the presence of a conotruncal heart defect. Other reported CVMs include ventricular septal defect, vascular ring, and atrial septal defect. Medially displaced and tortuous carotid arteries are common and need to be considered at the time of palatal surgery and/or tonsillectomy (9).

Central nervous system. Hypotonia of infancy and learning disabilities are common (70%–90%) (14,27). The learning disability often involves nonverbal skills, resulting in a wide verbal–nonverbal split on testing (25,26). The risk for psychiatric illness, including schizophrenia, bipolar disorder, and depression, appears to be increased in this disorder although the precise frequency is not fully delineated (22,23,27). Seizures occur but are usually associated with hypocalcemia, which may be present in infancy and occasionally has a later onset (18). Various brain malformations have been reported but are individually rare (2).

Musculoskeletal system. In childhood, 10% of patients have short stature and slow weight gain, with most individuals achieving a normal final height (6). Long and slender fingers are characteristic. A variety of anomalies such as umbilical or inguinal hernia, clubfoot, vertebral anomalies and/or rib anomalies, and scoliosis have been reported in large series of patients (11,14,16,18)

Immunologic findings. Frequent upper respiratory infections are common in early life. While evaluations may show immune defects such as decreased T-cell production and function, clinically significant immune dysfunction is uncommon (18,27). Juvenile rheumatoid arthritis occurs at a rate higher than in the general population (29).

Oral findings. Almost 70% of patients have a palatal abnormality, such as velopharyngeal incompetence (25%), bifid uvula (5%), submucous cleft palate (15%), or overt cleft palate (10%), while cleft lip with or without cleft palate is found in only 2% of patients (15). Adenoid pads are small to moderate in size (9). There is usually a history of delayed expressive speech and/or hypernasal speech requiring therapy.

Auditory system. Abnormalities of the external ears include protuberant, small, or overfolded helices; pits; tags; and narrow external auditory canals. Hearing impairment is found in 60% of patients; 25% have a sensorineural loss and 75% have a conductive loss (5). Palatal anomalies and velopharyngeal insufficiency are the likely cause of a high proportion of recurrent middle ear disease leading to hearing loss (5,17). One study noted that 23% of patients with normal hearing had tympanostomy tubes placed earlier in childhood, suggesting that aggressive management of chronic ear infections can reduce the rates of conductive hearing loss (24). Sensorineural or mixed hearing loss is seen in 5% to 15% of patients, often affecting the low frequencies more severely (17,24).

Because of the variability of clinical presentation in DiGeorge syndrome, patients with ear or palatal problems may come to the attention of otolaryngologists before being diagnosed with the syndrome. These would presumably be cases where cardiac, thymus, and/or parathyroid manifestations are mild (5). However, it would be important for the otolaryngologist to diagnose and test for the syndrome, not just to preempt future clinical problems of a more serious nature for the patient but also to screen for other family members who could have the same chromosomal deletion.

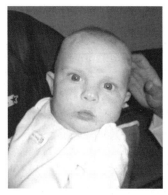
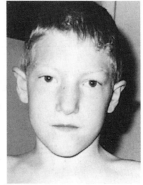
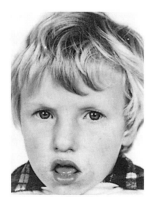

A　　　　B　　　　C

Figure 16–14. *Deletion 22q11 spectrum.* (A–C) Face appears long and myopathic. The nose is long and narrow with hypoplastic ale. There is a prominent nasal bridge and almond-shaped palpebral fissures. Note prominent ears in (A, B). [(A) courtesy of Rhonda Scanlon, E. Lansing, MI; (B,C) from AH Lipson et al., *J Med Genet* 28:596, 1991].

Cytogenetics. Most (85%–90%) DiGeorge/velocardiofacial syndrome cases have a common deletion of 3 Mb at 22q11.2. Eight to ten percent of cases have a 1.5 to 2 Mb deletion at the same band (8). A 3 Mb deletion is at the upper level of resolution by G-banded chromosomes, therefore only infrequently can a 22q deletion be detected on a routine karyotype. By using FISH with probes that hybridize to the commonly deleted region, almost all 22q deletions can be detected (1,20). In 10%–15% of cases, the deletion has been inherited from a parent (28).

Summary. Characteristics of this disorder are highly variable and can include (*1*) chromosome 22q11 deletion which may be inherited; (*2*) characteristic face; (*3*) cardiovascular malformation, typically conotruncal; (*4*) learning difficulties; (*5*) palatal abnormality; and (*6*) conductive or more rarely sensorineural hearing loss.

References

1. Berend SA et al: Dual-probe fluorescence in situ hybridization assay for detecting deletions associated with VCFS/DiGeorge syndrome I and DiGeorge syndrome II loci. *Am J Med Genet* 91:313–317, 2000.
2. Bird LM, Scambler P: Cortical dysgenesis in 2 patients with chromosome 22q11 deletion. *Clin Genet* 58:64–68, 1998.
3. Burn J et al: Conotruncal anomaly face syndrome is associated with a deletion within chromosome 22q11. *J Med Genet* 30:822–824, 1993.
4. Devriendt K et al: The annual incidence of DiGeorge/velocardiofacial syndrome. *J Med Genet* 39:789–790, 1998.
5. Digilio MC et al: Audiological findings in patients with microdeletion 22q11 (DiGeorge/velocardiofacial syndrome). *Br J Audiol* 33:329–334, 1999.
6. Digilio MC et al: Auxological evaluation in patients with DiGeorge/velocardiofacial syndrome (deletion 22q11.2 syndrome). *Genet Med* 3:30–33, 2001.
7. Driscoll DA et al: Deletions and microdeletions of 22q11.2 in velo-cardiofacial syndrome. *Am J Med Genet* 44:261–268, 1992.
8. Emanuel BS, Shaikh TH: Segmental duplications an "expanding" role in genomic instability and disease. *Nat Rev Genet* 2:791–800, 2000.
9. Ford LC et al: Otolaryngological manifestations of velocardiofacial syndrome: a retrospective review of 35 patients. *Laryngoscope* 110:362–367, 2000.
10. Giannotti A et al: Cayler cardiofacial syndrome and del 22q11: part of the CATCH22 phenotype. *Am J Med Genet* 53:303–304, 1994.
11. Goldberg R et al: Velo-cardio-facial syndrome: a review of 120 patients. *Am J Med Genet* 45:313–319, 1993.
12. Gripp KW et al: Nasal dimple as part of the 22q11.2 deletion syndrome. *Am J Med Genet* 69:290–292, 1997.
13. Lacassie Y, Arriaza MI: Opitz GBBB syndrome and the 22q11.2 deletion. *Am J Med Genet* 62:318, 1996.
14. Lipson AH et al: Velocardiofacial syndrome (Shprintzen) syndrome: an important syndrome for the dysmorphologist to recognize. *J Med Genet* 28:596–604, 1991.
15. McDonald-McGinn DM et al: The Philadelphia story: the 22q11.2 deletion: report on 250 patients. *Genet Couns* 10:11–24, 1999.
16. Ming JE et al: Skeletal anomalies and deformities in patients with deletions of 22q11. *Am J Med Genet* 72:210–215, 1997.
17. Reyes MR et al: Hearing loss and otitis media in velo-cardio-facial syndrome. *Int J Pediatr Otorhinolaryngol* 47:227–233, 1999.
18. Ryan AK et al: Spectrum of clinical features associated with interstitial chromosome 22 q11 deletions: a European collaborative study. *J Med Genet* 34:798–804, 1997.
19. Scambler PJ et al: Velo-cardio-facial syndrome associated with chromosome 22 deletions encompassing the DiGeorge locus. *Lancet* 339:1138–1139, 1992.
20. Shaffer LG et al: Molecular cytogenetics of contiguous gene syndromes. Mechanisms and consequences of gene dosage imbalance. In: *The Molecular and Metabolic Basis of Inherited Disease*, Scriver CR et al. (eds), McGraw-Hill, New York, 2001, pp 1291–1324.
21. Shprintzen RJ et al: A new syndrome involving cleft palate, cardiac anomalies, typical facies and learning disabilities: velo-cardio-facial syndrome. *Cleft Palate J* 15:56–62, 1978.
22. Shprintzen RJ et al: The velo-cardio-facial syndrome: a clinical and genetic analysis. *Pediatrics* 67: 167–172, 1981.
23. Shprintzen RJ et al: Late-onset psychosis in the velo-cardio-facial syndrome. *Am J Med Genet* 42:141–142, 1992.
24. Solot CB et al: Communication disorders in the 22q11.2 microdeletion syndrome. *J Commun Disord* 33:187–203, 2000.
25. Stevens CA et al: Di-George anomaly and velocardiofacial syndrome. *Pediatrics* 85:526–530, 1990.
26. Swillen A et al: Intelligence and psychosocial adjustment in velocardiofacial syndrome: a study of 37 children and adolescents with VCFS. *J Med Genet* 34:453–458, 1997.
27. Swillen A et al: Chromosome 22q11 deletion syndrome: update and review of the clinical features, cognitive-behavioral spectrum and psychiatric complications. *Am J Med Genet (Semin Med Genet)* 97:128–135, 2000.
28. Thompson PW, Davies SJ: Frequency of inherited deletions of 22q11. *J Med Genet* 39:789, 1998.
29. Verloes A et al: Juvenile rheumatoid arthritis and del (22q11) syndrome: a non-random association. *J Med Genet* 35:943–947, 1998.

Other cytogenetic rearrangements and hearing loss syndromes

There are dozens of syndromes associated with chromosome abnormalities. It is worth mentioning a few additional ones caused by known cytogenetic deletions or rearrangements that demonstrate external ear abnormalities and/or hearing loss as an occasional component. Mosaic trisomy 8 or mosaic trisomy 9, terminal deletions of 3p, 5p (cri-du-chat syndrome), 9p, or 11q, and duplications of 3q, 9q, or 10q all fall within this category. Fewer than 100 cases have been reported for some of these syndromes. Often ears are misshapen, malrotated, and/or low-set. Hearing acuity is only occasionally addressed in studies of these syndromes [reviewed in Jones (2)]. Because cytogenetic abnormalities often cause multiple congenital malformations and/or severe mental retardation, the unrecognized handicap of hearing impairment is not always the first system to be evaluated.

Unique cases

There are also numerous examples in the recent literature of unique chromosome rearrangements that appear to cause hearing loss. These include previously undescribed small deletions, duplications, inversions, and translocations.

Kelley et al. (3) described an adult male with learning disabilities, epilepsy, long fingers and toes, and bilateral sensorineural hearing loss of 65–70 dB. Cytogenetically, the individual had a duplication of the terminal long arm of chromosome 17, at 17q24–qter (3). Interestingly, the autosomal dominant nonsyndromic hearing disorders DFNA20 and DFNA26 both map to this region of 17q. It is possible that disruption of the copy number of a deafness gene in this interval led to the hearing loss in this individual.

Chen et al. (1) reported a woman of normal intelligence referred for minor facial anomalies, sterility, myopathy, scoliosis, and bilateral conductive hearing loss. This individual had a very unusual cytogenetic rearrangement in which no normal chromosome 1s were present. One chromosome 1 consisted of two copies of 1p (iso(1p)) and the other contained two copies of 1q (iso(1q)). All the genetic material that should be present from two normal chromosome 1s appeared to be included but rearranged. Significantly, all of the woman's chromosome 1 material was inherited from her father, not half from her father and half from her mother, as usually takes place. This finding suggests that genetic imprinting or one or more recessive mutations might account for the observed phenotype (1).

Kozma et al. (4) reported a female child with a de novo pericentric inversion of the long and short arms of a chromosome 2 (inv(2)(p13q11.2)). This child had minor craniofacial dysmorphism, hypotonia, developmental delay, and severe bilateral sensorineural hearing loss. The phenotype could be due to a submicroscopic deletion or duplication at one of the breakpoints, or to disruption of a gene required for embryonic central nervous system development.

Meschede et al. (5) described a male child with minor craniofacial anomalies, microcephaly, moderate mental delay, low-set, misshapen ears, and mixed hearing loss requiring hearing aids. Cytogenetically, the child had a submicroscopic deletion of terminal 14q that resulted from a de novo t(14;21)(q32.3;p11).

In each of the above examples, hearing loss is just one component of the patient's overall phenotype. It is possible that the noted hearing loss, or any other aspect of the phenotype, is not a direct result of the chromosome rearrangement but a coincidental finding. However, as more knowledge is gained about deafness genes and their locations in the genome, these unusual cases and their phenotypes may become interpretable and may even advance our understanding of molecular aspects of hearing and hearing loss.

References

1. Chen H et al: Uniparental isodisomy resulting from 46,XX,i(1p),i(1q) in a woman with short stature, ptosis, micro/retrognathia, myopathy, deafness, and sterility. *Am J Med Genet* 82:215–218, 1999.
2. Jones KL: *Smith's Recognizable Patterns of Human Malformation*, 5th ed. W.B. Saunders, Philadelphia, 1997.
3. Kelly BD et al: Dysmorphic features and learning disability in an adult male with pure partial trisomy 17q24–q25 due to a terminal duplication. *Am J Med Genet* 112:217–20, 2002.
4. Kozma C et al: Prenatal detection of de novo inversion of chromosome (2) (p13q11.2) and postnatal follow-up. *Prenat Diagn* 16:366–370, 1996.
5. Meschede D et al: Submicroscopic deletion in 14q32.3 through a de novo tandem translocation between 14q and 21p. *Am J Med Genet* 80:368–372, 1998.

Use of cytogenetics to identify hearing loss genes

Cytogenetics is used primarily as a diagnostic tool. One other extremely useful aspect of cytogenetics is that it can be employed to refine a disease locus. Individuals who have a cytogenetic rearrangement that disrupts or dysregulates a disease gene may manifest a disease. The breakpoints of the rearrangement can serve as landmarks to identify the disease locus. Described below is an example of successful use of this approach, to investigate potential genetic loci for Waardenburg syndrome.

Waardenburg syndrome is an autosomal dominant disorder characterized by deafness in 25% of affected individuals and by pigmentary anomalies of the skin, hair, and eyes. It is now recognized to be a phenotypically and genetically heterogeneous disorder, with four different types, WS1–4, caused by mutations in half a dozen different genes (see Chapter 14). The phenotype varies depending on the gene mutated and whether the mutation is heterozygous or homozygous.

Because of the genetic heterogeneity, early attempts at linkage analysis for Waardenburg syndrome were confounded; a possible locus at 9q34 was suggested (5). In 1989, Ishikiriyama and co-authors reported a Japanese boy with a phenotype consistent with WS1 (4). Significantly, this child had a small de novo chromosome inversion on the distal portion of one chromosome 2, with breakpoints at q35 and q37.3 (46,XY,inv(2)(q35q37.3)) (Fig. 16–15). Foy et al. (2) used this information to investigate genetic linkage of WS1 to distal 2q in a collection of Waardenburg syndrome families and found good evidence of close linkage. They suggested that WS1 might be homologous to the *Splotch* mouse, which mapped to a region of homologous synteny on

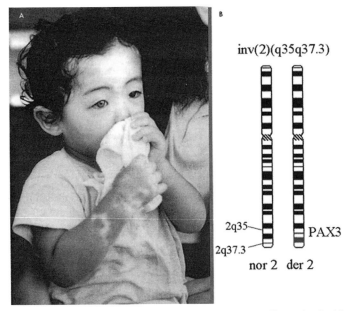

Figure 16–15. *Waardenburg syndrome type 1.* Ideogram of inversion 2 with breakpoints at 2q35 and 2q37.3.

mouse chromosome 1. The *Splotch* mouse has pigmentary changes consistent with Waardenburg syndrome but does not experience hearing loss. Mutations in the homeobox gene *Pax3* were identified as the cause of the *Splotch* phenotype in 1991 (1,3). Using heteroduplex analysis, Tassabehji et al. evaluated the human homolog, *PAX3* (designated *HuP2* in their report), as a candidate gene for WS1 in several families and found complete concordance. Sequencing of *PAX3* in these families identified the first WS1 disease-causing mutations (6). Since then, dozens of WS1 mutations have been identified in *PAX3*.

References

1. Epstein DJ et al: *splotch* (*Sp^{2H}*), a mutation affecting development of the mouse neural tube, shows a deletion within the paired homeodomain of *Pax3*. *Cell* 67:767–774, 1991.
2. Foy C et al: Assignment of the locus for Waardenburg syndrome type I to human chromosome 2q37 and possible homology to the Splotch mouse [see comments]. *Am J Hum Genet* 46:1017–1023, 1990.
3. Goulding MD et al: Pax-3, a novel murine DNA binding protein expressed during early neurogenesis. *EMBO J* 10:1135–1147, 1991.
4. Ishikiriyama S et al: Waardenburg syndrome type I in a child with de novo inversion (2)(q35q37.3). *Am J Med Genet* 33:505–507, 1989.
5. Simpson JL et al: Analysis for possible linkage between the loci for the Waardenburg syndrome and various blood groups and serological traits. *Humangenetik* 23:45–50, 1974.
6. Tassabehji M et al: Waardenburg's syndrome patients have mutations in the human homologue of the *PAX-3* paired box gene. *Nature* 355:635–636, 1992.

Index